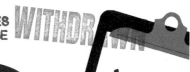

Chapters 22-37

Contemporary Dental Assisting

Contemporary Dental Assisting

DARLENE EATON NOVAK, CDA, EDDA, RDA, MA, EdS, EdD

Former Director, Office of Continuing Dental Education
  University of Louisville School of Dentistry
Louisville Kentucky;
Executive Director, Career Development Systems, LLC
Big Rapids, Michigan

with 1000 illustrations

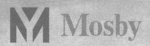 Mosby

St. Louis Baltimore Boston Carlsbad Chicago Minneapolis New York Philadelphia Portland
London Milan Sydney Tokyo Toronto

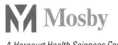

Mosby

A Harcourt Health Sciences Company

Publisher: John A. Schrefer
Senior Editor: Penny Rudolph
Project Manager: Linda McKinley
Senior Production Editor: Julie Eddy
Interior Designer: Elizabeth Young
Cover Designer: Bill Drone

NOTICE

Pharmacology is an ever-changing field. Standard safety precautions must be followed, but as new research and clinical experience broaden our knowledge, changes in treatment and drug therapy may become necessary or appropriate. Readers are advised to check the most current product information provided by the manufacturer of each drug to be administered to verify the recommended dose, the method and duration of administration, and contraindications. It is the responsibility of the licensed prescriber, relying on experience and knowledge of the patient, to determine dosages and the best treatment for each individual patient. Neither the publisher nor the editor assumes any liability for any injury and/or damage to persons or property arising from this publication.

Mosby, Inc.
A Harcourt Health Sciences Company
11830 Westline Industrial Drive
St. Louis, Missouri 63146

Printed in the United States of America

International Standard Book Number 0-8016-7732-7

01 02 03 04 05 GW/KPT 9 8 7 6 5 4 3 2 1

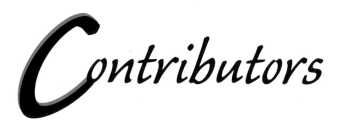

Contributors

LAWRENCE J. ABBOTT, DDS, MBA

Associate Professor
Department of Restorative Dentistry
University of Detroit Mercy
School of Dentistry
Detroit, Michigan

GAIL SANDERS D'ANDREA, CDA, EDDA, BS

Patient Care Coordinator
University of Louisville School of Dentistry
Louisville, Kentucky

STEPHEN M. FELDMAN, DDS, MSED

Associate Professor
Department of Periodontics, Endodontics, and
Dental Hygiene
University of Louisville School of Dentistry
Louisville, Kentucky;
Director of Dental Services
Jefferson County Health Department
Louisville, Kentucky

JOHN F. FRITZ, JR., BS PHARM, DMD, RPH

Instructor
Department of Diagnosis and General Dentistry
University of Louisville School of Dentistry
Louisville, Kentucky;
Private Practice
Lyndon Family Dental Center
Louisville, Kentucky

LINDA GAGEL, EDDA, CDT, COA

Private Practice
Louisville, Kentucky

C. BRENT HAEBERLE, DMD

Assistant Professor
Department of Diagnostic Sciences, Prosthodontics, and
Restorative Dentistry
University of Louisville School of Dentistry
Louisville, Kentucky

ZAFRULLA KHAN, DDS, MS, FACD, FACP

Professor
Department of Prosthodontics
J.G. Brown Cancer Center
University of Louisville School of Dentistry
Louisville, Kentucky;
Director
Dental Oncology and Maxillofacial Prosthetics
J.G. Brown Cancer Center
Louisville, Kentucky

DAVID L. LIEBETREU, DMD

United States Public Health Service
Eglin, AFB, Florida

MARK E. LIEBETREU, OD

Private Practice
Eye Health of Ft. Myers
Ft. Meyers, Florida

RICHARD L. MILLER, DDS, PHD

Professor
Department of Surgical/Hospital Dentistry
University of Louisville School of Dentistry
Louisville, Kentucky

THERESA M. MOONEY, CDA, EDDA

Department of Surgical/Hospital Dentistry
University of Louisville School of Dentistry
Louisville, Kentucky

ROBERT E. NOVAK, MBA, EDD

President
Career Development Systems LLC
Big Rapids, Michigan

M. MELINDA PARIS, DMD

Private Practice
Advanced Dental Care
Louisville, Kentucky

EDWIN T. PARKS, DMD, MS

Diplomat AAOMR, Diplomat ABOM
Associate Professor and Director
Division of Radiology
Department of Oral Surgery, Medicine, and Pathology
Indiana University School of Dentistry
Indianapolis, Indiana

ROBERT H. STAAT, PHD

Professor of Microbiology
Department of Molecular, Cellular, and
Craniofacial Biology
University of Louisville School of Dentistry
Louisville, Kentucky

JOHN N. WILLIAMS, DMD, MBA

Dean
University of Louisville School of Dentistry
Louisville, Kentucky;
Professor
Department of Periodontics, Endodontics, and
Dental Hygiene
University of Louisville School of Dentistry
Louisville, Kentucky

ANN M. WINDCHY, DMD

Associate Professor
Department of Diagnostic Sciences, Prosthodontics, and
Restorative Dentistry
University of Louisville School of Dentistry
Louisville, Kentucky

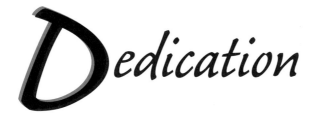

Dedication

This textbook is the accumulation of years of learning, teaching, and sharing among family, friends, and colleagues, all of whom have influenced the writing of *Contemporary Dental Assisting*. This book is dedicated to each of them.

To my husband Bob who still loved me when I was tired and withdrew into my computer and who I do not think I can adequately repay. To my children Mark, David, and Susan who supported me throughout the process of writing this textbook while I also completed doctorate studies. Special thanks to Appollonia, Anthony, Alessandra, Alexander, Abigail, Zachary, and Ethan; and to Ryan, Bradley, Colen, and Michael who are already searching for the answers of life and have the future ahead of them. To my grandmother, mother, father, sisters, and brothers: we recognize the value of family, education, responsible independence, and growth of character because we come from a long line of "builders."

To my friends and teachers at BRHS58, FSU, ULSD, and Spalding and especially to Pat and Dr. J. who were committed to excellence and lived it day by day. To practicing dentists who recognize the value of well-trained dental assistants and reward them for their efforts. To the state dental assisting president who left the podium and walked to the back of the auditorium to welcome this young dental assisting student and to the members and leaders of dental assisting organizations who support and encourage education, credentialing, and personal growth.

To my students who always delighted me and sometimes even frustrated me. To those who said, "it can't be done"; we showed them it could be done. To Sharon and Martha, dear friends and colleagues—"I'm ok, you're ok"—who kept their pens sharp and at times let me know it. To the contributing authors who hung on and supported our textbook; Sherry, our illustrator, and Ole, Dennis, Marian, and Tom, the photographers, who made us look good; and to Mosby, Harcourt Health Sciences, Penny, and Julie who gave us this writing opportunity, kept us on track, and supported our endeavors.

It is my pleasure to dedicate *Contemporary Dental Assisting* to the many people who support learning and express interest in becoming proficient dental assistants and find this textbook helpful in their studies. And to working dental assistants who seek to further their understanding of theory and advanced skills and recognize the value of continual learning and credentialing.

Preface

"Theory without experience is not learning." I believe that dental assistants must have a strong theory base on which to build clinical competency. It is also essential today to help students and working dental assistants become proficient in those skills that are part of their responsibilities in a shorter period. Recognizing the importance of work experience is particularly important because of the rapid technology changes in the practice of dentistry at this time. Also the varied range of clinical procedures that dental assistants are able to perform has increased and a growing need exists for well-trained chairside dental assistants who may also be educated in advanced functions to assume more decision-making responsibilities that can often affect the dental patient and other dental personnel. Because of this philosophy, I am dedicated to focusing on combining theory with clinical experience, proficiency, and self-evaluation of current and accepted dental procedures and techniques, thereby providing a textbook that can be used in the classroom and workplace.

Initially, being able to keep focused on the desired outcomes and accomplishing this combination concept was seen as a formidable task. The large volume of information needed to present theory and clinical skill processes essential for a broad-based contemporary dental assisting textbook, while attempting to include the most current principles and techniques necessary for advanced functions and specialty practice, was challenging. However, dental assistants, dentists, and educators with education expertise and clinical experience were selected from private practice and educational institutions to contribute to this textbook. The knowledge, experience, specialty expertise, and continual support of each of these contributing authors has allowed us to jointly assess accreditation standards, certification requirements, and advanced functions delegated to dental assistants nationally. Their effort has also helped us review current dental and education literature to accumulate and document the spectrum of knowledge and skills essential for dental assistants to become accomplished professionals in today's dental practice.

The contributing authors and I have maintained a reading level throughout *Contemporary Dental Assisting* that will help learners understand more difficult theories and concepts. Each chapter begins with a list of key points, a chapter outline, learning objectives, and key terms and ends with points for review, self-study questions, and suggested readings. These pedagogical aids will help the reader and instructor or supervisor identify needed information quickly and recognize important points and objectives in each chapter. They will also allow learners to work through each skill and evaluate their own progress.

In addition to receiving developmental support and photographs from dentists in private practice, faculty members, and manufacturers, 1000 photographs and computer-generated illustrations were developed by professional university medical illustrators and photographers for this textbook. These learning aids were created to help increase reader knowledge and comprehension level. Numerous step-by-step procedure boxes with related materials and equipment have been included throughout the textbook. Self-evaluation tables have been included to help the reader understand what is expected to accomplish each procedure. All of the teaching and learning support materials can be used in either the classroom or workplace. Each chapter represents a course of study that allows learners to read the material and answer self-study questions and, when appropriate, complete projects on their own. The comprehensiveness of each chapter and ease of reading with numerous support aids provides an opportunity for learners to prepare for certification or registration examinations.

Instructions for Use of Evaluation Tables   Readers of this textbook should understand what hands-on performance is expected and learn how to assess their own requirements. Evaluation tables are available for self-assessment and intermediary and final teacher evaluation. Following completion of the project or procedure, each skill can be evaluated by using the following numeric criteria:

4: Excellent (The task has been completed to the highest level with no error and within the appropriate allotted time.)

3: Good (The task has been satisfactorily completed within the allotted time but some improvement can be made.)

2: Below average (The task has been completed in an untimely manner and the project is usable but the skill needs to be improved.)

0: Unsatisfactory (The task has not been completed in the allotted time and the project is unusable.)

X: (Not able to evaluate.)

I begin the textbook by documenting key periods in dental history, recognizing the effect of organized dentistry and education and emphasizing the importance of career planning and professional development for the dental assistant. Basic management concepts and procedures that can be performed by the front office assistant or manager are presented with an emphasis on ethics and jurisprudence in today's technical but patient-oriented dental practice. I then integrate basic dental science theory with hands-on clinical skills, specialty techniques, and advanced clinic applications that can be practiced in the classroom or workplace of most dental offices with dentist supervision.

Unit I: Professional Dental Assisting Yesterday and Today This unit highlights three chapters. Chapter 1: *History of Dentistry and the Professional Environment Today* covers selective points in the evolution of dentistry and the role of allied dental personnel. Dental assisting education, credentialing, and the role of women in dentistry is emphasized, highlighting the various duties of dental assistants in contemporary dental practice and reinforcing membership in the dental assisting organization and credentialing. Dr. Malvin E. Ring, author of *Dentistry: An Illustrated History,* was instrumental in editing this chapter and supporting the textbook.

Chapter 2: *Career Planning for the Professional Dental Assistant* reinforces the need for career planning and employment preparation. Preparing proper correspondence and developing appropriate interviewing techniques are emphasized in this chapter. The American Dental Assistants Association has provided a sample employment agreement for reader review and use, photographs, and other pertinent information.

Chapter 3: *Dental Ethics and Jurisprudence* is one of the few detailed chapters written on this topic for dental assistants. It emphasizes the special nature of a profession as it relates to ethics and the laws that affect dentistry and identifies the basic behaviors required of the dentist and dental assistant in private practice. As the contributing author, Dr. Lawrence J. Abbott provided valuable new information in researching and documenting this detailed chapter.

Unit II: Practice Management Principles and Techniques This unit highlights four chapters. Chapter 4: *Managing Communications in the Dental Practice* reinforces the dental assistant's role in understanding and implementing the principles and functions of managing a dental practice and communicating effectively with the dental patient. This chapter evaluates listening skills and discusses the importance of office staff meetings. Two contributing authors provided their expertise to this chapter. Dr. John N. Williams provided up-to-date information on management techniques and Dr. Robert E. Novak, author of *Transitional Learning Relationships between Secondary and Postsecondary Schools,* provided

important information on how to recognize good communications and techniques that can be used to develop communication skills.

Chapter 5: *Managing Dental Office Information* discusses the use of computer record management and the role of the dental business assistant in managing appointment scheduling and maintaining appropriate accounts receivable, disbursement, and collection records. Dr. John N. Williams, contributing author, provided vital computer application and function management information and a list of on-line resources for this chapter.

Chapter 6: *Managing Dental Financial Records* focuses on making financial arrangements and presenting treatment and financial plans to the patient.

Chapter 7: *Dental Inventory Control* describes the role of the dental office assistant in inventory control and various considerations to be made in developing a functional inventory system with emphasis on ordering, receiving, tracking, and returning orders.

Unit III: Dental Sciences, Principles, and Techniques This unit highlights seven chapters. Chapter 8: *Anatomy and Physiology* describes the components of the 12 major systems of the body and their function. The tables and computer-generated illustrations are unequaled in many textbooks. They have been detailed especially for understanding difficult concepts. Dr. Melinda Paris, contributing author for this chapter, worked with the University of Louisville anatomy department and the medical and dental art illustrator to clarify and develop over 30 newly designed illustrations.

Chapter 9: *Oral Anatomy and Tooth Morphology* describes the identification techniques for permanent and primary teeth, the clinical and anatomic parts of the teeth, and the fundamentals of tooth form and function in detail with over 50 tables and illustrations. The newly developed photographs and computer-generated illustrations were designed to increase understanding and reinforce learning. The tables and illustrations provide learning reinforcement, which will help the reader understand difficult terms and concepts.

Chapter 10: *Microbiology for the Dental Assistant* covers microbial structure and function and the role of microorganisms in infectious disease. It details the control of infectious disease and identifies the infectious diseases that present occupational hazards and those that cause oral diseases. Dr. Robert Staat is the contributing author for this chapter. Original tables and illustrations were developed to help the learner understand microorganisms and the diseases they cause.

Chapter 11: *Oral and Maxillofacial Pathology and Oral Diseases* describes the team approach in detection, diagnosis, treatment, and prevention of patient disease. It documents the need for dental assistants to be familiar with common oral diseases and discusses oral disease as a localized disease or a manifestation of systemic diseases. Dr. Richard Miller, author of *General and Oral Pathology,* is the contributing author for this chapter. Twenty detailed pathology photographs have been included in this chapter.

Chapter 12: *Radiology and Radiation Safety* and Chapter 13: *Oral and Maxillofacial Radiography* cover x-ray production, image processing, image characteristics, and radiation biology and safety. These chapters also detail the production of acceptable dental radiographic surveys, intraoral and extraoral techniques, special needs, mounting radiographs, and radiographic anatomy. Dr. Edwin T. Parks, the contributing author for these two chapters, has completed an exceptional task of preparing this information and securing and developing in excess of 60 illustrations and tables.

Chapter 14: *General Pharmacology and Pain Control* covers the use of drugs as they relate to dentistry, effective pain control, and anesthesia. It also discusses the role of the dental assistant in pain control and the legal aspects of drug use and prescriptions. The three contributing authors who developed this chapter, Dr. John F. Fritz, Dr. Mark E. Liebetreu, and Dr. Wayne L. Olges, provided significant input from private practice, education, and research.

Unit IV: Clinical Principles and Techniques This unit highlights eight chapters. Chapter 15: *Dental Materials and Clinical Application* covers the physical and mechanical properties of dental materials, the primary types of dental materials used for dental treatment, the steps involved in manipulating each material, and important considerations for the selection and use of the materials. Many dental manufacturers supported this textbook by providing data and photographs for several chapters, particularly this chapter.

Chapter 16: *Nutrition and Dietary Counseling* provides a review of basic nutritional concepts. Dr. Stephen Feldman, the contributing author for this chapter, identified the influence of nutrition on general and oral health and explored a process of modifying the food habits of patients.

Chapter 17: *Preventive Dentistry and Advanced Oral Health Procedures* covers the rationale and scope of preventive dentistry, periodontal disease, and the etiology and prevention of dental caries. The contributing author, Dr. Stephen Feldman, identified the steps in patient education and discussed dental prophylaxis, pit and fissure sealants, systemic and topical fluorides, and the importance of maintenance recall programs.

Chapter 18: *Barriers to Disease Transmission* outlines the area of infection control and human health. It provides disinfectant and sterilization techniques, identifies proper instrument preparation, and provides the process for recycling the dental operatory for the best infection control. Dr. Robert Staat is the contributing author for this chapter.

Chapter 19: *Dental Instruments and Equipment* covers the identification and use of hand and rotary instruments and accessory dental instruments and equipment.

Chapter 20: *Current Concepts of Dental Chairside Assisting* is comprehensive, covering basic chairside assisting and advanced function operator techniques. It provides information on clinical dental auxiliary utilization, four-handed, sit-down dentistry, principles of work simplification, and practice efficiency methods. In consideration of advanced function personnel, this chapter includes a general guideline to assist the operator in gaining visibility and access in any area of the mouth while maintaining the principles of four-handed, sit-down dentistry. It covers operator, assistant, and patient positions and emphasizes retraction, finger rest, and suctioning techniques. Proper procedures for instrument grasp and transfer are also defined.

Chapter 21: *Oral Diagnosis and Treatment Planning* details the role of the dental assistant in securing patient history, treatment planning, and presentation. Gail S. D'Andrea, CDA, EDDA, BS, contributing author, identified the procedures and techniques used for clinical examination, diagnosis, and charting oral conditions.

Chapter 22: *Management of Dental Office Emergencies* covers the expectations and prevention of medical emergencies in dental practice and includes basic life support and CPR. Dr. Lawrence J. Abbott, contributing author for this chapter, identified the causes, signs, symptoms, and treatment of possible medical emergencies, highlighted occupational hazards, and emphasized the ethical and legal responsibilities related to medical emergencies in dental practice.

Univ V: Specialty Principles and Techniques This unit highlights ten chapters. Chapter 23: *Endodontics* describes the procedures involved in endodontic examination and treatment, root canal vitality testing, surgical procedures, and suture removal. It identifies endodontic instruments and tray setups.

Chapter 24: *Pediatric Dentistry* details child development and management of children's fear of the unknown and introduces the role of the dental assistant in providing pediatric dental procedures. It describes the physiologic processes of tooth and facial development, identifies the oral habits of children, and lists the types of correction mechanisms available.

Chapter 25: *Periodontics* covers the etiology of periodontal disease and identifies the periodontium and related anatomic structures. The signs and symptoms of periodontal disease are identified and the role of dental personnel in periodontal examination and therapy are discussed. Dr. Stephen Feldman, contributing editor, listed the essential periodontal instruments and provided illustrated periodontal surgery.

Chapter 26: *The Professional Orthodontic Assistant* covers the etiology of malocclusion and the types of orthodontic treatment available. It identifies the mechanism of realigning teeth, classifies occlusion and malocclusion, and lists the various types of orthodontic appliances and armamentarium. Linda Gagel, EDDA, CDT, COA, contributing author, also identified the rewards of a career in orthodontics, listed the qualifications of an orthodontic assistant, and included how to fabricate several basic orthodontic appliances.

Chapter 27: *Oral and Maxillofacial Surgery and Introduction to Hospital Dentistry* outlines preoperative and postoperative surgical considerations and pain and anxiety control. Oral surgery armamentarium is listed and the role of the dental assistant in oral surgery is described. Theresa M. Mooney, CDA, EDDA, contributing author, has identified and provided illustrations of several general and hospital oral surgery procedures, emphasizing emergency preparation.

Chapter 28: *Fixed Prosthetics and Temporary Crown and Bridge* discusses the effect of tooth loss and identifies the types of fixed prosthesis that are available to the patient. It identifies the role of the dental assistant in providing prosthodontic treatment and describes clinical and laboratory procedures.

Chapter 29: *Removable Prosthetics* covers the indications, contraindications, diagnosis, and treatment planning procedures. Dr. Ann M. Windchy, contributing author, has described the components of removable partial dentures and the construction and repair of removable partial dentures.

Chapter 30: *Complete Denture Prosthetics* identifies the indications, contraindications, diagnosis, and treatment planning for patients in need of complete dentures. Dr. Brent Haeberle, contributing author, has provided the procedures for the fabrication of complete dentures for edentulous and partially edentulous patients and the techniques for maintenance of complete dentures.

Chapter 31: *Dental Implantology* covers the indications for dental implants and describes consultation, diagnosis, and treatment planning techniques. Dr. Brent Haeberle, contributing author, has provided implant surgery cases and described maintenance procedures.

Chapter 32: *Dental Oncology and Maxillofacial Prosthetic Treatment* describes the treatment of oral cavity and dentition for patients receiving head and neck radiotherapy and chemotherapy. Dr. Zafrulla Khan, contributing author, described and illustrated the use of maxillofacial prostheses in the treatment of cancer, trauma, and birth defects affecting a patient's head and neck.

Unit VI: Advanced Operative Principles and Techniques This unit highlights five chapters developed with the following contributing authors and support staff: Dr. Kenneth W. Chapman and Dr. David L. Liebetreu.

Chapter 33: *Clinical Operative Procedures and Rubber Dam Isolation* discusses the preoperative and clinical procedures used for rubber dam isolation. This chapter also includes the assistant's role in caries removal, cavity preparation, and pulp protection. Cavity classification and nomenclature are also described.

Chapter 34: *Matrix Band and Retainer Assembly and Wedge Placement* identifies the use of matrix bands, retainers, and wedges. It describes the steps used for matrix band and retainer assembly and placement and wedge placement. A unique technique Dr. Chapman uses for large amalgam cores is also included.

Chapter 35: *Finishing and Polishing Dental Restorations* covers the finishing and polishing procedures used with hand instruments, rotary trimming and finishing instruments, and polishing devices using abrasive agents.

Chapter 36: *Clinical Application of Dental Amalgam Restorations* details the clinical application of dental amalgam restorations and the finishing and polishing techniques.

Chapter 37: *Direct and Indirect Composite Acrylic Resin Restorative Techniques* covers the clinical application of composite resin placement and the finishing and polishing techniques. Dr. Jane P. Casada provided an indirect composite resin technique for this chapter.

One of the challenges for dental assistants, practicing dentists, educators, and school counselors today is to recognize the dental assistant as a valuable team member and reach out and encourage women and men to consider dental assisting as a potential career choice. Dental assistants employed in practice today need to advance their knowledge and skills. Through the support of the dental community, they also need to realize that dental assisting can be an exciting long-term career. We must provide education and training opportunities for potential learners to become proficient members of the dental health team through alternative program planning. *Contemporary Dental Assisting* attempts to provide an education resource foundation for practicing dentists, learners, and educational institutions.

A fellow colleague from Russia recently told me that in teaching, "to share one's knowledge with another is the greatest gift one can give." In retrospect, I believe that when two or more dedicated teachers or learners come together, learning is always mutual and a welcomed gift. I thank him for his comment and hope you enjoy this textbook as much as we have enjoyed developing it. May you always experience the satisfaction of learning.

Darlene Eaton Novak, CDA, EDDA, RDA, MA, EdS, EdD

Contents

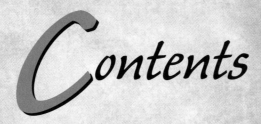

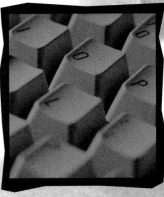

Unit II *Practice Management Principles and Techniques* 71

Chapter 4
Managing Communications in the Dental Practice 72

Chapter 5
Managing Dental Office Information 92

Unit III *Dental Sciences, Principles, and Techniques* **157**

Unit IV *Clinical Principles and Techniques* 349

Chapter 18
Barriers to Disease Transmission 434

Chapter 19
Dental Instruments and Equipment 458

Chapter 20
Current Concepts of Dental Chairside Assisting 486

Chapter 21
Oral Diagnosis and Treatment Planning 514

Chapter 28
Fixed Prosthetics and Temporary Crown and Bridge 740

Chapter 29
Removable Prosthetics 768

Chapter 30
Complete Denture Prosthetics 794

Chapter 31
Dental Implantology 812

Chapter 32
Dental Oncology and Maxillofacial Prosthetic Treatment 832

Unit VI *Advanced Operative Principles and Techniques* **847**

Chapter 33
Clinical Operative Procedures and Rubber Dam Isolation 848

Chapter 34
Matrix Band and Retainer Assembly and Wedge Placement 872

Unit I

Professional Dental Assisting Yesterday and Today

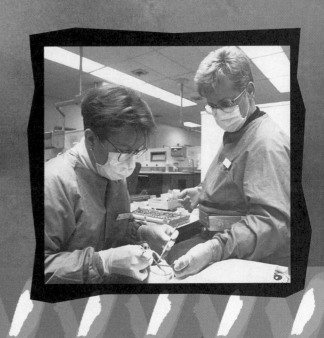

History of Dentistry and the Role of Dental Assisting

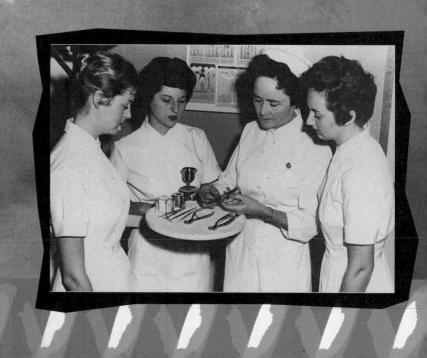

Chapter Outline

Evolution of Dentistry
   Early dentistry
   Modern dentistry
   Dental progress
History of Dental Education
   First schools in the United States
   First women of dentistry
Dental Organization and Regulation
   Early efforts at regulation
   Dental practice acts
Use of Allied Dental Personnel in Dentistry
   Early dental assisting
   American Dental assistants association
   The advancement of allied dental
     personnel education
Delivering Dental Care Today
Dental Practice
   General dental practice

Dental education
Dental examination
Professional dental organizations
Specialty dental practice
Dental public health
   U.S. Public Health Service
Use of Allied Dental Personnel
   The dental assistant
The Role and Responsibility of the Dental Team
The American Dental Assistants Association
Dental Assisting Education Programs
   Dynamic career opportunities in dental assisting
   Professional accrediting agencies
   Credentialing of dental assistants
   Certification

Learning Objectives

On completion of Chapter 1, the student should be able to do the following:

■ Define key terms.

■ Describe the evolution of dentistry.

■ Describe how the past has provided opportunities for professional growth and development for dental assistants.

■ Identify the various career opportunities available for dental assistants.

■ Describe the purposes and functions of professional membership organizations.

■ Describe why credentialing is important for dental assistants and which mechanisms are available.

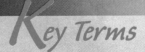

Key Terms

Accreditation	Certification	Registration
Allied Dental Personnel	Dentistry	Regulations
	Eligibility	Statutes
Apprenticeship		
	Licensure	Treatise

EVOLUTION OF DENTISTRY

Dentistry

The healing art and science of treating dental diseases and replacing the teeth and supporting structures of the oral cavity.

Dentistry is the restoration and maintenance of the normal health and function of the mouth and its associated structures. The delivery of quality dental health care has been an evolution of improved practice, education, organization, regulation, and allied dental personnel use.

Early Dentistry

Humans have strived through the ages to control disease, eliminate pain, and provide good health care. Dentistry evolved as part of the healing arts to relieve humans of the pain of toothache and to provide alternatives for missing teeth and oral structures. Although examination of early skeletons does not indicate restoration of the teeth, it does show the use of therapeutic ingredients to temporarily relieve pain (Figure 1-1).

Egyptian and Chinese records from as early as 5000 years ago indicate that specialists treated diseases of the teeth and gums, extracted teeth, and used gold wire to hold the teeth in place. The Egyptians replaced teeth only after death so that the corpse would be complete when interred.

The Greeks and Romans developed operative and orthodontic dentistry, the toothbrush and the toothpick, and many dental instruments. Greek history was influenced by Hippocrates (460-377 BC), the "father of medicine," who supported scientific reasoning in medicine rather than basing medicine on superstition and religion. The Oath of Hippocrates is the code of ethics for the U.S. medical and dental professions. Aristotle (384-322 BC), the "father of comparative anatomy," also referred to the human teeth and their differences in his writings. Cornelius Celsus (25 BC-50 AD), a Roman physician, described the treatment of jaw fractures and orthodontics. Although the Greeks did not produce dental restorations, their increased knowledge, skill, and new methods to alleviate dental pain gave these ancient practitioners a position of respect in dental health care.

In Alexandria, Egypt, in approximately 225 AD, Apollonia, the daughter of a leading judicial officer, suffered by having her teeth broken out and was burned alive because she refused to denounce Christianity. She was canonized in 249 AD and is recognized as the "patron saint of toothache sufferers and dentistry" (Figure 1-2).

Modern Dentistry

The fall of the Roman Empire and the coming of the Dark Ages began the decline in medical and dental progress for nearly 1000 years. However, the anatomic studies of Andres Vesalius (1514-1564) and Bartolommeo Eustacius (1520-1574), a pupil of Vesalius in Europe, helped introduce "modern dentistry." Vesalius advanced the understanding of anatomy and became known as the "founder of modern anatomy." He also recorded tooth articulation, which later helped in the study of orthodontics. Paracelsus (1493-1541)

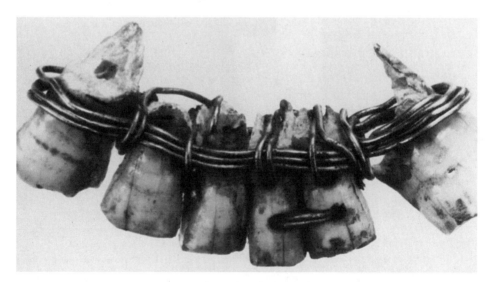

FIGURE 1.1

Phoenician fixed bridge, dated between the fifth and fourth centuries BC, which is made up of four human incisor teeth and two carved ivory teeth bound with gold wire. (Courtesy Muse's due Louvre, Paris.)

laid the foundation for pharmacology and was recognized for his great contribution of new drugs such as quinine sulfate and ipecac syrup.

Ambrose Paré (1517-1590), an experienced barber and surgeon to the French Court, had his writings published on the procedures to correct dental disorders, surgical procedures, simple bridges, and types of dental appliances. In 1580 the University of Paris admitted the first students for the study of dentistry. They received the title "operateur pour les dents" and were bound by ethical oath. Dentistry in France became regulated in 1699 when students were required to pass an examination given by the College of Surgeons and take an oath.

In these times of social change Europeans were settling the New World and people were distancing themselves from myths and religious restrictions. People were prospering economically, and personal appearance and esthetics became important. This change heightened new attitudes about health and appearance and led to new discoveries in dentistry.

In 1728, Pierre Fauchard (1678-1761), the "father of modern dentistry," established modern practice when he published his two-volume **treatise** *Le Chirurgien Dentiste (The Surgeon Dentist)* on dental information that described the character and scope of dentistry. Fauchard is recognized for the construction of full and partial dentures, tooth transplants, lead-filled root canals, scaling, and his dental instruments. He also noted that decay must be removed before filling the tooth. He was a strong advocate of oral hygiene and described scaling and polishing of teeth and devised many dentifrices. During this time an English surgeon, John Hunter (1728-1793), wrote his *Practical Treatise on the Diseases of the Teeth* and the *Natural History of the Teeth*. His scientific studies included dental infection, classification and description of the teeth, and complete removal of the pulp. He is often referred to as the "father of modern surgery."

Treatise

A study or outcome of a scientific investigation.

Dentistry in Colonial America

The Angel of Bethesda, the first medical information recorded in America, was written by Cotton Mather (1663-1728). He was a clergyman who wrote about the diseases of the mouth and listed folk remedies to relieve dental pain. Early Americans relied on these home remedies, and in 1736, Benjamin Franklin published *Every Man His Own Doctor*.

Dentists such as Robert Wooffendale in England and Josiah Flagg introduced advances in European dentistry to colonial America at the end of the Revolutionary War. Flagg was a private in the American army and studied under James Gardette, a French-trained dentist and naval surgeon. One of Flagg's contributions to dentistry was the invention of the dental chair. Another pioneer renowned for practicing dentistry in colonial America was John Baker (1732-1796), who claimed to have received medical training in England and settled in Boston around 1750. Baker trained Paul Revere (1735-1818), who took over the Boston practice when Baker left for New York to practice dentistry. Although Revere's interest in dentistry was brief, he is known for his prosthodontic work. Another student of Baker's was Isaac Greenwood, Sr. (1730-1803), who was the father of John Greenwood (1760-1819). In 1789, after the Revolutionary War, John Greenwood became the dentist for George Washington and is known for his study of the origin of tooth decay.

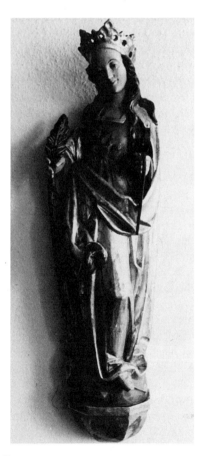

FIGURE 1.2

St. Apollonia, characterized in this Bavarian baroque eighteenth-century wood carving, balances on a globe carrying dental forceps and the palm of victory in her right hand. (Courtesy M.E. Ring, Rochester, NY.)

Dental Progress

In the past, dentistry consisted mainly of "pulling" teeth, and although much had been accomplished, unsatisfactory restorative materials, pain, and the cost of dentistry prevented most colonial citizens from seeking dental care. New innovations were tried and ideas progressed as America began to lead in the field of dentistry. The years following the

Revolutionary War in America provided some of the most important advancements in the history of modern dentistry.

James Morrison enhanced operative dentistry with the invention of the dental handpiece drill in 1871. The drill eliminated the removal of decay and hard tooth structure by hand and allowed for a more uniform cavity preparation. The introduction of the dental drill revolutionized dentistry. However, dentistry needed a restorative material that was less expensive than gold but with some of the same properties. A material called "silver paste" appeared to be the answer when Taveau introduced it in Paris, France, in 1826; however, no methods to prevent the expansion and shrinkage of the restoration were known. In 1833 the French Crawcour brothers introduced the silver paste in New York as "Royal Mineral Succedaneum" to replace the gold. Their improper methods of use and the material's shortcomings caused what was known to be the "Amalgam War."

After 20 years of controversy, investigations, and significant improvements, the dental community eventually accepted silver material known as amalgam. One of the leading dental scientists who contributed to its acceptance was Greene Vardiman (G.V.) Black (1836-1915). He perfected silver amalgam so that its negative properties were eliminated. His scientific investigations included study of the structure of tooth enamel, the requirements for retention of restorative materials, the considerations of forces of mastication, and the improvement and placement of amalgam materials. Greene Vardiman Black became known as "the grand old man of dentistry" because of his numerous scientific contributions to dentistry.

Numerous advances continued into the twentieth century. In 1895, Wilhelm Conrad Roentgen (1845-1923) revolutionized dentistry by discovering the x-ray beam. Dr. C. Edmund Kells is also famous for his contributions to dental radiography and was the first dentist to use radiographs in his office. Dr. Kells is specifically recognized and recorded for employing the first dental assistant. Nondentists such as Charles Goodyear (1800-1860) also contributed to the advancement of dentistry by inventing rubber vulcanite for denture bases in 1849. Vulcanite replaced gold and provided affordable dentures for many years until it was replaced by acrylic resin.

HISTORY OF DENTAL EDUCATION

Early dentistry was practiced by a medicine man or priests who were later replaced by physicians, surgeons, barbers, and traveling salesmen. Dental education, if provided at all, was limited to an apprenticeship with no formal course of study and consisted primarily of filling and pulling teeth. Many abuses took place, which caused a need for protection from malpractice and quackery.

In 1805 the Maryland Medical School amended its bylaws to grant a special license to dentists to practice. This was the first school to recognize dentistry as an independent specialty of medicine. The first trained dentist to receive a license was Horace H. Hayden, who was the originator of the idea of a dental school. He became the first dean of the first dental school in the United States, the Baltimore College of Dental Surgery.

First Schools in the United States

In 1827, Dr. Chapin Harris, a Bainbridge, Ohio, medical doctor who specialized in dentistry, offered to instruct a private class of medical students in the interest of dentistry. These classes represented the first formal attempt to teach dentistry in the United States. In November 1840 the first dental school, the Baltimore College of Dental Surgery, was founded. Although great strides were made in formal dental education, the profession was resisted by dentist who wanted to "profit from apprentice labors" and by physicians who held dentistry in low esteem. In 1867, Harvard University established a dental department that later became known as the Harvard Dental School.

Dental education gained respectability with the help and influence of Dr. Nathan Keep, Harvard's first dental dean, who recognized the professional standing of Harvard in the medical profession and assisted the dental department in the association with the medical department. A total of 13 dental schools came into existence between 1840 and 1867. Some were short lived but those that survived did so by becoming part of a university. Between 1867 and 1900, 57 dental schools were in operation. (Figure 1-3 shows changes at the University of Louisville.)

First Women of Dentistry

Women had been excluded from dentistry until the mid l800s. In 1854, Emeline Roberts married Dr. Daniel Albion Jones of Danielson, Connecticut, and assisted him until 1864 when he died. She took over his practice to support herself and children. It was not until 1893 that she was elected a member of the Connecticut State Dental Society. She practiced for 60 years.

During this time, Lucy Beaman Hobbs, a teacher from upstate New York, decided on a dental career. Although the dean of Ohio College of Dental Surgery told her that women were not admitted as students to dental school, she secured a preceptoral position in Cincinnati, Ohio, working until she opened her own practice in 1861 and later moved to Iowa. Her struggle was rewarded when the Iowa delegation to the American Dental Association (ADA) threatened to withdraw from ADA if Dr. Hobbs was not admitted to the Ohio College of Dental Surgery. She was admitted in 1865 and received her Doctor of Dental Surgery (DDS) degree on February 21, 1866, becoming the first woman in the world to graduate from a dental school. Other women, such as Dr. Olga Lentz of St. Paul, Minnesota, were beginning to practice dentistry (Figure 1-4).

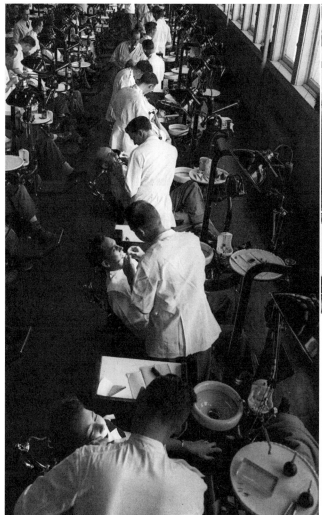

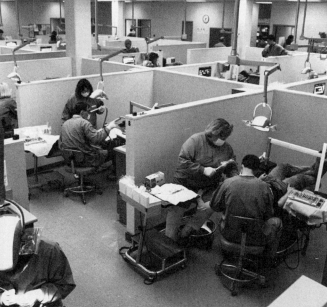

A

B

FIGURE 1.3

Changes in dental education, equipment, and facilities. **A**, University of Louisville in 1948. **B**, University of Louisville in 1999.

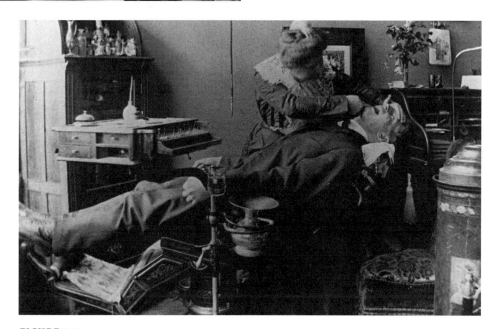

FIGURE 1.4

Dr. Olga Lentz, a dentist from St. Paul, Minnesota, was one of the few women who practiced dentistry around 1910. (Courtesy Albert Munson, Minnesota Historical Society, St. Paul.)

DENTAL ORGANIZATION AND REGULATION

In response to the lack of standardization in dentistry and inadequacies in education, practitioners Horace Hayden and Chapin Harris formed local and state associations and created journals to advance the interest of dental practice and education. Hayden was instrumental in developing the first national dental periodical in the world, the *American Journal of Dental Science*, and forming the American Society of Dental Surgeons in 1840, which was renamed the ADA in 1859. When the Civil War erupted, the Southern states broke away and formed their own organization, the Southern Dental Association. The ADA continued, however, and in 1895 the two groups decided to merge once more, with Southern dentists refusing to rejoin if the name continued as the ADA. Therefore the name of the merged organization was changed to the National Dental Association. In 1922 the name was changed to the original ADA, which has had an unbroken existence since 1859.

The ADA was responsible for the establishment of professional standards and provided a communications and lobbying mechanism. In 1923 the merger of several associations to unify dental education in North America formed the American Association of Dental Schools (AADS).

Early Efforts at Regulation

In ancient times, Egyptian practitioners were subject to dental regulation. In 1699 the French court passed the Edict of May, which required that dental experts be judged capable by members of the King's Court and by the faculty of medicine.

As dental organizations in the United States began to set criteria for the dental profession, laws were needed to regulate dentistry and to provide a mechanism for punishment of offenders. Active dentists encouraged the government to provide **regulations** to protect the profession and ensure that the public was protected through testing of graduates. These regulations gave states the right to grant dentists a license to practice and gave the profession the responsibility to certify that a dentist was fit to practice. In 1841, Alabama enacted a law requiring that a panel of physicians formally evaluate all practitioners of dentistry, and in 1868 the Kentucky Dental Association discussed the first dental law, which was passed by the General Assembly in 1878. The law required that all practitioners of dentistry in Kentucky have a diploma from a dental college or pass an approved examination. New York and Ohio followed with dental

Regulations

Criteria described in laws outlining what a practitioner can do under that act or statute.

laws establishing statutory requirements for the practice of dentistry. These laws gave the state the authority to issue licenses to dentists, after examination of competency, including those who had not graduated from dental school. By 1899 every state provided legislation to control the practice of dentistry.

Dental Practice Acts

Dental practice acts are part of the public acts, which provide **statutes** or laws that give authority or licensure to individuals to practice in a specific profession. Their primary purpose is to "protect the public." Furthermore, they require examination, regulation of the statutes, licensing, and **registration** of people engaged in the practice of dentistry and protect the profession against offenders of the provisions. State boards of dental examiners, appointed by governors of the state, were organized to implement the provisions of the acts. These boards have the power to make bylaws and necessary regulations for the fulfillment of their duties and to penalize practitioners for malpractice. Today, government regulation of dentistry serves to upgrade the quality of dental care provided to the public through the granting of a license to practice dentistry, while the profession is required to certify a dentist as fit to practice by establishing standards for the profession. This professional body, the Council on Dental Education of the ADA, was established in 1938 to develop educational policies and curriculum, set minimal standards, and inspect and accredit educational programs. In 1940 the council published the "Requirements for the Approval of a Dental School." The federal government agency the Bureau of Health and Human Resources is influential in providing funds for dental research to upgrade the quality of dental care.

Statutes

The laws that give authority or licensure for individuals to practice in a profession.

Registration

A record of people who are licensed to perform specific functions.

USE OF ALLIED DENTAL PERSONNEL IN DENTISTRY

Early Dental Assisting

Although some form of help was provided to those practicing dentistry, the first female dental assistants were found in Dr. Edmund Kells' New Orleans office in 1885. Gradually, people learned that women not only had the proper amount of intelligence but also could be of great assistance to the

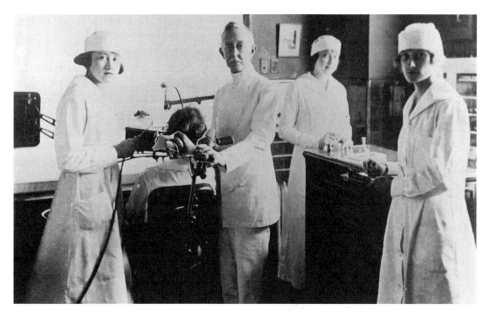

FIGURE 1.5

Dr. C. Edmund Kells and his dental assistants around 1900. (Courtesy the American Dental Assistants Association, Chicago.)

dentist. The presence of a female dental assistant made it respectable for a woman patient to enter the office without an escort (Figure 1-5).

The employment of women as assistants in dental offices and the ability of women to function as dentists was debated for years because many believed that the female's very form and structure unfit her for the duties of dentistry. The belief that a woman was inferior to men and lacked mechanicability also put women in the background of dental practice for many years. During this time, people were also fighting for recognition of nursing as a profession.

American Dental Assistants Association

Women such as Juliette A. Southard (Figure 1-6) organized dental assistants and formed the Educational and Efficiency Society in 1921, which was later known as the *American Dental Assistants Association (ADAA)*. In 1930 a curriculum committee was formed to draft courses of training to be used as educational guides. In 1943, members were required to have a high school education and in 1944 a Certification Committee was appointed to prepare standards and an examination for dental assistants. In 1947 a study course was adopted, and in 1948 the Certifying Board of the American Dental Assistants Association was established.

In 1950, 1- and 2-year dental assisting programs were established. In 1960 the ADA first approved "Requirements for Educational Programs for Dental Assistants" and the "Requirements for Approval of a Certifying Board for

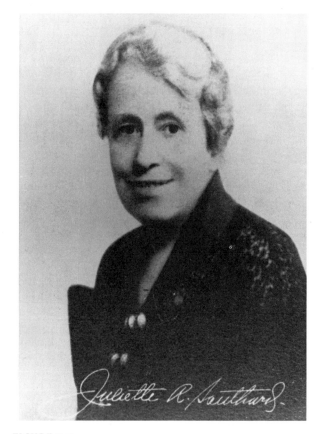

FIGURE 1.6

Juliette A. Southard organized dental assisting and in 1921 formed the Educational and Efficiency Society, which later became the American Dental Assistants Association. (Courtesy the American Dental Assistants Association, Chicago.)

Dental Assistants." On-the-job trained (OJT) dental assistants who had completed the special 104-hour study program before 1967 were eligible for examination until 1969. At this time, candidates for examination by the certifying board had to have completed an ADA accredited educational program.

The Advancement of Allied Dental Personnel Education

Intraoral Training for Dental Assistants

In the early 1900s, Dr. Alfred C. Fones began training his dental assistants to examine and polish teeth. He also started the first school for hygienists in his garage. In 1907, Dr. Fones and his friends assisted in amending the Connecticut dental law to permit specially trained dental assistants to examine, polish, and clean teeth, thus beginning the oral hygiene movement and dental hygiene education. In 1913 a school was established in Massachusetts, and in 1915, New York legalized a licensed dental hygienist. The specialized dental assistant was required to have a formal education and a **licensure** to perform intraoral procedures. The name "dental assistant" was changed to *dental hygienist* to reflect the nature of the services provided. In 1947 the ADA approved standards for dental hygiene, and state dental practice acts were revised to include specifically defined duties to be delegated to the hygienist. Several states have permitted the training of dental hygienists through preceptorship. The ADA also approved standards for dental technology education in 1948. The dental technician **certification** program was established in 1958 by the National Association of Dental Laboratories in cooperation with the ADA. The National Board for Certification administers the program.

Licensure

The legal document provided by a state law assuring that the practitioner is qualified to practice.

Certification

A credential assuring that a person has met a level of competency required for particular functions.

The 1950s and 1960s

While dentistry was evolving, society was changing. After World War II, America discovered poverty and injustice in a country of plenty. Studies showed the health effects of environment on family life and childhood development. Interest in health care increased in the 1950s; health insurance was established, death rates decreased, and postwar birth rates and income levels increased. The socioeconomic changes and technological advances caused the public to demand more and better medical and dental health services. These demands created an urgency to study ways to provide more production and better health care services.

Dental practice surveys performed by the Bureau of Economic Research and Statistics of the ADA between 1953 and 1956 showed that increased dental production and services could be improved through the use of trained dental auxiliaries. These surveys indicated that production could be 62% higher with 12% more services if auxiliary dental personnel were used. The Partnership for Health Act, the Comprehensive Health Planning bill, the Regional Medical Program, and the Hill-Burton bills were the first federal health care initiatives. These bills provided the financial initiatives necessary to support dental assisting education.

In 1961 a "Statement of Policy Regarding Experimentation in the Training and Utilization of Dental Hygienists and Dental Assistants" was adopted by the ADA. At this time, federal grants were awarded to dental schools to support programs for teaching dental students how to use dental auxiliaries efficiently. Dental auxiliary utilization (DAU) programs were successful in promoting improved delivery services through training both the dentist and the assistant in "four-handed dentistry." In 1963 the New York Academy of Medicine established a committee on social policy for health care in which they approved a policy statement on "The Role of Government Tax Funds in Problems of Health Care." In 1966 the first act of Congress directed specifically to allied health education, the Health Professions Educational Assistance Act, was passed. The act was designed to increase the opportunities for training allied health personnel and provided for the development of 1- and 2-year programs in proprietary and public colleges and universities (Figure 1-7).

Experimental expanded duty dental assisting (EDDA) and expanded function dental assisting (EFDA) programs were initiated to develop more skilled and technically trained dental personnel, especially in the underserved areas, and to contain anticipated increased dental care costs. These programs trained auxiliaries to perform tasks formerly completed by dentists, ensured that the quality of service would be maintained, and proved the training would take less time and money compared with training of dentists in designated procedures.

The Dental Manpower Development Center in Louisville, Kentucky, was a program established in 1964 through federal grants to study the quality and quantity of dental services that could be performed by expanded duty auxiliaries. The Navy Dental Corps, Indian Health Services, and Public Health Service also developed experimental programs, as did universities such as the University of Alabama and the University of Minnesota. Today, many states have modified their dental practice acts to include advanced functions for allied dental personnel.

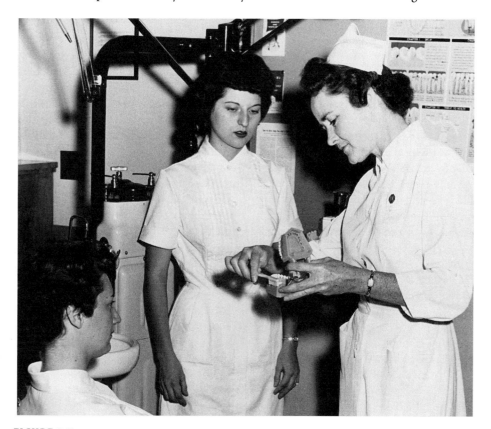

FIGURE 1.7

The 1950s represented Sputnik, a new emergence of scientific study and federal funding for allied health education programs. This photo represents the first 2-year dental assisting program (1958-1960) at Ferris Institute, now Ferris State University, Big Rapids, MI. The program was developed under the Partnership for Health Act, the Regional Medical Program, and the Hill-Burton Bill.

The 1970s

In 1970, the Council on Dental Education recognized the need to develop guidelines for delegating advanced functions and formed the Inter-Agency Committee on Dental Auxiliaries with representation from the AADS, the American Association of Dental Examiners, the ADAA, and the American Dental Hygienists Association (ADHA).

In 1971 the training in expanded auxiliary management (TEAM) grant program was initiated by the federal government to train dental students in the organization and management of a dental practice based on the concept of four-handed dentistry and use of a team of auxiliaries. Also in 1971, the health manpower educational initiative awards (HMEIA) section of the Comprehensive Health Manpower Training Act authorized the development of projects to improve the training of health personnel and expanded the health delivery system. In 1972, in response to this act, the Division of Dentistry of the Bureau of Health Manpower initiated the EFDA program to support basic and supplemental education. Formal training is required by many states for expanded functions, and examinations vary. The type of supervision during the performance of ex-

panded functions varies from direct to indirect, and functions also vary (see Chapter 2).

In 1974 the Comprehensive Health Planning, Regional Medical Program, and the Hill-Burton Acts were combined into the National Health Planning and Resources Development Act, Title XV, which identified health service areas and a health systems agency to improve the health of residents in designated areas. The ADA recognized the high priority of health planning and provided assistance to this agency.

The National Commission for Health Certifying Agencies (NCHCA), which is made up of the major health groups seeking credentials, was established in 1979 to research methods of credentialing.

DELIVERING DENTAL CARE TODAY

Research changed the practice of dentistry as humans tried to eliminate toothache and the misery of oral pain. Restorative dental care reduced the need to routinely "pull teeth," and research provided successful cost-effective results through methods used to decrease tooth decay. The use of fluoride, for example, along with good oral hygiene, toothbrushing, and flossing, helped in the prevention and control of caries and periodontal disease. In addition, more than l00 million people are covered by dental benefit plans that provide access to dental care.

Although the opportunity is available for good oral health and therefore good health, more than 43% of the U.S. population does not visit the dentist during the year. The need for dental care is significantly higher in homebound, homeless, chronically ill, disabled, aging, and other disadvantaged groups. The challenge for dentistry in the future will be to seek ways to provide access to dental care for all people.

Agencies such as the National Institute of Dental Research, National Institutes of Health, the National Center for Prevention Services, U.S. Centers for Disease Control, the American Fund for Dental Health, and other private groups are planning and initiating programs to fulfill these unmet needs and unrealized opportunities for dental health care (Box 1-1).

Each year, 30,000 cases of oral cancer are diagnosed and 8,600 individuals die from oral cancer. In the workplace, 20.9 million workdays are lost annually because of oral diseases or dental care, and more than $30 billion was spent nationally for dental care in 1990.

Although dental care is available and needs identified, the demand has not been present. People must value dental treatment and get dental care to prevent oral disease. Educational programs and community projects address the patient anxiety, fear, and pain associated with dentistry to encourage people to seek dental care.

Box 1.1

1992 Unmet Dental Needs in the U.S. Population

40%	have no access to fluoridated water
43%	receive no dental care
32%	of eligible Medicaid recipients receive dental care
50%	of homebound elderly people have not seen a dentist for more than 10 years
97%	of homeless people are in need of dental care
92%	of American children have not received dental sealants
84%	of 17-year-olds have experienced dental decay
25%	of all tooth surfaces in 40-44 year old adults have been affected by dental caries
25%	of people more than 45 years old are edentulous
41%	of 65-year-old or older people are edentulous
50%	of the total population experiences the gingival infection

Proceedings of the National Consortium Meeting on Oral Health 2000. Supported by the National Institute of Dental Research, National Institutes of Health, the National Center for Prevention Services, U.S. Centers for Disease Control, the American Fund for Dental Health, the American Dental Association, the American Trade Association, the American Association of Dental Schools, and Warner Lambert Company.

DENTAL PRACTICE

Dentistry has been cited as being the second most respected profession in America, and the dentist is recognized as one of the most highly trained practitioners in the health care profession, with high recognition for honesty and ethical standards from the public. Adult patients report being more satisfied with services received from dentists than from any other professional.

Government data have indicated that dentistry is sixth on a list of the 87 highest-paying careers in the United States. More than 140,000 dentists are active in the United States, and by the year 2000 more than 25,500 women will be active in dentistry.

General Dental Practice

Although fewer dentists go into solo practice after graduation, about 90% of them own their own business within 6 years. More dentists are forming partnerships and other group practices while working less than 40 hours a week on average. Although some dentists work more than 40 hours per week, other dentists have been in practice for many years and are limiting their office hours for treating patients, and many younger dentists maintain fewer hours while they are attempting to build a patient following.

Dental Education

Dental education consists of 2 or more years of science, liberal arts, business, or other degrees, with 3 or 4 years of dental school programming approved by the Commission on Dental Accreditation of the American Dental Association (CODA). This commission is recognized by the U.S. Department of Education and the Council on Postsecondary Accreditation to accredit dental schools, advanced dental specialties, dental assisting, dental hygiene, and dental laboratory technology educational programs. Programs that meet or exceed the basic **accreditation** standards are granted approval, and graduates of these programs are considered to be graduates of an accredited program.

Accreditation
The granting of approval by an official review board to an educational institution for meeting specific program or institutional requirements.

From 1982 to 1992, the number of women entering as first year dental students increased from 22.24% to 36.27% and minority enrollment increased from 17.17% to 31.01%. Many women entering dental school received their initial education in dental assisting or dental hygiene programs. Several dental schools have advanced placement for those high school students in accelerated programs.

Dental Examination

Graduates from dental school programs are granted either a Doctor of Dental Surgery (DDS) or a Doctor of Medical Dentistry (DMD). Dental specialization requires additional training in a specific graduate program. Dental graduates must pass a written and clinical examination by the state to receive a license to practice.

Professional Dental Organizations

Dentists may become members of their professional organization, the ADA, or the National Dental Association. The ADA provides a forum to present views and research and receive information on dental and other health care issues. The ADA is governed by bylaws, which define the rules of the organization, and is made up of councils and commissions that study specific problems and issues and recommend policies to the board of trustees and the house of delegates (Box 1-2).

Specialty Dental Practice

A dental specialist is a dentist who has received advanced education in one of the specialties recognized by the ADA and is limited to practice in that area of dental specialty. Each specialty has educational requirements also approved by the Council on Dental Education. For example, the dentist passing the examination of the American Board of Orthodontics is designated a "diplomat" of this board.

More than 19,847 dental specialists practice in the United States today, with approximately 60% in orthodontics or oral and maxillofacial surgery. The Council on Dental Education of the ADA recognizes that responsibilities among the recognized areas of dental practice overlap but stated in 1976 that specialists do not routinely provide procedures beyond the scope of that specialty (see Approved Specialties box, p. 14).

Dental Public Health

Dental public health is the science and art of preventing and controlling dental diseases and promoting dental health through organized community efforts. This form of dental practice serves the community as a whole rather than individuals. Dental public health is concerned with the dental health education of the public, applied dental research, the administration of group dental care programs, and the prevention and control of dental diseases on a community basis.

U.S. Public Health Service

The U.S. Public Health Service is part of the Department of Health and Human Services and is the primary health service for the federal government. The Public Health Service began in 1798 and currently includes eight agencies and

Box 1.2

American Dental Association Councils and Commissions

Council on Access, Prevention, and Interprofessional Relations
Council on American Dental Association Sessions and International Relations
Council on Communications
Council on Dental Benefit Programs
Council on Dental Education
Council on Dental Practice
Council on Ethics, Bylaws, and Judicial Affairs
Council on Governmental Affairs and Federal Dental Services
Council on Insurance
Council on Membership
Council on Scientific Affairs
Commission on Dental Accreditation
Joint Commission on National Dental Examinations
Commission on Relief Fund Activities

many programs from caring for the underserved population to regulating and researching the health care field (adopted May 1976).

USE OF ALLIED DENTAL PERSONNEL

The dental profession has used the term *dental auxiliary* for many years to refer to the dental assistant, dental hygienist, and dental laboratory technician. However, in 1990, because of the need for a more clear and acceptable term for these dental team members, the commission approved the use of the term **allied dental personnel** and *allied dental team members* to be used in commission policy statements, accreditation standards, reports, and other documents. The term *allied dental personnel* is used in this text when referring to dental assisting, dental hygiene, and dental laboratory technician. (Some acronyms and terms used in dentistry are listed in Box 1-3.)

Allied dental personnel

The staff associated with the practice of dentistry, for example, dental assistant, dental hygienist, and dental laboratory technician.

The Dental Assistant

Today, more than 200,000 dental assistants are employed in the United States, which represents approximately 2.5 dental assistants per dentist. Data indicate that acute shortages of

Approved Specialties

Endodontics

Endodontics is the branch of dentistry concerned with the morphologic, physiologic, and pathologic characteristics of the human dental pulp and periradicular tissue. The endodontic sciences include biology of the normal pulp and the etiology, diagnosis, prevention, and treatment of diseases and injuries of the pulp and associated periradicular conditions.

Oral and maxillofacial pathology

Oral pathology is the specialty of dentistry and discipline of pathology that involves the nature, identification, and management of diseases affecting the oral and maxillofacial regions. It investigates the causes, processes, and effects of these diseases. The practice of oral pathology includes research and diagnosis of diseases using clinical, radiographic, microscopic, biochemical, and other examinations.

Oral and maxillofacial surgery

Oral and maxillofacial surgery is the specialty of dentistry that includes the diagnosis and surgical and adjunctive treatment of diseases, injuries, and defects involving the functional and esthetic aspects of the hard and soft tissues of the oral and maxillofacial region.

Orthodontics and dentofacial orthopedics

Orthodontics is the area of dentistry concerned with the supervision, guidance, and correction of the growing or mature dentofacial structures, including conditions that require movement of teeth or correction of malrelationships and malformations of their related structures, the adjustment of relationships between and among teeth and facial bones by the application of forces, and the stimulation and redirection of functional forces within the craniofacial complex. The major responsibilities of orthodontic practice include (1) the diagnosis, prevention, interception, and treatment of all forms of malocclusion of the teeth and associated alterations in their surrounding structures; (2) the design, application, and control of functional and corrective appliances; and (3) the guidance of the dentition and its supporting structures to attain and maintain optimal occlusal relations in physiologic and esthetic harmony among facial and cranial structures.

Pediatric dentistry

Pediatric dentistry is an age-defined specialty that provides primary and comprehensive preventive and therapeutic oral health care for infants and children through adolescence, including those with special health care needs.

Periodontics

Periodontics is the specialty of dentistry that encompasses the prevention, diagnosis, and treatment of diseases of the supporting and surrounding tissues of the teeth or their substitutes and the maintenance of the health, function, and esthetics of these structures and tissues.

Prosthodontics

Prosthodontics is the branch of dentistry pertaining to the restoration of natural teeth and the maintenance of oral functions, comfort, appearance, and health of the patient by the replacement of missing teeth and contiguous oral and maxillofacial tissues with artificial substitutes.

Box 1.3

Acronyms Used in Dentistry

AADS: American Association of Dental Schools
ABHES: Accrediting Bureau of Health Education Schools
ADA: American Dental Association
ADAA: American Dental Assistants Association
ADHA: American Dental Hygienists Association
ADLA: American dental laboratory assistant
AMT: American medical technologists
ASAHP: American Society of Allied Health Professions
CDA: Certified dental assistant
CDPMA: Certified dental practice management assistant
CDXT: Certified in dental x-ray techniques
COA: Certified orthodontic assistant
COMSA: Certified oral-maxillofacial surgery assistant
DA Level I: Dental assistant category at level I
DA Level II: Dental assistant category at level II
DANB: Dental Assisting National Board
DAU: Dental auxiliary utilization

EDDA: Expanded duty dental assistant
EFODA: Expanded functions orthodontic dental assistant
EFDA: Expanded functions dental assistant
NADAD: National Association of Dental Assisting Directors
NAHCS: National Association of Health Career Schools
NATTS: National Association of Technical and Trade Schools
NRDA: National registry dental assistant
OJT: On-the-job trained
OSHA: Occupational Safety and Health Administration
QDA: Qualified dental assistant
RDA: Registered dental assistant
RDA-AMT: Registered dental assistant by the American medical technologist
RDAEF: Registered dental assistant in extended functions
TEAM: Training in expanded auxiliary management

dental assisting personnel will continue well into the turn of the century. These vacancies cost money, lower productivity, and affect patient morale significantly in the dental office. The demand for quality dental health care and new technological advances increase the need for hiring competent staff to assist with patient care.

Retention of well-trained staff is as critical as hiring dental assistants because of the many career options available in other fields. Although salaries have been much higher in many other career areas for women, the shortage in the number of qualified and trained dental assistants available to work has increased salary levels recently. In addition to making dental offices more productive, the delegation of expanded functions for dental assistants has provided higher salaries, potential upward mobility, and job satisfaction.

Role of the Dental Assistant

The dental assistant performs a variety of significant functions in the dental practice, which has been defined as follows:

> Dental Assistant Assists DENTIST engaged in diagnostic operative, surgical periodontal, preventive, orthodontics, removable and fixed prosthodontic, endodontic, and pedodontic procedures during examination and treatment of patients. Provides diagnostic aids including exposing radiographs, taking and recording medical and dental histories, recording vital signs, making preliminary impressions for study casts, and making occlusal registrations for mounting study casts. Performs clinical supportive functions including preparing and dismissing patients; sterilization and disinfecting instruments and equipment: providing postoperative instructions prescribed by DENTIST and preparing tray setups for dental procedures. Assists DENTIST in management of medical and dental emergencies. Assists in maintaining patient treatment records and maintaining operatory equipment and instruments. Performs such laboratory procedures as pouring, trimming, and polishing study casts; fabricating custom impression trays from preliminary impressions; cleaning and polishing removable appliances; and fabricating temporary restorations. Provides oral hygiene instruction such as conducting plaque control program. Performs basic business office procedures, including maintaining appointment control, receiving payment for dental services, and maintaining supply order.

The term *dental assistant* does not describe adequately who or what the dental assistant is as an individual because the duties performed are so broad in knowledge, skill levels, and functions. The categories of the dental assistant are often divided into chairside assistant, office assistant, expanded duty dental assistant, and laboratory assistant. In general, the essential duties of a clinical chairside assistant are to prepare the patient and work directly with the dentist in providing quality patient care promptly (Box 1-4). The office assistant (secretary, office assistant, or manager) fills a key position in the overall record and staff administration of the practice (Box 1-5).

Box 1.4

General Duties of the Chairside Assistant

Prepare and maintain operatory.
Greet and receive patient.
Prepare and dismiss patient.
Prepare, assemble, and sterilize instruments.
Assist in chairside procedure.
Perform proper instrument transfer.
Maintain proper seating positions.
Mix dental materials.
Take and record vital signs.
Record health information.
Chart oral conditions.
Maintain equipment and supplies.
Maintain infection control.
Prepare diagnostic aids.
Place, expose, process, and mount x-ray film.
Provide laboratory assistance.
Provide oral hygiene and diet counseling.
Provide cardiopulmonary resuscitation and emergency procedures.
Provide postoperative instruction.

Box 1.5

General Duties of the Office Assistant

Open the office and prepare for business day.
Greet and receive patients.
Handle telephone communication.
Schedule, confirm, and maintain appointment control.
File and pull records.
Prepare daily operatory appointment schedule.
Prepare patient statement.
Receive and record payment.
Maintain recall system.
Manage bookkeeping and control collections.
Prepare and maintain patient records.
Maintain supplies and inventory system.
Prepare insurance forms.
Prepare health history.
Manage office.
Schedule and manage personnel.
Present treatment plan.

Box 1.6

General Duties of the Laboratory Assistant

Pour impressions for study models.
Trim and finish study models.
Prepare working models for crown and bridge.
Construct custom trays.
Prepare base plates and occlusal rims.
Prepare space maintainers, orthodontic appliances, and occlusal guards.
Prepare temporary crowns and bridges.
Wash, invest, cast, and polish crowns and bridges.
Repair and polish dentures and removable appliances.

Box 1.7

Duties Delegated to the Expanded Duty Dental Assistant

Inspect the oral cavity.
Provide oral health instruction.
Expose radiographs.
Perform pulp vitality testing.
Make impressions for study casts.
Place and remove periodontal dressings.
Remove sutures.
Place and remove rubber dam.
Place and remove matrices and wedges.
Apply topical and anesthetic agents.
Apply topical anticariogenic agents.
Place and remove temporary restorations.
Apply cavity liners and bases.
Place, condense, and carve amalgams.
Polish amalgam restoration.
Place and finish anterior restorations.
Prepare enamel for etching and bonding.
Remove excess cement from coronal tooth surfaces.
Apply pit and fissure sealants.
Place and remove periodontal dressings.
Polish and scale coronal surfaces of teeth.
Monitor nitrous oxide analgesia.
Retract gingivae for impressions.
Take impressions for cast restorations, space maintainers, orthodontic appliances, and occlusal guards.
Cement bands and bonding brackets.
Bend archwires.
Prepare indirect patterns for endodontic posts and core castings.
Fit trial endodontic filling points.

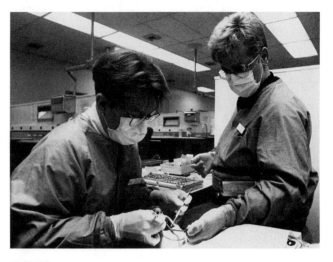

FIGURE 1.8

Expanded duty dental auxillary advanced training in expanded functions allows the dental assistant and dental hygienist to contribute to the productivity of the dental office and gives the potential for extended career mobility and increased salary.

The dental laboratory assistant performs functions that can be completed outside the clinical area and provides support in the completion of general laboratory procedures and fabrication of dental appliances (Box 1-6). These procedures contribute financially to the dental practice by reducing laboratory costs. The EDDA or EFDA provides direct patient care and therefore can increase dental services and provide a significant financial contribution to the dental practice (Figure 1-8 and Box 1-7).

Dental assisting has changed significantly over the past 20 years as health care providers recognized the ability of trained EFDAs to provide increased patient accessibility to dental services. This could reduce dental health care costs and increase dental health care delivery through the use of dental assistants in performing designated advanced dental functions. In addition to providing access to more patients, the EDDAs allow dentists to concentrate their expertise and time on those skills unique to the dentists' qualifications. Provisions in most dental practice acts and credentialing categories have allowed dental assistants to perform various intraoral procedures.

Education, testing, and licensure are required in some states for advanced trained allied dental personnel. The delegation of duties provided by dental practice acts varies from strict limitations to fairly broad provisions, and the use of terms such as *direct supervision*, *indirect supervision*, and *general supervision* also differs. Such variance provides flexibility for the dentist and the dental assistant who practices expanded duties.

The dental assistant has many career opportunities in the traditional dental practice and nontraditional settings. In addition to the roles described, the dental assistant can continue a career in dentistry through specialty practice, dental hygiene, dentistry, business management, sales, marketing, teacher education, and other areas such as the armed forces, government-sponsored programs, and international dental practice. The options are as expansive as the imagination. *The Dictionary of Occupational Titles* lists a variety of expanded career choices.

Dental Assisting Educators and Administrators

As the number of dental assisting programs increased, the need for well-trained educators and administrators also grew. Many allied health educators, which includes dental assisting, came directly from practice; few teacher education programs existed in the early 1950s when increased funding first became available to develop allied health training programs. Various federally funded workshops and institutes were developed to provide teacher training. As allied health teacher education programs increased, dental assistants who were interested in a career in education began completing baccalaureate degree programs. Dental assistants have entered many areas of higher education as teachers in various occupations of the dental assisting curriculum, such as related fields of allied health education and administrative educational positions within dentistry and in general education. They have assumed nontraditional roles such as owners of placement services, dental consulting, and political positions. Many dental assistants have become dental hygienists or dentists.

THE ROLE AND RESPONSIBILITY OF THE DENTAL TEAM

The role and responsibility of the dentist and dental personnel changed in the 1960s because of the need to increase dental services and the availability of funding through federal grants to improve the dental care delivery system. DAU programs provided for dentists and dental auxiliaries to be trained to work more efficiently together and EDDA and EFDA programs increased the skill level of dental personnel. In addition, the TEAM programs provided training in the organization and management of the dental work group or team, which included the dentist, one or more chairside and support assistants, expanded duty personnel, and the hygienist. This group became the efficient and organized team headed by the dentist. Although the dentist is responsible for all staff actions taken in the office, dental personnel also are individually responsible and liable for their actions. (See Chapter 3 for ethical considerations and Chapter 20 for clinical procedures.)

THE AMERICAN DENTAL ASSISTANTS ASSOCIATION

The ADAA is a membership organization that represents the profession of dental assisting. As the dental profession was evolving during the late eighteenth century and early nineteenth century, the profession of dental assisting was also emerging. As the demand for dental assistants became more evident and the numbers grew, the need for dental assistants to organize for the purpose of education and social interaction became apparent. Records from the ADAA document that in 1924, Juliette A. Southard brought the early associations together to establish a constitution and administrative bylaws and implemented the first election of officers of the ADAA.

Today, the ADAA is a national nonprofit corporation located in Chicago, Illinois, and has a tripartite membership with state associations and local societies. The ADAA provides many membership services including continuing education courses, publication of the *Dental Assistant Journal*, group insurance, human immunodeficiency virus test positive insurance, professional liability, a credit card program, financial planning, a member loan program, travel discounts for airlines and hotels, a rent-a-car program, and a discount health care products buying program. In addition, the ADAA provides employment data and other general information (Figure 1-9).

In 1967 the ADAA held the First International Dental Assistants Congress in Washington, D.C., and in 1993 sponsored the Second International Dental Assistants Congress in San Francisco, California. The purpose was to share educational and organizational information with international dental assistants and formulate the International Dental Assistants Federation, which provides continual communications and an international network for dental assistants.

The administrative body of the association, the board of trustees, comprises four elected officers (President, President-Elect, Vice President, Secretary/Treasurer), the immediate past president, and 12 district trustees who represent the state district areas. The administrative body is made up of all voting members of the association. The Executive Director is a member exofficial without the right to vote but, with the staff of central office, fulfills the operational responsibilities of the association. The board meets four times a year before and after the annual session and at least twice a year.

The house of delegates, which is the governing body made up of delegates from each state, meet during the annual session with the purpose of providing a membership forum to conduct business and provide an educational and social program for dental assistants on a national level. The annual sessions are held throughout the United States. Dental assistants have the opportunity to serve in local, state, and national organizational leadership

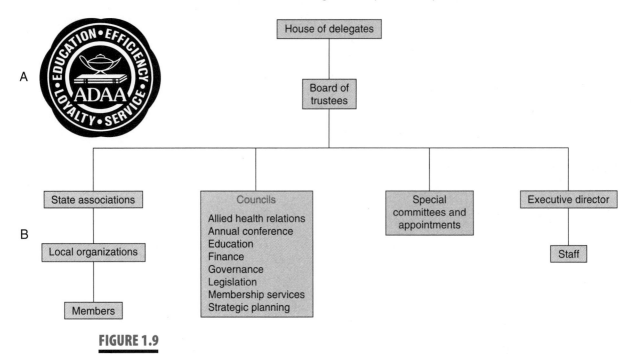

FIGURE 1.9

A, The ADAA seal. **B,** The American Dental Assistants Association organizational chart.

positions and on various committees. Members have an opportunity to make recommendations about policies affecting dental assisting, legislation, education, and credentialing and those supporting dentistry and the welfare of the public.

Today, dental assistants must see themselves as part of an active group of professional women and men because of the need for the profession of dental assisting to be involved in the changes taking place in health care delivery. The ADAA is the professional organization that represents all dental assistants and allows dental assistants to be proactive and take leadership positions within organized dentistry and the health care profession (Figure 1-10).

> **For more information, you can contact the following:**
> **American Dental Assistants Association**
> **203 North LaSalle Street**
> **Suite 1320**
> **Chicago, Illinois 60601-1225**
> **Telephone: (312) 541-1550**
> **Fax: (312) 541-1496**
> **Website: http://www.members.aol.com/adaa1/index.html**

DENTAL ASSISTING EDUCATION PROGRAMS

Dental assisting is one of the few health careers in which formal education is preferred but is not required for job entry. The most common method of entry into dental as-

sisting is through informal on-the-job training. In the past, this has often been referred to as **apprenticeship** training. Approximately two thirds of dental assistants entering dentistry do so through informal training in the office.

Apprenticeship
A specified term of study under the direct supervision of a professional practitioner.

The importance of a planned program of dental assisting education was recognized in 1923 when Juliette A. Southard, a dental assistant from New York City, organized the first local dental assistant society called the *Educational and Efficiency Society*. In 1924, she formed the first national dental assistants group, which was the original ADAA, with 200 members. In 1930 a curriculum committee was organized to develop courses, which was followed by self-study or correspondence courses. Since that time the ADAA and the Council on Dental Education of the ADA have been successful in developing high quality educational "Accreditation Standards for Dental Assisting Programs." These programs usually last 9 to 18 months.

Dynamic Career Opportunities in Dental Assisting

More recently, the ADA has reviewed current trends in dental assisting education and has taken steps to develop guidelines for innovative and flexible educational programs that are consistent with accreditation standards and also support

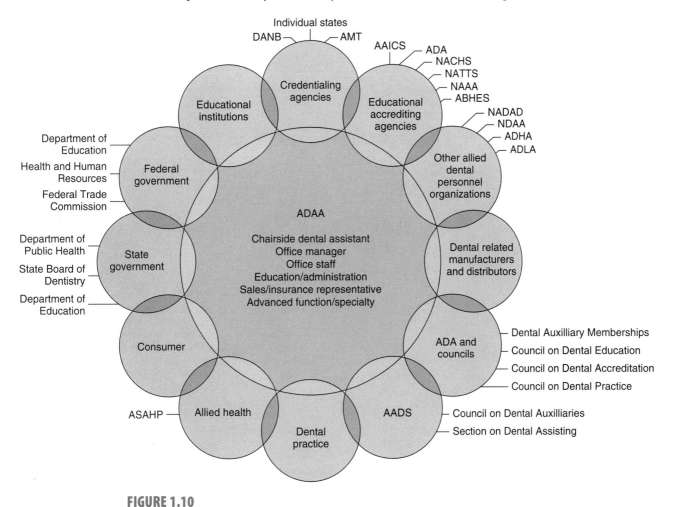

FIGURE 1.10

The American Dental Assistants Association's involvement with organized health care.

career growth for dental assistants and hygienists. Dentists and allied dental personnel have been active in encouraging legislation and pledging funding to increase enrollments in dental assisting and hygiene programs. These incentives and the increase in nontraditional education program options have promoted increased enrollment in these programs (Box 1-8).

Dental assisting programs have been established in the public and private sectors of education and are offered in high schools, vocational technical schools, community colleges, and universities. The duration of dental assisting programs ranges from 4 to 18 months, and these programs offer diplomas, certificates of completion, or associate degrees. Some institutions provide access or transfer tracks into advanced baccalaureate degree programs such as management, business, and teaching.

Current trends today indicate an even greater need for formalized dental assisting education because of regulatory health care concerns involving disease and infection control, radiation safety and other health and safety concerns for the dental staff and patient, hazardous material con-

tainment and disposal, and new technological advances in dentistry.

Professional Accrediting Agencies

Educational institutions are evaluated by specialized agencies called *accrediting agencies*, which assess and validate that the institution has met a prescribed standard of education. The role of accrediting agencies is to ensure that students are qualified to enter a specific discipline. Accreditation agencies may evaluate the entire institution or one or more of the programs offered.

Accrediting agencies that influence dental assisting educational programs are the CODA, the National Association of Health Career Schools (NAHCS), the Accrediting Bureau of Health Education Schools (ABHES), the American Association of Independent Colleges and Schools (AAICS), and the National Association of Technical and Trade Schools (NATTS). The Council on Postsecondary Accreditation (COPA) and the U.S. Department of Education recognizes these agencies.

Box 1.8

Careers in Dental Assisting Today

Career opportunities

Today, more than 200,000 dental assistants are active in the United States.

The shortage of dental assistants is increasing, and this employment need will remain through the year 2000.

Although dental assistants are employed primarily by general dentists, they are also employed by dental specialty offices and dental-related businesses.

Dentists employ an average of two to three dental assistants, and this number is rising.

Dental assistants can choose the number of hours they wish to work, and approximately 25% work part-time and sometimes in more than one office.

Dental assistants work in the same practice for approximately 5 years.

Career economics

Dental assisting salaries vary depending on responsibilities and geographic location.

Currently, the average national salary of a dental assistant is $9.90 per hour.

Dental assistants who have completed formal training or are employed in states requiring certification or registration receive higher salaries.

Benefits received by dental assistants include health and disability insurance, professional organization membership dues, uniform allowance, and paid vacations.

Education

Formal college-level education is encouraged, although dental assistants can find employment without a degree.

The American Dental Association's Commission on Dental Accreditation accredit approximately 232 dental assisting education programs in the United States.

Accredited dental assisting programs offer 9- to 11-month, full-time study, and some schools provide part-time curriculums or accelerated training.

Dental assisting careers are available to both men and women.

Dental assisting career opportunities are exceptional for minority students.

Dental assisting careers are excellent for nontraditional students, such as those who are 23 years of age or older, seeking a career change or job retraining, or culturally diverse or those who need a flexible schedule, often with evening hours.

Because of reductions in the number of students enrolled in dental assisting programs, employment demands for dental assistants are increasing to meet the growing need for dental services.

For additional information about dental assisting careers, you should call the American Dental Assistants Association (312-541-1550) or your state or local dental society.

Courtesy the National Career Guidance Program sponsored by the American Dental Association and The American Association of Dental Schools.

Credentialing of Dental Assistants

Because dental assisting did not follow the traditional education and credentialing lines as many other allied health professions did, dental assisting developed into a multiskilled profession. Therefore, credentialing is increasingly necessary because of the variety of skills dental assistants must perform; the increasing intraoral functions delegated to them; the need to provide infection control, radiation safety, biohazard disposal techniques, and medical emergency training; and the legal and ethical considerations of a dental health care environment. Dental assisting categories are evolving according to the essential skill levels being performed and the education and competency needed to complete the identified tasks. Credentialing of dental assistants has increased nationally.

A credential is a written letter, certificate, license, or other document that provides evidence of dental assistants' qualifications and gives them the authority to act. Dental assistants have several credentialing mechanisms. A letter of recommendation is often considered a type of credential giving an individual's opinion of the dental assistant's abilities or competency. The most commonly recognized formal methods are certification and registration.

Certification

Two independent certifying agencies for dental assistants are approved by the National Commission for Certifying Agencies of the National Organization for Competency Assurance. A certification credential is offered through the DANB (Figure 1-11), and a registration credential is offered through the American Medical Technologists (AMT) Association.

The DANB offers certified dental assistant (CDA) examinations for eligible candidates who meet the examination requirements for the CDA (general chairside-CDA), the certified oral and maxillofacial surgery assistant (COMSA), the certified dental practice management assistant (CDPMA), and the certified orthodontic assistant (COA). Applicants for these examinations must meet **eligibility** requirements for the pathway that they wish to pursue, complete an examination application, and pay an application fee. Examinations are offered periodically in designated areas throughout the United States. Certification is for 1 year and must be renewed annually. Recertification is acquired through completing continuing education and submitting a fee (Table 1-1).

Eligibility
The act of being qualified.

Dental assisting national board
Certified dental assistant

Pathway I	Pathway II	Pathway III
• Graduation from a dental assisting or dental hygiene program accredited by the ADA Commission on Dental Accreditation • Current Cardiopulmonary Resuscitation (CPR) Health Care Provider Level certification as prescribed by the American Heart Association or the American Red Cross	• High school graduation or equivalent • A minimum of 2 years full-time work experience (at least 3,500 hours accumulated over a 24-month period) as a dental assistant verified by dentist-employer • Current Cardiopulmonary Resuscitation (CPR) Health Care Provider Level certification as prescribed by the American Heart Association or the American Red Cross	• Previous DANB CDA certification with a lapsed status of 3 months or more and do not meet eligibility requirements for the CDA Reinstatement examination • Current Cardiopulmonary Resuscitation (CPR) Health Care Provider Level certification as prescribed by the American Heart Association or the American Red Cross

Certified dental assistant—reinstatement

To apply for the CDA Reinstatement examination, the candidate must document the following eligibility requirements:

1. Previous certification with expiration date occurring after December 31, 1986

2. Two years of full-time work experience (3,500 hours) as a dental assistant since January 1, 1995

3. Current Cardiopulmonary Resuscitation (CPR) Health Care Provider Level certification as prescribed by the American Heart Association or the American Red Cross

Certified orthodontic assistant

Pathway I	Pathway II	Pathway III	Pathway IV
• Work experience in an orthodontic practice setting, *plus* a CDA, RDH, or RDA credential • Current Cardiopulmonary Resuscitation (CPR) Health Care Provider Level certification as prescribed by the American Heart Association or the American Red Cross	• High school graduation or equivalent • A minimum of 2 years full-time work experience (at least 3,500 hours accumulated over a 24-month period) as an orthodontic assistant verified by dentist-employer • Current Cardiopulmonary Resuscitation (CPR) Health Care Provider Level certification as prescribed by the American Heart Association or the American Red Cross	• Completion of an orthodontic assisting preparation course at an institution having a dental assisting program accredited by the ADA Commission on Dental Accreditation plus the CDA credential • Current Cardiopulmonary Resuscitation (CPR) Health Care Provider Level certification as prescribed by the American Heart Association or the American Red Cross	• Previous DANB COA certification with a lapsed status of 3 months or more • Current Cardiopulmonary Resuscitation (CPR) Health Care Provider Level certification as prescribed by the American Heart Association or the American Red Cross

Certified oral and maxillofacial surgery assistant

Pathway I	Pathway II	Pathway III	Pathway IV
• High school graduation or equivalent • Successful completion of 500 hours of postsecondary education in oral and maxillofacial surgery assisting, *plus* 6 months of full-time work experience (875 hours) in an oral and maxillofacial surgery practice setting or the equivalent • Current Cardiopulmonary Resuscitation (CPR) Health Care Provider Level certification as prescribed by the American Heart Association or the American Red Cross	• Work experience in an oral and maxillofacial surgery practice setting, *plus* a CDA, LPN, RN, RDH, or RDA credential • Current Cardiopulmonary Resuscitation (CPR) Health Care Provider Level certification as prescribed by the American Heart Association or the American Red Cross	• High school graduation or equivalent • A minimum of 2 years full-time work experience (at least 3,500 hours accumulated over a 24-month period) as an OMS assistant verified by dentist-employer • Current Cardiopulmonary Resuscitation (CPR) Health Care Provider Level certification as prescribed by the American Heart Association or the American Red Cross	• Previous DANB COMSA certification with a lapsed status of 3 months or more • Current Cardiopulmonary Resuscitation (CPR) Health Care Provider Level certification as prescribed by the American Heart Association or the American Red Cross

Certified dental practice management assistant

Pathway I	Pathway II	Pathway III
• High school graduation or equivalent • Work experience in a dental practice setting verified by dentist-employer • Current Cardiopulmonary Resuscitation (CPR) Health Care Provider Level certification as prescribed by the American Heart Association or the American Red Cross	• High school graduation or equivalent • Completion of a practice management course at an institution having a dental assisting program accredited by the ADA Commission on Dental Accreditation • Current Cardiopulmonary Resuscitation (CPR) Health Care Provider Level certification as prescribed by the American Heart Association or the American Red Cross	• Previous DANB CDPMA certification with a lapsed status of 3 months or more • Current Cardiopulmonary Resuscitation (CPR) Health Care Provider Level certification as prescribed by the American Heart Association or the American Red Cross

FIGURE 1.11

Summary of DANB certified dental assistant and specialty component eligibility pathways.

Table 1.1

Dental Assisting National Board Certified Dental Assisting 1999 Recertification

Certification validity: Certification is valid for 1 year.
Recertification requirements: Affirm 12 hours of acceptable continuing dental education within 1 year from the following dental education sources.

Education	Hours
On-site lecture, course, seminar, table clinics, or exhibits	1 hour credit per hour of attendance annually
Home study courses	Preapproval
Reading activity	1 hour credit
Writing of a book and journal report	1 hour credit
Successful completion of Dental Assisting National Board examination	12 hours awarded
Community participation (2 hours)	1 hour for community service
Essay	1 hour for 250-word essay
College courses	12 hours
Cardiopulmonary resuscitation health care provider courses	4 hours
Scholarly activities such as teaching a professional dental course, authoring a published article, being a member of DANB test activity construction committee, submitting accepted examination items	3 hours for each
Electives such as professional development courses	3 hours maximum

Refer to the Dental Assisting National Board, Inc, *1999 Recertification Guidelines*, for more specific requirements in each area.

For more information, you can contact the following:

Dental Assisting National Board, Inc.
676 North St. Clair Street
Suite 1880
Chicago, Illinois 60611
Telephone: (800) FOR DANB
Fax: (312) 642-1475
Website: http://www.dentalassisting.com

The AMT is a certifying organization offering a registered dental assistant (RDA) RDA-AMT credential for those who fulfill the dental assisting requirements and successfully complete their examination. Applicants must meet the requirements for registration as a dental assistant, complete an application for examination, and pay an application fee. Examinations are offered three times a year, usually at the time of graduation or at designated sites. Registration is for 1 year and mst be maintained for a fee by completing continuing education requirements.

The certifying organizations that offer credentialing maintain that an individual meets certain educational prerequisites and experience requirements. However, certification does not mean that the dental assistant has complied with licensure or other state regulatory requirements. Today, most states allow some delegation of specific expanded functions to dental assistants and mandate some formal training and examination before dental assistants can be involved in expanded functions.

Many states recognize more than one category of dental assistanting and licensure, and registration programs are required for dental assistants in these states, particularly for dental assistants who wish to provide expanded functions. In addition, supervision requirements vary from state to state. Direct supervision requires that the dentist is in the office at the time of the procedure and examines the patient during the same visit. Indirect supervision requires that the dentist is in the office but may examine the patient at a later time. General supervision specifies that the dentist has authorized the procedure but may not necessarily be present in the office. Dental assistants must understand the dental practice laws of their state and should contact state and regional dental agencies for further information on any state law regulating dental assisting.

For more information, you can contact the following:

American Medical Technologists
710 Higgins Road
Park Ridge, Illinois 60068
Telephone: (847) 823-5169
Website: http://www.amt1.com/home.html

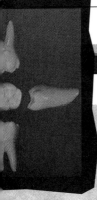

Points for Review

- Primary purpose of dentistry
- Historical events in the evolution of dentistry from its early foundation to modern times
- The early leaders who contributed to the advancement of dentistry
- The establishment of organized dentistry and the regulation of dentistry
- The role of allied dental personnel in dentistry
- The advancement of dental assisting in the practice of dentistry
- The role of the general dentist and dental specialists in the dental care delivery system
- The role and responsibility of allied dental personnel and the value of the dental team
- The opportunities for educating allied dental personnel and the role of accrediting and credentialing agencies especially as related to dental assisting education and career enhancement

Self-Study Questions

1. What is the ethical promise not to cause harm called?
   a. Edict of Mayo
   b. Oath of Hippocrates
   c. Code of medical and dental ethics
   d. b and c
2. Who was the "father of modern dentistry?"
   a. Aristotle
   b. Andres Vesalius
   c. Benjamin Franklin
   d. Pierre Fauchard
3. Who published the home remedy book *Every Man His Own Doctor*?
   a. Benjamin Franklin
   b. Pierre Fauchard
   c. Paul Revere
   d. Horace Wells
4. What did the use of the royal mineral succedaneum cause?
   a. The Edict of May
   b. The Amalgam War

c. The development of the x-ray machine
   d. The first laws to regulate dentistry
5. Who was the patron saint of dentistry?
   a. Aristotle
   b. Apollonia
   c. Andres Vesalius
   d. Pierre Fauchard
6. Who was the first woman in the world to graduate from a dental school?
   a. Juliette A. Southard
   b. Emeline Roberts
   c. Lucy Beaman Hobbs
   d. Olga Lentz
7. Who is recognized as hiring the first female dental assistant?
   a. Horace Hayden
   b. Edmund Kells
   c. Chapin Harris
   d. Nathan Keep
8. What was the first dental school in the United States?
   a. Baltimore College of Dental Surgery
   b. Maryland Medical School
   c. Northwestern University
   d. University of Louisville
9. Who organized the Educational and Efficiency Society?
   a. Juliette A. Southard
   b. Charles Goodyear
   c. Chapin Harris
   d. Horace Hayden
10. What document showed that increased dental production and services could be improved through the use of trained dental auxiliaries?
    a. The Partnership for Health Act
    b. The Comprehensive Health Planning Bill
    c. The Hill-Burton Bill
    d. The ADA Bureau of Economic Research and Statistics dental practice survey of 1953 to 1956
11. What key program or programs were funded that advanced dental assisting functions?
    a. DAU
    b. EDDA/EFDA
    c. TEAM
    d. All of the above
12. What agency researches methods of credentialing?
    a. The NCHCA
    b. The ADA Bureau of Economic Research and Statistics

c. The Health Systems Agency

d. All of the above

13. What is the main cause for people not seeking dental treatment?

a. Lack of access

b. Success of sealant usage

c. Aspects of anxiety, fear, and pain

d. All of the above

14. How can accessibility to dental care be effectively increased?

a. Use of EFDA

b. Successful marketing

c. Use of third party payors

d. All of the above

15. Under what type of supervision do most dental assistants operate?

a. None

b. Indirect

c. Direct

d. None of the above

16. Dental assistants are legally and ethically responsible for their own actions in the dental office.

a. True

b. False

17. Approximately 92% of American children have received dental sealants.

a. True

b. False

18. The ADAA represents the profession of dental assistants.

a. True

b. False

19. Credentialing agencies assess and evaluate dental assisting programs to determine whether they meet a prescribed standard of education.

a. True

b. False

20. What agency certifies dental assistants?

a. The DANB

b. The ADAA

c. The ADA

d. Only state agencies

21. Certification means that a dental assistant has complied with all licensure, registration, and other state regulatory requirements.

a. True

b. False

22. The functions that dental assistants can perform legally are the same in all states.

a. True

b. False

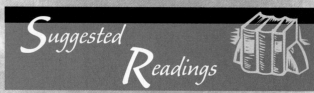

Suggested Readings

American Dental Assistants Association: *Special credentialing project*, Chicago, July 1988, Steering Committee Report to the American Dental Assistants Association Board of Trustees.

American Dental Association: *Innovative dental assisting and dental hygiene programs*, Chicago, 1992, Council on Dental Education and Council on Dental Practice.

American Dental Association: *Legal provisions for delegating functions to dental assistants and dental hygienists*, Chicago, April 1990, Department of Educational Surveys, Division of Education.

American Dental Association: *Trends in dental assisting education*, Chicago, 1992, Department of Educational Surveys, Division of Education.

American Dental Assistants Association: *ADAA endorses federal guidelines for radiologic technologists qualifications*, Chicago, 1981, update newsletter.

American Dental Association: *Accreditation standards*, Chicago, 1980, Commission on Accreditation of Dental and Dental Auxiliary Educational Programs.

American Dental Association: *A compilation of facts related to the teaching of expanded functions*, Chicago, Council on Dental Education Report.

American Dental Assistants Association: *The history of the American dental assistants association, the first fifty years 1924-1974*, Chicago, 1974, ADAA.

American Dental Association: *Legal provisions for delegating expanded functions to dental hygienists and dental assistants*, Chicago, 1977, Council on Dental Education, Division of Educational Measurements.

American Fund for Dental Health: *Oral health 2000*, Chicago, 1990, Proceedings of the National Consortium Meeting.

American Medical Technologist: *Dental assistant certification*, Park Ridge, Ill, 1999.

Bluegrass Regional Health Planning Council: *Health systems agency on the rise*, Frankfort, Ky, The Health Planning and Resources Development Act of 1974.

Breitbart AR, Aftoora PC: *A brief history of dentistry and dental education*, Champaign, Ill, 1979, Cal, CoLaboratories.

Council on Dental Health: *Dentistry's participation in the national health planning and resources development act*, Chicago, 1976, ADA.

Council on Public Higher Education: *Dentistry*, Phase 1 Rep, Frankfort, Ky, 1975, Comprehensive Planning for Higher Education, Kentucky and Health Sciences Education.

Council of State Governments: *Dental health care delivery systems*, A background paper prepared for the National Task Force on State Dental Policies, Lexington, Ky, 1978, National Headquarters.

Council of State Governments: *Manpower utilization*, A background paper prepared for the National Task Force on State Dental Policies, Lexington, Ky, 1978, National Headquarters.

Council of State Governments: *Organization and function of state dental boards*, A background paper prepared for the National Task Force on State Dental Policies, Lexington, Ky, 1978, National Headquarters.

Dental Assisting National Board: *Membership information*, Chicago, 1999.

Dunbar WF: *The Michigan record in higher education*, Detroit, 1963, Wayne

State University Press.

Frost JC: *Your future in dental assisting*, New York, 1964, Richard Rosen Press.

Galambos EC: *Implications of lengthened health education: nursing and the allied health fields*, Manpower and Education Rep, Atlanta, 1979, Southern Regional Education.

Gies WJ: *Dental education in the United States and Canada*, The Carnegie Foundation for the Advancement of Teaching, Bulletin Number 19, New York, 1926, McGraw-Hill.

Greenberg DS: Health-care colossus, *The Washington Post*, Dec 18, 1979.

Guerini V: *A history of dentistry: from the most ancient times until the end of the eighteenth century*, Pound Ridge, NY, 1969, The Milford House.

Hawkins NG: Medical health, welfare, and social science, *Choice* 19:12, 1973.

Hixson JS, Mochniak N: *Forecasts of employment in the dental sector to 1995*, Washington, DC, 1980, US Department of Health, Education, and Welfare, Public Health Service, Health Resources Administration, Bureau of Health Manpower, Division of Manpower Analysis, US GPO.

McCluggage RW: *A history of the American dental association*, Chicago, 1959, ADA.

Michigan, State of: *Annual Reports, 1913-1924*, Board of Dental Examiners, Presented to Governor Woodbridge N. Ferris, 1913-1924.

Michigan, State of: *Public acts in the legislature: 1907-1978*, State Publishing, 1907-1978.

Newman JF, Larsen Arne: *A decade of dental service utilization*, Hyattsville, Md, 1974, US Department of Health and Human Services, Public Health Service, Health Resource Administration, Bureau of Health Professions, Division of Dentistry, Chase, Rosen, and Wallace.

New York Academy of Medicine: *The role of government tax funds in problems of health care, closing the gaps in the availability and accessibility of health services*, New York, 1965, 41:12, Health Conference.

Novak DE: Dental assisting update, *J Am Dent Assist Assoc* 1:4, 2:1 1993.

Novak DE: *Dental auxiliary education in the US*, Ann Arbor, 1982, University of Michigan, (dissertation).

Novak DE: *Dental auxiliary evolution: a historical perspective*, *J Am Dent Assist Assoc* (53) 5:17-22, Sept/Oct 1984.

Novak DE: *Dental assisting manpower complexity: practice, education, need, and credentialing*, Boston, 1988, Annual Meeting, American Public Health Association.

Novak DE: *Adult and continuing education in the United States: the role of program design*, Ann Arbor, Mich, 1982, University of Michigan, Adult and Continuing Education, Research study EdS.

Novak DE: *Dental auxiliary education in the United States: new program design and implication for practice*, Ann Arbor, Mich, 1982, University of Michigan, Adult and Continuing Education, Research study EdS.

O'Rourke JT, Miner LMS: *Dental education in the US*, Philadelphia, 1941, WB Saunders.

Paul A: *Improve dental health care delivery*, Lansing, Mich, 1975, Capital Corridor, House of Judicial Committee.

Ring ME: *Dentistry: an illustrated history*, St Louis, 1992, Mosby.

Sheppard HJ, Grover AC: Testimony presented to the Council of State Government's National Task Force on State Dental Policies, San Francisco, 1978, Federal Trade Commission.

US Department of Health, Education, and Welfare, Public Health Service, Health Resources Administration: *Expanded function dental auxiliary (EFDA) training grant programs*, Washington, DC, 1978, Program Guide.

Weinberger BW: *An introduction to the history of dentistry*, St Louis, 1948, Mosby.

Chapter 2

Key Points

- ▪ Career planning
- ▪ Employment preparation

Career Planning and Interview Techniques for the Professional Dental Assistant

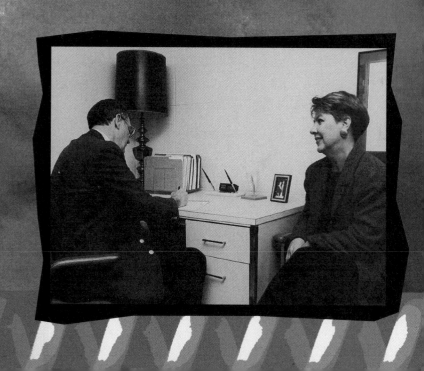

Chapter Outline

Career Planning
Preparing for a Career in Dental Assisting
    Education and training
Finding the Right Job
    Initial considerations in seeking
    employment

Resources for job opportunities
Preparing a resumé and cover letter
Preparing for the interview
Interviewing
Employment Agreement
Employment Privileges and Rights

Learning Objectives

On completion of chapter 2, the student should be able to do the following:

- Define key terms.
- Describe the importance of career planning and self-assessment in making career decisions.
- List the personal qualities that a dental assistant should possess.
- Develop a personal resumé and cover letter.

- List the qualities essential for good interview techniques.
- List the primary areas to be discussed with an employer during an interview.
- Develop a personal budget based on your projected income and expenses.
- List the provisions appropriate for a desirable employment agreement.

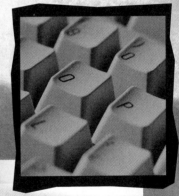

Key Terms

Apprenticeship	Discrimination	Probation
Benefits	Interview	Reference
Career	On-the-Job Training	Resumé

CAREER PLANNING

Career success depends on how you focus your talents. Ask yourself the following questions: What is important to you? What do you like doing? What do you believe in? Because

Career

A chosen occupation and pursuit in professional advancement.

imagining what you want to do for the next 5 to 20 years of your life is difficult, choosing the right **career** and job employment becomes extremely important and necessitates self-assessment (Box 2-1).

Think about and list the things that interest you, what you like and do not like in a work environment, and the skills that you have. After thinking about your personal needs, consider how you can best prepare for your career.

Career opportunities, advancement potential, and salaries for dental assistants have increased significantly in the last few years because of the rise in the number of dentists, shortage of dental assistants, and growth in the functions that can be delegated to dental assistants. The accelerated number of the elderly population, the "new baby boom," increased health insurance coverage, and other factors are raising the need for dental assistants. Surveys indi-

cate that 50% to 76% more qualified dental assistants and up to 400% more basic entry-level dental staff or dental office aides will be needed nationally by the year 2000.

PREPARING FOR A CAREER IN DENTAL ASSISTING
Education and Training

The more than 300,000 dental assistants in the United States have entered the profession in one of several ways. The largest number of dental assistants are informally trained, or receive **on-the-job training**. Formally educated dental assistants receive their education through high school programs or colleges and universities.

On-the-job training

A type of informal training that takes place in the workplace rather than through an academic educational program of study.

The largest number of women and men entering the dental assisting field have not completed a formal dental assisting educational program. These dental assistants are being trained on-the-job by the dentist or a staff member. This type of training is also referred to as in-office training, preceptorship, or **apprenticeship** training. One advantage of this route is that it provides immediate job entry for people who cannot take time to complete a formal educational program. The untrained person entering directly into certain dental staff positions may have other credentials, ex-

Apprenticeship

A specified term of study under the direct supervision of a professional practitioner.

periences, or education that pertain to that job. For instance, a person with experience in banking, secretarial work, or other related backgrounds can perform in a reception or business office position. A good attitude and personality influence the acceptability of a person for employment, often over education and experience. An employee who can help with training is a benefit to the practice and assistant so that the dentist can continue normal work production. Proper training takes time, and preparation of a new dental assistant can result in loss of productivity for the dentist and potentially for decreased knowledge and skill levels for the dental assistant. However, some dentists prefer to train their own dental assistants and are able to take the time to train them adequately, but the majority prefer dental assistants who are already trained and have several years of experience.

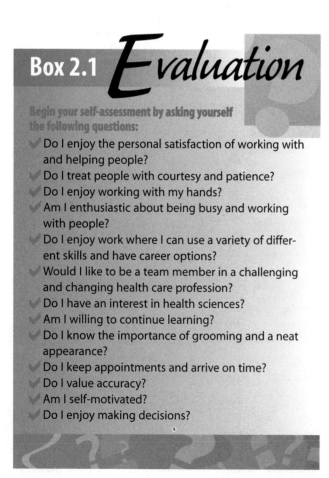

Box 2.1 *Evaluation*

Begin your self-assessment by asking yourself the following questions:

- Do I enjoy the personal satisfaction of working with and helping people?
- Do I treat people with courtesy and patience?
- Do I enjoy working with my hands?
- Am I enthusiastic about being busy and working with people?
- Do I enjoy work where I can use a variety of different skills and have career options?
- Would I like to be a team member in a challenging and changing health care profession?
- Do I have an interest in health sciences?
- Am I willing to continue learning?
- Do I know the importance of grooming and a neat appearance?
- Do I keep appointments and arrive on time?
- Do I value accuracy?
- Am I self-motivated?
- Do I enjoy making decisions?

Continuing Education

On-the-job training can be supplemented through continuing education course offerings, night school, or correspondence courses. An increasing number of schools and private training programs provide short-term courses for working dental assistants. Dentists often provide financial support for their dental assistants to take continuing education courses after they have been employed for a period. These usually short-term courses provide additional information to the assistant's knowledge base, so these programs may not provide the basic information necessary for entry-level staff members. The dentist is responsible for informing the new staff member of the hazards of the work environment and the laws that affect the employee's work practices. The dental assistant is responsible for inquiring about health care information when entering the dental practice. People are ethically and legally responsible for their own actions or lack of action (see Chapter 3).

Formal education provides the standardized training essential to teach the basic knowledge and skills necessary for competent and qualified dental assistants. Today, many educational institutions provide alternative dental assisting programs. These programs have revised curriculum design, program length, and admission requirements to meet the needs of a broader range of students. The programs also provide part-time, evening, and weekend courses, satellite courses or outreach locations, and advanced standing and independent or self-study. Although these programs are replacing some traditional programs, the number of new programs has not increased enough to replace the ones that have closed recently. The decrease in the number of dental assisting programs has occurred at a time when the need for quality trained and educated personnel is increasing.

- What kind of practice am I interested in: large, small, group, solo, partnership, general dentistry, specialty practice, military, public health, and so on?
- Do I know anyone who works for this dentist or knows the dentist who might be able to give me a **reference**?

Answering these questions could, for instance, help you select an area to work that may best suit your needs or prepare you to discuss problems with the potential employer associated with your travel to and from work. Answering the questions may also help you select an employer who best fits your personality and needs because you may spend as much time with your employer as you do your family.

Reference
A person who is in the position to recommend another person for a job.

Resources for Job Opportunities

Once you have reviewed your career plans, identified and made your career preparation, and considered some initial work preferences, you are ready to find a job. The dental assistant and dentist need to make sure that they are comfortable with each other and with other staff in the office. Do not take it for granted that you will find the right job in your first search or on the first interview. Do not get discouraged. You have many options to help find employment. (Box 2-2 shows where to start your job search.)

Some dentists require a written application be submitted before an interview. If the employer wants the application to be sent to a post office address, you will not have the street

FINDING THE RIGHT JOB

At some point, you are going to be looking for the "right job." As you search for a job, remember that the dentist is also looking for the "right" employee. Because the dentist, you, and other office personnel make up the "team," you and the dentist should meet each other's expectations and employer and employee needs.

Initial Considerations in Seeking Employment

Successful job application begins with careful preparation. Knowing what you want in a position is as important as finding a job. Before you begin looking for employment or meeting with potential employers, you may want to ask yourself the following questions:

- What jobs are available?
- What area of the city or town do I want to work?
- Is the office accessible to public transportation or near my home?

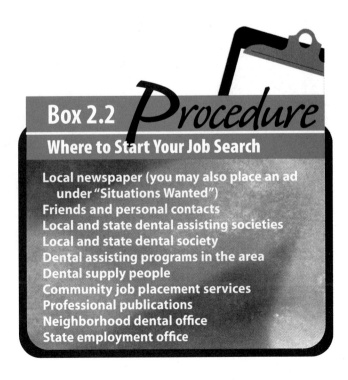

Box 2.2 *Procedure*

Where to Start Your Job Search

Local newspaper (you may also place an ad under "Situations Wanted")
Friends and personal contacts
Local and state dental assisting societies
Local and state dental society
Dental assisting programs in the area
Dental supply people
Community job placement services
Professional publications
Neighborhood dental office
State employment office

Box 2.3

Procedure

Style Sheet for the Chronologic Resumé

1. Center your name with appropriate credentials. You may wish to use *capital letters* with *boldface type*.
2. Your address and telephone number should follow your name. Be certain to add your zip code and telephone area code. If you are difficult to reach, add a telephone number of a relative or friend who can be contacted easily and will give you the message.
3. *Capitalize* key headings followed by a colon. You may wish to use *boldface type* for these headings also.
4. If you are sending your resumé to one office, you may wish to state a *specific objective* for a position. However, if you are planning to send a single resumé to several different positions, you should not include a specific objective because your potential to be considered for certain jobs may be limited. A *career* objective may be used stating your *general* interest in a position. A specific objective or objectives is effective when you know the employment needs of the dentist.
5. Provide an *education* category listing the educational institution, degree, and date the degree was awarded. List your most recent education first.
6. Provide a *continuing education* category, if appropriate, listing the provider, title of the course, and date the course was taken. You should list this especially if you have not had formal education since your last year in high school, high school graduation, or completion of a graduate equivalency degree (GED). List the most recent course first.
7. List any *credentials* (*license and certification*) you may have earned.
8. List any educational, academic, or professional *honors* or *awards* that you have received.
9. Provide a *work experiences* category, listing your most recent experience first. Provide the *employer's* name, *position* you held, *duties* performed, and *dates* of employment. If you are a recent dental assistant graduate, you may wish to list the type of work you performed while on externship. These experiences help the potential employer understand your capabilities. You may also

wish to list any nondental experiences, which indicate your experience with people or other areas of business.
10. *Equipment experience* is an additional category that provides information about the clinical, laboratory, and office equipment you can operate. List this information by machine name and the processes you can perform on this equipment.
11. Include a *professional membership* category, if appropriate, listing the *organization* or *organizations* you belong to, *date* of membership, and *activities* you were involved in. You can also list committee chair or officer positions.
12. Provide a *special professional activities* category to list the other types of activities that you were involved with such as presentations, writing projects, publications, or research projects.
13. *Hobbies* categories are often added to emphasize other interests that you may have.
14. An *other information* category will provide you with an area to list information that might be important to an employer and not found in the above categories.
15. *References* are usually listed at the bottom of the resumé or provided on request. Always receive permission from people you plan to list as references so that they can be prepared to answer questions that the potential employer may ask. Because of the legal implications of giving references today, you may be asked to provide written authorization for your reference to provide employment information. Do not feel offended if your reference does not wish to provide a referral for you. They support you and wish you the best in your job search, but legal controversy about the liability of referrals exists. Not discussing referrals with your references can lead to embarrassment and often reflects negatively on you if your references prefer not to give a response to a potential employer. The typical questions asked of references involve dates of employment, dependability, initiative, cooperation, relationships with other staff members, and job skills. Questions about personality and attitude are as important as skills to most dentists.

address, but if an office mailing address is given, you can identify the office location. Often a telephone number is given. You can call and request additional information about the job, perhaps even a job description, before you spend your time and effort pursuing a lead in which you have no interest. Be sure to identify yourself and give your reason for calling. Learn as much as you can about the employer and the working environment before the interview.

Questions such as salary and **benefits** are not usually discussed on the telephone. Do not hesitate to ask questions.

Benefits

Entitlements or advantages that enhance the well-being of an employee and that are part of an employment agreement.

For example, you can ask for information such as the location of the office, name of the dentist, correct spelling of the dentist's name, professional designation (for example, DMD or DDS), type of office, and number of work days and hours. Remember that the first telephone conversation may be an "interview," which can give you the opportunity to get information that may help you decide whether the job meets your needs and is worth pursuing. Although you may not be able to speak with the dentist, the receptionist may be able to answer some of your questions.

Preparing a Resumé and Cover Letter

Resumé

A record of one's personal history and experiences provided for job application.

If you have not had an opportunity to speak with the dentist on the telephone, your **resumé** and cover letter is the first impression that the potential employer will receive.

Resumé

How neatly you prepare your resumé, the format you use, and the information you give represent you. Your resumé is an investment into your career. It should be clear, concise, and preferably one page in length. A chronologic resumé represents education and work experience. It may not be the best type of resumé for the dental assistant just beginning a career. The skills resumé may be better. You may wish to write both resumés to see which one suits you more.

If you do not have the ability to prepare your resumé in a professional format, you can have it prepared by a commercial service available in most communities. Box 2-3 is a style sheet for the chronologic resumé. All information on the resumé should be correct, and you should be prepared to answer specific questions regarding your resumé and your experiences. Soft-white, ivory, or light-gray paper with black

type is preferred for a resumé. Using the same paper stock for your resumé and cover letter are more acceptable. According to Title VII, Civil Rights Act of 1964, you do not have to include personal information such as age, marital status, pregnancy status, whether you have children, height, weight, religion, habits, or disabilities (Figure 2-1).

The following guideline represents the skills resumé (Figure 2-2):

1 Center your name with appropriate credentials. You may wish to use *capital letters* with *boldface type*.
2 Your address and telephone number should follow your name. Be sure to add your area and zip codes.
3 You may also wish to state a *specific objective* for a particular position on a skills resumé. However, as with the chronologic resumé, you should not include a specific objective if the resumé is to be sent to more than one office. Again, a *career* objective may be used to state a *general* position interest.
4 List your various *skills* such as *clinical, office, administrative, laboratory, advanced function*, and so on as separate categories.
5 Provide *references* or list "On request."

Cover Letter

The purpose of a cover letter is to respond to the job advertisement and express your interest in the position. The cover letter is placed on top of the resumé and gives the dentist an opportunity to focus attention on your key qualifications and experiences. The cover letter may be the first impression of you and your first communication with the potential employer. The cover letter should be one page in length and typed, with well-written information that is clear and to the point and attracts the employer's attention (Box 2-4). Correct spelling and grammar are important and may be a key factor in your getting the job. The letter should be well balanced on the page and spaced. Do not staple the cover letter to the resumé. You must make sure that the potential employer's name, title, and address are correct. This shows your appreciation of accuracy and indicates a level of enthusiasm, organization, responsibility, and professionalism (Figure 2-3).

Preparing for the Interview

Preparing for an **interview** is often as important as the actual meeting. You should know what type of position you are looking for, what financial restrictions you have, and what you need to know to make a decision.

Find out if you will be interviewing with the office manager or the dentist and

Interview

A conversation between an employer and a potential employee for the purpose of assessing the qualifications of a person for a job.

if a second interview will take place, particularly if the first

Text continued on p. 35

SUSAN ADAMS, CDA, RDA
1826 Browns Lane
Anytown, USA 00001
(502) 465-6184

EDUCATION:

Jefferson State School	Dental Assisting Diploma	1989
Middleview High School	Diploma	1988

CONTINUING EDUCATION:

University of Louisville	AIDS/HIV	1989
KDAA	Radiation Safety	1990
University of Louisville	EDDA	1991

LICENSE/CERTIFICATION:

Certified Dental Assistant	1989 - Current
Registered Dental Assistant	1991 - Current

HONORS/AWARDS:

Community Dentistry Student Award	1989

WORK EXPERIENCE:

Dr. John Sheldon	Internship Chairside Assistant	1989
Dr. Kenneth James	Internship Office Assistant	1989
Dr. Larry Penny	Part Time Chairside Assistant	1990 - Current
(List types of procedures you		
performed in these positions)		

EQUIPMENT EXPERIENCE:

Computer	Word Perfect Correspondence

PROFESSIONAL MEMBERSHIP:

ADAA	Member	1990-93
KDAA	Member	1990-93
LDAS	Education Committee	1990-93

SPECIAL PROFESSIONAL ACTIVITIES:

KDAA Annual Meeting	Table Clinic

HOBBIES: Sailing, swimming, and skiing
REFERENCES: On request

FIGURE 2.1

Chronologic resumé sample.

SUSAN ADAMS, CDA, RDA
1826 Browns Lane
Anytown, USA 00001
(502) 465-6184

Objective

To obtain a challenging position where I will be able to contribute successfully to the dental practice, provide a service to dental health care delivery, and use my education and experience.

Skills

Clinical   Knowledge and skills in all phases of chairside dental assisting, including infection control, radiation safety, taking vital signs, health history, CPR, and advanced function restorative application.

Office   Working knowledge and practical skills in the operations of the reception area, telephone techniques, computer operation, and appointment and records management.

Laboratory   Hands-on skills in pouring, trimming, and finishing study models, pouring working impressions, making baseplates and bite rims, polishing and repairing dentures, and other appliances.

References   On request

FIGURE 2.2

Skills resumé sample.

SUSAN ADAMS, CDA, RDA
1826 Browns Lane
Anytown, USA 00001
October 27, 1999

Dr. Samuel Crawford
1921 Broadway
Louisville, Kentucky 40284

Dear Dr. Crawford:

I am responding with interest to your advertisement in the October 25, 1999 Courier Journal News. The enclosed resume provides an overview of my education and experience as a dental assistant.

I developed my skills through the Dental Assisting Program at the Jefferson State School and I am a Certified and Registered Dental Assistant.

I believe that I am able to meet your stated requirements for the position and will be able to contribute successfully to your practice.

I look forward to the opportunity of meeting you and your staff and to discussing my qualifications with you. Please feel free to call me at (502) 465-6184.

Sincerely yours,

Susan Adams, CDA, RDA

Enclosure

FIGURE 2.3
Cover letter sample.

Box 2.4

Procedure

Suggested Format for an Acceptable Cover Letter

1. Center your name with appropriate credentials. You may wish to use *capital letters* with *boldface type*.
2. Your address and telephone number should follow your name. If you are difficult to reach, add a telephone number of a relative or friend who can be contacted easily and will give you a message.
3. The date should follow.
4. The name of the dentist and address of the office, including city, state, and zip code, should be typed on the left margin. If you use "Dr.," you do not also use the title (DDS or DMD, and so on). However, you may use the name without "Dr." and then use the title.
5. The salutation should begin "Dear Dr. _____:" with a colon after the last name. *Do not use the first name.*
6. The content of the letter should follow with an *interest* statement and where you heard about the position. Also state that you are enclosing your resumé. You may wish to make a statement about where you obtained your skills and if you are credentialed. You may also add a brief statement about how you can meet the needs of the position, with an ending statement expressing your interest in the opportunity of an interview.
7. One of the most common closures used is, "Sincerely yours," followed by your full name and credentials.
8. The word "Enclosure" is used because the cover letter will be sent with a resumé.

interview is not with the dentist. Preferably, plan your interview with the dentist at the beginning of the day or at the end of the day to minimize changes in the schedule and interruptions. Usually the office manager, whose impressions will be as important as the dentist's observations, will have more time for the interview.

If the position you are seeking is a clinical chairside assisting position, find out if you will be assisting more than one person. If you are going to be assisting more than one dentist or practicing staff member, such as an expanded function assistant or dental hygienist, you should also have an opportunity to meet and talk with them. If you are offered the position, you should meet the other staff members and have an opportunity to walk through the office to observe the equipment and facility. Your satisfaction with a new position is often as much determined by the work environment and other staff members as by your relationship with the employer.

In addition to being prepared to answer questions about your resumé and work experiences, you should be ready to ask questions about the dental practice, work expectations, and other employees. *Do not be afraid to ask questions.* Interviewing the dentist is as important as the employer interviewing you. This position may be a major part of your future career.

Make a list of your career and personal goals. Do the needs and goals of the dentist and your goals and expectations match, and if not, will they in the near future? A dentist who has recently graduated may not be able to provide the salary, benefits, or job opportunity that you are looking for at this time, but you may be able to grow with the practice and develop a long-term employment relationship. A more established dentist may be able to offer you greater options at the time of initial employment, but the long-term growth options may not be as satisfying.

Interviewing

To be at your best during the interview, make sure that you slept comfortably the night before and do not have any other appointments near the time of your job interview. Relieve yourself of unnecessary stress, give yourself plenty of time to get to the office, and be in the reception area at least 10 minutes early. You may even want to drive by the office before the day of the interview if you live in a large city or need to observe traffic at the time of your interview. Being on time is crucial. The few extra minutes that you have before the interview gives you an opportunity to observe the office atmosphere, staff attitude, and staff and patient relationships. Some employers will ask you to fill out a job application or take a personnel test before the interview. Follow the directions, write neatly, and give accurate information.

Your personal hygiene, dress, and overall appearance reflect your professionalism, organizational skills, personal habits, and work ethic. Select clothes that are comfortable yet professional, clean, and ironed. Be sure that undergarments do not show through outer clothing or hang below the hemline. Do not wear excessive jewelry and do not chew gum. Heavy makeup is also not appropriate in the health care practice. A clean face, skin, hair, hands, and fingernails also reflect good grooming habits.

The initial impressions that the interviewer receives will be based on your attitude and ability to communicate clearly. Take a pencil and note pad, extra resumé, and your list of questions. Also take a briefcase or portfolio folder for your materials that is organized and professional and keeps your materials together. Greet the interviewer by name and with a strong handshake. Introduce yourself and wait to be offered a seat. Once the interview begins, speak clearly and be positive and honest. Relax and be yourself. Maintain good eye contact, smile, and provide the requested information clearly. Do not be vague or too lengthy in your answers. Explain your skills, experience, and accomplishments.

Explain how you can contribute to their dental practice. Do not hesitate to use your resumé as a guide to help organize your thoughts as you speak. Find out what the employer's goals are for the practice and what would be expected of you. Discuss your strengths and weaknesses as they relate to job expectations. Ask if a job description is available for you to review; but if one is not available, be prepared with specific questions about the job. If the position is clinical, ask about the dentist's chairside assisting expectations, x-ray responsibilities, or the number of patients seen daily. Listen carefully, ask for clarification if you do not understand a comment, be sensitive about interrupting in midsentence, and be enthusiastic and show interest. Exchange thoughts on how your career goals may match that of the employer. Answer questions and do not be afraid to ask questions relating to your interview. Show self-confidence, be truthful, and give clear answers that relate to the question.

You are also interviewing the employer to find out if you are compatible. Your interview will give you an opportunity to make an informed decision. An interested employer may share the office personnel policies with you to review and clarify what the practice has to offer you.

Interview Guidelines

The following topics represent a guideline of employment information to consider when interviewing. This employment information should help you develop a list of questions that may be important to your particular needs when preparing for an interview. The topics are not prioritized and do not represent other information that you may wish to ask the employer. You will need to decide what employment information is important to you and what will make the difference in whether you accept the position.

Job Description

Dental assistant is a broad term that refers to allied dental personnel who have a variety of skills. Find out exactly what the job requirements are and what the employer expects, especially if several staff members are working in the same area. Job descriptions usually include the following information:

1 Employer's name, address, and telephone number
2 Title of the position
3 Education level required such as high school diploma or equivalency, college education or degree, or continuing education
4 Professional credentials required
5 Previous work experience required
6 Position status such as permanent full-time, part-time, or temporary
7 Number of workdays or hours and whether work hours include weekends or evenings
8 Type of supervision required and supervisor's name
9 Work factors such as primary, secondary, and incidental duties
10 Equipment, machines, and instruments used and frequency of use
11 Special physical or mental requirements of the position (vision, hazards, temperature, lifting)
12 Critical decisions made in this position and frequency of these decisions
13 Types of personal contacts to be made within and outside office
14 Critical responsibilities assumed in this position such as collection of money, proper functioning of equipment, and so on
15 Necessity of accuracy and effects of errors

Work experience may or may not be necessary depending on educational background. Some employers will hire personnel with little or no experience and others require several years of experience. Salary and benefits are usually based on work experience, skills, and education. You should know what the minimum level of education is for the job and what credentials are required. Depending on state regulations, an educational degree, course requirements, or credentials may be required to perform certain functions. Continuing education is mandatory in a number of states. Be sure to find out what those regulations are, how you can meet the requirements, and who will be responsible for the costs. Continuing education is often considered a benefit in dentistry and is paid for by the employer. Additional responsibilities may also be required such as filling in during other employees' absences and cross training. If you are trained on the job, find out if your skills meet the needs of the new employer or if you are required to take additional courses.

Staff Meetings

You may be interested in whether regularly scheduled staff meetings occur. These meetings provide an opportunity to improve office operations and patient service and allow the dentist and staff to promote good working relationships.

Performance Reviews

You should ask about formal performance reviews or periodic evaluations developed for employees. Usually, performance reviews are scheduled at the end of 3 months of employment, 6 months, and then annually. Performance and salaries are reviewed at this time. The 3-month period is usually considered the "probationary" period. At this time you can decide if the job is suitable to you, and the dentist can also decide if the working relationship should continue.

Probation

The trial period during which one has to prove the ability to carry out the responsibilities of the job.

The review period will give employees an opportunity to clarify questions they may have after working in that office environment. During the **probation** period no sick leave or absences are usually allowed. Employees may be released from employment if they do not have the ability to handle work assignments, have inadequate work habits such as in punctuality, appearance, or attitude, or are not behaviorally suited for the position.

A performance review should be considered a positive aspect of the work environment because it is a good overview of the new staff member's accomplishments and it also allows the employee an opportunity to ask questions, seek performance information, and perhaps learn to improve skills in designated areas. This review time gives the staff and dentist a chance to check individual goals and revise or update the goals or work plans for the office. The evaluation can lead to innovative approaches to office operations and patient care.

If after the probationary time an employee's performance is unsatisfactory, an employer may give the employee a 2-week's notice, or pay may be given in place of the 2-week's notice. Employees can also be released immediately for just cause for disciplinary reasons such as excessive, unexcused absences, behavior problems with staff or patients, violation of rules, or misconduct.

Performance reviews are based on a level of individual accomplishment and may include employee dependability, initiative, interpersonal skills, and job achievement. Performance review documents may contain the following information and criteria.

Dependability Dependability is the responsibility an employee takes for actions such as being on time and rarely being absent. The employee realizes that tardiness and absenteeism can affect the production of the office and morale of other employees. A responsible employee plans vacations or time off well in advance and makes proper adjustments and completes work assignments on time.

Initiative Initiative is the willingness of the employee to accept additional responsibilities and creativity the employee uses to complete strenuous assignments and solve difficult tasks, often beyond expectations.

Interpersonal Skills Interpersonal skills are represented by the employee who is sensitive and courteous to others and willing to cooperate and help coworkers in building a team relationship to make the office run effectively.

Job Achievement Job achievement is based on the results of performance and whether the employee met or exceeded job requirements. The employer evaluates quality and quantity of work and the ability of the employee to complete assignments willingly and without constant supervision from the employer.

Working Hours

You should have a clear understanding of what working hours mean: the number of work hours required; whether working overtime, on weekends, or in the evenings is part of the job; and what days the office is closed. The work schedule may affect the ability of a working parent to accept a position. The average work time for employees per week is 36 to 40 hours.

Salary

Before the interview, you should review your personal financial needs and decide what type of salary and benefits you must have to meet your personal living expenses (Box 2-5). You also need to think about the type of salary increase you expect and how and when you become eligible for these increases and benefits. Often the interviewer will ask you what you expect in salary and increases, so you should be prepared with a salary based on realistic needs (Figure 2-4). Salary increases are often connected with performance evaluation periods and results.

The starting base-rate salary for dental assistants varies greatly from state to state and from one office in a city to another office in the same city or even next door. However, education, experience, a positive attitude, and skill levels are

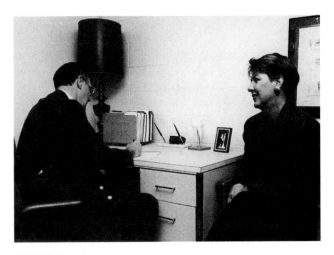

FIGURE 2.4

Careful review of your financial needs will help you to negotiate your employment agreement and decide if you are able to accept the job offer.

Box 2.5

Personal Living Expenses

The following budget categories will help you determine your salary needs:

Income

Salary
Other

Expenses

Housing mortgage or rent
Taxes
Insurance
Utilities
Telephone
Car transportation
   Gas
   Maintenance
   Insurance
Public transportation
Food
Clothing
Entertainment
Household
Personal insurance
Donations
Loans
Charge accounts
Vacation
Savings
Insurance
   Health
   Life
   Liability
   Disability
Professional dues
Education
Publications
Miscellaneous

usually factors that affect salary. Salaries may be higher in group practices and public clinics compared with solo practices. The kinds and amounts of benefits provided to the employee also influence the base-rate salary. Salaries are confidential between employee and employer.

Deductions from salary will include those required by law, city, state, and federal income and social security tax. You may have voluntary deductions to cover your insurance, retirement, and so on. However, you must give written authorization before the deduction is made.

You should find out if the salary is based on an hourly, weekly, or monthly rate and how often you are paid and on what day. Pay periods are usually semimonthly and end on the fifteenth and thirtieth of the month or every 2 weeks. Semimonthly paychecks provide you with 24 pay periods, and 2-week paychecks give you 26 pay periods.

Some dentists offer a bonus or profit sharing at the end of the year as a benefit to employees if the office meets a certain production level. The employer may also provide a commission to expanded duty dental assistants above the base-rate salary based on production. Time worked more than 40 hours is *overtime* and is paid at a rate of time and a half as designated by employment law. Time worked over regular hours is often taken as *comp* time or time off by employees rather than pay.

Benefits

Benefits are an important part of the employment package and need to be taken into consideration as part of the salary. For instance, the employer may pay 100% of the employee medical, life, disability, liability, and retirement contribution, premium, or coverage. Therefore the employee may be able to accept a lower starting salary than if the expense is shared with the employer or if the employee is self-insured. Salary is usually negotiable. Because of the shortage of dental assistants, salary levels and benefit programs have increased and provide the opportunity for dental assistants to enter into better-paying positions. The following benefit information will give you some general considerations that may help you with questions you may wish to discuss with the interviewer (Figure 2-5).

Professional Services Professional services are often provided to full-time employees and their immediate families at no charge. The employee usually pays any lab fee, and if a spouse has dental coverage, the insurance carrier may be billed.

Holidays Holidays are optional. However, the most common paid holidays are Independence Day, Thanksgiving, Labor Day, Christmas, and New Years Day. Other religious holidays may be observed in certain areas of the country. Personnel policies often state that unauthorized absence on the day before or the day after a holiday may cancel pay for that holiday and also for the day missed. Be sure that you understand these conditions of employment.

Professional Organization Activities Professional organization activities are often recognized and supported by the dentist through payment or partial payment of membership dues, registration fees, and meeting expenses. The dentist may also contribute to the cost of maintaining continuing education, certification, or licensure. You should find out if a policy called *request for leave* exists that defines any advance notice requirement.

Health Insurance Health insurance options (medical, disability, liability, and so on) vary from office to office and are usually based on full-time employment and a defined amount of service such as 6 months to 1 year. Employees may have an option to cover their families through regular paycheck deductions. No consideration for extra salary may occur if the option is declined. Dental assistants should secure liability if the dentist does not cover it, especially if direct patient care is provided.

Staff benefits will vary from one dental office to another. The following options represent the diversity of these benefits.

Professional services	Primarily for full-time employees and their families at no charge. Laboratory fees are usually paid for by employee or insurance.
Holidays	Although optional, the most common paid holidays are Independence Day, Labor Day, Thanksgiving, Christmas, and New Years Day. Various religious holidays may be observed in certain areas of the country. Often unauthorized absences on the day before or the day after may cancel pay to that holiday and also for the day missed.
Professional organization activities	Dentists may provide payment or partial payment of membership dues, registration fees, and meeting expenses. They may also contribute to the cost of maintaining continuing education, certification, or licensure. Advance notice or a request for leave may be essential to participate.
Health insurance	Medical, disability, liability, and so on may vary and are usually based on full-time employment and a defined amount of service such as 6 months to 1 year. Employees may have an option to cover their families through regular paycheck deductions. There may be no consideration for extra salary if the option is declined. Dental assistants secure liability insurance if it is not covered, especially if direct patient care is given by the dental assistant.
Personal days	If provided, personal days include 1 or 2 extra days of leave in addition to holiday, vacation, and sick time after a designated period. Additional days may be added after defined periods of employment. Requests for leave usually have to be coordinated with the office schedule so sufficient notice should be given. Personal days usually cannot be accumulated after 2 years.
Vacation	Vacation time varies and is often coordinated with the dentist's vacation time. Vacation time is often dependent upon number of years worked. For example, 1 year of employment allows 1 week vacation, 3 years allows 2 week's vacation, and 8 years allows 3 week's vacation.
Sick time	Sick time may not be paid unless personal days and vacation days are used first. Contact the dentist or office manager immediately if you are sick. If illness continues, provide a physician's certification of illness as soon as possible with date of return. Sick time can often be made up or it may be deducted from the employee's pay.

FIGURE 2.5

Sample staff benefit options.

Continued

Bereavement leave	Bereavement leave is provided in case of death of immediate family (father, mother, brother, sister, husband, wife, child) and usually will not exceed 3 days.
Maternity leave	Maternity leave may be taken at the time the employee feels it is necessary or medically required by a doctor. 6 weeks is the normal time taken and usually personal, vacation, and sick days are integrated for pay.
Family and medical leave	The Family and Medical Leave Act of 1993 applies only to employers with 50 or more employees. Dental employers will have provisions for sick time, emergency leave, maternity leave, and emergency surgery leave.
Emergency surgery leave	Usually 6 weeks is provided for emergency surgery leave, and personal, vacation, and sick days are integrated for pay. If the emergency, accident, or illness result from employment, it must be reported immediately to receive proper treatment.
Military leave	Military leave is granted and may be charged the same as vacation and personal days. If the tour of duty is extended, the office may reinstate the employee to a comparable position if one is available.
Jury duty	Jury duty release time is mandatory unless there is an emergency. The dentist may pay full salary during the time the employee is gone, or pay may be the difference between the jury pay and regular salary.
Disability insurance	Disability insurance may be provided or may be available by payroll deduction. The policy may be long-term or short-term.
Group term life insurance	Group term life insurance may be provided after a defined length of employment such as 6 months. The policy will usually provide a base coverage (for example, $10,000).
Pension plan	A pension plan may be provided only after defined years of service. Depending upon the plan, vesting could occur over a period such as 1 year and would allow the employee to be 20% vested, 2 years to be 40% vested, 3 years to be 60% vested, 4 years to be 80% vested, and 5 years to be 100% vested.
Profit sharing	Profit sharing is often provided to long-term (5 or more years) employees to encourage employment retention or to provide an incentive to share or increase work productivity. This is especially attractive in dental practices that use expanded function auxiliaries.

FIGURE 2.5—Cont'd

Sample staff benefit options.

Personal Days Personal days are provided by some employers. This includes 1 or 2 personal days in addition to holiday, vacation, and sick time after a certain amount of months of employment. Employers may also add extra days after a certain period. A request for leave usually has to be coordinated with the schedule, so you should give sufficient notice. Personal days can not usually be accumulated after 2 years because they are intended to help the employee when a personal need arises and are not to be used as vacation time.

Vacation Vacation time varies depending on the number of years of employment and is often coordinated with the dentist's vacation time. Some options include the following:

Employment	Vacation
1 year	1 week
3 years	2 weeks
8 years	3 weeks
Or	
1 year	6 days
2 years	10 days
3 years	13 days
5 years	15 days

Sick Time Sick time is provided for employees but may not be paid unless personal days and vacation days are used first. The dentist or office manager must be contacted as soon as possible, and if you are not able to return right away, you will probably need a physician's certification and an approximate date of return. Sick time can often be made up or is deducted from the employee's pay.

Bereavement Leave Bereavement leave is provided in case of death of immediate family (parents, brother, sister, husband, wife, child) and usually does not exceed 3 days.

Maternity Leave Maternity leave may be taken at the time the employee feels time off is necessary or medically required by a doctor. Approximately 6 weeks is the normal time taken, and usually personal, vacation, and sick days are integrated for pay.

Family and Medical Leave Act of 1993 The Family and Medical Leave Act applies to employers with 50 or more employees. Dental employers have provisions for sick time, and emergency, maternity, and emergency surgery leave.

Emergency Surgery Leave Emergency surgery leave usually includes 6 weeks, and personal, vacation, and sick days are also usually integrated for pay. If the emergency, accident, or illness occur on the job, they must be reported immediately to receive proper treatment.

Military Leave Military leave is granted and may be charged the same as vacation and personal days. If the tour of duty is extended, the office may reinstate the employee to a comparable position if one is available.

Jury Duty Jury duty release time is mandatory unless an emergency arises. The dentist may pay you full salary during the time you are absent, or pay may be the difference between the jury pay and regular salary.

Disability Insurance Disability insurance may be provided or may be available by payroll deduction. The policy may be long-term or short-term.

Group Term Life Insurance Group term life insurance may be provided after a defined length of employment, such as 6 months. The policy usually provides a base coverage (for example, $10,000).

Pension Plans Pension plans may be offered by the dentist but will usually be provided only after defined years of service. Depending on the plan, vesting could occur over a 5-year period:

Year	Vested
1 year	20% vested
2 years	40% vested
3 years	60% vested
4 years	80% vested
5 years	100% vested

Other Concerns

During the interview, additional topics may include questions about smoking prohibition if you are a smoker, the office dress policy, or how staff problems are handled. You should be prepared to discuss your employment needs. Let the dentist know what employment areas are important to you and explore the possibility of agreement on those issues that are not normally part of that office's employment package.

Inform the dentist if you are interested in the position or why you may not be able to accept the offer. If you are given an acceptable offer, let the interviewer know you accept and give a firm handshake. Thank the interviewer for the time and interest provided to you. Follow up the interview with a brief, formal note thanking the employer for the time spent with you and the courtesy shown. This will allow you another opportunity to put your name forward if several people are interviewed for the position.

If you have had several interviews and a position is offered to you, evaluate the offer, compare it with other options that you are considering, and let the interviewer know your decision as soon as possible. If you do not hear from an interviewer about a position that you are interested in within 8 to 10 days, call and ask if the position has been filled. And if the position has been filled, ask the employer to provide you with the names of other potential employers.

EMPLOYMENT AGREEMENT

You should be provided with a written employment agreement at the time you begin a new job. The agreement should include the provisions that have been negotiated and agreed on. Negotiations also reflect federal and state laws. The agreement provides you with a clearer understanding of what is expected of you and the employer and can be either an informal letter of agreement that you may provide based on your understanding of your employment at the dental office or a more formal employment agreement or contract. The American Dental Assistants Association has developed a sample employment agreement for dental assistants, which can be helpful in clarifying your employment relationship.

The employment agreement may include the following components:
- Names of the employee and employer
- Starting date
- Address or office location
- Responsibilities of the dental assistant in accordance with the State Practice Act
- Responsibilities of the dentist
- Terms of employment, days, regular hours, and overtime hours
- Salary, method of compensation, and increases
- Legal obligations

- Health and safety measures
- Infection control mechanisms
- Benefits
- Performance evaluation and salary review
- Termination procedures and compensation
- Severability of agreement
- Signature and date of employee and employer

Once you have discussed employment conditions, this information should be presented in writing to clarify the employee's and employer's understanding of what has been agreed on. Whichever type of employment agreement is decided on, formal or informal, it should be clarified between both parties and reviewed independently. The agreement should then be discussed at a second meeting before either party signs it to clarify any information or answer any questions or discrepancies of either party. A short form for the employment agreement may be used (Box 2-6) or the dentist may use a more comprehensive form (Box 2-7).

Box 2.6

Employment Agreement: Short Form

Name _____ Date _____
Address _____
City/state_____ Zip code _____
Phone _____ Social security number _____
Emergency contact_____
Job title _____ Classification _____
Duties and responsibilities (see attached copy)

Salary and benefits

Starting rate:_____
Provisions for increase: Annual review will be on or near anniversary date.

Benefits: See Personnel Policy Manual

Uniform requirements

Name tag and personal protective equipment will be provided by the employer (see Infection Control Policy).

Conditional period of employment

The first 3 months of employment are considered a conditional period. During this time, the employee may leave or be dismissed with 24-hours notice.

Certifications

The employee must provide the practice with documentation of all pertinent certifications, registrations, and information.

Termination

The employee is expected to give at least 2 weeks notice (longer if possible).
I acknowledge that I have read the Personnel Policy Manual and Employee Agreement and will adhere to its policies and procedures.

_____   _____
Employee   Employer

Box 2.7

ADAA Sample Employment Agreement

This agreement is entered into by_____, hereinafter referred to as dentist or employer, and_____, hereinafter referred to as dental assistant or employee, on this _____ day of _____, 19_____.

Whereas the employer is a duly licensed dentist in the state of _____, and the employee is a dental assistant in the state of _____, and the parties are desirous of entering into an employment agreement on the terms and conditions set forth below.

Therefore the following is agreed on:

(1)   The dentist hereby employs the dental assistant effective the _____ day of _____, 19_____, to perform the services of a dental assistant in the dental office at _____, whose services shall be consistent with the provisions of the dental practice act of the state of _____ and any rules and regulations pursuant thereto and shall include the following:
_____
_____
_____

and shall *not* include the following:
_____
_____
_____

The dental assistant hereby accepts such employment and agrees to perform the foregoing services in a professional manner.

Regular hours

(2)   The dental assistant shall work _____ regular hours per day between the hours of _____ and _____, with 1 hour off for lunch. The dental assistant shall work _____ days per week for a total of _____ hours per week.

Overtime hours

(3)   In any one day, the dental assistant may work beyond the specified _____ hours. However, the dental assistant may not work more than _____ hours in any one day. For those hours of work beyond the regular _____ hours per day, the dental assistant will receive compensation equal to one- and one-half times the regular salary agreed to be paid under paragraph 4 of this agreement.

Salary

(4)   For the services rendered by the dental assistant, the dentist shall pay the dental assistant the following:
A salary of $_____ per year, payable in equal twice-monthly installments of $_____. These installments shall be paid on the first and fifteenth day of each month.
A salary of $_____ per hour, payable in twice-monthly installments on the first and fifteenth day of each month.

Legal obligations

(5)   At all times during the course of the dental assistant's employment, the dental assistant shall adhere strictly to all laws, rules, and regulations regarding the practice of dental assisting and to all office practices established by the dentist that are consistent with these laws, rules, and regulations. In no instance should the dentist compel the dental assistant to perform illegal duties or functions.

Health and safety

(6)   The dentist shall comply with all federal and state occupational safety and health laws and should undertake all reasonable measures to provide a safe and healthful working environment. Likewise, the dental assistant shall comply with all safety and health laws.
Recognizing that the modern dental office environment harbors a number of biohazards such as ionizing radiation, anesthetic gases, mercury vapor, and infectious diseases that can cause fetal and reproductive damage, the dentist will take all reasonable measures to safeguard the health of female dental assistants of childbearing age.

Continued

Box 2.7—Cont'd

ADAA Sample Employment Agreement

Infection control

(7)   The centers for disease control (CDC) have issued specific guidelines for dental personnel who come in contact with dental patients. The guidelines are effective in preventing hepatitis B and other infectious diseases including AIDS and should be used routinely in the care of all dental patients. The dentist will ensure that the latest CDC-recommended infection control procedures are implemented in the dental office and used routinely on all dental patients. The dentist will agree not to dismiss or otherwise penalize or reprimand the dental assistant if he or she refuses to work in the absence of such procedures.

Paid sick leave

(8)   One month after the commencement of the dental assistant's employment, the dental assistant shall be entitled to a paid sick leave of 1 day per month. Paid sick leave may be accumulated to a maximum of 12 days.

Holidays

(9)   The dental assistant shall be entitled to the following paid holidays:

_____

_____

_____

Vacation

(10)   Six months after the commencement of the dental assistant's employment, the dental assistant shall be entitled to a paid vacation of _____ days. The time of the vacation shall be agreed upon by the parties. The amount of pay during the vacation shall be equal to the average daily earnings during the 30 working days before the vacation.

Unpaid days off

(11)   The dentist may direct the dental assistant to take up to _____ unpaid days off per year. If the number of directed days off exceeds _____, the excess directed days off shall be treated as regular working days, and the dental assistant shall be entitled to the usual pay for said excess directed days off.

Health insurance

(12)   The dentist shall provide fully paid health insurance for the dental assistant.

Workmen's compensation

(13)   The dental assistant shall be covered by state industrial accident and workmen's compensation insurance or equivalent insurance.

Disability benefit insurance

(14)   The dentist shall provide a disability benefit program for the dental assistant.

Pension plan

(15)   The dental assistant shall be covered by a pension plan that shall include provisions for vesting and voluntary contributions by the dental assistant.

Professional liability insurance

(16)   The dentist shall reimburse the dental assistant up to $_____ per year for professional liability insurance.

Additional employee benefits

(17)   The dentist shall reimburse the dental assistant for annual dues payments to the American Dental Assistants Association.

(18)   The dental assistant shall receive a uniform allowance in the amount of $_____ annually.

(19)   The dental assistant shall be entitled to _____ days leave with pay each year to attend courses, institutes, workshops, seminars, or other meetings of an educational nature if the following occurs:

    (a) The dental assistant applies at least 30 days in advance in writing, specifying the educational program he or she wishes to attend, the sponsoring organization, the fee, and how participation will benefit the employee.

    (b) The dental assistant obtains permission from the dentist.

    (c) Such leave shall not interfere with the operation of the dental office.

Box 2.7—Cont'd

ADAA Sample Employment Agreement

Periodic performance and salary review

(20)   Periodic evaluation of the dental assistant's professional performance and review of the compensation provisions set forth in this agreement will be undertaken by the dentist with the dental assistant at least once a year.

Termination

(21)   The term of employment of the dental assistant shall be 1 year from the effective date of the dental assistant's employment (see Paragraph 1). This term shall be automatically renewed from year to year, unless terminated by either party. This agreement shall be terminable without cause and for any reason whatsoever, by either party upon 30 days before written notice to the other party.

(22)   In the event that either party violates any of the provisions of this agreement, upon notice to the other party, this agreement shall at once terminate and neither party shall be under any further obligation to the other. However, the dentist shall pay to the dental assistant any compensation due up to the time of such termination.

Entire agreement

(23)   This agreement constitutes the entire agreement between the parties and contains all of the agreements between the parties with respect to the subject matter hereof. This agreement supersedes any and all other agreements, either oral or in writing, between the parties hereto with respect to the subject matter hereof.

(24)   No change or modification of this agreement shall be valid unless the same is in writing and signed by the dentist and the dental assistant. No waiver of any provision of this agreement shall be valid unless in writing and signed by the party to be charged.

Severability

(25)   If any portion or portions of this agreement shall be, for any reason, invalid or unenforceable, the remaining portion or portions shall nevertheless be valid, enforceable, and carried into effect, unless doing so would clearly violate the present legal and valid intention of the parties hereto.

_____

Dentist

_____

Date

_____

Dental assistant

_____

Date

EMPLOYMENT PRIVILEGES AND RIGHTS

Employers offer certain privileges or benefits that are provided to those employed in that office. These privileges are usually identified and negotiated at the time of the interview and are detailed in the employment agreement. The potential employee and the employer should have an understanding and agreement of each other's needs before beginning employment.

Assured rights exist that are also guaranteed by law. Although many federal laws relate to large businesses such as the Family and Medical Leave Act of 1993, which pertain to employers who employ 50 or more employees, employer's should also understand the laws that interest the dental assistant.

Sex Discrimination

Title VII of the Civil Rights Act of 1964 covers workers by making certain things unlawful: discrimination on the basis of sex, race, color, religion, or national origin when hiring or firing, providing wages or benefits, or classifying, referring, assigning, or promoting employees. The Equal Employment Opportunities Commission enforces this act. The act provides protection in training, retraining, or apprenticeship opportunities. The act also makes labeling jobs as women's jobs or men's jobs or to advertise as such a violation of the law.

Sexual Harassment

Title VII also makes unlawful requesting sexual favors, making unwelcome sexual advances, or exhibiting other verbal or physical sexual actions when submission is a condition of a worker's employment, affects employment decisions, or interferes with work performance by creating a hostile work environment. The employer is also responsible for the acts of supervisory employees, coworkers, and potential patients and related dental agents.

Pregnancy Discrimination

In 1978, Title VII was amended to prohibit **discrimination** because of pregnancy. The act protects women from not being hired, fired, or penalized because of pregnancy. A woman cannot be forced to leave at a certain time and has reinstatement rights that include credit for previous service, seniority rights, and accrued retirement benefits.

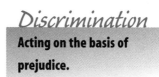

Discrimination

Acting on the basis of prejudice.

Maternity leave is a benefit provided in the employment agreement, and leave time is based primarily on a doctor's release to work with no restrictions. This law also prohibits the employer to discriminate against a woman because she has exercised her abortion rights. The Family and Medical Leave Act of 1993 only relates to these issues if the company has 50 or more employees and under certain guidelines.

Occupational Safety and Health

Safe and healthful working conditions are ensured by the 1970 Occupational Safety and Health Act (OSHA). The employer is responsible for being familiar and complying with OSHA standards and must provide a workplace free from recognized hazards that can cause death or serious physical harm (see Chapter 3 and Chapter 18).

Age Discrimination

The Age Discrimination in Employment Act (ADEA) of 1967 was amended to prohibit discrimination in hiring, discharging, or compensating workers on the basis of age, which includes persons between 40 and 70 years old. This act is enforced in businesses with 20 or more employees. Advertisements indicating age preference, such as 25 to 55, may exclude qualified applicants and is therefore illegal. Involuntary retirement of workers is also not permitted.

Minimum Wages and Overtime Pay

Minimum wage and overtime pay is covered under The Fair Labor Standards Act (FLSA) often called the *Federal Wage and Hour Law*. It does not apply to businesses grossing less than $362,500 annually, and therefore minimum wage does not usually pertain to professional employees. This law does not limit the number of hours employees 16 years and older can work but the law entitles most workers to one and one-half times their regular rate of pay for more than 40 hours worked.

Equal Pay

The Fair Labor Standards Act was amended by the 1963 Equal Pay Act includes professional workers and prohibits unequal pay for women and men performing jobs in the same work place that require equal skill, effort, and responsibility. Jobs do not have to be identical to meet this requirement. Job descriptions should indicate the "essential functions" of the job to clarify difference or likeness. Pay also includes overtime, uniforms, travel, education, and other benefits, and these related payments cannot be reduced for any employee for the purpose of eliminating illegal salary differences. Pay equity laws are being developed as questions and complaints of undervalued and underpaid female occupations are being tested. For instance, a job may contain different content but require the same or more educational preparation, experience, skill, and responsibility as a male job receiving higher pay.

Pensions

The Employee Retirement Income Security Act of 1974 does not require companies to provide pension plans but it does set up an insurance system to cover certain defined benefit pension plans that terminate without enough money to pay the benefits. The act also prohibits an employer from discharging a worker to avoid paying pension benefits.

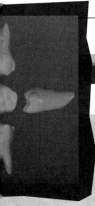

Points for Review

- Difference between informal on-the-job training and formal education
- Considerations in seeking employment and career planning
- How to write a resumé
- Importance of a cover letter
- Parts of an employment package
- Important parts of an employment agreement

Self-Study Questions

1. Self-assessment helps people better understand what is important to their happiness and thus assists them in finding a job that will fulfill their needs.
   a. True
   b. False

2. Which sources provide job opportunity information?
   a. Newspapers
   b. Friends and personal contacts
   c. Suppliers
   d. All of the above

3. Why is a professional-appearing resumé important?
   a. Shows that the interviewee is interested in the job
   b. Provides the first impressions of the interviewee
   c. Provides a personal introduction to the interviewee
   d. None of the above

4. The purpose of a cover letter is a response to the job advertisement and an expression of the interviewee's interest in the position.
   a. True
   b. False

5. What is the key reason to prepare for the interview?
   a. To understand what you are looking for in a job
   b. To know your financial restrictions
   c. To assist in making a well thought out decision
   d. All of the above

6. What is the best way to relieve stress when preparing for an interview?
   a. Getting rest the night before
   b. Having no other appointments at that time
   c. Having extra time to get to the office
   d. All of the above

7. What are the key points a dental assistant should be prepared to address during an interview?
   a. Employer expectations and job description
   b. Salary and benefits
   c. Employee expectations and employee agreement
   d. All of the above

8. The primary importance of the employment agreement is to provide a job description.
   a. True
   b. False

9. The Civil Rights Act of 1964 makes discrimination on the basis of gender, race, color, religion, or national origin when hiring or firing unlawful.
   a. True
   b. False

10. The Employee Retirement Income Security Act requires the employer to provide a pension plan.
    a. True
    b. False

Suggested Readings

American Dental Assistants Association: *Sample employment agreement*, Chicago, 1987, ADAA.

American Dental Association, Council on Dental Education: *Council on Dental Practice: innovative dental assisting and dental hygiene programs*, Chicago, 1992.

Dental Hygiene Employment Reference Guide, American Dental Hygienists Association, 1990.

Educational Testing Service: *Dental assisting occupation, system of interactive guidance and information* (SIGI PLUS), Princeton, NJ, 1993.

Jefferson State Vocational Technical School: *Training our health care workforce*, Frankfort, Ky, 1995, Kentucky Department of Education.

Johnson DW: *Reaching out: interpersonal effectiveness and self-actualization*, Englewood Cliffs, NJ, 1996, Prentice-Hall.

Lyons S: Climbing higher: results of the dental assistant's readership survey, *Dent Assist J*, 58(4):30, 1989.

Novak DE: *Hiring allied dental personnel*, Louisville, Ky, 1995, University of Louisville.

Solomon ES, Gray CF: Trends in dental assisting and dental laboratory technology, *J Dent Educ* 53:3, 1989.

United States Department of Health and Human Services: *The employee retirement income security act of 1974*, Baltimore, Md, Social Security Administration.

United States Department of Labor: *Labor statistic reports*, Washington, DC, 1995, Labor-Management Services Administration.

United States Department of Labor: *Family and medical leave act of 1993*, Washington, DC, Labor-Management Services Administration.

United States Department of Labor: *Occupational safety and health act of 1970*, Washington, DC, Occupational Safety and Health Administration.

Chapter 3

Dental Ethics and Jurisprudence

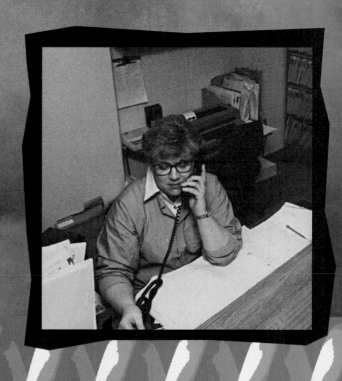

Chapter Outline

Ethics, Jurisprudence, Professionalism, and Dentistry
  The special nature of a profession
  Ethics and jurisprudence
Ethics
  Basic principles of ethics
  Professional ethics
  General principles of ethics in dentistry
Jurisprudence
  Jurisprudence and laws affecting dentistry
Legal Duties and Responsibilities in the Dentist and Patient Relationship
  Standards of care
  Credentials
  Knowledge, skill, care, and judgment
  Standards
  Personnel
  Consent
  Abandonment
  Fees
  Legal actions

  Information
  Referral
  Complete dental treatment
  Treatment outcome
  Guarantees
  Records
  Confidentiality
  Code of ethics
Implied Duties of the Patient
Termination of the Doctor and Patient Relationship
Liabilities in Dentistry
  Defamation of character
  Personal liabilities from office hazards
  Breach of contract
  Misrepresentation, deceit, or fraud
  Breach of confidentiality
  Medical professional liability or malpractice
Preventing Professional Liability Claims in Dentistry
  Actions to prevent or minimize malpractice claims

Learning Objectives

On completion of chapter 3, the student should be able to do the following:

- Define key terms.
- Describe the special nature of a profession.
- Describe the nature of ethics and jurisprudence and their differences.
- Describe the role of ethics and jurisprudence in professional behavior.
- Describe the ethical and legal principles that affect the dental profession.
- Describe the basic behaviors required for the dentist and dental assistant.

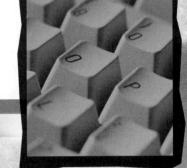

Key Terms

Autonomy

Consent

Contract

Ethics

Implied Consent

Informed Consent

Justice

Liability

Malpractice

Negligence

Paternalism

Reciprocity

Statutory Law

Tort

ETHICS, JURISPRUDENCE, PROFESSIONALISM, AND DENTISTRY

Dentistry is a profession, which means it is different from most commercial enterprises. People working in a profession, whether they are the professional practitioner or trained support personnel, are bound by a code of conduct above and beyond ones that apply to a nonprofessional. Codes apply specifically to different professions and have internal and external sources. Internally, the code is based on the personal **ethics** of the individual and the collective ethics of the profession. Externally, the code comes from the various laws that apply to that particular profession.

Ethics

The branch of philosophy that encompasses moral conduct (right and wrong behavior), good and evil, duty, and judgment.

For practicing dental assistants to understand the principles of dentistry, they should know something about the special nature of a profession, the basics of ethics and jurisprudence, and the application of ethics and jurisprudence to a profession and dentistry.

The Special Nature of a Profession

Society has traditionally given certain occupations, such as the healing arts, law, and clergy, special status compared with other occupations. These special occupations are referred to as *professions*. Society has made professions special for several reasons (Box 3-1).

These standards and obligations, not seen in other occupations, originate from a set of ethical principles that apply to that profession. Those same standards and obligations also make the professional dental assistant vital to the dental profession.

Ethics and Jurisprudence

Ethics and jurisprudence are not the same. Behavior can be unethical and still be legal but it cannot be illegal and still be ethical. As a general rule, an ethical standard is usually considered to be of a higher order than a legal standard.

Ethics is the branch of philosophy that deals with moral conduct (right and wrong behavior), good and evil, duty, and judgment. Ethics is a systematic, reasoned, and disciplined theory that might support specific moral judgments or behaviors. It concerns matters of right and wrong,

Box 3.1

Nature of a Profession

Professions provide certain values that society considers essential and unique.

Values are essential and unique and they cannot be provided without special knowledge and training.

Specialized knowledge and training are not only essential to society but also exclusively possessed only by those who have successfully completed the necessary training and demonstrated the necessary competence.

Because a profession is unique, and its practice is so exclusive, a mutual recognition of special expertise exists among those who practice.

Because of the essential, unique, and exclusive knowledge of professionals, society grants *autonomy* to the members of a profession. These professionals are given the privilege of self-regulation because the expertise of a professional can only be compared with or challenged by other professionals.

Because of the special privileges and power associated with a profession, a practitioner of that profession is bound by a special set of standards and obligations

that are not seen in other occupations. The professional should abide by the following rules when working with a client or a patient:

The profession (and the professional) exists primarily to serve the needs of chief client or clients.

The relationship between the professional and client or patient is expected to be *ideal*.

The client's and patient's well-being is expected to come ahead of the professional's well-being.

The professional is expected to maintain the competence to perform professional tasks.

The professional is expected to uphold and maintain the *central values* of the profession.

Central values are essential to the proper practice of a profession.

The professional is expected to relate to coprofessionals respectfully, collegially, and honorably.

The professional, by virtue of unique knowledge, expertise, and power, also has the responsibility to serve the larger community and society.

founded on personal or cultural standards and defines a *maximum* level of conduct.

Ethics seeks to answer two fundamental human questions as follows:

1 *What* should I do?
2 *Why* should I do it?

Ethics refers to what one *should* do, not what one *must* do.

Jurisprudence is the law or science or system of laws and is based on a code of laws governing human behavior. Those laws can be either written or established by legal precedent. Jurisprudence defines a *minimum* level of conduct.

Jurisprudence refers to what one *must* do, not what one *should* do.

ETHICS

Basic Principles of Ethics

Justice

> **The principle of fairness in the distribution of goods and deprivations and treating people fairly and equitably.**

Ethical principles and problems are present in every part of our lives. They include the way we treat and relate to ourselves, human beings, living creatures, society, and the environment and workplace. Over time, four basic and universal principles of ethics have been identified as follows:

1 Regard for self-determination (respect for autonomy)
2 Avoidance of doing harm (nonmaleficence)
3 Promotion of well-being (beneficence)
4 Fairness in the distribution of goods and deprivations (**justice**)

Autonomy

> **The ethical principle of respect for the individual and of the individual's right to pursue life, liberty, and welfare, as long as such decisions and actions do not adversely affect the life or welfare of others.**

Autonomy is the basis for the right to privacy, freedom of choice, and the acceptance of responsibility for one's own actions. It supports one's freedom to think, judge, and act independently without undue influence.

Nonmaleficence may be paraphrased by Hippocrates' admonition, "above all, do no harm." This principle relates to all levels of human interpersonal, social, and environmental behavior and is the foundation for most, if not all, criminal jurisprudence.

Beneficence is based on the idea that actions are moral or good, as long as they enhance the common good. Whereas

nonmaleficence is the avoidance of doing something harmful, beneficence is the obligation of doing something positive and good.

Justice contains two related ideas as follows:

1 Treating people fairly.
2 Giving people what they deserve and are entitled to receive.

Personal ethical standards are based on the four ethical principles described earlier. Almost without realization, we apply our personal ethical principles to every facet of our lives. For example, an *ethical decision* or action might include the following:

- Returning excess change incorrectly given to you by a sale's clerk: *Principle of justice.*
- Respecting the beliefs of others, even if you do not agree with those beliefs: *Principle of autonomy.*
- Offering assistance to those in need, such as helping someone whom has car trouble: *Principle of beneficence.*
- Avoiding behavior that will physically or psychologically hurt someone, such as spreading false gossip about a fellow worker or student: *Principle of nonmaleficence.*

Examples of an *unethical decision* or action might be the following:

- Cheating when providing goods or services, such as selling 4 lb of produce for the same price as 5 lb of produce: *Principle of justice.*
- Not allowing a patient to choose between more than one appropriate treatment: *Principle of autonomy.*
- Not providing assistance, such as offering an elderly person a seat on a crowded bus: *Principle of beneficence.*
- Harming another person, such as giving alcohol to someone who is known to be an alcoholic: *Principle of nonmaleficence.*

In studying these and other examples of ethical and unethical behavior or decisions, more than one ethical principle could possibly be involved at a time. Although not all unethical actions are illegal, all illegal actions are unethical.

Professional Ethics

Similarly, the four principles of ethics are present in the practice of the professions. Because the professions are special occupations and practitioners of the professions are granted unusual privileges, powers, and obligations, each of the professions today have developed a formalized and written *code of ethics*. A professional code of ethics is the standard of moral principle and practice to which a profession abides by.

Everyone practicing in a profession, in any capacity, is expected to comply with the profession's code of ethics. The standards and behaviors described are voluntary; they are *not* laws. They originate from the ethical principle of autonomy and privilege granted to a profession to regulate and police itself, and enforcement of the code is handled within

The spirit of the Golden Rule should be the guiding principle of conduct for dental assistants. In all contacts with the dental profession and society, dental assistants should maintain honesty, loyalty, and a desire to serve to the best of their abilities, employers, and patients.

The dental assistant should give the employer the cooperation needed to serve patients capably and efficiently. Dental assistants will hold in confidence the details of professional services rendered by employers and should refrain from performing any service for patients that requires the professional competence of the dentist, or which may be prohibited by the dental practice act of the state in which the dental assistant is employed. Additionally, dental assistants should avoid making disparaging remarks about the conduct of the employer's treatment of patients.

Dental assistants have an obligation of increasing skills and efficiencies by availing themselves of educational opportunities provided by the American Dental Assistants Association (ADAA) and its state and local groups. Dental assistants should support the efforts of the state associations and local organizations to improve their educational status and should support this Code of Ethics.

A

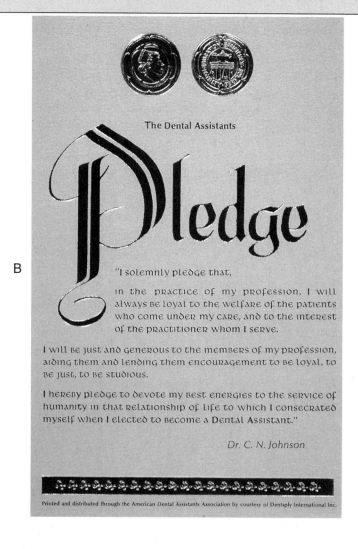

B

The Dental Assistants

Pledge

"I solemnly pledge that,

in the practice of my profession, I will always be loyal to the welfare of the patients who come under my care, and to the interest of the practitioner whom I serve.

I will be just and generous to the members of my profession, aiding them and lending them encouragement to be loyal, to be just, to be studious.

I hereby pledge to devote my best energies to the service of humanity in that relationship of life to which I consecrated myself when I elected to become a Dental Assistant."

Dr. C. N. Johnson

Printed and distributed through the American Dental Assistants Association by courtesy of Dentsply International Inc.

FIGURE 3-1

A, American Dental Assistants Association code of ethics. **B**, Dental assistant's pledge by Dr. C.N. Johnson.

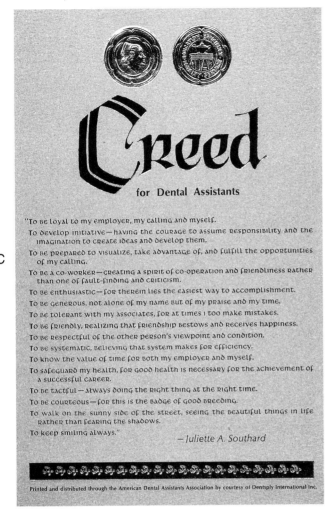

C

FIGURE 3-1—Cont'd

C, Creed for dental assistants by Juliette A. Southard.

the professional organization. The code of ethics of the American Dental Association (ADA), the American Dental Hygienists Association (ADHA), and the American Dental Assistants Association (ADAA) are available on request. The ADAA's code of ethics (Figure 3-1, *A*), the *Dental Assistant's Pledge* by Dr. C.N. Johnson (Figure 3-1, *B*), and the *Creed for Dental Assistants* by Juliette A. Southard (Figure 3-1, *C*) are the codes of conduct that will guide the rest of your career in dentistry.

When applying ethics to a professional practice, practitioners must not only employ their own code of ethics but they also must employ the codes established by the profession. If and when these codes are contradictory, the potential for internal conflict on the part of the practitioner may exist.

General Principles of Ethics in Dentistry

The general principles of ethics in dentistry originate from one or more of the basic principles of ethics described previously. I will describe these principles and discuss specific examples of their application in the professional practice of dentistry, especially as they relate to the dental assistant.

Patient Rights

Autonomy

The principle of autonomy states that a competent individual has the right to freely make those decisions that affect life or welfare, provided those decisions or actions do not adversely affect the life or welfare of others. Thus in the delivery and practice of health care services, patients have the right to choose the care they receive and do not receive.

In the practice of dentistry, neither the dentist, hygienist, nor dental assistant may provide any service or treatment that has not been previously approved by the patient, either implicitly or explicitly. Therefore to avoid violating this ethical principle, the dentist and dental assistant must do the following:

- The dentist must provide only those treatment services authorized by the patient.
- The dental assistant must provide only those services authorized by the dentist and previously approved by the patient.

The principle of autonomy also applies to practitioners. It gives the providers of health care services the right to recommend appropriate care and decline services requested by the patient or guardian that in their professional judgment should not be provided. *For dental assistants this also means that they have the ethical right and responsibility to decline performing a task that in their judgment or conscience is inappropriate.* This should occur rarely, but unfortunately does happen. An example of an assistant refusing to perform a task might be if the dentist told the assistant to do something that violates the state dental practice act, such as performing a scaling and prophylaxis. A dentist may also instruct the dental assistant to use materials incorrectly, not sterilize instruments properly, or falsify third-party insurance claims. These situations create a dilemma for the assistant. To follow the dentist's instructions would clearly be unethical and not right but to follow one's conscience would probably mean losing a job. No simple answer to this problem exists.

Informed Consent

Informed consent

Expressed consent, always at least verbal and usually written, that is freely given and based on a reasonable presentation and understanding of the facts.

Closely related to the principle of autonomy is the concept of **informed consent**. The basic ethical principle of autonomy means that health care providers, such as the dentist or dental assistant, have a duty to allow people to make informed decisions about matters affecting their health. People must have good information before they can make decisions regarding their health and welfare.

When patients appear for an examination or emergency

Implied consent

Nonverbal and nonwritten consent given by one person to another by external actions and behavior. For example, a person who comes to the dentist for a checkup gives the dentist implied consent to conduct a standard dental examination.

service, they have given you **implied consent** by their presence and request to conduct an examination, touch their body (if that is a necessary part of an adequate examination), and give an opinion and report. This is the initial **consent** given by new patients in any health care service. Neither the dentist nor the dental assistant should do anything to or for new patients at this stage of the relationship that exceeds this level of consent.

After the examination, the doctor is responsible to give the patient an opinion and possibly a recommendation, which is the informed part of informed consent. The doctor must give the patient the findings and opinion and what the natural outcome of the findings will be. The doctor must also give the patient a list of possible and recommended treatments, the advantages and disadvantages, risks of all

Consent

Permission given to someone to do something.

treatments (including doing nothing), and where and how these treatments might be performed. The doctor should give this information in such a way that the patient understands it. As will be discussed in the next section, the patient is assumed to be competent to understand this information and act on it. Only after the patient has evaluated all of this information and has given the doctor and health care team specific permission, always verbally but usually also in writing, can treatment for the condition begin. This is called *explicit* consent.

In addition to doing nothing beyond authorized services, during the examination stage, dental assistants must be careful about what is said to patients regarding the problem. Often patients are scared or confused. They may want a second opinion, and the closest and most convenient second opinion may be that of dental assistants. Although assistants are an integral and essential part of the professional practice, they are not the health care professional. To comment on the findings, outcomes, or treatments would be a violation of the ethical principle of justice. Assistants would be giving patients information they are not qualified to give. In addition, they would be in violation of the law because to comment on the dental nature of the case can be considered practicing dentistry without a license.

Competency

Also related to the principle of autonomy is the concept of competency, which refers to the idea that all people are not completely autonomous. Young children, mentally ill, or disabled people are not considered qualified or competent to make decisions about their lives or welfare completely on their own.

A broad range of competency exists, from the completely incompetent, such as an infant or comatose individual, to those who are almost completely competent or autonomous, such as a mature, intelligent teenager. In the latter case, although teenagers may possess the intelligence to make all of their own personal decisions, they often do not have the experience or maturity to make such decisions responsibly. For that reason, society does not grant them this privilege until they have reached the age of legal maturity.

In the delivery of health care services, when the person being treated is not completely competent, the individual responsible for the patient's welfare, such as the parent, legal guardian, or state that acts as the patient's surrogate in these circumstances, must approve consent for treatment.

In dental practice, treating people without their consent is unethical. It is also unethical to treat people who cannot or may not give consent for themselves, unless the consent of the parent, guardian, or state has been previously obtained. Violation of this principle is usually illegal and unethical. Thus everyone in the dental practice, such as the dentist, assistant, and other support staff, needs to ensure that proper consent is always obtained for all patients. If patients cannot provide proper consent, then consent must be obtained from those who are responsible for their welfare.

The two exceptions to the requirement of informed consent before treatment that dental assistants should be aware of include the following:

1 A true emergency situation in which grave risk of either permanent damage or loss of life to a patient who does not possess decision-making abilities occurs. (The patient is unconscious, a minor, or suffering from a mental disorder, which might be the result of a head injury or drug or alcohol overdose.) In these circumstances, consent is not necessary to begin initial treatment. However, reasonable efforts must be made to obtain permission from an appropriate surrogate. Fortunately, this problem is seldom seen in dentistry.

2 To come on the scene of an accident and find a seriously injured person. In this instance, people with health care training, including dental assistants, have a moral and ethical obligation, under the principle of beneficence, to provide whatever assistance they can. In providing such emergency care, health care providers are not practicing their specialty; instead they are providing high-quality first aid at the site of the accident. In addition, *most states have enacted what are called Good Samaritan laws that protect the **liability** of health care providers who are providing emergency care to their patients.*

Liability

A legal obligation and responsibility.

Paternalism

Somewhat related to the issue of competency is the concept of **paternalism**. This means that if people are not competent to decide or act on their own behalf, someone else is authorized to make decisions on behalf of the incompetent individuals. As noted earlier, this is usually the parent, legal guardian, or state.

Paternalism

Authorized decisions or actions on behalf of another person.

For health care professionals, paternalism can be a real problem and risk. Because dentists, and usually everyone on the staff including the dental assistant, know more about dentistry than patients, they can fall into the trap of thinking they know best and make treatment decisions for patients. This is unethical and violates patients' autonomy. Professional information regarding the problem and treatment should come only from the dentists. Coercing patients, however unconsciously, and making specific decisions are paternalistic and unethical.

Right of Refusal

Patients have a right to refuse treatment. Unless the patients' problem can affect others, such as having a contagious disease that can be spread to others in the course of normal contact, they have the right to decline recommended treatment. This right exists even if declining treatment results in serious illness or even death. Dental assistants must recognize and respect this right.

In the cases of a parent or guardian declining recommended services for incompetent individuals, such as children, and if the consequences are so serious that they cause permanent and significant injury or even death, the ethical issues become complex. Such ethical issues are beyond the scope of this text and will seldom, if ever, affect dental assistants directly in the course of their work.

Hippocrates' Principle

The basic ethical principles of beneficence and nonmaleficence dictate that the objectives of the practice of dentistry are "doing good and avoiding harm." No health care services are completely risk free. Whether the service is an examination or a specific treatment, a chance of risks are involved. However, in performing any health care service, all staff members involved assume that the potential for good outweighs the potential for harm. This assumption implies that all people involved in the service are qualified and competent. Thus everyone on the health care team, including dental assistants, *have the ethical responsibility to attain and always maintain a level of competency so that harm to patients is minimized.*

Dental assistants have numerous opportunities to help or harm patients. Some duties of dental assistants include taking radiographs, making impressions and preparing materials, sterilizing or transferring instruments, or carrying out instructions from dentists. Dental assistants are therefore ethically responsible to ensure they are always capable of performing their assigned tasks. To be unqualified, or even temporarily impaired, is unethical.

If dental assistants find themselves not qualified to accomplish a task, even temporarily, they are ethically bound to refrain from even attempting the task if it places any additional risks for the patients.

Fidelity Obligations

Trust

When people seek the services of dentists, a key feature of the relationship is *trust*. Patients must be able to trust dentists for the following reasons:

1 Professionals have a special role in society and unique training to fulfill that role.

2 Professionals have knowledge and skills not possessed by patients.

3 Patients are vulnerable, unable to help themselves in dental situations, and depend on professionals.

4 Professionals are in a position of power in the relationship, which must not be abused.

In trusting dentists, patients must also be able to trust the staff, including the dental assistant. Expectations of this trust include the following:

- The dentist and dental assistant will exercise the highest level of skill, care, and concern in the treatment of patients.
- The dentist or dental assistant will not take advantage of patients, either personally, psychologically, financially, or sexually.

Trust between patients and providers is sacred. Dental assistants are an integral part of that trust and violating that trust would be a major breach of professional ethics.

Dental assistants are also involved in a trusting relationship between themselves and their employer. In this relationship, *both parties must trust each other completely and not take advantage of the other in any way*. In this relationship, the assistant, as an employee, is usually in the more vulnerable position. However, the dentist must also trust the assistant to be dependable, loyal, competent, and discrete. The dentist must be able to trust the dental assistant to use that knowledge correctly and not abuse it.

Confidentiality

Another part of trust is *confidentiality*. A large part of professional ethics involves the confidentiality between patients and practitioners including the professional support staff, such as the dental assistant.

Patients being treated by a professional such as a dentist must often disclose personal information. Telling whether they have or had a specific disease or allergy is necessary for treatment to be successful. According to the ethical principle of autonomy, which includes respect for the individual, information learned during the treatment *must* be kept absolutely confidential.

Information can be released to someone not involved in this specific treatment only with expressed written permission of the patient. In the course of dental practice, the dental assistant learns a great deal about the patient, including information about the patient's finances, medical and sexual history, emotional state, and so on. Although such information may be gossip, especially if the patient is a prominent member of local society, it must be kept absolutely secret. Such information should not be a topic of conversation *anywhere*, either within or outside of the office. The information should only be used when it is an essential part of the patient's treatment. A good rule to follow might be as follows: *What is learned in the office, said in the office, and done in the office, stays in the office.*

Violation of professional confidentiality is a serious breach of professional ethics. Such violations can cause the dentist to be disciplined and the dental assistant to be dismissed.

Honesty

Another part of autonomy is the principle of *honesty*, also called *truth telling* or *veracity* and closely related to trust. These virtues are essential in a relationship based on mutual respect. The relationship between the professional and patient must be based on honesty and truth, otherwise respect for the other person is compromised and the outcome of treatment could be unsuccessful. The dentist and dental assistant must always be honest and truthful in dealing with the patient. In this instance, however, the principle of beneficence complicates matters because occasions may arise when total candor can harm the welfare of the patient. This can occur when the patient's mental state is essential to the treatment or its success. For example, a child patient may be terrified of receiving a shot. The dentist, using topical anesthetic, good technique, and distraction, could accomplish the injection without the patient even knowing it. Another patient who is terrified of cancer might come to the office with a suspicious mouth lesion.

In these examples *how* people say or do something is as or more important than *what* they say or do. However, in engaging in such bits of deception, the dentist and dental assistant must be careful not to fall into the trap of paternalism. Thus honesty in dealing with patients becomes an essential but difficult balancing act. The dentist and dental assistant must always exercise careful and considerate judgment as they honor the spirit of honesty and truthfulness, without harming the overall well-being of the patient.

Besides the patient, the dental assistant must also work honestly and truthfully with the dentist or employer. Deceiving an employer about basic issues of employment is unethical and dishonest. Matters of employment include demographic information, (name, social security number, residence, and so on) credentials, references, availability, and abilities. The dentist must also be honest and truthful with the employee about terms, conditions, and expectations of employment. Without honesty and trust, the relationship will fail and the effectiveness of care will be diminished.

Promise Keeping

The dentist and dental assistant have an ethical obligation of *promise keeping*, usually implied and expected, to the patient and each other. A broken promise is a broken trust, which compromises the doctor and patient relationship, the employer and employee relationship, or both.

Promise keeping can involve almost any aspect of the practice. For dentists it means essentially to "deliver the goods," that is, accomplishing what they said they would. It can also mean providing after-hours emergency care, which is an implied promise of the practice and expectation of the patient, when needed. For the dental assistant, most promise keeping occurs in the satisfactory performance of normal and expected duties. Those duties will affect the patient and dentist directly and indirectly, and failure to perform them adequately is a broken promise to the patient and dentist.

Fairness and Equity in Dental Practice

Justice

Justice means treating people fairly and equitably. Most justice issues within a dental practice involve treating people (patients, doctors, coworkers) fairly and without discrimination. Discrimination on the basis of age, gender, race, national origin, beliefs, and so on is unethical and illegal. Prohibiting discrimination is an accepted part of our society today. However, within the practice, justice means that all patients must be treated with the same standard of judgment, consideration, and skill. However, all patients will not receive the same treatment. Treatments for identical problems may vary based on values, financial resources, medical conditions, and mental or emotional conditions. *All* patients must be given the same standard of care and concern.

Ethics in Third-Party Financing

Much of dental practice today involves third-party financing, which is full or partial payment for dental care by a third party, such as an insurance company or the state. Because large amounts of money are involved in such financing, some people may be tempted to cheat or commit fraud, which is not only illegal but also unethical. Cheating violates the principle of justice because the insurance company and all of its policyholders are not treated fairly. Therefore making a fraudulent claim to an insurance company is unethical for the dentist, staff, or patient. The temptations are many and may include the following:

- Performing an unneeded or unjustified service.
- Providing a lower cost or value service and claim or charge for a higher cost.
- Overcharging for a service.
- Lying about key dates, such as dates of injury, previous services, or current services.
- Waiving the patient portion of the copayment.

All of these actions are fraudulent and unethical. Dental assistants must be careful not to become involved in such activity. To do so could theoretically make them an accomplice to a crime.

Ethical Responsibilities Toward Incompetent, Dependent, or Impaired Colleagues

The dentist and dental assistant have a primary obligation to the patient. As members of one of the healing professions, they also have an obligation to maintain and support the overall standards and special nature of the profession. When dentists suspect colleagues of being incompetent, dependent, or impaired, ethical review boards exist within the professional dental society and state board of dentistry to help the compromised dentists and protect the public. *Dental assistants have an obligation to the patient and dentist.* Should a colleagues or even another dentist on the staff be impaired, *dental assistants have an obligation to discuss the problem with them first and recommend that they seek outside help*. If that effort is not successful, the information should be reported in a confidential and considerate manner to the senior dentist in the practice. The senior dentist becomes responsible for evaluating the information and acting appropriately. In taking this action, the dental assistant maintains a trust with the practice, patients, and dentist.

Ethical Responsibilities Toward the General Public

Because of special knowledge, the dental assistant has certain responsibilities to the general public. This occurs because of the dental assistant's knowledge of dental health care, first aid, and cardiopulmonary resuscitation (CPR). CPR is now a common requirement for most dental assistants, making them responsible for using the knowledge they have properly should the need ever arise. *If called on, the trained dental assistant must be willing and able to provide CPR.*

The dental assistant also has the responsibility to participate in appropriate dental education programs sponsored by the local dental assisting society, dental society, dental practice, community college, or university. This is an important public role for the dental assistant, who will usually be working with other dentists, hygienists, and assistants.

Violations of Professional Ethical Principles

Because ethics are internal standards, the consequence of ethical violations is handled within the profession by the profession. The ethics committee of the professional dental society usually handles ethical violations by a dentist. Such violations by a dentist may result in the following:

- The loss of respect by colleagues
- Specific disciplinary action by the committee, which might include the following:
  1 Censure, an official reprimand, or professional disapproval
  2 Suspension or temporary loss of membership
  3 Expulsion and complete loss of membership

Ethical violations by the dental assistant are the responsibility of the employer. The consequences are usually dismissal.

JURISPRUDENCE

Jurisprudence and Laws Affecting Dentistry

Law is a rule or code of conduct that is imposed and binding on society by a sovereign external authority. Without laws governing human behavior, a civilized society becomes impossible. Jurisprudence is the philosophy or science of law. Dental jurisprudence is the philosophy or science of law concerned with dentistry. The two types of law that affect dentistry and all of society are called *statutory law* and *common law*.

Statutory Law

Statutory law

> **Law that is written and imposed by the legislature of various sovereign (lawful) governments.**

Statutory law or legislative law is written and imposed by various sovereign governments. Statutory law can override the common law. A violation of a statutory law is often a minor crime or misdemeanor.

Federal Law

In dentistry, several statutory laws affect the nature of dental practice and are imposed by federal and state governments. *Federal law* controls the use of prescription drugs, medicines, and narcotics. A dentist must have a federal narcotics license to prescribe, or authorize a pharmacist to dispense, narcotics or dangerous drugs.

State Law

State law controls the practice of dentistry within that state and is called *the State Dental Practice Act*. To enforce the State Dental Practice Act, a State Board of Dentistry is usually created through various regulations and administrative decisions. Other federal and state laws affecting the dentist include labor law and laws regulating environmental safety and hazardous waste.

Common Law

Contract

> **A voluntary agreement between two or more competent people involving the exchange of a specified service or product in return for a specific compensation (usually money).**

Tort

> **Wrongful conduct that violates common law but does not involve a contract. In law, the person who commits a tort is responsible to compensate the victim of the tort with damages to "make the victim whole."**

Common law is also called *case law*, *precedent law*, or *judge-decided law*. Common law derives its authority from the courts, not from a particular written statute. The law is made up of court decisions in such areas as **contracts**, **torts**, property, trusts, and other areas in which the legislature has not specifically spoken. Common law is obtained from judicial precedents in which a court makes a decision based on rational reasoning and human morality to provide peace, order, and justice in the community. Judicial decisions by the courts that interpret written laws (statutes) also make up a part of the common law. Because common law originates from the court, it can only be amended by appeal to a higher court. A violation of common law can result in a civil lawsuit in which a wronged individual seeks justice and compensation through the court system from the person who has caused a wrong that is not specifically a crime. This process is called a *lawsuit*.

Common law primarily affects relationships with patients. Contracts and torts are two large areas of common law that affect the dentist and patient relationship.

Statutory Laws Affecting Dentistry

Federal Narcotics Law

As mentioned previously, federal narcotics laws control the use, prescription, and dispensing of drugs. To be eligible for a narcotics license, dentists must possess a valid state dental license and have no criminal convictions that might disqualify them from possessing such a license.

State Dental Practice Act

The practice of dentistry is regulated in each state by the State Dental Practice Act. The main purpose of this state law is to protect the public from being harmed by unqualified or incompetent practitioners. To achieve that purpose, this act sets limits and restrictions on *who* and *how* dentistry may be practiced in that state. This is done in the following ways:

- Defining what constitutes the practice of dentistry
- Defining whom is eligible for licensure
- Creating an administrative board, usually called the *State Board of Dental Examiners*, to oversee the practice of dentistry, the process of licensure of qualified applicants, and the discipline of those who violate the act or public trust regarding the practice of dentistry

Reciprocity

> **The granting of a license by credentials only, without the dentist having to take the usual examination.**

- Defining grounds for suspension, revocation, or **reciprocity** of license
- Defining the legitimate duties that may be delegated to auxiliaries

Definition of Dental Practice The State Dental Practice Act usually presents a definition for the practice of dentistry in the following way:

> The practice of dentistry is the diagnosis, treatment, prescription, or operation for any disease, pain, injury, deficiency, deformity, or physical condition of the teeth, mouth, jaws, or adjacent structures. Activities which fall within this type of description constitute the practice of dentistry, and anyone who performs such activities must have a license.

License The State Dental Practice Act makes provisions for the granting of a license to practice dentistry. A *license* is the legal permission of people to engage in a specific profession or business. To obtain a dental license, an applicant must meet the educational and moral requirements and pass a written and practical examination. The requirements for dental licensure usually include the following:

1 Graduating from a dental school or allied dental personnel school approved by the State Board of Dental Examiners and the Council on Dental Education of the ADA
2 Passing a theoretical and practical examination given by the State Board of Dental Examiners
3 Having good moral character
4 Not committing a crime involving moral turpitude (base depravity, corruption, or immorality)
5 Not being addicted to chemical substances, such as drugs or alcohol

Minimum age and residency requirements for licensure may also exist. To maintain a license, licensees must usually pay an annual fee; publicly display the license at their practice; and complete some professional continuing education each year.

State Board of Dental Examiners   The State Board of Dental Examiners, created by the State Dental Practice Act, is empowered to manage the licensure process within the state. This includes administering an appropriate examination, granting or revocation of licenses, and disciplining those convicted of practicing dentistry without a license. Violation of the State Dental Practice Act is a crime. Depending on the wording of the act, possible penalties for practicing dentistry without a license can include court restraining orders, fines, and imprisonment.

Practicing Dentistry Without a License   People who practice dentistry without a license can include dentists whose licenses are inactive or revoked, unlicensed denturists, and dental personnel who perform tasks beyond the scope of the law or their credentials. *People practicing dentistry without a license are responsible for their illegal acts.* If licensed dentists knowingly permit staff to perform an illegal function under their direction and supervision, the dentist and staff member are responsible for the illegal acts and legal liability that may result. Such action by the dentist may also be grounds for the revocation of the dentist's license. A dental license can be revoked for a variety of reasons including the following:

1 Conviction of a felony, including murder, rape, narcotics violations, and similar crimes of moral turpitude
2 Unprofessional conduct that can include permitting an unlicensed person to perform dentistry; permitting staff to perform tasks not specifically permitted by state law; deceiving the public through false and misleading advertising; giving or receiving rebates; and repeated and intemperate chemical abuse
3 Gross incompetence or personal incapacity that may be because of an accident, disease, or age

Reciprocity   Reciprocity is the granting of a license by credentials and occurs when one state grants a license based on licensure granted by another state. The details of obtaining licensure by reciprocity vary from state to state. The granting of the second license is done either without any additional examination or by taking only part of the normal examination. However, applicants must usually present and verify their credentials to the state board when reciprocity is requested.

Regulation of Allied Dental Personnel   The regulation of the activities of auxiliaries may either be spelled out in the Dental Practice Act or left to the discretion of the board of examiners. Dental personnel who perform certain tasks may be required to either register or be certified (see Chapter 2).

When expanded duties are employed in a dental practice, the dentist and expanded duty auxiliary should be perfectly clear about what may and may not be permitted by the State Dental Practice Act.

The Law and the Dentist and Allied Dental Personnel Relationship

In common law, when one individual authorizes and controls the action of another, such as an employer and employee relationship, the employee becomes an *agent* of the employer. In this relationship, *both* the employer and employee are responsible for the acts of the employee, based on the legal principle of *respondeat superior*, which means "let the higher one answer." However, the reverse is not true; the employee is not responsible for the acts of the employer.

The dentists are the licensed professionals and have the ultimate responsibility for everything that occurs in the practice. This includes not only what they do but also the actions of all employees *that are carried out in the performance of assigned duties.* For example, when a dental hygienist performs a prophylaxis for a patient or a dental assistant takes radiographs, these actions are performed under the direction and authorization of the dentist. The auxiliary is acting on behalf of and as the agent of the dentist. Although this principle makes the dentist and employer responsible for the authorized acts of their assistant and employee, it does *not* relieve employees of responsibility for their acts. Should the auxiliary harm the patient while performing authorized services, the auxiliary and dentist are liable, and the patient can sue them for damages.

The dentist would not be responsible for those acts of the employee that are either not authorized, personal, and not related directly to the practice.

LEGAL DUTIES AND RESPONSIBILITIES IN THE DENTIST AND PATIENT RELATIONSHIP

Standards of Care

A contract relationship exists between the doctor, staff, and patient based on common law. Unless specific written terms have been expressed, the courts have identified several basic and implied duties owed to the patient. These implied duties of the dentist are collectively known as the *standard of care.*

All practicing dentists and allied dental personnel are held to this standard. In accepting the contract with the patient, the dentist accepts certain duties and obligations.

Credentials

The dentist must be properly licensed, registered, and meet all other legal requirements to practice dentistry in that state. *The patient and public have the right to expect that the dentist and staff are properly licensed and credentialed and comply with all of the laws related to the practice of dentistry. Thus if required by state law, the auxiliary must be licensed or registered. The auxiliary is also responsible for performing only those duties allowed by state law and not performing any duties not permitted by state law.*

Knowledge, Skill, Care, and Judgment

Dental health care providers must exercise reasonable knowledge, skill, care, and judgment according to the standards of care provided by similar practitioners in the same community or specialty of practice. Knowledge is an understanding of a subject or topic; skill is knowledge plus the ability to use such knowledge; care is the level of consideration and attention used in applying that skill; judgment is the process of deciding which treatment to use. The dentist and the auxiliary are legally bound to possess and use these traits *at a level ordinarily possessed and used by similar dentists and personnel in the same community and under similar conditions.* This includes the expectation to take all necessary precautions, consistent with the patient's medical history, in the treatment of the patient. *Presently, the courts also include certification in CPR among reasonable skills expected of dentists and staff.*

Standards

Standard techniques, materials, drugs, and treatments should be used in dentistry. At the least, the dentist can use those methods employed by a respectable minority of practitioners in the community or a similar community. Experi-

Box 3.2

Situations in Which Consent Must Be Given in Writing

If new drugs are used
If experimentation or clinical testing is involved
If a patient's identifiable photograph is used
If a general anesthetic is used
If minor children are treated in a public program
If the treatment takes more than 1 year to complete

mental methods or drugs cannot be used in the course of normal treatment.

Personnel

Competent support personnel must be employed and proper supervision must be maintained. The dentist is in charge of employing only competent personnel and training and supervising them properly. Support personnel are responsible for performing competently and should only perform tasks they are trained to do.

Consent

Informed consent must be obtained before beginning an examination or treatment. The law makes binding the ethical principle of obtaining only *valid, informed* consent before proceeding with treatment. Valid consent is giving permission for someone to do something. For the consent to be valid, the following requirements must be met:
- The one giving consent must be legally competent.
- The consent must be informed.
- The consent must be for a specific action or series of actions.
- The consented action must be legal.
- The consent must not have been obtained by deceit or trickery (fraud).

Informed consent is given only when the patient has enough information to make a rational choice. Therefore the patient must understand the following:
- The nature of the problem
- The recommended treatment of the problem
- The risks involved, including the following:
1 The failure of treatment
2 The results of no treatment
- The alternative choices of treatment

Implied consent is given by the actions of patients, such as sitting in the chair and opening their mouth.

Expressed consent is given either verbally or in writing for a specific procedure.

For those not qualified to give legal consent such as a child or incapacitated adult consent must be given by the parent or legal guardian only, either verbally or in writing. In a true emergency in which life or permanent harm is threatened, implied consent may be presumed (Box 3-2).

Abandonment

Although dentists or other health professionals have the right to decline to treat people who are not their patients, once dentists accept people as patients (the dentist and patient contract) they must treat those needs specifically agreed on; to not do so becomes a *breach of contract.*

Abandonment is the desertion of a patient and termination of care before treatment is completed; it may also be the refusal to treat a patient of record. Abandonment occurs when the practitioner is not available to a patient of record when the patient may reasonably expect to require assistance. If the dentist is going to be temporarily away from the office and unable to provide care, the dentist is responsible for arranging another qualified dentist to provide services during the absence to avoid a charge of abandonment. If the dentist is not able to complete the patient's treatment, the dentist must also refer the patient to a dentist who can complete the work.

Fees

A reasonable fee for services should be charged, based on community standards. An essential element of the dentist and patient contract is a fair charge by the dentist for the services provided to the patient. To avoid misunderstandings, the dentist should present the fee to the patient and get agreement from the patient at the presentation of the treatment plan.

Even if the dentist agreed to provide a service or services at no charge, a binding dentist and patient contract is still considered to exist in law.

Legal Actions

Related to the responsibilities of licensure, dentists must not allow anyone acting under their direction or supervision to perform an illegal act while providing care. As stated previously, if a staff member performs an illegal act, the staff is responsible, and the dentist is also responsible under the doctrine of respondent superior.

Information

The dentist should provide adequate instructions to patients, keep them informed of the progress of treatment, and advise them of any possible untoward incidents that may occur during the treatment. The dentist must give adequate instructions to the patient for any postoperative care, routine self-care, or any follow-up observations or care. The dentist should make sure that the patient understands the instructions. If the patient is a child, an incapacitated adult, or recovering from a general anesthetic, the dentist must give instructions to the parent, guardian, or person responsible for accompanying the patient to the office.

Referral

No one can do everything. Dentists will usually refer unusual cases, or those beyond their scope of training, to a specialist. In so doing, the dentist must advise the patient that services are needed that cannot be properly performed in the office. If possible, the dentist should assist the patient in finding an appropriate specialist who can provide the needed services.

Complete Dental Treatment

The dentist is obligated to start and complete care and treatment in a reasonable period: 1 year. Complex cases, such as orthodontics, implants, or reconstruction, may take considerably longer. If so, the treatment time should be discussed when the case is presented and accepted.

Treatment Outcome

To fulfill their part in the dentist and patient contract, dentists must achieve a reasonable outcome of treatment. Failure to do so is a breach of the standard of care and contract with the patient. However, the outcome does no have to be ideal or even exactly as anticipated at the beginning of treatment. Neither biology nor human behavior are completely predictable. Unexpected outcomes are always possible. Part of informed consent is to advise the patient of the possibility of alternative and less-desirable outcomes.

Guarantees

Because an outcome cannot be completely predicted, the dentist should never guarantee one or give promises. A dentist making a promise or claim about the outcome of care, which could be interpreted by the patient as a guarantee, is unethical, illegal in some areas, and foolish. Just as heart surgeons cannot and do not guarantee the hearts they transplant, dentists cannot guarantee the results of their dental work.

Records

The dental assistant should keep accurate, complete, and secure records of the diagnosis and treatment of the patient. Keeping records is a professional obligation to the patient and to other dentists who may later treat the patient.

Confidentiality

All dental personnel must maintain confidentiality of information obtained from the patient or as a result of treatment. The same expectations of patient confidentiality and privacy that exist in the ethical obligation to the patient also exist in law. Dental personnel must abide by the following rules:

- No information of any kind (health, finances, behavior, address, phone number, and so on) about the patient obtained during the treatment may be released to *anyone* without the patient's *written* permission.
- The patient must sign a release of information to submit claims to an insurance company; such a release is usually a part of the claim form.
- No observers may be in the operatory during treatment without the patient's permission.
- Written permission is needed if photos of the patient are to be published, even if the patient cannot be identified.

Code of Ethics

Dental assistants must practice in a manner consistent with the code of ethics of the profession. The law recognizes the profession's code of ethics and holds the practitioner to that standard.

IMPLIED DUTIES OF THE PATIENT

Just as the dentist and patient contract contains duties and obligations for the dentist, the patient also has duties and obligations. Failure to abide by these duties and obligations is considered a breach by the patient and breaks the contract with the dentist and the dentist's corresponding obligations to the patient. In accepting the contract for care, the patient accepts the following duties:

- Keeping appointments: Failure to keep scheduled appointments makes it impossible for the dentist to provide the necessary care in a timely manner and complete the treatment.
- Cooperating in care: Most health care treatments require certain behaviors and expectations of the patient for the treatment to be successful. Just as the heart patient must stop smoking and start exercising, the dental patient must follow the various instructions by the dentist. A lack of necessary cooperation by the patient can easily nullify the efforts of the dentist and break the relationship.
- Paying a reasonable fee and making timely payments: Part of the contract includes the charge of a reasonable fee for the service agreed on. Failure to pay the fee, or make payments in a timely and reasonable manner, assuming dentists have kept their part of the contract, is a breach by the patient.
- Notifying the practitioner of any changes in health status: In providing a health care service, the dentist must be made aware of any changes in the patient's health. Such information can have a serious affect on the outcome of care. Lack of new information could compromise the outcome of treatment and make success impossible. If so, the fault would be with the patient, not the dentist, and the patient would be the one to break the contract that they agreed on.

TERMINATION OF THE DOCTOR AND PATIENT RELATIONSHIP

The doctor and patient relationship does not last forever. The contract between the doctor and patient may be ended by the following circumstances:

- Death: Either party dies. Obviously the contract is terminated because one of the principal parties is no longer available.
- Cure: The patient is cured of the specific disease for which the patient sought treatment. If the specific problem for which the patient sought help is resolved, care is no longer needed and the relationship may be terminated.
- Mutual agreement: The doctor and patient mutually agree to end the relationship. Occasionally, the doctor and patient mutually agree that ending the relationship is best for everyone. If this occurs, the patient must still pay for services provided to that date. The dentist must cooperate with any future doctor who might provide care for the patient. This cooperation must be done with the patient's permission.
- Patient decision: The patient ends the relationship. At any time the patient can dismiss the doctor. When that happens, the relationship ends.
- Doctor decision: The doctor ends the relationship. The doctor can also unilaterally end the relationship but not as easily as the patient can. To legally withdraw from caring for a patient of record and terminate the relationship, doctors must do the following:
  1 Notify the patient in writing of their intent to withdraw, and the following actions must be taken:
  2 A specific withdrawal date must be stated (usually 30 days from the date of the letter) to allow the patient adequate time to find another dentist.
  3 The need for future care, if needed, must be stated.
  4 Send a notice to the patient by registered or certified mail with a return receipt requested.
  5 Place that receipt in the patient's dental record.
  6 Dental care cannot be discontinued at a time when the patient's health may be compromised.
  7 Cooperate in the future care of the patient by making all necessary records, radiographs, and so on available to the new dentist (with the patient's permission).

Termination of the relationship by the dentist because the patient has not paid the agreed on fee is neither legal nor ethical. The dentist is obligated to either complete all procedures that have been started or assist the patient in finding a dentist who can complete those procedures. If the patient is not financially able to continue treatment, the dentist is not required to begin new procedures that are not an emergency. The usual custom in these circumstances is to temporarily suspend treatment by mutual agreement until the patient can resume treatment. During this period, the dentist and patient are still bound by their contractual relationship, and the dentist must provide at least emergency services until treatment either resumes or formally ends.

LIABILITIES IN DENTISTRY

A *liability* is a legal obligation and responsibility. To be *liable* is to be accountable, responsible, and legally required to compensate for any loss or damage. In dentistry, the dental personnel are exposed to professional and criminal liabilities in their relationship with the patient. *Crimes* are acts that are considered to harm the public, instead of injuring one specific individual (although that may occur as part of the crime). In dentistry, the most common major crimes include:

- Narcotic violations
- Income tax evasion

Negligence

An unintentional tort (wrongful conduct not involving a contract).

- **Negligence** that causes injury or death

Conviction of a major crime usually results in the suspension or revocation of the dentist's license and punishment for the crime. However, the majority of liabilities in dentistry are professional and related specifically to the practice of dentistry. Dentists can incur a professional liability if they violate the rights of others or fail to perform their legal duties. Such an action is a civil wrong (tort), not involving a contract, which results from a breach of duty for which the dentist is liable and legally responsible.

If a tort is committed, the dentist is obligated to compensate the injured party, usually in the form of money. This is called *payment of damages*. If personnel (agent) cause a tort, the staff member and dentist, under the doctrine of respondent superior, may be held liable. The most common torts in dental practice include the following:

Malpractice

Any professional misconduct or any unreasonable lack of skill, care, or judgment in the performance of professional duties. The word means "bad practice."

- Defamation of character or maligning a patient
- Personal liabilities, such as office hazards
- Breach of contract
- Deceit or fraud
- Breach of confidential information
- Medical professional liability or **malpractice**

Defamation of Character

Defamation of character includes the following:

- *Malign* is *saying* or *writing* something that will defame a character and harm a reputation.
- *Slander* is *saying* something that will harm a reputation.
- *Libel* is *writing* something that will harm a reputation.

The dentist and the auxiliary must be careful what they say or write about a patient, regardless of what they think about the patient personally. For example, suppose the patient does not follow home-care instructions. To tell patients that they are bad, stupid, or irresponsible for not following recommended home-care instructions in a tone that could be overheard by others in the office is not only bad manners but also is *slander*. To write similar comments in the patient's record is *libel*. Both violations are torts in which the dentist has defamed the character of the patient, and the dentist could be sued for damages.

The correct way to handle this situation would be to objectively advise the patients that their home-care efforts are thus far inadequate and explain the biological consequences of poor home care. The entry in the patient record should note the patient's present home-care efforts and that the patient has been advised. At no time should anyone in the office, either dentist or staff, make any character judgments about a patient.

Personal Liabilities from Office Hazards

Everyone who has a home or place of business is responsible for any injury that may occur there. This is called *personal liability*, and the dentist and the staff must always be alert to identify and eliminate such possible hazards, including the following:

- Slipping on a wet floor
- Tripping on a torn carpet
- Being struck by a faulty x-ray head

If a patient is harmed in any way from an accident described earlier, the dentist is personally responsible because as the professional, the dentist is accountable for everything that occurs in the office.

Breach of Contract

Most medical professional liability (malpractice) actions are from a breach of duty to maintain the standard of care. However, if dentists promise to perform a certain service, or guarantee a certain result (discussed previously and definitely *not* recommended) and either does not perform the service or achieve the result, they could be guilty of breach of contract.

Misrepresentation, Deceit, or Fraud

If a dentist withholds information from patients about either the status of their health or progress of treatment and their health is jeopardized, the dentist is guilty of *deceit*. The dentist may withhold information about fractured and retained root tips or endodontic files; this is called a *tort* and can be a costly mistake, in which the dentist may be sued. *Fraud* can occur in third-party claims if claimed services were not provided or completed. In cases of insurance fraud, the insurance company may initiate either a civil or criminal action against the dentist.

Breach of Confidentiality

Confidential information may be released only with the expressed *written* permission of the patient. The only exception is the requirement to report certain communicable diseases to the appropriate government authorities. When patients accept referral to a specialist, they give implied consent for the referring dentist to provide appropriate information to the specialist. In some jurisdictions, information related to the sexual activity of a minor may not be revealed to the parent without the minor's consent. A breach of this nature may bring civil and criminal actions.

Medical Professional Liability or Malpractice

Malpractice can be defined as any professional misconduct or any unreasonable lack of skill, care, or judgment in the performance of professional duties. It is also practice contrary to accepted standards. A dentist may be sued for malpractice if patients feel they were detrimentally affected or injured by the treatment or the diagnosis was incorrect.

Medical professional liability can be defined as treatment that is wrong, bad, or poorly conceived and executed, which results in injury, unnecessary suffering, or death to the patient. Poor treatment is a result of ignorance, carelessness, lack of proper professional skill, disregard of established rules or principles, neglect, or a malicious or criminal intent. Dentists incur a civil liability by any professional act, or by a failure to properly perform their duties, if that failure results in injury to the patient. Both terms mean almost the same thing; they imply a breach of the duty to apply skill, care, and judgment, resulting in harm to the patient.

Admissions against interest is a statement made by people that harms their interest. The patient can use a statement against the dentist in court, for example if a dentist or auxiliary were to say, "I'm sorry, it was my fault" after an accident that injures the patient. Any statements that are "part of the action" may be used against the dentist. Regardless of what happens, the dentist and assistant must be careful about what they say. *Rather than accepting fault or blame, the dentist or staff should acknowledge the fact of the incident and attempt to correct the problem.* When in doubt, say nothing.

Common Causes of Dental Malpractice

Lack of Informed Consent
To treat patients without their informed consent is a violation of the standard of care. To provide any service without prior approval by patients is considered malpractice.

Assault, Battery, and Unjustified Restraint
In law, one person may not touch another person without permission or if the touch is not permitted by social custom. In our society, shaking hands or tapping someone on the shoulder is customary. However, touching beyond these customs is usually not acceptable. To threaten to touch someone without permission, especially in a harmful manner, is called *assault*. To actually touch someone without permission, whether harm occurs or not, is called *battery*. Assault and battery are criminal offenses. The civil equivalent is civil trespass.

For dental personnel to physically restrain an uncooperative child to provide care, without the understanding and permission of the parent or guardian, is *unjustified restraint* and a breach of the duty to inform.

Failure to Diagnose
Failure to diagnose is a breach of the use of professional knowledge, skill, care, and judgment. Failure to diagnose, or incorrectly diagnose a problem that the typical practitioner would be expected to correctly diagnose, such as periodontal disease, or a nonhealing oral lesion, is called *negligence*.

Related to the failure to diagnose, is the failure to use normal diagnostic tools correctly. For example, the failure to either take normal diagnostic radiographs, or to take them incorrectly when they are needed to obtain a correct diagnosis, is negligence. However, sometimes a patient refuses to allow the dentist to take recommended radiographs or any other diagnostic tests that the dentist thinks is needed to correctly determine the patient's problem. If this happens, the dentist should have the patient sign a release (either as a separate form, in the patient record, or both) confirming that the patient has declined this recommended test. This places the assumption of risk on the patient and will help to defend the dentist against a charge of failure to diagnose.

Failure to Refer
An average dentist is expected to properly refer cases that they cannot properly handle, which might include complex oral surgery, orthodontics, endodontics, periodontics, or pediatric dentistry. To fail to do so is a breach of duty.

Failure to Exercise Universal Precautions
Universal precautions, such as sterilization of all instruments, use of barrier products, and so on are now accepted as standard practices of the profession. To fail to do so is a breach of the standard of care.

Errors in Judgment
Dentists are expected to exercise a reasonable level of judgment consistent with the standard of care in the community. Not doing this may result in a claim of negligence if the result is an undesired outcome. For example, to not use a rubber dam during endodontic treatment would be an error in judgment and a violation of the standard of care. However, an error in judgment is not negligence if the decision was the best that could have been made at the time. For example, if a patient were to have an unexpected allergic reaction to a medication, not anticipated by the history, negligence did not occur.

Foreign Body Left in the Mouth
The breakage of root tips, anesthetic needles, or endodontic files occasionally occur in the practice of dentistry. Such accidents by themselves are not necessarily negligence because

they are a legitimate risk in dentistry. However, dentists are negligent in the following circumstances:

- If they do not inform the patient that the accident has occurred
- If they fail to make every effort to correct the problem
- If they fail to refer the patient to a specialist when they cannot resolve the problem, which makes them vulnerable to a charge of malpractice. Dentists are not negligent when they have an accident, but their response could be considered malpractice.

Failure to Inform the Patient

Most malpractice suits are a result of a failure to communicate. No one likes unpleasant surprises. If dentists do not keep the patient informed of the findings, prognosis, and progress of treatment, they could easily be charged with negligence and failure to inform. For example, failure to inform could occur if patients are surprised to learn in the middle of treatment that they have periodontal disease.

Instrument Slippage

An accident, such as the slippage of an instrument, is in the same category as a broken instrument. It is a risk of dental practice. However, if the dentist does not deal with the occurrence properly, the result could be a malpractice claim.

Swallowing or Aspirating a Foreign Body

The standard of care dictates that rubber dams, throat packs, or extreme care be used if a risk of swallowing or aspiration exists. To fail to do so is negligence. Should such an incident occur without these precautions, the dentist is liable.

Anesthetic Accidents

The administration of local and general anesthetics pose risks to the patient. These risks include allergic reactions, permanent or temporary numbness, or complications with existing medical conditions. For example, the dentist is expected to use a local anesthetic that does not contain epinephrine if the patient has a heart condition. To use the incorrect anesthetic would make the dentist liable.

Incorrect Use of Medications

Dentists are expected to prescribe and use medications properly. To use drugs in ways that complicate the patient's condition, or compound a known addiction, is malpractice.

Fracture of the Jaw

Fracture of the jaw is also a risk in certain dental procedures. To avoid malpractice, the dentist must advise the patient of the risks in advance and exercise extreme care.

Unsatisfactory Dentures or Bridges

If a dentist were to make a denture, bridge, or appliance that is grossly inferior to the standards of care in the area, the dentist could be guilty of malpractice. However, if despite the best efforts of the dentist, the desired result is not obtained, an unfortunate result could occur but not necessarily malpractice. Malpractice exists only if the four requirements for malpractice, listed previously, are met. Patients may sue for malpractice if they have unrealistic expectations of the treatment. Such expectations can be minimized by proper communication with the patient that emphasizes a reasonable outcome.

PREVENTING PROFESSIONAL LIABILITY CLAIMS IN DENTISTRY

Malpractice prevention is based on a combination of attitudes and actions in the dental office. The primary attitude is one of *genuine caring*, and the primary action is *communication*. The role of the dental assistant is critical if caring and communication are to become a reality in the practice. People who are angry, humiliated, embarrassed, or surprised file most malpractice claims. Rightly or wrongly, they feel that they have been treated unfairly and improperly. They want justice, and the only way for them to receive it is through a malpractice lawsuit.

Genuine caring is the first step in preventing these powerful negative emotions from appearing. Such caring is nothing more than the golden rule, in which every patient is treated the same way the dentist and assistant would want to be treated. Responding to patients in this manner helps to satisfy their basic emotional needs, because all patients want to be treated as a human being with dignity and respect. Patients who are treated in this way will like and trust the dental staff, even if they do not like dental treatment. Patients who like and trust the people in the office, are respected, and are made to feel welcome and important are unlikely to file a malpractice claim against the dentist or anyone in the office.

Communication is the next active step in preventing malpractice actions. Patients want no surprises; they want to know what has happened to their dental health, what is happening during the treatment, and what will happen when treatment is completed. Patients who understand what is happening and why will be an active and understanding participant in their own treatment, and treatment is more likely to be successful.

Actions to Prevent or Minimize Malpractice Claims

In addition to the generalizations of caring and communication, the dental assistant can perform many specific actions, related to the causes of malpractice discussed earlier, to prevent or minimize a malpractice claim that a patient might bring against the practice.

Avoid Admission

The dental assistant should avoid admissions against interest. If an unfortunate event occurs in the office, such as the breakage of an instrument, the dental assistant must acknowledge the event and deal with the consequences but not assume responsibility for it. Above all, the dental assistant should try to avoid saying something spontaneously that will compound the problem, such as "Oops, my fault." With training and anticipation, such statements become less likely to occur.

Perform Legal Functions

Perform only those tasks that you can legally complete and for which you are adequately trained.

Patient Records

Guard zealously the accuracy, completeness, legibility, and security of the patient's dental record. The records should contain the following:

- Demographic and necessary personal data
- Current medical and dental history
- Chief complaint or initial request for care
- Examination findings
- Diagnostic tests, including radiographs and results
- The diagnosis
- Consultation requests and responses
- Recommended treatment plan or plans
- Consent for care
- Detailed records of services provided, which should include date, vital signs that day, type and quantity of medications administered or prescribed, specific procedures performed, normal and unusual observations, treatment outcomes, and instructions provided
- A log of broken or failed appointments
- Copies of all correspondence with the patient

Do *not* place financial information or account statement in the patient's treatment record. Financial account information is separate from and not part of the treatment record.

The record should be kept clean, neat, legible, and unaltered. If an inadvertent entry has been made, that entry should *not* be erased or blocked out. Simply draw a single line through the entry. So it is still readable, write "error" above it, enter your initials and the date, and make the correct entry on the next line.

The law states the record, including the radiographs, are the legal property of the doctor. Do not release the record or let anyone else look at it without the doctor's permission. If the patient is transferred to another doctor, do *not* give the record to the patient or send the record to the new doctor. You must obtain written permission from the patient to *copy* the record and radiographs and send those copies to the new doctor. To not do so would make the dentist liable for releasing confidential information without the consent of the patient.

The original record must stay with the practice. Do not make any subjective or character judgments about the patient in the record. Such comments could be considered libel. State objective facts or observations only. The record is your best defense against a malpractice action. It can contain information regarding the patient's assumption of risk for a specific treatment or possible contributory negligence for not following instructions. Protect it in a secure and fireproof environment.

State laws may vary on how long an inactive record (the patient has not seen in more than 3 years) must be stored. In many states an inactive record is 5 to 7 years since the last visit or past the age of 21 if the individual was a child when treatment began. Several legal experts now advise the doctor to keep records as long as the practice exists.

Comments

Do not criticize or comment on the work of another dentist. One cannot know the conditions under which those dental services were delivered. Negative comments of previous dentists and their work do not enhance the patient's perception of this practice. Rather, they diminish the reputation of dentistry in general. Such unnecessary comments can also lead to unjustified lawsuits, which harm the entire profession. Make sure that appropriate consent is obtained for all elective services, especially surgery, that require specific written consent. For many emergency and examination services, implied consent may usually be assumed.

To avoid misunderstandings, all postoperative instructions should be given to the patient verbally and in writing. A verification that those instructions have been given should be entered in the progress notes of the patient record.

Do everything possible to keep the office meticulously clean, neat, and organized. All equipment should be working properly, and any potential hazard should be corrected. Such an environment gives the patient an impression of competence and consideration. If patients think that the office is proficient, they will be less likely to sue for malpractice.

Skills Performance

Perform all of your duties to the best of your ability. Maintain and upgrade your skills by inoffice training and continuing education. In addition to caring and communication, clinical excellence is your best protection against a lawsuit.

Scrupulous

Dental personnel must be careful to avoid anything that could be interpreted as practicing dentistry. This includes opinions about dental problems; recommendations on treatment, medications, or dosages; predictions of outcomes; refilling prescriptions without the dentist's authorization, and so on.

Financial Arrangements

Fees should be explained and understood before treatment begins. Financial misunderstandings can cause claims.

Accurate Claims

All insurance claims and forms must be accurately and completely filled out. Inaccurate insurance forms can be used against a dentist in a legal action.

Confidentiality

Never violate the principle of confidentiality.

Advise Dentist

If patient dissatisfaction is sensed in any way, advise the dentist immediately (Box 3-3).

Box 3.3

Role of the Dental Assistant in Preventing Malpractice

Avoid admissions against interest.

Perform only those tasks that are legal and for which you are trained.

Ensure that the patient record is accurate, complete, legible, and secure.

Do not criticize the work of another dentist.

Ensure that appropriate consent is obtained for all procedures.

Present all postoperative instructions in writing.

Keep the office meticulously clean and safe.

Maintain the highest level of professional skill and always perform to the best of your ability.

Avoid doing anything that might be considered the practice of dentistry (e.g., refilling prescriptions).

Make sure that two people are present in the operatory during treatment.

Make sure that the patient understands the fees before treatment begins.

File all insurance claims accurately and completely.

Never violate the principle of confidentiality.

Inform the dentist immediately if the patient is unhappy about the dental care.

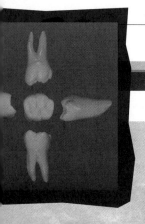

Points for Review

- The role of ethics in dental practice
- The meaning of ethics and jurisprudence
- Informed consent
- Trust as the key feature in a professional or personal relationship
- The ethical principle of autonomy and confidentiality
- The importance of good communications in the dental office
- Your State Dental Practice Act

Self-Study Questions

1. What principle deals with right and wrong behavior, evil, duty, and judgment?
   a. Ethics
   b. Res ipsa loquitur
   c. Jurisprudence
   d. Beneficence
2. What principle describes a minimum level of personal conduct?
   a. Common law
   b. Ethics
   c. Jurisprudence
   d. Statutory law
   e. Civil law
3. What standard of moral principles and practice should professionals follow?
   a. The professional code of ethics
   b. The State Professional Practice Act
   c. The regulations of the state board of the profession
4. What principle deals with decisions regarding the welfare of another?
   a. Respondent superior
   b. Paternalism
   c. Res ipsa loquitur
   d. Beneficence
5. Which violation occurs if a dentist or dental assistant falsifies third-party insurance claims?
   a. Ethics

   b. Jurisprudence
   c. a and b
   d. None of the above
6. What is the basis of dentistry's present position regarding patients with HIV and their providers?
   a. The 1990 Americans with Disabilities Act
   b. The ADA's ethical position on this issue
   c. The effectiveness of universal precautions
7. What is the legal permission called that allows a person to engage in a specific profession or business?
   a. Licensure
   b. Registration
   c. Certification
   d. Reciprocity
8. If a dentist allows an auxiliary to perform a dental function not permitted by the State Dental Practice Act, who is responsible?
   a. The dentist
   b. The auxiliary
   c. a and b
9. Which offense causes a dentist's license to be suspended or revoked?
   a. Narcotics violations
   b. Conviction of a felony
   c. Gross incompetence
   d. Permitting an auxiliary to perform illegal tasks
   e. All of the above
10. What do dentists do when they accept patients into their care?
   a. Enter into a contract relationship with the patient
   b. Accept the duties and obligations contained in the standard of care
   c. Accept the profession's code of ethics
   d. All of the above
11. What condition occurs if a patient fails to keep appointments or follow instructions?
   a. Admissions against interest
   b. Res ipsa loquitur
   c. Liability
   d. Contributory negligence
12. How can a malpractice claim be defended?
   a. The statute of limitations
   b. The patient's assumption of risk
   c. The patient's contributory negligence
   d. All of the above

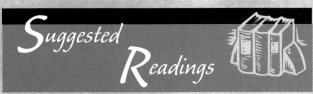

Suggested Readings

American Dental Association: *Principles of ethics and code of professional conduct,* Chicago, 1997.

Davison JA: *Legal and ethical considerations for dental hygienists and assistants,* ed 1, St. Louis, 2000, Mosby.

Ebersold LA: *Malpractice: risk management for dentists,* Tulsa, Okla, 1986, Pennwell.

Erlich A: *Ethics and jurisprudence: fundamentals for dental auxiliaries,* Champaign, Ill, 1978, Colwell.

Howard WW, Parks AL: *The dentist and the law,* St Louis, 1973, Mosby.

Motley WT: *Ethics, jurisprudence, and history for the dental hygienist,* ed 3, Philadelphia, 1983, Lea & Febiger.

Morris WO: *Dental litigation,* Charlottesville, Va, 1972, Michie.

Ozar DT, Sokol DJ: *Professional ethics at chairside: professional principles and practice applications,* St Louis, 1994, Mosby.

Pollack BR, editor: *Handbook of dental jurisprudence and risk management,* Littleton, Mass, 1987, PSG.

Rule JT, Veatch RM: *Ethical questions in dentistry,* Chicago, 1993, Quintessence.

Schafler NL: *Medical malpractice: handling dental cases,* Colorado Springs, 1985, Shepard's/McGraw-Hill.

Seear J, Walters L: *Law and ethics in dentistry,* ed 3, Oxford, 1991, Wright.

Weinstein BD: *Dental ethics,* Philadelphia, 1993, Lea & Febiger.

Willig SH: *Legal considerations in dentistry,* Baltimore, 1971, Williams and Wilkins.

Unit II

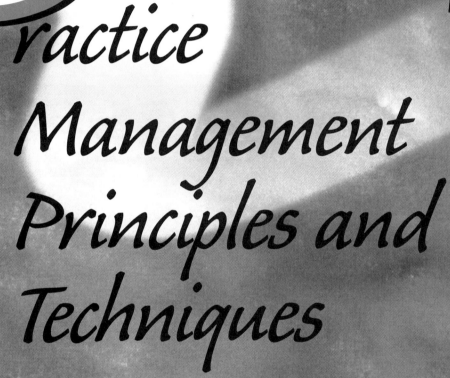

Practice Management Principles and Techniques

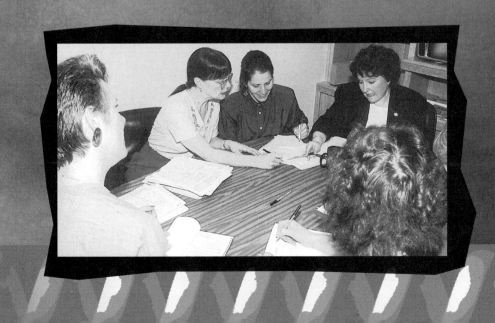

Chapter 4

Managing Communications in the Dental Practice

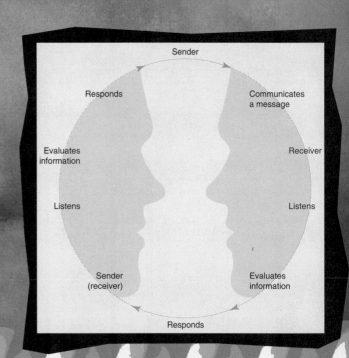

Chapter Outline

Management Principles for the Dental
    Assistant
    Elements of the management process
    Managerial basics
Dental Practice Environment
    Internal environment
    External environment
    Dentistry as a service business
Organizational and Legal Forms of Dental
    Practice
    Sole proprietorship
    Partnership
    Corporation
    Multipractitioner arrangements
Management Functions in a Dental Office
    Dental assistant's role in practice
    management
Dental Office Communications
    Communications defined

    Communication process
    Basic forms of communications
Developing Effective Relationships
    Physical dimensions
    Behavioral dimensions
    Interactional dimensions
    Environmental dimensions
    Other dimensions
Reception Techniques
    Personal appearance
    Promptness
    Greeting the patient
Telephone Techniques
    Answering the telephone
    Placing telephone calls
Written Communications
    Business letter format
    Return address and date

Learning Objectives

On completion of Chapter 4, the student should be able to do the following:

- Define key terms.
- Describe the relationship among the management processes of planning, organizing, leading, and evaluating.
- Explain the communication process.
- List methods for resolving conflict in the workplace.
- Identify how to manage stress.
- List the steps in the decision-making process.

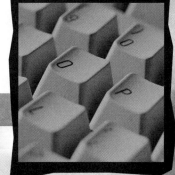

Key Terms

Dimension	Interaction	Organizing
Evaluation	Leadership	Planning
Goals	Motivation	Policies
Hierarchy	Objectives	Procedures

MANAGEMENT PRINCIPLES FOR THE DENTAL ASSISTANT

Goals

General statements that translate the mission statement or philosophy of an institution into an attainable objective.

Objectives

Further defines the goals by making them specific, measurable, and timely.

Policies

A course of action, guiding principle, or procedure designed to influence and determine decisions and actions.

Procedures

A set of established forms or methods for administering the activities of a business.

A dental practice does more than provide professional dental care services for patients; it is a small business. As such, it must be organized and managed by its leader and the management team to achieve the **goals** and **objectives** of the practice. The dental assistant is an important part of the dental office management team. Responsibilities include performing duties consistent with the **policies** and **procedures** for the office and advancing the goals and objectives for the practice.

Dental assistants may be in charge of many of the business functions within a dental office. In some larger offices, one dental assistant may be designated as the full-time business manager or dental practice administrator of the office. This role requires a thorough knowledge of management principles and office policies and procedures. Although a complete presentation of detailed business principles is beyond the scope of this text, the basics of management principles are presented in this chapter to introduce the dental assistant to these concepts.

Elements of the Management Process

Planning

A process to formulate a program to accomplish specific goals or objectives, such as what the dental practice wants to accomplish.

Management of any activity is an ongoing process. Plans must be made, the business needs to be organized, activities have to be evaluated, and changes should be made to the business to improve it. Four elements, **planning**, **organizing**, leading, and evaluating, make up the management process.

Large and small businesses follow the same basic process. In a large company such as General Motors the plans are much more complicated because of the size and complexity of the business. A small business such as a dental office uses the same concepts but is easier to manage because it is less complex, has fewer employees, and concentrates on dental care (Figure 4-1).

Planning

The process of planning encourages the dental practice to formulate a program to accomplish a goal or an objective. A plan provides direction, and without it, the staff is disorganized and the dental practice is not efficient. To have a good business, the dental practice must have a plan.

Plans can be simple or complex. Planning where to locate a dental practice is complicated and requires research. Planning to add a computer system to the office is a simpler decision. Plans are developed to outline a strategy for an action.

Planning permits a dentist and the staff to discuss their goals and contemplate possible options on paper before they make changes. Planning allows them to think through a variety of options and select the best one based on practice goals and available resources, such as money, space, and staff.

Organizing

After plans are made, the process of becoming organized is used to arrange the necessary resources to implement these plans. Purchasing an office computer system requires deciding where it will be located in the office, how it will be paid for, which staff members will be responsible for operating it, and so on. Specific tasks should be assigned to the staff to ensure that the plan becomes reality.

A good plan without proper organization is doomed to failure. An example of poor organizing would be scheduling a dinner party and going to the grocery store to buy the food but forgetting to bring any money. Careful organization is necessary for smooth implementation of a plan.

Leading

Much has been written in the management literature about **leadership**. In its simplest form, leading involves guiding and supervising personnel in carrying out their assigned job duties. In most

Organizing

A process to identify resources necessary to implement a plan, such as how business will achieve goals and objectives.

Leadership

A process of guiding office personnel to accomplish tasks. Leadership requires effective communication, instruction, and motivation skills.

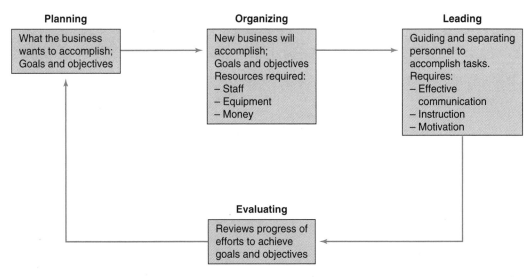

FIGURE 4.1

Elements of the management process.

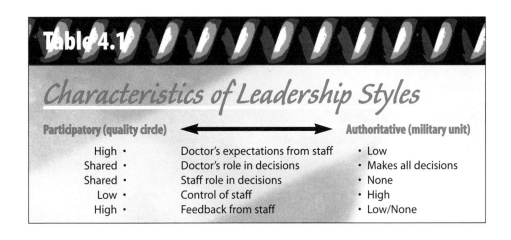

Motivation

The ability to incite or impel oneself or others to action.

dental practices, the dentist is the leader.

Leading consists of communicating effectively, providing clear instructions, and **motivating** office personnel to perform their jobs. For example, if a computer is going to be purchased for the office, effective leadership would consist of providing adequate instructions on how the computer works and encouraging employees to use the computer to improve office efficiency.

Styles of leadership in a dental office may range from authoritarian to participatory (Table 4-1). Authoritarian leaders do almost everything themselves, delegate very little to other staff members, expect little from employees, share little information, and tend to determine all office policy. Participatory or democratic leadership is the opposite of authoritarian leadership. The leader invites staff to help make decisions, encourages feedback from staff, and allows staff to determine many of their own daily work routines. Other types of leadership styles exist between these two extreme positions, which combine elements of the two types of leaders.

Evaluating

Evaluation is the final step in the management process. This action reviews the activities to date and compares what is happening with what was planned. For example, if after 10 months of purchasing a computer, practice information such as patient and financial data is being lost, someone needs to evaluate this. If staff members do not understand how to store information in the computer, immediate steps should be taken to train them to use the proper methods.

Evaluation

A process used to review past efforts to achieve goals and objectives.

Failure to evaluate the planning and organization processes can also have disastrous effects on the dental practice.

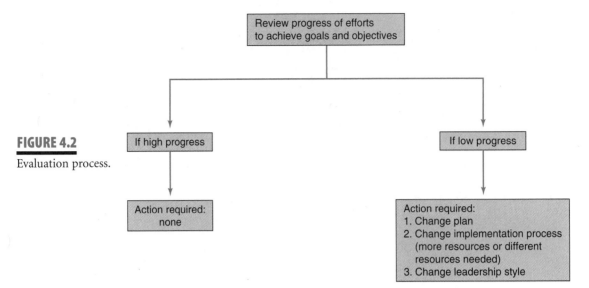

FIGURE 4.2

Evaluation process.

If minimal progress has been made toward achieving a goal or objective, results of the evaluation should be used to change the plan or organization. Conversely, if great progress has been made, then no action is required. In either case, the evaluation process provides the necessary feedback to improve practice performance (Figure 4-2).

Managerial Basics

The five basic elements of the managerial process can be applied to the development of office policies and procedures. For effective management to occur, the dental office must have goals and objectives that are implemented through consistent office policies and procedures. The failure of a dental practice to set goals and objectives can cause confusion and lack of direction for the practice. The development of office policies includes the following:

1 Practice mission or philosophy: The mission or practice philosophy statement is a general declaration of the dentist's personal and professional values and attitudes and beliefs toward patient care, staff, business practices, and community involvement.

2 Goals: Goals translate the mission of the practice into something more meaningful for the office. The doctor and staff create goals to communicate the areas of emphasis and priorities for them to follow.

3 Objectives: Objectives further define the goals by making them more specific, measurable, and timely. The development of objectives is critical to achieving the practice goals and therefore accomplishing the mission or philosophy of the dental practice.

4 Policies: Policies describe how the practice will handle various situations in a standardized manner. Policies can be written for a number of subject areas, such as personnel, patient, or doctor. Examples could include vacation or sick-day policies and a policy on how to handle telephone solicitations. Policies are essential to the dental office for several reasons: (1) they help ensure that problems are handled systematically and quickly. For example, the office billing policy might state that all people with unpaid accounts over 30 days are to be sent a reminder notice; (2) policies result in fairness in dealing with employees and patients; and (3) policies increase office efficiency by making training new employees easier and keeping morale high because the staff have duties.

5 Procedures: Procedures help the office personnel tell the staff what should be done more precisely in specific situations. A dental office may have procedures for making appointments for new patients or filing and tracking insurance claims. Procedures clarify office tasks by communicating to all personnel what is expected of them. Procedures should be established for all activities in the office. They should be based on actual need, easily understood by all staff, revised only when necessary, and given to the staff in written form.

Some offices may assemble these five components into an office manual to be shared with office personnel and patients. The patients generally will see the office philosophy and goals statements. Having responsibility for the daily office operations, the staff will see and use the objectives, policies, and procedures portion of the manual. The use of a manual improves the flow of office tasks because all personnel know the goals and objectives of the practice in advance.

DENTAL PRACTICE ENVIRONMENT

A dental practice operates in an environment that has a direct influence on how the practice will grow and develop. As detailed in Figure 4-3, this environment can be divided into

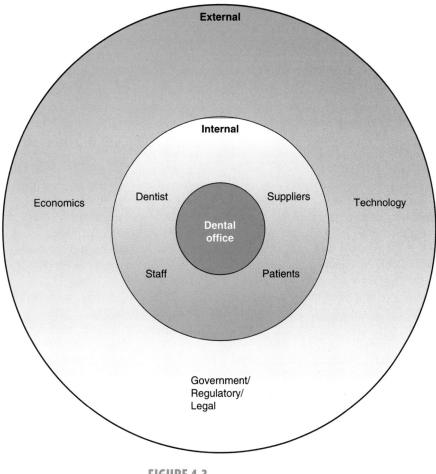

FIGURE 4.3

Dental practice environment.

an internal environment, within the practice, and an external environment, outside of the daily practice activity. Although changes in the internal environment can have an immediate effect on the practice, changes in the usually more subtle external environment must also be considered if a practice is to survive.

Internal Environment

The internal environment includes patients, the staff and doctor, and suppliers of goods and services to the practice. If the internal environment is stable and well organized, the practice will grow. If patients keep their appointments, arrive on time, and receive treatment with all doctors, staff, and supplies available, a positive **interaction** between the patients and practice has occurred. The patients will probably return for continuing care.

Interaction

The activity or behavior that takes place between people or things.

The absence of any one element (patient, appropriate dental supplies, doctor, and staff) can have a bad result for the practice, and the patients may seek dental care elsewhere.

Dental care decisions of patients are influenced by the way that the doctor and staff treat them. Everyone responds favorably to politeness, good grooming, and respect for another person.

Office policy and procedure manuals are used to provide consistency and stability for the internal environment. They describe how staff should handle various patient interactions, such as making appointments or greeting patients. They may also outline office policies about vacation, attendance, and continuing education. These manuals can be changed periodically by the dental practice to better meet the needs of the internal environment of the office.

External Environment

The external environment exists outside of the direct influence of the dental practice. The dentist and staff usually cannot determine what happens in it. Economic conditions, technology changes, and governmental, regulatory, and legal influences have an effect on the dental practice in much more subtle ways than those factors of the internal environment.

Economic Conditions

If the local economy is depressed because of factory layoffs or closings, people who are unemployed might postpone regular dental treatment. If these people also had an employer-paid dental insurance program, they may no longer be a part of the plan. Changing economic conditions can have a major effect on a dental practice.

One concern in the 1990s is the development of managed care contracts among employers, insurance companies, and dental offices. These contracts attempt to reduce the cost of dental care by negotiating a fixed, or contract, price for a variety of dental services. If a dental practice is located in a community with a large number of managed care contracts but does not participate in these contracts, many of their patients may change to a practice that participates in a managed care contract.

Technology

Innovations for the diagnosis and treatment of dental diseases are offered on the commercial market continually. Some of these new technologies can improve office efficiency. A growth in computer applications has occurred, ranging from digital x-ray equipment to computerized patient records and billing and accounting practice management software. New technology can be expensive. A dental practice has to constantly evaluate the available technology to determine which items should be purchased for the practice.

Government, Regulatory, and Legal

The government has much to say about the operation of a dental practice. In addition to the legal requirement that all dentists, dental hygienists, and in some states dental assistants be licensed to practice their professions, government influences the practice through laws and regulations at the federal, state, and local levels. Mandatory continuing education, periodic HIV and AIDS courses, the use of ionizing radiation (x-rays), disposal of solid waste and waste water from the dental office, and use of nitrous oxide scavengers are a few things regulated by the government in various states.

The state medical assistance program is a government-sponsored health care program that provides dental treatment for people with low incomes. Periodically, these programs are changed to expand or reduce coverage for certain age groups or certain dental procedures. If the practice does not stay informed about anticipated changes in the publicly financed programs, these changes can have bad influences on it.

Continual monitoring of the internal and external environments is necessary for the dental practice to survive. The dental assistant is important in both areas. Attention to detail within the office to ensure proper patient flow, inventory control, and regular employee attendance are part of the internal environment. The assistant should read dental articles on the latest technology and news articles on economic conditions and government changes and think about ways to improve the practice.

Dentistry as a Service Business

A dental office is typically a small business that provides a wide range of general or specialized dental services to patients. As a service business, the dental practice shares several traits in common with other service businesses. Examples of other service businesses include repair shops, hotels, banks, insurance companies, and accounting firms.

Special characteristics of service businesses include the following:

- No merchandise inventory: Dental offices provide patient services but do not sell products. Therefore only the supplies necessary to render services and manage the dental office are required. A lot of money is not tied up in merchandise inventory as in a hardware store.
- Limited market: Dentistry is difficult to deliver to patients. Generally, the patients must come to an office to receive the services of a dentist. Therefore dental offices usually have patients coming from a small geographic area in the office neighborhood.
- Specialized skill: A dentist provides a specialized skill that requires extended education and training, enabling the dentist to provide expert patient care. This skill is much more important than having a large amount of money to start the business.
- Labor costs predominate: Because no products are sold, the basic business cost of dental service is labor. In some cases, the fee dentists charge may seem to the patient to be high compared with the small amount of time spent rendering the care. However, the fee reflects the skill of the dentist and staff and cost of the supplies required to provide the service. Dental fees have increased in recent years because of the rising costs for providing more extensive infection control measures in the dental office.

ORGANIZATIONAL AND LEGAL FORMS OF DENTAL PRACTICE

From a business perspective, a dental practice can be one of several different organizational and legal types: sole proprietorship, partnership, and corporation. The dental assistant should understand the basic characteristics of each type, because tax reporting, dentist ownership, and employee benefit plans vary from one type to another.

Sole Proprietorship

Sole proprietorship is by far the most popular form of dental practice ownership. Approximately 80% of dentists practice alone. This is a business owned and managed by one individual dentist.

It is one of the easiest business organizations to start. After obtaining a dental license and any necessary local business licenses, a dentist may begin treating patients.

The sole proprietorship is generally the least expensive form of ownership to establish. The dentist does not need to file legal papers, reducing the amount of governmental reporting to tax agencies.

Because dentists are in total control of the practice, they can respond quickly to changes needed in the practice. They do not need to consult a partner or group practice management board to make decisions. The dentist may use a participatory leadership style, which includes other office personnel in the decision-making process.

Partnership

A partnership is an association of two or more dentists who engage in dental practice as coowners of the business. In a partnership, the coowners share the ownership of everything, including the debts of the business. They also share the profits, if any, according to the terms of a partnership agreement entered into before establishing a partnership dental practice.

A partnership is best established after a legal understanding has been reached. The agreement states clearly the exact status and responsibility of each member in the partnership. Too often dentists think they know what they have agreed to only to find later that this is not the case. A partnership agreement states in writing all the terms of the partnership, therefore preventing any misunderstandings.

Corporation

A corporate form of dental practice is the most complex of the three major forms of business ownership. The corporation is a business that is a separate legal entity. One dentist can establish a professional service corporation (PSC) in most states. The corporation owns the practice assets, hires the staff, and is taxed on its profits. A corporation may be sued and hold property. Individual dentists, employees, or a combination of both may own a corporation. A corporation may have extensive staff benefit plans, such as health, life and disability insurance, profit sharing, and retirement plans.

Multipractitioner Arrangements

Although 80% of dentists practice alone, the other 20% practice in a multipractitioner arrangement. These are organizational practices that offer flexibility to their participant dentists and include group practice, associateship, and space sharing.

Group Practice

A group practice is a dental practice in which more than two dentists work together in business. This group may be a corporation but it does not have to be. A group practice generally reduces the amount of control by an individual dentist who gives up a portion of decision-making authority and responsibility to other members of the group. The benefits of a group arrangement include professional consultation, referral of patients within the group, reduced overhead costs for individual dentists, and greater flexibility in time off from work. A group may be made up of two or more dentists, and some groups employ as many as 75 dentists. A group may consist of generalists or a mixture of generalists and specialists.

Associateship

Associateships are popular in dental offices. Generally, an established dentist hires an associate to work in the owner's practice. The associate may work on salary or commission or may function as an individual contractor within the practice. The associate does not own any of the dental practice. An associateship agreement, which is a legal contract, is recommended to clarify the duties and obligations of the owner dentist and associate.

Office Space Sharing

Another popular arrangement is called *office space sharing*. In this arrangement an owner dentist may lease space to another dentist during hours in which the owner is not present. Space sharing arrangements can vary from having two dentists occupy a large space to having only one dentist in an office at a time. Therefore the office can remain open 70 to 80 hours per week. Space sharing improves the efficiency with which office space and expensive dental equipment are used.

MANAGEMENT FUNCTIONS IN A DENTAL OFFICE

Because a dental office is a service business, it has several standard management functions in common with all businesses. These functions include the following:
- Managing information
- Communications (written and oral)
- Dental office records
- Dental payment plans
- Inventory control

A dental assistant must understand these basic management functions to work in or manage a dental office. These functions are described and discussed more fully in the chapters that follow.

Dental Assistant's Role in Practice Management

A dental assistant may be employed to assume much or all of the management of a dental office. This responsibility requires knowledge of general office duties, technical skills, strong communication abilities, and knowledge of basic management functions. Much is demanded of the dental assistant who performs business management functions in a dental office. The better the assistants understand basic business functions, the better able they will be to do the job.

DENTAL OFFICE COMMUNICATIONS

Communications is one of the most critical areas in the treatment of patients and managing the dental practice. All dental personnel must be able to communicate appropriately with the patient, dentist, other staff members, vendors, and other associated individuals. Each member of the dental team represents the dentist, practice, and profession of dentistry. Although the business assistants have a major responsibility to coordinate and manage formal office communications, everyone in the office must try to create a good impression that reflects favorably on the dentist and dental profession and provides a good working environment.

Communications Defined

Communication is a purposeful exchange of meanings between individuals, groups, and society. Whether personal or professional, communication is constant and important in our lives and is our way of expressing attitude, feelings, mood, and expectations.

Communication Process

A communication process refers to the procedures that are used to get a message across to a listener (Figure 4-4). Every communication process has a sender. This sender can be a person, sound, silence, movement, or any source that has the ability and capacity to communicate information. For example, if you were alone in a room and could look out outside, many types of senders could be communicating messages. The senders could be well-dressed people walking by and seemingly in a hurry. They could also be automobiles, trucks, bicycles, birds, or other small animals. A sender could also be the weather. One glance outside could communicate a lot of information, and this information would be continually changing. These illustrations provide us with messages and tell us what is happening, and we interpret that message according to our experience, knowledge, or psychologic readiness. *Psychologic readiness* is the state of mind one is in to receive, interpret, and act on a message or action.

The receiver can be anyone who is in the listening range. In this range, the receiver must listen to the entire message. A partial or misunderstood communication will fail to allow the receiver to respond appropriately or intelligently. If you have ever listened and heard only part of a message or walked in on the end of a discussion, you may have interpreted the message wrong. If you were expected to reply, you may not have had enough factual information to respond correctly.

FIGURE 4.4

The communication process. The sender or speaker communicates a message to the receiver or listener who then evaluates the information and responds or answers. The communication process may continue if further discussion is necessary.

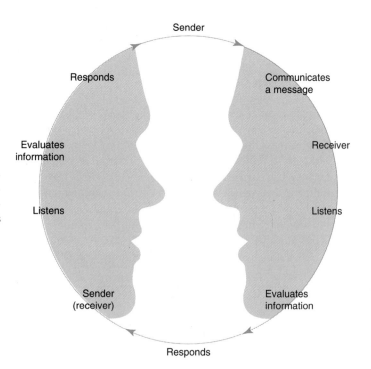

Listening is a critical component to good communication, requiring practice and concentration. To be an effective listener, people must be able to clear their thoughts and listen. Listening means to hear, evaluate, understand, and respond to the person communicating. Communication expands beyond verbal communications. People may be communicating in many ways. For instance, their body posture or facial expression may be nonverbally telling you something different than what is said.

Maintaining eye contact is important when people are speaking. People will visually receive communications about the intensity or sensitivity of the people speaking. For example, the speakers may look nervous or tense or have difficulty finding the right words. They may use certain words that are inappropriate for the situation they are discussing and they may not be speaking clearly. They may garble their words or run them together without pausing for emphasis to highlight certain words important to the conversation.

Once received, the message must be evaluated for content. Properly evaluating the information that is received involves understanding what has been said, how it was said, and the circumstances (where, when, why) under which the words or actions were spoken. Ask yourself the following questions:
- Does the message require a response?
- Does the message require a judgmental opinion?
- Should the response be verbal or nonverbal?
- Does the message require an immediate answer to resolve a concern, or can an answer be given after more facts have been gathered?

The evaluation of the message is critical because an appropriate response is necessary. The listener can put the speaker at ease, cause concern, or even require more information. In addition, and even worse, the response given may cause the sender of the message to lose trust or confidence in the receiver or respondent. Properly evaluating a message will help to place the proper importance on the information and the communication process.

After the evaluation phase is completed, the receiver will then communicate back to the sender who is the original communicator. Sometimes the dental assistant will ask a question or series of questions to be certain the message has been properly received. If receivers believe they understand the message but question the purpose or reason for the message, they can ask for clarification by replying, "Why do you ask?" or "What do you mean by that?" Simple questions can resolve a potential misunderstanding between the sender and receiver. If the listener has properly listened to and evaluated the message, the response will potentially have meaning and credibility.

The communication process may not be concluded after the initial response because the response may cause a need for further discussion. The entire process may take seconds or longer. However, if the process is completed successfully, a purposeful exchange of meanings will occur.

Basic Forms of Communications

Three basic forms of communications include the following:
1. The language of words
2. The language of behavior
3. The language of systems

Language of Words

Words can be spoken or communicated nonverbally. The choice of words, how they are spoken, and the environment in which they are spoken are vital to successful communication. The dental assistant may be the initial contact with patients. Greeting patients in a friendly, positive manner will cause patients to respond in a similar way. Speak clearly, keep eye contact, and listen to responses from the patient or other staff members. This will help in understanding how communication is being received.

What is being said may be difficult to understand. For instance, if patients are concerned about the cost of the dental treatment, they may not communicate this directly. They may have difficulty in relating to a discussion or condition because they are still questioning the cost or wondering how they will be able to pay for the prescribed treatment. They may be in a hurry, without mentioning it, and be pressured about the time the dental treatment is taking. They may actually be trying to speed the process by saying, "Yes that feels fine," when it does not, or "Are you finished now?" when the procedure appears to be slowing.

Understanding the communication process (what is really happening here and now) especially in a busy dental practice requires good listening skills and attention to what is really taking place. The dental assistant should check with the patient immediately if any questions about what is being said or not said are asked. Follow up can help build patient relationships and increase the dental assistant's value as a professional member of the dental team.

Language of Behavior

The way people behave or express themselves is learned to satisfy needs, and behavior is motivated by these needs. Abraham Maslow's **hierarchy** of needs (Figure 4-5) establishes five levels of need satisfaction that range from basic life maintenance to self-actualization and include the following:

Hierarchy

A system of arranging people or things in order of rank or importance; for example, from basic concepts to complex situations.

- Basic survival: The first basic need is learning how to survive in the environment through the satisfaction of human physical needs, such as food, water, shelter, and reproduction.
- Safety: Once the basic need of survival is accomplished, protection and comfort become important. A safe envi-

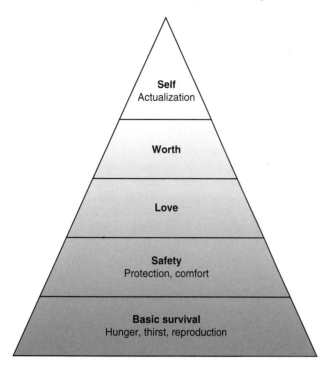

FIGURE 4.5

Maslow's hierarchy of needs.

ronment is necessary to help us feel secure about ourselves and our surroundings. How we are treated and how we treat others affect our safe and comfort levels and involve our interpersonal relationships.

- Love or social affection: People have a need to be loved, cared for, or included in a group. Love involves reaching out to others and having the ability to be a loving and caring person by listening and having empathy for the feelings of others.
- Worth: Esteem and recognition are human needs. Feeling worth is developed through our interrelationships with others, such as our families, friends, coworkers, and so on. Doing a task well is accomplished by developing good skills, knowledge, and a positive attitude.
- Self-actualization: Self-actualization is the highest level of human need. Achieving a level of maturity and responsibility for making decisions in our personal and professional lives is part of being a whole, responsible person.

Language of Systems

A *system* is a group of elements that make up a whole unit and can be interrelated or have independent elements that function as a unit. For instance, the body is a unit or system that is made up of many subsystems. Systems have a definite vocabulary associated with them, for example, dentistry has a special vocabulary and conditions that are not necessarily understood if used by other systems.

A language of systems represents the many parts or variations that make up what is called *communication*. Most communication is developed to understand a variety of systems, such as our educational, legal, and health care systems. The dental practice is a system that varies in practice and specialty because of the nature of each individual practice. However, the language of dentistry remains the same.

Meeting someone for the first time causes all of our communication styles or communicative languages to contribute to how we interact with others. Some people may prejudge others or a situation and instantly like or dislike them. Judgments are based on our background and perceptions. We may stereotype characteristics of people and therefore people themselves, which is called *first impressions* or *stereotyping*. Stereotypes may limit our relationships if we do not understand our interpersonal processes.

Each person has needs that must be satisfied. In a dental practice, establish a patient-provider relationship with every patient and a colleague relationship with office personnel, which reflects the professionalism of the dental practice. These relationships may be for a short time or extend over many years, and even this variable determines how people interact.

DEVELOPING EFFECTIVE RELATIONSHIPS

Developing good communication skills and effective relationships also involves understanding what motivates our behavior and the conditions that influence our behavior. These conditions are called *interactional dimensions* and include the following:

Dimension
The extent or size of an object or situation that is measurable.

1 Physical dimensions
2 Behavioral dimensions
3 Interactional dimensions
4 Other dimensions

All of these dimensions shape our values and affect our behavioral actions, decisions, communication, and often control how we behave in our relationships with others.

Physical Dimensions

People often develop a communication style with children or young people that may be different from conversations with older people. However, one can not assume older people have a greater comprehension of what is communicated than younger people or that younger people can not understand the words or vocabulary used when discussing a topic on the adult level. Some people are more comfortable speaking with a man rather than a woman or vise versa. Patients may be more comfortable speaking to the dental assistant rather than the dentist because they may think they are interrupting a busy schedule or their question may be too trivial. Our interactions with people depend on perceptions that we have developed and learned throughout our lives. A goal in communications is to try to understand personal perceptions, feelings, and reactions, and if the behavior is inappropriate, to be able to recognize and change those actions to improve communication skills and successfully accomplish the task.

Behavioral Dimensions

Quiet people can offer a special challenge to our listening skills. If they do not ask questions or make listening signs, such as nodding the head or uttering a sound, we cannot assume they understand or agree with what is being stated. Talkative people may verbalize a great deal, which can convey they understand when they really do not. If a person is perceived as honest or confidential, the communication may be different than if the person is perceived to be dishonest. Friendly people may make us feel good just to be in their presence, and we may choose to model or emulate their behavior. Aloof people may not appear to be serious about everything that is happening around them. However, their behavior may be influenced by a lack of confidence in themselves or in the situation.

Interactional Dimensions

The ability for individuals and diverse groups to communicate depends on each unique situation. For example, friends are those people we feel most comfortable with. We can share our feelings and know we will receive support in return. Our relationship with peers, supervisors, and subordinates may be different.

Environmental Dimensions

The environment we are communicating in may affect how we react. For instance, communication in the work environment would most likely be different than in a social environment. The schedule of a busy dental practice may influence the amount of time that can be spent educating or explaining a procedure to a patient.

Other Dimensions

Examples of the other dimensions that affect communications are attitudes, psychologic perspective, and conceptual thinking. The attitude of a person, whether the sender or receiver is the dentist, dental assistant, or patient, greatly affects how people behave during communications. People with good attitudes, even in difficult and stressful situations, will be received in a more positive manner. Dental personnel who respond in a friendly but direct manner with an angry patient can often turn that person into an understanding, although not always agreeable, patient. The psychologic perspective of how a person is feeling or the degree of understanding they have will often determine if the conversation is positive and free-flowing.

Dealing with an Angry Person

Many types of anger exist. Small babies can express anger when they have a need that is not being satisfied or they are not receiving appropriate attention. Adults often express anger for the same reason. However, the basic reason for anger is often a lack of clear communication.

A dental assistant may have to deal with an angry patient. People who are angry are not always willing to listen to anyone they feel does not understand their needs. Respond to angry people by controlling your own emotions. Anger sometimes seeks support and often times anger is expressed to provoke a rebuke so the speaker can justify their anger.

When dealing with an angry patient, lower the volume in your voice and try to articulate every word you speak. Angry people have difficulty challenging someone who will not support their anger. Do not tell people to calm down and lower their voice; this only gives them a reason to continue; listen to determine what may be the cause of the anger. Angry people often need to express what they are feeling, and someone willing to listen is all they need to calm down. Silence and patience are also often required to be a good listener.

Listening is a valuable resource for handling anger. Once what is causing the anger is known, one can act appropriately. Attempt to neutralize the situation by asking a question, "You seem to be upset. Would you like to talk about it?" Lowering the voice, using direct eye contact, and exhibiting a pleasant expression can encourage conversation and may help to neutralize hostility and anger. Do not attempt to debate an issue. Be positive in offering to help someone. If they appear to have multiple questions or problems, answer them one at a time. Be understanding and say, "Now you have expressed this situation, is that correct?" Once agreement is reached, get confirmation on the solution and move on to the next question. You may not be successful in every situation. However, keeping a calm, positive response to your patient or coworker can create a willingness to cooperate.

Listening Skills

Listening is an art; it is a learned skill. It takes practice and patience to hear what people are saying, but more importantly, what they mean. Listening requires concentration and time to form a response, especially if a question is asked. It requires conscious attention to what is being said. One cannot talk and listen at the same time because the mind can only think about one of these details at a time. The listener

Table 4.2

Evaluating Your Listening Ability

How good of a listener are you?	Yes	Sometimes	No
Would you rather talk than listen?	3	2	1
Do you enjoying listening only to people you like?	3	2	1
Are you easily bored when other people talk?	3	2	1
Do you paraphrase what others are saying?	3	2	1
Do you maintain eye contact with someone who is speaking?	3	2	1
Do you give the speaker your undivided attention or do you find something else to do?	3	2	1
Do you often ask people to give examples of what they mean?	3	2	1
Do you often try to get others to see your point of view?	3	2	1
Do you let people finish what they are saying or do you finish sentences for them?	3	2	1
Do you continue to listen even though you know what people are going to say?	3	2	1
Do you smile, nod, or use nonverbal signs to let people know you are listening?	3	2	1
If people mispronounce words, do you correct them?	3	2	1
Can you listen objectively without forming an opinion until you are certain you know what the person speaking really means?	3	2	1
Do you keep your emotions under control when listening to an angry person?	3	2	1
Do you patronize someone who you do not like?	3	2	1
Do you pause and use silence to help someone find the right words to speak?	3	2	1
Do you ask questions of the speaker often?	3	2	1
Do you assume when people do not ask questions they understand everything you have said?	3	2	1
If people omit information do you ask them for it?	3	2	1
If someone looks to you for support of their anger do you listen for the cause of their anger?	3	2	1
Your score			

If you scored 58, you are an excellent listener.
If you scored 32, you are an average listener.
If you scored 10 or below, you are not listening.

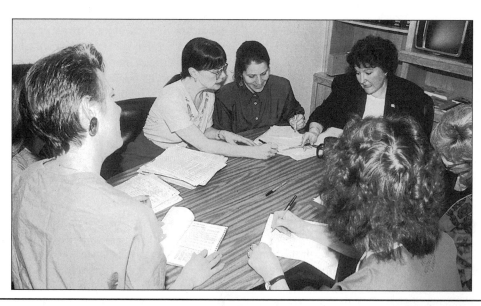

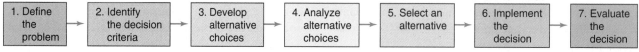

FIGURE 4.6

Decision-making process.

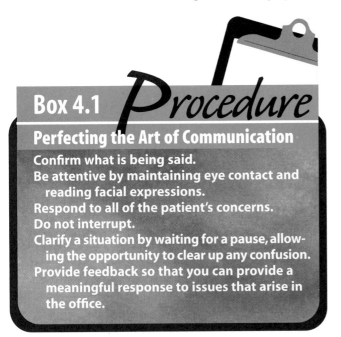

Box 4.1 *Procedure*

Perfecting the Art of Communication

Confirm what is being said.
Be attentive by maintaining eye contact and reading facial expressions.
Respond to all of the patient's concerns.
Do not interrupt.
Clarify a situation by waiting for a pause, allowing the opportunity to clear up any confusion.
Provide feedback so that you can provide a meaningful response to issues that arise in the office.

must concentrate visual and mental attention to the speaker. They must keep their mind receptive to what is being said and try to grasp the speaker's meaning and feeling while avoiding any negative opinion of the other person. Box 4-1 and Table 4-2 review the important steps in the listening process and evaluate your ability.

Making Decisions

One requirement of all dental assistants is the ability to make decisions. Decisions to be made may be minor, such as where to go for lunch, or they may be major, such as deciding what type of car to buy. Regardless of the type of decision, the process of decision-making must be structured and orderly. After the decision-making process is learned, it may be used in a variety of situations regardless of the issue being decided. The process consists of seven steps (Figure 4-6).

Decision-Making Process

Define the Problem The decision-making process begins with the existence of a problem. Suppose that the dental office needs to decide whether to buy a new intraoral camera. Because this is not a routine decision, follow the decision-making process to arrive at the best decision.

First, one must decide that the camera is necessary and can add some benefit to the office. If this point is not considered, a problem may not exist. The first step, therefore, is to carefully define the problem.

Develop Alternative Choices Once the problem has been identified, the criteria for making a decision needs to be known. The dentist and office staff might include criteria such as price, model, portability, manufacturer, warranty, or product reviews. Whether stated or not, every decision-maker has criteria that guides the decision.

Develop Alternative Choices This step requires the decision-maker to list the possible product alternatives that could be bought to solve the problem. Perhaps three different kinds of intraoral cameras would meet the criteria defined when identifying the decision criteria.

Analyze Alternative Choices After listing the alternatives, the products must be analyzed in terms of strengths and weaknesses. These ratings could be done by numerically grading (1,2,3, and so on) or by making judgments of good, better, and best.

Select an Alternative A choice of the best alternative is now made. When products are alike, knowing which is the best is difficult. Careful analysis and enough time to consider the alternatives are helpful to the process.

Implement (Act On) the Decision Buy one of the cameras.

Evaluate the Decision Some anxiety always exists after a purchase decision. Evaluate the decision by determining if the product, the intraoral camera, meets the expectations as described.

The decision-making process outlined previously is an effective management tool for identifying problems and seeking the appropriate solutions. A dental assistant who masters this technique will be an outstanding member of the dental care team.

Group Process and the Dental Team

A dental practice consists of people representing a variety of skills and talents who join together to perform as a team. Through daily interactions and face-to-face communications with each other, people identify common interests and form groups based on these interests.

The dental practice team forms standards of behavior or rules of conduct after time, which are shared by members of the team. Although these rules are often unwritten, all members of the team recognize them.

The degree of cohesiveness in a dental team determines how much influence team members have over one another and how much people want to remain together as a group. Highly cohesive dental office teams remain together for many years, accept individual differences, and achieve a great deal for the practice and patients.

Conflict exists within every group of people and can arise over team member roles, authority, and limited resources. When managed appropriately, conflict can be productive to the dental practice. These conflicts can involve questions about the facts of a situation, the best method to resolve an issue, and the goals and objectives of the practice. When conflict arises, discussion and resolution needs to occur. Ignoring conflict causes stagnation, which decreases office morale and productivity.

The dental assistant is a member of the management team and functions as a group member. Being aware of group rules of conduct, cohesiveness, and conflict are vital aspects to maintain and improve roles on the management team.

RECEPTION TECHNIQUES

Try to remember your first impression when you entered the dental office. Start at the beginning and think where the office was geographically located in your community. Was the office on a busy street with heavy traffic and easy to locate? Was parking simple to find or was it a challenge to find the correct building and park? Whatever your encounters, some patients may have similar occurrences. Discussing your feelings may help the patient relax, realizing someone else had a similar experience. Continue to recall your thoughts as you opened the door to the office. What did you see, hear, and smell? What object or feeling caught your attention? In most instances the same office situation is still there. On a planned basis, ask patients what their impression of the office may be.

Personal Appearance

Dental personnel represent the practice. Appropriate dress should always be neat, clean, and reflect a professional health care office. People in the dental practice must exercise care in their personal appearance.

Promptness

Be prepared to receive patients and answer the telephone before the office is scheduled to open. When staff members are late and patients cannot enter the office or contact anyone about office hours, lack of commitment is indicated to the patient and gives the message that timeliness does not matter. Being conscientious and dependable is not only a common courtesy to the patients but also indicates the dependability and professionalism of the office. Office policies should assure patients that someone is always prepared to treat them when the office is closed and when the dentist is out of town.

Electronic mail is useful for providing and receiving messages when the office is closed. The variety of electronic devices today helps the health care provider communicate with patients for emergencies on short notice. Messages can be recorded through electronic mail in the office or by pager and accessed by the dentist or assigned personnel from home.

The dentist develops office policy for handling emergencies when the office is closed. All messages should be retrieved by the business assistant on arrival at the office and recorded with the callers telephone number on a telephone log, returning calls as soon as possible. The date, time, and response should also be noted on the log for future reference if needed.

Greeting the Patient

First impressions are important. Be warm and friendly and know and use the patient's names. Greet the patient promptly and pleasantly. Two basic cornerstones for any relationship to succeed are trust and respect. One of the greatest acts a human being can do for another is to respect their feelings, concerns, and sensitivities. Withholding your human presence from another person is to totally reject that person. Understanding or being empathetic to another's feelings results in a respect that flows between people.

Dental personnel represent the office in which they work and the profession of dentistry. Whether in the office or attending a meeting or social function, kindness offered that is sincere is appreciated. Practice being kind and polite to patients and staff. A "thank you" to the patient and among the dental team for small events creates a good working environment for everyone in the office.

Address new and regular patients by their name, always giving them your complete attention. Keep eye contact to make their appointment time as important to them as it is to the practice. If patients are new to the office, introduce them to the dentist and other office personnel. No matter how many times patients have been in the office, a good first impression creates a successful practice.

Golden 10 Minutes

The time right after you first say "hello" to the patient is called the *golden 10 minutes*. This is the time when you can build patients' confidence in the dental practice and share their expectations of dentistry. If you use this opportunity wisely, you will create the best possible environment in which to begin a long and positive relationship with patients.

The golden 10 minutes is your opportunity to capitalize on this initial appointment. You will not get a better opportunity to tell them specifically what they can expect as patients in your practice. You will get the first chance to influence new patients before they develop any preconceived notions or negative attitudes regarding dentistry or your practice. Make the most of the time.

The key to the golden 10 minutes presentation is highlighting a few, specific, key expectations; not giving a laundry list of what to do and not to do. Your objective is to impress patients with the importance of correcting any immediate problem. Defining what that problem is and expressing your desire to resolve it is meaningful to patients. Concentrate on being certain that you and your patients understand what is being said. All your efforts should be spent on making patients feel as though the treatment the dentist is about to give is the best solution for taking care of their immediate problem and any future problem they may have. Your welcome can begin as follows:

1 Open with a positive statement: "We want to thank you (name of patient) for selecting our office for your dental needs. We will do everything we can to assure that your problems will be professionally taken care of. I know we will enjoy working with you. We will explain what is taking place as you are being treated. Do you have any questions before we begin?"

2 Get a commitment on cooperation: "We know you are interested in taking care of your teeth, and sometimes we put off things that we think are going to take care of themselves, that is understandable, but we know you want what is best for you. Isn't that right . . . . ? Good, I thought so. We will set another appointment for you as quickly as possible."

"(Name of patient), our practice is best suited to help you and your family with any dental problems that may occur. I know you want the best dental care available for you and your family....right? Certainly, we all do. Feel free to call anytime you or anyone in your family has a problem or questions about your teeth. I look forward to working with you at any time."

3 Make it good: This cannot be done hit or miss. You should use this information as a model and prepare a presentation in language natural to you. Be sure not to expand this into a long, complex speech. When you have written it, practice. Rehearse and drill yourself until you can say it smoothly and sincerely so that you will establish the mood of understanding and trust you need for this to be effective.

You have to be believable to the new patient on these three objectives. The more you practice, the better you will become. The better you are in the golden 10 minutes, the better your dental practice will be.

TELEPHONE TECHNIQUES

The methods used to receive the patient by telephone are as important as receiving the patient in person. Interacting with the patient over the telephone is more difficult because we lose some of the nonverbal relationships such as the handshake, a smile, or the nod. Therefore the business assistant must be able to project some of these nonverbal skills in other ways (Box 4-2).

When you smile naturally, the tone of your voice reflects a more enjoyable tone and even your behavior becomes more relaxed and contented, therefore, smile as you speak on the telephone. Speak natural but at a moderate speed that is low in pitch. Pronounce each word distinctly. Be expressive, pleasant, and alert.

Answering the Telephone

Answer the telephone promptly and speak directly into the mouthpiece. Identify the practice immediately, "Good morning, Dr. Coyne's office. May I help you?" Or you can say, "Good afternoon, Dr. Coyne's office, Jamie speaking." If the patient must be put on hold, excuse yourself and return by thanking the patient for waiting. Use the patient's name frequently. Sometimes the caller will ask to speak with the dentist. Try to avoid interrupting the dentist. Explain that the dentist is with a patient and ask if you can help. If the

Box 4.2

Telephone Techniques

1. Smile as you speak over the telephone.
2. Speak naturally but at a moderate speed.
3. Speak in a low pitch.
4. Pronounce each word distinctly.
5. Be expressive, pleasant, and alert.
6. Answer the telephone promptly.
7. Speak directly into the mouthpiece.
8. Identify the practice immediately.
9. Greet the caller and ask how you may help.
10. Do not put the patient on hold unless absolutely necessary and thank the patient for waiting.
11. Use the patient's name frequently.
12. Avoid interrupting the dentist.
13. Take accurate written messages.
14. Plan for emergency telephone calls or special situational calls.
15. Do not discuss fees over the telephone.
16. Limit personal calls.

caller insists on talking with the dentist, explain that the dentist is treating a patient but will call back as soon as possible. Ask for a name and telephone number if you do not already have them. Complete the conversation politely and keep an accurate written message, making sure to let the dentist know about the call.

Often a patient in pain feels the need to talk with the dentist. Question the patient thoroughly about the location of the sensitive area and ask about the duration of the discomfort. Ask if there is swelling or bleeding. If patient has a record at the office, retrieve the chart, and try to set up an appointment. If it is not possible to set up the appointment without talking with the dentist, write the patient's name on a piece of paper and show it to the dentist out of sight of the patient being treated. Some operatories have a call light or electronic signal on the operatory-based computer to signal the doctor when these emergencies occur. These situations should be discussed with the dentist in advance so that you will know exactly how to handle special problems, emergencies, and calls. Remember to not discuss fees over the telephone.

The dentist will want to talk with certain people, such as their spouse, children, other dentists, and physicians, when they call. Let the dentist know when you receive these calls as inconspicuous as possible. The patient should never feel they are any less important than the incoming caller. Interruptions are timely and cause mental fatigue so the dentist should be interrupted as little as possible. Personal calls for the dentist should be written down on a telephone message form for later return whenever possible. Be sure to understand how the dentist wants to handle these special calls.

Return address

Jamie J. Coyne, D.M.D.
454 Bishop Lane
Louisville, KY 40000
(502) 456-0000

Date

November 20, 1996

Letter address

Carol A. Eaton
202 Meade Rd.
Louisville, KY 40200

Salutation

Dear Ms. Eaton:

I would like to take this opportunity to thank you for your cooperation in recently completing your dental treatment.

Body of letter

Restoring the patient to a higher level of dental health is our goal. After initial diagnosis and necessary appointments have been made, it is a source of satisfaction and accomplishment for both the patient and the doctor.

Your cooperation and personal responsibility for this is greatly appreciated. With conscientious home care and periodic dental examinations, we will look forward to maintaining your dentistry for many years to come.

Complimentary close

Kindest regards,

Signature

Jamie J. Coyne, D.M.D.

FIGURE 4.7

Sample block letter style.

Placing Telephone Calls

A number of routine calls are made daily and weekly to insurance providers, vendors, pharmacies, and laboratories. Keep a list of the names and telephone numbers regularly called near the telephone with emergency numbers for convenience and easy access. Make sure your thoughts are organized and you know what you are going to say. Make a note for yourself if needed to clarify what you plan to discuss. This may only be necessary when you are responsible for giving and receiving telephone calls. Have the correct number, the name of the person in which you need to talk, and any paper, file, or material necessary in which to refer. Always keep extra paper and pencils ready for taking notes or transcribing. Identify yourself promptly and courteously. Personal calls should not made frequently.

WRITTEN COMMUNICATIONS

Letters also project an image of the dental office. Therefore letters should be neat, simple, to the point, and formatted on the paper in an attractive manner. Grammar, spelling, and punctuation must be correct. Do not rush or wait until the last minute to write letters. A rough draft of the letter should be written clearly, listing key points in logical succession. Select words carefully, making sure they are spelled correctly. If you are using a computer be sure to run a spell-check. A variety of preprinted or electronic form letters are available, such as welcome, referral, appreciation, confirmation, collection, congratulation letters, and recall notes that can be customized to meet the needs of the dental practice.

Business Letter Format

Business letters should look well-placed on the paper. The left and right margins and the top and bottom margins should be set so the letter is centered evenly on the paper. Letters are usually prepared in block style (Figure 4-7) or modified block with indented paragraphs. The block style letter is typed with the return address, date, letter address, salutation, body of the letter, complimentary close, and signature all flush with the left margin. The modified block letter is flush with the left margin except the following needs to be done:

1 The date is placed on the left margin.
2 Each new paragraph in the body of the letter is indented five spaces.
3 The complimentary closing begins in the center of the page.
4 The signature is centered with the complimentary closing.

The style will need to be decided before beginning the letter. Whatever style is selected, all future business letters should follow the same format for consistency and uniformity. Business assistants will usually type their initials in small letters flush with the left margin.

Return Address and Date

Dental business letters will usually be typed on letterhead stationary or notepaper that includes the name of the dentist, address, telephone number, and sometimes the Fax number for the dental office. If the stationary has a letterhead, the date should be typed two spaces below the letterhead. If no letterhead appears on the letter, a return address 12 to 13 lines from the top of the paper with the date on line 14 immediately following the address should be typed in. The return address and date the letter is written is flush with the left margin if the letter is block style or in the center or flush with the right margin if the letter is modified block style.

Letter Address

No less than three or four blank lines or more than eight or nine lines between the date and the letter address should be present. The letter address should always include at least three lines even if the city and state are on separate lines. The zip code should follow a comma after the state name.

Salutation

The salutation is the greeting. It should be flush with the left margin and a double space added before and after the salutation. When addressing a patient use Mr., Mrs., Miss, or Ms. with the last name.

Body of the Letter

The placement of the letter on the sheet will be determined by the number of words in the letter. A short letter will usually have between 50 to 100 words, an average letter 101 to 200 words, a long letter 201 to 300 words, and a two-page letter will be needed if over 300 words appear. Margins will be set according to these classifications. As stated, letters should be neat, simple, and to the point. Rambling just confuses the reader and often loses the meaning.

Complimentary Close

The first word of the complimentary closing should be capitalized and placed two spaces below the final line of the letter. Complimentary conclusions can include: "Very truly yours," "Sincerely yours," or "Sincerely."

Signature

The writers name should be typed at least four lines below the closing to leave room for a signature. Use a pen with blue ink for signatures to reflect that the letter is not a form letter. Hand-signed signatures are often considered more personal and meaningful.

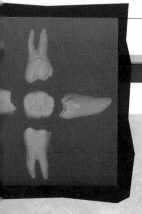

Points for Review

■ Importance of planning, organizing, leading, and evaluating

■ Successful leadership styles

■ How policies and procedures standardize practice and describe various situations

■ Differences and advantages of sole proprietorship, partnership, corporation, group practice, and associateship

■ The dental assistant's role in practice management, dental office communications, the communication process, basic forms of communications, and written communication

■ Developing effective communication, relationships, interpersonal, and listening skills

■ Dealing with an angry person

■ Reception and telephone techniques

Self-Study Questions

1. What is the role of the dental office manager?
   a. Requires no knowledge of any dental procedures completed in the dental office.
   b. Requires complete knowledge of every dental procedure that a dentist performs.
   c. Requires the manager to control every business function performed in a dental office.
   d. Requires a thorough knowledge of management principles and office policies and procedures.

2. In what order should the four elements of the management process occur?
   a. Leading, organizing, planning, and evaluating
   b. Organizing, leading, evaluating, and planning
   c. Planning, organizing, leading, and evaluating
   d. Evaluating, leading, planning, and organizing

3. Which of the following is a complete list of components that contribute to the development of office policies?
   a. Practice mission or philosophy of practice and goals
   b. Practice mission or philosophy of practice, goals, and objectives

   c. Practice mission or philosophy of practice, goals, objectives, and policies
   d. Practice mission or philosophy of practice, goals, objectives, policies, and procedures

4. What are the general statements about the dentist's personal and professional values, attitudes, and beliefs toward patient care, staff, business practices, and community involvement called?
   a. Objectives
   b. Goals
   c. Mission statement or practice of philosophy
   d. Goals and objectives

5. Which of the following has a direct influence on the external environment?
   a. Economic conditions
   b. Technology
   c. Government, regulatory, and legal
   d. Economic conditions, technology and government, regulatory, and legal

6. Approximately how many dentists are general practitioners in the United States today?
   a. 80%
   b. 70%
   c. 60%
   d. 50%

7. Which type of business represents a separate legal entity?
   a. Sole proprietorship
   b. Partnership
   c. Corporation
   d. Associateship

8. What is the multipractitioner arrangement in which more than two dentists work together for business reasons?
   a. Group practice
   b. Associateship
   c. Space sharing
   d. Specialty practice

9. What is the first step in the process of decision making?
   a. Making a decision
   b. Analyzing alternative choices
   c. Evaluating the decision
   d. Defining the problem

10. A dental practice is a service business. Which of the following is *not* a characteristic of a service business?
    a. Labor costs predominate
    b. Carries large inventories

c. Limited market

d. Specialized skill

11. Abraham Maslow developed a better understanding of human needs through which of the following conditions?

    a. Language of words

    b. Language of systems

    c. Language of behavior

    d. Forms of communications

12. Which of the following represents a human's highest level of human need?

    a. Self-esteem

    b. Self-actualization

    c. Love and social affection

    d. Survival

13. Relationship spectrum refers to which of the following?

    a. How we create an atmosphere to gain new relationships

    b. How we are influenced by those close and distant to our lives

    d. Our hierarchy of needs

    d. How we gather information

14. Interactional dimensions refer to which of the following conditions?

    a. Physical, behavior, interactional, and environmental relationships

    b. The language of words, behavior, and systems

    c. Motivation

    d. Sending, receiving, listening, and evaluating

15. The way in which we relate to family, friends, and people with whom we associate refers to which of the following?

    a. Motivation

    b. Communicative language

    c. Forms of communication

    d. Interactional dimensions

16. The cornerstone of any relationship is which of the following?

    a. Influencing and helping others

    b. Trust and respect

    c. Expectations

    d. Love and social affection

17. People who constantly complain are often seeking which of the following?

    a. Problem resolution

    b. Attention

    c. Role clarification

    d. Someone to listen

18. What should you do when dealing with angry people?

    a. Make them listen to your point of view

    b. Agree with them

    c. Listen and attempt to neutralize the situation

    d. Try to express a sense of humor

19. As a good listener, you should do which of the following?

    a. Help the sender finish their statement if you are aware of what they are going to say

    b. Smile, nod, and use nonverbal signs to let people know you are listening

    c. Correct words that are not pronounced appropriately

    d. Relax eye contact and look away occasionally

Suggested Readings

Ailes R: *You are the message*, New York, 1989, Dell Publishing Co.

Coleman B: *The small business survival guide: a handbook*, New York, 1984, WW Norton.

Decker B: *You've got to be believed to be heard*, New York, 1992, St. Martin's Press.

Finkbeiner BL, Finkbeiner C: *Practice management for the dental team*, ed 5, St Louis, Mosby (in press).

Frank MO: *How to get your point across in 30 seconds or less*, New York, 1986, Simon & Schuster.

Goldhaber GM: *Organizational communication*, St Louis, 1990, WC Brown.

Hersey P, Blanchard KH: *Management of organizational behavior*, Englewood Cliffs, NJ, 1993, Prentice Hall.

Johnson DW: *Reaching out: interpersonal effectiveness and self-actualization*, Englewood Cliffs, NJ, 1981, Prentice Hall.

Robbins SP: *Management*, ed 2, Englewood Cliffs, NJ, 1988, Prentice Hall.

Scarborough NM, Zimmerer TW: *Effective small business management*, ed 2, Columbus, Ohio, 1988, Merrill.

Williams JN, Willis DO et al: *Practice growth through partnerships, group practices and shared office arrangements: dental practice library*, Chicago, 1992, ADA.

Williams LF, Hopps JG: *On the nature of professional communication: publication for practitioners*, Washington, DC, 1988, National Association of Social Workers.

Weisbord MR: *Productive workplaces*, San Francisco, 1987, Jossey-Bass.

Chapter 5

Managing Dental Office Information

Key Points

- Management of dental information
- Use of the computer for record management
- Role of the dental business assistant
- Record management

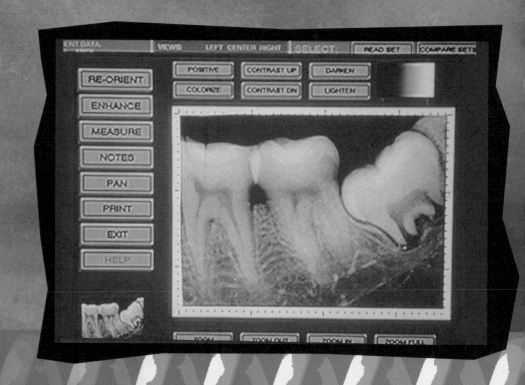

Chapter Outline

Computer Information Systems
- Computer use in dental practice
- Computer literacy, not computer programming
- Components of a personal computer system
- How personal computer systems work
- Dental office computer systems
- Future applications

Dental Office Records

Role of the Dental Business Assistant in Recordkeeping

Appointment Determination and Scheduling Format
- Units of scheduling time
- Schedule lay out

Appointment Entry
- Regular appointment scheduling
- Special scheduling arrangements
- Scheduling changes
- Scheduling and confirming appointments
- Call list
- Periodic recall appointments

Maintaining Patient Records
- Types of filing systems
- Retrieving patient records

Accounts Receivable Records
- Electronic financial recordkeeping
- One-write pegboard manual system
- Adjustments
- Banking procedures
- Record control
- Checking account deposits

Disbursements
- Writing checks
- Check register
- Balancing the bank statement
- Miscellaneous cash fund

Collections
- Collection letters
- Telephone follow up
- Collection agency

Learning Objectives

On completion of Chapter 5, the student should be able to do the following:

- Define key terms.
- List the three software applications used most for the dental practice.
- List the elements of a personal computer system.
- Describe how a computer system can improve dental practice performance.
- Identify how appointments are determined and entered and how schedules are formatted.
- List the types of accounts receivable records used in the dental office.
- Enter data into the accounts receivable records.
- Make disbursements by writing checks, entering data into the check register, and balancing the bank statement.
- Identify methods for collecting accounts.

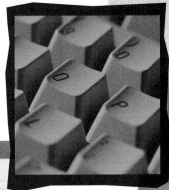

Key Terms

Adjustments	Gigabyte	Receipt
CD-ROM	Hardware	Reconcile
Disbursements	Internet	Software
Disk Operating System (DOS)	Recall	Statement

COMPUTER INFORMATION SYSTEMS

The ability to efficiently manage information is critical to the success of a business. A dental practice must manage a wide variety of information in the course of rendering patient care. Chapter 4 highlighted management principles and the elements of managing information. Dental patient records, inventory systems, and accounting and billing are examples of dental practice information. In short, the practice of dentistry relies on information, and efficient management of information will be even more critical for a dental practice.

Computer Use in Dental Practice

Before 1980, only a few dental practices were using or had access to a computer. The machines that were used were large and inefficient by today's standards. The computers were primarily used for accounting and billing functions for the office. Service bureaus and account processing companies used mini or mainframe computer systems to provide billing services for a dental office. A dental practice rarely owned its own computer. Computer services were purchased from one of these companies.

In the 1980s, growth of the *microcomputer* or *PC* (personal computer) occurred. The PC was much smaller than a mini or mainframe computer but performed many of the same information management functions of the larger machines. IBM introduced the first personal computer in 1981, which provided small businesses and individuals access to computing power that had previously only been available to large corporations. Individuals could now electronically type letters and documents (word processing), manage data (database management), and communicate with other computers over telephone lines (telecommunications). The first PC had little storage, a small working memory, used floppy disk drives, and lacked good video screen resolution. Unlike today's computers, microcomputers were slow and expensive.

In contrast, the 1990s is the decade of networking and telecommunications. The PCs are extremely fast, have high capacity storage, provide high-resolution video images in color, and can do a multitude of functions. Many of these computers are used on a local area network (LAN), providing access to information for all individuals in an office regardless of location. PCs on LAN networks are able to deliver computerized information not only to the front office but also to each dental operatory.

Hardware

Computer equipment such as the monitor, keyboard, printer, or light pen.

The American Dental Association estimated that in 1984, only 11% of dentists had a computer in their primary practice but by 1997, 79.5% of dental offices had a computer. These computers were used by dental practices for patient written information, scheduling, office newsletters, accounting, diagnosing and monitoring of treatment, maintaining patient treatment records, insurance form processing, and record-keeping management. Approximately half of these offices has the necessary **hardware** and **software** to communicate with other computers. This function of a computer is called *telecommunications*.

Dentists who use telecommunications do so to send electronic insurance claims, order supplies by computer, access electronic bulletin boards to exchange information with other computer users, and conduct information searches. Computers used in dentistry in the future will include storage and display of digital radiographs (x-rays), digital photographs made by an intraoral camera, and use of electronic patient charts.

Computer Literacy, Not Computer Programming

Computer education used to emphasize learning how to write programs for the personal computer. Some people still equate computer literacy with being a good computer programmer. Today, knowing how to program a computer to use it productively is not necessary.

Computer literacy is the ability to use personal computer hardware and software to accomplish tasks. It requires a basic knowledge of how hardware works, what software can do, and how to make hardware and software function together to manage information.

Components of a Personal Computer System

A personal computer system is made up of hardware and software. Hardware is the physical equipment one can touch, such as the keyboard, computer video monitor, or the system box. Software is the set of instructions, or a computer program, that tell the hardware what to do. Software is used in operating system software and applications software.

Hardware

Hardware can be divided into input, output, and storage devices (Figure 5-1) and are described in the following ways.

Software

Generic term to describe the program instructions given to the computer. Software can be either (1) operating system software such as the disk operating system (DOS) or (2) application software such as word processing, database, electronic spreadsheet, graphics, or telecommunications.

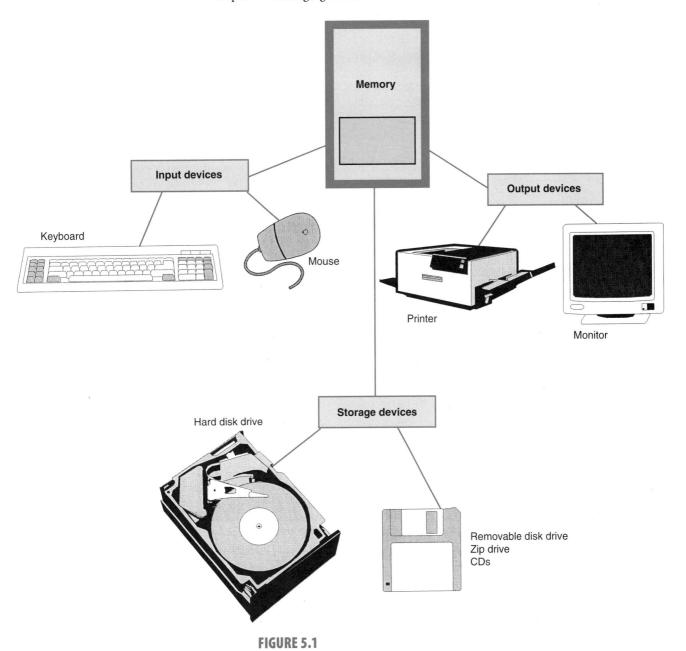

FIGURE 5.1

Input, output, and storage devices.

Input devices are hardware components that permit data or instructions to be taken into the computer. Examples of input devices are keyboards, light pens, a mouse, and bar code reader.

Output devices are hardware components that display data after they have been processed. Output devices include monitors and printers.

Storage devices allow the storage of data when the computer is off. Storage devices are generally known as *disk drives* and are available as either floppy or fixed (hard) disk drives. Hard drives store more information than floppy drives. Other examples of high capacity storage devices include tape drives and compact disks (**CD-ROM**). Tape drives are used to back up files for the entire computer system.

CD-ROM

Compact disk-read only memory. The disk resembles an audio CD and stores large amounts of data.

Software

The operating system software is necessary to permit the hardware components to work with one another and directs the movement of data through the input and output devices to storage areas. These data move through the memory and central processing unit (CPU) components of the hardware.

Disk operating system

Operating system software that functions as a supervisor of a computer and is essential before any application software can run on a computer. The disk operating system is the program first loaded into a computer at boot-up and controls other applications programs used. It also controls the printer, monitor, disk drives, and other equipment attached to the computer.

For example, the operating system software informs a word processing program what directions to follow when a word-processed document on a disk needs to be stored in the computer.

PCs use several different types of operating systems. The most popular systems are Microsoft disk operating systems (MS-Windows 98, MS-Windows 95, MS-Windows NT, and Linax and the Macintosh operating system (Apple Computers). These **disk operating systems** come in different versions and are designated by number; the higher the number, the more recent the release of the operating system software. Currently, MS-Windows 98 (ed 2) is the most recent version available.

Application software is a computer program written to perform specific functions. For example, word processing programs function to turn a personal computer into an electronic typewriter with additional options. An application software program requires hardware and DOS to perform. Without these two elements, an application software program will not function.

Application software is used for a variety of office functions, including typing (word processing), filing (database management), using the telephone (telecommunications), doing calculations (electronic spreadsheets), drawing pictures (graphics), and managing a dental practice (specialized database management software). A number of different software programs are available to perform the various office tasks (Table 5-1).

How Personal Computer Systems Work

Combining the hardware and operating system and application software of a personal computer system allows the computer to manage information. When the hardware is turned on, the operating system software is first loaded into the working memory of the hardware. The operating system software inspects the other hardware components such as disk drives, monitor, and printer to ensure readiness.

Second, an application software program is loaded into memory usually from the storage device (floppy or hard drive), and the computer system is ready to manage information. Startup takes less than a minute. Some computer systems automate much of the access to application software by using a windows program with a menu selection screen to simplify the process of gaining access to a variety of computer application software functions.

Uses of Application Software in the Dental Office

Application software enables computer hardware and DOS to do useful work. Most dental practices are more interested in what computers can do rather than how they do it. Five basic types of information management exist that all personal computer systems can perform. Dental offices most frequently use the first three applications in the following list:

Word processing
Database management
Telecommunications
Graphics
Electronic spreadsheets

A PC can simply be converted from word processing to a graphic device. The application software contains a set of instructions that tell the computer how to handle data from the keyboard or another input device and how to manipulate and eventfully display the pictures on a screen and printer.

Table 5.1

Selected Application Software

Office Function	Application	Software Brand Names
Typing	Wordprocessing	Voice Pilot-Naturally Speaking
		WordPerfect
		Wordstar
		Microsoft Word
		MS-Word
Filing	Database management	Paradox
		dBase III/IV
Telephone	Telecommunications	MS-Office 2000-Outlook
		ProCom
		Lap-Link
		PC Anywhere
		MS-Office 2000-(Web-Based)
Calculations	Electronic spreadsheet	Lotus 123
		MS-Excell
		MS-Office 2000-CAK
Drawing pictures	Graphics	Print Shop
		Coral Draw
		Powerpoint (MS-Office 2000)
Dental office management	Specialized database management and wordprocessing	Practice Works
		SoftDent
		Easy Dental
		MS-Office 2000-Access

Word Processing

Word processing is a category of application software used to create, manipulate, and print text materials such as letters, documents, **recall** notices, or written reports. Word processing is replacing typewriters because it allows more flexibility to produce written documents.

Word processing application software has many different titles and prices (see Table 5-1). In general, the more features a word processing software program has, the more expensive the product. The majority of commercially available word processors use a screen-orientated technique feature known as *WYSIWYG*, an acronym for "what you see is what you get." Text on screen will appear the same in a printed document.

Word processing application software contains a basic set of operations that are similar regardless of manufacturer. Although the specific commands are different, the same basic operation occurs. For example, almost all packages contain a command to center text on a line. In one word processor software program, the centering command may occur when you type the "F2" key, and in another word processor product the centering function may happen when you hold the control key and press the "c" key.

General operations are the main set of word processing commands. These word processing commands depend on the use of files. In a computer, a *file* designates a collection of related information in a storage area. General operations for using word processing software include creating or retrieving a file, saving a created file to a storage device, printing a file, stopping work in one file and doing something else to another file, and terminating the word processing program to engage in another PC function. Other commands control editing and printing documents.

Some word processing application software contains functions to assist with spelling. Spelling checkers include a routine that will read through a document and search for misspelled words. This feature saves time and improves the accuracy of printed documents.

Word processors today have become extremely powerful and contain numerous additional functions. The transition from text-based documents to those generated in a graphical

---

Recall

A periodic patient appointment scheduled after initial treatment for preventative measures.

user interface (GUI) such as Windows or on a Macintosh computer provide much greater flexibility to create, edit, format, and print documents.

A specialized form of word processing application software is known as *desktop publishing*. Desktop publishing permits the user to include not only text in a variety of typestyles and fonts but also allows pictures and graphics to be included in a document. The resulting document can have a professional printed appearance. Desktop publishing is used in some dental offices to produce office brochures or newsletters.

Database Management

Database application software is the main software program for medical and dental practice management software. An information management software program enables a dental office to organize patient data into files and process the data quickly.

For example, you may first use the database software to search and print the names of all patients who have the same last name. It can also select all patients who have birthdays in a certain month. Database management software enables the user immediate access to data that could be stored in several different locations within the PC.

The basic elements of database management software include records, fields, and files. Think of a paper filing system when trying to picture the electronic database management software. A paper file folder is just like the electronic file; they both contain information of a related nature. A field contains a unique identifier for each record such as last name, address, or telephone number. These assembled fields make one record. A collection of records comprises a file.

A file of patient names and addresses consists of a separate record for each patient. A file may contain thousands of patient records. In addition, each record contains unique information about that patient. The computer uses the unique features of a patient's name and address record to sort, search, and retrieve patient information. This powerful tool helps a dental office manage its information quickly and efficiently.

The database management software contains instructions to create records, edit records, and then index, sort, retrieve, and store information for future use. Like the word processor, it will also allow you to print information although it does not provide as much flexibility in formatting the printed information. Dental practice management software is simply a specialized use of the database management application.

Telecommunications

Communication that occurs between two computers by telephone is called *telecommunications*. A hardware device and software application program are necessary for these computers to "talk" to each other.

The computer must have a hardware component called a *modem* to engage in telecommunications. It directs data through the telephone line by converting the computer's digital data into a data form that can be transmitted over a telephone line. A modem on the receiving computer converts the data back into digital data.

Application software is also needed in this process. It provides a set of instructions to the computers about how to control the data flow over the telephone lines and functions to activate the modem to send and receive the data from the computers.

Telecommunication is used to send and receive data between two computers and is the basis of electronic claims transmission that transmits financial data from a dental practice to an insurance processing center. Other examples of telecommunications include communicating with local or national bulletin boards, information services (Internet service provider, AOL, Compuserv, MS-Network), or the **Internet**. The Internet contains information about many topics and displays the data as text or pictures. Several dental information sites are available on the Internet including the American Dental Association, many dental schools, and several dentists' offices (Box 5-1).

Internet

A massive integrated network of computer connections throughout the world that permits electronic communications with a PC.

A specialized application of telecommunications is the *facsimile machine*, or *fax*. Many dental offices use fax machines to send and receive written information through telephone lines. The principles are the same as using two computers, but two fax machines are necessary. The fax machine sending information converts the written document into an electronic image and sends it over the telephone line to a receiving fax that converts the electronic image into written form and prints it on paper.

Many of today's PCs are equipped with fax capability, permitting computer-to-fax machine telecommunications and improving the information management of the dental practice.

Dental Office Computer Systems

A dental office computer system is an example of how PCs can be used to help the practice manage information. The system consists of hardware and operating and application software. Dental practice management application software is a specialized adaptation of database management software with the addition of a word processing and perhaps telecommunication software. It permits patient information to be stored and managed with the computer system.

Box 5.1

On-Line Sources for Information on Dental Assisting

Dental-related sites

Alpha Omega International Dental Fraternity
    www.ao.org
American Dental Association
    www.ada.org/prac/careers/fs-dass.html
American Dental Hygienists Association
    www.adha.org
Canadian Dental Hygienists Association
    www.cfc-efc.ca/cdha
Careers in Dentistry: Dental Assisting
    www.dent.unc.edu/careers/cid04.html
Dental Gnome
    www.appledore.co.uk/d_gnome1.html

Dental libraries

Government Employment: Dental Assisting
    www.federaljobs.net/overview.html
Northwestern University-Galter Health Sciences
    Library
    www.galter.nwu.edu/hw/dent
University of California Los Angeles Periodontics
    Information Center
    www.dent.ucla.edu/pic
University of North Carolina Dental School
    www.dent.unc.edu
Waldmann Dental Library Home Page
    www.nyu.edu/dental/library/homepage.html

Private and government organizations

Academy of General Dentistry
    www.agd.org
Academy of Periodontology
    www.perio.org
Alliance for the Best Clinical Practices in Dentistry
    www.omfr.health.ufl.edu/ABCPD/index.html
American Association of Public Health Dentistry
    www.pitt.edu/~aaphd
American Dental Assistants Association
    www.adaa.org
American Dental Hygienists Association
    www.adha.org
American Dental Association
    www.ada.org
American Medical Association
    www.ama-assn.org
American Public Health Association
    www.apha.org
CDC-Oral Health Division
    www.cdc.gov/nccdphp/oh

Bridges of particular interests for dental professionals

Dental Cyber Web: Related Links
    www.netsville.com/dental-web/bridges.html

A dental computer system will have input, output, and storage devices. Input devices are generally keyboards or a pointing device known as a *mouse*. These input devices are used to place information into a computer.

Output devices are typically monitors and printers. Printers can be either dot matrix, ink jet, or laser depending on the quality of print desired. Laser printers produce high-quality print that is generally easier to read than a dot-matrix printer.

The storage device will be a hard disk drive whose capacity is measured in megabytes (MB), where mega equals 1000 bytes. Dental office computer systems commonly have a 10 to 30 **gigabytes** (GB) hard disk drive. In addition, the practice data will be stored on back-up files on a large capacity tape back-up system to provide a duplicate copy of the dental practice information. This is critical in the event some electronic information is lost and must be restored.

PCs are a common sight in many dental offices today. Initially, they were purchased to improve the office manage-

Gigabyte

A measure of capacity for disk drive storage.

ment tasks of patient accounting and billing, especially dental insurance. Expanded use of this technology includes appointment scheduling, electronic claims submissions, and using the PC to expand the practice through marketing.

Today, the computer most used in a dental office is a single or networked personal Windows 95 or 98, Celeron II or III, and K6-2 Athlon computer systems. The system is composed of a keyboard, monitor, central processing unit (CPU) speed of 500 MHZ processor TM, one or two types of printers (dot matrix or laser), and perhaps a modem. All computer systems must have two types of software: 1) DOS and 2) a dental management application software program (specialized database management software program), word processing, and telecommunication software if a modem is present.

A dental office computer system is no different than any other computer system used in business. It consists of identical components although some systems may have a few more advanced features than other systems. However, when it is turned on, the dental management application software program takes control and allows you to do dental office management and financial and word processing functions (Box 5-2).

Accounting and Billing

Accounting and billing functions are used most commonly in a dental office computer system. Like a manual system where financial information is recorded on ledger cards or perhaps a peg-board system, the computer receives data from the keyboard regarding dental procedures rendered and the charges for them.

Once the data is entered electronically, it can be used by the computer to generate a patient bill (**statement**) for payment at the time services are rendered or print an insurance form for submission to an insurance carrier. Some computer systems permit the telecommunication function of electronically transferring this data over the telephone lines to an insurance carrier.

Statement

A letter or form providing the patient with a description of services, payments, and the balance owed on the accounts.

Charge and payment transactions are handled the same way. The computer retrieves the patient's account by identification of the patient's last name, and the transaction is recorded. Credits and other **adjustments** are also done electronically.

Adjustments

A modification or change on a bill.

Management of accounts receivable is greatly simplified with a computer. Transactions are recorded along with the date of the transaction. Because most computers have an internal clock and calendar, the date information is used from the computer and compared with the transaction type and date to generate a report on accounts that are past due. Most dental management software programs then categorize the accounts into ones that are 30, 60, or over 90 days past due.

Insurance Management

Closely related to the accounting and billing function, is the management of dental insurance. With the growth in the number and types of dental insurance plans available, the task of managing a variety of plans is streamlined by using a computer. Dental management software will record transactions using ADA insurance codes and a predefined office fee schedule and print an insurance claim form.

The printing is done one of two ways. Using a preprinted standard insurance form, a dot-matrix printer will fill out the form by printing the required information in each section. Obviously, the computer cannot print information it does not have so a preliminary step is necessary to set up the insurance carrier and patient information (name, address) in the dental management software.

The other type of printing is done using a laser printer. It uses blank paper and prints the entire insurance form and information needed by the insurance company directly on the paper, done at one time. Laser printers provide higher-quality print than dot-matrix and impact printers.

Appointment Scheduling

Another function that has traditionally been done manually is appointment scheduling. Several dental management systems have appointment scheduling as one of their functions. Computers can be used to schedule appointments by recording the patient's name, procedure, and amount of time necessary to complete the procedure. Patients on recall or follow-up care may be scheduled automatically by the computer for appointments 1 week or 6 months in advance.

The electronic schedule can be printed for posting throughout the office. Holidays and other times the office is closed are electronically blocked out just as in a manual system. The benefits of computerized appointment scheduling are improved organization of the appointment book and the ability to locate patient appointments quickly using the computer. A computerized appointment system is particularly helpful in offices with multiple locations or dentists (Figure 5-2).

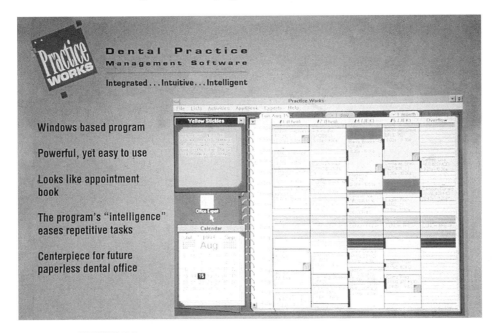

FIGURE 5.2

Computerized appointment schedules have replaced paper scheduling.

Reports

The collection and processing of information is important but the ability to review the practice activity in greater detail is fundamental to effective decision making and management of the dental office. All dental management systems have the ability to generate reports. Reports provide a wide variety of information to the user. Accounting and financial information and patient tracking and other measures of productivity are available.

A powerful report feature is *ad hoc* reporting. This feature permits the dentist or staff members to create their own types of reports from the various data elements (name, address, dental procedures) contained in the database management software. The use of the report function is essential to provide a realistic picture of what is happening in the practice.

Future Applications

Dental informatics describes a spectrum of computer technologies with applications for dental education, research, and practice. Dental informatics is the application of computers to dental practice and represents the blending of information management and automatic processes that a computer can do. PCs now form the basis of support for a variety of future technologies that are being used in the daily practice of some dental offices. These technologies include digital radiography (x-rays), intraoral digital photography, and an electronic patient chart.

Digital Radiography

Traditionally, patient radiographs have been taken using ionizing radiation and silver-coated film packets to permit the diagnosis of dental conditions. The use of radiation, no matter how slight, presents some risk to the patient. As technology has evolved, dental radiographs can be made using substantially less radiation exposure to the patient.

Film has been replaced by an electronic device that is inserted into the patient's mouth, and when exposed to an x-ray, converts an image into a digital picture (Figure 5-3). This digital image is displayed immediately on a computer screen for review; no developing time is needed. This technology also permits the computer to make enhancements to the original digital radiograph for improved evaluation and diagnosis.

The advantages of digital radiography include faster exposure and display of radiographs, decreased radiation exposure for the patient, and the ability to use one radiograph to analyze a dental condition in greater detail through computer enhancement.

Intraoral Photography

Using fiberoptics and a computer, dental office personnel are able to photograph patient conditions and display this information on a color television monitor within the operatory. These color photographs range from a single tooth to an entire arch. Full facial profiles are also available. These images can be converted to digital images for storage in a computer system. Intraoral photography provides a visual

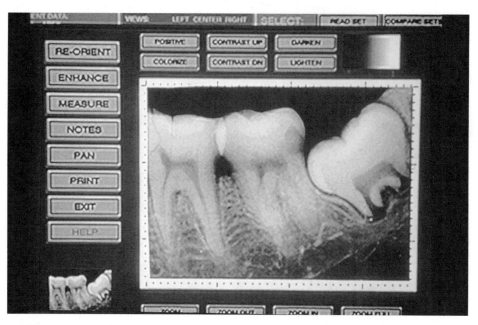

FIGURE 5.3

A dental radiograph produced using a computer (digital radiography) rather than traditional film.

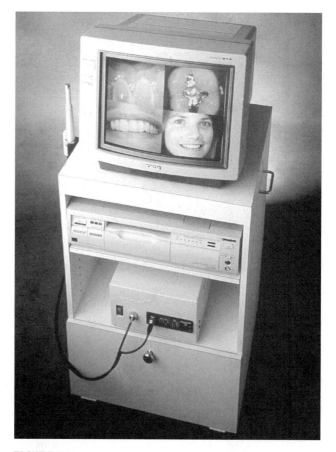

FIGURE 5.4

Intraoral photography provides visual information on individual teeth, an entire dental arch, or a patient's face.

record of a patient's dentition or facial profile to document existing dental conditions (Figure 5-4). Using pictures instead of words is also helpful to educate patients about their dental condition and need for treatment.

Electronic Patient Chart

Some dental practice management software programs permit the linking of intraoral photographs and radiographs to a patient's dental record. Refinement of these technologies will permit the development of a complete electronic patient chart. The future dental records will probably be a combination of medical and dental histories and dental chartings and digital radiographs linked and available to staff members at any location within the office on a computer terminal.

Telecommunications permits the movement of this information anywhere in the world in a matter of seconds. Although technical and legal barriers still remain, this possibility is near.

These future applications of imaging and computers are a few exciting new applications under development. Others include voice-activated systems to record patient information, expert decision support systems to assist in diagnosis, development of CD-ROM high-capacity storage disks for use in patient and staff education, and vastly expanded use of the telecommunications components of the Internet for transmission and retrieval of information to enhance the delivery of patient care. Since 1995, the use of computers with CD-ROMS has increased from 45.7% to 81.4% in 1997, and use of modems has increased from 61.7% to 69.1%. Furthermore, 81.4% of all dentists had access to CD-ROM drives and modems at work and home.

Dental informatics is the next innovative creation for dentistry as computer technology is used as a tool to improve the quality of patient care. The computer or PC has progressed in a few, short years and will be accomplishing more in the future than simply adding numbers and printing letters to patients.

DENTAL OFFICE RECORDS

Electronic and bookkeeping programs have made office recordkeeping less complex and easier to manage. However, planning, organizing, and evaluating the financial management system are still needed for an efficient and effective business.

ROLE OF THE DENTAL BUSINESS ASSISTANT IN RECORDKEEPING

To have a smooth-running business record system, the dental business assistant must have knowledge of various business systems, knowledge of dentistry, skills to carry out the daily activities involved in the dental business office, and the ability to work with the patient and various people involved in business operations. Records must be accurate and completed in a timely fashion.

The term *business assistant* encompasses the receptionist, secretary, business record or bookkeeper, office manager, and dental assistant. Often a single dental assistant with business skills implements each of these roles on a daily basis in a solo practice. However, the size of the dental practice does not matter; the business assistant must be accurate when developing a record system and maintaining dental records.

APPOINTMENT DETERMINATION AND SCHEDULE FORMAT

The purpose of the appointment book is to identify the daily operational schedule for the dentist and staff members. Arranging the appointments and determining the schedule enables the dental practice to run effectively. Once the appointment book system is decided, the decisions for making appointments on a daily basis should remain the responsibility of one person, usually the business assistant.

Dental appointments can be entered into an appointment book or a computerized appointment system. The complexity of the appointment schedule will be determined by the number of operatories used by the dentist and dental personnel. Two operatories are usually planned and prepared for the dentist. For instance, a dental practice with one dentist, chairside assistant, and dental hygienist will need an appointment schedule with three columns, if the hygienist is scheduled in the operative appointment book. An appointment schedule for the hygienist may be maintained separately from the dentist's appointment schedule. If this appointment system is used, a two-column schedule would be satisfactory for the dentist's appointments. A dental practice with five or six operatories employing two advanced function dental assistants and a dental hygienist would need an appointment schedule with multiple columns (Figure 5-5). Most dentists and business assistants prefer the "Week-at-a-Glance" appointment schedule. A daily appointment schedule is sometimes used in a new or first-time dental practice that is building its practice or a smaller office setting. Although some appointment schedules are set up in 10-minute intervals, the most common unit of time is 15 minutes set in 1-hour blocks. Appointment books and computerized appointment schedules are available with the dates already identified on the schedule.

Units of Scheduling Time

The dentist determines how much time is needed for the various procedures based on the treatment plan and identifies that time as units. The treatment plan designates the units of time necessary to complete specific procedures. The

Monday,
December 20, 1999

	Operatory A	Operatory B	Operatory C	Operatory D-DH	
8:00		Evelyn Brook		Susan Mann	**8:00**
8:15		RC-fin fill/#3		587-1212	8:15
8:30		587-6600		↓	8:30
8:45				Pat Johns	8:45
9:00	Bob Maines	Vern Herde		486-6265	**9:00**
9:15	244-6788	Adj. dent.		Premed-N2o/02	9:15
9:30	C-bldup/cr. #30	↓		↓	9:30
9:45				Pan Tang	9:45
10:00		Nina Ross		486-7986	**10:00**
10:15		624-8766			10:15
10:30		Am adj.	Pan Tang	Tracy Hass	10:30
10:45	↓		Post & core	624-7892	10:45
11:00	Barbara DeSoto	John Wilson	Crn. prep.	Deanne Gill	**11:00**
11:15	239-0767	Adj. part.		587-0214	11:15
11:30	Repair bridge			↓	11:30
11:45					11:45
12:00	LUNCH				**12:00**
12:15					12:15
12:30					12:30
12:45					12:45
1:00	OFFICE MEETING				**1:00**
1:15					1:15
1:30	Rick Rearson	James Snider		Robin Hunter	1:30
1:45	Cr. prep.	N.P. 466-4073		486-6821	1:45
2:00	566-1861			↓	**2:00**
2:15				Sealants	2:15
2:30		Gail Thorpe		Richard Hanes	2:30
2:45	↓	Emerg.		↓	2:45
3:00	Tim Sellek			Dana Young	**3:00**
3:15	566-8924			486-4411	3:15
3:30	RC				3:30
3:45	↓			↓	3:45
4:00	Steve McDonald			David Armstrong	**4:00**
4:15	239-6841			587-2011	4:15
4:30	AMS				4:30
4:45	↓			↓	4:45
5:00					**5:00**
5:15					5:15
5:30					5:30
5:45					5:45
6:00					**6:00**
6:15					6:15
6:30					6:30
6:45					6:45
7:00					**7:00**
7:15					7:15
7:30					7:30
7:45					7:45
8:00					**8:00**

Monday, December 20, 1999

FIGURE 5.5

Multiple appointment schedule with designated entries. The arrows pointing down after a patient's name indicate the time needed by the professional assigned to the patient. The angled arrow indicates the patient will have an appointment with the dental hygienist and continue treatment with the dentist. The cross marks at the bottom indicate "time not available" (5 to 8 p.m.) by any professional.

most common unit of time is 1 unit equals 15 minutes. Therefore 2 units of 15 minutes each equals 2 hour, and 4 units equals 1 hour.

Some dentists provide a guideline for the number of units for the most routine treatment provided in the office. For instance, a single-surface amalgam or composite may be 1 unit and a three-surface restoration may be 2 units. A posted guideline helps the business assistant make decisions regarding scheduling when one is not noted on the patient's record. In a short period, the experienced business assistant will know how much time to schedule for various treatments. The business assistant will also have the responsibility of controlling the appointment book by determining the following:

1 The number and type of patients seen daily
2 Any special scheduling needs
3 The schedule of operational personnel
4 Productivity
5 Potential stress factors

If the dental practice schedules expanded function personnel, indicating the dentist's and expanded functions dental assistant's units of time is necessary. Many methods are used to indicate the multiple use of a time block. A simplified method is to identify "D" for dentist and "A" for assistant in a column to the left of the time block, which provides a clear indication of who is treating the patient.

If an appointment book is used, the appointment schedule should provide enough space to write clearly and the paper texture should allow for erasures. Spiral-bound appointment books or inring binders permit the book to be folded or opened flat on the desk. A flat, solid surface to write on provides for neat penmanship, making writing in the appointment book easier.

Schedule Lay Out

Before planning the lay out for the appointment schedule, several simple techniques can be used for identifying times not available for appointments, multiple units of time, and abbreviations or symbols.

Times Not Available

Diagonal lines "\" or an "X" can be placed across time units that appointments are not available for such activities as lunch or staff meetings. Felt-tip markers can also be used to designate the lunch schedule or staff meetings (see Figure 5-5).

Multiple Units of Time

Arrows "↓" can be used to represent the amount of units that will be needed for each patient. After the patient's name is clearly entered in the scheduling space, an arrow is drawn from the time the appointment begins to when it ends. This will plainly indicate the number of units needed for a particular appointment. Some dentists and patients prefer longer appointments to complete defined procedures in a shorter period, and others prefer to treat patients for a longer period.

Abbreviations or Symbols

Because of the minimum space available to write in the appointment book, abbreviations and symbols, similar to charting to designate certain concepts, are used. For example, "H" refers to home telephone number and "B" refers to the business number. New patients are often designated with an "N," and red checks "✓" express the confirmation of a patient's appointment. The use of a diagonal or angled arrows "↙" or "↘" indicates a same-day continued appointment with the dental hygienist or advanced function dental assistant and dentist (see Figure 5-5).

APPOINTMENT ENTRY

Appointment entries should include the patient's first and last name, home and work telephone numbers, procedure to be completed, and the patient's account number. *Write all entries in pencil so that they can be erased. Make sure information is complete and legible. Do not cross names out and rewrite them.* An appointment schedule is a record of the operation of the dental practice. Therefore maintaining a well-kept schedule is important.

Several appointment considerations should be made before scheduling patients. These considerations include decisions such as managing regular appointment scheduling, making special scheduling arrangements, and scheduling changes. These decisions can be included as part of the office policy manual.

Regular Appointment Scheduling

Schedule patients so that procedures can be completed within the time allotted. Having too much time between patients or scheduling patients so close that the dentist and personnel are rushed and under unnecessary stress is inefficient.

People have times in the day when they feel most energized. Therefore, identify the time of day that the dentist feels most energized and ready to take on extended treatment procedures. The dentist may prefer to schedule specific treatment on defined days of the week. The key to good appointment planning is not to schedule all difficult procedures at one time. Scheduling should include a mix of different procedures to avoid stressful situations. For instance, a simple alloy or composite restorative appointment could follow a 2-hour crown and bridge preparation. Scheduling an unruly child before or after a long, complex appointment should not be done.

Children

Preschool children are most rested, easier to work with, and more cooperative in the early morning. If the child is in school, scheduling an appointment before school or after school is better. If a child misses school, provide a doctor's note for the teacher's record. Most offices have preprinted cards to handle this task.

Older Adults

Older adults are usually retired, have a flexible schedule, and are often willing to come in midafternoon, during the times that may be harder to fill. Do not confuse older adult patients by changing their appointments and confirm their appointment the day before they are scheduled for treatment. Appointments that are scheduled on the same week day and time also help patients remember them.

Short Appointments

Short appointments are sometimes needed for suture removal, replacement of a denture tooth, or a denture adjustment. These short appointments can often be integrated, or dove-tailed, into the regular schedule.

Treatment Plan Appointment Series

After the treatment plan has been accepted, the necessary appointments will need to be scheduled. Consider time between appointments for healing if surgery has occurred or laboratory work needs to be complete. If the patient has designated a convenient time for an appointment, schedule them on the same day and during the same time.

Special Scheduling Arrangements

In addition to preparing the schedule for lunch and routine times the office is closed, special scheduling events also need to be noted.

Buffer Units

A buffer unit is usually 1 unit, or 15 minutes, scheduled once in the morning and once in the afternoon during the busiest time to provide flex-time. This buffer time helps alleviate stress when an emergency patient needs to be treated, if the patient or doctor is late, or other unforeseen events happen.

Emergency Appointments

Emergencies such as a child falling, causing a tooth to become loose or knocked out can occur at any time. Other emergencies include a recent toothache or the loss of a denture tooth for a businessperson. The patient should be seen immediately in urgent situations. However, most offices will schedule a buffer time for emergencies, and patients should be encouraged to come in during these times. If this is not possible, most scheduled patients will understand if the dentist has to take care of the emergency.

The business assistant should find out the nature and severity of the emergency by asking how long the patient has been in pain, if the pain is sharp or dull, or if a fever exists. If a child has lost a tooth, make sure the tooth is wrapped in a damp cloth and brought to the office. Sometimes patients need to be seen for an emergency after office hours. Usually the dentist will see them. An evening emergency procedure should be set up for staff assistance if necessary.

Holidays

Holidays recognized and observed by the dentist need to be marked on the appointment schedule.

Professional Meetings

Occasions arise when appointments will not be scheduled because the dentist is attending professional meetings. Some professional organizations and continuing education offices provide convenient typed adhesive labels for the business assistant to place in the schedule.

Staff Meetings

The dentist and staff should schedule meetings once or twice a month to discuss operations and concerns and share any ideas they have to improve office efficiency. These meetings help personnel feel more involved with the business and therefore more supportive of its success.

Scheduling Changes

The dentist must at times make a change in the schedule because of illness or other occasions. These changes should not happen often but when they do, the patient should be called immediately to explain the situation and reschedule the appointment. A follow up letter should be sent thanking the patient for making the change and a confirmation call should be made the day before the new appointment to remind the patient of the change.

Late Patients

Patients are occasionally late. Therefore if this becomes routine the dental assistant should explain in a pleasant but firm manner that the time scheduled is essential to complete their treatment. If the patient continues to be late, the dental assistant can reschedule the patient rather than treating the patient at that time or charging a late fee. Late fee charges should be explained first during treatment planning time to emphasize the importance of being on time for all appointments.

Open Door Policy

An increasing number of dental clinics see patients on an unscheduled basis. These clinics usually have more than one dentist and often advanced function auxiliaries to help treat patients. However, general dental practices will occasionally have nonscheduled patients come in. If the patient has an emergency, identify the severity of the emergency and schedule the patient, or try to work the patient into the buffer time. In a nonemergency situation, schedule the patient for another time. This will help eliminate recurrences from the same patient or friends. Accommodating a patient who is new to the neighborhood could lead to the practice acquiring a new patient or family. The dentist should provide some guidance to the business assistant on preference for unusual scheduling events.

Rescheduled and No-Show Appointments

Patients need to reschedule an appointment at certain times. However, if this continues repeatedly, remind the patient that the dentist is unable to complete treatment if appointments are not kept. Another appointment can only be scheduled if the office is confident the patient will keep ap-

pointments in the future. All broken appointments must be noted on the patient's record and a letter should be sent to the patient confirming the next appointment (Figure 5-6). A fee may be charged for the broken appointment.

Scheduling and Confirming Appointments

When scheduling appointments, find out if the patient prefers coming to the office in the morning or afternoon and provide the patient with two options, if available. If a second appointment is being scheduled, ask the patient if the same

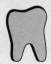

Jamie J. Coyne, DMD
454 Bishop Lane
Louisville, KY 40000
(502) 456-0000

January 14, 2000

Anna M. Suttles
1123 Elmira Drive
Louisville, KY 40204

Dear Ms. Suttles:

I appreciate having the opportunity to talk with you on Friday, January 11, 2000 about rescheduling your appointment. We understand that there are times when unforeseen circumstances arise that interrupt our planned schedules. However, this is the second time we have had to reschedule this appointment for you. Dr. Coyne is concerned about your dental health and the need to complete your treatment if you do not keep your appointment.

After talking with you, we feel confident that you intend to keep your next appointment scheduled for January 25, 2000 at 9 a.m. However, as you know and we discussed, our policy requires a $20.00 rescheduling fee when more than two appointments have been missed. This fee will be charged the next time an appointment is not kept.

We will look forward to seeing you on *January 25, 2000 at 9 a.m.*

Sincerely yours,

Ms. Carol A. Eaton
Business Assistant

FIGURE 5.6

Sample confirmation letter for broken appointment.

Call list					
Name	Date	Telephone number	Preferred time	Treatment	Time units

FIGURE 5.7

Using and maintaining the call list gives patients with unpredictable schedules more time options and helps the dentist fill unused time slots.

time is preferred and check for the next opening. Usually patients prefer the same time and day of the week because of memory and availability.

Many types of appointment cards exist. They provide business information for the patient by documenting the dentist's name, address, and telephone number. They also tell who the appointment is for and appointment date. Some appointment cards provide small maps that locate the dental office in a high-traffic area. Write legibly on the appointment card. If an electronic system is used to schedule appointments, a written appointment may also be processed through the computer.

Call List

The primary purpose of a call list is to provide an opportunity for patients to make earlier appointments but are unable to do so at the time because of a full dental schedule. Business people with busy schedules often prefer to be put on a call list for short notice appointments. This may also be an advantage for the patient who is often late or unable to keep regularly scheduled appointments or misses appointments but wishes to remain a patient. A call list helps fill in appointment times as they become available and provides a mechanism to keep the practice productive (Figure 5-7). The list should include the patient's name, telephone number, date added to the call list, time preference, treatment, units of time for the appointment, and dates the patient was called.

Periodic Recall Appointments

Periodic recall appointments are scheduled as part of the preventive maintenance program to follow up patient treatment, assess patient home care, and motivate the patient to maintain good oral health. This can best be accomplished by periodically evaluating and treating the patient. After patients finish treatment, they are usually placed on a 3- or 6-month recall schedule to be seen by the dental hygienist.

The recall appointment system is separate from the regular scheduling system. The recall appointment is usually made in the dental hygienist's schedule, preferably at the time of the patient's last treatment appointment. When a patient is finished with treatment the following can occur:

- The name is entered into the computer for automatic retrieval at the designated time or a written recall appointment system can be used by the following:
- Placing an appointment card into a chronological (monthly) recall file
- Recording the new recall date in a monthly recall binder

Reminder letters or cards may be sent to the patient before the appointment date or the patient may be contacted by telephone close to the recall time (Figure 5-8). A recall card addressed by the patient is an excellent way to remind the patient of the follow up appointment.

When the patient returns for periodic recall, the dental hygienist will update the patient's health history, vitals, medications, and complete a preop chart. The hygienist will then perform a soft- and hard-tissue examination and complete periodontia and caries charting. Radiographs may be taken, and a toothbrush demonstration will often be given if needed. The hygienist will then complete the prophylaxis treatment. If no further operative treatment is necessary, the date for the next recall appointment will be placed in the recall system and on the treatment plan.

MAINTAINING PATIENT RECORDS

Patient dental records include the office registration form, medical and dental records, treatment plan, radiographs, and any correspondence. Patient records must be complete and accurate because they are legal documents (see Chapter 3). *These records belong to the dentist, and only the patient has the right to review that record unless authorized by the patient in writing.* If the patient wishes to transfer the record,

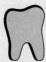

Jamie J. Coyne, DMD
454 Bishop Lane
Louisville, KY 40000
(502) 456-0000

January 14, 2000

Donn P. Suttles
1123 Elmira Drive
Louisville, KY 40204

Dear Mr. Suttles:

   Your recall appointment is set for January 25, 2000 at 9 a.m. We look forward to seeing you again and checking the condition of your teeth.

Dear Mr. Suttles:

   It is time for you to make an appointment for treatment follow up and cleaning. Please call our office soon so we can work you into our schedule.

Dear Mr. Suttles:

   We missed seeing you this month for your checkup and cleaning. Please call our office right away so we can set an appointment for you.

Dear Mr. Suttles:

   We have not seen you since July, 1994 when you had your dentures and oral tissue checked. As we discussed, changes can occur in the hard and soft tissue of your mouth that can affect the fit of your dentures. It is important that your mouth is checked for any abnormal physical conditions affecting these supporting oral tissues.

Sincerely,

Leslie M. Eaton, RDH

FIGURE 5.8

Sample recall letters.

the dentist has the option to do so. If approved, written authorization by the patient must be obtained. Only a copy of the record and duplicate films should be sent. Because dental records are permanent legal records of the dental practice, they must be preserved in a safe file and storage system where they can be easily retrieved for future needs. *Only the dentist can determine when inactive patient records of the practice can be discarded.*

Types of Filing Systems

Increasing numbers of dental practices are using computers to maintain patient dental records, eliminating the need for other types of filing systems. However, because many dental practices still manage their records by traditional filing systems, several types of filing systems will be discussed.

Patient records can be maintained in file folders to preserve and protect them. These files are labeled clearly by typing the following:

1 The patient's surname first
2 The first name second
3 The middle name
4 Any degree or seniority (for example, Eaton, Leslie, Mariton, II, or Senior)

The patient's home and work telephone numbers and account number are often listed on the label for easy access. The label is placed on the file folder according to the type of filing system used.

Although many types of file systems exist, the most common files used in dental practice are the vertical, lateral, and lateral open-shelf. The lateral open-shelf filing system provides an easy filing and retrieval method that allows for color-coding of the folders (Figure 5-9). Lateral track files with open shelves are used in large dental clinics. Some dental offices use the Rolodex file for easy access to patient names, addresses, and telephone, account, and other important numbers.

Alphabetical Filing

Many dental management systems file patient charts and account records alphabetically. Alphabetically labeled index cards can be used to divide patient charts in the file for easy retrieval.

Color-Coded Filing

Color-coded labels with the first two letters of the patient's last name and active date of treatment can be placed on the patient's file folder to make retrieval faster and easier.

Chronologic Filing

Recall records are usually filed by the month and date the patient is returning to the dental office for preventive care. This type of filing system is called *chronologic.*

Numerical Filing

Dental offices using computers usually have patient records listed by a coded account number for easy access. An alphabetical list of patient names is necessary to cross-reference the account numbers.

Subject Filing

Routine business records are usually placed in a folder and labeled and filed by subject. Often, these records will also be separated with alphabetical index cards. For instance, information on "equipment" may be placed in a folder and filed after the letter "E."

Retrieving Patient Records

Usually the business assistant will retrieve the records for the following day and call each patient to confirm appointments. Each record should be checked to make sure radiographs are available, the patient chart is up-to-date, and any laboratory work needed is ready. Patient account records should be checked for any late payment. If the payment is not up-to-date, the dentist should be notified and the business assistant should be prepared to discuss the account with the patient, if necessary. When treatment is completed, the records should be filed as soon as possible.

ACCOUNTS RECEIVABLE RECORDS

The business assistant is responsible for maintaining the accounts receivable record. (See Chapter 6 for the methods of payment and insurance plans.) The accounts receivable record is an accounting of all payments accepted for dental

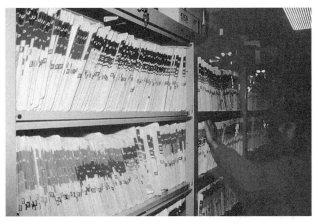

FIGURE 5.9

Proper use of the established filing system and use of color coding makes it easier to retrieve patient information whenever needed.

Jamie J. Coyne, D.M.D.
Family patient history

Page: 1
10-31-99

#00002   Family balance   0.00
John Jones   Family contracts   0.00
101 Cherokee Dr.
Louisville, KY 40000
Home phone: (502) 424-0000
Work phone: (502) 524-0000

Date	Name	Date of srvc. Tth./Sfc.	Dr.	Transaction/procedure	Debit	Credit
04-30-98	John		2	01110 Adult prophy	30.00	
04-30-98	John		2	00274 Bitewings – Four fi	22.00	
04-30-98	John		1	00120 Periodic oral exami	15.00	
05-22-98	John			Insurance pmt. Ck #039167		67.00
08-16-98	John		2	01110 Adult prophy	30.00	
08-16-98	John		1	00120 Periodic oral exami	15.00	
09-13-98	John			Insurance pmt. Ck #14625		0.00
10-15-98	John			Patient pmt. Ck #1718		45.00
11-09-98	John			Insurance pmt. Ck #081693		0.00
11-11-98	John			Insurance pmt. Ck #081693		0.00
02-07-99	John		1	00120 Periodic oral exami	16.00	
02-07-99	John		2	01110 Adult prophy	35.00	
03-09-99	John			Insurance pmt. Ck #1211		51.00
08-01-99	John		1	00120 Periodic oral exami	16.00	
08-01-99	John		4	00274 Bitewings – Four fi	24.00	
08-01-99	John		4	01110 Adult prophy	35.00	
08-04-99	John			Patient pmt. Ck #1950		75.00
12-15-99	John		3	00120 Periodic oral exami	16.00	
12-15-99	John		2	01110 Adult prophy	35.00	
12-15-99	John			Patient pmt. Ck #2039		51.00

Monthly statement sent and insurance filed dates and amounts

Date	Name	Amount
	No monthly statement sent dates available.	
	No insurance filed dates available.	

FIGURE 5.10

Sample electronic accounts receivable record. Ledger sheet.

services. Accounts receivable records include completing the following activities:

1 Receipt: As payments are received for dental services, the patient will be given a **receipt** that includes the charge for services, any credits, and the balance.

2 Ledger sheet: A patient's ledger sheet is the official patient financial record.

Receipt

A slip given to the patient when a payment is received for services.

It is filled out with the patient's name, address, date, service, charge, credits, and balance. The ledger sheet is not placed in the patient's file; but maintained in a separate ledger file or tray (Figure 5-10).

3 Statement: The ledger card can be copied and used as a statement or a separate statement can be typed. The statement is a request for payment and informs the patient of service fees, payments, and account balance. Most statements are sent in the middle or end of the month (Figure 5-11).

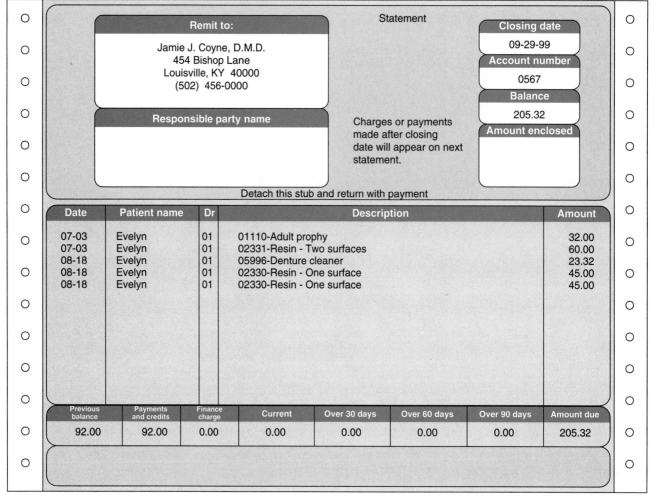

	Statement		Closing date
Remit to:			09-29-99
Jamie J. Coyne, D.M.D.			**Account number**
454 Bishop Lane	Charges or payments		0567
Louisville, KY 40000	made after closing		**Balance**
(502) 456-0000	date will appear on next		205.32
Responsible party name	statement.		**Amount enclosed**

Detach this stub and return with payment

Date	Patient name	Dr	Description	Amount
07-03	Evelyn	01	01110-Adult prophy	32.00
07-03	Evelyn	01	02331-Resin - Two surfaces	60.00
08-18	Evelyn	01	05996-Denture cleaner	23.32
08-18	Evelyn	01	02330-Resin - One surface	45.00
08-18	Evelyn	01	02330-Resin - One surface	45.00

Previous balance	Payments and credits	Finance charge	Current	Over 30 days	Over 60 days	Over 90 days	Amount due
92.00	92.00	0.00	0.00	0.00	0.00	0.00	205.32

FIGURE 5.11

Sample electronic accounts receivable record. Statement.

4 Daysheet: The fee charged, service rendered, amount received, any adjustments, and the balance will be entered onto a daysheet or daily log that includes all accounts receivable for the day (Figure 5-12).

5 Deposit slip: A deposit slip will be filled out with all daily receipts to be deposited in the bank.

Electronic Financial Recordkeeping

Electronic financial recordkeeping is simple with less paper being used. As the treatment is completed and the payment data is entered, the computer electronically enters the payment into the accounts receivable section, provides the patient with a receipt of payment, and enters the receipt into the daily log. An advantage of an electronic system is the ability to retrieve accounts receivable reports any time. These reports provide account information by the day or month, and a receivables summary report can be generated from the data to summarize production and net collections.

One-Write Pegboard Manual System

The one-write pegboard manual accounts receivable system has been a method of receipts and **disbursements** in dental offices for many years and continues to be used. No matter which system is used, the accounts receivable ledger must be accurate and legible. The one-write pegboard manual system is made up of the following:

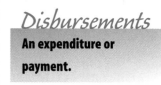
Disbursements
An expenditure or payment.

1 Patient receipt
2 Charge slip
3 Ledger or statement on the left side of the accounting section
4 Daysheet
5 Deposit form

As part of the system, the right side of the accounting section will contain a daysheet and may include a deposit

Jamie J. Coyne, D.M.D.
Daysheet

Page: 1
10-28-99

Pat. no.	Fam. no.	Patient name	Prov.	Trans/proc	Tooth/ surface		Debit amount	Credit amount
0073	0073	Morgan, A Tom	2	Periodic oral exa			24.00	
0073	0073	Morgan, A Tom	5	Bitewings – Two f			26.00	
0073	0073	Morgan, A Tom	5	Adult prophy			42.00	
0073	0073	Morgan, A Tom		Compdent credit				92.00
0325	0306	Bali, I Ear	1	1 Surface poster i	3	F	114.00	
0325	0306	Bali, I Ear	1	1 Surface poster i	5	F	114.00	
0054	0054	Roberts, A Wil	2	OFFICE VISIT ONLY			0.00	
0204	0204	James, C Roy	2	Amalgam – One sur	18	B	53.00	
0204	0204	James, C Roy	2	Seat crown	19		0.00	
0204	0204	James, C Roy		Compdent credit				31.00
0204	0204	James, C Roy		Pat. chk. #1839				203.62
0312	0312	Pope, H Tim	2	Periodic oral exa			24.00	
0312	0312	Pope, H Tim	5	Bitewings – Two f			26.00	
0312	0312	Pope, H Tim	5	Adult prophy			42.00	
0312	0312	Pope, H Tim		Compdent credit				92.00
0057	0057	Framer, O Dan		Pat. chk. #1355				25.00
0077	0077	Muller, A Mary		Pat. chk. #5482				40.00
0347	0347	Silver, W Brad	2	Initial oral exam			31.00	
0347	0347	Silver, W Brad	5	Child prophy			36.00	
0347	0347	Silver, W Brad		Compdent credit				67.00
0391	0391	Knast, L Tom	1	Three canals (exc	19		485.00	
0391	0391	Knast, L Tom		Misc. credit adju				485.00
0310	0310	Krum, C Mel	1	Resin – Three sur	10	MFL	118.00	
0310	0310	Krum, C Mel	2	Restorative liner	10		28.00	
0310	0310	Krum, C Mel		Compdent credit				118.00
0310	0310	Krum, C Mel		Pat. chk. #3289				28.00
V 0227	0227	Sound, J Julie	2	OFFICE VISIT ONLY			0.00	
V 0946	0946	Sully, P Mark	2	Periodic oral exa			24.00	
0946	0946	Sully, P Mark	5	Bitewings – Two f			26.00	
0946	0946	Sully, P Mark	5	Adult prophy			42.00	
0946	0946	Sully, P Mark		Compdent credit				92.00
0105	0105	Head, Lauri	1	OFFICE VISIT ONLY			0.00	
0348	0348	Low, K Brad	2	Initial oral exam			31.00	
0348	0348	Low, K Brad	5	Panoramin film			66.00	
0348	0348	Low, K Brad	5	Adult prophy			42.00	
0348	0348	Low, K Brad	5	Perio charting			36.00	
0348	0348	Low, K Brad		Compdent credit				170.00
0326	0326	Hurn, O Bev	1	OFFICE VISIT ONLY			0.00	

*   V = Voided transaction

* * * Today's totals * * *

Balance forward	0.00	Credit balance forward	0.00
Office visit	945.00	Cash payment	0.00
Finance charge	0.00	Check payment	296.62
Late payment charge	0.00	Insurance payment	0.00
NSF check	0.00	Charge card payment	0.00
Return check charge	0.00	Insurance bulk payment	0.00
Balance refund	0.00	Tmt. applied to contract	0.00
Initial contract charge	0.00	Bad debt charge-off	0.00
Monthly contact charge	0.00	Finance charge credit	0.00

FIGURE 5.12

Sample electronic accounts receivable record. Daysheet.   *Continued*

Jamie J. Coyne, D.M.D.
Daysheet

Page: 2
10-28-99

Pat. no.	Fam. no.	Patient name	Prov.	Trans/proc	Tooth/ surface	Debit amount	Credit amount
		Initial contract agreeme		0.00	Late charge credit		0.00
		Contract interest charge		0.00	Overcharge credit		0.00
		Insurance refund		0.00	Patient referral credit		0.00
		NSF debit		0.00	Payment credit adjustmen		0.00
		Compdent check debit		0.00	Amount moved to contract		0.00
		Put in wrong debit		0.00	Patient discount credit		0.00
		Ins. reimbursement debit		0.00	Insurance credit		0.00
		Balance forwarded debit		0.00	Compdent credit		662.00
		* * * Sales tax * * *		0.00	Kenpac credit		0.00
		Misc. debit adjustment		0.00	Randmark credit		0.00
					Wrong account credit		0.00
					Coupon credit		0.00
					DMO credit		0.00
					Bankruptcy credit		0.00
					Misc. credit adjustment		0.00

Increase in A/R $945.00   Decrease in A/R $958.62

Yesterday's A/R balance: $170,795.13
Your accounts receivable decreased by: – $13.62   today.

Today's accounts receivable balance: $170,781.51

Month-to-date patient charges: $98,350.74
**   Month-to-date payments: $50,197.88

* * * Today's total payments * * *

$296.62

* * * Provider production * * *

	Productions	Collections
Provider #1. Jamie J. Coyne, D.M.D.	$346.00	296.92
Provider #2. Jamie J. Coyne, D.M.D. DMD CODENT	$215.00	0.00
Provider #5. Hygiene - compdent	$384.00	0.00

* * This is not a total of your month-to-date collections.

FIGURE 5.12, cont'd

Sample electronic accounts receivable record. Daysheet.

form. To prepare the account, attach the patient receipt to the left margin over the daysheet with the ledger sheet or statement positioned between the patient receipt and daysheet. The carbon copy allows the business assistant to do the following:

1 Post (enter) the date
2 Describe the service
3 List the total fees
4 Record the payment
5 Make any adjustments
6 Provide a balance

By entering this data just once, the information is transferred to all three records. The amount of the payment is then recorded on the deposit form on the right side of the accounting section. This multientry system reduces errors and increases efficiency.

Adjustments

Adjustments are made occasionally for checks that may be returned, in which case the amount of the check is added to the balance to represent the increase in the account balance or amount the patient still owes. If a returned check is received from the bank, the patient can be called and arrangements can be made to redeposit the check. In this situation, write "redeposit of NSF" (nonsufficient funds) with the patient's name on a separate deposit slip and resubmit it. The amount of the returned check should be added to the balance on the patient's ledger sheet until the check clears. At the time the check clears, the amount can again be deducted from the patient's balance. This will prevent any confusion later. Discounts are subtracted to denote a decrease in the balance.

Banking Procedures

In most instances, banking procedures will have already been established by the dentist. The business assistant's banking responsibilities usually include writing checks, making deposits, reconciling the bank statement, and identifying errors. In large dental practices, reconciling bank statements, providing payroll checks, and completing monthly accounting procedures may be controlled by a business agent or accountant.

Record Control

Deposits should be made daily from accounts receivable. The accounts receivable records are audited frequently to check for accuracy. Receipts given to patients should be numbered, and checks should be stamped "for deposit only." This may help protect the business assistant in case of financial concerns and also protects the dental practice from embezzlement.

Checking Account Deposits

Checking account deposit tickets are customized with the dentist's name and address. The amount of currency and coins are counted and documented on the first two lines. Each check must be endorsed and listed separately on the numbered lines of the deposit ticket. When the front of the deposit ticket is filled, it can be turned over for additional space. The total from the back of the ticket is placed on the front, and the two amounts are added for a total of all checks. The total amount of deposits is also listed on the ledger and checkbook. Deposit tickets are available with duplicate copies retained as part of the office accounts receivable record.

Bills and checks should be bundled together. The money, deposit slip, and bankbook are placed in the deposit bag. If a carrier makes the deposit, the bank will return the duplicate deposit slip stamped. Carrier deposits and night deposits are often used when the day deposit cannot be made. Banks will provide mail deposit slips and envelopes if deposits are made by carrier. If this method of deposit is used, the payee should sign the check; the business assistant should stamp the check for deposit only; and the authorized office party should endorse the check. The night depository can be used after hours to drop the deposit bag that contains the deposit ticket and accounts receivable deposit. The bag will be picked up for next-day deposit.

DISBURSEMENTS

The business assistant will also have the responsibility of maintaining the accounts payable and disbursing checks. The dentist may want to review payments before mailing them. All statements or invoices should be maintained in the accounts payable file folder for safekeeping. Usually checks are made out twice a month unless the invoice reflects a discount for early payment. Each invoice must be checked against items received at the time of delivery to ensure that everything ordered was received (see Chapter 7). Verifying that the receipt is valid is necessary because some distributors and magazine marketing strategies use ordering and subscription advertisements that look like invoices.

All invoices from one distributor should be stapled together to ensure proper payment. All disbursements should be made by check to provide proof of payment. Once the check is made out, the business assistant should write or stamp on the invoice, "paid," with the date and check number. The invoice may be perforated so that a portion can be mailed with the payment, and the portion can be retained for the record. Be sure to follow the instructions on the invoice. The invoice should be is maintained for tax purposes. After the check is made out and the invoice is properly marked, the invoice is placed into the proper folder and kept on file.

Writing Checks

Checks are used to handle the majority of all dental office financial transactions. The dental practice will have personalized business checks for routine payments. Checks can be written in ink, typed, or prepared through a electronic system but should never be written in pencil or erasable ink. This will help prevent altering the amount of the check. If an error is made, void the check and retain it for accounting purposes. Be certain the account balance is sufficient before writing checks. As with other legal documents, checks must be written accurately and legibly. The following information should be written on the check:

- Current date
- Full name of the person or company with the payee's address
- Correct payment amount
- Legal authorized signature

Retain the checks in a safe place until the dentist can sign them. The business assistant should never sign the dentist's name and can only sign checks if the dentist has approved legal signature authority through established banking procedures.

If a regular business checkbook is used, enter the date, name of the payee, amount of the check, and the account balance onto the check stub. Anytime a new page is used, the account balance must be carried over onto the new sheet.

If the pegboard system is used, special pegboard checks are placed over a check register sheet on the pegboard (similar to the pegboard accounts receivable transactions). When the check is filled out, the information is transferred to the check register sheet. Align the check properly over the first blank line of the register. Special payroll forms can be placed under the check, and the entry will be transferred directly from the check to the personnel payroll records.

Check Register

A check register is used to record the dates, check numbers, transactions, checks, and deposits. The register can be completed manually or electronically to acquire the up-to-date balance and help **reconcile** the bank statement.

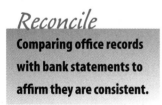

Reconcile

Comparing office records with bank statements to affirm they are consistent.

Balancing the Bank Statement

The written statement provided by the bank will provide the following information:

- Account number
- Beginning and ending dates of the statement
- Taxpayer ID number

- Beginning balance
- Total deposits and credits
- Checks and debits
- Ending balance

All dates for deposits and checks with check numbers transacted during the statement period will be listed individually. Balancing or reconciling the bank statement should be completed in a quiet, private area away from the distractions of the office activities. A comfortable spot where the deposit receipts, checks, and statements can be spread out is best.

The following manual guideline and illustrated forms will provide the procedures needed for balancing the bank statement (Figure 5-13):

1 Compare the deposit receipts with the deposits shown on the statement. Be sure to add any balance interest or other credits shown on the statement to the checkbook or register.
2 List any deposits made but not shown on the statement onto *Form A*.
3 Check the statement's list of checks or withdrawal against the business checkbook and mark each check returned.
4 Be sure that any other charges shown on the statement is also deducted from the checkbook or register balance.
5 List all outstanding checks and withdrawals not shown on the statement onto *Form B*.
6 Enter the ending balance from the statement onto line l, *Form C*.
7 Enter the total unlisted deposits on line 2, *Form C*.
8 Total lines l and 2 and enter on line 3, *Form C*.
9 Enter the total outstanding checks and withdrawals on line 4, *Form C*.
10 Subtract line 4 from line 3 and enter on line 5, *Form C*.
11 Enter checkbook or register balance on line 6, *Form C*. This should agree with line 5.
12 If the checkbook or register balance do not agree with the resulting balance, repeat the process to make sure each figure has been entered correctly and the math has been completed accurately.

Miscellaneous Cash Fund

Do not keep large amounts of cash in the dental office. However, cash will be needed at times to make change for patients who pay cash. Only a minimum amount of money should be retained in the office, and this amount should be placed in a safe after hours. Whenever cash is removed from this fund, a check or voucher should also be made out for the total amount. The check or voucher also should be dated, signed, and placed with the cash fund. When additional cash is needed, the vouchers are totaled, the amount is entered into the accounts payable, and a check is written for the amount needed.

Big City

Big City Bank, Kentucky

Louisville, Kentucky 40000

The money statement

Jamie J. Coyne, D.M.D.
454 Bishop Lane
Louisville, KY 40000
(502) 456-0000

00009
45186466

Page 1 of 2

| Business checking account |

Account number	32198745	Beginning balance	5,112.06
Beginning date	August 21, 1999	Deposits/credits	1,631.01
Ending date	September 19, 1999	Checks/debits	1,588.56
Taxpayer ID number		Ending balance	5,154.51

Form A

Unlisted deposits

Date	Amount
9/05/99	836.00
9/10/99	2005.50
9/18/99	1560.00
Total (2)	4401.50

Form B

Outstanding checks

Number	Amount	
1126	1106	50
1150	592	50
1173	153	25
1180	205	00
1191	1643	50
Total (4)	3699	75

Form C

Beginning balance	$5154.51 (+)	(1)
Unlisted deposits	$4401.50	(2)
Total	$9556.01 (−)	(3)
Outstanding checks	$3699.75	(4)
Total	$5856.26	(5)
Balance check book	$5856.26	(6)

FIGURE 5.13

Reconciling the bank statement.

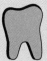

Jamie J. Coyne, DMD
454 Bishop Lane
Louisville, KY 40000
(502) 456-0000

January 14, 2000

John B. Stanley
821 Spring Garden Drive
Louisville, KY 40204

Dear Mr. Stanley:

I appreciate having the opportunity to talk with you on Tuesday, January 8, 2000 about your account, which is past due. Your account indicates your last payment was on November 8, 1999. We will expect this payment of $150.00 by Friday, January 18, 2000 as we discussed.

Dear Mr. Stanley:

Please refer to our past correspondence. Your account is currently 2 months past due. There has been no response to our requests for payment of $150.00. As we discussed, our policy states that all accounts past 60 days will be referred to our attorney for collections as necessary. This action may require the account to be turned over to the Credit Bureau. Payment in full must be received in our office no later than Monday, January 28, 2000. Thank you for your cooperation. If you have any questions concerning this matter, please do not hesitate to call our office.

Dear Mr. Stanley:

We have made every effort over the last several months to satisfactorily resolve this payment problem and have received no response from you regarding your overdue account in the amount of $150.00. We have been more than fair in trying to work with you concerning this matter. YOUR ACCOUNT WILL BE FORWARDED TO OUR ATTORNEY FOR COLLECTION ON THURSDAY, JANUARY 30, 2000. IF PAYMENT IN THE AMOUNT OF $150.00 OR PAYMENT OF ACCOUNT IN FULL HAS NOT BEEN RECEIVED IN OUR OFFICE, YOU WILL INCUR A FEE OF $20.00 FOR COLLECTION.

Sincerely yours,

Ms. Carol A. Eaton
Business Assistant

FIGURE 5.14

Sample collection letters. *Top*, First month late. *Middle*, Second reminder. *Bottom*, Final letter.

COLLECTIONS

The success of collections often depends on the time taken for treatment planning and financial presentation with the patient. If the patient understands the need for the treatment and agrees with the financial arrangements, trust and a willingness to follow through with payments should happen. Some patients may be unintentionally late with payments, making for collection problems. The business assistant is then responsible, with approval from the dentist, to develop a collection procedure. Uncollected accounts prohibit the growth of the dental practice, prevent the dentist from paying business accounts, and hinders other office responsibilities.

When accounts are not paid, they become late and may begin to age. If billing is completed electronically, the computer will automatically identify the bills not paid and the date of the last payment. Some dental offices age late accounts manually by color coding late accounting ledgers by month or placing late accounts on a monthly outstanding account list for follow up. Collection procedures include sending collection letters, making telephone calls, and sometimes transferring accounts to a collection agency. Whichever method or combined system is used, a collection procedure must be initiated to maintain up-to-date accounts.

Collection Letters

Personal letters are better to use for collection. However, personalized form letters are available that represent different collection problems. Collection letters should be brief, contain accurate account information, and lead to a positive outcome. The patient should be motivated to cooperate by sharing an understanding that payments may be late at times. However, this should be followed by firmly stating the date when the payment will be expected (Figure 5-14).

Telephone Follow Up

Collection letters should be followed by a telephone call if no response is received. This provides the business assistant and patient with an opportunity to discuss and resolve any difficulty or misunderstanding. The business assistant can use the following guidelines for telephone collection:

- Make the call in a private area.
- Have all account information available before calling the patient.
- Speak only to the person responsible for the account.
- State politely the nature of the call.
- Do not criticize the patient; instead be understanding and positive.
- Seek understanding and commitment.
- Document the date and amount of payment to be sent, repeating the arrangement with the patient.
- Call the patient rather than leaving a message requesting a return call.
- Send a follow up letter confirming the arrangements recommended.

Collection Agency

The business assistant, with the dentist's permission, may contact a collection agency for help with the account if all endeavors fail. The business assistant should not send further statements to the patient after arrangements have been made and accounts have been sent to the collection agency. The ledger sheet should reflect the date the account was transferred to the agency, and all future calls from the patient about the account should be referred to the collection agency. If any payment is received after the transfer of records has been made to the collection agent, the business assistant should notify the agency as soon as possible.

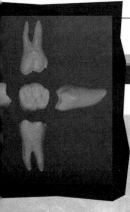

Points for Review

- Use of PCs to provide small businesses and individuals access to computing power
- Use of word processing, database management, and telecommunications in contemporary dental practices
- Understand terms such as *field*, *record*, *file*, and *modem*
- Importance of Internet and other electronic computer networks to the practice of dentistry
- Dental informatics, digital radiograph, intraoral radiography, and electronic patient charts offer a new spectrum of computer technologies with applications in dental practice
- Role of the business assistant in managing dental records
- Techniques used for scheduling and entering appointments
- Accounting and billing techniques

Self-Study Questions

1. During what decade did the PC appear?
   a. 1960
   b. 1970
   c. 1980
   d. 1990
2. Approximately what percentage of dental offices had an inoffice computer in 1997?
   a. 25.5%
   b. 55.5%
   c. 79.5%
   d. 89%
3. How was the computer primarily being used for offices with PCs in 1997?
   a. Games
   b. Electronic spreadsheets
   c. Accounting
   d. Internet access
4. What is having a basic knowledge of how hardware works and what software can do called?
   a. Computer programming
   b. Computer literacy

   c. Telecommunications
   d. Modem
5. What is the hardware device of a PC system that stores data called?
   a. Input
   b. Output
   c. Storage
   d. Memory
6. What is computer hardware?
   a. The physical equipment one can touch
   b. A computer program
   c. Telephone transmission of information
   d. A set of instructions
7. What are the two major types of computer software called?
   a. Application and integration
   b. Operating system and integration
   c. Application and operating
   d. Telecommunication and database management
8. What are the three most commonly used application software programs in a dental office?
   a. Games, DOS, and word processing
   b. Word processing, telecommunications, and database management
   c. Telecommunications, faxes, and games
   d. Database management, word processing, and DOS
9. What are the two future applications of computer technology in dental practice?
   a. Hardware and software
   b. Electronic patient chart and intraoral photography
   c. Modems and faxes
   d. Printers and monitors
10. What is the method for developing radiographs that uses less radiation and permits display of an x-ray on a computer screen called?
    a. Conventional radiography
    b. Digital radiography
    c. Analog faxing
    d. Telecommunications
11. What type of application software program permits communication between a computer and modem and a fax machine?
    a. Telecommunications
    b. Database management
    c. Graphics
    d. Word processing

12. What determines the complexity of the appointment schedule format?
    a. Number of patients
    b. Number of operatories
    c. Time of day
    d. Number of minutes in each scheduling unit

13. What is usually the best time to schedule appointments for children?
    a. Early morning
    b. Midmorning
    c. Early afternoon
    d. Midafternoon

14. What is buffer time?
    a. Scheduled time for staff meetings
    b. Lunch time
    c. Flextime for emergencies
    d. Time when the office is closed

15. What mechanism is available to the business assistant to schedule short notice appointments?
    a. Periodic recall
    b. Call list
    c. Reminder letters
    d. All of the above

16. Dental office records belong to the patient.
    a. True
    b. False

17. What kind of file system is organized by the month?
    a. Numerical
    b. Subject
    c. Alphabetical
    d. Chronologic

18. What record is given to patients when they complete treatment?
    a. Daysheet
    b. Ledger sheet
    c. Receipt slip
    d. Voucher

19. What is used to maintain the patient's official financial record?
    a. Daysheet
    b. Ledger sheet
    c. Receipt slip
    d. Pegboard

20. What is the one-write manual accounts receivable system called?
    a. Daysheet
    b. Ledger sheet
    c. Receipt slip
    d. Pegboard

21. What is the best way to minimize collection problems?
    a. Sending personalized collection letters
    b. Following up collection letters with a telephone call
    c. Taking time for treatment planning and financial presentation
    d. Transferring aged accounts to a collection agency

Suggested Readings

Abbey LM, Zimmerman JL: *Dental informatics: integrating technology into the dental environment*, New York, 1992, Springer-Verlag.

ADA Survey Center: *Survey of Current Issues in Dentistry*, Chicago, 1995 and 1997.

Chasteen JE: A computer database approach for dental practice, *J Am Dent Assoc* 123: 27-33, 1992.

Eisner J et al: *The computer-based oral health record: a new foundation for oral health information systems*, Chicago, 1993, American Fund for Dental Health Monograph.

Finkbeiner BL, Finkbeiner CA: *Practice management for the dental team*, ed 5, St Louis, Mosby (in press).

Kiser T, Nash K: Computers in dentistry on the rise, *J Am Dent Assoc* 123:106-107, 1992.

Murray K: *Introduction to personal computers*, ed 2, Carmel, Ind, 1991, Que Corporation.

Parker CS: *Computers and theory applications*, New York, 1988, Holt, Rhinehart and Wilson.

Seltzer S: *High tech zone: digitized dentists enter hyperoral space*, Academy of General Dentistry Impact Newsletter, 23 (5): 13-18, 1995.

Williams JN: The basics of practice management software, *Preview* 3 (2): 24-26, 1994.

Zimmerman JL, Ball MJ, Petroski SP: *Computers in dentistry*, Philadelphia, 1986, Dental Clinics of North America.

Chapter 6

Managing Dental Financial Records

Key Points

- Financial arrangements
- Presentation of treatment and financial arrangements
- Alternative dental care delivery systems

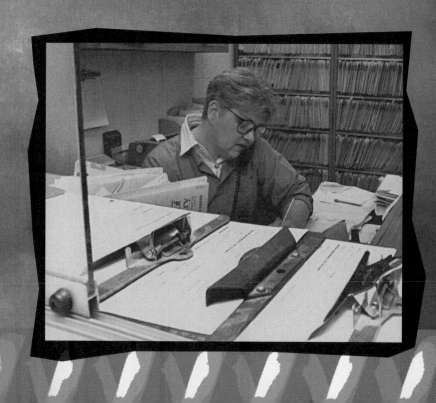

Learning Objectives

On completion of Chapter 6, the student should be able to do the following:

- Define key terms.
- Define various financial arrangements.
- Present treatment and financial options.

- Identify alternative dental delivery systems.
- Determine fee coverages.
- Identify types of service.
- Prepare and file insurance claims.

Key Terms

Alternative Dental Care Delivery Systems

Benefits

Deductible

Deferred Payment Plan

Indemnity Program

Insurer

Insured

Premium

Schedule of Benefits

Third-Party Coverage

FINANCIAL ARRANGEMENTS

One of the key components to any successful dental practice is having people skills or good verbal and nonverbal communication abilities (see Chapter 4). Good people skills are especially important when making financial arrangements with patients. A positive attitude and willingness to invest in dental treatment begins the first day patients enter the dental office and continues as they complete treatment and maintain a long-term relationship with the practice. Office personnel should secure personal history and medical and dental history of their patients (see Chapter 21). The patient acquaintance form provides personal and family data such as name, address, Social Security number, and employer and may include who is responsible for the account and the name of the insurance company if they are to cover the dental treatment (Figure 6-1).

Many dental offices find it beneficial to provide the person responsible for financial arrangements with a letter describing the financial policies of the dental office. This letter describes the methods of payment that the dentist accepts. When establishing financial policies for the dental practice, acknowledge the philosophy and goals of the dentist and the **alternative dental care delivery systems** available in the area in which the dental office is located. Financial policy should be based on established business principles and should include payment options for patients. Established financial policies should be presented in written form to patients so that they will know the various options that are available.

Alternative dental care delivery systems

Various choices or options for paying for dental care.

Presentation of Treatment and Financial Options

Several key procedures must be accomplished before making the financial arrangements. After the initial appointment, the dentist must establish a treatment plan with a fee structure. The treatment schedule or number of appointments anticipated to complete treatment must be identified. Once this is completed, the information must be presented to patients and financial arrangements made.

Although the dentist establishes dental fee structures and financial policies, presentation of this information to patients may vary. Many dentists choose to present the treatment plan including the fee structure and treatment schedule to the patient, and others choose to briefly discuss the fees with patients and have the business assistant or office manager make the financial arrangements and set the treatment schedule (see Chapter 24).

In some dental practices, after the dentist establishes the treatment plan, fee structure, and number of appointments necessary, the presentation of this financial information to patients is delegated, along with the financial arrangements and treatment schedule, to a skilled and prepared business assistant. Developing this relationship between the dentist and the business assistant involves open communications, skill, and trust. Many dentists who are temperate or easy going wish to leave financial arrangements to the business assistant. They find delegation a rewarding arrangement and many times the business assistant is able to present this information in a more appropriate environment to give patients time to agree on a satisfactory payment plan. Patients can sign a consent form agreeing on treatment at this time. If patients are a minor or cared for by an adult, a consent form must be signed by the caregiver. The person who has legal custody or power of attorney to approve the treatment and pay for the dental services should sign the form.

Alternative Dental Care Delivery Systems

Although financing dental treatment varies, several types of financial arrangements have been established for dental treatment.

Cash for Service

Some dental patients will pay in full by cash or check immediately following treatment. However, the ability to pay cash will depend on the cost of the dental treatment rendered. The dentist provides treatment on a fee-for-service basis. This means the dentist must charge a fee, based on cost, of the treatment that is provided for the patient. Usually payment is due at the time services are rendered unless other arrangements are made before treatment. Payment in full within a specified time, often no more than 30 days of receipt of the statement, is usually considered cash.

If extensive treatment is planned that includes office expenses and laboratory fees, the patient should understand that if treatment is to be paid by cash, these fees must be paid at the time treatment is initiated or other arrangements must be made. Cash arrangements will often require that all treatment involving laboratory fees include a down payment of 30% to 50% with the balance paid on delivery. When the patient prefers cash, payment should be made before completion of the treatment. Some dental practices provide cash incentives. For instance, for cash treatment of $500.00 or more some dentists will provide a percentage (10%) courtesy discount for full cash or check payment at the beginning of treatment.

Another popular method of paying cash is the use of credit cards. Patients can use a credit card to cover fees at the time of treatment or cover the entire cost of major treatment. The credit card should be processed appropriately.

James D. Eaton, D.M.D.
Patient Acquaintance Form

Page: 1
10-28-99

Name _____ Address _____

City _____ State _____ Zip _____ Home phone _____

Work phone _____ Sex (m/f) _____ Marital status _____

Birthdate _____ Social security # _____

Name of responsible party _____

Billing address _____

Insurance (y/n) _____ Employer name _____ Phone _____

Address _____ City _____ State _____ Zip _____

Insurance company name _____ Phone _____

Referred by _____

Does your medical history include any of the following?

1. Do you have a physician? _____ Phone _____ _____ Yes _____ No
2. Have you had a complete physical? .... Date _____ _____ Yes _____ No
3. Are you under any medical treatment? .... _____ Yes _____ No
4. Have you had any major operations? ..... List .... _____ Yes _____ No
5. Have you had any adverse response to any drugs? .... _____ Yes _____ No
6. Are you allergic to any medications? ..... List .... _____ Yes _____ No
7. Are you in good general health? .... _____ Yes _____ No
8. Have any wounds healed slowly? .... _____ Yes _____ No
9. Are you pregnant? .... _____ Yes _____ No
10. Do you have anemia? .... _____ Yes _____ No
11. Do you have a heart ailment (heart murmur, mitral valve prolapse)? .... _____ Yes _____ No
12. Do you have high blood pressure? .... _____ Yes _____ No
13. Do you have respiratory disease? .... _____ Yes _____ No
14. Do you have diabetes? .... _____ Yes _____ No
15. Do you have rheumatic fever? .... _____ Yes _____ No
16. Do you have rheumatism or arthritis? .... _____ Yes _____ No
17. Do you have tumors or growths? .... _____ Yes _____ No
18. Do you have any blood disease? .... _____ Yes _____ No
19. Do you have any liver disease? .... _____ Yes _____ No
20. Do you have any kidney disease? .... _____ Yes _____ No
21. Do you have any stomach or intestinal disease? .... _____ Yes _____ No
22. Do you have any venereal disease? .... _____ Yes _____ No
23. Do you have AIDS? .... _____ Yes _____ No
24. Do you have yellow jaundice or hepatitis? .... _____ Yes _____ No
25. Do you have any problems that need to be treated now? .... _____ Yes _____ No
26. What is the approximate date of first dental visit? .... _____ Yes _____ No
27. Is your mouth sensitive to hots, colds, or sweets? .... _____ Yes _____ No
28. Do you clench your teeth at night? .... _____ Yes _____ No
29. Do your gums bleed? .... _____ Yes _____ No
30. Have you ever had local anesthetic? ...... Any problems .... _____ Yes _____ No
31. Have you had any difficult extractions in the past? .... _____ Yes _____ No
32. Have you had instructions in brushing and flossing? .... _____ Yes _____ No
33. When was your last full mouth x-ray taken? .... _____ Yes _____ No
34. Have you ever had convulsions or epilepsy? .... _____ Yes _____ No
35. List drugs you are presently taking _____

_____

36. Pharmacy name _____ Phone _____
37. In case of emergency, notify: _____ Phone _____

_____
Patient signature   Date

FIGURE 6.1

Electronic patient acquaintance form.

Patients may anticipate receiving an amount of unearned income during dental treatment (income tax refund) from which to pay for the dental treatment. Although patients may have good intentions, the dental practice should not accept this type of cash proposal unless a signed payment plan is part of the arrangement. A financial agreement should be provided for all patients involved with extended treatment, regardless of the payment method.

A follow-up system should be established if patients agree to pay cash and do not following treatment. This system may include a late fee if payment is not received by the due date or within a specified period. Be firm but polite when discussing financial arrangements with patients. If a past check has been returned, a returned check fee should be established.

Extended Payment Plans

Deferred payment plan

Payment plan for dental services in place of fee for service.

Dental practices usually provide an extended payment plan for dental treatment, such as a **deferred payment plan.** Financial arrangements can also be provided through a financial institution such as a bank or credit agency.

Dental Deferred Payment Plans

Most deferred payment plans provided by the dentist will include a down payment of 30% to 50% with the balance in equal payments. The down payment may be less if the patient is a patient of record and has made payments on time in the past. Payments can be scheduled weekly, monthly, biannually, or at specific times of the year when they may be receiving cash.

A credit report can be obtained for a fee from the local retail merchants to review patients credit records and used to consider the down payment and consecutive payments. The agency will need the patients complete name, spouse's name, address, employment, Social Security number, and any other identified creditor. If credit is denied, the Fair Crediting Report Act requires the dental practice to notify patients, who then have an opportunity to contact the agency for further information on the denial.

Dental practices are required by federal law, through the Truth and Lending Act, to provide patients with a financial agreement statement, referred to as a *Truth in Lending Statement*, when financial arrangements involve four or more payments. This verifies that a payment agreement exists between the provider and patient.

The statement can be in the form of a financial letter or statement format. All financial arrangements must be dated and signed by the patient or responsible party. The statement should include the following:

1 Name of the provider

2 Name of the patient

3 Total amount agreed on

4 Amount of the down payment

5 Balance after initial payment

6 Amount of installments

7 Date of installments

8 Finance charges

The patient should understand that if unforeseen treatment is necessary, the treatment and any additional fees will be discussed and agreed on before initiating any changes in treatment or fees.

Installment Payment Plans

In addition to general cash receipt records, the assistant should maintain an individual installment payment record. The record should contain the patient's name, address, telephone number, down payment, balance, and consecutive payments. This record is maintained with the financial agreement.

Patients can be provided with an installment payment book that includes the same information for their personal recordkeeping and a perforated statement to send with their check to the dental office. To ensure the success of whatever treatment and payment plan is appropriate for the dental office, the patient should understand and agree with the financial arrangements. The dentist may want the business assistant and patient to sign the treatment plan and financial arrangement form.

Bank Payment Plan

If the patient chooses a bank payment plan, the business assistant will be responsible for helping the patient fill out all necessary forms and submitting them to the agency. If the account is authorized, the dentist may receive fees up front from the agency, and all payments will be made directly to that agency; the bank buys the debt for a fee. The business assistant and patient can work out payments that may also be made on a designated time schedule.

A bank draft system may also be used to pay dental fees. After authorization has been received and signed, the appropriate number of checks are typed and filed with the bank draft authorization card. This authorization permits the dentist to deposit the designated check on the date that payment is due, eliminating the business assistant's time to send monthly statements and the patient having to remember to send a check. The business assistant will need to send a payment book to the patient, confirm all arrangements, deposit the check as designated, and post the check in the patient record.

Today, patients can use electronic fund transfer to authorize the bank to debit their checking or savings account for the amount of payment and transfer that amount into an established dental account. This electronic transfer is done by the bank for a nominal fee and eliminates personal transfer of funds.

PREPAYMENT AND INSURANCE PLANS

A prepayment or insurance plan is a written contract or agreement between the **insurer** (administering agent) and

Insurer

The administering agent who provides the prepayment coverage.

Insured

The patient or person covered by the plan benefits.

Benefits

The types of procedures and treatment a plan will cover.

Premium

The charge paid for service or treatment.

insured (patient), agreeing to cover full or partial payment of scheduled services. These services are agreed on in advance and are called *benefits*. The insurer collects **premiums** from the insured and pays for the service or treatment as claims are presented. The premium is the charge that is paid for the service or treatment and the claim is the formal written request for payment of a benefit.

If the insured pays the entire amount of the premium, the program is called a *noncontributory plan*, but if the premium is paid in part or in full by the employer it is a *contributory plan*.

Accurate and detailed patient records should be maintained and all patient records should be kept confidential. The dentist and office personnel must understand the legal implications of these claim forms and should behave ethically. They can be sued, fined, and incarcerated for fraudulent records. Fees must be listed correctly, treatment must be correct, and claims must be billed only on completion of the treatment. Although the business assistant may not be aware of every insurance plan available, the dentist and business assistant should have some knowledge of the insurance programs.

Increasing numbers of employers offer dental insurance coverage as a benefit of employment. The patient should check the extent of their dental coverage with the insurance company before beginning treatment. This will help patients understand what is covered by their insurance policy and if necessary the portion of the dental fee they may need to supplement. It will also give the patient an opportunity to secure the necessary insurance forms.

The business assistant may help the patient complete and file the dental insurance forms but patients are responsible for paying for their dental treatment. The business assistant should be aware of and have knowledge of insurance programs in that geographical area and is able to fill out the insurance claim forms. The dental office will submit the insurance claim form after the treatment plan has been approved and financial arrangements have been agreed.

Methods of Prepayment

Third-Party Coverage

Third-party coverage provides partial payment of dental fees directly to the insured. The third party is the carrier or insurer of the insurance or payment policy. Usually third-party providers are insurance companies, such as Comp Dent, Delta Dental,

Third-party coverage

The carrier or insurer.

Blue Cross/Blue Shield, Aetna, Partners, and any other insurance company that has a dental component.

The State and Federal Government Dental Insurance

The state and federal government dental insurance benefits are also considered third-party coverage, but Medicare and Medicaid will be mentioned separately. Medicare is an insurance program under the Social Security Administration that provides medical care for the elderly. Medicaid is a jointly funded program by the state and federal government, which provides medical aid for people who are unable to finance their own medical expenses. Each state administers its own Medicaid program.

Coinsurance

For coinsurance, the insurance carrier pays a portion of the dental fees and the insured pays the balance.

Direct Reimbursement

Direct reimbursement is a benefit in which the employer pays the insured employee a portion of or the total cost of dental fees on submitting a receipt for the dental treatment. A cap may be placed on the total amount the employer will cover. Fees may be paid intermittently as treatment is completed or paid in full on completion.

Managed Health Care Programs

Managed health care programs are often called *health maintenance organizations* (HMOs). These organizations provide insurance coverage and manage the services provided. Participating dentists receive allowable fees, and employees must choose from the provider's list of dentists or group clinics.

Individual Practice Associations (IPSs)

Individual practice associations (IPSs) are organized groups of dentists who provide dental treatment on a capitation basis to patients who participate in the program. Each participating dentist files a claim and receives a percent of the predetermined fee for service. The remaining percentage is held in reserve to provide the balance of payment at the end of the period if the capitation was sufficient to cover cost.

Corporate Dental Practice

A corporate dental practice is the dental care facility that is owned and operated by a company that provides services to their employees and often families. Employees may choose other dental providers but to receive benefits they must use the company's providers.

Determination of Fee Coverage

Many insurance companies offer prepaid dental programs to employers, which vary according to the treatment fee coverage the employer is able to provide as an employee benefit. The amount of coverage or compensation provided by the insurance company is determined by the following:

1. Usual, customary, and reasonable fees (UCR)
2. Fixed fees
3. Closed panel
4. Table of allowance
5. Capitation

Usual, Customary, and Reasonable Fees

Usual, customary, and reasonable fees are based on what is a prevailing fee or usual charge for that particular geographical area. These fees will then be used by the insurance company to base their schedule of fees and process claims. The schedule of fees is a list of the benefits and fees that are covered by the plan.

Fixed Fee Schedule

A fixed fee schedule is a predetermined list of fees that will be charged for particular types of treatment. Dentists providing service must accept the established and agree on fees.

Closed Panel

The closed panel insurance plan provides agreed on fees with participating dentists and requires that members covered by the plan receive dental care only from the participating dentists. The dental office that accepts this type of fee arrangement is called the *contract practice*.

Table of Allowance

Indemnity program

A table of allowance or the set fees provided for specific treatment.

A table of allowance, sometimes called an **indemnity program**, provides participants with an allotment or set fee for specific dental treatment. Some programs require a copayment or **deductible**. The patient must pay noncovered charges, or those fees not included in the plan. Some dental programs offer a percentage reimbursement for defined services such as preventive, diagnostic, and minor and major services. For instance, the percentage can range from 100% to 50% for the different types of services and can be capped at a set amount. The dentist agrees to accept the allowable amount as payment-in-full for the covered services.

Capitation

Capitation is represented by a fixed group fee. The participating dentist must agree to provide dental treatment for all members of that group over a given period at the specified group rate.

General Insurance Information

Deductible

The amount that the insured must pay.

Insurance companies provide certificates of coverage. The certificate is not a legal document although it is issued in accordance with the provisions of the state standard. The certificate is a guarantee that means the following:

1. The coverage cannot be denied on the basis of health conditions.
2. The coverage must be renewed except for nonpayment of premium, fraud, or misrepresentation, noncompliance with plan provisions, or if the health maintenance organization ceases to do business in that state.

The plan document that is maintained by the group is the legal contract, and the certificate is subject to the terms and conditions of the plan. These conditions are referred to as *general provisions*. General provisions refer to the following:

1. Who is eligible for coverage and when changes in enrollment may be made
2. How benefits are paid
3. How and when coverage terminates
4. What privileges exist when coverage terminates

If a conflict arises, the provisions of the plan document will prevail over the certificate. The insured should read the certificate and plan carefully.

Schedule of Benefits

The general information found in standard health insurance programs include the schedule of benefits. This schedule will describe the type of service, the covered benefits, the innetwork coverage, and the out-of-network coverage (Table 6-1).

Types of Service

The type of service in a standard health insurance program includes such categories as the following:

1. Hospital care
2. Outpatient services
3. Emergency services

Table 6.1

Schedule of Benefits and Subscriber Copayments*

ADA code	Procedure	Patient pays	ADA code	Procedure	Patient pays
Appointments			**Space maintainers**		
9430	Office visit (normal hours)	$5.00	1510	Fixed, unilateral	$55.00†
9430	Emergency visit (regular hours)	$20.00	1515	Fixed, bilateral	$55.00†
9440	Emergency visit (after hours)	$35.00	1520	Removable, unilateral	$85.00†
0999	Broken appointments		1525	Removable, bilateral	$85.00†
	(without 24 hr notice, per 15 min)	$10.00	1550	Recementation of space maintainer	$10.00
	Maximum $40 per broken appointment.		**Restorative (fillings)**		
	No charge will be made because of		2999	Sedative base (under fillings)	No charge
	emergencies				
Diagnostic			AMALGAM (SILVER)		
0140/0150/0160	Oral evaluation	No charge	2110/2140	One surface	$12.00
0120	Periodic oral evaluation	No charge	2120/2150	Two surfaces	$18.00
0470	Diagnostic casts (study models)	No charge	2130/2160	Three surfaces	$25.00
0999	Diagnosis and treatment plan		2131/2161	Four or more surfaces	$35.00
	presentation	No charge			
9310	Consultation (second opinion) as		RESIN RESTORATION (INCLUDING ACID ETCH,		
	provided by participating dentist	$15.00	GLASS IONOMER LINER)		
0460	Pulp vitality tests	No charge	2330	Anterior one surface	$35.00
Radiographs (x-rays)			2331	Anterior two surfaces	$40.00
			2332	Anterior three surfaces	$45.00
0210	Intraoral - complete series	No charge	2510	Inlay - metallic - one surface	$85.00
0220	Intraoral - periapical - first film	No charge	2520	Inlay - metallic - two surfaces	$95.00
0230	Intraoral - periapical - each		2530	Inlay - metallic - three or more surfaces	$120.00
	additional film	No charge	2940	Sedative filling	$15.00
0270	Bitewings - single film	No charge	**Crown & bridge**		
0272	Bitewings - two films	No charge			
0274	Bitewings - four films	No charge	2930	Prefabricated stainless steel - primary tooth	$50.00
0330	Panoramic	No charge	2790/2791/2792/6790/6791/6792	Full cast crown	$270.00
Preventive			2750/2751/2752/6750/6751/6752	Porcelain	
1110/1120	Prophylaxis			fused to metal crown	$275.00
	(routine, once very 6 months)	No charge	2810	Three quarter cast crown	$270.00
1110/1120	Additional prophylaxis	$18.00			
1201/1203	Topical application of fluoride		PONTICS		
	(up to 16 years of age)	No charge	6210/6211/6212	Full cast pontic	$270.00
1351	Sealant - per tooth	$10.00	6240/6241/6242	Porcelain fused to metal pontic	$275.00
1330	Oral hygiene instruction	No charge	2950	Core build up	$45.00
			2951	Pin retention - per tooth	$12.00

The above copayments do not include the additional cost of precious and semiprecious metal.

All procedures listed may not be performed by the participating general dentist you select. The copayments shown apply to those company participating general dentists who do perform those services and are not applicable for services performed by a specialist. Therefore you are encouraged to discuss availability of the scheduled services with your participating general dentist. Procedures not listed on the schedule of benefits that are performed by the selected participating general dentist will be charged at that participating general dentist's usual and customary fee less 25%.

Should you need a specialist, (Endodontist, Orthodontist, Oral Surgeon, Periodontist, Prosthodontist, Pediatric Dentist), you may be referred by your participating general dentist or you may refer yourself to any participating specialist from our directory. On identification of yourself as a company member, you will receive a 25% reduction from usual and customary fees for services performed. Specialist services are available only in areas where the dental plan has a participating specialist.

When crown or bridgework exceeds six consecutive units, the patient may be charged an additional $25.00 per unit.

*Because these fees change please note that these fees do not necessarily represent actual benefit or copayment costs.

†Plus laboratory fees when applicable.

Continued

Table 6.1—cont'd

Schedule of Benefits and Subscriber Copayments*—cont'd

ADA code	Procedure	Patient pays
PONTICS—cont'd		
2952	Cast post and core	$95.00
2954	Prefabricated post and core	$80.00
2910/2920/6930	Recement inlay/onlay/crown/ bridge (per unit)	$15.00

Endodontics

ADA code	Procedure	Patient pays
3220	Therapeutic pulpotomy	$30.00
ROOT CANALS		
3310	Anterior	$120.00
3320	Bicuspid	$195.00
3330	Molar	$250.00
3410	Apicoectomy (anterior only)	$110.00

Periodontics (gum treatment)

ADA code	Procedure	Patient pays
4210	Gingivectomy/gingivoplasty - per quadrant	$130.00
4211	Gingivectomy/gingivoplasty - per tooth	$40.00
4220	Gingival curettage, surgical - per quadrant	$75.00
4341	Periodontal scaling and root planning - per quadrant	$45.00
4355	Full mouth debridement	$38.00
4381	Localized delivery of chemotherapeutic agents (two teeth)	$45.00
4910	Periodontal maintenance procedures	$45.00

Prosthodontics

Standard complete dentures (includes adjustments within 30 days)

ADA code	Procedure	Patient pays
5110	Complete maxillary (upper)	$280.00
5120	Complete mandibular (lower)	$280.00
5130	Immediate maxillary (upper)	$300.00
5140	Immediate mandibular (lower)	$300.00
Partial dentures (includes adjustments within 30 days)		
5211/5212	Maxillary/mandibular partial - resin base (with two clasps)	$300.00
5213/5214	Maxillary/mandibular partial - cast metal with resin base (with two clasps)	$400.00
5410/5411	Adjust complete - maxillary/mandibular	$15.00

ADA code	Procedure	Patient pays
5421/5422	Adjust partial denture - maxillary/ mandibular	$15.00
5999	Additional clasps	$30.00

Repairs to prosthetics

ADA code	Procedure	Patient pays
5510/5610	Repair broken resin denture base	$20.00†
5520/5640	Replace missing or broken teeth (each tooth)	$15.00†
5520/5640	Each additional tooth	$15.00†
5630	Repair or replace broken clasp	$20.00†
5650	Add tooth to existing partial denture	$30.00†
5850/5851	Tissue conditioning, maxillary/ mandibular	$30.00
5730/5731/5740/5741	Relining (chairside)	$45.00
5750/5751/5760/5761	Relining (laboratory)	$35.00†

Extractions oral surgery

ADA code	Procedure	Patient pays
7110	Single tooth	$15.00
7120	Each additional tooth (per visit)	$15.00
7130	Root removal - exposed roots	$20.00
7210	Surgical extraction of erupted tooth	$40.00
7220	Soft-tissue impaction	$45.00
7230	Partially bony impaction	$65.00
7240	Completely bony impaction	$90.00
7250	Surgical removal of residual tooth roots	$25.00
7310	Alveoloplasty in conjunction with extractions - per quadrant	$25.00
7320	Alveoloplasty not in conjunction with extractions - per quadrant	$60.00

Anesthesia

ADA code	Procedure	Patient pays
9215	Local anesthesia	No charge
9230	Analgesia (nitrous oxide - per 15 min)	$15.00

Adjunctive services

ADA code	Procedure	Patient pays
9951	Occlusal adjustment - limited	$25.00
9952	Occlusal adjustment - complete	$150.00

Orthodontics

Benefits for orthodontics for adults and children are available from Participating Orthodontists at their usual fee less 25%.

4 Preventive services
5 Substance abuse care
6 Mental health care
7 Other services

Covered Benefits

Covered benefits are those types of procedures and treatment the insurance plan will cover. Exclusions are those services that are not covered by the plan. Cosmetic dentistry is not covered because it is a personal option and not essential treatment. In standard health insurance programs, all covered benefits are listed. Dental coverage is usually listed under the heading "other services."

Innetwork Coverage

Innetwork coverage refers to the amount (copayment or coinsurance) of costs that are covered if the insured uses the providers and services within the network or organization. If the plan is offered by a preferred provider organization, maximum benefits will be provided only if the insured uses participating providers.

Out-of-Network Coverage

Some programs will cover a lower amount of service fees if the insured uses an out-of network provider or service. This refers to a provider that is not part of the network. However, many of these types of managed care programs will not pay any of the fees if they are not provided by their participating providers or will only pay a portion if the provider coverage is available.

Types of Deductibles

Insurance programs may cover all fees at 100%. However, with the rising cost of health care, increasing numbers of programs have payment options. Many programs today apply a deductible, except for specific designated services, which must be satisfied before expenses are paid (Box 6-1). The benefits may be based on a single or family deductible. Coverage will also be determined on whether the service has been provided innetwork or out-of-network. Deductibles are sometimes called *surcharges*.

Some covered services will list the amount that the insured pays before the provider pays any expenses. This amount, which is a percentage of expenses, may be identified as *coinsurance*. The amount may be a copayment, which is represented as a specific dollar amount that the insured (patient) is responsible to the provider (dentist) for eligible expenses. A copayment must be paid at the time treatment is rendered. Missed appointments are not eligible expenses.

The **schedule of benefits** may also identify *out-of-pocket limits*, which is the total amount of the fees that the insured must pay before the insurance program will pay any fees. This limit will also be based on whether the benefits cover a single or family plan and if services are provided innetwork or out-of-network.

Schedule of benefits

The type of service, benefits, and innetwork and out-of-network coverage.

Insurance Cards

An insurance card is the patient's ID card. It must be presented to the provider whenever care is received. The card will list the member and group number, names of the family members if covered, and the effective eligibility date. The eligibility date is when the insured is covered by the benefits. Each family member will receive a card. In addition to the general information, the card will also list benefit and copayment information and often the local or toll-free telephone number of the insurance company. An ID card does not mean that the holder is entitled to benefits. The business assistant should check to make sure that the card is properly presented. If the patient is not entitled to use the services and presents the card, this is fraud. If a card is lost or found, it must be reported immediately.

Box 6.1

Summary of Dental Benefits

Deductible   Waived for preventive care and orthodontic
Single: $100
Family: $200

Preventive care   100% of allowable amount

Oral examinations
Cleaning and scaling
Fluoride treatments
Sealants
Bitewing x-rays (1 x-ray per 6 months)
Full mouth (1 x-ray per 2 years)

Prosthetic and restorative services   80% of allowable amount

Fillings, extractions, oral surgery, and space maintainers
Treatment of gums, tissues, and bone that supports teeth
Endodontics, root canal therapy
Antibiotics, tests, lab, emergency pain treatment
Repair and replacement of chipped, broken, or extracted teeth
Inlays, crowns, repair, and installation of full or partial bridgework (subject to limitations)
Oral surgery

Orthodontic treatment   50% (limited to $500 per person per lifetime)

Please refer to the summary plan description for a full disclosure of benefits.

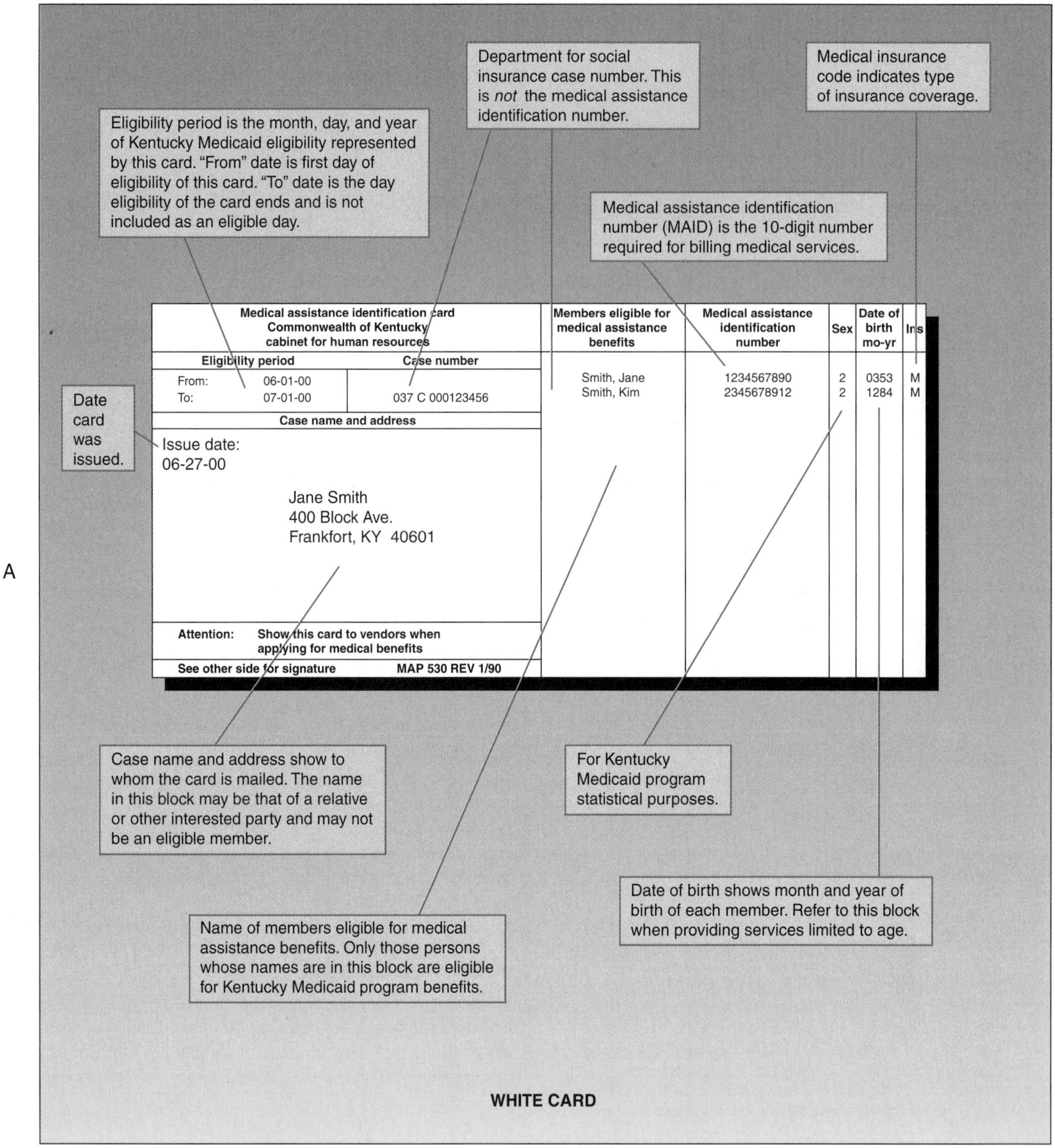

Eligibility period is the month, day, and year of Kentucky Medicaid eligibility represented by this card. "From" date is first day of eligibility of this card. "To" date is the day eligibility of the card ends and is not included as an eligible day.

Department for social insurance case number. This is *not* the medical assistance identification number.

Medical insurance code indicates type of insurance coverage.

Medical assistance identification number (MAID) is the 10-digit number required for billing medical services.

Date card was issued.

Medical assistance identification card Commonwealth of Kentucky cabinet for human resources			Members eligible for medical assistance benefits	Medical assistance identification number	Sex	Date of birth mo-yr	Ins
Eligibility period		Case number	Smith, Jane	1234567890	2	0353	M
From: 06-01-00 To: 07-01-00		037 C 000123456	Smith, Kim	2345678912	2	1284	M
Case name and address							

Issue date:
06-27-00

Jane Smith
400 Block Ave.
Frankfort, KY 40601

Attention: Show this card to vendors when applying for medical benefits

See other side for signature   MAP 530 REV 1/90

A

Case name and address show to whom the card is mailed. The name in this block may be that of a relative or other interested party and may not be an eligible member.

For Kentucky Medicaid program statistical purposes.

Name of members eligible for medical assistance benefits. Only those persons whose names are in this block are eligible for Kentucky Medicaid program benefits.

Date of birth shows month and year of birth of each member. Refer to this block when providing services limited to age.

WHITE CARD

FIGURE 6.2

Kentucky medical assistance identification (MAID) card. **A,** Front of card.

Information to providers. Insurance identification codes indicate type of insurance coverage as shown on the front of the card in "Ins" block.

Providers of service

This card certifies that the person(s) listed hereon is/are eligible during the period indicated on the reverse side, for current benefits of the Kentucky medical assistance program. The Medical assistance identification number must be entered on each billing statement precisely as contained on this card in order for payment to be made.

Questions regarding provider participation, type, scope, and duration of benefits, billing procedures, amounts paid, or third-party liability should be directed to:

Cabinet for Human Resources
Department of Medicaid Services
Frankfort, KY 40621-0001

Insurance identification

A-Part A. Medicare only
R-Part A. Medicare premium paid
B-Part B. Medicare only
C-Both parts A & B Medicare
S-Both parts A & B Medicare
   premium paid
D-Blue Cross Blue Shield
E-Blue Cross Blue Shield
   major medical

F-Private medical insurance
G-Champus
H-Health maintenance organization
J-Unknown
K-Other
L-Absent parent's insurance
M-None
N-United Mine Workers
P-Black lung

Recipient of services

1. This card may be used to obtain certain services from participating hospitals, drug stores, physicians, dentists, nursing homes, intermediate care facilities, independent laboratories, home health agencies, community mental health centers, and participating providers of hearing, vision, ambulance, nonemergency transportation, screening, and family planning services.
2. Show this card to the person who provides these services to you whenever you receive medical care or have prescriptions filled.
3. You will receive a new card at the first of each month as long as you are eligible for benefits. For your protection, please sign on the line below and destroy your old card. Remember that for anyone to use this card is against the law except the persons listed on the front of the card.
4. If you have questions, contact your eligibility workers at the county office.
5. Recipient temporarily out of state may receive emergency Medicaid services by having the provider contact the Kentucky Cabinet for Human Resources, Department for Medicaid Services

_____
Signature

Recipient of services: You are hereby notified that under state law, KRS 205. 624, your right to third-party payment has been assigned to the cabinet for the amount of medical assistance paid on your behalf.
Federal law provides for a $10,000 fine or imprisonment for a year, or both, for anyone who willfully gives false information in applying for medical assistance, fails to report changes relating to eligibility, or permits use of the card by an ineligible person.

Notification to recipient of assignment to the Cabinet for Human Resources of third-party payments

Recipient's signature is not required.

B

FIGURE 6.2, cont'd

Kentucky medical assistance identification (MAID) card. **B,** Back of card.

In Kentucky, the Medicaid program provides a medical assistance identification (MAID) card, which is issued monthly to recipients with ongoing eligibility (Figure 6-2). The card shows a month-to-month eligibility period. Therefore the business assistant should check the card for eligibility even if the patient has been in the office previously. A copy of the card should be kept on file with the patient records. The local agency in each state will be able to provide eligibility information to providers.

Preparing Insurance Claims

When patients call to make an appointment, the business assistant should ask patients if they have dental coverage. If they are covered, they will need to bring the insurance information with them. This will give the assistant and patient an opportunity to review the insurance program. If appointments are requested for a family, the business assistant should find out if the insurance program covers only the certificate holder or the entire family. If custody of children is involved or a power of attorney, the business assistant should also clarify the arrangements and receive copies of necessary documents to keep on file.

Most medical health insurance plans do not include dental coverage. They will usually cover oral and maxillary surgery if the services relate to accidental injury to the jaws, sound teeth, mouth, or face. Some medical conditions that cause loss of oral structures and prohibit the patient from eating (catastrophic disease such as cancer) may be covered. Injury resulting from chewing or biting is usually not considered an accidental injury.

Completing the Claim Form

The business assistant usually completes the claim form. The patient should provide necessary signatures during the first dental appointment. The pretreatment estimate will not be

Check one:
☐ **Dentist's pretreatment estimate**
☐ **Dentist's statement of actual services**

Carrier name and address
Delta Dental of Kentucky
9901 Linn Station Road
Louisville, KY 40223

| 1. Patient name first   m.i.   last | 2. Relationship to employee ☐ Self ☐ Child ☐ Spouse ☐ Other ____ | 3. Sex m f | 4. Patient birthdate MM DD YYYY | 5. If full-time student School City |

| 6. Employee/subscriber name and mailing address | 7. Employee/subscriber soc. sec. or I.D. number | 8. Employee/subscriber birthdate MM DD YYYY | 9. Employer (company) name and address | 10. Group number |

| 11. Is patient covered by another dental plan? Yes No If yes, complete 12-a. Is patient covered by a medical plan? Yes No | 12-a. Name and address of carrier(s) | 12-b. Group no.(s) | 13. Name and address of other employer(s) |

| 14-a. Employee/subscriber name (if different than patient's) | 14-b. Employee/subscriber soc. sec. or I.D. number | 14-c. Employee/subscriber birthdate MM DD YYYY | 15. Relationship to patient ☐ Self ☐ Parent ☐ Spouse ☐ Other ____ |

I have reviewed the following treatment plan. I authorize release of any information relating to this claim.

▶ _____
Signed (patient or parent of minor)   Date

16. Name of billing dentist or dental entity	24. Is treatment the result of occupational illness or injury?	Yes No	If yes, enter brief description and dates.
17. Address where payment should be remitted	25. Is treatment result of auto accident?		
City, state, zip	26. Other accident?		
18. Dentist soc. sec. or T.I.N.	19. Dentist license no.	20. Dentist phone no.	27. If prosthesis, is this initial placement?	(If no, reason for replacement)	28. Date of prior placement
21. First visit date current series	22. Place of treatment Office Hosp. ECF Other	23. Radiographs or models enclosed? No Yes How many?	29. Is treatment for orthodontics?	If services already commenced enter: Date appliances placed Mo. treatment remaining

Identify missing teeth with "x"

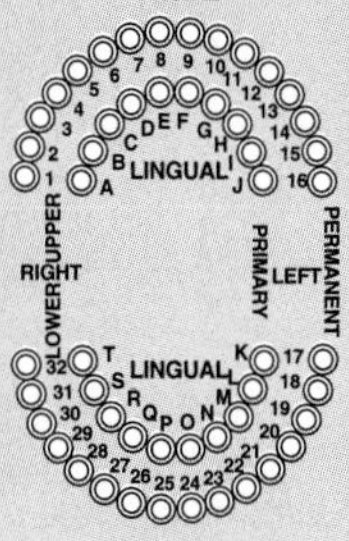

30. Examination and treatment plan. List in order from tooth no. 1 through tooth no. 32. Use charting system shown.

Tooth # or letter	Surface	Description of service (including x-rays, prophylaxis, materials used, etc.)	Date service performed Mo Day Year	Procedure number	Fee

31. Remarks for unusual services

I hereby certify that the procedures as indicated by date have been completed and the fees submitted are the actual fees I have charged and intend to collect for those procedures.

▶ _____
Signed (treating dentist)   Date

32. ☐ Send supply of forms
☐ Have representative call

Total fee charged	
Max. allowable	
Deductible	
Carrier %	
Carrier pays	
Patient pays	

FIGURE 6.3

Delta dental claim form.

approved without the patients signature on the form unless the insurer will accept a signature on file. If the plan is not available and the patient intends on submitting proposed treatment for benefit payment, have the patient provide a social security number and employer name to request insurance information from the employer.

All insurance companies have their own claim forms (Figure 6-3). However, the information included on the various claim forms is similar. The American Dental Association (ADA) has developed a standardize form that is used in dental offices and accepted by many insurance carriers. Most of the information on this standardized form is self-explanatory. However, several items and sections will be clarified.

ADA Standard Claim Form

The form is divided into the patient and dentist sections. When filling out the form, be sure to check if the information represents the dentist's pretreatment estimate or actual services. The carrier's name and address will need to be printed on the upper right-hand corner.

Patient Section

As identified in the patient section, if the patient is not the employee, called the *certificate holder*, the relationship will need to be identified in item 3. The employee's Social Security number should be written correctly. If the patient is covered on another insurance plan, the name and address of the second carrier must be identified along with that group number. Often, the second carrier is associated with the spouse's employer. If this is the case, identify that employee's name and Social Security number for coordination of benefits. Coordination of benefits refers to the identification of the primary and secondary payor. The primary plan will pay first, and the secondary will pay the balance.

The middle left-hand side of the form must be signed by patients to acknowledge the following:

1 They have reviewed the treatment plan
2 They authorize claim information to be released
3 They are responsible for all costs incurred for dental treatment

In addition, patients may choose to prepay for treatment in which they will be reimbursed by filing the claim or they may rather assign the benefits to the provider, called an *assignment of benefits*. If patients have an assignment of benefits, they will need to sign and date the right-hand column to authorize payment directly to the dentist.

Dentist Section

The dentist section must also be filled out carefully. The dentist's Social Security number or tax identification and license numbers must be accurate. The place of treatment, office, hospital, extended care facility, or other facility must be documented. The rest of the information in the dentist section is self-explanatory.

Examination and Treatment Plan Section

The examination and treatment plan must be listed according to the universal numbering system and in order by tooth numbers, 1 to 32. The surface of the tooth and a description of the service must be noted. Make sure to list the correct procedure number and fee.

Dental Procedure Codes

A list of dental procedure codes has been approved by the ADA. The five-digit code numbers identify each dental procedure and service (Table 6-2). Each digit is significant and indicates the following:

1 The procedure is dental
2 The category of service
3 The class of the procedure
4 The subclass

The digit is also used if additional code digits are needed.

Each treatment category corresponds with a numerical code series. For instance, the code series for diagnostic service is 00100-00999, and the code series for orthodontic service is 08000-08999. The business office assistant must have the current code list to accurately complete the claim form and should be aware of changes. Some offices create their own in-office code forms to simplify this process (Figure 6-4).

Table 6.2

CDT-2 Five-Digit Coding System

	Category of service	Code series
I.	Diagnostic	00100-00999
II.	Preventive	01000-01999
III.	Restorative	02000-02999
IV.	Endodontics	03000-03999
V.	Periodontics	04000-04999
VI.	Prosthodontics, removable	05000-05899
VII.	Maxillofacial prosthetics	05900-05999
VIII.	Implant services	06000-06199
IX.	Prosthodontics, fixed	06200-06999
X.	Oral surgery	07000-07999
XI.	Orthodontics	08000-08999
XII.	Adjunctive general services	09000-09999

Code

1. The first number is always "0" indicating a dental procedure.
2. The second number is the type of dental procedure, for example "02" is restorative.
3. The XII adjunctive general services "09" code series is not classified and includes emergency treatment.

CDT code 1995

| Return this form to the receptionist | To file insurance: Complete the personal information on your insurance claim form. Attach this copy and mail to your insurance company. This copy contains all of the information the doctor is required to supply. | Name 0674 |

Diagnostic Fee

☐ 0110 Initial exam ____
☐ 0210 Intraoral - Complete ____
☐ 0220 Intraoral - First film ____
☐ 0230 Intraoral - Each additional # _____ ____
☐ 0272 Bitowing - Two films ____
☐ 0274 Bitowing - Four films ____
☐ 0330 Panoramic film ____
☐ 0470 Diagnostic models ____
☐ 0471 Diagnostic photos ____

Preventive

FLOSSERCIZE™ - A dental health program for a lifetime of healthy smiles

☐ 1110 Prophylaxis - Adult ____
☐ 1351 Sealants - Per tooth @$ _____
____ / ____ / ____ / ____

Restorative

☐ 2140 Amalgam 1 surface p. @$ _____ ____
MODBL MODBL MODBL MODBL
☐ 2150 Amalgam 2 surface p. @$ _____ ____
MODBL MODBL MODBL MODBL
☐ 2160 Amalgam 3 surface p. @$ _____ ____
MODBL MODBL MODBL MODBL
☐ 2161 Amalgam 4 surface p. @$ _____ ____
MODBL MODBL MODBL MODBL
☐ 2330 Composite 1 surface p. @$ _____ ____
MIDFL MIDFL MIDFL MIDFL
☐ 2331 Composite 2 surface p. @$ _____ ____
MIDFL MIDFL MIDFL MIDFL
☐ 2332 Composite 3 surface p. @$ _____ ____
MIDFL MIDFL MIDFL MIDFL
☐ 2335 Composite 4 or more surface p. @$ ___ ____
MIDFL MIDFL MIDFL MIDFL
☐ 2385 Resin 1 surface p. @$ _____ ____
MODBL MODBL MODBL MODBL
☐ 2386 Resin 2 surface p. @$ _____ ____
MODBL MODBL MODBL MODBL
☐ 2387 Resin 3 surface p. @$ _____ ____
MODBL MODBL MODBL MODBL
☐ 2740 Crown-Ceramic @$ _____ ____
____ / ____ / ____ / ____
☐ 2750 Crown-Proc./gold @$ _____ ____
____ / ____ / ____ / ____

Restorative - Cont. Fee

☐ 2790 Crown-Gold @$ _____ ____
____ / ____ / ____ / ____
☐ 2950 Crown buildup-pin retalged @$ _____ ____
____ / ____ / ____ / ____
☐ 2951 Pin retention @$ _____ ____
☐ 2952 Post & core (cast) @$ _____ ____
☐ 2960 Bonding @$ _____ ____
☐ 2962 Ceramic veneer @$ _____ ____
____ / ____ / ____ / ____

Endodontics

☐ 3110 Direct pulp cap @$ _____ ____
____ / ____ / ____ / ____
☐ 3120 Indirect pulp cap @$ _____ ____
____ / ____ / ____ / ____
☐ 33___ Root canal _____ @$ _____ ____
____ / ____ / ____ / ____

Periodontics

☐ 42___ Surgery _____
____ / ____ / ____ / ____
☐ 4341 Scale & root plane (per quad)
UR UL LL LR @$ _____ ____
☐ 4345 Periodontal scaling ____

Prosthodontics - Rem.

☐ 5110 Complete upper ____
☐ 5120 Complete lower ____
☐ 5130 Immediate upper ____
☐ 5140 Immediate lower ____
☐ 5211 Partial upper acrylic ____
☐ 5212 Partial lower acrylic ____
☐ 5213 Partial upper chr ____
☐ 5214 Partial lower chr ____
☐ 54___ ___Adjust ____
☐ 57___ ___Reline ____
☐ 58___ ___Temporary dentures ____

Prosthodontics - Fixed (pontics)

☐ 6240 Proc. w/gold @$ _____ ____
____ / ____ / ____ / ____

Date of service ___ _____
Patient Fee

Prosthodontics - Fixed (pontics) Cont.

☐ 6241 Proc. w/metal @$ _____ ____
____ / ____ / ____ / ____

Prosthodontics - Fixed (retainer)

☐ 6545 Bonded bridge retainer @$ _____ ____
____ / ____ / ____ / ____
☐ 6750 Proc. w/gold retainer @$ _____ ____

Oral surgery

☐ 7120 Extraction - 1 _____ @$ _____ ____
☐ 7120 Extraction - each additional @$ _____ ____
____ / ____ / ____ / ____
☐ 72___ Surgical extraction @$ _____ ____
____ / ____ / ____ / ____
☐ 7310 Alveoloplasty per quad
UR UL LL LR @$ ____ per quad ____

General

☐ 9310 Consultation _____ ____
_____ ____
☐ 9630 Drug/medication ____
☐ 9910 Dosonsit _____ ____
☐ 9940 Occlusal guard ____
☐ 9950 Occlusal analysis (mounted) ____
☐ 9951 Occlusal adjustment (limited) ____
☐ 0000 Broken appointment ____

Overcoming dental anxiety sm • A behavioral control program for those persons desiring to overcome their fear of the dental environment

☐ Other _____ ____
_____
_____
_____
_____
_____

☐ This is a pretreatment ☐ Statement of actual cost estimate
Total charges $ _____

I hereby certify that the procedures indicated have been completed.

Signature _____ Date _____

Assignment and release:
I hereby authorize my insurance benefits to be made directly to the doctor and I am financially responsible for noncovered charges. I also authorize the doctor to release any information required.

Signature _____ Date _____

ID# _____ S.S.# _____
MA Prov. # _____ KY. Lic. # _____

Carol A. Eaton, DMD
Medical building

FIGURE 6.4

An adapted inoffice code form.

Specific Codes

The correct code should always be used. This can be difficult when crowns, bridges, or partial dentures are part of the treatment. The type of metal used in the alloy to fabricate the prosthodontic appliance must be identified by a specific code number. The specific code number relates to the amount of noble metal used in the alloy. Gold, platinum, and palladium are considered noble metals and tin; lead and zinc are base metals. Therefore the name high noble is associated with the higher amounts of noble metal. For example, a full cast crown coded as gold high noble would be 02790 and a full cast crown with noble metal (predominantly a base metal) would be 02792. Each type of casting is coded differently, therefore the business assistant should ask the dentist for clarification if any particular case is not clear.

Filing the Insurance Claim

Dental radiographs may need to be sent with the pretreatment estimate. Do not send the original radiographs. The x-ray mount should be labeled plainly with the patient's name, date, and dentist's name and address. Treatment can be started once the pretreatment estimate is sent to the carrier if the dentist feels assured that treatment will be covered by the patient or the insurance organization. Claims must be filed within 12 months from the date of service. Claim forms will need to be mailed or sent by computer. Electronic transmission can speed receipt of payment and eliminate paper work. The patient's signature should also be kept on file if electronic transmission is used because of the inability for signature authority on the claim form. Scanners are available now that will make this possible.

Once the claim forms are received, the carrier will send the patient and dentist an explanation of benefits. This statement will describe the services provided by the provider and the benefits the carrier has provided. The patient or dentist can contact the carrier if they have any questions. If the claim forms are not sent within the 12-month period, the insurer has the right to refuse payment within 30 days from receipt of the claim.

Medicaid and Medicare Claims

Medicaid and Medicare claims must be filed on state-approved forms and often may be submitted electronically, also using state-approved codes. When claims are submitted electronically, the original form must be submitted as soon as possible. The copy is retained with the patient records. The business assistant must be familiar with the individual state forms.

The Cabinet for Human Resources, Department for Medicaid Services administer the Kentucky Medicaid program. The Medicaid Program, identified as Title XIX of the Social Security Act, was enacted in 1965 and operates according to a state plan approved by the U.S. Department of Health and Human Services. The program is monitored through postpayment review.

The program provides payment for certain medical and dental services provided to Kentucky recipients who lack sufficient income or other resources to meet the cost of medical and dental care. The cabinet sets a reasonable fixed upper limit for all covered services. Reimbursement for covered services by a participating provider must be accepted as payment in full. The patient may not be charged the difference but if a nonparticipating provider treats the patient, the patient is responsible for the services. Also, if the patient agrees to services that are not covered under the KMAP plan, the patient is responsible for charges incurred. Payment is limited to the dental benefit schedule and includes the following:

1 Diagnostic
2 Preventive
3 Oral surgery
4 Endodontics
5 Operative
6 Crown
7 Prosthetics
8 Orthodontics
9 Other services

The Kentucky Medicare program provides services to people who are 65 years of age or older and some disabled people under that age. Dental services are covered under a limited plan. These services cover the treatment of the oral cavity if a life-threatening disease such as cancer is present. The plan will also provide treatment for people who have received trauma to the face or mouth but their primary care physician must refer them and have a documented case of the disease or injury. The services must be filed on the American Medical Association forms using the ADA and international classification of disease (ICP) codes (Figure 6-5).

Past Due Claims

Developing a file system to follow up on the predetermined and payment pending past due claims is necessary. This should be a traditional or electronic alphabetical file with intermittent tracking schedules at 30-, 60-, and 90-day intervals. A telephone call may take care of late reimbursement but a formal written letter, fax, or electronic mail may be necessary. Some insurance carriers have special provider inquiry forms available. The business assistant should become familiar with insurance organization representatives.

Adjustment Requests

The occasion may occur when an adjustment needs to be requested on the original claim. When making an adjustment, make sure the original claim or control number, patient's name, and the dentist's name and address are listed correctly. The business assistant will also need to be specific about what is to be adjusted on the claim and the reason for the adjustment. A copy of the original claim and remittance advice or explanation of benefits will need to be attached. The sample adjustment request form provides a good outline to follow for making an adjustment.

A

1. Recipient last name	2. First name	3. M.i.	4. Medical assistance I.D. number

5. If patient was in any kind of accident, check box: ☐	6. If patient has health insurance, enter the name and address of company and the policy number.

7. If claim required a prior authorization, enter the prior authorization number here:	8. If services were provided because of a screening exam, check box: ☐	9. If patient was referred to you, enter the name of the referring practitioner.	10. Leave blank

11. Universal tooth identification *(Use in coding column 18)*

1	2	3	4	5	6	7	8	9	10	11	12	13	14	15	16	Upper	A	B	C	D	E	F	G	H	I	J
32	31	30	29	28	27	26	25	24	23	22	21	20	19	18	17	Lower	T	S	R	Q	P	O	N	M	L	K

Right — Left Right — Left

12. Line no.	13. Date of service Mo. Day Yr.	14. Procedure description	15. Procedure code	16. Units of service	17. Place of service note (1)	18. Tooth number	19. Charge	20. Leave blank
1								
2								
3								
4								
5								
6								
7								
8								

Note:(1) Place of service codes:

11-Doctor's office	22-Outpatient hospital	52-Day care facility (Psy)
12-Patient's home	24-Ambulatory surgical center	52-Night care facility (Psy)
21-Inpatient hospital	32-Nursing facility	99-Other locations

Total claim charge	21.	22. Leave blank
Less amount from health insurance	23.	
Net claim charge	24.	

26. Provider certification and signature

This is to certify that the foregoing information is true, accurate, and complete and that any subsequent transactions that alter the information contained therein will be reported to the Medicaid program. I understand that payment and satisfaction of this claim will be from federal and state funds and that any false claims, statements or documents, or concealment of a material fact may be prosecuted under applicable federal or state laws.

Signed

27. Provider name and address	28. Provider number	25. Invoice date Month Day Year

31. Name and address of inpatient facility	32. Leave blank	33. Clinic number	29. Leave blank	30. Invoice number 0698644
			34. Leave blank	

FIGURE 6.5

A, Sample Medicaid statement for dental claim.

Block no.	Item name and description

1 Recipient last name
Enter the last name of the recipient exactly as it appears on the current medical assistance identification (MAID) card.

2 First name
Enter the first name of the recipient exactly as it appears on the current (MAID) card.

3 M.I.
Enter the middle initial of the recipient.

4 Medical assistance I.D. number
Enter the recipient's identification number exactly as it appears on his current MAID card. The number consists of 10 digits and all of them must be entered.

5 Accident
Check box provided if the treatment provided to recipient was necessitated by some form of accident.

Note: When billing, Procedure D0130 Block #5 shall be marked to indicate patient was in an accident.

6 Health insurance
If recipient has any kind of health insurance other than Medicare, enter the name and address of the insurer and the policy number.

7 Prior authorization
If the service provided required prior authorization by the department, enter the authorization number assigned by the department for Medicaid services.

8 Screening related services
Check box provided if the treatment provided was a referral from an early and periodic screening, diagnosis and treatment examination.

9 Referring practitioner
If the recipient was a referral, enter the name of the practitioner who referred the recipient.

10, 11, 12 No entry required

Note: Blocks 13 through 19 must be completed for each line of service being billed.

13 Date of service
Enter the date on which each service was provided in month, day, and year sequence and in numeric format. For example, January 2, 1996, would be entered as 01 02 96. Zeros shall precede single digits.

14 Procedure description
Enter a brief description of the service provided to the recipient.

Note: The extraction of supernumerary teeth shall be billed listing the adjacent tooth number with suffix A. Enter this tooth number in the procedure description block (#14) on the MAP-6 form. The procedure description shall also indicate the type of extraction (i.e., simple extraction or impaction).

A description of complexity is also necessary when billing for the exposure of an unerupted or impacted tooth for orthodontic reasons (i.e., soft tissue, partially bony or fully bony).

When billing procedures involving quadrants, please indicate quadrant billing by using quadrant abbreviations (i.e., LLQ, LUQ, RUQ, RLQ). When treatment involves all four quadrants please indicate by writing "Full mouth."

Intravenous sedation billing shall list the medications used and the time sedation was intiated and ended in procedure description block (#14).

B

FIGURE 6.5, cont'd

B, Instructions for use of Medicaid claim form.   *Continued*

15   Procedure code
Enter the HCPCS procedure code (from the codes specified in Section IV) that identifies the service performed.

16   Units of service
Enter the total number of times per line the procedure was performed on the recipient on this date. A maximum of four tooth numbers may be billed per line. When billing the same procedure code for the same date of service, use only one line, when possible, listing the total number of units under Item 16.

Note: When billing for IV sedation the actual sedation time shall be entered in minutes in the units of service block (#16).

17   Place of service
Enter the two-digit code number from the list on the face of the invoice that identifies where the service was provided.

18   Tooth number
Enter up to four tooth identification numbers (from the universal tooth chart shown in block 11) for teeth treated by the service billed on this line. Zeros shall precede single numbers, (e.g., 01). If more than four teeth were treated, additional lines must be used to bill for services. Procedures not requiring tooth identification numbers are: D0110, D0131, D0220, D0230, D0270, D0272, D0274, D0330, D0340, D1110, D1201, D1205, D4210, D4341, D5610, D5620, D5750, D5751, D5931, D5932, D5936, D7260, D7310, D7430, D7510, D7520, D7530, D7880, D7910, D7960, D7999, D8110, D8120, D8370, D9110, D9240, D9310, D9420, and W0725.

Note: Two digit tooth numbers shall be entered in one block only.

19   Charge
On each line, enter the total usual and customary charge for the service listed on that line. Do not enter the dollar sign ($).

20   No entry required

21   Total claim charge
Enter the total of the individual procedure charges listed on lines 1 through 8. Do not enter the dollar sign ($).

22   No entry required

23   Health insurance reimbursements
Enter the total amount (if any) received from other health insurance sources for services billed on this invoice. Do not enter the dollar sign ($).

FIGURE 6.5, cont'd
B, Instructions for use of Medicaid claim form.

Cash Refund Documentation

An occasion might arise when a refund will be necessary. This may occur because payment has been received from another source or for the following reasons:
1 Health insurance, auto insurance, or Medicare payment
2 Billing was in error
3 Duplicate payment was received
4 Processing error or overpayment
5 Paid to wrong provider
6 Money was requested
7 Other

Appeal Procedures

If a claim has been denied, the patient may call a customer service representative who is trained to answer any questions about the plan. The patient has an appeal procedure to follow if resolution is sought. If the customer service representative is not able to resolve the concern satisfactorily, the pa-

---

24   Net claim charge
Subtract the amount in block 23 from the total claim charge in block 21 and enter the remainder. Do not enter the dollar sign ($).

25   Invoice date
Enter the date in month, day, and year numeric format (e.g., 01 02 96) on which this invoice was completed. Zeros shall precede single numbers (e.g., 01). This date shall not precede the date of service.

26   Provider certification and signature
A delegated or authorized signature shall be acceptable. A delegated or authorized signature shall be the name of the dentist who provided the service followed by the name or initials of the person authorized or delegated to sign the claim forms. Stamped signatures shall not be accepted.

27   Provider name and address
Enter the complete name and address of the provider performing the services being billed on this invoice. Use of a rubber stamp shall be permissible for the name and address but not for the signature.

28   Provider number
Enter the eight-digit Kentucky Medicaid provider number assigned to the provider.

29, 30   No entry required

31   Name and address of inpatient facility
If the services were provided in an institutional setting (place of service codes 4, 5, and 7), enter the name and address of the facility; otherwise, leave blank.

32   No entry required

33   Clinic number
If the services were provided by a member of a group or clinic to which payment should be sent, enter the Medicaid clinic provider number assigned for your group or clinic. If clinic number is omitted, payment shall be made to the dentist whose name and provider number appear on the claim.

34   No entry required

FIGURE 6.5, B, cont'd

B, Instructions for use of Medicaid claim form.

---

tient can make a detailed formal written complaint to the second level of response. A written complaint is usually acknowledged within 10 days, with a determination of the case within 30 days.

When review of a written complaint is unsatisfactory to the insured, a formal written complaint can be sent to an appeals committee. At this time an appeals representative will review the grievance with individuals associated with the case and attempt to resolve the issue. If this cannot be accomplished, the appeals committee will review all material and the patient will be given an opportunity to appear at a committee meeting. An appeals committee hearing is not a legal hearing; therefore legal representation is not invited. If the decision is not acceptable, a second level appeal can be made. Emergency appeals procedures are also provided in case of serious medical consequences. The final level of appeal is arbitration. The appeal is final and binding, and costs are shared by both parties.

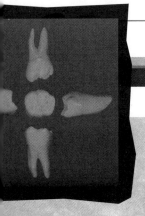

Points for Review

- Financial arrangements
- Presentation of treatment and financial arrangements
- Alternative dental delivery methods
- Preparing the insurance claim
- Filing the insurance claim

Self-Study Questions

1. What is completed before making the financial arrangements?
   a. Determination of the type of insurance available
   b. Treatment plan and fee structure
   c. Claim forms
   d. Provider inquiry form
2. What form should be signed before treating a child?
   a. Custody form
   b. Extended payment plan form
   c. Consent form
   d. Credit card form
3. To what does deferred payment refer?
   a. Insurance plan
   b. Credit report
   c. Cash for service
   d. Credit card
4. What should all patients sign before treatment?
   a. Financial arrangements
   b. Insurance application
   c. Claim forms
   d. All of the above
5. What is the insurance term for the administering agent?
   a. The insured
   b. The insurer
   c. The carrier
   d. b and c

6. What is the insurance term for the patient?
   a. The insured
   b. The policy holder
   c. The claimant
   d. All of the above
7. What is the charge that is paid for services called?
   a. Claim
   b. Benefit
   c. Premium
   d. Plan
8. Does a managed health care program refer to an HMO?
   a. Yes
   b. No
9. What are prevailing fee schedules based on?
   a. Fixed fee schedule
   b. Prevailing fees
   c. Table of allowance
   d. None of the above
10. What term or terms relate to fixed fees?
    a. Capitation
    b. Varying fee schedule
    c. Indemnity program
    d. a and c
11. What is often included in a schedule of benefits?
    a. Type of service
    b. Covered benefits
    c. Code
    d. All of the above
12. What type of coverage does the term *participating providers* refer to?
    a. Out-of-network
    b. Innetwork
    c. Deductible
    d. Surcharge
13. What does the insurance term *provider* mean?
    a. Patient
    b. Carrier
    c. Dentist
    d. Certificate holder
14. What does assignment of benefits mean?
    a. Payment is made directly to the dentist
    b. The patient will need to authorize direct payment
    c. The dentist will be directly reimbursed
    d. All of the above

15. How are dental procedures indicated on the claim form?
    a. By procedure codes
    b. By specific codes
    c. By tooth number
    d. All of the above
16. What does Title XIX of the Social Security Act of 1965 regulate?
    a. Insurance fraud
    b. Only Medicaid
    c. Only Medicare
    d. Medicare and Medicaid
    e. None of the above

Suggested Readings

American Dental Association: *Council on dental care programs*, Chicago.

Colwell Systems, Inc, Champagne, Ill.

CompDent Dental Plan, Louisville, Ky.

Delta Dental Plan of Kentucky, Inc, Louisville.

Dental Assistance Plan, Utica, NY.

Dental Plan Incorporated: *Easy dental software*, Dallas.

Finkbeiner BL: *Practice management for the dental team*, ed 3, St Louis, 1990, Mosby.

ICDC: *Guide to health claims*, Insurance Career Development Center, St Louis, 1994, Mosby.

Medical Assistance Identification: *Commonwealth of Kentucky*, Cabinet for Human Resources.

Mosby's Medicode: *Reimbursement strategies*, St Louis, 1994, Mosby.

Prudential Health Care Dental Support, Louisville, Ky.

Chapter 7

Dental Inventory Control

Dental associates
Supply requisition

5. No. SR-28590

1. Date ordered   9-24-99

Please type or print with blue or black ball point pen.
Do not enter more than one item per line.
Do not write in shaded areas.
Do not return items on this form.
After completion retain part 4-associate copy send parts 1, 2, and 3 to dispensary; part 3 will be returned with merchandise.

6. Associate   A. Anthony D.M.D.

2. Account no. |__|__|__|__| 0 | 8 | 4 | 0 | 1 | 2 |

3. Ordered by Susan Liebetreu

4. Approved by A. Anthony

7. Room no. C-310   8. Phone ext. 4688

13. Date order filled |__|__|__|__|

9. Quantity ordered	10. Unit	11. Description	12. Stock number	14. Quantity shipped	15. Action
2	Btl	Zinc cement, liquid, flick by mizzy	1 0 0 8		
2	Btl	Zinc cement, powder, fleck by mizzy	1 0 0 9		
3	Btl	Zoe, liquid, caulk	1 0 1 0		
3	Btl	Zoe, powder, caulk	1 0 1 1		
1	Btl	Temp. cement kit, CADCO	1 0 4 9		

16. No. of pkg delivered ▢

17. Received by _____   18. Filled by _____

Computer copy

Action
1. Item temporarily out of stock. It will be held on back order and delivered as soon as as received. If this is urgently needed please contact the buyer at 588-0000.
2. Item not carried in dispensory. Please reorder on a purchase requisition and forward to purchasing.
3. Stock numbers and description do not agree. Please check stock catalog and reorder.
4. Partial shipment-balance will be shipped as soon as received.

Chapter Outline

Learning Objectives

On completion of Chapter 7, the student should be able to do the following:

- Define key terms.
- Identify the role of the dental office assistant in inventory control.
- List the important components of a successful inventory control system.
- Identify the types of materials included in dental inventory.
- Identify storage considerations.
- List ordering and payment methods.

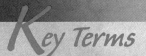

Key Terms

Back Order	Invoice	Storage Guidelines
Discount	Reorder Point	Supplies
Inventory	Requisition	Vendor

IMPORTANCE OF INVENTORY CONTROL

Supplies

Equipment, instruments, and clinical, laboratory, and office materials needed to operate the dental practice.

Inventory

A detailed list of all equipment and dental materials in stock.

Dental offices, like other businesses, must be able to control the large amount of **supplies** they stock for use in the practice. **Inventory** is the quantity or amount of all dental clinic, laboratory, and business office supplies. The materials and equipment dental offices have in stock are part of the assets or value of the dental practice. Inventory control is the system developed and implemented in the dental office to manage the inventory or stock to minimize the amount of supplies in stock and increase other financial opportunities. To do this a dental practice must have a detailed inventory list.

A crisis would occur in the dental office if the doctor needed amalgam and none was stocked. Every dental office should have an effective method of supply control. Whether the dentist or dental assistant is at chairside, in the laboratory, or in the business office, nothing is more frustrating or potentially critical than running out of essential materials. To keep track of stock, one person should be responsible for maintaining the inventory list and ordering needed supplies. However, cooperation of everyone is essential to make sure nothing is taken from inventory without following proper inventory procedures. Developing and maintaining the inventory control system is often the responsibility of the business office assistance.

ESTABLISHING AN INVENTORY SYSTEM AND PURCHASING SUPPLIES

When establishing an inventory system, one must identify all expendable, nonexpendable, and capital items that comprise the dental practice and develop a record or inventory list of those items. Expendable supplies include items that are consumed or used, such as impression materials, x-ray film, cements, cotton rolls, anesthetic, brochures, and paper products. Nonexpendable supplies include items that are not consumed, such as dental instruments, burs, and instrument cassettes. Capital items include costly equipment that is used over a period, such as the dental chair, dental units, autoclave, computer, model trimmer, lathe, and radiographic equipment.

Inventory Record

An inventory record can be designed separately for expendable and nonexpendable supplies and capital equipment. Often expendable and nonexpendable supplies are grouped together and may be divided into clinical and office supplies. The inclusion and design of an inventory system will be determined by the dentist and designated inventory control person.

Large amounts of dental supplies are not kept in stock because of investment costs, the rate of use, storage space, product expiration date, and product change. The availability of suppliers to provide quick delivery will determine the necessity of carrying large amounts of supplies. However, considering the possible price breaks on quantity or larger orders is important. Nonexpendable and capital equipment are only ordered as they break or wear.

Capital Equipment Inventory Record

A capital equipment inventory record should include the name of each piece of equipment in the dental practice, model number, and cost when purchased. The record should also include the name, address, and telephone number of the manufacturer, purchase date, servicing or repair date, type of repair, and name, address, and telephone number of the repairperson. If an outside **vendor** repairs the equipment, an **invoice** or bill will be provided that should be maintained with the capital inventory system. The manufacturer's equipment manual should also be included in a capital equipment inventory file. This information will save time when a piece of equipment breaks and must be repaired or ordered quickly. The inventory information will also identify the depreciation of equipment for tax purposes.

Vendor

The manufacturer's sales representative who sells dental products.

Invoice

The detailed list of goods shipped or services provided and an accounting of all costs.

Expendable and Nonexpendable Supply Inventory

Expendable supplies must be ordered more frequently than nonexpendable items. Therefore the expendable and nonexpendable supply inventory records will require more managed control. A basic alphabetical inventory list of expendable and nonexpendable supplies, whether typed, computerized, or included in a card file, should contain the name of the item, manufacturer, and supplier; the maximum quantity stocked; the minimum amount on hand; cost and reorder date.

When starting an inventory system, a restocking point or reorder level must be established. To establish a reorder level, several things must be considered. Economics will help guide purchasing. The financial outlay needed to buy in bulk or to order costly items will also play a major role in what and how many supplies and equipment are purchased. The person responsible for reordering will need to know the supply budget limitations and control purchases as designated by the dentist.

Rate of Use

Identify the rate of use for each item allowing for potential increase in use, for example how much amalgam is used in 1 day or 1 week and whether school or vacation schedules are beginning. Seasonal changes and holiday vacations can affect the rate that supplies are used or consumed.

Storage

Determine the amount of storage space available. Although dental offices often have a limited amount of space for storage, all supplies should be stored in an organized manner providing quick and easy retrieval. Supplies should also be organized to allow for new materials to be placed toward the back and older materials brought forward. This keeps materials rotating so that older supplies can be used first.

Too many bulky supplies should not be ordered at one time unless plenty of storage space is present. Special attention should be given to supplies such as x-ray film that must be refrigerated or gypsum that should be stored in a dark, cool, or dry area. The storage space should be well lighted to help in finding smaller items quickly. Supply shelves and bins should be clearly labeled to make items easier to find.

OSHA Guidelines

Personnel responsible for handling storage of supplies have an awareness of the Occupational Safety and Health Act (OSHA), the federal **storage guidelines** regarding the use and storage of materials used in the dental office. Dental offices are required to have material safety data sheets on file that contain product information including the following:

1 Name, address, and emergency telephone number of manufacturer who makes the chemical or material
2 Hazardous ingredient data (permissible exposure limits)
3 Physical and chemical data that includes boiling and melting points, evaporation rate, vapor pressure, and water solubility
4 Fire and explosion hazard data such as flash point, flammable limits, and extinguishing media
5 Reactivity data that includes stability and conditions to avoid, incompatibility, and any hazardous byproducts
6 Health-hazard data such as eye, skin, and respiratory protection, routes of entry, carcinogenicity, signs and symptoms of exposure, and emergency and first aid procedures

7 Precautions for safe handling and work practices such as handling and storing precautions, waste disposal methods, and normal clean up
8 Control measures such as respiratory protection, ventilation needs, protective clothing or equipment, and safe work practices

OSHA makes the ultimate decision when disposing hazardous materials. However, local and state laws also govern the disposal of medical waste. The regulations identified by OSHA regarding medical waste or biohazards are outlined in Box 7-1.

Storage guidelines
The proper methods followed when storing and dispensing supplies.

Material safety data sheets can be obtained by writing to the following:
Business and Legal Reports
64 Wall Street
Madison, Connecticut 06443-1513
Telephone: (203) 245-7448

Controlled Substances

Controlled substances must also be handled carefully and should be securely locked as soon as they are received. Because first aid kits often include drugs, they must also be secured in a safe place out of patients' sight and reach. Many dentists have all drugs locked in an office safe with a limited number of staff able to unlock it. This protects the patient, dental personnel, and dentist.

Box 7.1
OSHA Guidelines

1. Sharps such as needles, burs, and scalpel blades, must be separated from paper and fluid products and placed into separate containers.
2. The weight of the biohazard waste must be determined.
3. The waste containers must be leak and puncture proof, inflexible, and sealed tightly.
4. The containers must be labeled as "biohazard." Biohazard labels are available for this purpose.
5. Waste containers must be stored or refrigerated in a controlled area to safeguard and protect from odors.
6. The date and contents must be marked on the container with the dentist's and transporter's names, address, and code number.
7. Disposal can be made to a biohazard processing station by the dentist, designated staff, OSHA-approved transporter, UPS or other mail or pick-up service, depending on local and state regulations.
8. Biohazard waste must be documented with the dentist's and transporter's names, signature, address, state permit, date of shipment, and amount of waste. The record must be maintained for 3 years.

Expiration Limits

Identify the expiration limits of the material, shelf life, length of time material is usable, and storage requirement (for example, some dental materials must be refrigerated).

Delivery Time

Define the delivery time needed, making sure to allow extra time for items that may often be more difficult to get during a normal delivery turn around time.

Special Purchase Rates

Identify items that are often on special and the best quantity for the price. For instance the best value for the money may be 1000 items for $19.95. Although local dental suppliers may be convenient, large **discount** or wholesale suppliers may provide better rates and faster service through electronic mail ordering. Catalogs, listing products and often special prices, are provided by all suppliers. The person designated with ordering responsibilities must keep up with current prices and new materials. Decide how sales representatives are to be scheduled and if the dentist will speak to a representative who comes by the office.

Discount

A reduction in the cost, quantity, or value of products.

Laundry

Clinic scrubs and uniforms should be kept clean and laundered. Many dental practices provide uniforms for all office personnel and contract with a commercial laundry to clean the uniforms or provide a weekly uniform rental service.

Financing

Economics will help guide purchasing. The financial outlay needed to buy in bulk or order costly items will also play a major role in what and how much supplies and equipment are purchased. The person responsible for reordering will need to know the supply budget limitations and control purchases as designated by the dentist.

Inventory Record Systems

Inventory records can be typed as a list on paper and kept in a binder, recorded in a card file index, or entered into a computerized program. Most supplies will be ordered from dental representatives but some items such as medications and drugs are ordered from the local pharmacy. Business office and cleaning supplies are usually purchased from local business suppliers or ordered through the mail. Cost and service will also be a consideration when ordering office supplies.

Card File Inventory System

A card file inventory control or retrieval system will require a separate file card to be completed and filed alphabetically for each stocked item listed on the master inventory list. The same information will be needed for each item in the inventory regardless of what system is used. A card file will usually include the primary section identified as the "inventory" (Figure 7-1). As items are needed, the card is retrieved, the

Item name:	Zinc Cement-Liquid	Card number: 949
Brand:	Fleck's #605-1400	Manufacturer: Mizzy
Vender:	Aims Dental Supply	Telephone: (616) 796-0000
Address:	816 Grant Street Big Rapids, MI 49307	Fax: (616) 796-1000

Maximum stocked	Minimum on-hand	Unit	Unit price	Amount ordered	Date ordered	Date received
4	2	BTL	5.25	2	9/24/99	9/30/99

FIGURE 7.1

Sample inventory card file system.

Back order

An unfilled order that will be available at a later date.

items are ordered, and the card is placed in the ordered section. Items may not be available at the supply center immediately. If this happens, the supply center will notify the office and the card will need to be placed in a **back order** section for follow up. Red tags may be used to flag the back order so that it will not be forgotten (Box 7-2).

Inventory List System

An inventory list contains much of the same data as found in the inventory file card system except that the items are entered into a continuous alphabetical listing. This list can be typed or computerized. The inventory list is usually designed into category columns using a supplier code number instead of the supplier's name, address, and telephone and fax numbers (Figure 7-2). Because of the space needed for this amount of information, the suppliers are listed alphabetically on another form with a code number that corre-

---

Box 7.2

Procedure

Procedure for Initiating and Maintaining an Inventory File Card

1 Secure file box for cards and have the formatted or designed index cards printed.
2 Fill out the top of the card for each expendable and nonexpendable item, including the name of the item brand, supplier, address, telephone and fax numbers, and manufacturer name.
3 Note the maximum amount of stock you plan to keep in inventory and the minimum amount essential for operations.
4 List the unit price for the item.
5 Note the maximum amount to be ordered.
6 Decide the date to reorder stock.

7 Place red flag reorder label on low stock items.
8 If an item and reorder label are removed from the shelf, give to appropriate person initiating the ordering of supplies.
9 Place the reorder label with the file card and note the date and quantity ordered on the card and file under ordered.
10 When the new items arrive, place the reorder label on the minimum amount bottle.
11 Record the date and amount received on the file card. (This should bring the maximum amount to the desired level.)

	Dental associates								
Initial date: 9/15/99	inventory supply list								
For October, 1999			All doctors						
Supplier code #	Item name	Brand	Manuf	Maximum stocked	Minimum needed	Amount on-hand	Reorder date	Item cost	Date received
949	Zinc cement	Fleck Liq	Mizzy	4	2	2	9/24/99	5.25	9/30/99
949	Zinc cement	Fleck Pwd	Mizzy	4	2	2	9/24/99	5.25	9/30/99
949	ZOE	ZOE Liq	Caulk	6	3	3	9/24/99	5.50	9/30/99
949	ZOE	ZOE Pwd	Caulk	6	3	3	9/24/99	5.50	9/30/99
541	ZONE	Temp	CADCO	2	1	1	9/24/99	14.90	9/30/99

FIGURE 7.2

Sample computerized inventory supply list.

sponds with the code number on the inventory list. In addition to the supplier code number, the inventory list includes columns for the name of the item, brand, manufacturer, maximum quantity stocked, minimum amount needed in supply, reorder date, and cost of the item.

Box 7-3 details the procedure for entering data into an inventory list. This information can be easily accessed, particularly if the inventory and supplier lists are in the computer. Today, a needed item can be identified on the computer and sent directly by electronic mail to the supplier. Overnight delivery and 1-day service make reordering and delivery convenient and eliminates the need for large amounts of inventory and cash output.

Master Inventory List

A master inventory list can be designed to document all office, clinical, laboratory supplies, and instruments and equipment used in that dental practice. This list is not necessarily used for ordering but for having a comprehensive list of all inventory. Many dental practices initiate this data and enter it into a computer for access to weekly, monthly, and yearly inventory references. This information usually includes the name of the program (for example, prg INV915), page number, date, and time the inventory was retrieved from the computer program (Figure 7-3). The columns can include the item number, description of the item, unit or abbreviation for how the item is packaged, for example, bottle (btl), box (bx), each (ea), amount on hand, unit price, and extended price (total price of all like items).

The *ADC office set-up guide* provides a comprehensive list of dental office supplies including the following:

- Business office supplies
- Laboratory equipment, supplies, and accessories
- Operating room equipment, instruments, and accessories
- Surgical supplies and accessories
- Filling materials and supplies
- Prosthetic supplies and accessories
- X-ray film processing supplies and accessories
- Paper and cotton goods

This list can be used to develop an individualized office inventory system.

In addition to a master inventory list, the inventory system may include a computer-generated inventory master maintenance report. This maintenance report identifies each item

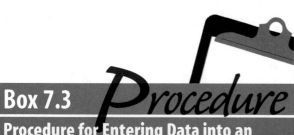

Box 7.3 Procedure

Procedure for Entering Data into an Inventory List

1 Inventory programs are available for the computer but easily programmed into the computer by the office assistant who has some basic computer skills.
2 The described data will need to be gathered and placed on the typed list or computer list in appropriate columns.
3 The item identified at the minimum supply level will be identified with the red flag reorder label.
4 As supplies are needed, the reorder label is attached to the typed list or keyed into the computer as ordered.
5 Back orders can be noted on the list.
6 The computer inventory list can be cross-referenced so that current orders or back orders can be identified or a list of supplies purchased or supply costs for that month or year can easily be obtained.

Run date	11/16/99	Dental associates		Prg name Inv915
Run time	16/11/45	inventory master list		Page 1
Location - 1				

Item number	Description	Unit	On-hnd	U-price	Ext-price
1859	Accufilm II, black/red	BX	5	10.00	50.00
1443	Accufilm II, black/red	PAC	2	14.00	28.00
1	Acetone	BT	5	3.92	19.60
3	Acrilustre, 5 oz.	EA	2	2.60	5.22
199	Adhesive, hold spray-on tray 2.7 oz.	CN	29	7.25	210.25
325	Adhesive, permlastic	BT	2	8.15	6.30
507	Aiming ring - anterior & bite wing	EA	4	1.98	7.92
508	Aiming ring - posterior	EA	4	1.98	7.92
1759	Air techniques starter	BTL	3	5.50	16.50
89	Alcohol dena red	AL	2	5.98	1.76

FIGURE 7.3

Sample working dental office master inventory list.

Reorder point

The point at which a dental item needs to be reordered to maintain a certain level of supplies.

stocked in an individual file from which reports can be generated as needed. The report may include the item number, description, costs, vendor number, **reorder point**, and maximum inventory. The report may also include command codes.

Reorder Point

Establish and record the reorder point for each item by making the following observations and decisions:

1 Identify the maximum amount of stock you plan to keep in stock or inventory.
2 Determine the minimum or low amounts of each item essential for operations.
3 Affirm the unit price for all items.
4 Decide the amount that should be ordered to bring stock to maximum inventory.
5 Determine the date for recordering stock.

The reorder point will need to be marked on the supplies in reserve. This can be done with red flag reorder labels (tape or tag). This reorder label should be placed on the item that represents the minimum number to be kept on hand or the reorder point. The reorder labels should be placed on the items at the time the inventory system is established. For instance, if six bottles of ZOE cement represents the maximum amount to be stocked and two is the minimum amount needed, the reorder label is placed on bottle number two. When bottle number two with the label is removed from the shelf, the reorder label is given to the person designated to complete the ordering of supplies. As soon as the item is ordered, the reorder label can be placed with the file card and the date and quantity ordered entered onto the card and filed under "ordered." When the new items arrive, the reorder label can again be placed on the bottle that represents the minimum amount

on hand or bottle number 2. At this time, the date and amount received can be placed on the file card or inventory list. This should bring the maximum amount to the desired level.

A computer program can be designed to provide a detailed inventory reorder report. The described inventory reorder list provides the item number, description, total on hand, reorder point, and amount below the reorder point. This type of computer print out provides a detailed and up-to-date list of what stock needs to be reordered at any time (Figure 7-4).

In addition to the reorder report, the dentist may wish to identify what and how many specific supplies have been ordered from a particular vendor. This information can be retrieved through the use of a computer-generated ordering analysis report. This report can identify the vendor number, name of the vendor, telephone and fax numbers, item number, description, vendor item number, category, unit, packaged account, reporting months, amount on hand, how many used or sold, price, and quantity ordered.

ORDERING SUPPLIES

The person responsible for ordering supplies must be informed of new products and ideas. The staff person should also be alert and aware of special savings, such as seasonal savings, convention specials, or supply house specials. They should also review the inventory periodically, know what is needed, how much of it is needed, and must be able to supply all the correct information necessary to identify and order the product. Supply catalogs must be kept up-to-date. The ordering person should have a working relationship with supply distributors and area representatives because they can provide information on new products, let the office know of any specials, and answer specific questions the dentist and personnel may have about a particular product or piece of equipment.

Run date	10/07/99	University of Louisville			Prg name Inv925
Run time	9/50/43	inventory reorder list			Page number 1
Locations - 1					

Item number	Description	Tot on-hnd	Reorder point	Below reorder
223	Bags, isolation-red, 20″ × 18″ × 45″ − *1	1	1	
884	Bags, poly (10 × 10 × 24 − .001) bulk - 1000	3	8	5
510	Bars (arms) - bite wing		4	4
445	Brush, bridge & clasp	1	1	
1580	Bur, curbide #703 hp	70	100	30
921	Bur, diamond #813 - 018 fg		6	6
686	Burnisher, brittman #1 - *3	4	6	2
1617	Denture orientation kit	10	12	2
91	dh kit w/311 brush, floss, & mouth mi	12	64	52
138	Finishing & polishing strips	1	2	1
151	Floss threaders (10 env./pkg.)	7	10	3
1072	Ion, ow, pol rb #10	2	10	

FIGURE 7.4

Inventory reorder list.

Supply Requisition

Requisition
A formal written request for something needed.

A dental supply **requisition** is a formal written request for clinical, office, or laboratory supplies. Requisitions are not purchase orders but are requests for supplies, and often preauthorization or approval is needed before retrieval from the stock room or purchase from an outside vendor. These requisitions are often used for accounting purposes. The use of a preapproved requisition is important in an educational institution or dental clinic in which several associate dentists have a centralized storage area or dispensary. Centralization of supplies in a stock room for several dentists provides the financial benefit of ordering larger quantities of stock at reduced cost.

The stockroom requisition will let the dispensary staff know that the item needs to be retrieved from existing stock for that particular dentist. It will also initiate an order for the purchaser (dispensary manager, office manager, or purchasing agent). At this point, needed items can be ordered to fill low inventory. When the stockroom requisition is authorized and signed in duplicate, the item or items may be retrieved from dispensary stock. The duplicate is usually returned with the items requested. This type of requisition can be used as the first step in requesting supplies or approving a request and then ordering the items. If a requisition is used as the initial request, it must be followed by a purchase order.

General Supply Requisition Information

Information on a supply requisition will include general data, signature authority, and specific ordering requirements. Figure 7-5 provides a sample of a supply requisition with the following ordering data:

1 Date ordered
2 Account number assigned to a particular associate dentist
3 Name of person placing the order
4 Name of person approving the order
5 Supply requisition (SR)
6 Name of associate dentist
7 Room or clinic number to be delivered
8 Telephone extension

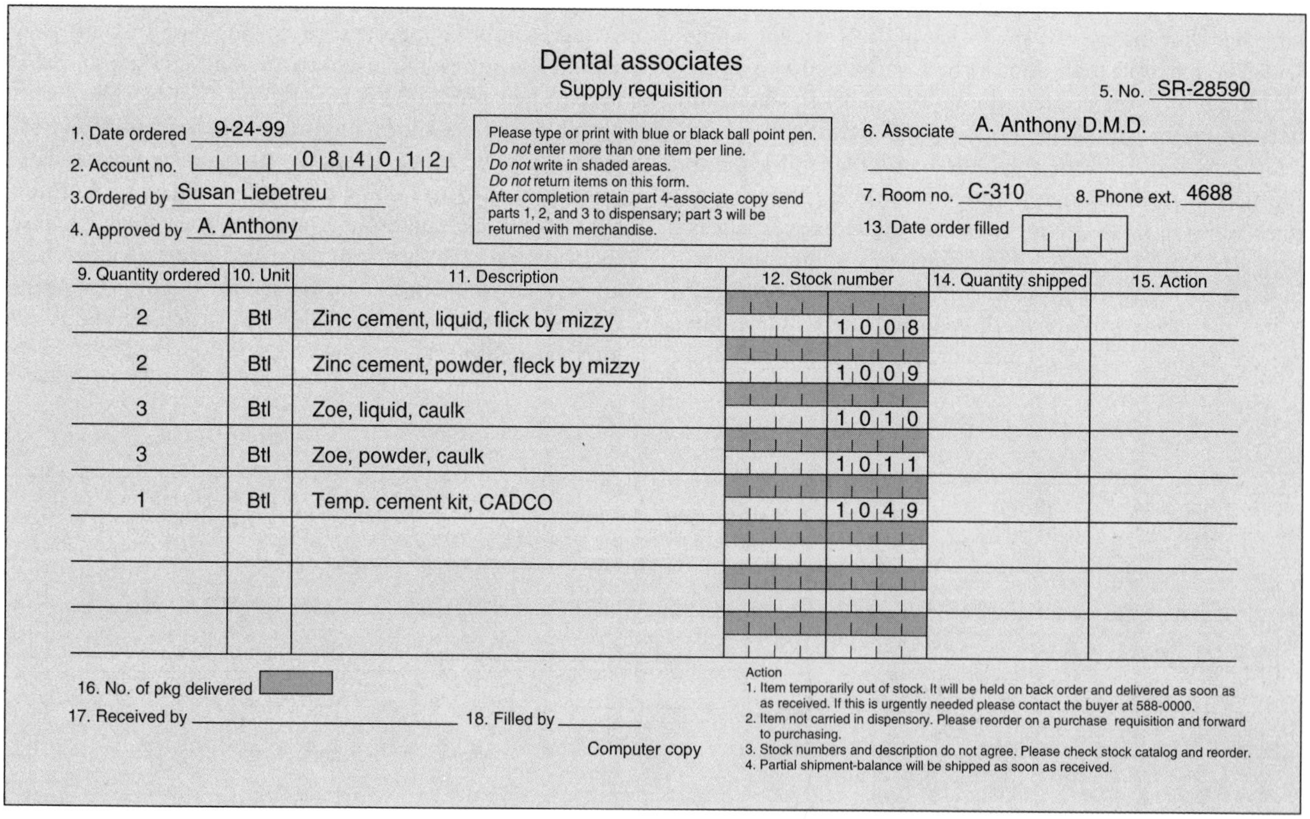
Dental associates
Supply requisition

5. No. SR-28590

1. Date ordered 9-24-99
2. Account no. 0 8 4 0 1 2
3. Ordered by Susan Liebetreu
4. Approved by A. Anthony

Please type or print with blue or black ball point pen.
Do not enter more than one item per line.
Do not write in shaded areas.
Do not return items on this form.
After completion retain part 4-associate copy send parts 1, 2, and 3 to dispensary; part 3 will be returned with merchandise.

6. Associate A. Anthony D.M.D.
7. Room no. C-310 8. Phone ext. 4688
13. Date order filled

9. Quantity ordered	10. Unit	11. Description	12. Stock number	14. Quantity shipped	15. Action
2	Btl	Zinc cement, liquid, flick by mizzy	1008		
2	Btl	Zinc cement, powder, fleck by mizzy	1009		
3	Btl	Zoe, liquid, caulk	1010		
3	Btl	Zoe, powder, caulk	1011		
1	Btl	Temp. cement kit, CADCO	1049		

16. No. of pkg delivered
17. Received by ____ 18. Filled by ____
Computer copy

Action
1. Item temporarily out of stock. It will be held on back order and delivered as soon as as received. If this is urgently needed please contact the buyer at 588-0000.
2. Item not carried in dispensory. Please reorder on a purchase requisition and forward to purchasing.
3. Stock numbers and description do not agree. Please check stock catalog and reorder.
4. Partial shipment-balance will be shipped as soon as received.

FIGURE 7.5
Sample supply requisition information.

Stock Information

The dental office assistant should be specific and provide correct stock information when ordering each item. This data can include the following:

9 Quantity or amount ordered
10 Unit (box, bottle, and package)
11 Item description
12 Dispensary stock numbers (corresponds to the master inventory list)

The account number, store requisition number, date the order is filled, stock number, and quantity shipped is keyed for computer entry. This computer data system provides the practice with up-to-date information on inventory.

Confirming Requisitions for Delivery

Once the order is filled, the following information is confirmed on the requisition:

13 Date order is filled
14 Quantity shipped
15 Action
16 Number of packages delivered
17 Received by
18 Order filled by

The word *action* in the lower right corner refers to what has happened if the complete order is not delivered. For instance, if the item is temporarily out of stock, not carried in dispensary, an error exists in stock number and description, or partial shipment has occurred. If an item is not carried in dispensary, it will need to be reordered from an outside vendor on a purchase requisition.

Purchase Order

A purchase order is used to order supplies from vendors. A signed purchase order and assigned purchase order number (PO) is the promise or obligation (OB) to pay for the items shipped. These PO or OB numbers let the person requesting the items and distributor know the items being ordered are approved for payment. The approved purchase order may then be sent to the appropriate vendor by the person requesting the items or the purchasing agent. The person responsible for ordering supplies can use purchase forms provided by distributors or vendors or they can use order forms that have been designed by the dental practice. The methods of ordering include placing orders directly by mail, telephone, fax, other methods of electronic mail, or automatically as designated by the date on inventory. A purchase order is usually prepared in duplicate. One copy is returned with the items ordered. An invoice may be returned with the order instead of the purchase order copy.

Remember the difference between the supply requisition and the purchase order. The supply requisition is used to obtain purchase approval and a PO number and provide data on delivery of the supplies (numbers 13 through 18). The purchase order is the actual obligation to pay for the listed items. Purchase orders will usually include the following general information:

1 Name of dental practice with address and telephone and fax numbers
2 Date items were ordered
3 Account number (if established and approved)
4 Who ordered the items
5 Dentist signature
6 Quantity ordered
7 Unit
8 Description of each item
9 Catalog number (may include page number)
10 Price per item
11 Total price
12 Delivery charge (if appropriate)

RECEIVING SUPPLIES

When supplies are received, the date of the receipt should be stamped or written on the invoice in case of future questions. The person ordering for the dental practice should be aware that difficulties are occasionally encountered with delivery of the supplies. Sometimes a partial shipment will be sent with the balance to follow, or large orders may be sent in separate packages. Items may be temporarily out of stock through the distributor and will be held for back order and delivered as soon as the item is in stock. If this happens, the distributor will notify the office immediately.

If a back order is a problem for the dental practice and an item is needed at once, the person responsible for ordering supplies in the dental office can contact the distributor, immediately on receiving the back order, and work with a sales representative to identify a local source for the item. The manufacturer representative and local sales representative are important to the dental office. Most representatives provide information and samples of new products and are usually willing to show office staff how to mix materials or operate new equipment. They will also help identify equipment problems and find solutions for office inefficiencies. Most representatives know the dental community and are willing to help dental practices.

The person who requisitions supplies should document all essential order information carefully so that descriptions are accurate and stock numbers and descriptions are the same.

Packing Slips and Invoices

Each package received in the dental office will contain a packing slip (or list), an invoice, or both. A packing slip lists the items in the package, but an invoice will list the contents, price of each item, and total charge. A packing slip will often have a perforated section that will be removed by the delivery service on receipt of the package. An invoice is often provided in place of a statement of charges or the bill. Invoices may have a general, simple form or they may be detailed. When a supply order copy is used as the invoice, the delivery duplicate is usually returned with the package.

The person receiving the delivery should check to make sure that each item on the invoice has been delivered and the bill is accurate before signing for the order or paying for the delivery, if appropriate.

If an item is back ordered, it must be noted and entered on the inventory card. After the invoice has been verified, place it in the "to be paid" file or if paid, in the "paid" file. New supplies will need to be stored and entered in the inventory system. If the invoice is not paid at the time of delivery, a statement will usually be received at the end of the month or designated time. *Do not pay* an invoice or statement without checking for accuracy first.

Tracking Orders

Tracking an order may include following up on a purchase not received or may entail keeping an inventory system of items that have been sold or delivered on a routine basis. Occasions may arise when tracking or checking an order is necessary because the order is late, a change or substitution in the order is needed, or a question arises about the product. If this happens, have the purchase order, account, and stock numbers, date the item was ordered, and description in hand when contacting the vendor. Following up a verbal conversation with written communications to clarify the discussion or confirm what has been said may also be necessary. Sometimes several calls have to be placed to clarify the question or problem and also resubmitting the order with a request for confirmation of receipt has to occur.

In large dental facilities, as part of the inventory system, identifying which clinic (customer) received the dispensed items is essential. A computerized tracking system can provide this information easily. A tracking report can indicate the item number, a description of the item, the invoice date, the quantity sold, and the customer or clinic number.

Returning Orders and Receiving Credit

Sometimes a whole order or items in an order need to be returned to the dental supplier for credit. Occasionally an item may be broken or damaged. The item should be returned to the supplier immediately for replacement, and return a copy of the invoice with the item or items to assure proper credit. If this happens, the supplier will send a credit memo or credit slip to the office to confirm the transaction (Figure 7-6, *A*). Credit will usually appear on the following month's statement from the supplier (Figure 7-6, *B*).

A

Credit memorandum

Dental Supply
14 West Sixth Street
Louisville, KY 40204

Telephone: (502) 895-0000
Fax: (502) 895-1111

No. 084012

Date 10/1/99

To: Dr. J. J. Coyne
454 Bishop Lane
Louisville, KY 40000

Your account has been credited for: Original

Quantity	Description	Cat. no.	Unit price	Amount
2	BTL zink cement, liquid fleck by mizzy	1008	5.25	10.50

Date 12-14-99

Statement of account

To: Dr. J. J. Coyne
454 Bishop Lane
Louisville, KY 40000
Telephone (502) 466-2222
Fax (502) 466-2000

Dental Supply
14 West Sixth St.
Louisville, KY 40204
Telephone (502) 895-0000
Fax (502) 895-1111

Date	Code	Charges	Credits	Balance due
9-15-99	802	87.50		
10-1-99	802		10.50	
				77.00

FIGURE 7.6

A, Credit memorandum form. **B,** Statement of account.

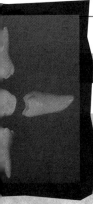

Points for Review

- Importance of dental inventory control
- Establishing an inventory system and purchasing supplies
- Importance of Internet and other electronic computer services
- Identifying inventory record systems
- Ordering supplies
- Delivery of dental supplies

Self-Study Questions

1. What is the quantity or amount of all dental supplies, materials, and equipment called?
   a. Expendable supplies
   b. Nonexpendable materials
   c. Inventory
   d. Capital equipment

2. What are dental instruments, burs, and instrument cassettes called?
   a. Expendable supplies
   b. Nonexpendable materials
   c. Capital equipment
   d. All of the above

3. Which of the following should be considered when establishing a reorder level for supplies?
   a. Rate of use
   b. Storage
   c. Special purchase rates
   d. All of the above

4. What act is responsible for how hazardous materials are handled?
   a. Occupational Safety and Health Act
   b. Employee Protection Act
   c. Dental Practice Act
   d. None of the above

5. What must be handled carefully and locked as soon as they are received?
   a. Medications
   b. Controlled substances
   c. Hazardous materials
   d. All of the above

6. Which of the following indicate how a reorder point for supplies is established?
   a. Identify the maximum amount needed
   b. Determine the minimum amount needed
   c. Shelf life of the item
   d. All of the above

7. What is a formal written request for supplies called?
   a. Purchase order
   b. Supply requisition
   c. Back order
   d. Invoice

8. What is the name given to a written obligation to pay for listed items?
   a. Purchase order
   b. Supply requisition
   c. Back order
   d. Invoice

9. What form will often be included in a delivered package to act as a statement of charges?
   a. Purchase order
   b. Supply requisition
   c. Back order
   d. Invoice

10. What is included with an order if an item is out of stock?
    a. Purchase order
    b. Supply requisition
    c. Back order
    d. Invoice

Suggested Readings

American Dental Cooperative, Inc. *ADL office set-up guide*, St Louis, 1996.
Finkbeiner BL, Finkbeiner CA: *Practice management for the dental team*, ed 5, St Louis, Mosby (in press).

Unit III

Dental Sciences, Principles, and Techniques

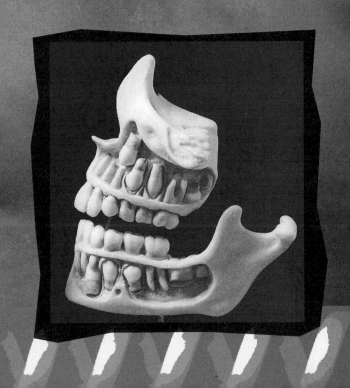

Chapter 8

Anatomy and Physiology

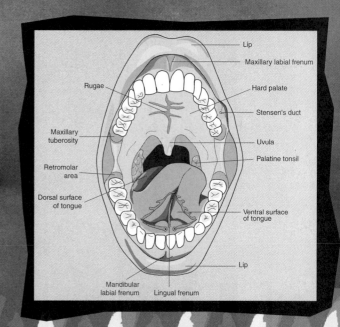

- Lip
- Maxillary labial frenum
- Rugae
- Hard palate
- Stensen's duct
- Maxillary tuberosity
- Uvula
- Retromolar area
- Palatine tonsil
- Dorsal surface of tongue
- Ventral surface of tongue
- Lip
- Mandibular labial frenum
- Lingual frenum

Chapter Outline

Anatomy and Physiology
    Terminology of anatomy
    Structural units of the body
The Skeletal System
    Functions of the skeletal system
    Structure of bone
    Joints
    Appendicular skeleton
The axial skeleton
    Bones of the skull
    Bones of the middle ear
    Bones of the face
The Muscular System
    Structure of muscle
    Types of muscle
    Muscle activity
    Muscle origin and insertion
    Major muscles of facial expression
    Major muscles of mastication
    Muscles of the floor of the mouth
    Muscles of the tongue
    The pillars of fauces
    The temporomandibular joint
The Nervous System
    Neuron
    Central nervous system
    Peripheral nervous system
The Circulatory System
    Blood
    Heart

Arteries of the face and oral cavity
    Major veins of the face and oral cavity
The Lymphatic System
    Lymph fluid
    Lymph vessels and capillaries
    Lymph nodes
    Tonsils
    Spleen
    Thymus
The Respiratory System
    Lungs
    Diaphragm
    Bronchi
    Trachea
    Larynx
    Pharynx
    Nose
The Digestive System
    The oral cavity
    Accessory structures of the digestive
      system
    Phases of swallowing
The Urinary System
    Kidneys
The ureters, bladder, and urethra
The Reproductive System
    Female
    Male
The endocrine system
Skin
Composition of Skin

Learning Objectives

On completion of Chapter 8, the student should be able to do the following:

- List the 12 major systems of the body and describe their main functions.
- Identify the anatomic landmarks of the maxilla and mandible.
- Describe the functions and locations of the major muscles of facial expression, mastication floor of the mouth, and muscles of the tongue.
- List and describe the special senses of the peripheral nervous system and discuss the innervation of the oral cavity.
- List the arteries and veins of the face.
- Describe the main function and components of the lymphatic system.

- Describe how the AIDS virus affects the immune system.
- List the components of the respiratory system and their functions.
- List the accessory structures of the digestive system, with special emphasis on the salivary glands.
- List the structures of the urinary system and their functions.
- Describe the components of the female and male reproductive systems.
- List and describe the seven glands of the endocrine gland, their locations, and their functions.

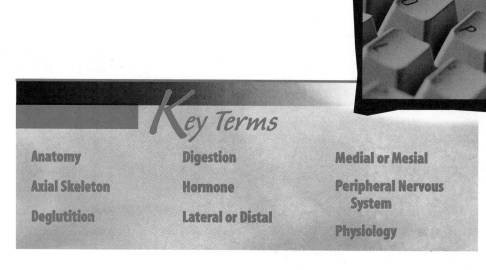

ANATOMY AND PHYSIOLOGY

Anatomy
The study of the body and its parts.

Physiology
How the body functions.

The human body is comprised of many parts. The study of the body and its parts is called *anatomy*. **Physiology** is how the body and its parts function or work.

This chapter is divided in the following manner:

1 Terminology of anatomy
2 Structural units of the body
3 Systems of the body

Terminology of Anatomy

To understand anatomy and physiology, certain terms must be learned. This section is divided into the terminology of body direction and body planes.

Body Directions

The terms of body directions are as follows:

1 *Superior* or *cephalic* is that portion of the body that is toward the head, upper.
2 *Inferior* or *caudal* is that portion of the body that is toward the feet, lower.
3 *Anterior* or *ventral* is that portion of the body that is toward the front.

4 *Posterior* or *dorsal* is that portion of the body that is toward the back.
5 ***Medial*** or ***mesial*** is that portion of the body that is toward the middle.
6 ***Lateral*** or ***distal*** is that portion of the body that is toward the side.

Body Planes

Medial or mesial
The portion of the body that is toward the midline.

Lateral or distal
The portion of the body that is toward the side.

The *anatomic position* is the standard position of the body from which all terminology is based. In this position the body is upright, the head is forward, the feet are forward and slightly apart, and the arms are at the side with palms forward. The body planes are as follows:

1 The *sagittal plane* is any vertical plane that divides the body into right and left sides. The sagittal plane divides the body at the midline into equal halves (Figure 8.1, *A*).
2 The *frontal plane* is sometimes referred to as *coronal plane*. It divides the body into front and back or anterior and posterior sections (Figure 8.1, *B*).
3 The *transverse plane* is also known as the *horizontal plane*. It divides the body into upper and lower or superior and inferior sections (Figure 8.1, *C*).

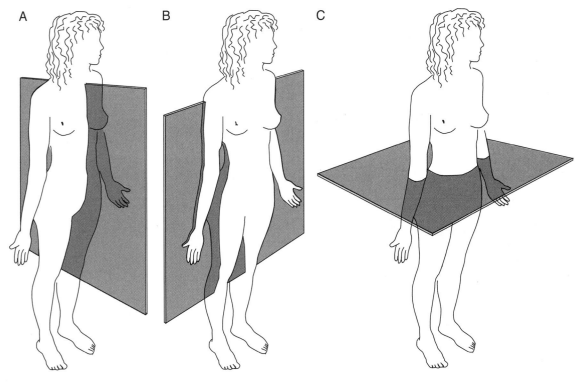

FIGURE 8.1

Body planes. **A**, Midsagittal plane. **B**, Frontal (coronal) plane. **C**, Transverse (horizontal) plane.

Structural Units of the Body

Cells

The basic structural unit of the body is the cell. Cells are grouped together in a specialized manner to form tissues. Tissues organize themselves into organs. Organs group themselves together to form systems. Cells are composed of the nucleus, plasma membrane, and cytoplasm.

The *nucleus* is the brain of the cell. It controls all cellular activity. Within the nucleus is stored the body's genetic material or DNA (deoxyribonucleic acid).

The *plasma membrane* or cell wall encloses the cell and contains the cell's contents. This membrane is important in maintaining the fluid volume of a cell.

The *cytoplasm* is the cellular material between the plasma membrane and nucleus. The cytoplasm contains many specialized organelles that carry out specific cellular functions. Most cellular activity occurs within the cytoplasm.

Cells are classified according to their shape and arrangement. *Squamous* cells are flat or scalelike. *Cuboidal* cells are cube shaped. *Columnar* cells are columnar shaped. *Simple* cells are the thickness of a single cell layer and have the same shape. *Stratified* cells are many layers thick and of the same shape.

Tissues

When groups of similar cells specialize for a common function, a tissue is formed. Some of the tissues discussed are ep-ithelial and connective. Muscular and nervous tissues are discussed in their respective systems.

Epithelial tissue makes up the internal lining, glandular tissue, and external covering, or skin, of the body. Epithelial tissue is classified according to the shape and arrangement of the cells.

Simple squamous epithelium has cells that are a single layer of flat cells. An example of simple squamous epithelium is the alveoli of the lungs.

Stratified squamous epithelium has flat cells that are several layers thick. Skin and mucous membranes are examples of stratified squamous epithelium.

Connective tissue is the most abundant tissue of the body. This tissue has a rich blood supply (with the exception of tendons, ligaments, and cartilage) and a nonliving "matrix." Bone, cartilage, fibrous, fat, and hemopoietic (or blood-forming) tissue are all types of connective tissue.

Organs

An *organ* is defined as a group of different tissue types organized for a specific function. The organization of organs to perform specific functions is called a *system*.

Systems

The remainder of this chapter will discuss the various systems of the body. Table 8.1 lists the major systems of the body, their component parts, and their functions.

Table 8.1

Major Systems of the Body

System	Components	Functions
Skeletal	206 bones	Support protection, blood formation, mineral storage
Muscular	Smooth muscle	Movement of the body
	Striated muscle	Movement of fluids
	Cardiac muscle	Production of heat, communication
Nervous	Central nervous system	Stimuli coordinating
	Peripheral nervous system	Stimuli receiver
	Sense organs	Stimuli transmission
Circulatory	Blood	Nutrition of cells
	Blood vessels	Waste elimination
	Heart	Cellular respiration
Lymphatic	Lymph fluid, vessels, nodes	Defense mechanism
	Tonsils, thymus, spleen	Fluid return to blood vascular system
Respiratory	Nose, sinuses, pharynx, epiglottis, larynx, trachea, bronchi, and lungs	Provides framework for and supplies oxygen to the cells, eliminates carbon dioxide
Digestive	Oral cavity, pharynx, esophagus, stomach, small and large intestines, and accessory organs	Digestion and absorption of food, excretion of solid wastes
Urinary	Kidneys, ureters, bladder, and urethra	Production and elimination of urine
Reproductive	Female: ovaries, fallopian tubes, uterus, vagina Male: testes, penis	Production of offspring
Endocrine	Adrenals, parathyroids, pancreas, pituitary, thymus, thyroid, gonads	Body maintenance, regulation of growth
Integumentary	Skin, nails, hair, sebaceous and sweat glands	Protection, regulation of fluids and temperature

THE SKELETAL SYSTEM

Axial skeleton

The portion of the skeleton composed of the vertebral column, thorax, and skull.

The skeletal system is composed of 206 bones (Figure 8.2). This section will briefly discuss the functions of the skeletal system, structure of bone, types of joints, and appendicular and **axial skeleton**. The bones of the skull will be discussed in more detail.

Functions of the Skeletal System

The human skeleton is the framework of the body. The muscles are attached on this framework. The shortening and elongation of muscles produces movement. Because of their hard dense structure, bones are excellent protectors of vital organs. The ribs protect the heart and lungs, and the skull provides protection for the brain. Bone also serves to store minerals in the body. The minerals stored within bone are removed and replaced as needed. Bone is also important in blood formation or hemopoiesis.

Structure of Bone

Bone is a hard connective tissue composed of both organic and inorganic components. The organic portion of bone consists of cells and matrix. Inorganic minerals stored within bone give it its strength. The two main types of bone are *cancellous bone* and *cortical bone.*

Cancellous bone is also called *spongy bone.* This type of bone is less dense than cortical bone because of its sponge-like arrangement. This spongy matrix of cancellous bone is formed by numerous bony extensions called *trabeculae.* The red bone marrow is housed along these trabeculae. The red bone marrow produces red blood cells, white cells, and platelets. Yellow bone marrow is found in the central portions of long bones; in adults, it is composed of mostly fatty tissue.

Cortical bone is sometimes referred to as *compact bone* because this portion of bone is hard, dense, and strong. Cortical bone is located between the periosteum and cancellous bone.

The *periosteum* is the fibrous connective tissue covering of bone. The periosteum functions to protect, repair, and feed the bone. It also aids in bone growth.

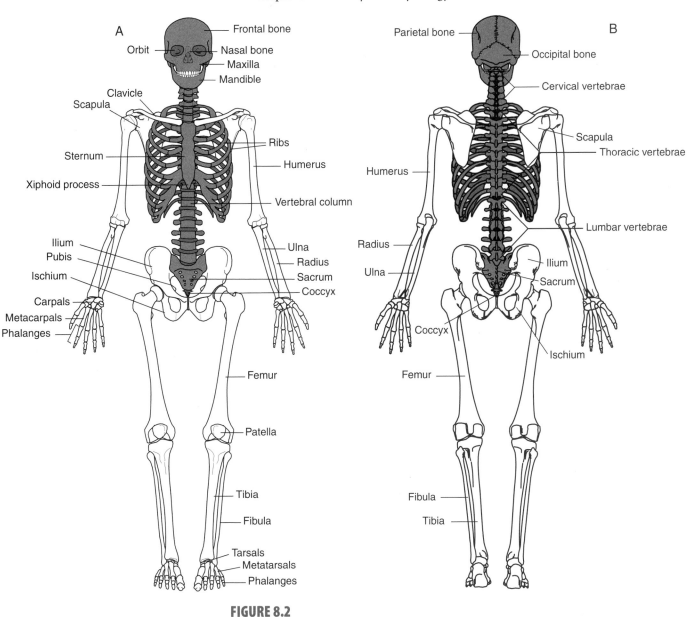

FIGURE 8.2

Skeletal system. **A**, Anterior view. **B**, Posterior view.

Joints

A joint is an area where two or more bones come together. Any union of bones in this manner is called an *articulation*. The three main types of joints include the following:

1 Fibrous
2 Cartilaginous
3 Synovial

The joining of bones of the skull is called a *suture* or *fibrous joint*. No movement occurs at a fibrous joint (Figure 8.3, *A*).

Bones that are connected by cartilaginous tissue form a symphysis. An example of a cartilaginous articulation is the pubic symphysis. These joints permit only slight movement (Figure 8.3, *B*).

The synovial joint is the type of joint that allows free movement (Figure 8.3, *C*). Fibrous connective tissue surrounds the synovial joint, forming a sac called the *joint capsule*. The articular cartilage covers the ends of each of the joining bones and provides protection. The synovial membrane lines the synovial cavity and secretes a fluid that lubricates the joint cavity. Types and examples of synovial joints include the following:

1 Ball and socket: Hip and shoulder
2 Hinge: Elbow and knee
3 Gliding: Vertebra

Appendicular Skeleton

The skeletal system has two divisions: the appendicular and the axial. The appendicular skeleton is composed of the

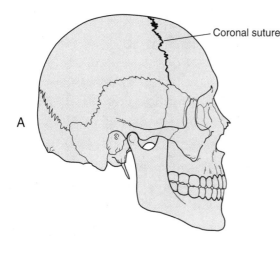

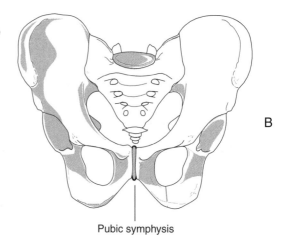

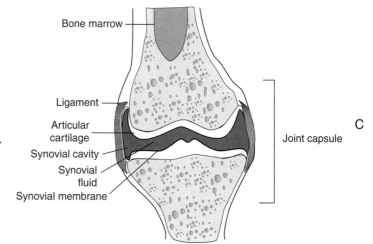

FIGURE 8.3

Types of joints. **A**, Fibrous. **B**, Cartilaginous. **C**, Synovial.

bones of the upper and lower extremities (shoulder girdles; arms, wrists, hands, and pelvic girdle; hip, legs, and feet) (Table 8.2).

The Axial Skeleton

The axial skeleton is composed of the vertebral column, thorax, hyoid bone, and skull (See Figure 8.2).

Vertebral Column or Spine

The spine is a series of separate interconnecting bones called *vertebrae*. The vertebrae are designed to allow the spinal cord to lie protected within its center. This central opening is called the *vertebral foramen*. The vertebral column is composed of the following:

1 Cervical vertebra (7): Neck region
2 Thoracic (12): Rib area
3 Lumbar: Lower back
4 Sacrum (1): Hip area
5 Coccyx (1): Tail bone

Thorax

The thorax, or chest, consists of 24 ribs, the sternum (breastbone), and 12 thoracic vertebrae. The bones of the thorax function to protect the heart, lungs, and upper digestive tract.

Hyoid Bone

The hyoid bone is attached to the styloid processes of the temporal bone of the skull by the stylohyoid ligaments and is suspended between the larynx and mandible. It is horseshoe shaped and serves to support the tongue and various other muscles.

Bones of the Skull

The bones of the skull are divided into the following groups:

1 The cranium, which is made up of 8 bones
2 The middle ear, which has 6 bones
3 The 14 bones of the face

Cranium

The cranium is the portion of the skull that protects and is immediately adjacent to the brain. It is composed of the following bones (Figures 8.4 and 8.5):

1 Frontal (1)
2 Parietal (2)
3 Temporal (2)
4 Occipital (1)
5 Sphenoid (1)
6 Ethmoid (1)

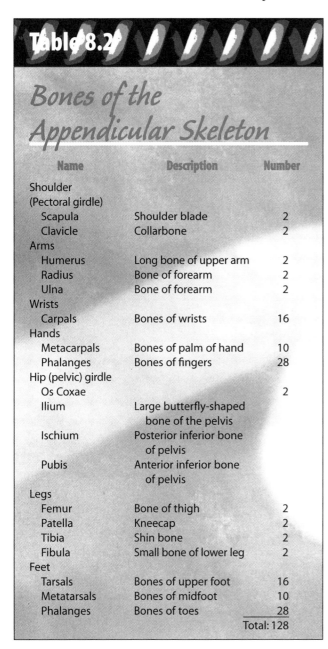

Table 8.2

Bones of the Appendicular Skeleton

Name	Description	Number
Shoulder (Pectoral girdle)		
Scapula	Shoulder blade	2
Clavicle	Collarbone	2
Arms		
Humerus	Long bone of upper arm	2
Radius	Bone of forearm	2
Ulna	Bone of forearm	2
Wrists		
Carpals	Bones of wrists	16
Hands		
Metacarpals	Bones of palm of hand	10
Phalanges	Bones of fingers	28
Hip (pelvic) girdle		
Os Coxae		2
Ilium	Large butterfly-shaped bone of the pelvis	
Ischium	Posterior inferior bone of pelvis	
Pubis	Anterior inferior bone of pelvis	
Legs		
Femur	Bone of thigh	2
Patella	Kneecap	2
Tibia	Shin bone	2
Fibula	Small bone of lower leg	2
Feet		
Tarsals	Bones of upper foot	16
Metatarsals	Bones of midfoot	10
Phalanges	Bones of toes	28
		Total: 128

Frontal Bone

The frontal bone of the forehead forms a portion of the floor of the cranium and upper portion of the eye sockets, or orbits. The frontal sinuses are located within the frontal bone, toward the midline and superior to the orbits (see Figure 8.5).

Parietal Bones

The two parietal bones are located on the top of the skull and posterior to the frontal bone (see Figure 8.4). The suture line, which joins the frontal bone and the parietal bones, is called the *coronal suture*. This is the area called the *fontanelle* or "soft spot" on the infant's skull. The juncture between these three bones does not close completely until approximately 18 months of age.

Temporal Bones

The two temporal bones are located in the temple region (see Figure 8.4). The temporal bones form the external and internal structure of the ear. Also, these bones form the mastoid process, which contains the mastoid sinuses behind the ear. The styloid process is an extension of the temporal bone and is important in muscle attachments.

Occipital Bone

The occipital bone forms the base of the skull and is the most posterior portion of the cranium (Figures 8.4 and 8.6). The foramen magnum is located within the occipital bone. The spinal cord exits the skull through this opening.

Sphenoid Bone

The sphenoid bone forms the central portion of the cranium floor. It joins the occipital, frontal, and ethmoid bones. The pituitary gland is located in the sella turcica of the sphenoid bone. The pterygoid process of sphenoid bone plays an important role in muscle attachment. The sphenoidal sinuses are located within this bone (see Figure 8.4).

Ethmoid Bone

The ethmoid bone is located between the orbits and forms the upper portion of the nasal septum. The ethmoid sinuses are located in the ethmoid bone (see Figure 8.4).

Bones of the Middle Ear

The six bones of the middle ear are the malleus, incus, and stapes.

- Malleus: Hammer (2)
- Incus: Anvil (2)
- Stapes: Stirrup (2)

These bones are located within the temporal bone and will be discussed in more detail later in this chapter.

Bones of the Face

The 14 bones of the face include the following (see Figures 8.4 and 8.5):

Zygomatic (2)
Maxillary (2)
Palatine (2)
Nasal (2)
Lacrimal (2)
Vomer (1)
Inferior conchae (2)
Mandible (1)

Zygomatic Bones

The two zygomatic bones join the frontal bone and form the zygomatic arches, or cheek bones. These bones form a portion of the lateral walls and floor of the orbits (see Figure 8.4).

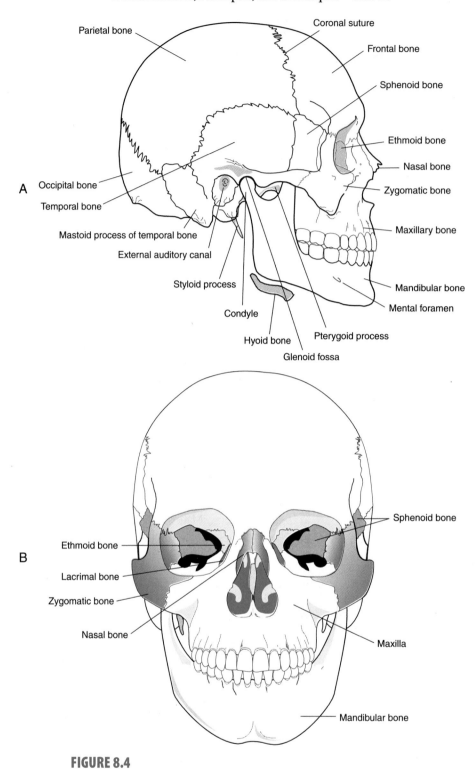

A, Lateral view of the skull. **B,** Frontal view of the skull bones of the orbits.

Maxillary Bones

The two maxillary bones form the upper jaw. The alveolar process supports the maxillary teeth. These two bones also help to form the roof of the mouth, floor of the orbit, and sides and floor of the nose. The maxillary bones contain the maxillary sinuses (see Figures 8.4 and 8.5).

Palatine Bones

The two palatine bones form the most posterior portion of the hard palate. They also form a part of the floor and sides of the nose and floor of the orbit (see Figure 8.6).

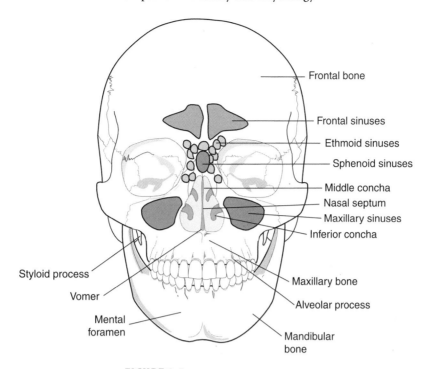

FIGURE 8.5

Frontal view of the skull and sinuses.

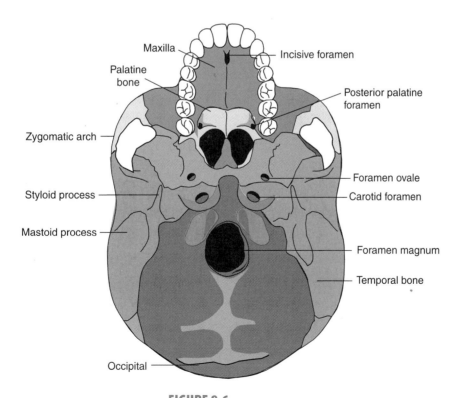

FIGURE 8.6

Inferior view of the skull.

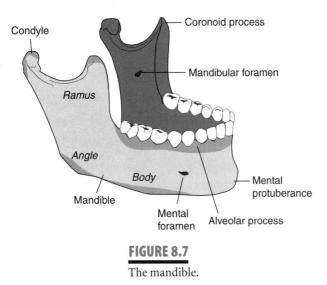

FIGURE 8.7

The mandible.

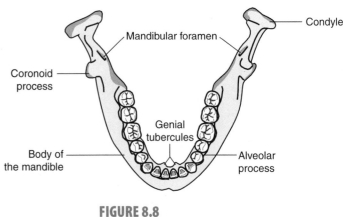

FIGURE 8.8

Superior view of the mandible.

Nasal Bones

The bridge of the nose is formed by the two nasal bones (see Figure 8.4).

Lacrimal Bones

The small lacrimal bones form the anterior medial wall of the orbit and side walls of the nose (see Figure 8.4).

Vomer

The vomer, a single flat bone, forms the base of the nasal septum (see Figure 8.5).

Inferior Concha

The two inferior concha bones lie just under the superior and middle conchae bones of the ethmoid (see Figure 8.5). These are fragile, scroll-shaped bones located on the lateral surfaces of the nose. They function to increase the surface area of the nasal chamber.

Mandible

The mandible is the strong, horseshoe-shaped inferior bone of the skull (Figure 8.7). The mandibular condyle articulates in the glenoid fossa of the temporal bone. This joint is called the *temporomandibular joint*, or TMJ. The temporo-mandibular joint will be discussed in more detail later. Other anatomic landmarks of the mandible include the following:

1 Alveolar process: The area where the mandibular teeth are supported
2 Mental protuberance: The chin
3 Ramus: The upright portion of the mandible
4 Coronoid process: The anterior portion of the ramus
5 Mandibular foramen: The opening for nerves and blood vessels located on the lingual surface of the ramus
6 Body: The major portion of the mandible
7 Mental foramen: Located on the facial surface of the body of the mandible

8 Angle: Located between the body and ramus of the mandible
9 Genial tubercles: Small, raised, bony protuberances located on the lingual surface of the mandible at the midline (Figure 8.8)

THE MUSCULAR SYSTEM

The primary purpose of the muscular system is to give movement to the systems of the body. The skeletal muscles are specifically designed to move the bones of the body through contraction and relaxation. The cardiac muscle gives the heart its great strength to force blood to all parts of the body.

Muscles move food through the digestive system. Figure 8.9 illustrates some major muscles of the body.

Structure of Muscle

Each muscle is composed of long slender fibers known as *muscle fibers*. These muscle fibers are composed of many smaller fibers or cells called *myofibrils*. Myofibrils consist of thick and thin filaments. During muscle contraction, these

Types of Muscles

Striated	Voluntary
1. Skeletal	1. Skeletal
2. Cardiac	
	Involuntary
Smooth or Visceral	1. Smooth
1. Digestive	2. Cardiac
2. Blood vessels	
3. Urinary tract	

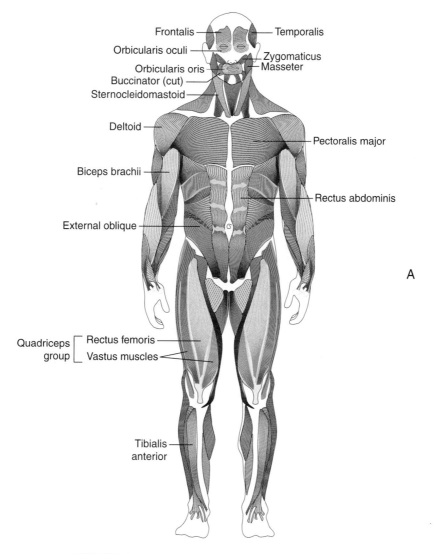

Frontalis — Temporalis
Orbicularis oculi — Zygomaticus
Orbicularis oris — Masseter
Buccinator (cut)
Sternocleidomastoid

Deltoid — Pectoralis major

Biceps brachii —

Rectus abdominis

External oblique —

A

Quadriceps group — Rectus femoris
— Vastus muscles

Tibialis anterior

FIGURE 8.9

Major superficial muscles of the body. **A**, Anterior view.
Continued

tiny filaments pull on each other to shorten the muscle. Muscles are covered by a protective fibrous connective tissue called *fascia*. The fascia of muscles form tendons that attach muscles to bone.

Types of Muscles

Striated muscles are so named because of their striped or striated appearance. These stripes are because of the dark and light bands of the thick and thin filaments, or sarcomeres, of muscle fibers. Striated muscles are capable of producing strong quick contractions. Skeletal and cardiac muscles are both striated.

Smooth or *visceral muscles* are found in the lining or viscera of the body. The digestive system, blood vessels, and uri-

nary tract are examples of body systems containing smooth muscles. Smooth muscles do not contain the striations found in skeletal or cardiac muscles, and therefore their contraction is much slower.

Voluntary muscles are muscles that we can control. Skeletal muscles are voluntary muscles.

Involuntary muscles are muscles that we cannot control consciously. Smooth muscles and cardiac muscles are involuntarily controlled by the autonomic nervous system.

Muscle Activity

A group of muscle fibers stimulated by a single nerve fiber or motor neuron is called a *motor unit*. When the motor neuron is stimulated the motor unit contracts or tightens. When

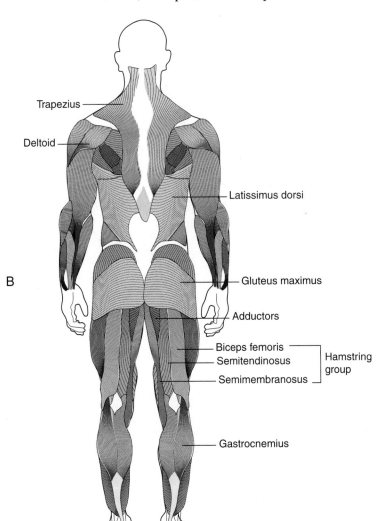

B

Trapezius

Deltoid

Latissimus dorsi

Gluteus maximus

Adductors

Biceps femoris
Semitendinosus   } Hamstring group
Semimembranosus

Gastrocnemius

FIGURE 8.9, cont'd

Major superficial muscles of the body. **B,** Posterior view.

the stimulus is removed the muscle relaxes or returns to its original shape.

The energy necessary for muscle contraction and relaxation is stored within the muscle in the form of glycogen. The breakdown of glycogen within muscles produces heat. It is this chemical breakdown within muscle tissue that produces the heat needed to maintain our 98.6°F body temperature.

Muscle Origin and Insertion

The *origin* (O) of a muscle is where the muscle begins. A muscle's origin is located on a bone that remains fixed (does not move). Where a muscle ends is called the *insertion* (I). The insertion is the end of a muscle that draws the bone toward the origin. Many muscles are named according to their origin and insertion. The origin portion is listed first, and the insertion portion is listed last. An example is the palatoglossus muscle. The soft palate is its origin and the tongue, or glossus, is its insertion.

Major Muscles of Facial Expression

The major muscles of facial expression are the buccinator, orbicularis oris, zygomatic major, and mentalis (Figure 8.10). These muscles acting together allow us to express our emotions through facial movement. By the action of these few muscles we can convey happiness, sadness, anger, fear, surprise, and so on.

1 Buccinator
   Function: Compresses cheeks and retracts angle the corners of the mouth

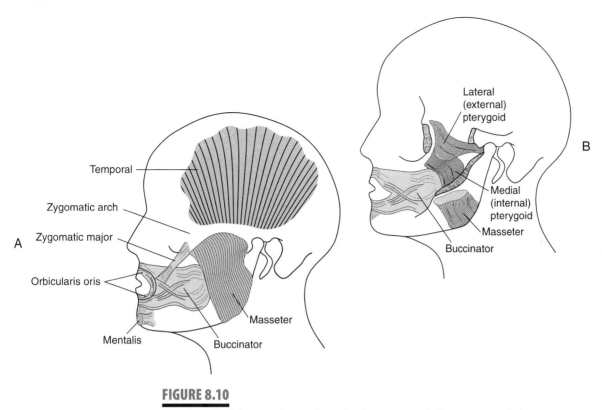

FIGURE 8.10

Muscles of facial expression and mastication. **A**, Lateral view. **B**, Internal view.

Location: Maxilla and mandible (O) to orbicularis (I)
2 Orbicularis oris
   Function: Protrudes and closes lips
   Location: Encircles mouth
3 Zygomatic major
   Function: Draws corners of mouth up and back, as in smiling or laughing
   Location: Zygomatic bone (O) to orbicularis oris (I)
4 Mentalis
   Function: Raises and protrudes lower lip
   Location: Mandible (O) to skin to chin (I)

Major Muscles of Mastication

The major muscles of mastication are the masseter, temporal, lateral pterygoid, and medial pterygoid. These muscles function to close, retrude, and move the mandible from side to side. Through the action of these muscles, mastication or chewing occurs (see Figure 8.10).
1 Masseter
   Function: Closes the jaw
   Location: Zygomatic arch (O) to angle and ramus of mandible and coronoid process (I)
2 Temporal
   Function: Closes the lower jaw; retrudes mandible

Location: Temporal fossa of temporal bone (O) to coronoid process of mandible (I)
3 Lateral (external) pterygoid
   Function: Opens, protrudes, and moves the mandible from side to side
   Location: Greater wing of sphenoid bone and lateral surface of pterygoid plate of sphenoid bone (O) to condyle of mandible and into disc and ligament of TMJ (I)
4 Medial (internal) pterygoid
   Function: Closes jaw
   Location: Lateral pterygoid plate of sphenoid bone, palatine bone, and tuberosity of maxilla (O) to the ramus of the mandible (I)

Muscles of the Floor of the Mouth

The floor of the mouth is formed by the following muscles: the digastric, mylohyoid, geniohyoid, and stylohyoid (Figure 8.11). The action of these muscles moves the hyoid bone and tongue and aids in opening the mouth. Their location also aids in supporting the floor of the mouth.
1 Digastric
   Function: Opens jaw and moves hyoid back

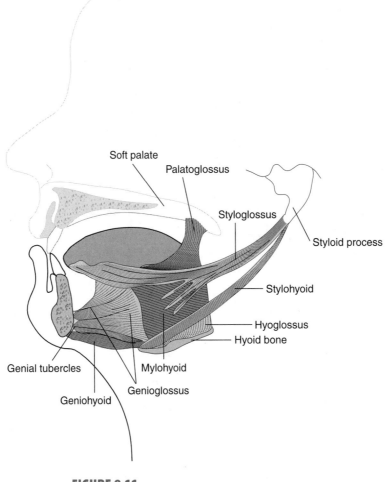

FIGURE 8.11

Muscles of the tongue and posterior of the mouth.

Location: Lower border of mandible and mastoid process of temporal bone (O) to body of hyoid bone (I)

2 Mylohyoid

Function: Opens jaw, rises tongue, and supports floor of mouth

Location: Lingual surface of mandible (O) to hyoid bone (I)

3 Geniohyoid

Function: Draws hyoid and tongue forward

Location: Lingual midline of mandible (O) to hyoid bone (I)

4 Stylohyoid

Function: Retrudes and raises hyoid bone

Location: Styloid process of temporal bone (O) to hyoid bone (I)

Muscles of the Tongue

The muscles of the tongue are the hyoglossus, styloglossus, and genioglossus. These muscles move the tongue down, up, back, and forward.

1 Hyoglossus

Function: Depresses tongue

Location: Hyoid bone (O) to lateral border of the tongue (I)

2 Styloglossus

Function: Draws tongue back and up

Location: Styloid process of temporal bone (O) to side and entire lower surface of tongue (I)

3 Genioglossus

Function: Lowers and moves tongue forward

Location: Lingual midline of mandible (O) to hyoid bone and lower surface of tongue (I)

The Pillars of Fauces

The posterior portion of the mouth is formed by two arches called the *pillars of fauces* (Figure 8.12). The anterior pillar of fauces is formed by the palatoglossus muscle. The posterior pillar of fauces is formed by the palatopharyngeus muscle.

The palatoglossus and palatopharyngeus muscles act to narrow the pillars and aid in closing off the nasopharynx.

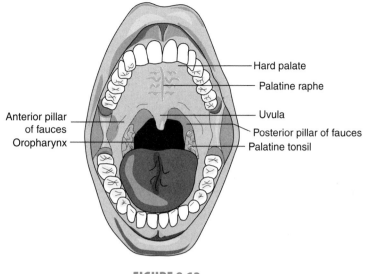

FIGURE 8.12

The pillars of fauces.

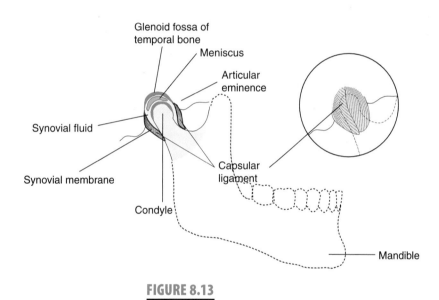

FIGURE 8.13

The temporomandibular joint.

The palatine tonsils are located between the anterior and posterior pillars of fauces.

The Temporomandibular Joint

The temporomandibular joint (TMJ), as the name implies, is the joint between the temporal bone of the skull and the mandible (Figure 8.13). The TMJ is actually two joints that move as one. The right and left side must move in unison to produce the specialized movements of chewing, swallowing (**deglutition**), and speech. The TMJ is both a hinge and gliding syn-

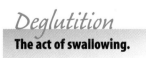

Deglutition

The act of swallowing.

ovial joint. Some movements of this joint use a hinge-only action, and some are a combination of hinge and gliding actions (Figure 8.14).

The condyle of the mandible fits within the glenoid fossa of the temporal bone. The articular eminence, which is located just anterior to the glenoid fossa, plays an important part in the TMJ's gliding movements.

The TMJ is surrounded by a dense, fibrous, connective tissue capsule. This capsule is composed of the capsular ligament, meniscus, and synovial membrane and fluid. The capsular ligament connects the temporal bone with the mandibular condyle. The meniscus, or disc, cushions the condyle in the glenoid fossa. The capsule is lined with synovial membrane, which secretes synovial fluid. The synovial

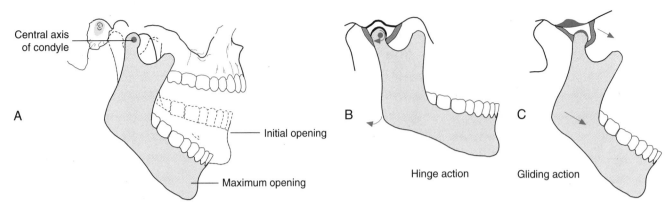

FIGURE 8.14

The hinge and glide action of the temporomandibular joint (TMJ). **A,** Initial and maximum opening of the TMJ. **B,** Hinge action of the TMJ. **C,** Glide action of the TMJ.

fluid lubricates the capsule and allows free movement of the meniscus.

The initial stage of jaw opening uses a hinge-only action. In Figure 8.14, *A* and *B*, the muscles that open the mandible (the lateral pterygoid, digastric, and mylohyoid) pull the jaw downward. The condyle of the mandible actually rotates around its central axis, and little or no anterior or downward movement of the condyle occurs. This movement produces initial opening of the mandible.

The second stage of the jaw opening involves the gliding action (Figure 8.14, *A* and *C*). When the lateral and medial pterygoid muscles contract, the condyle rides along the articular eminence in a downward and forward motion. When the medial and lateral pterygoid on the same side contract, they produce a protrusive mandibular movement. Maximum mandibular opening is achieved by this gliding movement. When the medial and lateral pterygoid alternate contraction from one side to the other, lateral or chewing movements occur.

THE NERVOUS SYSTEM

The nervous system includes the brain, spinal cord, nerves, and sense organs of the body. The brain and spinal cord comprise the central nervous system or CNS. All nerves of the body are referred to as the **peripheral nervous system** (PNS).

Peripheral nervous system

All nerves of the body.

Neuron

The neuron is the main cell of the nervous system. It is composed of a cell body, dendrites, and the axon. The cell body contains the nucleus and cytoplasm. Dendrites are fingerlike projections that bring impulses to the cell body. The axon is a tail-like projection that carries impulses away from the cell body.

The axon is covered in a protective sheath of myelin. Myelin is composed of Schwann's cells and is white in appearance. Nerves of the peripheral nervous system are covered with myelin and are called *white matter*. The brain and spinal cord of the CNS contain portions of nerves that are uncovered, which are called *gray matter*.

Neurons are classified according to the direction in which they transmit impulses. Sensory neurons carry impulses from the body to the CNS, and motor neurons carry impulses from the CNS to the body.

Central Nervous System

The brain is the body's control center. The spinal cord is actually an extension of the brain stem. All sensations of the body enter the spinal cord or brain directly, where they are stored or processed into motor actions (muscle movements).

The brain and spinal cord are protected by the skull and vertebrae column of the axial skeleton. The CNS is also protected by strong fluid-filled membranes called *meninges*. The fluid, found within the meninges, acts to cushion the brain and cord against injury and is called *cerebrospinal fluid*.

Peripheral Nervous System

The peripheral nervous system, or PNS, is divided into the following three types of nerves:

1 The *cranial nerves* consist of 12 pair of peripheral nerves of the brain and are named for the area or function they serve. They are listed as Roman numerals.
2 The *spinal nerves* consist of 31 pair of peripheral nerves of the spinal cord.
3 The *autonomic nervous system* is the involuntary portion of the nervous system that controls the cardiovas-

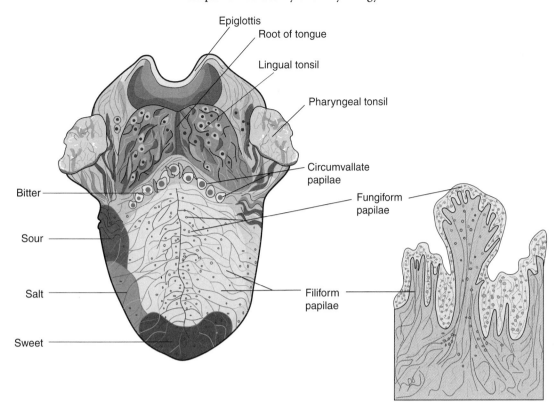

FIGURE 8.15

Regions of the tongue sensitive to various tastes.

cular and gastrointestinal systems, smooth muscles, and glandular secretions.

Special Senses of the Peripheral Nervous System

The five special senses of the PNS are sight, smell, hearing, touch, and taste.

Sight

The eye is the sense organ of sight or vision. It contains rods and cones within the retina. Rods allow us to see at night. Cones give us day vision as well as the ability to see color.

Smell

The receptors for the sense of smell are called *olfactory receptors*. They are located in the upper portion of the nasal cavity. Odors that we smell are dissolved in the mucous membrane lining of the nose and transferred to the olfactory receptors. The olfactory receptors identify the odor and then transmit this information to the brain.

Hearing

The organ of hearing (and balance) is the ear. The portion of the ear we can see is called the *external ear*. The middle ear contains the malleus (hammer), incus (anvil), and stapes (stirrup). Sound causes the eardrum to vibrate, which in

turn causes these three small bones to move against the inner ear. The inner ear receives these sound waves and transmits these nerve impulses to the brain.

Touch

The skin contains receptors that interpret touch as pain, pressure, and temperature. The skin will be discussed in more detail later in the chapter.

Taste

The receptors for taste are the taste buds. They are located within the many small projections, or papillae, on the top of the tongue. The tongue has three principle types of papillae. The *fungi form* papillae are the most numerous and are mushroom shaped, as the name implies. The *filiform papillae* are sharp and flame shaped. The *circumvallate papillae* are large taste buds that from a V-shape in the posterior portion of the tongue. They are similar in shape to the fungi form papillae and are surrounded by a ring of tissue.

The primary tastes sensations are sweet, sour, salty, and bitter. Figure 8.15 illustrates the part of the tongue that is sensitive to these various tastes.

Innervation of the Oral Cavity

The primary nerve of the oral cavity is the *trigeminal nerve*. It subdivides at the semilunar ganglion (a ganglion is a group of nerve cells bodies in the PNS) in this manner.

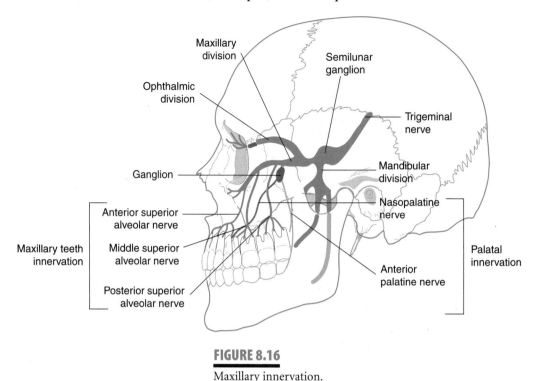

FIGURE 8.16

Maxillary innervation.

Ophthalmic Division	
Maxillary Division	
Anterior superior alveolar	**Innervation of maxillary teeth**
Middle superior alveolar	
Posterior superior alveolar	
Nasopalatine	**Innervation of palate**
Anterior palatine	
Mandibular Division	
Buccal	**Innervation of mandibular teeth**
Lingual	
Inferior alveolar	
Mental	

The Maxillary Division of the Trigeminal Nerve

The maxillary division of the **trigeminal nerve** can be further subdivided into palatal innervation and innervation of the maxillary teeth (Figure 8.16). The two branches of the maxillary division of the trigeminal nerve that serve the palate are the nasopalatine and anterior palatine nerves. The nasopalatine nerve exits the maxilla at the incisive foramen and innervates the anterior palate. The anterior palatine nerve exits the maxilla at the

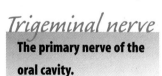

Trigeminal nerve

The primary nerve of the oral cavity.

posterior palatine foramen and gives sensation to the major portion of the palate.

The maxillary teeth are served by three branches of the maxillary division of the trigeminal nerve. The anterior superior alveolar nerve innervates the maxillary anterior teeth (the centrals, laterals, and canines). The middle superior alveolar nerve serves the maxillary premolars and mesiobuccal root of the maxillary molar. The posterior superior alveolar nerve serves the maxillary molars.

The Mandibular Division of the Trigeminal Nerve

The mandibular division of the trigeminal nerve is made up of the buccal, lingual, and inferior alveolar branches (Figure 8.17).

The buccal nerve supplies the mucous membranes of the cheek and the mucoperiosteum (periosteum of bone with a mucous-secreting membrane) of the maxillary and mandibular molars.

The lingual nerve serves the anterior two thirds of the tongue and tongue membranes. The inferior alveolar nerve enters the mandible at the mandibular foramen located on the lingual surface of the ramus of the mandible and innervates all of the mandibular teeth, alveolar process, and periosteum of the mandible. The inferior alveolar nerve ends as the incisive nerve. This nerve innervates the mandibular incisors. The mental nerve branches off from the inferior alveolar nerve and exits the mandible through the mental foramen to serve the chin and lower lip.

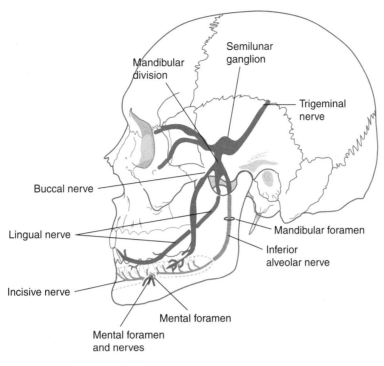

FIGURE 8.17

Lingual and buccal innervation of the mandible.

THE CIRCULATORY SYSTEM

The blood, blood vessels, and heart are the three main components of the circulatory system. Every cell of our body is constantly in need of food and cleansing. The blood is the fluid that carries food toward and waste away from the cells. Blood is pushed through the blood vessels by the force of the heart.

There are two major divisions of the circulatory system. The pulmonary circulation is the blood flow through the lungs. Systemic circulation is the blood flow to all other body systems. Figure 8.18 illustrates some of the principle arteries and veins of the systemic circulation.

This section will discuss the blood, blood composition, blood cells, blood groups, Rh factor, blood clotting, blood vessels, heart, blood pressure and pulse, and major arteries and veins of the face and oral cavity.

Blood

The composition of blood is approximately 52% blood cells and 48% plasma. Blood plasma is 91% water and 9% plasma proteins, albumin, and globulin. Blood serum is plasma minus its clotting factor.

Blood Cells

There are three main types of blood cells: erythrocytes or red blood cells, leukocytes or white blood cells, and thrombocytes or platelets. The leukocytes are further divided into neutrophils, monocytes, lymphocytes, and basophiles.

Erythrocytes, which contain the blood protein hemoglobin, are important in the transport of oxygen to the body. The neutrophil and monocyte leukocytes are necessary to the body's immune defenses. The lymphocytes produce antibodies and regulate antibody production. The basophiles are important in the inflammatory response. Thrombocytes are required for blood clotting.

Blood Groups and Rh Factor

Because of disease or blood loss, transfusions are necessary at times. A person's blood type and Rh factor must be known and crossmatched to determine compatibility with other blood. A fatal reaction could occur if a person receives incompatible blood.

The Rh factor is said to be positive (Rh+) if it contains a certain antigenic compound within the erythrocytes. If a person's blood does not contain this antigenic compound, it is Rh negative. Rh+ individuals must receive Rh+ blood and vise versa. Blood groups are determined by antigens and antibodies found within blood. The following are the major blood types and their compatibility with other blood types.

1 Type AB is the *universal recipient*. This means type AB individuals can give blood to AB individuals and receive blood from all blood groups.

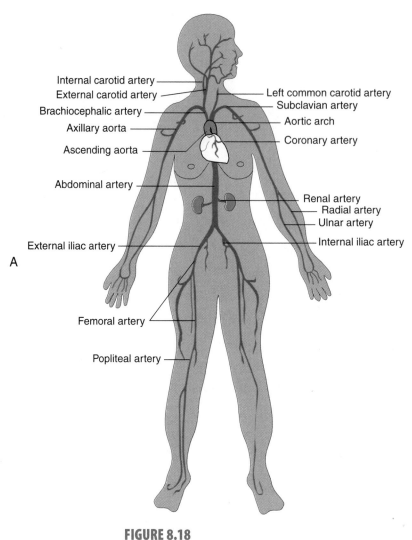

Internal carotid artery

External carotid artery

Brachiocephalic artery

Axillary aorta

Ascending aorta

Abdominal artery

External iliac artery

A

Femoral artery

Popliteal artery

Left common carotid artery

Subclavian artery

Aortic arch

Coronary artery

Renal artery

Radial artery

Ulnar artery

Internal iliac artery

FIGURE 8.18

Circulatory system. **A,** Major arteries.

2 Type O is the *universal donor*. These individuals can give blood to all blood types but can only receive blood from type O.

3 Type A individuals can donate blood to types AB and A and receive blood from types O and A.

4 Type B individuals can donate to types AB and B and receive blood from types O and B.

Blood Clotting

The ability of the body to control bleeding is called *hemostasis*. Five important events must occur to complete hemostasis, as follows:

1 Platelets stick to the injured area, forming a platelet plug.

2 Platelets release serotonin, which causes the blood vessel to constrict.

3 Thromboplastin is released, causing the clotting cascade.

Thromboplastin + prothrombin = thrombin

Thrombin + fibrinogen = fibrin

4 Fibrin produces a meshlike net to trap red blood cells, plasma, and platelets. The clot forms.

5 Blood serum (plasma minus its clotting factor) is squeezed from the clot. The wound's edges are drawn closer together.

Blood Vessels

Arteries, veins, and capillaries are the three main types of blood vessels of the body.

Arteries have a thick, smooth muscle layer over an elastic layer. This gives them the ability to constrict and relax and aids in blood distribution throughout the body. Arteries carry oxygenated blood to all parts of the body.

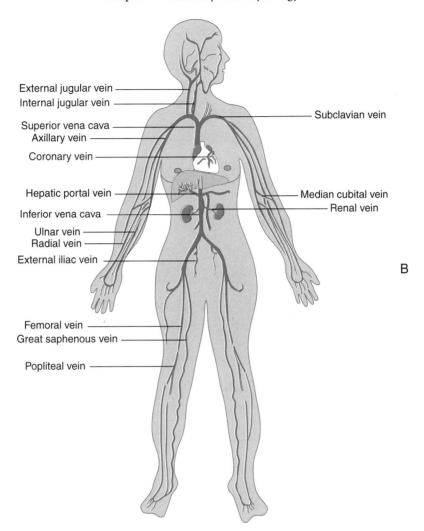

External jugular vein
Internal jugular vein
Superior vena cava
Axillary vein
Coronary vein
Hepatic portal vein
Inferior vena cava
Ulnar vein
Radial vein
External iliac vein
Femoral vein
Great saphenous vein
Popliteal vein
Subclavian vein
Median cubital vein
Renal vein
B

FIGURE 8.18, cont'd

Circulatory system. **B,** Major veins.

Veins are similar to arteries but have much thinner walls and contain one-way valves. Veins carry carbon dioxide—rich blood to the heart.

Because the pressure within the veins is much lower than that within the arteries, blood could have a tendency to flow backward between heartbeats. The valves prevent this from happening.

Capillaries are the tiny microscopic vessels that connect the arteries and veins. The endothelium is the innermost lining of both the arteries and veins and is only one cell layer—thick. Capillaries are comprised only of endothelium. Glucose, oxygen, and carbon dioxide wastes can easily be exchanged between capillaries.

Heart

The heart is the body's pump. This strong muscle provides the power needed to force the blood to all systems of the body.

The heart (Figure 8.19) is divided into four chambers: two atriums, or upper chambers, and two ventricles, or lower chambers. The atriums and ventricles are also divided into right and left atrium and ventricle.

The outer membrane of the heart is called the *pericardium*. The pericardium is as thick as two fibrous tissue layers, with a fluid-filled central space between the layers. These two layers slip against each other without friction to protect the heart . Blood flows through the heart in the following manner:

1 CO_2 blood from the head and body enters the right atrium.
2 O_2 blood from the lungs enters the left atrium.
3 CO_2 blood from the right atrium enters the right ventricle.
4 O_2 blood from the left atrium enters the left ventricle.
5 The right ventricle pumps CO_2 blood to the lungs.
6 The left ventricle pumps O_2 blood to the body.

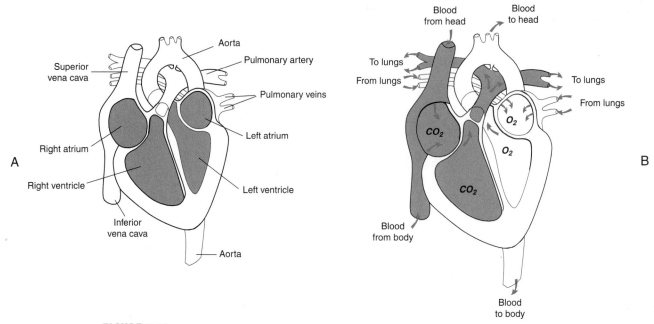

FIGURE 8.19

The heart. **A**, Anatomy of the heart. **B**, Blood flow through the heart. CO_2 = Carbon dioxide; O_2 = Oxygen.

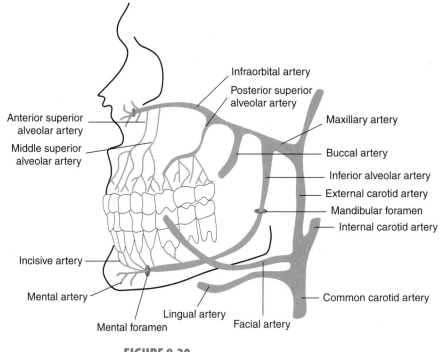

FIGURE 8.20

Major arteries of the face and oral cavity.

Blood Pressure and Pulse

The pressure of the blood on the walls of the blood vessels is termed *blood pressure. Systolic pressure* is the pressure exerted when the ventricles contact. It is the highest or strongest pressure. Normal systolic pressure is 120 mmHg. *Diastolic pressure* is pressure on the vessel walls when the heart is relaxed. Normal diastolic pressure is 80. A normal blood pressure is written 120/80 mm Hg.

Each beat of the heart forces blood through the vessels. This pulsation within the vessels can be felt when a finger is placed over an artery near the surface of the body. Taking the pulse is a valuable clinical tool. It can give information about

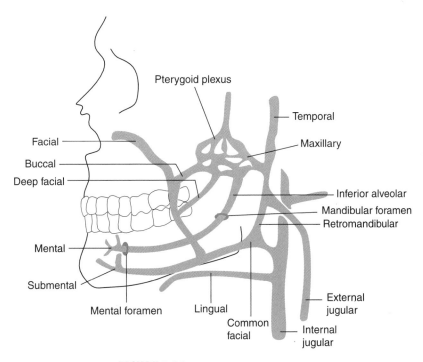

FIGURE 8.21

Major veins of the face and oral cavity.

the strength, rate, and regularity of the heartbeat. A normal pulse rate is about 72 beats per minute.

Arteries of the Face and Oral Cavity

From the left ventricle of the heart the aorta ascends to form the common carotid artery. The common carotid artery branches into the internal and external carotid arteries. The external carotid artery branches into the lingual, facial, and maxillary arteries supply the face (Figure 8.20).

The maxillary artery further subdivides into the inferior alveolar, buccal, and posterior superior alveolar arteries. The maxillary artery terminates as the infraorbital artery. From the infraorbital artery the anterior superior alveolar artery and middle superior alveolar artery branch to supply blood to the maxillary incisors and canine teeth.

The buccal artery supplies the cheeks and the posterior superior alveolar artery supplies the maxillary molars. The inferior alveolar artery enters the mandible at the mandibular foramen and terminates within the mandible as the incisive artery. The portion of the inferior alveolar artery that exits the mandible at the mental foramen is called the *mental artery*. Table 8.3 lists these arteries and their distribution.

Major Veins of the Face and Oral Cavity

The major veins of the face and oral cavity approximate the arteries (Figure 8.21). However, veins drain or return blood

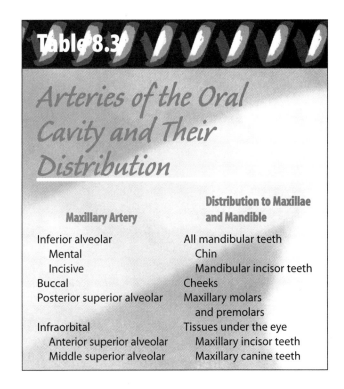

Maxillary Artery	Distribution to Maxillae and Mandible
Inferior alveolar	All mandibular teeth
Mental	Chin
Incisive	Mandibular incisor teeth
Buccal	Cheeks
Posterior superior alveolar	Maxillary molars and premolars
Infraorbital	Tissues under the eye
Anterior superior alveolar	Maxillary incisor teeth
Middle superior alveolar	Maxillary canine teeth

Table 8.3

Arteries of the Oral Cavity and Their Distribution

so that the blood flow through them is described in reverse of the arteries.

The pterygoid plexus branches into the maxillary, buccal, deep facial, and inferior alveolar veins. The inferior alveolar vein enters the mandible at the mandibular foramen, branches to the mental vein, and closely contacts the sub-mental vein.

The facial vein starts at the side of the nose. It passes over the cheek area, around the angle of the mandible, and enters the common facial vein.

The maxillary vein joins the temporal vein to form the retromandibular vein. The retromandibular vein connects the common facial and external jugular veins. The lingual vein terminates in the internal jugular vein.

THE LYMPHATIC SYSTEM

The main function of the lymphatic system is to protect the body against disease (Figure 8.22). The components to the lymphatic system are as follows:

1 Lymph fluid
2 Lymph vessels and capillaries
3 Lymph nodes
4 Tonsils
5 Spleen
6 Thymus

Lymph Fluid

The fluid of the lymphatic system is very similar to blood plasma. Lymph fluid nourishes and cleans areas of the body that are not supplied by blood. By filtration in tissue spaces, this fluid accumulates and is carried through the lymphatic system until it eventually empties into the venous circulation by way of veins in the neck.

Lymph Vessels and Capillaries

The lymph capillaries are delicate thin-walled tubes that carry lymph fluid from the tissue spaces to the lymph vessels. The

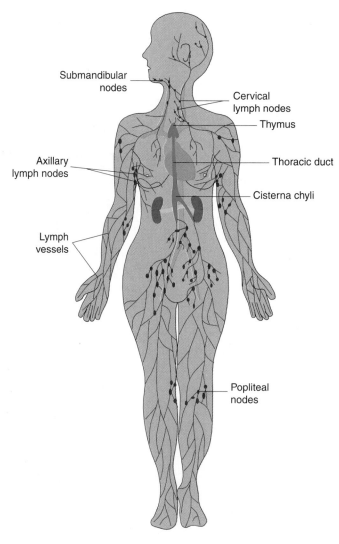

FIGURE 8.22
The lymphatic system.

lymph vessels are similar to veins of the circulatory system in that they have valves that permit lymph fluid to flow in one direction only. The lymph vessels eventually drain into the *thoracic duct*. From the thoracic duct the lymph is stored in the *cisterni chyli* until it is emptied into the venous circulation.

Lymph Nodes

Lymph nodes are small round or oval structures found along the lymph vessels. They function in two important ways: 1) they act to filter out harmful bacteria and abnormal cells; and 2) they form white blood cells or lymphocytes to fight infection.

By filtering out bacterial and other atypical cells and by lymphocyte formation, lymph nodes prevent infections from spreading. Products formed by the filtration process can produce swollen tender nodes at certain points of the body. Physical palpation of swollen nodes is a good indicator of disease or infection. The axillary or "armpit" nodes are important in the diagnosis of breast cancer. Figure 8.23 shows the major lymph nodes of the head and neck.

Tonsils

The tonsils form a protective ring of lymphoid tissue surrounding the posterior oral cavity. Arranged in this manner, as seen in Figure 8.24, the tonsils protect the entrance of the respiratory and digestive systems from invading microorganisms. The palatine tonsils are located on each side of the throat. These are visible in the mouth during an oral examination and are commonly referred to as the "tonsils". The *lingual tonsils* are located at the base of the tongue. The *pharyngeal tonsils* or adenoids are located in the posterior opening of the nasal cavity.

Spleen

The spleen is located between the stomach and diaphragm and is protected by the lower ribs on the left side of the body. It is the largest lymphoid organ of the body and has the following functions:

1 Blood filtration
2 Blood storage
3 Destruction of old red blood cells
4 Prevention of iron destruction
5 Production of cells important in the immune response

Thymus

The thymus is found posterior to the upper portion of the sternum and extends into the neck (see Figure 8.22).

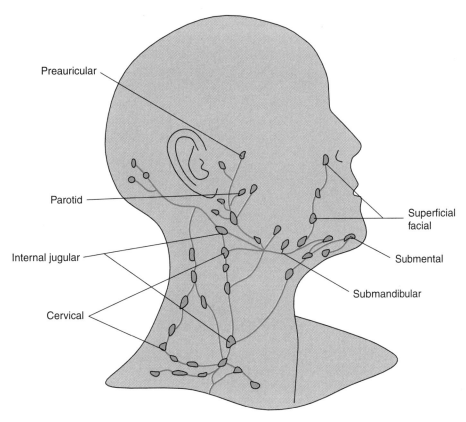

FIGURE 8.23

Major lymph nodes of the head and neck.

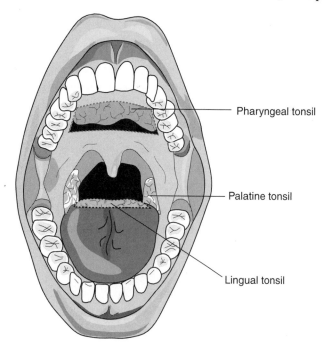

FIGURE 8.24
Tonsils.

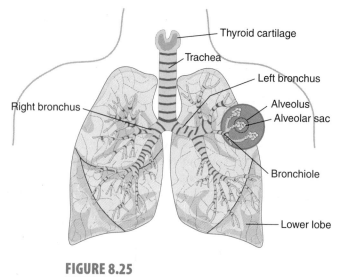

FIGURE 8.25
The lungs, bronchi, bronchioli, and alveoli.

T-lymphocytes or "T-cells" are produced by the thymus and are important cells of the immune response. The thymus is largest and most active in the fetal stage through puberty. After puberty it diminishes in size but is still a vital lymphatic organ in the adult immune system.

THE RESPIRATORY SYSTEM

The respiratory system's main function is to supply oxygen to and remove carbon dioxide and other wastes from the cells of the body. The components of the respiratory system include the lungs, diaphragm, bronchi, trachea, larynx, pharynx, and the nose.

Lungs

The lungs are the two largest primary organs of the respiratory system (Figure 8.25). They lie within the thoracic cavity and are protected by the ribcage. The right lung has three lobes and the left lung has two lobes.

The outer covering of the lungs is called *pleura*. Pleural fluid secreted by this membrane covering permits the lungs to move freely within the thoracic cavity during breathing.

The lungs contain many branching tubules called *bronchioles*. Bronchioles branch and subdivide and eventually end as *alveoli* or air sacs. It is here within the alveoli that gas exchange occurs with the blood of the lungs. This gas exchange is termed *external respiration*. *Internal respiration* occurs in the circulatory system. Capillaries exchange gases with tissue cells.

Diaphragm

The diaphragm separates the thoracic cavity from the abdominal cavity. It is a dome-shaped muscle with its convexity toward the lungs.

During *inspiration*, the diaphragm contracts and the thoracic cavity is pulled downward. This movement of the diaphragm increases the space within the chest, and the lungs are filled with air. During *expiration*, the diaphragm relaxes, the thoracic space is decreased, and air is forced out of the lung. Inspiration and expiration are the processes of pulmonary ventilation, or breathing.

Bronchi

The right and left bronchi are formed by the division of the trachea. Bronchi are the large air tubes that enter the lungs. The right bronchus is larger and straighter than the left bronchus.

Trachea

The trachea is more commonly called the *windpipe*. It is the connecting tube between the larynx and the bronchi. The trachea is reinforced with C-shaped bands of cartilage. This C-shaped arrangement of cartilage allows the trachea to be flexible where it abuts the esophagus, yet rigid enough to keep the trachea open.

Larynx

The larynx (voice box), located just above the trachea, is composed of four major cartilages. The largest cartilage is known as the thyroid cartilage or "Adam's apple." The vocal cords are short fibrous bands that pass over the laryngeal opening. These vocal cords vibrate with air passage to produce speech sounds.

The epiglottis, which is also cartilage, is positioned just above the larynx and acts as a trapdoor. During swallowing, the epiglottis closes and prevents food from entering the respiratory system.

Pharynx

The pharynx, or throat, can be divided into the following three sections:

1 The *nasopharynx*: The uppermost portion of the pharynx just behind the nasal cavities
2 The *oropharynx*: Directly behind the mouth and extends to the epiglottis
3 The *laryngopharynx*: From the epiglottis to the larynx

The pharynx is lined with a mucous-secreting membrane and contains lymphatic tonsillar tissue. The pharyngeal tonsils, or adenoids, are located in the nasopharynx. The palatine and lingual tonsils are located in the oropharynx.

Nose

The nose functions to warm, filter, and moisten air. The nose is divided into two nasal cavities by the nasal septum. The nasal cavities are lined with mucous membranes. The secretions of these membranes provide the fluid necessary to moisten and filter the air we breathe. The *conchae* located within each nasal cavity increases the surface area of the nose.

The sinuses are also lined with mucous membranes and therefore function to aid the nasal cavity by providing mucous. The sinuses also function to lighten the skull and aid in sound production. The sinuses have already been discussed in the skeletal system (see Figure 8.5).

THE DIGESTIVE SYSTEM

The two major purposes of the digestive system are to break down ingested food into particles small enough to be absorbed into the blood and also eliminate solid wastes. *Digestion* and *absorption* are two ways in which food is processed in the digestive system.

> *Digestion*
> **The breaking down of ingested food into particles small enough to be absorbed into the blood.**

Digestion changes the food we eat by both mechanical and chemical actions. Through mastication, swallowing, and peristaltic action, food is broken down into smaller parts. Chemical actions (enzymes) further reduce food to their basic component. Now food can be absorbed and transported by the blood to all cells of the body.

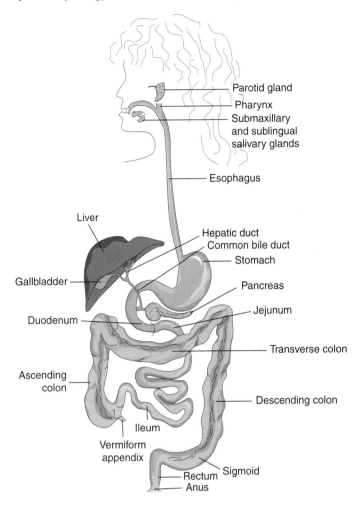

FIGURE 8.26
The digestive system and its accessory structures.

The digestive system, or the *alimentary canal* as it is sometimes called, is a continuous hollow tube about 27 feet in length. It begins at the mouth and ends at the anus. The component parts of the digestive system include the oral cavity, pharynx, esophagus, stomach, small intestine, and large intestine (Figure 8.26).

Several glands and organs are also associated with the digestive system. These accessory structures of the digestive system are the salivary glands, liver, gallbladder, and pancreas. The secretions from these glands and organs enter the digestive tract and play an important part in digestion.

The Oral Cavity

The oral cavity consists of the lips, cheeks, tongue, hard and soft palates, and teeth (Figure 8.27). The lining of the oral cavity is one of three types of mucous membranes: lining mucosa, specialized mucosa, or masticatory mucosa.

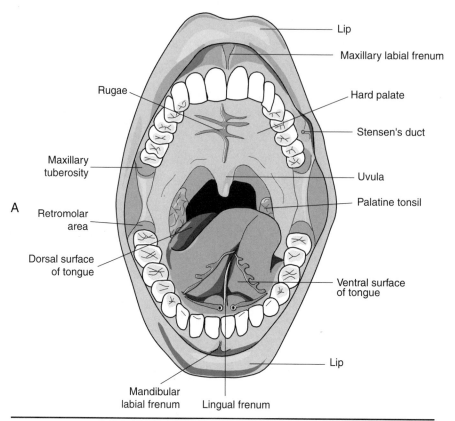

A

- Lip
- Maxillary labial frenum
- Rugae
- Hard palate
- Stensen's duct
- Maxillary tuberosity
- Uvula
- Palatine tonsil
- Retromolar area
- Dorsal surface of tongue
- Ventral surface of tongue
- Lip
- Mandibular labial frenum
- Lingual frenum

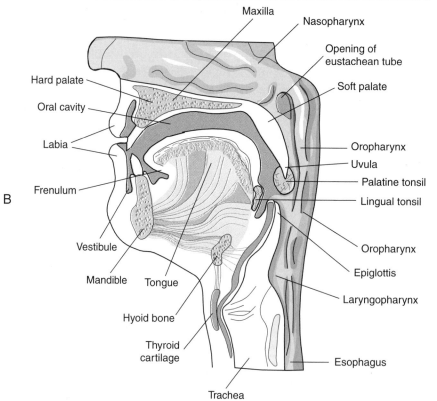

B

- Maxilla
- Nasopharynx
- Opening of eustachean tube
- Hard palate
- Soft palate
- Oral cavity
- Labia
- Oropharynx
- Uvula
- Frenulum
- Palatine tonsil
- Lingual tonsil
- Vestibule
- Oropharynx
- Mandible
- Tongue
- Epiglottis
- Hyoid bone
- Laryngopharynx
- Thyroid cartilage
- Esophagus
- Trachea

FIGURE 8.27

Structures of the oral cavity. **A,** Frontal view. **B,** Lateral view.

The lining mucosa is a thin layer of epithelium with mucus-secreting properties. Mucus is a thick film that allows the membranes to remain moist. Just beneath the lining, mucosa is a layer of submucosa. The submucosa is a layer of connective tissue that contains the blood vessels and nerves. The lining mucosa covers the inside of the lips and cheeks, vestibule, bottom portion of the tongue, and soft palate.

Specialized mucosa, as the name implies, is mucosa that is specialized for a specific function. In this case the special purpose is taste. This type of mucosa is found on the top of the tongue in the form of taste buds.

Masticatory mucosa is found covering the gingiva and hard palate. The tissues covering these areas must withstand the forces associated with masticating or chewing food. This mucosa is therefore a thicker, tougher epithelium.

Lips

The lips provide the anterior protection of the oral cavity. They are both skin externally and mucous membrane internally. The vermilion border or red portion of the lips is the transition between skin and mucous membrane.

The lips help maintain teeth in their position, are important in speech, serve as a seal to prevent food and saliva from escaping and also prevent foods that are too hot or too cold from entering the mouth.

The area between the teeth and the lips is called the *labial vestibule*. The lips have two important frenums, or attachments, that anchor them to the gingiva. The upper lip is attached to the gingiva at the midline by the maxillary labial frenum. The lower lip is attached to the gingiva at the midline by the mandibular labial frenum.

Cheeks

The side walls of the mouth are the cheeks. A large portion of the cheeks is comprised of the buccinator muscle. The cheeks, like the lips, hold the position of the teeth and aid the chewing process by holding food against the teeth. The *buccal vestibule* is the area between the cheek and teeth. The *buccal frenum* connects the cheek to the gingiva in the maxillary premolar area.

Tongue

The tongue is skeletal muscle with a specialized epithelial covering that contains the taste buds. The posterior area of the tongue is attached to the bones of the skull and hyoid bone, but its anterior portion is freely movable. The lingual frenum attaches the midtongue to the floor of the mouth. The tongue serves an important function in chewing, swallowing, and speech production.

Hard Palate

The hard palate is the anterior portion of the roof of the mouth. A series of ridges that occur in the front portion of the hard palate just behind the maxillary anterior teeth is referred to as *rugae*. These rugae, plus the tough fibrous tissue of the hard palate, aid the tongue in crushing certain food before swallowing. Although the hard palate is a hard, dense tissue, it is still very sensitive and aids to protect the oral cavity from hot or very coarse foods.

Soft Palate

The soft palate is the posterior portion of the roof of the mouth. It is comprised of mostly muscle that ends in the free pendulated *uvula*. The soft palate functions to close off the nasopharynx during swallowing. The soft palate contains the *pillars of fauces*, which were explained in the musculature system. The *gag reflex* is located in the posterior area of the mouth (Figure 8.28). Stimulation of the pillars of fauces or at times the posterior tongue can produce a protective reflex of gagging or vomiting.

Teeth

The primary function of the maxillary and mandibular teeth is to grind and tear food. Their secondary function to aid in swallowing and speech. The anatomy and physiology of the teeth will be discussed further in dental anatomy.

Pharynx

The pharynx aids in both respiration and digestion. During swallowing, the nasopharynx is sealed by the soft palate and the laryngeal entrance is closed by the epiglottis. To protect the respiratory system the bolus of food moves downward and posteriorly to the esophagus.

Esophagus

This muscular, mucus-lined tube connects the pharynx and stomach. It is approximately 10 inches long. The esophagus lies posterior to the trachea and anterior to the vertebrae. It uses gravity and muscular or peristolic waves to propel food into the stomach.

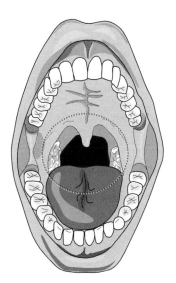

FIGURE 8.28
Area of the gag reflex.

Stomach

The stomach lies just beneath the diaphragm in the abdominal cavity. The stomach is very expandable; when empty, it is not much larger than a large sausage. The contraction of smooth muscles in the stomach mixes food with gastric juices (hydrochloric acid and enzymes) to form a half-solid, half-liquid mixture known as *chyme*.

The stomach functions to store food and also regulates the release of chyme into the small intestine. This regulated release of chyme allows for proper digestion and absorption in the small intestine. No absorption of nutrients occurs within the stomach.

Small Intestine

The upper portion of the small intestines is called the *duodenum*. The *pyloric sphincter* muscle controls food passage from the stomach to the duodenum. The small intestine is approximately 18 feet in length. It begins at the distal portion of the pyloric sphincter and ends at the beginning of the large intestine.

The lining of the small intestine consists of many tissue folds called *plicae*. The plicae are covered with tiny fingerlike villi, which serve to increase the surface area of the small intestine and therefore allow for greater absorption. The majority of food absorption into the blood occurs in the small intestine.

Movement in the small intestine is through peristolic waves and segmentation, or short segments of rhythmic contractions along the small intestine.

Large Intestine

The large intestine is only about 5 feet in length. It has no villi and is much less muscular than the small intestine. As the name implies, it is much larger in diameter than the small intestine. Undigested food passes through the *ileocecal valve* and enters the large intestines. Bacteria within the large intestine have important functions. The bacteria that act upon the undigested material from the small intestine can release certain nutrients that have not been absorbed. Bacteria are also responsible for vitamin K synthesis, which is important in blood clotting. After this vitamin is formed, it is absorbed into the blood in the large intestine. Although the large intestine absorbs water, salts, and vitamins, it is not designed to handle absorption as well as the small intestine.

Accessory Structures of the Digestive System

The accessory structures of the digestive system are the salivary glands, liver, pancreas, and gall bladder. All these structures secrete their products into the digestive system and aid in digestion.

Salivary Glands

The three pairs of the salivary glands are the parotids, submandibulars, and sublinguals (Figure 8.29). The 2 to 3 pints of saliva secreted by these glands each day acts to moisten the mouth and food and aids in swallowing. Saliva cleans the

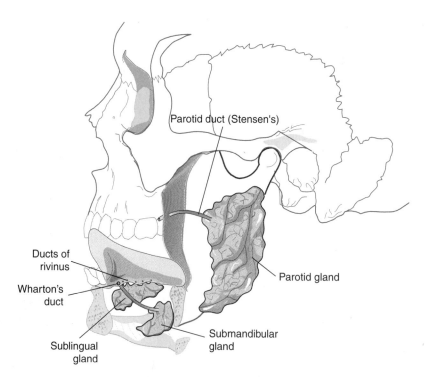

FIGURE 8.29

The salivary glands and ducts.

mouth of food debris and aids in digestion. The enzyme *ptyalin* is present in saliva. This enzyme acts on starch to reduce it to a less complex form.

Parotid Salivary Glands

The parotid glands are the largest of the salivary glands and are located in front of and below the ear subcutaneously. The duct or tube that drains the saliva of the parotid gland is called *Stensen's duct* (see Figure 8.29). It empties into the oral cavity through the cheek just opposite of the maxillary molars.

Sublingual Salivary Glands

The sublingual glands are the smallest of the salivary glands and are located in the floor of the mouth just beneath the tongue. Their secretions enter the mouth through tiny sublingual *Rivinus ducts* and a larger duct located just behind the lower anterior teeth.

Submandibular Gland

The submandibular gland is larger than the sublingual gland and is located posteriorly and inferiorly to the sublingual gland.

Wharton's duct empties the submandibular gland's saliva into the floor of the mouth just behind the mandibular incisors.

Liver and Gallbladder

The largest organ of the body is the liver. It is located on the upper right side of the abdominal cavity. The liver functions to produce bile, antibodies, and plasma proteins, destroy red blood cells, and aid in detoxification and lymph formation.

Bile emulsifies fat and therefore is very important in digestion. Bile enters the small intestine through the hepatic duct.

The gallbladder is the small green sac located on the inferior surface of the liver. Its main function is to store bile. It empties into the small intestine through the common bile duct.

Pancreas

The pancreas is located behind the stomach in the C-shaped concavity of the duodenum. It is both an exocrine and endocrine gland. It secretes *pancreatic juices* and endocrine **hormones**. The pancreatic juices are the most important of the digestive juices. The enzymes in pancreatic juices digest all food types.

Pancreatic secretions follow the major pancreatic duct and empty into the duodenum along with bile.

Hormone

> A chemical substance formed in one part of the body and transferred through the blood to affect another part of the body.

Phases of Swallowing

Swallowing is also termed *deglutition*. It is a very coordinated effort by the muscles and structures of the oral cavity. There are three phases of swallowing. The first phase is voluntary and the last two phases continue involuntarily (Figure 8.30).

- Phase I: the bolus of masticated food is collected on the top of the tongue. The bolus is transferred from the tongue to the oropharynx. In this phase the lips are closed, the teeth are together, and the tip of the tongue touches the rugae of the palate. The upper esophageal sphincter is constricted.
- Phase II: the bolus is passed through the pharynx to the esophagus. Respiration ceases momentarily as the epiglottis seals the larynx and trachea. The upper esophageal sphincter is relaxed and the esophagus is opened.
- Phase III: the bolus of food passes through the esophagus into the stomach. The soft palate is lowered and the epiglottis moves off the larynx. The upper esophageal sphincter is constricted, closing the esophagus. The respiratory passage is opened and breathing is continued.

THE URINARY SYSTEM

The urinary system filters the waste products from the blood and excretes them as urine. In this process the body's fluid balance is maintained. The structures of the urinary system are the kidneys, ureters, bladder, and urethra.

Kidneys

The kidneys are a pair of bean-shaped organs located slightly above the waist on both sides of the vertebrae column in the posterior abdominal cavity. Because the kidneys act as filters to remove metabolic waste from blood, they receive 20% of the total blood volume of the body.

The concave surface of the kidney is called the *hilum*, where the renal artery, vein, and nerve enter. The outer portion of the kidney is called the *cortex* and the inner portion is called the *medulla*. The calyx are the fan-shaped extensions of the enlarged renal pelvis.

The basic functioning unit of the kidney is located in the cortex and is called the *nephron*. The kidneys contain about 2 million of these units. The nephron is a capillary tuft called a *glomerulus*, surrounded by the renal tubular system called the *glomerular capsule* or *Bowman's capsule*. Together these comprise the renal corpuscle. At the renal corpuscle the blood is filtered and waste (urine) is reabsorbed into the glomerulus capsule. The urine then flows through the kidney's collecting tubules in the medulla and out the ureters.

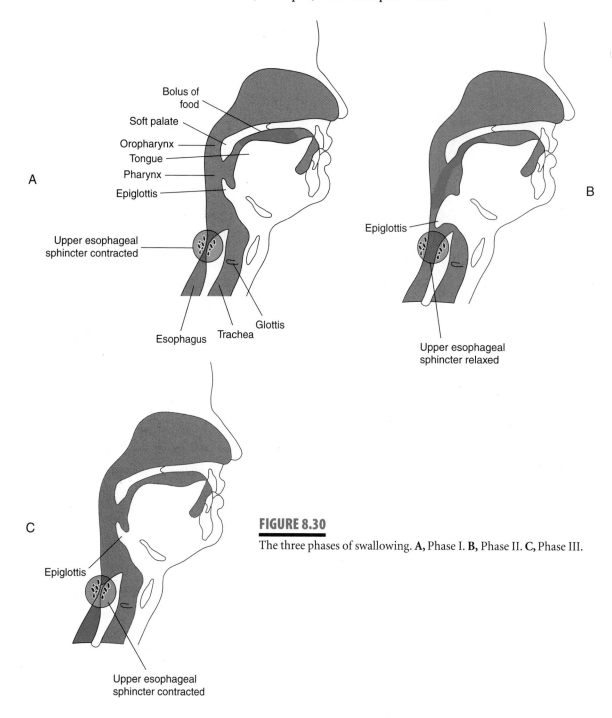

FIGURE 8.30

The three phases of swallowing. **A,** Phase I. **B,** Phase II. **C,** Phase III.

The Ureters, Bladder, and Urethra

Urine flows from the ureters into the bladder, where it is stored. The bladder is located within the pelvis just posterior to the pubic symphysis. The urethra carries urine from the bladder to the exterior of the body.

THE REPRODUCTIVE SYSTEM

The primary function of the reproductive system is the production of offspring. Male sperm and female ovum fuse to produce a single-celled zygote, which develops into a new individual.

Female

The principle structures of the female reproductive system are the ovaries, fallopian tubes, uterus, and vagina. The menstrual cycle will also be discussed in this section.

The ovaries are paired, almond-shaped gonads. They are found on the lateral walls of the pelvis and held in place by numerous ligaments. The ovaries function to develop and expel *ovum*, or eggs, and to produce *estrogen*, the female sex hormone.

The fallopian tubes are two hollow tubes that extend from the ovaries to the top portion of the uterus. The uterus is a hollow, pear-shaped, muscular organ. It is located between the bladder and rectum; similar to the ovaries, it is held in place by numerous ligaments. The lining of the uterus is called the *endometrium* and it is here that the fertilized egg implants itself. The uterus supports and nourishes the fetus until birth. If the ovum is not fertilized and does not embed in the endometrium, then this endometrial lining is shed during menstruation. The cervix forms the base of the uterus.

The vagina is a muscular tube that connects the uterus to the vulva or external genital organs. The vagina has a mucous membrane lining and is very distendible. It serves as the birth canal during childbirth.

The mammary glands, or breasts, are considered supportive sex glands. They are located over the pectoral muscle of the chest and are sweat glands modified to produce human milk.

Menstrual Cycle

The menstrual cycle is normally 28 days in length. Each cycle has 3 phases: the menstrual phase, the postmenstrual phase, and the premenstrual phase.

The menstrual phase is the time during which the endometrial lining of the uterus sheds itself. It is an average of 1 to 5 days in duration.

The postmenstrual phase is also called the *proliferative* phase because during this time the uterine lining proliferates or rebuilds itself. This phase occurs on or about days 6 to 13. At the end of this phase, or day 14, ovulation (release of the egg) occurs.

The premenstrual phase, or secretary phase, occurs between days 15 and 28. It is during this phase that the uterine lining or endometrium prepares itself for implantation of the fertilized ovum. If fertilization and implantation does not occur, then the endometrium sheds itself and the cycle is repeated.

Fertilization is the joining of the 23 chromosomes of the sperm with the 23 chromosomes of the ovum to form an individual zygote of 46 chromosomes. Fertilization usually occurs within the fallopian tubes. The *zygote* travels down the fallopian tubes and embeds in the uterine lining to begin its growth.

Male

The principle structures of the male reproductive system are the testes, seminal vesicles, prostate gland, urethral gland, and penis.

The testes, or testicles, are paired gonads. They are located in the scrotum and function to produce *sperm* and *testosterone*.

Semen is the fluid that carries the sperm. Semen is produced by the seminal vesicle, prostate gland, and bulbourethral gland. The sperm-containing semen is ejaculated through the urethra. The penis is the external male reproductive organ and is designed to deliver sperm to the female reproductive system.

THE ENDOCRINE SYSTEM

The endocrine system regulates the body through the use of hormones. Hormones control and maintain metabolism, growth and development, reproduction, and the defense system, as well as controlling water, nutrient, and electrolyte balance in blood.

The system is termed *endocrine* because it does not secrete its product into ducts as do exocrine glands. This ductless system relies on the blood to distribute its hormone production.

The endocrine system is composed of the following glands: pituitary, thymus, thyroid, parathyroids, pancreatic islets, adrenals, and the gonads (Figure 8.31). Table 8.4 lists the glands of the endocrine system, their locations, and their functions.

SKIN

The skin is the primary organ of the integumentary system. It is the largest organ of the body, weighing approximately 6 pounds, which is about twice the weight of the liver or brain. The skin is one of the most important organs of the body and its functions are numerous. Skin protects the body and retains the body's fluids. The skin is sensitive to pain, temperature, and touch, and it regulates the body's temperature through sweat glands.

Composition of Skin

The outer layer of skin is called the *epidermis*. This layer is composed of stratified, squamous epithelial cells. The pigment layer lies within the epidermis.

The dermis lies directly under the epidermis and is composed mostly of connective tissue. Within the dermis are found the hair follicles, sebaceous (oil) gland, and sweat glands.

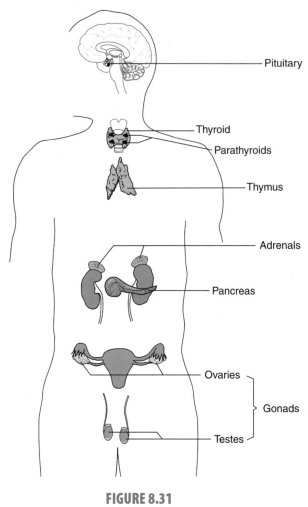

FIGURE 8.31

The endocrine system.

Table 8.4

The Glands of the Endocrine System

Gland	Location	Function
Pituitary	Sella turcica of sphenoid bone	Regulates other endocrine glands, and growth and development
Thymus	Upper thorax behind sternum	Regulates immune system
Thyroid	Anterior neck over trachea	Regulates metabolism, growth development, and sexual maturity
Parathyroids	Posterior to thyroid lobes	Regulates calcium
Pancreatic Islets (Islets of Langerhans)	Pancreas	Produces insulin and regulates carbohydrate metabolism
Adrenals	Top of kidneys	Produces adrenalin (epinephrine) for "fight or flight" response
Gonads	Sex hormones: Androgens	
	Ovaries: Female pelvis	Estrogen production
	Testicles: Scrotum	Testosterone production

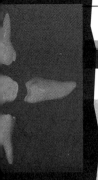

Points for Review

- The parts of the body and how they function
- The basic structural units of the body
- Identification of the systems of the body: bone, muscles, nerves, circulatory system, lymphatic system, respiratory system, digestive system, and glands
- Identification of the structures of the oral cavity

Self-Study Questions

1. What are the bones of the face called?
   a. Frontal, clavicle, radius and femur
   b. Zygomatic, lacrimal, vomer and palatine
   c. Maxillary, mandible, tibia, and phalanges
   d. Nasal, palatine, sternum, and clavicle
2. What are the muscles of mastication called?
   a. Masseter
   b. Masseter and temporal
   c. Lateral and medial pterygoid
   d. All of the above
3. What are the special senses of the peripheral nervous system called?
   a. Sight and smell
   b. Sight, smell, and hearing
   c. Sight, smell, hearing, touch, and taste
   d. None of the above
4. What is the primary nerve that innervates the oral cavity?
   a. Ophthalmic
   b. Trigeminal nerve
   c. Mandibular division nerve
   d. Posterior superior alveolar nerve
5. What does the lymphatic system include?
   a. Thymus, spleen, stomach, and tonsils
   b. Thymus, spleen, lymph nodes, and tonsils
   c. Thymus, spleen, stomach, tonsils, and lungs
   d. None of the above
6. What are the components of the respiratory system?
   a. Diaphragm, bronchi, trachea, and tonsils
   b. Diaphragm, bronchi, trachea, larynx, and spleen
   c. Diaphragm, lungs, bronchi, trachea, larynx, pharynx, and nose
   d. All of the above
7. The major functions of the digestive system are digestion and absorption.
   a. True
   b. False
8. What do the accessory structures of the digestive system include?
   a. Liver, pancreas, gallbladder, and salivary glands
   b. Liver, pancreas, gallbladder, salivary glands, and stomach
   c. Liver, kidneys, stomach, and gall bladder
   d. None of the above
9. What are the principle structures of the female reproductive system?
   a. Testis, urethra, ovaries, uterus, and vagina
   b. Ovaries uterus, vagina, and urethra
   c. Ovaries, fallopian tubes, uterus, and vagina
   d. None of the above
10. The pituitary gland of the exocrine system is called the *master gland*.
    a. True
    b. False

Suggested Readings

Grant J: *An atlas of anatomy*, Baltimore, 1972, Williams & Wilkins.

Gray H: *Anatomy of the human body*, Philadelphia, 1973, Lea and Febiger.

Hollinshead WH: *Textbook of anatomy*, Hagerstown, Md, 1974.

Jacob WS: *Structure and function of man*, Philadelphia, 1970, WB Saunders.

Marieb EN: *Essentials of human anatomy and physiology*, Redwood City, Calif, 1984, Cummings.

Thibodeau GA: *Structure and function of the body*, St Louis, 1997, Mosby.

Torres HO, Ehrlich A: *Modern dental assisting*, Philadelphia, 1999, WB Saunders.

Oral Anatomy and Tooth Morphology

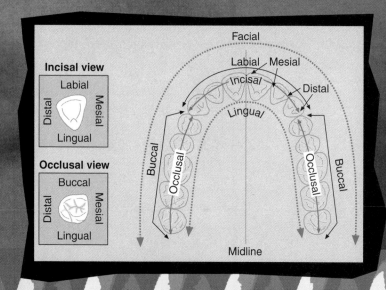

Chapter Outline

Learning Objectives

On completion of Chapter 9, the student should be able to do the following:

- Define key terms.

- Identify primary and permanent teeth, including importance, number, names, position, function, numbering systems, and eruption dates.

- Identify and locate the clinical and anatomic parts and surfaces of the teeth and supporting structures.

- Discuss the fundamentals of tooth morphology including centric contacts, proximal contacts, interproximal spaces, embrasures, tooth contour, alignment, and geometric shapes.

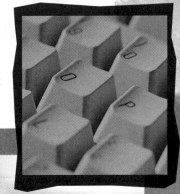

Key Terms

Interproximal Space

Midline

Parallel

Perpendicular

Primary (Deciduous)

Proximal

Secondary
(Permanent)

UNDERSTANDING ORAL ANATOMY AND TOOTH MORPHOLOGY

Tooth morphology is the study of the form and function of teeth. A dentist spends at least 50% of operating time restoring parts of teeth that have been destroyed by disease or accident. Being able to restore teeth requires the operator to form a mental picture of the missing tooth structure and then apply digital skills to replace the missing tooth structure. Because dental assistants function in clinics as chairside assistants and operative personnel in expanded-function positions, they must have varied levels of knowledge and skills. The level of knowledge needed depends on the position held by the dental assistant and the skills necessary to function in that position. For example, an office assistant generally needs to understand tooth morphology as it relates to answering patient questions and keeping records. A chairside assistant should have an overall understanding of dental anatomy and tooth morphology to assist the dentist in charting and restoring the teeth. Generally speaking, a dental hygienist needs a level of knowledge and skill related to providing a prophylaxis and interpreting conditions of the oral cavity for patient records. On the other hand, the expanded-function dental assistant, depending on the state's dental statutes and regulations, needs a higher level of knowledge and understanding of tooth morphology as well as the psychomotor skills necessary to complete complex intraoral procedures such as restoring teeth to normal form and function. A dental assistant who is educated in restorative dentistry would spend the majority of operating time restoring tooth structures destroyed by caries or accident. Therefore working knowledge of anatomic landmarks, tooth form, and occlusion is essential.

The delegation of advanced restorative functions require dental personnel to have the ability to recall a mental picture of what the tooth looked like, as well as the coordination essential to reproduce the missing tooth structure after the dentist has removed the caries and prepared the tooth for restoration. Expanded-function dental personnel must restore the missing parts of the teeth as effectively as the dentist. Therefore it is essential that advanced-function clinical dental personnel are instructed in tooth morphology and receive in-depth training in restorative dentistry.

INTRODUCTION TO TOOTH MORPHOLOGY

Teeth are important to the physical and mental well-being of the human body. They affect the processes of mastication and speech and are important to esthetics. Although teeth can be "repaired" and artificial teeth can be fabricated, these are not ideal. Patients must be educated as to the value and importance of their teeth. This is another important function that the dental assistant can provide to humanity and the dental profession.

Mastication

The teeth are part of the initial process of breaking down food for digestion. Because large pieces of food must be broken down into swallowing sizes, the teeth are designed for specific purposes related to cutting, tearing, pulverizing, and grinding. This process is called *mastication*. The four types of teeth related to these processes are the incisors, cuspids, premolars, and molars, described as follows:

- Incisors have thin "incising" and wedge-shaped surfaces designed to cut and separate food pieces.
- Cuspids have a large point or cusp and are thicker with long stable roots that allow for food to be pulled between the upper and lower cuspids and torn.
- Premolars are often called *bicuspids*. They are broader and have more than one cusp for breaking down the food and pulverizing it into smaller particles.
- Molars are larger than premolars. They have multiple cusps that provide a broad occlusal surface, which intercusps with opposing teeth to grind the larger pieces of food into smaller, digestible pieces.

Speech

The teeth, tongue, and other oral structures allow for proper pronunciation of words and speech patterns. Speech defects are caused by such physical conditions as brain damage, cleft palate, diseases of the larynx, or deafness. The teeth play an important part in this physical and emotional speech development. An edentulous patient may have difficulty forming clear concise words, and the child who has lost the "two front teeth" may lisp.

Esthetics

Esthetics (or aesthetics) pertains to a sense of beauty, art, and good taste. Teeth are the center of our smile and reflect our well-being. They provide personal characteristics that are recognized as an individual's perceived self. Because *self* is important to self-esteem, self-confidence, and self-actualization, our emotional and psychologic well-being can be affected by the condition of our teeth or the lack of teeth. Although there are certain genetic characteristics over which we have little control, quality dental treatment and health care can improve a persons appearance. Today's marketing techniques emphasizing the "beautiful smiling person" indicate the importance of teeth and esthetics to human society.

PRIMARY AND SECONDARY TOOTH DEVELOPMENT

The correct dental term for *baby teeth* is **primary** or **deciduous** teeth. The accurate term for adult teeth is sec-

Primary (deciduous)
Children's teeth.

Secondary (permanent)

Adult teeth.

Midline

The imaginary line that divides the right and left sides of the body.

ondary or **permanent** teeth. Both primary and permanent teeth are aligned into two arches called the *maxillary arch* on the top and the *mandibular arch* on the bottom. The arches are divided into right and left quadrants by an imaginary line called the *median line*, **midline**, or *midsagittal line*. The arches are also divided into anterior and posterior teeth. The anterior teeth include the central incisors, lateral incisors, and the cuspids. The posterior teeth include the premolars and molars. Anterior teeth have incisal or cutting and tearing working surfaces, whereas posterior teeth have occlusal or chewing surfaces.

When charting the teeth, remember that you are looking at the patient, making the patient's right and left side opposite yours. Both the maxillary and mandibular arch and the right and left quadrants contain the same number of teeth; the number of teeth in the primary dentition differs from the number of permanent teeth.

Primary Teeth

There are 20 teeth in the primary dentition, as follows:
8 incisors: 4 central incisors and 4 lateral incisors
4 cuspids
8 molars: 4 first molars and 4 second molars

Primary Tooth Eruption

The teeth erupt into the oral cavity at different times. The first primary tooth to erupt is usually the mandibular central incisor at approximately 6 months of age, and the last tooth to erupt is usually the maxillary second molar at approximately 24 months. The average *eruption* dates are designated in Figure 9.1. These eruption dates are just averages because children grow and develop in different time frames, and these figures should only be used as estimated eruption dates. Often parents express concern to the dental assistant when their child's teeth are not erupting as quickly as another child's teeth. Parents should be assured this is normal.

Developmental Spacing

As the child grows the head and jaws also become larger. Once the teeth erupt they do not grow in size, therefore spaces appear between each tooth. This is called *developmental spacing*. This space will allow room for the permanent tooth to erupt.

Attrition

As the child grows older, another phase takes place called *attrition*. This is the normal wearing down of the working or chewing surface of the teeth. Attrition is also part of the aging process and normal tooth wear of the adult dentition. The rate of attrition varies in relation to diet and the type of abrasive foods eaten. During this process the teeth will lose the fine detail of the cusps and incisal edges and often become smooth and flat.

Resorption

As the permanent teeth begin erupting, they press against the roots of the primary teeth. This pressure causes *resorption*

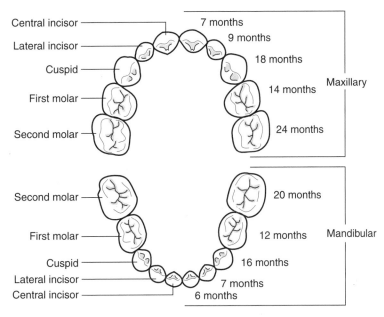

FIGURE 9.1

Names of the primary teeth and general eruption dates by month.

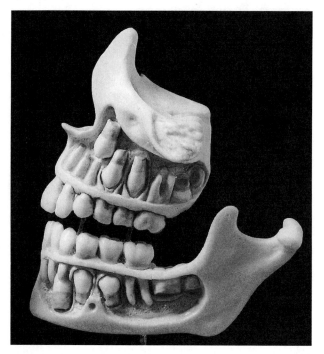

FIGURE 9.2

Mixed dentition of a 6-year-old child may include all primary teeth plus first permanent molars.

of the root of the primary tooth. Resorption is the wearing away or absorption of the primary root caused by the eruption of the permanent teeth. A similar process also occurs during orthodontic treatment when the teeth apply pressure to the alveolar bone through the use of orthodontic appliances. The pressure causes resorption of the alveolar bone as the teeth are moved into a corrected position.

Exfoliation

During the eruption and resorption process, the primary root is resorbed and the tooth becomes loose. Finally the tooth comes out or is *exfoliated,* and the permanent tooth moves into the open space.

Succedaneous

The permanent teeth that replace the 20 primary teeth are called *succedaneous teeth* because these permanent teeth succeed or follow into the space left by the primary teeth (Figure 9.2). The succedaneous teeth are the permanent incisors, cuspids, and premolars.

Mixed Dentition (6 to 12 Years)

During the eruption phase when a child has primary and permanent teeth in the mouth at the same time, a period exists around 6 years of age when the permanent mandibular

Table 9.1

Chronology of Primary, Mixed, and Permanent Dentition

Age	Development
Utero	
5 to 6 weeks in utero	Earliest sign of dental development: dental lamina formation.
14 to 19 weeks in utero	Calcification begins in all primary teeth.
	Permanent first molars begin initial calcification.
Primary dentition	
3 to 5 months	Permanent anterior teeth (central, laterals, canines) begin calcification, with exception of maxillary lateral incisor (10 to 12 months).
6 to 8 months	First primary teeth erupt (mandibular centrals).
11 months	All primary teeth have completed calcification.
1.5 years	Primary centrals, laterals, and first molars have erupted.
2.5 years	All primary teeth erupted. Remaining permanent teeth except third molars begin calcification. Second premolars may not begin until 8 or 9 years.
3.5 years	All primary teeth in occlusion and apices closed.
Permanent (mixed) dentition	
6 to 8 years	First molar, centrals, and laterals begin to erupt.
8 to 10 years	Lower cuspids erupt.
10 to 13 years	Second premolars, upper cuspids, and second molars erupt.
7 years	All permanent teeth except second and third molars completed calcification (centrals, laterals 4 to 5 years).
8 to 10 years	Third molars begin calcification. Second molars completed calcification.

first molar erupts. This is called *mixed dentition* and is explained further in Table 9.1 and Figure 9.2).

Supernumerary Teeth

Sometimes there can be more than the normal number of teeth. These additional teeth are called *supernumerary teeth.*

Secondary Teeth

There are 32 teeth in the secondary dentition, as follows:
8 incisors: 4 central incisors and 4 lateral incisors
4 cuspids
8 premolars: 4 first premolars and 4 second premolars
12 molars: 4 first molars, 4 second molars, and 4 third molars

Unlike the primary dentition, the permanent dentition has eight premolars and four third molars.

Secondary Tooth Eruption

As with the primary teeth the secondary teeth erupt into the oral cavity at different times. The first secondary tooth to erupt is usually the mandibular first molar at approximately 6 years of age, and the last teeth to erupt are maxillary third molars around the age of 16 years. Because the third molars usually erupt as the teenager is entering adulthood they are often referred to as the *wisdom teeth*. Refer to Figure 9.3 for eruption dates.

TOOTH IDENTIFICATION SYSTEMS

The primary teeth are positioned in each quadrant with the central incisor proximal or next to the median line, followed by the lateral incisor, cuspid, first molar, and second molar (Figure 9.4, *A* and *B*). Remember that the identification systems and charting methods are used as if you were looking at the patient. Therefore the patient's left is on your right and the patient's right is on your left.

There are several ways to properly identify a tooth. The tooth can be completely described by identifying the following: 1) if the tooth is located in the primary or secondary dentition; 2) in which arch it is located; 3) in which quadrant (right or left) it is positioned; and 4) the type of tooth (e.g. primary, maxillary, right, central incisor or primary, mandibular left, first molar). However, this becomes cumbersome when attempting to record and identify a patient's dental condition. Therefore several uniform numbering systems have been developed to identify the individual teeth: the universal system, the Palmer system, and the Federation Dentaire Internationale system.

Universal Numbering System

In 1968 the American Dental Association adopted the universal numbering system. This system has become the most

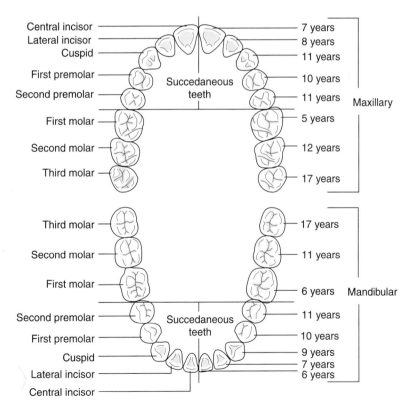

FIGURE 9.3

Permanent teeth eruption. Note the general eruption dates of the permanent teeth are listed in years; the term *succedaneous teeth* refers to only the permanent teeth that replace the primary teeth.

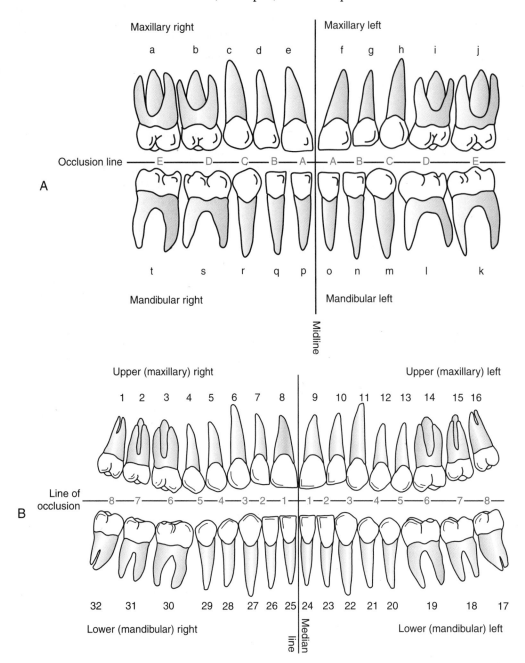

Universal and Palmer tooth identification systems. **A,** Primary. **B,** Secondary. The universal system numbers (permanent) and letters (primary) used for identification are highlighted in black. The Palmer system is identified in blue. The Palmer system relies on the quadrant symbol to complete identifying a tooth.

widely used method for dental offices, dental schools, and insurance companies. This method uses the letters of the alphabet to identify the primary teeth and Arabic numbers to identify permanent teeth.

When identifying primary teeth, the universal system corresponds the letter *A* with the maxillary right second molar and proceeds around the arch to *J*, the maxillary left second molar. At this point the letter *K* then drops down to the mandibular left second molar, proceeds around, and ends with T, or the mandibular right second molar (Figure 9.4, *A*).

When identifying permanent teeth, the universal system uses numbers instead of letters. It begins with the number 1 to represent the maxillary right third molar, 16 for the maxillary left third molar, 17 for the mandibular left third molar, and 32 for the mandibular right third molar (see Figure 9.4, *B*).

Palmer Numbering System

The Palmer system also uses letters of the alphabet to identify primary dentition and numbers to identify permanent dentition. However, this method is based on the four quadrants of the dentition. The intersection of the midline and the occlusion line forms the method for labeling each quadrant. For instance _/ represents the maxillary right, _ represents the maxillary left, \\ represents the mandibular right, and /‾ represents the mandibular left. These intersecting lines are used in conjunction with letters for the primary teeth and numbers for the permanent teeth. For example, when labeling the primary teeth, *A* represents the four central incisors, *B* represents the four lateral incisors, *C* represents the four cuspids, *D* represents the four first molars, and *E* represents the four second molars. These letters are placed within the intersecting brackets to represent, for instance, the maxillary right central incisor A| or the mandibular left second molar |E (see Figure 9.4, *A*).

The Palmer method used for identifying the permanent dentition is the same, except numbers are used instead, and of course there are more teeth in the permanent dentition. Each quadrant is labeled 1 through 8 with the number 1 representing the central incisors and 8 representing the third molars. The numbers are placed within the intersecting brackets to represent a particular tooth. For example, the

maxillary left cuspid would be |3 and the mandibular right second premolar would be 5| (see Figure 9.4, *B*). Chapter 21, "Oral Diagnosis and Treatment Planning," will describe the use of these systems for charting the teeth.

Federation Dentaire Internationale (FDI) System

The FDI system uses a two-digit number system for both the permanent and primary dentition. The first number represents the quadrant and the second number represents the tooth. The quadrants of the permanent dentition, represented by the first number, are numbered from 1 to 4, and the quadrants of the primary dentition are numbered from 5 to 8. The individual teeth are represented by the second number; the permanent dentition is numbered from 1 to 8, and the primary dentition is numbered from 1 to 5. The number 24, for example, would be the permanent, maxillary, left, first premolar. The 2 represents the permanent, maxillary, left quadrant, and the 4 represents the first premolar (Figure 9.5).

CLINICAL AND ANATOMIC PARTS OF THE TEETH

The tooth, in general, is made up of three anatomic structures: the crown, neck, and root (Figure 9.6). The crown of the tooth is referred to as the *coronal* portion of the tooth.

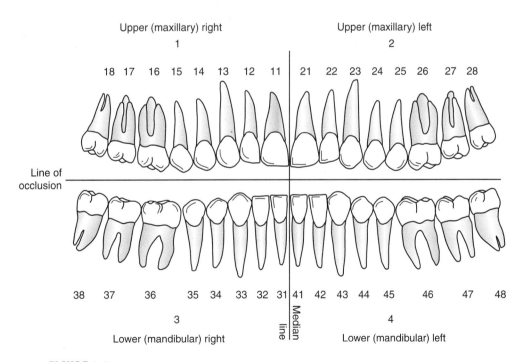

FIGURE 9.5

Federation Dentaire Internationale (FDI) tooth numbering system for permanent teeth.

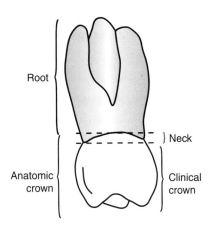

FIGURE 9.6

Identification of tooth parts.

The portion of the crown that can be seen when examining a normal healthy mouth is called the *clinical crown*. It is the supragingival portion of the crown because it is above the gingival margin. The *anatomic crown* refers to the whole crown. Because the neck of the tooth is normally covered with free gingival, only the clinical crown can be seen. However, the crown of a tooth extends below the gingival margin or subgingivally, approximately 1.5 to 2 mm.

The neck of the tooth is that part of the tooth where the enamel of the crown meets the cementum covering the root portion of the tooth. This area is referred to as the *cervical line* or *cementoenamel junction*.

The root of the tooth is that portion of the tooth that lies within the alveolar bone and helps to secure the tooth in position. Teeth have varying numbers of roots, which will be discussed later. The anatomic division forming more than one root is called a *furcation*. If a tooth has two roots the separation is called a *bifurcation* and if three roots are formed the separation is called a *trifurcation*. The tip of the root is called an *apex*.

HARD AND SOFT TOOTH TISSUE AND SUPPORTING STRUCTURE

In addition to the three anatomic structures—crown, neck, and root—the tooth is composed of specific hard and soft tooth tissues and supporting structures.

Tooth Structure

The hard tooth tissues consist of enamel and dentin. The soft tissue refers to the pulp. Cementum may be considered one of the hard tooth tissues or a supportive structure.

Enamel

Enamel is the translucent white substance which covers the anatomic crown of the tooth. The translucency depends on the thickness of the enamel, and the white shading varies from a light yellow to a gray color. The enamel is that part of the tooth exposed to the oral cavity. Although enamel is the hardest substance in the human body and can withstand the biting and chewing forces of mastication, it is also brittle and subject to decay. The problem is that enamel cannot regenerate itself and therefore must be artificially replaced or restored if damaged.

Enamel is thickest on the working surfaces of the crown and thinnest around the neck of the tooth. Enamel is formed by ameloblasts and composed primarily of the minerals calcium and phosphorus. Enamel is not structurally solid; it is made up of enamel rods or prisms that are encased in rod sheaths and bonded together by an interred substance. These rods are aligned **parallel** and extend in a **perpendicular** line along the dento-enamel junction.

Parallel
Side by side or an equal distance apart.

Perpendicular
A line or plane at right angles or vertical to a given horizontal position.

Dentin

Dentin is the yellowish portion of tooth that makes up the main body. Dentin is covered by the enamel on the coronal portion and by the cementum on the root portion. The dentin contains the pulp chamber or cavity. It is harder than cementum but not as hard as enamel.

Dentin is formed by odontoblasts that continue to exist in the dentin next to the pulp chamber. The dentin developed during tooth formation is called *primary dentin*. Unlike enamel, dentin is a living tissue that reforms itself regularly and is able to repair itself in response to trauma or irritants. This reformed dentin is called *secondary dentin*.

Dentin is a porous tissue that contains many tiny canals called *dentinal tubules*. These tubules evolve from the surface of the dentin to the pulpal chamber. They are filled with sensitive, living tissue called *dentinal fibers*. These fibers contain odontoblasts that stimulate secondary dentin formation. Because of the sensitivity of the dentinal fibers and their active part in secondary dentin formation, the dentinal tubules must be sealed or covered during restorative procedures.

Pulp

Each tooth has a pulp chamber that is located in the coronal portion of the crown (Figure 9.7 and 9.8, *A*) and pulp canals or root canals located in the root portion of the

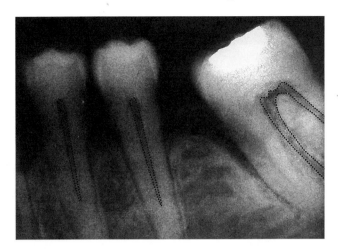

FIGURE 9.7
Radiograph delineating actual dental tissues with the dental pulp highlighted.

tooth. The pulp chamber has pulp horns that correspond to the cusps of each tooth. Dental pulp is the sensory soft tissue of the tooth located within the chamber and canals. It extends through an opening, the *apical foramen*, in the apex of the tooth root to connect with the nerve, blood, and lymphatic systems. Pulp consists of arteries and veins, nerve and lymphatic vessels, and connective tissues that nourish and protect the tooth. The nerves, for instance, produce a physiologic reaction by responding to pain, thus aiding in stimulating blood flow, odontoblasts, and fibroblasts. This process aids in the production of the secondary dentin, which helps to protect the tooth from injury. When extensive trauma occurs the pulp may become devital or dead. Root canal therapy is discussed in Chapter 27, "Endodontics."

Supporting Structures

The supporting tooth structures, or the periodontium, refers to those tissues that support the tooth and includes the gingivae, cementum, periodontal ligament, and alveolar bone.

Gingivae

The gingivae is soft oral tissue that covers the alveolar bone and attaches to the teeth. It blends into the soft flexible oral mucosa that lines the cheeks, lips, vestibule (the space between the alveolar ridge and the lips or cheeks), soft palate, floor of the mouth, and undersurface of the tongue (Figures 9.8, *A* and *B*.

Cementum

Cementum is the thin layer of mineralized bonelike substance that covers the root portion of the tooth. Cemen-

tum is softer than enamel and dentin. Cementum is thinner in the cervical or cementoenamel junction area of the tooth, where it may barely overlap the enamel. However, cementum is slightly thicker on the apex of the root. The purpose of the cementum is to provide an attachment for the periodontal fibers or ligaments that hold the tooth firmly in the tooth socket or alveolus. There are cellular and acellular, cementum-forming cells called *cementoblasts*. Cellular cementoblasts are located on the apex of the root and continuously reform and reinforce tooth attachment throughout a person's lifetime. This reformation is often stimulated in response to trauma or the need to reinforce the periodontal ligaments (see Figure 9.8, *A*).

Periodontal Ligaments

Periodontal ligaments are fibers embedded in the cementum. These fibers, called *Sharpey's fibers*, aid in attaching the tooth to the alveolus and holding it in proper position; they also cushion the tooth in response to trauma or normal forces of mastication. The predominate periodontal fibers are the apical, interradicular, transseptal, oblique, horizontal, and alveolar crest (Figure 9.8, *A* and *C*).

Alveolar Bone

The teeth are also supported by alveolar bone, which is often called the *alveolar bone proper*. Each tooth is positioned in a tooth socket or alveolus. The alveolus is lined with compact bone or plate, called the *lamina dura*, which can be seen on a radiograph as a light line encircling each tooth root. The periodontal fibers that are attached to the cementum also attach to this lamina dura and provide support for the tooth (see Figure 9.8, *A*).

Bone is formed by osteoblasts and absorbed by osteoclasts. This process is particularly important in orthodontic treatment. Teeth are moved in a particular direction as pressure is applied to the tooth and against the bone. This causes the bone to absorb but also reform and fill in the space as the tooth moves.

TOOTH SURFACES AND ANGLES

Several standardized systems of identifying the teeth and tooth surfaces have been developed. These systems are important because they aid in recording and charting dental health conditions in a precise manner so information can later be interpreted, understood, and communicated to other practitioners or groups such as insurance agencies. As discussed previously, each tooth is identified by the use of a number or letter. Each tooth also has five surfaces, identified according to the direction it faces. The surfaces of the anterior teeth are mesial, distal, labial, lingual, and incisal. The surfaces of the posterior teeth are mesial, distal, buccal, lingual, and occlusal.

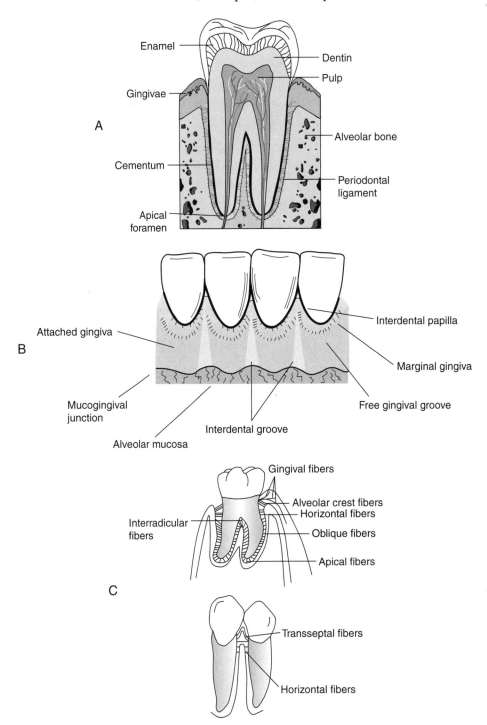

FIGURE 9.8

A, Parts of the posterior tooth. **B,** Gingivae tissues. **C,** Periodontal fibers.

These tooth surfaces are classified as follows:

Mesial surface (M) is the surface of the tooth that faces the midline.

Distal surface (D) is the surface of the tooth that faces away from the midline and is opposite the mesial surface.

Labial surface (LA) is the surface on the anterior teeth that faces the lips.

Buccal surface (B) is the surface on the posterior teeth that faces the cheeks.

Facial surface (F) is the term used to refer to both the labial surface and the buccal surface.

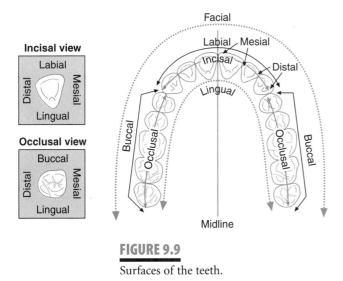

FIGURE 9.9

Surfaces of the teeth.

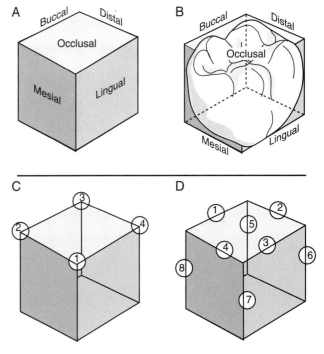

FIGURE 9.10

Point and line angles. **A,** Surfaces. **B,** Tooth surfaces. **C,** Point angles: *1* Mesiolingu-occlusal point angle; *2* Mesiobucco-occlusal point angle; *3* Distobucco-occlusal point angle; *4* Distolingu-occlusal point angle. **D,** Line angles: *1* Bucco-occlusal line angle; *2* Disto-occlusal line angle; *3* Lingu-occlusal line angle; *4* Mesio-occlusal line angle; *5* Distobuccal line angle; *6* Distolingual line angle; *7* Mesiolingual line angle; *8* Mesiobuccal line angle.

Lingual surface (L) is the surface of all teeth that faces the tongue.

Incisal surface (I) is the working surface or cutting and tearing surface of the anterior teeth. The terms *incisal ridge* or *incisal edge* also refer to this surface.

Occlusal surface (O) is the working or chewing surface of the posterior teeth (Figure 9.9).

A procedure using the universal numbering system involving a single surface, such as the mesial of the permanent maxillary right lateral incisor, would be recorded as 7M. A multiple surface, such as the mesial, occlusal, and distal of the permanent mandibular right second premolar, would be recorded as 29MOD. Note that the surfaces are written from mesial to distal (MOD) and *not* in reverse (DOM) or (OMD).

Angles

Be sure to classify or identify specific areas of the teeth to document the area of the crown in which an operative procedure is being completed or to identify and record a dental anomaly (a condition that is not normal). To accomplish this, *line angles* and *point angles* are used to divide the tooth crown.

Line angles describe where two surfaces of the tooth crown come together or meet. The name of the line angle is determined by the name of the two surfaces that meet. For instance, the line angle in which the mesial surface and the occlusal surface meet on a posterior crown is called the *mesio-occlusal line angle*. The suffix *al* is dropped and replaced by *o* when combining surfaces. Therefore the mesial and occlusal line angle are described as the mesio-occlusal line angle.

Point angles describe three surfaces of the tooth crown come together or meet. The name of the point angle is determined by the name of three surfaces that meet. For instance, the point angle in which the mesial, lingual, and occlusal surfaces meet on a posterior crown is called the *mesiolinguo-occlusal point angle* (Figure 9.10).

Thirds

To visualize the shape and form of the teeth, it is necessary to understand the concept of the division of the tooth into thirds. The separation of the teeth into thirds help to locate specific areas on the tooth such as the height of contour or contact area. Thirds also help to comprehend angles such as the mesioincisal angle and the distoincisal angle (Figure 9.11, *A* and *B*).

Both the crown of the tooth and the root are divided into thirds. A tooth can be viewed from the labial, buccal, lingual, mesial, distal, occlusal, or incisal surface. The thirds are identified according to the aspect from which the tooth is viewed and may include identifying the thirds horizontally or vertically (axial or with the long axis of the tooth).

Each third is named after the area in which it is located. For instance, from the facial view the distal third is located

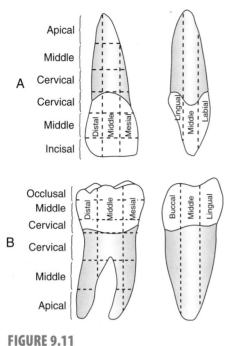

FIGURE 9.11

Tooth thirds. **A,** Anterior view. **B,** Posterior view.

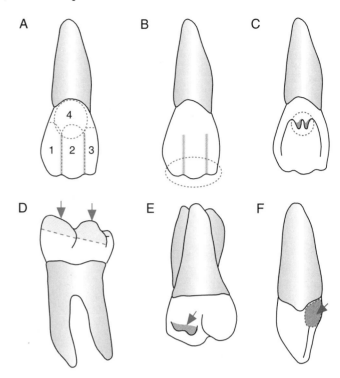

FIGURE 9.12

Developmental landmarks. **A,** Lobes. **B,** Mamelons. **C,** Tubules. **D,** Cusps. **E,** Cusp of carabellin. **F,** Cingulum.

on the distal surface of the tooth and the mesial third is located on the mesial surface. The space between the distal and mesial third is called the *middle third*. If an anterior tooth is viewed from the mesial, the axial thirds become lingual, middle, and labial, and the horizontal thirds would be incisal, middle, and cervical (gingival).

A tooth viewed from the occlusal aspect would show the mesial, middle, and distal third and the buccal, middle, and lingual third. Likewise the labial aspect of a root would include a cervical, middle, and apical third and a mesial, middle, and distal third.

ANATOMIC LANDMARKS

The dental assistant must be familiar with the anatomic structures or landmarks of the teeth to record and communicate properly with the dental team and patients. The dentist and the clinical dental assistant who performs advanced restorative procedures spend at least 50% of their operative time restoring the parts of teeth that have been destroyed by caries or fracture. Therefore they need to have a working understanding of these structures. These anatomic terms are described with greater detail for restorative dentistry in Chapter 36 and 37.

The surface of each tooth is made up of elevated areas and depressions. These anatomic areas or landmarks are formed during the stages of tooth development and each structure is identified and described in detail according to the tooth surface on which they are found. The following terms are related to tooth developmental elevations and depressions. Figures 9.12 to 9.18 describe these developmental elevations and depressions from simple terms to complex combinations of terms reflecting the locations of these structures.

Developmental Elevations and Ridges

Developmental elevations are raised structures located on the individual surfaces of teeth and are described as follows:

Lobes: Segments of teeth formed as the stages of tooth development take place. These lobes come together to form a crown. However, these segments do not come together smoothly, leaving visible structures such as cusps, mamelons, grooves, and ridges (Figure 9.12, *A*).

Mamelon: Raised, rounded projections on the incisal edge of recently erupted incisors. Mamelons will usually wear away through attrition. (Figure 9.12, *B*).

Tubules: Tubular projections on the lingual surface of anterior teeth extending from the cingulum (Figure 9.12, *C*).

Cusps: Rounded projections or raised areas on the occlusal surface of posterior teeth and cuspids. The number of cusps vary on different teeth (Figure 9.12, *D*).

Cusp of Carabelli: An auxiliary or additional cusp, considered the "fifth" cusp, located on the lingual of the mesiolingual cusp of the maxillary first molars (Figure 9.12, *E*).

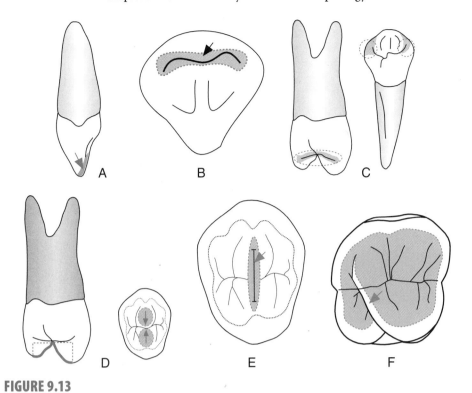

FIGURE 9.13

Developmental ridges. **A,** Incisal "edge". **B,** Cusp ridge. **C,** Marginal ridge. **D,** Triangular ridge. **E,** Transverse ridge. **F,** Oblique ridge.

Cingulum: A rounded, raised area on the lingual cervical third of anterior teeth (Figure 9.12, *F*).

Ridges

Ridges are linear elevations on the occlusal surface of posterior teeth and lingual surface of anterior teeth. Ridges are named after the surface on which they are found. (Figures 9.13, *A–F*, and Figure 9.14).

Incisal ridge: The rounded linear elevation on the linguoincisal surface of central and lateral incisors referred to as the cutting or biting incisal edge (Figure 9.13, *A*).

Cusp ridge: The rounded linear elevations on cusps, sometimes referred to as the *cusp arm*, extending from the marginal ridge to the tip of the cusp and from the buccal, lingual, or distal developmental grooves to the cusp tip. Each cusp ridge is named after the surface and cusp to which it relates, such as mesiobuccal cusp ridge or mesiolingual cusp ridge (Figure 9.13, *B*).

Marginal ridge: The rounded linear elevation on the mesiocclusal or distoclusal surfaces of posterior teeth or the mesiolingual or distolingual surfaces of anterior teeth. Marginal ridges form the mesial and distal borders on all teeth (Figure 9.13, *C*).

Triangular ridge: A triangular-shaped linear elevation on the occlusal surface of posterior teeth and the lingual surface of cuspids extending from the tip of the cusp and widening to the central area or developmental groove. The ridge is named after the cusp on which it is positioned, such as mesiobuccal triangular ridge (Figure 9.13, *D*).

Transverse ridge: A linear elevation on the occlusal surface of posterior teeth, made up of two triangular ridges that extend directly across from the tip of the buccal cusp to the center of the tooth and the tip of the lingual cusp in a somewhat continuous ridge (Figure 9.13, *E*).

Oblique ridge: A linear elevation on the occlusal surface to maxillary molars extending in an oblique direction from the mesiolingual cusp tip to the distobuccal cusp tip (Figure 9.13, *F*).

Developmental Depressions and Fossa

Developmental depressions are grooves or shallow depressions on the surfaces of teeth. Grooves are linear depressions or developmental grooves formed by the merging of the lobes and ridges during crown development. Grooves are named after the area in which they form. The key grooves are described as follows (Figures 9.15, *A–F*, and 9.16):

Central groove: A linear depression positioned in the middle third of the occlusal surface and extending from the mesial to the distal surfaces of the crown (Figures 9.15, *A*).

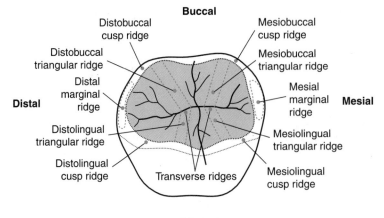

FIGURE 9.14

Ridges found on a molar.

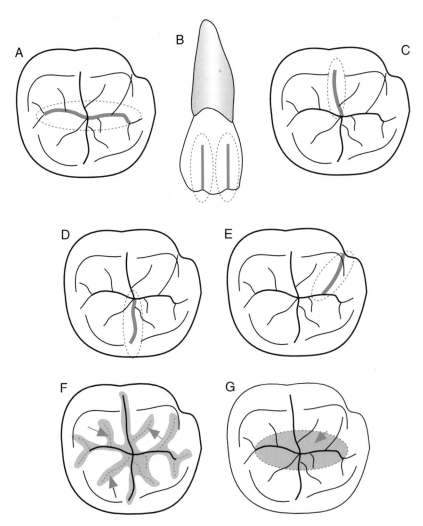

FIGURE 9.15

Developmental grooves. **A,** Central groove. **B,** Labial groove. **C,** Buccal groove. **D,** Lingual groove. **E,** Distal groove. **F,** Supplemental grooves. **G,** Sulcus

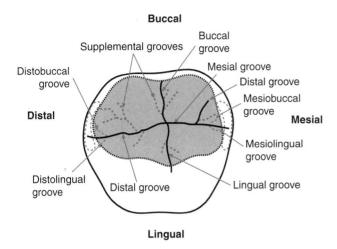

Buccal

Supplemental grooves

Buccal groove

Distobuccal groove

Mesial groove

Distal groove

Mesiobuccal groove

Distal

Mesial

Mesiolingual groove

Distolingual groove

Distal groove

Lingual groove

Lingual

FIGURE 9.16

Developmental grooves are named after the surface on which they are located.

Labial groove: Linear depressions on the labial surface of anterior teeth extending from the middle third to the incisal edge, often emphasizing the mamelons if visible (Figure 9.15, *B*).

Buccal groove: A linear depression extending from the middle third of the buccal surface to the central developmental groove between the mesiobuccal and distobuccal cusps. The lingual groove of the maxillary molars extends obliquely following the angle of the elevation of the oblique ridge (Figure 9.15, *C*).

Lingual groove: A linear depression extending from the middle third of the lingual surface to the central developmental groove between the mesiolingual and distolingual cusps (Figure 9.15, *D*).

Distal groove: A linear depression extending from the buccal surface of the distobuccal cusp to the central developmental groove between the distobuccal and distal cusp (Figure 9.15, *E*).

Supplemental groove: A less distinct, shallow, and irregular linear depression that produces wrinkled surface characteristics on the occlusal surface of the teeth (Figure 9.15, *F*).

Sulcus: A linear depression on the occlusal surface that has a developmental groove at the center (Figures 9.15, *G*, 9.17, *E*, and 9.17, *G*).

Fossa

Fossa are rounded irregular depressions located on the occlusal or lingual surface of the crown and are described as follows (Figure 9.17, *A*–*G*):

Central fossa: The rounded depression on the central occlusal surface of posterior teeth (Figure 9.17, *A*).

Lingual fossa: The shallow, rounded, spoon-shaped depression on the lingual surface of anterior crowns (Figure 9.17, *B*).

Triangular fossa: The rounded depression on the occlusal surface of posterior teeth and the lingual surface of ante-

rior teeth found adjacent to and below the mesial and distal marginal ridges (Figure 9.17, *C*, *D*, *F*, and *G*).

Developmental Faults

Developmental faults are defects in a fossa or developmental groove caused from the failure of the lobes to come together tightly during development and are described as follows:

Pit: A rounded fault or defect in the lingual, central, or triangular fossa area (Figure 9.17, *D*, *F*, and *G*).

Fissure: A linear fault or defect along the developmental groove (Figures 9.17, *E* and *G*).

FUNDAMENTALS OF TOOTH MORPHOLOGY

In addition to the anatomic landmarks of the teeth, there are identifiable curvatures of teeth that serve to provide protection to the periodontal tissues and aid in mastication (Figure 9.18). Both the anatomic landmarks and contours of the teeth are physiologic in nature and must be replaced to provide proper tooth form, alignment and occlusion. The protective functions of tooth form include the following:

1 Proximal contact
2 Interproximal space
3 Embrasures
4 Tooth contour
5 Occlusion

Proximal Contact

The two primary functions of contact areas are 1) to keep food from packing between the teeth, resulting in inflammation and potential breakdown of the periodontium, and 2) to assist in stabilizing the tooth's position to maintain the dental arches (Figure 9.19, *A*–*C*). Each tooth contacts adjacent teeth on the **proximal** (adjacent) surface, except the distal of the third molars and the

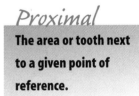

Proximal

The area or tooth next to a given point of reference.

mesial contact between the two central incisors. The term *contact point* is often used to refer to the contact area. However, the term *contact area* is preferred. Age and wear often cause the contact areas to broaden.

When restoring the teeth the proper location of the contact area is very important. In addition to maintaining a tight contact, the contact area must also be properly located in an occlusocervical and buccolingual direction. The following information will help in locating the proper contact area:

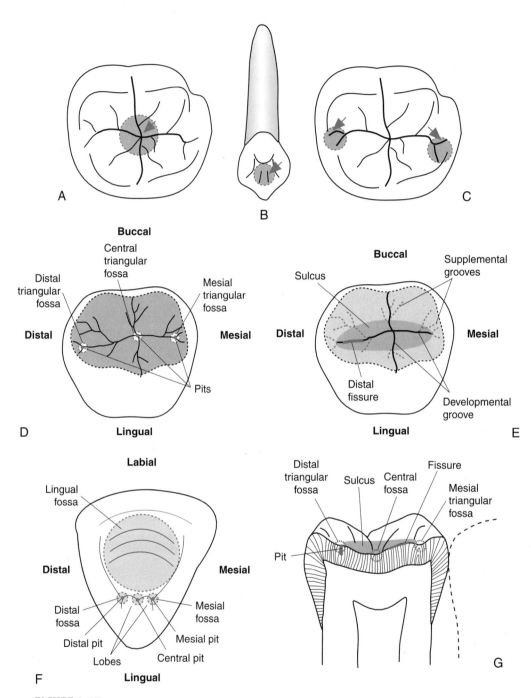

FIGURE 9.17

Fossas, sulcus, and faults. **A,** Central fossa. **B,** Lingual fossa. **C,** Triangular fossa. **D,** Fossa and pits. **E,** Grooves and fissure sulcus. **F,** Anterior tooth with fossas, pits, and lobes. **G,** Posterior tooth with fossas, pit, fissure, and sulcus.

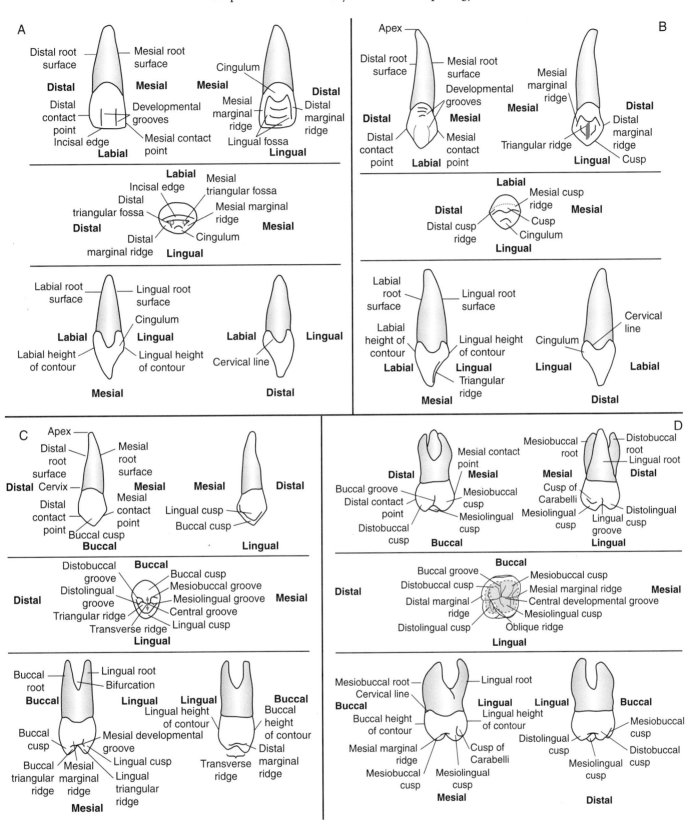

FIGURE 9.18

Each tooth has identifiable anatomic landmarks. **A,** Maxillary central incisor. **B,** Maxillary cuspid. **C,** Maxillary first premolar. **D,** Maxillary first molar.

Continued

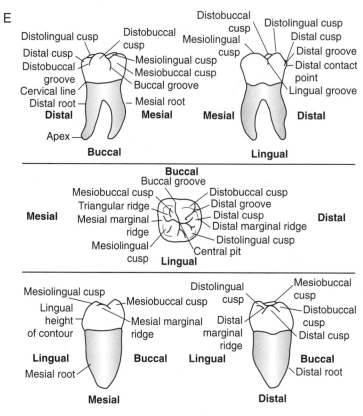

FIGURE 9.18, cont'd

Each tooth has identifiable anatomic landmarks. **E,** Mandibular first molar.

1 The contact areas become more cervically located from anterior to posterior in each quadrant.

2 The distal contact area is usually located more to the cervical than the mesial contact area.

3 The size of the contact areas increase from anterior to posterior in each dental arch.

4 The contact areas from an incisal/occlusal view are toward the labial dimension on anterior teeth.

5 The contact areas are usually located slightly to the buccal of center in the buccolingual dimension on posterior teeth.

Interproximal Space

The **interproximal space** is the triangular-shaped area be-

Interproximal space

The area or space between the teeth.

tween adjacent teeth in the same arch that is cervical to the contact area (Figure 9.19, *A*). This space can be seen best by looking at the teeth from the facial aspect. The interproximal space is filled by gingival tissue

called the *interdental papilla.* The triangular interproximal area is formed by a cervical base of alveolar bone, the sides are formed by the proximal surfaces of contacting teeth, and the apex is formed by the contact area of the adjacent teeth.

The shape of the interproximal space will vary with the form of the contacting teeth and the position of the contact area. The interproximal space is filled with gingival tissue except where gingival recession occurs some of the interproximal spacing may be visible.

Proper restoration of the teeth should occur to maintain the correct contact and alignment of adjoining teeth to prevent attachment of food around and between the teeth. The general triangular shape of the interproximal space should be maintained when placing a restoration to aid in self-cleaning.

Embrasures

Embrasures are open **V**-shaped spaces between the proximal surfaces of two adjacent teeth in the same arch. Embrasures have three primary purposes: (1) to provide "spillways" for food to escape during mastication; (2) to provide self-cleansing of the teeth; and (3) to provide protection and stimulation of the periodontium. Remember when complet-

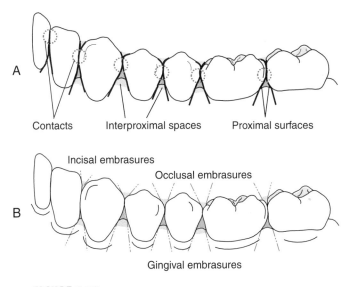

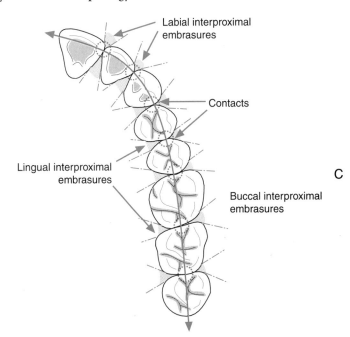

FIGURE 9.19

A, Facial view of proximal surfaces, interproximal spaces, and contact areas. **B,** Facial view of incisal, occlusal, and cervical (gingival) embrasures. **C,** Incisal/occlusal view of embrasures and contacts.

ing restorative procedures that proper embrasure form is restored. Embrasures that are too large may cause lack of protection and result in overstimulation of the periodontium and tissue breakdown. Embrasures that are too narrow may cause overprotection and result in lack of stimulation and tissue breakdown.

The contact area is surrounded by the embrasures and interproximal area. The embrasures diverge from facial to lingual and from incisal or occlusal to cervix from the contact area due to the contouring or rounding of these surfaces.

Embrasures are named for their location and depend on the aspect from which the teeth are viewed. An incisal or occlusal view (see Figure 9.19, *C*) shows the labial or buccal and lingual interproximal embrasures caused by the space that widens out from the contact area toward the labial, buccal, and lingual surfaces of the teeth. A facial or lingual view (see Figure 9.19, *B*) shows the incisal or occlusal and gingival embrasures. Some general rules to remember in regard to embrasure forms are as follows:

1 From the facial or lingual aspect the incisal or occlusal embrasures increase in relative size from the anterior teeth toward the posterior.
2 From the facial or lingual aspect the gingival embrasures decrease in relative size from anterior to posterior.
3 From the incisal aspect the labial and lingual embrasures are nearly equal in size in anterior teeth.
4 From the occlusal aspect the lingual embrasure is normally larger than the buccal embrasure in posterior teeth.

5 When one side of an embrasure has a certain contour (for example, convex) the other side of the embrasure will have a similar contour.

Tooth Contour

The contour of the teeth is another important part of tooth form and function. For instance, the location of the height of contour or crest of curvature helps protect the periodontal tissue. The height of contour is the greatest area of curvature on the facial and lingual surfaces of the crown and is best seen when viewed from the proximal surfaces or mesial and distal aspects (Figure 9.20, *A* and *B*). The contact area on proximal surfaces represents the crest of curvature of the mesial and distal surfaces, and the height of contour represents the crest of curvature on the facial and lingual surfaces. Just as embrasures and contacts protect and stimulate the gingival tissue, the height of contour also carries out this function. These contours must be replaced during restorative procedures for the tooth to function properly. Likewise there are curvatures on the crown of the tooth in which the curve is *concave.* This means the curvature is inward rather than outward or *convex* (Figure 9.20, *C*).

Remember when restoring a tooth that any excess bulge or overhang represents overcontouring caused by an undercarved restoration. Likewise a restoration that is overly flat or underfilled is undercontoured or overcarved (Figure 9.20, *D*). The following general rules are helpful when restoring the tooth:

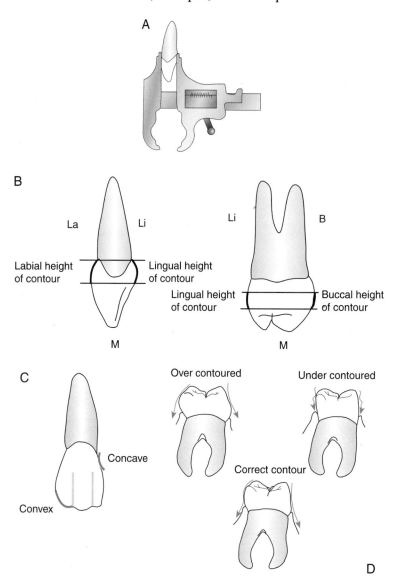

FIGURE 9.20

Height of contour. **A,** Boley gauge measuring height of contour. **B,** Height of contour identifies the greatest curvature on the facial and lingual surfaces compared with correct contour. **C,** Example of a concave and convex surface. **D,** Overcontoured and undercontoured surfaces.

1 The height of contour on the labial and lingual of anterior teeth is located in the cervical third.
2 The height of contour of the buccal surface of posterior teeth is located in the cervical third.
3 The height of contour of the lingual surfaces of posterior teeth is located in the middle or occlusal third.

The shape of the teeth are also represented by several geometric shapes: triangle, trapezoid, rhomboid, rectangular, and oval or round. These tooth forms must also be consid-

ered when restoring tooth contour, form, and function (Figure 9.21, *A–D*).

Occlusion and Alignment

The relationship of the mandibular arch as it occludes with the maxillary arch is called *occlusion*. The muscles of mastication, teeth, and temporal mandibular joint (TMJ) all de-

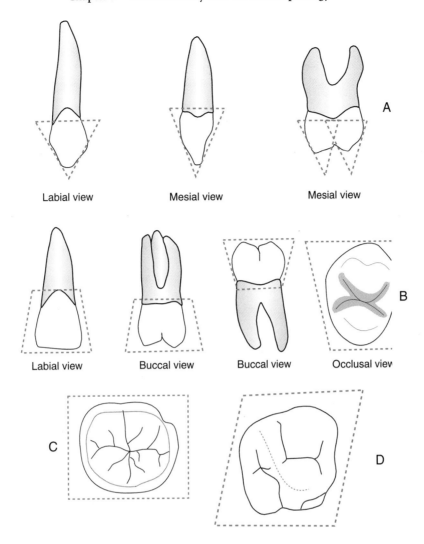

Labial view   Mesial view   Mesial view   A

Labial view   Buccal view   Buccal view   Occlusal view   B

C   D

FIGURE 9.21

Tooth formation and geometric shape. **A,** Triangle. **B,** Trapezoid.
C, Rectangle. **D,** Rhomboid.

termine occlusion. Occlusion functions to bring the jaws into centric occlusion (rest position) and also to provide lateral (side to side) movement and protrusive (lower jaw forward) movement. Poor occlusion can cause malocclusion and result in TMJ dysfunction or bruxism (grinding the teeth).

Basically, the two arches do occlude and the cusps of the teeth should interdigitate. Each tooth should have two opposing teeth, except for the mandibular central incisors and the maxillary third molar, which have only one opposing tooth. The facial cusps and incisal edges of the maxillary arch should overlap the facial cusps and incisal edges of the

mandibular arch for the teeth to be esthetically matched. For further information on occlusion refer to Chapter 30, "Orthodontics."

OUTSTANDING CHARACTERISTICS OF THE SECONDARY TEETH

Outstanding characteristics of the teeth, such as the number of cusps or roots, help identify individual teeth (Table 9.2). Other characteristics relate to the size, shape, and detail (Box 9.1).

Table 9.2

Cusp and Root Identification

Tooth	Cusps		Roots	
	Maxillary	Mandibular	Maxillary	Mandibular
Cuspid	1	1	1	1
First premolar	2 (1B/1L)	2 (1B/1L)	2 (1B/1L)	1
Second premolar	2 (1B/1L)	3 (1B/1L)	1	1
First molar	4 + 1 (2B/2L/ 1ML)	5 (2B/2L/1D)	3 (2B/1L)	2 (1M/1D)
Second molar	4 (2B/2L)	4 (2B/2L)	3 (2B/1L)	2 (1M/1D)
Third molar	4 (2B/2L)	4 (2B/2L)	Varies	Varies

Box 9.1

General Characteristics of Individual Teeth

Incisors

Maxillary central incisors

Universal numbering: right = 8, left = 9
Palmer numbering: right = 1/, left = \1
Widest mesiodistally of anteriors
Labial surface is broad and flat
Labial is square or rectangular shape
Nearly straight incisal edge
Nearly straight incisal edge
Mesial incisal angle is 90 degrees
Distal incisal angle is more rounded
Mesial aspect is wedge-shaped or triangular
Root is cone-shaped with blunt apex

Maxillary lateral incisors

Universal numbering: right = 7, left = 10
Palmer numbering: right = 2/, left = \2
Smaller than central incisor in all dimensions except
    root length
Crown is smaller than central incisor and more curved
Outline is more rounded than central incisor

Mandibular central incisors

Universal numbering: right = 25, left = 24
Palmer numbering: right = 1\, left = /1
Smaller mesiodistal dimensions than any tooth
Smaller than the lateral incisor
Sharp mesial and distal incisal angles
Labial surface is smooth and flattened

Mandibular lateral incisors

Universal numbering: right = 26, left = 23
Palmer numbering: right = 2\, left = /2
Somewhat larger than central incisor
Distal is slightly more contoured

Cuspids

Maxillary cuspid

Universal numbering: right = 6, left = 11
Palmer numbering: right = 3|, left = |3
Longest tooth in the dental arch
Large, well-defined single cusp
Root tips distally
Large cingulum

Mandibular cuspid

Universal numbering: right = 27, left = 22
Palmer numbering: right = 3\, left = /3
Same length or longer than maxillary cuspid, but
    smoother and more slender
Cusp not as well-developed as maxillary cuspid
Labiolingual aspect is thinner, resembling the incisors

Premolars

Maxillary first premolar

Universal numbering: right = 5, left = 12
Palmer numbering: right = 4|, left = |4
Two cusps
Buccal cusp is 1 mm longer than lingual cusp
Very well-defined cusps with well-defined grooves
Usually two roots
Trapezoid shape
Centrally located central groove

Maxillary second premolar

Universal numbering: right = 4, left = 13
Palmer numbering: right = 5/, left = \5
Form similar in all aspects to first premolar
Cusps equal heights
Sulcus is more shallow
Occlusal surface appears more wrinkled
One root

Box 9.1—cont'd

General Characteristics of Individual Teeth

Mandibular first premolar

Universal numbering: right = 20, left = 28
Palmer numbering: right = 4̄\, left = /4̄
Two cusps
Buccal cusp is more developed, large, and pointed
Single root
Lingual cusp is half the height of the buccal cusp
Occlusal aspect is circular in outline

Mandibular second premolar

Universal numbering: right = 29, left = 20
Palmer numbering: right = 5\, left = /5
Three cusps
Buccal cusp is shorter than first premolar
Mesiolingual cusp is shorter than distolingual cusp
Rectangular in shape

Molars

Maxillary first molar

Universal numbering: right = 3, left = 14
Palmer numbering: right = 6|, left = |6
Largest tooth in the mouth
Rhomboid in outline
Four well-developed cusps
Cusp of Carabelli on mesiolingual cusp
Oblique ridge from distobuccal cusp to tip of
   mesiolingual cusp
Three roots
Mesiobuccal cusp width is greatest

Maxillary second molar

Universal numbering: right = 2, left = 15
Palmer numbering: right = 7|, left = |7
Similar to first molar but smaller in dimensions
Similar to first molar but smaller in dimensions
Four cusps but shorter
Three roots but closer together
No fifth cusp

Rhomboid (smaller)
Oblique ridge is not as detailed

Maxillary third molar

Universal numbering: right = 1, left = 16
Palmer numbering: right = 8|, left = |8

Maxillary third molar—cont'd.

Called *wisdom tooth*
Much smaller than first and second
Many variations of form
1 to 8 roots, may be fused together
Usually three cusps: two buccal and large lingual cusp
Usually poorly developed

Mandibular first molar

Universal numbering: right = 30, left = 19
Palmer numbering: right = 6̄\, left = /6̄
Five cusps: mesiobuccal cusp larger
Small distal cusp
Rectangular shape: may be more trapezoidal
Buccal cusps are almost same width
Lingual cusps are longer than buccal
Two well-developed roots

Mandibular second molar

Universal numbering: right = 31, left = 18
Palmer numbering: right = 7̄\, left = /7̄
Four cusps: outline is smaller than the first
Occlusal surface are square or rectangular shape
Two roots: smaller than first
No distal cusp

Mandibular third molar

Universal numbering: right = 30, left = 17
Palmer numbering: right = 8̄\, left = /8̄
Undeveloped and irregular shape
Similar to the second molar but smaller

Comparing Anatomic Differences

Use Figure 9.22 and Box 9.1 to compare the individual anatomic differences of the following:

1. Compare the individual anatomic differences between the maxillary central and lateral and the mandibular central and lateral incisors.

Note that the mandibular teeth are positioned upright to easier compare with maxillary teeth.

2. Compare the individual anatomic differences between the maxillary and mandibular cuspids (Figure 9.23).
3. Compare the individual anatomic differences between the maxillary first and second premolars and the mandibular first and second premolars (Figure 9.24).
4. Compare the individual anatomic differences between the maxillary first, second, and third molars and the mandibular first, second, and third molars (Figure 9.25).

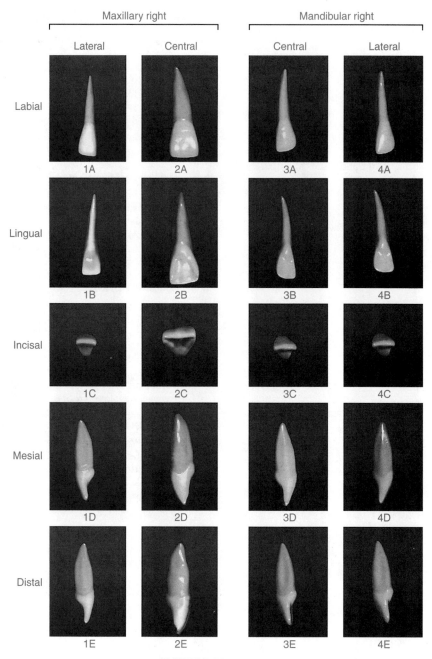

FIGURE 9.22

Incisor characteristics.

Maxillary
right

Mandibular
right

Labial

Lingual

Incisal

Mesial

Distal

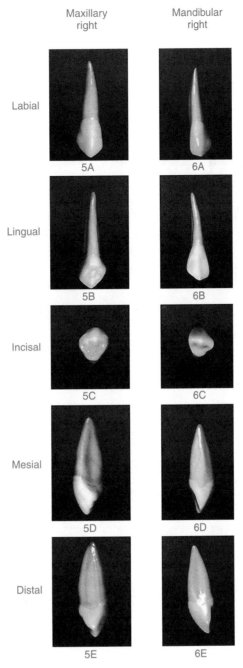

5A   6A

5B   6B

5C   6C

5D   6D

5E   6E

FIGURE 9.23

Cuspid characteristics.

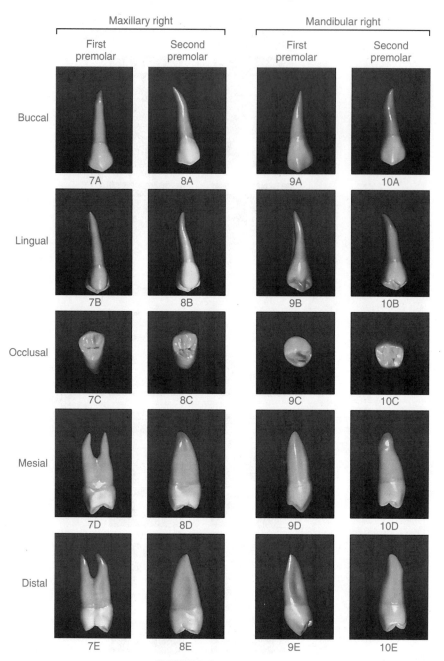

FIGURE 9.24

Premolar characteristics.

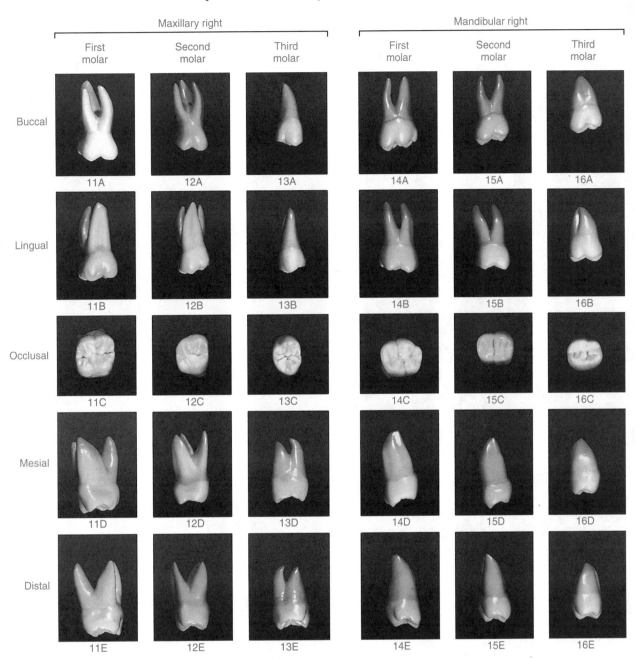

FIGURE 9.25

Molar characteristics.

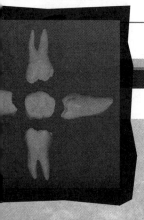

Points for Review

- Primary and secondary tooth development
- Tooth identification systems including both the universal and Palmer systems
- Hard and soft tooth tissue and supporting structures
- Tooth surfaces and angles
- Anatomic landmarks
- Fundamentals of tooth morphology
- Characteristics of permanent teeth

Self-Study Questions

1. What is the imaginary line called that divides the right and left side of the body?
   a. Parallel line
   b. Proximal line
   c. Midline
   d. Line angle

2. What is the proximal surface of a tooth called that is farthest from the midline of the dental arch?
   a. Lingual surface
   b. Mesial surface
   c. Distal surface
   d. Incisal surface

3. What is the hardest substance in the body?
   a. Cementum
   b. Bone
   c. Dentin
   d. Enamel

4. What is the ridge called that diagonally crosses the occlusal surface of a maxillary molar?
   a. Marginal ridge
   b. Oblique ridge
   c. Transverse ridge
   d. Triangular ridge

5. What is the depression called that is formed when the lobes of a tooth come together?
   a. Central fossa
   b. Developmental groove
   c. Supplemental groove
   d. Triangular fossa

6. What ridge is formed when a buccal and a lingual triangular ridge join together?
   a. Buccal ridge
   b. Oblique ridge
   c. Marginal ridge
   d. Transverse ridge

7. What are the rounded ridges called that form the mesial and distal borders on the occlusal surfaces?
   a. Oblique ridges
   b. Marginal ridges
   c. Transverse ridges
   d. Buccal ridges

8. Where is the contact area on the mesial surface of the maxillary permanent central incisor located?
   a. Occlusal third
   b. Gingival third
   c. Middle third
   d. Incisal third

9. Which symbols are used when charting the permanent dentition using the universal system?
   a. A through J
   b. 1 through 20
   c. A through E
   d. 1 through 32

10. What are additional teeth to the normal dentition called?
    a. Edentulous teeth
    b. Succedaneous teeth
    c. Supernumerary teeth
    d. Secondary teeth

11. What is the center of calcification that forms a cusp called?
    a. Mamelon
    b. Lobe
    c. Cusp
    d. Tubercle

12. What is the name of the bonelike substance that covers the roots of the teeth?
    a. Dentin
    b. Enamel
    c. Cementum
    d. Pulp

13. How many premolars are in a full complement of permanent teeth?
    a. Two
    b. Four
    c. Six
    d. Eight

14. At what age does the first permanent tooth erupt?
    a. 6 years
    b. 7 years
    c. 10 years
    d. 6 to 8 months

15. How many cusps does the mandibular first molar have?
    a. Four
    b. Five
    c. Four plus one auxiliary cusp
    d. Two

Suggested Readings

Brand RI: *Anatomy of orofacial structures*, vol 6, St Louis, 1998, Mosby.
Wheeler RC: *Wheeler's atlas of tooth form*, Philadelphia, 1984, WB Saunders.

Chapter 10

Microbiology for the Dental Assistant

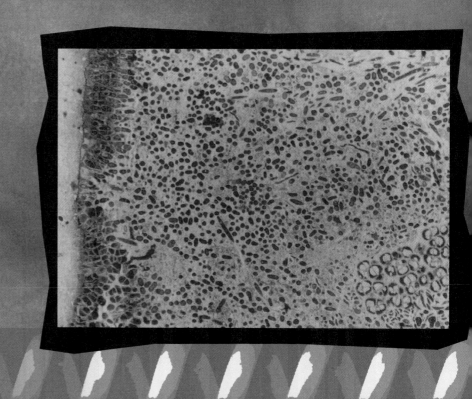

Chapter Outline

Microbiology
Characteristics of Microorganisms
   Bacteria
   Viruses
   Antibiotics
Immunology
   Nonspecific host defenses
   Specific host defenses

Infectious Diseases
   Viral diseases
   Bacterial diseases
Oral Microbiology
   Dental plaque
   Periodontal disease
   Dental caries

Learning Objectives

On completion of Chapter 10, the student should be able to do the following:

- Define key terms.
- Characterize procaryotic and eucaryotic cells.
- Describe the fundamental components of a typical bacterial cell.
- Describe the structure of typical viral particles.
- Discuss bacterial replication and growth.
- Discuss viral replication and growth.
- Discuss the conceptual philosophy of antibiotic therapy.

- Describe the specific and non-specific body defense systems.
- Describe in general terms the function of T-cell and B-cell immunity.
- Discuss the general reactions of hypersensitivities and allergies.
- Have an understanding of infectious diseases that pose occupational hazards.
- Discuss the microbes associated with different forms of dental disease.

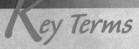

Key Terms

Allergy	Disease	Pathogens
Antibiotics	Flora	Virulence
Antigen	Infectious	

MICROBIOLOGY

The biologic world is divided into five kingdoms. Plants and animals are easily defined or recognized. The other three kingdoms contain organisms that are associated with causing **disease** and often difficult to identify. They are the fungi, the protists that include protozoans, and the moneria

Disease

A condition of the body that displays a characteristic pathology.

that contain the bacteria. Microbiology is the study of these three later groups of organisms. Because several microorganisms cause disease in animals, including human beings, the study of resistance to disease, or immunology, is a division of microbiology.

Little progress was made toward understanding the true causes of disease until the late 1600s, when Anton van Leeuwenhoek, an optical lens grinder, built a microscope capable of magnifying objects about 200 times. This simple microscope opened a new world of science, because van Leeuwenhoek was able to describe organisms too small to be seen with the unaided eye. One of the first places he searched for these animalcules was the dental plaque from his own mouth. From those observations, he described the three common shapes of bacteria: rods, spheres, and spirals.

Although those in science had become aware of microscopic life, most considered these tiny organisms to have developed spontaneously from inert (nonliving) material. It took almost 200 years for scientists such as Louis Pasteur to prove spontaneous generation did not occur on a continuing basis. The period from 1870 to 1900 proved to be the "golden age" of microbiology. Louis Pasteur developed the pasteurization process and the rabies vaccine, and about the same

Infectious

Capable of transmitting organisms that cause disease.

time Robert Koch advanced his postulates for demonstrating that bacteria cause many **infectious** diseases. Koch's postulates have proved invaluable in researching diseases, but they can be applied only to certain bacterial diseases; they do not explain most viral diseases or some other bacterial diseases, such as periodontitis. Many other brilliant microbiologists also contributed to our understanding of diseases during this period.

Antibiotics

Chemical compounds that can inhibit or kill microorganisms by blocking some aspect of metabolism or growth.

Although a number of causative agents (antigens) of disease exist, infectious diseases are caused by microorganisms (Box 10.1). However, disease-producing microbes are greatly outnumbered by those that

Box 10.1

Causative Agents (Antigens) of Disease

1 Microorganisms such as bacteria or viruses can cause disease, known as *pathogens*.
2 Abnormal cells of the body can cause disease such as cancers.
3 Poisons from insects, animals, or chemicals can harm the body and stimulate the immune system.
4 Pollens can affect the body and produce an immune response called an *allergy*.
5 Medicines can stimulate antibody production resulting in severe sickness.
6 Transplanted organs can trigger the immune response causing organ rejection.

coexist with and often benefit other forms of life. For example, intestinal bacteria provide human beings with vitamin k; many foods, such as cheese, pickles, and meat, are enhanced by microbes. Many disease-fighting **antibiotics** are microbial products, and even nature uses microorganisms to cleanse the beaches after a crude oil spill.

CHARACTERISTICS OF MICROORGANISMS

The fundamental characterization of microbes involves organization of the genetic material. In simple or less developed cells, including bacteria, the genetic material is not arranged in typical chromosomes, but rather is loosely organized in the cytoplasm of the cell. These simple cells are called *prokaryotes*. In more advanced cells, such as fungi, protozoa, and higher systems, including human beings, the genetic material of chromosomes is confined within the cytoplasm by a nuclear membrane. These cells are called *eucaryotes*. microscopically, eukaryotic cells are characterized by the presence of a defined nucleus; prokaryotes have no detectable nucleus. Most microorganisms, significant to dental assistants, are either procaryotic cells or viruses. Viruses are not considered cells because they cannot reproduce independently of other living material.

Bacteria

Size and Shape

Bacteria vary considerably in size and shape. Typically, spherical (coccus) bacteria measure approximately 1 micron (μm) in diameter (a micron is one millionth of a meter). Some microbial cells can be as small as 0.2 μm in diameter, and some rod (bacillus) forms can approach 60 μm in length. For comparison, a red blood cell is about 7 μm in diameter. Other size comparisons are shown in Figure 10.1.

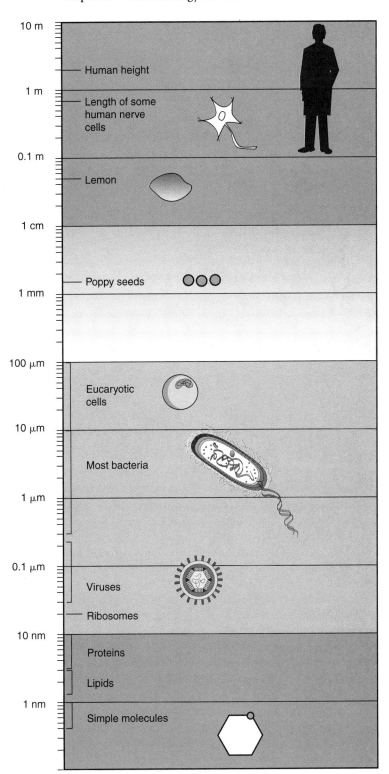

FIGURE 10.1

Size comparison of molecules. One nanometer (l nm) equals 0.000000001 of a meter.

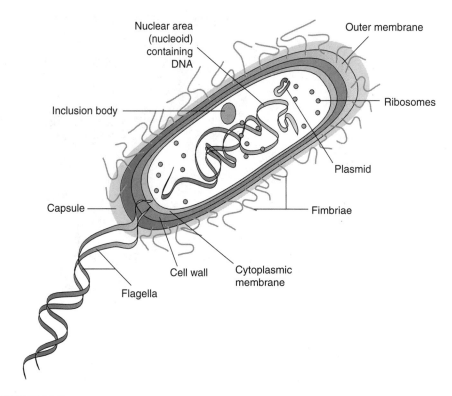

FIGURE 10.2

Cross section of a bacterial cell. The presence of an outer membrane indicates that this is a gram-negative cell.

Subcellular Structure

Figure 10.2 depicts a cross section of a bacterial cell. The bacterial *cytoplasm* is confined by the outer covering layers of the cell, which constitute the *cell envelope* or wall. The *cytoplasmic membrane* is the essential structure of the envelope. This membrane is flexible and serves the cell in numerous ways. It is selectively permeable, allowing certain molecules to pass through whereas others are blocked. It performs active transport of specific chemicals. In this process, cellular energy is used to overcome osmosis and to concentrate molecules in the cell from lower concentrations outside the cell. The cytoplasmic membrane also serves as an attachment point for several molecules inside the cell, the nucleoid including deoxyribonucleic acid (DNA), and the cellular appendages.

Outward from the cytoplasmic membrane is the bacterial *cell wall.* This structure is rigid and determines the cell's shape. The cell wall also protects the cytoplasmic membrane from physical damage and from severe changes in osmotic pressure. Technically, the cell wall is composed of long chains of sugar molecules *(glycans)* cross-linked by short chains of amino acids *(peptides);* the resulting molecule is called a *peptidoglycan.*

Although all bacteria have cell envelopes, two distinct types are found in nature, and these two types define gram-positive and gram-negative cells. Gram-positive and gram-negative cells were recognized long before the cell wall structure became known because of an elegant cell staining procedure called a *Gram's stain.* Gram-positive cells have a thick, tough cell wall that, after a wash with alcohol, retains the iodine-crystal violet complex of the Gram's stain. The gram-negative cell wall, however, is much thinner and cannot retain the dye complex. Microscopically, gram-positive cells are vivid blue to violet, and gram-negative cells usually appear red because of a counterstain that is applied to the alcohol-washed, clear cells.

The outermost portion of the cell envelope of gram-negative cells is a second membrane called the *outer membrane.* Endotoxin, which triggers inflammation in a human host, is a major component of this membrane. Gram-positive cells do not have a similar layer.

Viewed simply, a gram-positive cell has a thick, two-layer cell envelope; a gram-negative cell has a much thinner cell envelope with three distinct layers.

Other surface structures, such as a *capsule,* may be found on some bacteria. A bacterial capsule is not required for microbial growth; rather, its primary function is to help the bacterial cell avoid detection or entrapment by white blood cells. Capsules may form on the outside of either gram-positive or gram-negative cells. Another feature found on some bacteria is whiplike *flagella* that extend outward from the envelope. The flagella give the bacteria the capability of directed movement. However, no clear relationship has been established between the presence of flagella and the ability to cause disease.

Inside the cell envelope, several structures can be identified in the cytoplasm. The *nucleoid* is an area of concentrated DNA. Unlike with higher forms of life, bacterial DNA does not combine with other molecules to form chromosomes. Because each cell has only one copy of DNA, bacteria are *haploid cells* and do not exhibit dominant and recessive characteristics.

In order to grow and reproduce, bacteria require the synthesis of proteins, a process that is carried out by *ribosomes.* The major molecules that make up ribosomes are the *ribonucleic acids (RNAs).*

Most bacteria have a very limited ability to survive exposure to harsh environments. However, two gram-positive, rod-shaped bacteria, members of the *Bacillus* and *Clostridium* genera, produce highly resistant intracellular bodies *(endospores).* For years endospores may endure conditions unsuited to the growth of typical bacteria; they are the life form most resistant to destruction. Endospores do not reproduce because cellular multiplication does not occur. During the formation of an endospore (Figure 10.3), the cellular DNA is compacted and covered by a cortex layer and then by the spore coat. The single endospore has virtually no metabolic activity. In favorable conditions, the endospore germinates and grows into a typical cell capable of reproduction. Endospores are not significantly affected by heat (boiling water), drying (desert conditions), chemicals (for example, alcohol), or radiation (ultraviolet rays or x-rays).

Growth Conditions

Growth and reproduction are essential to all living cells. In order for these processes to occur, a cell must have sources of energy and chemical components to build cellular material. *Metabolism* is the term used to describe the chemical reactions within the cell that provide energy and synthesize cellular components. Many bacteria can use simple sugars, such as glucose (grape sugar), for all metabolic reactions. The microbes extract energy and structural building blocks from the sugars through a series of reactions. In many ways, the process is comparable to burning a piece of paper, which is also made of sugars:

$$C_6H_2O_6 \; + \; 6O_2 \; + \; fire \; = \; 6CO_2 \; + 6H_2O \; + \; Energy$$

Glucose	Oxygen		Carbon	Water	Heat
(paper)			dioxide		

In this process the fire and the amount of heat given off are uncontrolled; however, in the living cell the process is closely controlled by several enzymes. *Enzymes* are proteins that catalyze or facilitate reactions between molecules. The enzymes of metabolism act in sequence and cause the energy to be captured in a chemical form rather than lost as heat. *Adenosine triphosphate (ATP),* the high-energy chemical form created by most cells, is used to power the syn-

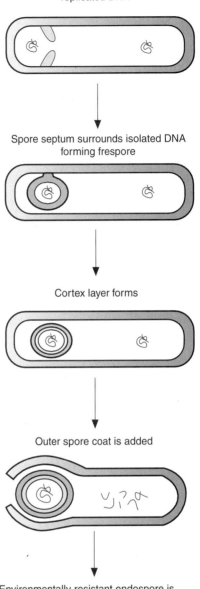

Spore septum begins to isolate newly replicated DNA

Spore septum surrounds isolated DNA forming frespore

Cortex layer forms

Outer spore coat is added

Environmentally resistant endospore is freed from disintegrating cell

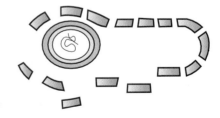

FIGURE 10.3

Formation of environmentally resistant bacterial endospores. Note that one bacterial cell yields just one endospore; bacterial sporulation therefore is not a form of reproduction.

thesis of cell parts and to support other functions that require energy. The key to understanding bacterial metabolism can be stated in this way: cells use enzymes to break down sugars in a stepwise, regulated fashion that results in the capture of the released energy in a chemical form rather than loss of the heat energy produced when sugars are burned. In addition, as the stepwise breakdown of glucose and other sugars proceeds, some of the partly digested molecules are drawn away from energy production and used by the cell as building blocks to form the larger molecules needed for cell growth.

Microorganisms reproduce in a wide variety of environments. Many must have oxygen readily available for metabolism; these are referred to as *aerobic organisms.* For other microbes, oxygen is toxic; these are *anaerobic organisms.* Most microorganisms found on the human host can live in either the presence or absence of oxygen; these are *facultative organisms.* Aerobic cells produce carbon dioxide (CO_2) and water (H_2O) as end products. Because of the lack of oxygen, anaerobic microorganisms cannot completely break down sugars to CO_2; rather, they "pollute" their environment with by-products such as ethyl alcohol or lactic acid. The lactic acid produced by specific oral bacteria causes the breakdown of tooth enamel, which results in the disease called "tooth decay."

In addition to nutritional elements, the physical environment determines which microbial cells grow and if they thrive. These environmental factors include the acid, or pH, level; disease-producing cells prefer to grow around the neutral point of pH 7. Notable exceptions are the *acidophilic* (acid-loving) bacteria found in decaying teeth. Similarly, most microbes of dental interest grow best at 37° C, the normal human body temperature.

Reproduction

Traditional biology textbooks devote significant space to the life cycles of various organisms. However, the life cycle of bacteria and other procaryotic cells is quite simple. The cells undergo asexual *binary fission* (Figure 10.4), which is literally a splitting in half of the cell. The resulting daughter cells are exact copies of each other. The time it takes for this to occur is the doubling, or generation, time. Under ideal laboratory conditions, a cell may double every 30 minutes or less, but in the real world doubling rates of several hours are common. Some cells may require many days per generation. As bacteria continue their simple division, a population of identical cells is created. If left undisturbed, these cells continue to reproduce indefinitely. However, to reproduce, the cells must use nutrients and release end products; by this process the surrounding environment is changed and growth is altered.

When the development of a bacterial population is graphed, a typical bacterial growth curve emerges. To illustrate a growth curve, a single bacterial cell can be introduced into a new environment that will support microbial growth. The cell gradually responds to the new surroundings and be-

gins to divide at a slow rate; this is the *lag phase.* Once the cells have adjusted to the available nutrients and conditions, they begin doubling at the optimal rate; thus two cells become four, four become eight, and so on in an exponential or *logarithmic phase.* If this were to continue for any length of time, the earth would quickly be covered with identical microorganisms. Fortunately for us, either depletion of available nutrients or excess accumulation of by-products occurs, and the cells are forced to enter a *stationary phase,* in which they are alive but not reproducing. If no change occurs in the environment, the cell population either starves or is poisoned and enters the *death phase.* At this point the cells can no longer reproduce.

Invasive Products

Bacterial growth by itself is not necessarily bad for the host. Rather, the by-products of growth cause the damage. Microbes capable of damaging the host are called **pathogens.** The degree to which they are invasive or inflict damage is the **virulence** of the microbe.

Typical microbial compounds that cause pathologic changes in tissues include exotoxins.

Pathogens
Organisms capable of causing disease in a host.

Virulence
The relative ability of an organism to cause disease.

Endotoxins, and enzymes. *Exotoxins* are proteins excreted from bacteria (Figure 10.5); they range from the deadly neurotoxin of tetanus to the toxin that causes the rash of scarlet fever.

Endotoxins are lipopolysaccharides that are found only on the surface of gram-negative bacteria (Figure 10.5). They generally have very little direct effect on individual host cells but induce fever in the host by interacting with parts of the immune system. Microbial *enzymes* that contribute to bacterial pathogenicity include those that break down host collagen or proteins.

Viruses

Essential structures

Viruses are simple creatures compared to bacteria. They range in size from 0.03 μm to about 0.2 μm. Structurally, viruses can be visualized as a protein shell *(capsid)* that is stuffed with a nucleic acid. Depending on the type of virus, the protein shell may be covered with other proteins, carbohydrates, or lipids. The nucleic acids are either DNA or RNA, but the two are never found together. Because a virus does not have both nucleic acids, it cannot reproduce independently; thus viruses depend on living cells to provide the metabolic systems to support their replication.

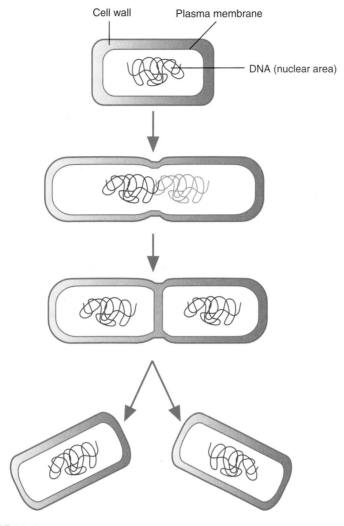

Cell wall   Plasma membrane

DNA (nuclear area)

FIGURE 10.4

Binary fission of bacteria, which yields identical copies of the original (parent) cell.

Replication

Because viruses are not complete cells, they cannot undergo even simple binary fission; rather, they rely on a host cell for replication (Figure 10.6). Once a virus finds a susceptible cell, the viral nucleic acid enters the cytoplasm and takes command of the metabolic processes. The host cell's normal cellular functions stop, and all subsequent cellular activity is directed toward making new viral components. Numerous copies of nucleic acid are synthesized, protein shells are formed, and then whole viral particles are assembled from the parts. Once assembled, hundreds or thousands of these new particles are released from the host cell at one time. They do not replicate again until they find a healthy, intact cell that can be invaded and used to produce and assemble viral parts.

It should be clear from the above discussion that viruses need healthy host cells to survive. It is this dependence on host cells that makes attacking viral infections with antibiotics so difficult. Blocking viral replication requires blocking a host's cellular function; thus by killing the virus, the host also is killed. For this reason, the old adage, "There is no cure for the common cold," is still true.

Scientists have not yet been able to provide a thorough explanation of the way in which viruses extensively damage the host. What is known is that viruses cause obvious changes within a cell, changes known as *cytopathic effects*. These changes may range from lethal effects on the cell to essentially no observable consequence. To date, no secreted products similar to bacterial toxins have been detected for viral infections.

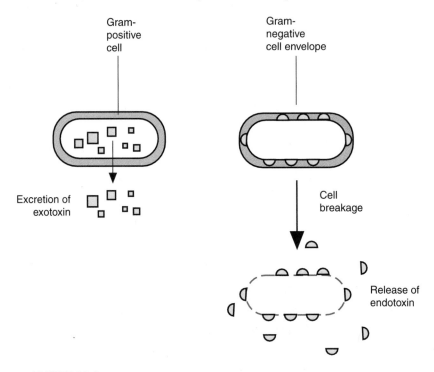

FIGURE 10.5

Release of toxic products by gram-positive and gram-negative bacterial cells.

Antibiotics

Mechanism of Attack

Protein molecules most essential to the immune system are antibiotics and complements. Antibiotics combine with antigens to alter the antigens so that they are no longer harmful to the body. This antigen and antibiotic binding is called the *immune reaction* (See Figure 10.8). A major reason for studying the structure and function of microorganisms is to determine what part of the organism might be susceptible to attack by biochemicals, or *antibiotics*. Not only must the antibiotic kill or inactivate the microbe, it also must not harm the host. Researchers therefore are constantly looking for antibiotics that interfere with microbial functions that are different from those found in higher animals, including human beings. Thousands of antibiotics have been discovered, but just a few are safe enough for human use. Although fungi or other bacteria are the source of most antibiotics, several antibiotics recently have been developed solely in the laboratory.

Microbial structures that have little in common with animal cells include the bacterial cell wall, the ribosome, and the membrane of cells such as the yeast *Candida*. Perhaps the most studied antibiotics are those of the penicillin group. These antibiotics prevent synthesis of peptidoglycan, which forms the cell wall, and without a complete cell wall, the bacteria are at the mercy of host defenses. Erythromycin and the tetracycline-type antibiotics bind only to bacterial ribosomes, effectively stopping protein synthesis and, consequently, growth of the bacterial cells. Obviously, without the ability to reproduce, bacteria soon are overpowered by host defenses. The antibiotic nystatin stops the growth of yeasts. It binds to the cytoplasmic membrane of the yeast cells, causing them to leak essential metabolites and thus eventually to die.

The idea that no antimicrobials are available to fight viruses is only partly true. One group of antiviral drugs is the nucleic acid analogs. These molecules look and act very much like the real nucleic acid building blocks but have minute differences. The nucleic acid analogs are incorporated into the virus during synthesis. However, when the virus infects a second cell, the cellular enzymes cannot identify these analogs, and viral replication stops. Unfortunately, most of these drugs also inhibit animal cells, therefore the analog drugs are often restricted to localized or topical application. There is hope that as more is learned about replication of unique viruses (such as the human immunodeficiency virus, which forces cells to produce enzymes that function differently from those found in animal hosts), antimicrobial drugs will be found that block replication of the virus but have little effect on the host.

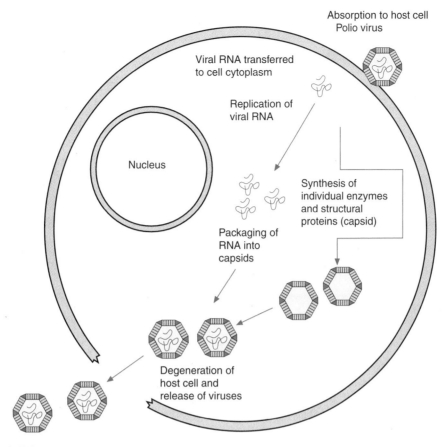

Absorption to host cell
Polio virus

Viral RNA transferred
to cell cytoplasm

Replication of
viral RNA

Nucleus

Synthesis of
individual enzymes
and structural
proteins (capsid)

Packaging of
RNA into
capsids

Degeneration of
host cell and
release of viruses

FIGURE 10.6

Replication of polio viral particles, starting with adsorption of the virus to the host cell and ending with release of new viral particles from the cell.

Microbial Resistance

Many bacteria have developed a resistance to antibiotics. Microbes use two basic mechanisms to fight off antibiotics: they either produce an enzyme that will destroy the antibiotic, or they alter the microbial structure under attack so that the antibiotic no longer interferes with the function. The real question is, how can these resistant microorganisms become established so quickly in a population? The answer is simply that it takes just a single microbe in a population of perhaps a trillion or even more to acquire resistance. All but this one resistant cell will be killed, but the process of logarithmic growth then starts with the one resistant cell, and the trillion or more microbes soon are back and resistant to antibiotics.

A single, resistant microbial cell is not the only means of quickly reestablishing a population. The microorganisms occasionally release small sections of DNA, called *plasmids,* or *resistance factors ("R" factors).* These pieces of DNA can carry the gene that enables the microbe to resist the effects of the antibiotic. Nonresistant bacteria may assimilate these "R" factors and convert to resistant strains. If this happens

repeatedly, multiple antibiotic–resistant strains develop; the most notable in today's health literature are the drug-resistant strains of *Mycobacterium tuberculosis,* which causes the disease tuberculosis.

IMMUNOLOGY

Nonspecific Host Defenses

Microbiology is the study not only of microbes, but also of the ways in which the human host defends the body against these invaders. This is accomplished through the immune system that gives us immunity or enables us to resist disease. This system relies on molecules and cells to accomplish its tasks. The body is protected by two basic defensive systems (Box 10.2). The first system of defense is a generalized response to all foreign invaders. Because all invaders are challenged, the response is called a *nonspecific* one because the body does not attempt to distinguish the type of

Box 10.2
Major Host Defenses

Nonspecific host defenses

First line of defense
Intact skin
Mucous membranes
External secretions (e.g., sweat, tears)

Second line of defense
Nonspecific phagocytic blood cells
Inflammation
Antimicrobials (e.g., interferon)

Specific host defenses

Third line of defense
Circulating antibodies (B-cell products)
Targeted phagocytic cells (T-cells)

---

bial molecules must be large and complex, and they must be foreign, or dissimilar, to any compounds produced by the host. If a molecule fits this general description, it is called an **antigen.** Most protein molecules and many carbohydrate molecules are good antigens.

Antigen

A foreign substance capable of inducing an immunologic response.

When a microbe breaches the body's mechanical barriers, the scavenger cells, such as PMNs and macrophages, work hard to eliminate the intruder. However, the immune system recognizes the need to supplement the body's first line of defense and starts the process of mounting a successful defense against the specific microbes. Through a series of cellular signals and rearrangements of host molecules, the body creates immune system molecules *(receptors),* which fit very tightly to the contours of the microbial antigen. The functional concept is analogous to a locksmith who is given a lock (the antigen) and is asked to make a key to fit (the immune receptor). Once made, the key fits the lock perfectly; however, just as the key fits only the one lock, an immune receptor fits only the microbial antigens that caused the specific receptors to be formed. Because the body responds to the foreign material and creates a new response, this is referred to as *acquired immunity.*

The acquired immunity system has two components. One is associated with certain lymphocytes (white blood cells) formed in bone marrow and called *stem cells.* These white blood cells are called *T-lymphocytes* or *T-cells* (thymus-dependent), or cellular, response. Lymphocytes circulate in the body fluid and large numbers are found in the thymus, spleen, and other lymphatic tissue. The other involves the immunoglobulin, or antibody fraction of blood plasma, and is known as the *B-lymphocytes* or *B-cell* (bursa-dependent), or humoral, response. B-cells produce antibiotics for specific antigens. B-cell production of antibiotics is regulated by T-cells. T-cells that increase antibody production are called *helper cells,* and T-cells that decrease antibody production are called *suppressor cells.* Both types of response use specific immune receptors to recognize foreign material.

The T-cells generally attack microbes that live successfully inside host cells, including viruses and certain bacteria, such as *M. tuberculosis.* B-cell derived antibodies are more effective in neutralizing extracellular microbes and their toxic products. Macrophages are large, white blood cells that are also produced in the bone marrow. Macrophages function to engulf and digest, producing substances by a process called *phagocytosis.* Large numbers of macrophages are found in the spleen and lymph nodes.

microorganism trying to gain access to the host. The most obvious portion of this defensive system is the body's mechanical barrier, which is composed of the skin and other surface linings, including mucosal tissue. These barriers prevent most microbes from establishing infections by blocking entrance to susceptible tissues.

To bolster the physical barrier established by the skin and intact mucous membranes, the body reinforces these tissues with glandular secretions, such as sweat and saliva. These fluids contain antimicrobial compounds. Stomach acids, skin oils, and enzymes that attack bacteria are examples of these compounds. When these barriers are broken down, even by something as simple as a tiny cut on the finger, the body relies on scavenger white blood cells, polymorphonuclear leukocytes (PMNs), and macrophages to keep the injured tissue free of infection. These cells are capable of *phagocytizing,* or engulfing, the foreign invader. Once taken up, the invading microbes usually are digested by the cells. This process often is accompanied by the development of inflammation around the injured area, characterized by redness, heat, and the formation of pus, which is the accumulation of white cells, microbes, and cellular debris.

Specific Host Defenses

Antigens

Complementing the nonspecific system is the body's *specific* host defense system, which is a response to individual microbes when they breach the mechanical barriers. This specific defense is the body's acquired immune response. Specificity is achieved because the body can effectively distinguish between the different molecules found in and on microbes. Two overriding criteria govern such recognition: the micro-

T-cells

T-cells are divided into many types, or subgroups (Table 10.1), each having a specific function. The three subgroups that have the greatest impact are the cytotoxic T-cells, the

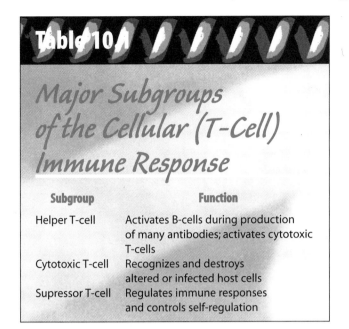

Table 10.1

Major Subgroups of the Cellular (T-Cell) Immune Response

Subgroup	Function
Helper T-cell	Activates B-cells during production of many antibodies; activates cytotoxic T-cells
Cytotoxic T-cell	Recognizes and destroys altered or infected host cells
Supressor T-cell	Regulates immune responses and controls self-regulation

T-helper cells (CD4 cells), and the T-suppressor cells (CD8 cells). *Cytotoxic T-cells* are the cells directly responsible for eliminating foreign material from the body. The most important factor in this process is the T-cells' ability to recognize antigenic foreign matter. Once identified by the specific receptors, cytotoxic T-cells engulf and destroy the antigen. The *T-helper cells* help to coordinate antibody formation by B-cells, and *T-suppressor cells* prevent the body from recognizing self-antigens. *Self-antigens* are the unique antigens found on all host cells. Without T-suppressor cells, the host would quickly destroy itself.

B-cells

Antibodies

Antibodies, which are also called *immunoglobulins*, are produced by plasma cells that come from B-lymphocytes. Five classes of antibodies are found in blood plasma, all based on the fundamental immunoglobulin molecule. The major player in disease resistance is immunoglobulin G(IgG), which is found exclusively in blood plasma. The oral cavity is protected by an immunoglobulin produced in conjunction with saliva (and other secretions); this immunoglobulin is called secretary immunoglobulin A (sIgA). Table 10.2 lists the immunoglobulins and their functions.

In contrast to cytotoxic T-cells, immunoglobulins are molecules and have no way of engulfing foreign antigens. Instead, antibodies attach themselves to antigens, often on a microbial surface. At this point very little, if anything, happens to inhibit or damage the microbe. However, a major consequence to microbes coated with antibody is that the microbes do not readily stick or adhere to tissues that normally provide a good growth environment for the invaders. By remaining suspended, the microbe either is targeted for

destruction by circulating PMNs or is swept from the body. For example, swallowing saliva effectively eliminates countless bacteria coated with sIgA from the oral cavity. A second consequence is that PMNs phagocytize most antigens much more effectively if the antigen or microbe is coated with antibody, a process referred to as *opsonization*.

Many bacteria coated with IgG or IgM are also susceptible to the action of complement. *Complement* is a series of enzymes found in blood plasma that destroys bacteria by "boring" holes in the cytoplasmic membrane cell wall, ultimately killing the cell. The unique aspect of complement is that the enzymes are not active in the bloodstream; that is, they do not act on membranes under normal circumstances. However, an antibody bound to a microbial antigen in the presence of complement triggers the transformation of (activates) the complement proteins into active enzymes, which attack the invader.

To summarize, antibodies generally do not affect microbial antigens directly; however, by coating antigens, they set in motion the following processes:

1 Antigen attachment to tissues is diminished.
2 Phagocytosis of antigens is enhanced.
3 Destruction of microbial membranes by complement is initiated.

When the specific response is functioning (be it the T-cell or the B-cell response), systemic chemicals, called *lymphokines,* are released by the cells into the bloodstream. Lymphokines act as messengers and recruit other defensive white blood cells to the area, such as PMNs and macrophages. The process of inflammation accompanies the accumulation of these cells as they clean up and dispose of the foreign or invading microbe.

Antibody Synthesis

The production of antibodies to specific antigens is not as simple as might be inferred from the preceding material. The antigen must undergo significant processing by individual cells before the host can synthesize immunoglobulins to match it. This process is summarized in Figure 10.7. The initial step in antibody synthesis is capture of the antigen by a nonspecific scavenger cell, usually a macrophage. In most cases the macrophage passes the antigen to a T-helper (CD4) cell. The T-helper cell partly digests the antigen and prepares to pass it to a B-lymphocyte. Once the B-lymphocyte receives the T-cell processed antigen, it differentiates into either a plasma cell or a memory B-lymphocyte. Plasma cells are dedicated to producing antibodies only to the antigen that caused the process to begin. Memory B-lymphocytes do not make antibodies but retain the information on what antibody to produce for future use. Over time, antibodies and the plasma cells disappear from the bloodstream; however, the memory B-cells remain. If the antigen enters the body at a later time, the memory B-cells convert to plasma cells and begin producing specific antibodies. Activation of memory B-cells is called the *anamnestic response.* This response is the

Table 10.2

Major Classes of Antibody (B-Cell) Immune Response

Immunoglobulin	Percentage of Serum	Function
IgG	80	Promotes phagocytosis through PMNs production; detoxifies or neutralizes toxins, viruses, and maternal antibodies of newborns
IgM	5-10	Tends to agglutinate (stick together) antigens; first antibody produced to counter new antigen
IgA	10-15	Prevents microbial attachment to surfaces
sIgA	0	Found only in secretions; prevents infection of mucosal tissues
IgD	0.1-0.2	Unknown
IgE	0.001-0.1	Reduces allergic reactions by causing release of histamine and lysis of parasitic protozoa

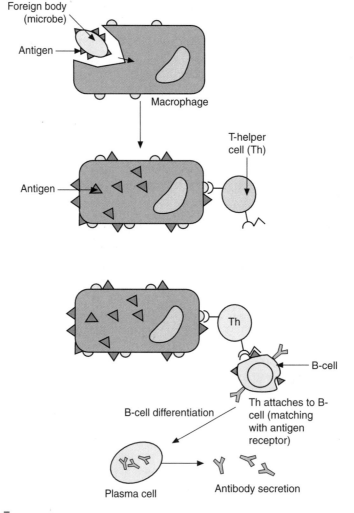

FIGURE 10.7

The stepwise process of antibody formation, starting with recognition of foreign material (antigen) and then passage of the material to T-helper cells and on to the antibody-secreting plasma cells.

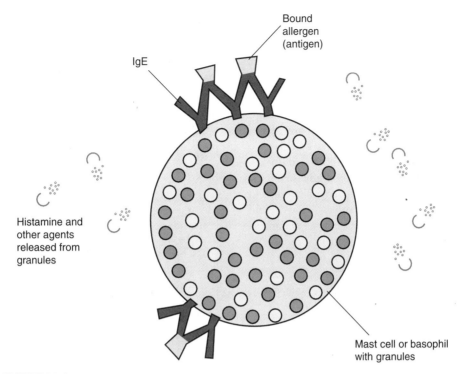

FIGURE 10.8

Hypersensitivities, including hay fever and asthma, are caused by the degranulation of mast and basophilic cells, which is caused by the binding of antibody and antigens.

basis of lifelong resistance to diseases such as mumps, hepatitis, and polio after the host has been initially exposed to the antigen through disease or vaccination.

Interference with the antibody formation process leads to severe diseases, including acquired immunodeficiency syndrome (AIDS), which is caused by the human immunodeficiency virus (HIV). HIV stops antibody formation by infecting T-helper cells, thereby blocking antigen processing and consequently paralyzing a major component of the body's specific defense system.

Hypersensitivities

The major function of the immune response is to protect the host from invading microbes. Unfortunately, the immune response sometimes carries things too far and causes damage to the host. The most common example of this situation is the development of allergies.

An **allergy** actually is a hypersensitive response to antigens that develops only after exposure to the antigens. Hypersensitivities mediated by antibodies produced by B-lymphocytes are known as immediate reactions, and these often occur within minutes of exposure. Most cases of hay fever, asthma, and food allergy are typical of the immediate hypersensitivity response. These common allergies are called *atopy,* and the symptoms are caused by local anaphylactic reactions.

During the sequence of an atopic allergy attack (Figure 10.8), the antigen (for example, plant pollen), which often is called an *allergen,* enters the host and matches with an immunoglobulin of the IgE class specific for the particular plant pollen. This antigen-antibody complex causes host mast cells in the vicinity of the complex to degranulate, releasing biologically active compounds, including histamine. The principal effect of histamine on the surrounding tissues is vasodilation, which causes blood vessels not only to swell but also to become leaky, with fluid flowing into surrounding tissues. Smooth muscle also contracts. Although uncomfortable, the host generally does not have significant problems with these atopic, localized reactions.

On the other hand, allergens with more direct access to the bloodstream of highly sensitized individuals (for example, through injections or insect bites) can induce these same reactions throughout the body, resulting in systemic anaphylaxis. In severe cases epinephrine must be given to counter the causes of the anaphylactic reaction, or severe shock sets in because of the lack of smooth muscle activity.

Atopic allergies are best controlled by avoiding the offending allergen. If this is not practical, *desensitization* (through allergy shots) often is achieved by allowing the body to generate antibodies of the IgG class directed against the allergens. When the specific IgG complexes with the

Allergy

A hypersensitivity to immunogenic substances.

complementary allergen, the allergen is readily inactivated or removed from the body. Consequently, no allergen remains that could bind with IgE and trigger an allergy attack. If initiation of atopic allergies cannot be stopped, the symptoms can be eased by drugs, including antihistamines and antiinflammatories such as aspirin.

Other immediate hypersensitivities do not involve IgE but instead work through IgG. As mentioned previously, when an antigen combines with IgG, a series of enzymes, called complement, is activated. A major outcome of this reaction is the production of a localized inflammatory reaction at the site of the antigen. The process generally results in elimination of the antigen, but quite often damaged and scarred host tissues remain. Examples of this type of damaging immediate hypersensitivity reaction include rheumatic fever, glomerulonephritis, and transplant tissue rejection.

Allergies caused by the host's cellular (T-lymphocyte) response are called *delayed hypersensitivities.* Unlike atopy, symptoms generally develop a day or two after contact with the antigen. The primary symptom is inflammation, often followed by vesicle formation that results in oozing blisters at the contact site. Tissue damage is the result of nonspecific destruction by macrophages and other scavenger cells. Delayed hypersensitivity reactions can be caused by the oils of poison ivy and poison oak and occasionally by the talc and latex in clinic gloves. The skin test for exposure to tuberculosis also relies on the cellular immune response.

Because hypersensitivity reactions are triggered by specific antigens, the host's response to the initial exposure is to produce either T-cells or antibodies with matching specific receptors. Few if any symptoms are seen on initial exposure, but all future contact with the antigen will cause symptoms typical of the hypersensitivity.

INFECTIOUS DISEASES

Viral Diseases

Scientists have known for more than 100 years that infectious diseases are caused by microorganisms. To list all the known diseases and their causes is beyond the scope of this chapter. However, certain infectious diseases are occupational hazards for the dental assistant. Viral diseases generally are given the most notoriety, and hepatitis, HIV infection, and herpes are the most meaningful hazards.

Hepatitis

Hepatitis is an inflammatory disease of the liver. Hepatitis can be caused by infectious viruses (types A, B, and C), drugs and medications (isoniazid and acetaminophen), toxins and poisons (ethyl alcohol, chloroform), and immune reactions (Box 10.3). Clinical symptoms of hepatitis frequently include jaundice, anorexia, nausea, fever, and abdominal pain. It is important to recognize that all patients with a history of

Table 10.3

Consequences of Liver Disease

Defect	Symptom
Decrease in glycogen	Low blood sugar
Decrease in clotting factor formation	Bleeding
Decrease in conjugation of bilirubin	Jaundice
Decrease in drug and chemical detoxification	Poisoning
Decrease in breakdown of ammonia	Brain damage
Failure of blood protein synthesis	Edema

hepatitis or jaundice are not necessarily infectious. In fact, they may never have had infectious hepatitis at all. On the other hand, some forms of viral hepatitis are subclinical, showing few signs and symptoms. Still other patients are asymptomatic carriers. For these reasons, patients who have no history of hepatitis may be contagious to dental personnel or other patients unless infection control techniques are followed.

A history of hepatitis has an important impact on the dental treatment plan in three respects: (1) hepatitis may be caused by dental preparations, prescriptions, and agents; (2) viral hepatitis may be spread in a contaminated dental setting; and (3) a patient with hepatitis may have disease of sufficient severity to compromise routine dental care. For example, both the phenols and the aldehydes used in dental disinfection and preparations have been reported to cause hepatitis. In addition, several known instances of transfer of hepatitis B virus to both patients and personnel have occurred within a dental practice. Finally, because the liver is important in drug and chemical detoxification, blood clotting, infection control, and sugar regulation, problems with any or all of these systems might be expected in association with dental treatment of a patient with hepatitis or cirrhosis (Table 10.3).

Numerous viruses can cause hepatitis. We shall briefly discuss hepatitis virus type A (HAV), type B (HBV), and type C (HCV).

Hepatitis A

Hepatitis A is caused by the hepatitis type A virus. This contagious disease usually is spread by fecal contamination of

Table 10.4

Types of Viral Hepatitis

Type	Mode of Transmission	Chronic Form	Consequences
Hepatitis A (HAV)	Contaminated food or water	None	Resolves
Hepatitis B (HBV)	Blood	5%–7% of those infected	Cirrhosis, carcinoma
Hepatitis C (HCV)	Blood	50% of those infected	Cirrhosis, carcinoma

food or water resulting from unsound sanitary practices. Outbreaks also have been reported after ingestion of tainted food in restaurants or from sewage-fouled water systems. The disease is not spread in a dental setting. The resultant hepatitis manifests acute clinical signs and symptoms typical of liver disease (for example, fatigue and jaundice). The incubation period, which follows recovery from the acute onset, is short (2 to 6 weeks), and almost all patients recover completely after 2 to 5 weeks. There is no carrier state and no chronic form of the disease (Table 10.4). Only patients with active acute disease are considered a minor dental risk. Blood tests can help detect active disease and confirm a history of past disease.

Hepatitis B

The hepatitis B virus usually is transmitted by blood products from contaminated instruments used by drug addicts or in a unhygienic medical practice. The virus also can be transmitted sexually. Most infected individuals develop asymptomatic disease. Those who become symptomatic develop hepatitis after a longer incubation period (6 to 20 weeks). Acute hepatitis B shows symptoms similar to other forms of hepatitis and therefore is difficult to distinguish by clinical presentation alone. In most instances the acute hepatitis resolves without sequelae. In a minority of cases (5% to 7%) the infection persists as chronic disease and may cause long-term symptoms that are quite debilitating (see Table 10.4), such as chronic fatigue, jaundice, and a distaste for food. Some patients may be severely affected, whereas others may be able to function normally. Chronic hepatitis B may lead to total scarring of the liver (cirrhosis) and resultant liver failure. Some patients recover from chronic hepatitis B. Individuals with a history of hepatitis B or posthepatitic cirrhosis have a greater chance of developing liver cancer.

Carrier States of Hepatitis B Occasionally the hepatitis B infection is not apparent, but the HBV persists. Such individuals are considered carriers and may unknowingly infect others through risky situations. Several blood tests are available to help determine infectivity (HB_sAg) and an individual's type of infection and immunity status (anti-HB_s). Vaccination for HBV is highly successful and useful. All dental personnel who come into contact with patient's blood should be vaccinated. Blood transfusion products are routinely screened for the virus.

Hepatitis C

The hepatitis C virus usually is transferred through blood transfusion or blood-contaminated sharps (hypodermic needles), and less commonly by sexual means. Blood products and transfusion materials are now screened for this virus. The incubation period after infection is 4 to 22 weeks, and primary infection usually is a subclinical condition. When symptoms occur, they are similar to those caused by other viral and chemical hepatitides and do not distinguish HCV from other types. Unlike the other viral forms, HCV infection often progresses to chronic and carrier disease forms (see Table 10.4). For this reason, even though the incidence of HCV infection is far smaller than that of HAV or HBV, consequences are much more likely to develop. These consequences commonly include chronic hepatitis, cirrhosis and, in rare cases, cancer of the liver. Hepatitis C is one of the most frequent causes of cirrhosis in the United States. Tests are now available to detect evidence of HCV in the blood. However, currently we do not know if a positive test result indicates whether a patient is infective or immune. No vaccine is available. Vaccination for hepatitis B does not impart immunity for hepatitis C, therefore thorough infection control standards must be observed in a dental practice.

Cirrhosis

Cirrhosis develops after destruction of liver cells and resultant scarring of the liver. The term refers specifically to scarring of the liver and is not used for scarring of any other organ. Some of the common causes of cirrhosis are chronic alcoholism, HBV or HCV infection, obstruction of the bile ducts (for example, by stones or inflammation), and heart failure. Alcoholism is the most common cause, but most patients with cirrhosis are not alcoholics.

Effects of Cirrhosis

Cirrhosis has two major consequences: hepatocellular failure and portal hypertension. The destruction of liver cells (*hepatocellular failure)* results in such consequences as bleeding tendencies, edema and swelling of tissues, inability to detoxify drugs and chemicals, and jaundice, among other problems. These problems, which arise because of diminished liver function, can have a profound impact on dental therapy.

Portal hypertension occurs because the scar tissue in the liver blocks the normal return of blood from the intestines, stomach, and spleen through the liver to the vena cava and the heart. This blood backs up into the portal vein supplying the liver and must find an alternate route of circulation back to the heart. The increased pressure in the portal system and the hepatocellular failure allow fluid (edema) to back into the abdominal cavity (Figure 10.9). This leakage is called *ascites*. Ascites fluid predisposes the individual to abdominal infection. In addition, the spleen becomes congested with blood and destroys red cells, platelets, and white cells more quickly. Because of this, patients with cirrhosis who have portal hypertension are susceptible to bleeding (platelet deficiency), infection (white cell destruction), and anemia (red cell destruction). Finally, portal hypertension causes veins

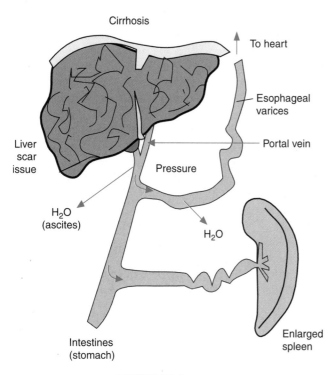

FIGURE 10.9

Portal hypertension.

within the esophagus to dilate markedly *(esophageal varices)* in order to return blood to the heart by an alternate route. These esophageal varices are extremely susceptible to acute and chronic hemorrhage after such minor irritation as eating. This can lead to anemia, acute hemorrhage, and death. It's easy to see that patients with hepatitis and cirrhosis have numerous problems that can affect dental treatment or that may be complicated by dental treatment. All dental personnel must clearly understand the status of these patients.

Herpes

The herpes simplex virus (HSV) causes the typical "cold sore" found on the lips of many people. Most people are infected with this virus at an early age through contact with an infected person. HSV is a DNA type of virus and is subdivided into HSV type 1 (HSV-1) and HSV type 2 (HSV-2). HSV-1 is found most commonly on the upper part of the body, whereas HSV-2 is associated with genital infections. Upon initial infection the HSV-1 lesion may be of little consequence or may cause gingival stomatitis, a severe swelling of the gingival tissues accompanied by lesions on the oral mucosal tissues. The major difficulty with HSV-1 or HSV-2 is that the virus inhabits neurons, where it remain *latent* (silent) for months or years. During times of stress in the host, the virus can travel down the neuron and cause a secondary or recurrent infection. Because dental professionals may work close to herpetic lesions, they are at risk, and the risk is not limited to the mouth; it includes the eye (from splatter) and the area around the finger nail (herpetic whitlow) from direct contact with saliva.

Human Immunodeficiency Virus and Acquired Immunodeficiency Syndrome

The human immunodeficiency virus is an RNA virus that causes AIDS. HIV is a *retrovirus,* meaning that the host synthesizes DNA from a viral RNA template; this is just the opposite of normal cell operations. This unique characteristic offers a possible target for antimicrobial therapy. AIDS, first reported in the United States in 1980, is of major importance to the dental team for the following reasons:

1 The infection is very common, with an estimated incidence of 1 in 300 individuals.

2 HIV can be spread through blood and perhaps saliva, common components of dental treatment.

3 The disease is relentless and usually fatal.

4 AIDS develops in healthy carriers at an early but infectious stage.

5 Patients with HIV and AIDS take new and experimental medicines that may interact with dental therapeutics or affect dental therapy.

6 Early signs and symptoms of HIV-related diseases often are present in the oral cavity.

7 Individuals with HIV can be expected to develop oral diseases and complications secondary to immune suppression.

Mechanisms of HIV Infection and AIDS

HIV is spread through sexual contact or exchange of blood products, or from infected mother to fetus. The virus preferentially infects the immune system specifically, where it initiates destruction of the CD4 (T-helper) immune cells (Figure 10.10). A few weeks after infection, the individual develops flulike symptoms but quickly recovers. After 6 months to 2 years without clinical signs or symptoms, the person begins to develop multiple opportunistic fungal, protozoan, and bacterial infections. These organisms are very common but seldom cause serious disease or any disease at all in immunocompetent individuals. Often one of the earliest diseases to appear in AIDS is thrush, an intense inflammation of the mouth caused by the yeast *Candida albicans.* Such common diseases as oral herpes, shingles, tuberculosis, pneumonia, histoplasmosis, blastomycosis, toxoplasmosis, pneumocystis, and others can be fatal in immunosuppressed patients (Figure 10.11).

As T-helper cells are depleted by the virus, the immune system deteriorates further and the individual may develop multiple severe infections and characteristic cancers, such as Kaposi's sarcoma and non-Hodgkin's lymphoma. Once certain specific life-threatening infections and cancers develop or after the CD4 blood count falls below 200, the person has the terminal disease AIDS (see Figure 10.11). The average life expectancy once AIDS develops is approximately 3 years.

Dental Implications

HIV survives poorly outside human tissues, is relatively difficult to transmit, and is easy to inactivate. For these reasons, there is little risk of transferal to patients or dental personnel if sound hygienic precautions, good sterilization procedures, antisepsis, barrier controls, cleanliness, and good sharps,

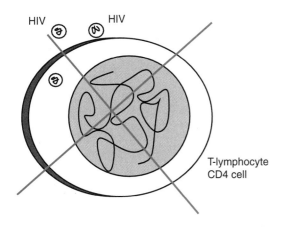

FIGURE 10.10

Oral disease that has occurred secondary to T-lymphocyte (CD4) deficiency.

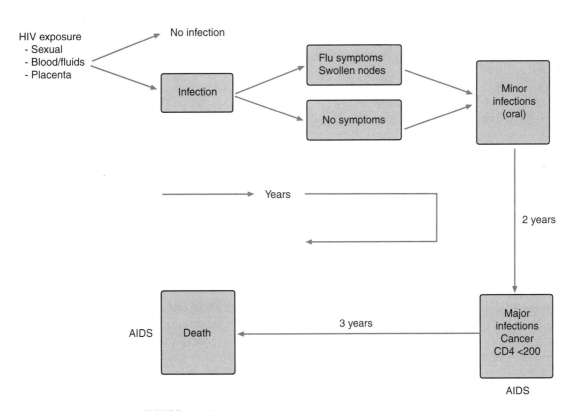

FIGURE 10.11

Course of human immunodeficiency virus (HIV) infection.

hygiene are followed. Patients with HIV should not be feared if infection control measures are sound. Since many individuals infected with HIV are asymptomatic and have not been tested for the virus, all patients should be regarded as possibly infectious, and sound infection control (universal precautions) should always be practiced.

Patients with HIV, and especially those with AIDS, are immunosuppressed, often have numerous infections and tumors, are frequently taking many and new medications, and have other functional disorders (for example, dry mouth and bleeding). Such factors put these patients at risk for complications from rather routine dental procedures. They therefore require special dental treatment, prophylaxis, frequent consultation with a physician, and modified dental treatment plans for optimal care.

Bacterial Diseases

Tuberculosis

As mentioned before, tuberculosis (TB) is a bacterial disease caused by *Mycobacterium tuberculosis.* This contagious organism is most commonly spread by inhaled droplets from coughing or sneezing or by contaminated instruments. Because dentistry involves both the creation of atomized droplets and the contamination of instruments, the risk of spreading tuberculous bacteria in the dental setting may be considerable. Pulmonary tuberculosis was a major cause of disease and death in the United States before 1950. During the past half century, the disease has been controlled (but not eliminated) through the development of effective drugs and sound public health practices, such as testing and early detection. However, tuberculosis is still a major cause of death in underdeveloped countries. Also, the incidence of tuberculosis in the USA has risen recently because of the emergence of multidrug-resistant tuberculosis (MDRTB) strains and the increase in the number of high-risk patients, such as individuals infected with HIV. The disease tends to occur in populations living in crowded conditions (for example, prisons and military camps) and in lower socioeconomic groups. Geographic areas where such conditions exist and where immigration from third world countries is common, such as Southern California and South Florida, are especially affected.

Primary Tuberculosis

Tuberculosis usually occurs as a pulmonary disease. Upon initial (primary) exposure to the TB organism, the immune response is a chronic granulomatous inflammation. The infection usually involves the outer middle portion of the lungs (Figure 10.12), and the lesions often spread to the central (hilar) lymph nodes of the lungs. These peripheral and central granulomas often can be seen on a chest x-ray. This primary stage usually is asymptomatic. The inflammatory/immune process neutralizes and isolates the organism, and in most cases the individual never becomes ill.

Secondary Tuberculosis

Secondary tuberculosis also usually develops initially in the lungs. An individual with primary TB lesions acquires more organisms, either from the environment (reinfection) or through escape of "dormant" organisms from the primary lesions as a result of immunosuppression. The immune system reacts to the reinfection by producing numerous large, proliferative, inflammatory nodules (granulomas) that in themselves can damage the lung tissue. These granulomas can erode into a bronchus or vessel and occasionally thereby spread the organism throughout the lungs or even the entire body. A person with pulmonary secondary tuberculosis often has fever, night sweats, malaise, a chronic cough with blood-tinged sputum, and marked weight loss. The sputum is highly infective, with occasional reports of infection of the gingiva or tongue in these patients, resulting in chronic ulcerated lesions of the oral mucosa.

Miliary Tuberculosis

In rare instances, but more often in immunocompromised patients, TB organisms can be disseminated throughout the body after either primary or secondary infection (miliary spread) (see Figure 10.12). Because this condition can cause the destruction of several organs, the symptoms are diverse, depending on the systems involved.

Tuberculosis Testing

Testing and early diagnosis have been instrumental in controlling tuberculosis. The tuberculin test (that is, the purified protein derivative [PPD] test) is a skin test in which noninfective protein antigen is injected into the skin. An individual who has had a TB infection will show an immune reaction at the test site, with resultant inflammation. Uninfected individuals show no reaction. A positive result on the TB skin test indicates only previous infection; it does not distinguish active disease from dormant disease or from immunity to the organisms. Other useful tests for TB include sputum cultures for organisms, chest x-rays to detect lesions, and biopsy and culture of tissue from lesions to detect organisms.

Spread in the Dental Office

Dental personnel must be aware of a patient's TB status. Barrier techniques and sound sterilization practices help diminish the spread of the organisms. It is appropriate to delay elective dental procedures if a patient has active tuberculosis.

Other Common Bacterial Hazards

Other occupational hazards posed by bacteria are more of a nuisance than a serious health risk. Skin eruptions often are caused by staphylococci and streptococci and can be transmitted by direct contact. One common but often overlooked disease is "pink eye," caused by a gram-negative rod bacterium, *Haemophilus aegyptius.* This disease is highly contagious, and minor contact with the face of an infected person is sufficient to spread the disease.

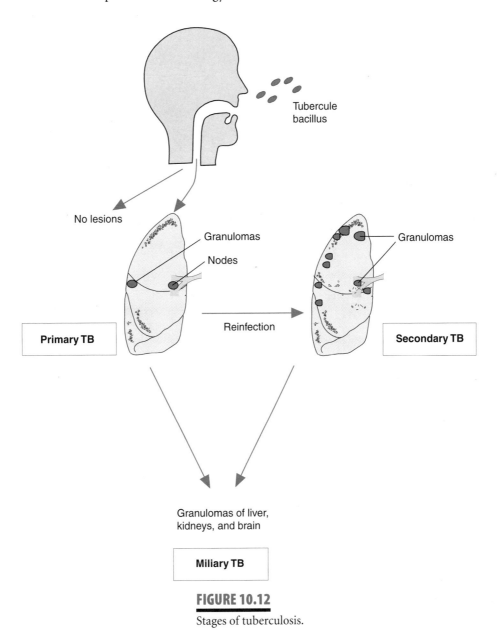

Tubercule bacillus

No lesions

Granulomas

Nodes

Primary TB

Reinfection

Granulomas

Secondary TB

Granulomas of liver, kidneys, and brain

Miliary TB

FIGURE 10.12

Stages of tuberculosis.

This partial list of microbial occupational hazards may not offer dental assistants the greatest comfort, but knowledge of these diseases and adherence to strict infection control standards, regardless of the patient, will protect dental personnel from contracting diseases in the workplace.

ORAL MICROBIOLOGY

Dental Plaque

The mouth is a very good place for microorganisms to grow. Most oral microbes do no harm to the host and are referred to as the normal oral **flora.** No one can state ex-

actly how many different types of microbes are in the mouth, but 350 is a good estimate. The highest concentration of microbes is found in dental plaque (Figure 10.13). *Dental plaque* is defined as the accumulation of bacteria and associated salivary constituents that adheres firmly to the tooth surface. If dental plaque is allowed to develop over several days, the normal flora changes in composition by shifting from the gram-positive facultative microbes to gram-negative anaerobic microbes. As the flora shifts away from the gram-positive bacteria, *gingivitis,* or inflammation of gingival tissue, starts to

Flora

Organisms that reside in a particular area.

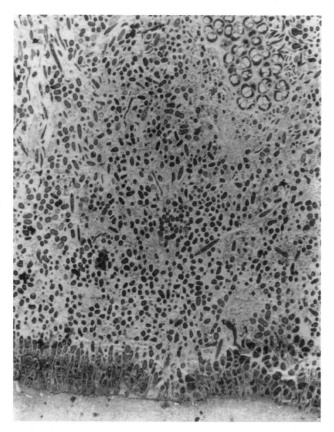

FIGURE 10.13

Cross section of human dental plaque, showing the variety and number of bacteria found on the surface of a normal tooth.

develop adjacent to the accumulating dental plaque. Removal of the plaque buildup allows the gingival tissues to quickly revert to a healthy condition. Because no single microbe causes gingivitis, it is known as a *nonspecific disease.* The other microbial diseases of the mouth have been described well enough that specific microbial types can be identified as the causative agent or agents.

Periodontal Disease

Diseases of the periodontium can occur any time teeth are present in the mouth. Several species of bacteria cause the different types of periodontitis (Table 10.5), but all the pathogenic strains have common characteristics: they are gram-negative, rod-shaped bacteria with little or no tolerance for oxygen (anaerobic).

Diseases of the periodontium generally are considered to develop slowly, and many refer to them as *chronic (persistent)* diseases. A notable exception is *acute necrotizing ulcerative gingivitis (ANUG).* Young adults under stress and individuals infected with HIV are the groups at greatest risk for development of this disease. The disease lesions start on the interdental papillae. These lesions are filled with the bacteria

Table 10.5
Bacteria Associated with Major Types of Periodontal Disease

Disease	Bacteria
Adult periodontitis	*Porphyromonas gingivalis, Prevatilla intermedia, Bacteroides forsythus*
Juvenile periodontitis	*Actinobacillus actinomycetemcomitans, Capnocytophaga*
Acute necrotizing ulcerative gingivitis (ANUG)	*Prevatilla intermedia* gram-negative spirochetes

Prevatilla intermedia and with microbes. This disease is effectively treated by mechanical cleansing of the lesion and improved oral health care, and antibiotics can be used if needed.

In the more typical adult periodontitis, the pathogen that causes the most damage is

Porphyromonas gingivalis. This bacterium produces enzymes that attack the collagen of the periodontal ligament and the proteins of the individual cells. In addition, the endotoxin found on the outer surface of the bacterium greatly diminishes the ability of PMNs to defend the area.

P. gingivalis is not the only bacterium that may cause adult periodontitis (see Table 10.5), but it best fits the bacteriologic and immunologic data. The disease responds to mechanical therapy, but complete instrumentation around the tooth root surfaces is virtually impossible, and antibiotics usually are given to help eliminate the periodontal pathogens.

Juvenile periodontitis is a rapidly progressive destruction of periodontal tissues in children. The cause, *Actinobacillus actinomycetemcomitans,* is routinely found in patients this age. *A. actinomycetemcomitans* survives in the host by aggressively attacking the defense system found in gingival tissues. The organism kills PMNs with a powerful toxin, destroys macrophages with endotoxin, and stimulates T-suppressor cells, which diminishes the synthesis of antibodies. If these effects are not enough, *A. actinomycetemcomitans* invades the periodontal tissues, making it impossible to clear the infection mechanically with dental instruments. Fortunately, antimicrobial therapy effectively stops progression of the disease and provides healthy tissue as long as good oral hygiene is maintained. *A. actinomycetemcomitans* can be found in about one third of adults with periodontitis, and the microbe is considered a major periodontal pathogen.

Dental Caries

Tooth decay, or *dental caries,* is another major infectious disease found in the oral cavity. Caries is a simple disease from one standpoint: acidic by-products of bacterial growth dissolve the tooth enamel. When this activity continues for an extended period, a "cavity" develops.

Research has shown that most cavities are started by a species of bacteria known as *Streptococcus mutans.* In addition to the bacteria, dietary *sucrose,* or common table sugar, is required. The sucrose requirement is significant because *S. mutans* forms glucans only from sucrose (Figure 10.14). The glucans reinforce *S. mutans'* ability to remain on the surface of the tooth. Once established, *S. mutans* produces acidic by-products and provides an environment favorable to the growth of *Lactobacillus* bacteria. The lactobacilli thrive in acidic environments and continue the decay process started by *S. mutans.*

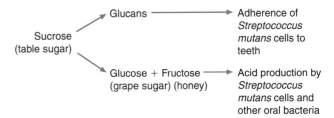

FIGURE 10.14

Metabolism of sucrose (table sugar) by the bacterium *Streptococcus mutans,* which causes tooth decay. Glucans, which can be made only from sucrose, appear to be required for the development of caries.

The incidence of tooth decay is declining, primarily because of fluoride prevention programs and the increasing use of nonsucrose dietary sweeteners. Fluoride reduces tooth decay either by diminishing the bacteria's ability to produce acid or by altering the tooth enamel structure, making it less sensitive to bacterial acid. Without dietary sucrose, *S. mutans* cannot solidify itself in the structure of dental plaque and therefore is swept away from the tooth before irreparable damage can be done.

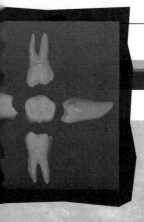

Points for Review

■ The structure of bacterial cells and the function of subcellular components

■ The structure and composition of viruses

■ The way the body protects itself from disease

■ How dental assistants can avoid the occupational hazards of infectious diseases

■ The role of microorganisms in dentistry's two major diseases

Self-Study Questions

1. How can a procaryotic cell be identified?
   a. It has no membranes.
   b. It has no nucleus or nuclear membrane.
   c. It has a characteristic type of cell wall.

2. Why do bacteria stop reproducing and enter the stationary phase?
   a. Nutrients have run out.
   b. End products have become toxic.
   c. Either a or b

3. What are bacterial endospores?
   a. Reproductive cells
   b. A preservation stage
   c. A more metabolically active form than the parent cell

4. Which of the following groups is in the proper order if descending size (largest to smallest) is the criterion?
   a. Virus, RBC, bacteria
   b. RBC, virus, bacteria
   c. RBC, bacteria, virus

5. Which of the following is a major difference between hepatitis A (HAV) and hepatitis B (HBV)?
   a. HAV contains only RNA and HBV contains only DNA.

   b. Only HBV attacks the liver.
   c. Infection with HAV produces lifelong immunity, but infection with HBV does not.

6. What do vaccines to most diseases induce?
   a. Antibodies
   b. Specific T-cells
   c. Complement

7. What term describes a large molecule that causes a specific immune response?
   a. Vitamin
   b. Antigen
   c. Immunoglobulin

8. What is the function of the T-helper cells?
   a. To kill invading foreign cells
   b. To process most foreign molecules in the development of a specific immune defense system
   c. To produce immunoglobulins

9. What results in lifelong immunity to many diseases?
   a. Production of memory cells, or the anamnestic response
   b. The function of T-suppressor cells in keeping microbes in check
   c. Strong public health measures

10. What causes acquired immunodeficiency syndrome (AIDS)?
    a. Long-term infection with the human immunodeficiency virus (HIV)
    b. Killing of plasma cells
    c. Infection with the tuberculosis organism

11. After the initial infection, where can the herpes virus be found?
    a. On the surface of the affected skin or tissue
    b. In the nerve supplying the affected tissue
    c. Always circulating in the blood of infected people

12. What bacterium initiates dental caries?
    a. *Streptococcus mutans*
    b. *Mycobacterium tuberculosis*
    c. Species of *Lactobacillus*

13. What bacterium is most closely identified with adult periodontitis?
    a. *Porphyromonas gingivalis*
    b. *Prevotella intermedia*
    c. *Actinobacillus actinomycetemcomitans*

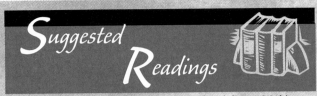

Genco R et al: *Molecular pathogenesis of periodontal disease*, Washington, DC, 1994, ASM Press.

Harris NO, Christen AG: *Primary preventive dentistry*, ed 4, East Norwalk, Conn, 1995, Appleton & Lange.

Nisengard RJ, Newman MG: *Oral microbiology and immunology*, ed 2, Philadelphia, 1994, WB Saunders.

Tortora GJ, Funke BR, Case CL: *Microbiology: an Introduction*, Redwood City, Calif, 1995, Benjamin/Cummings Publishing.

Chapter 11

Oral and Maxillofacial Pathology and Oral Disease

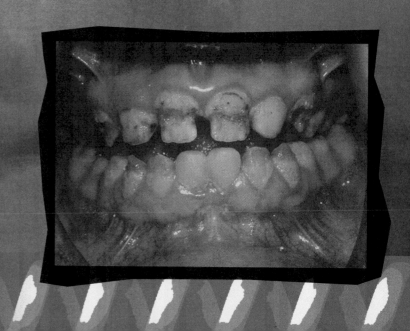

Chapter Outline

Learning Objectives

On completion of Chapter 11, the student should be able to do the following:

- Identify key terms.
- List the functions of the oral cavity.
- Describe a systemic method of oral examination for disease.
- List the cause, diagnosis, treatment, and intervention for common oral diseases.

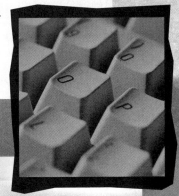

Key Terms

Abscess	Granulocytopenia	Ulcerations
Aphthae	Malignant	Varicose vein
Cyst	Oral assessment	

THE ORAL CAVITY

The mouth is a unique and important area of the body. It originates and participates in several vital physiologic and psychologic functions. Physiologically, the oral cavity begins the first step in the process of digestion. It provides not only a passive channel for delivery of food to the digestive tract but also the first components of digestion such as chewing, sucking, and chemical breakdown of foodstuffs. The mouth also functions as a major point of entrance for the process of gas exchange and respiration. Another important oral function includes the modification of sound by the tongue, teeth, and lips necessary for speech and vocalization. The oral cavity also provides one of the first components of body defense. Such neurologic oral functions as taste, touch, temperature, and pain act as a warning system for injurious substances. The saliva and mucous membranes contribute toward a physical protection system, and the secretion of antibacterial chemicals and antibodies in saliva serve as an antimicrobial defense mechanism.

Psychologically, the oral cavity provides us with such esthetic gratifications as visual beauty but also odor or bad breath (halitosis). Indeed billions of dollars per year are spent on lipstick, mouthwash, and esthetic dental products to provide this satisfaction. Many individuals experience oral satisfaction from such activities as smoking, drinking, taste, and food appreciation beyond functional needs.

An interruption of these functions by disease can lead to devastating physiologic or psychologic consequences and affect the physical and psychosocial components of both the dental treatment plan and overall health.

DETECTION OF ORAL DISEASES

The dental assistant aids the dentist in detection of oral diseases. Some diseases may originate in the oral cavity and occur as highly specific lesions, which must be recognized, diagnosed, and treated by the dental team. Other diseases may be indicators or barometers of systemic conditions. The presence of these diseases may warrant medical consultation and testing. In addition some oral disease may be infective and pose a risk of transfer to other patients and members of the dental team unless properly managed. The outcome of oral and systemic or oral diseases may be fatal. Therefore the early detection of these conditions is necessary to ensure quality patient care.

The dental assistant, as part of the dental team, assumes responsibility for detection and recognition of oral disease and for appropriate consultation with other members of the team leading to diagnosis, treatment, and prevention. Therefore the dental assistant should be familiar with common oral diseases and the causes, clinical course, prognosis, and prevention of these diseases.

The techniques used for proper oral examination, which include visual observation, palpation, jaw positioning, tissue reflection, and observation of smell, are simple and easily accomplished. Special techniques such as dental x-rays, instrument-assisted probing, and electrical pulp testing are useful and are usually best performed by the dentist. A simple **oral assessment** technique is described in Chapter 21.

Oral assessment

An examination of the oral cavity for the purpose of detecting and diagnosing pathologic lesions.

Stained Teeth

Dental stains and discolorations may be from internal (intrinsic) or external (extrinsic) nature. Extrinsic discolorations such as tobacco tars, beverage pigments, and heavy metal salts may render the teeth brown or black. Green teeth are often noted in children who practice poor oral hygiene and accumulate dental plaque containing chromogenic bacteria. Intrinsic discoloration occurs in teeth that incorporate tetracyclines or high concentrations of fluorides in teeth during tooth development and in teeth that lose their vitality.

Signs and Symptoms

Both intrinsic and extrinsic discolorations may cause unsightly appearance. The teeth and surfaces involved, the color of stain, and the surface deformation or malformation in tooth structure should be noted and recorded.

Diagnosis

Enamel hypoplasia is a common condition in which areas of the teeth appear pitted and stained. Frequently these stains are clinically apparent as a linear horizontal defect in enamel formation and represent a period of arrested enamel development secondary to a childhood exanthemas (rash-like) disease, prolonged fever, or other systemic disturbance during tooth formation (Figure 11.1).

Rarely individuals express hereditary enamel hypoplasia (amelogenesis imperfecta) of all teeth in both dentitions. The discoloration results from either exposed dentin or exogenous pigment trapped in the defective pits of the enamel. This condition is sometimes difficult to distinguish from dental caries, with location enamel hypoplasia frequently affecting self-cleansing surfaces and linear pattern important considerations in diagnosing hypoplasia.

Occasionally single teeth will manifest enamel hypoplasia in cases of local trauma or infection to the area during tooth development. Excessive fluoride during tooth development causes a specific enamel hypoplasia called mottled enamel, in which the enamel appears brown-white and frequently pitted. The levels of fluoride added to public water supplies

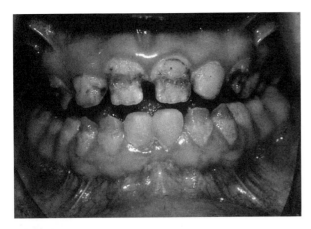

FIGURE 11.1

Enamel hypoplasia is the linear pitting and staining of the enamel of the anterior teeth.

do not cause this condition. The clinical extent of mottled enamel is proportional to the concentration of fluoride and the duration of the patient's drinking excessively fluoridated water (usually well water).

Tetracyclines administered during tooth development may cause a brown-yellow discoloration of teeth, usually without pitting. Because tetracyclines pass the placental barrier, the primary dentition may be stained if the drug is given to the pregnant mother. Tetracyclines should therefore not be given electively to pregnant women or to children under 10 years of age.

Individual teeth that have lost their vascularity appear darker and grey or brown because of changes in the organic composition of the dentin or residual blood pigment deposited in the dentin. These dead teeth are not pitted but are especially susceptible to fracture, even after root canal therapy (endodontics).

Extrinsic stains are frequently noted in the smooth surfaces of teeth, especially about the gingiva. A careful patient history usually will unearth the causative substance. Certain dental preparations such as chlorhexidine are notorious for causing brown staining of teeth and mucous membranes. Heavy smoking, coffee drinking, and certain medicines will frequently cause exogenous pigmentation of both the teeth and dorsal tongue.

Treatment and Intervention

Intrinsic stains are sometimes temporarily treated by dentists with bleaching or permanently by crowning or veneering the teeth. Enamel hypoplasia is treated aesthetically with crowning or plastic fillings or may be left untreated. Extrinsic stains usually can be removed by cleaning and polishing by a member of the dental team. Tooth staining and pitting must be distinguished from dental caries by probing, x-ray, history, and other means. Extrinsic staining gives some indication of patient habits and hygiene.

Dental Caries

Dental caries is defined as the infective disease process that results in demineralization of hard tooth structures. Dental caries usually results in unsightly cavities and tooth breakdown and, if left untreated, acute and chronic infections of the pulp and of the alveolar bone.

Causes

Three components of caries must exist: the infectious bacteria, carbohydrate substrate, and a susceptible tooth surface. Some bacteria of dental plaque ferment carbohydrates of the diet and produce acid byproducts at the surface of the teeth. These byproducts dissolve the mineralized structure of the teeth and create softened areas within the dental hard tissue (cavities). When this demineralization process progresses to the dental pulp, the oral bacteria infect and destroy the dental pulp (pulpitis). The infection spreads to the apical periodontium and bone. Numerous oral bacteria can cause dental caries with *Streptococcus mutans,* seemingly one of the most infectious (see Chapter 10).

Signs and Symptoms

Only about one third to one half of carious lesions are visible in relatively early stages. Early-stage lesions appear as chalky white to white-brown somewhat roughened areas on the enamel. Later-stage lesions are more brown, and usually the surface pit or fissure becomes soft or breaks down, forming a cavity. Finally, whole portions of crown crack away and large cavities result. Whole crowns break away, leaving only infected roots embedded in the gingiva.

Symptoms of deep caries include acute or chronic toothache, often after stimulation with cold or sweets, and perceived sharpness of teeth. Pulpally infected teeth may give acute or chronic toothache, sensitivity when eating, and swelling of associated soft tissues and bone when the infection spreads to the bone about the root of the tooth. Frequently a sinus tract forms at the apex of an infected tooth and drains to the gingiva or alveolar mucosa through a parulis (gum boil). The parulis will appear as a red-yellow, soft, raised lesion of the gingiva from which pus can frequently be expressed with pressure (Figure 11.2).

Diagnosis

The process of caries involves primarily the pits and fissures of the occlusal (chewing) surfaces of teeth and smooth surfaces between teeth. Early lesions of pits and fissures resemble stained pits and are difficult to diagnose visually. Probing with a pointed instrument (explorer) is necessary. Early lesions between teeth may be impossible to see, and therefore dental x-rays are necessary for diagnosis.

Treatment and Intervention

The location and severity of dental caries is recorded. Caries is best treated by total removal of the infected tooth material and

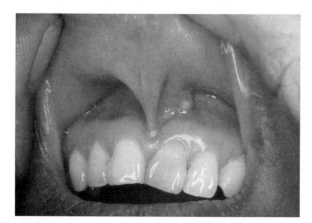

FIGURE 11.2

Parulis is a red gum boil that drains the infected carious tooth adjacent to it. Note the discoloration of the associated dead central incisor.

replacement with inert filling material. Adjunctive antibiotic and analgesic therapy, tooth extraction, or root canal filling (endodontics) may be necessary when pulpal or periapical infections exist as a consequence of caries. Caries are prevented by removal of any one of the three necessary components. Plaque control by brushing and flossing helps eliminate bacteria. Fluorides in dentifrice and public water strengthen susceptible tooth surface, making it more caries resistant. Plastic coating materials (sealants) are used to fill pits and fissures and protect tooth surfaces from the bacteria and acids. Dietary sugar control and sugar substitutes reduce the substrate necessary for bacterial growth adherence and acid production.

Gingivitis

Inflammation of the gingiva is extremely common, is seen in all ages of patients, and is caused by a number of factors or combinations of factors. The most common causes are dental plaque and calculus on the teeth, local irritation (mouth breathing, desiccation), lack of gingival stimulus, trauma, pregnancy and puberty, and more rarely very serious conditions such as anemias, leukemia, agranulocytosis, and vitamin C deficiency. Certain infectious childhood diseases that can cause gingivitis are discussed later.

Signs and Symptoms

The gingiva usually appears bright red and somewhat swollen. Pain and bleeding may occur. In pregnancy gingivitis, the gingiva becomes especially red and swollen and occasional "pregnancy tumors" of the gingiva form. These "tumors" bleed easily and spontaneously and may be painful.

Diagnosis

This is based on the clinical signs and symptoms and the absence of associated systemic conditions. A history of preg-

nancy or puberty, habits, and oral hygiene help distinguish the cause.

Treatment and Intervention

The cause of gingivitis should be determined. If plaque or irritative factors are determined as the cause, the irritant is removed or alleviated and oral hygiene is reinforced or assisted. If the patient is forced to breathe through the mouth because of nasal obstruction or habit, the gingiva may be protected or lubricated with petrolatum. Hygienic reinforcement such as brushing and use of gingival stimulants may be necessary for debilitated patients. Pregnancy gingivitis in its severest form is caused by poor oral hygiene. Because the gingiva is sore and bleeds easily, the patient tends to avoid proper hygienic procedures, which can lead to more severe manifestations, such as inflammatory periodontal destruction (periodontitis).

Oral hygiene must therefore be reinforced. It is important that any unexplained or marked gingivitis be immediately brought to the attention of the dentist; it may represent leukemia, **granulocytopenia**, a consequence of HIV infection, or a manifestation of one of the anemias.

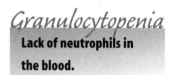

Granulocytopenia
Lack of neutrophils in the blood.

Acute Necrotizing Ulcerative Gingivitis

Also known as trench mouth or vincent's infection, this acute gingival infection is caused by spirochetes and fusiform bacteria. It is apparently not communicable (the causative bacteria are found in most mouths) but is closely associated with 1) poor oral hygiene and dental care, 2) lowered patient resistance, 3) smoking, or 4) agranulocytosis, leukemia, or HIV infection.

Signs and Symptoms

The trench mouth patient usually demonstrates fever and malaise, cratered **ulcerations** of the interpapillary gingiva between the teeth, a metallic taste, hypersalivation, pain, and bleeding of the gingiva. The breath has a particular fetid odor in these patients.

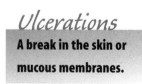

Ulcerations
A break in the skin or mucous membranes.

Diagnosis

Diagnosis is based on clinical signs and symptoms and history and absence of associated systemic conditions.

Treatment and Intervention

Treatment consists of cleaning the teeth with supportive topical anesthesia, antibacterial rinses, and systemic antibiotics. A patient who has trench mouth of long duration (more than 3 weeks) or recurrent episodes must be carefully evalu-

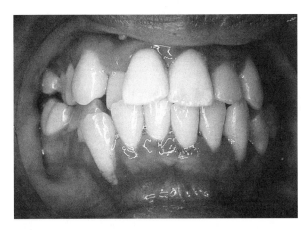

FIGURE 11.3

In cases of both gingivitis and chronic periodontitis, the teeth appear elongated and the gingiva appears red and swollen.

ated for agranulocytosis, leukemia, anemias, or immune disorders.

Periodontitis

Periodontitis is a very common oral disease that involves the inflammatory degeneration of the gingiva, periodontal ligament, supporting alveolar bone, and tooth cementum. This disease is most often caused by toxins elaborated by the bacteria of subgingival dental plaque and the resultant inflammatory destruction of the tooth supporting tissues. Local irritation and smoking causes and contributes to the disease. Periodontal disease is the most common cause of tooth loss after age 30.

Signs and Symptoms

Clinically, periodontitis is usually first apparent as a red, swollen inflammation of the gingiva (gingivitis). It is not particularly painful and therefore given little attention. As the disease progresses, the gingiva may become firm and scarred and begin to recede; that is, the roots of the teeth are exposed, making the teeth appear longer (Figure 11.3). The patient usually notes bleeding of the gingiva and perhaps a peculiar taste (pus) while brushing or chewing. As the disease further progresses, the periodontal ligament and cementum are destroyed and the gingival attachment progressively moves apically, causing "pocket" formation. The alveolar bone disappears, resulting in loosening and migration of the teeth. Occasionally, local **abscesses** of the periodontium can cause considerable pain and swelling, but usually the patient notes only occasional low-grade pain of the tooth-supporting areas.

Abscess

A local accumulation of pus, usually from a bacterial infection.

Diagnosis

Periodontitis is frequently of more severe and early onset in uncontrolled diabetics, individuals with blood dyscrasias such as agranulocytosis and anemias, and in females during pregnancy and puberty. Severe oral and systemic diseases such as gingival carcinoma, metastasis, Langerhans cell histiocytosis, and tuberculosis can closely mimic periodontitis. These must be distinguished by examination of patient history, biopsy, and specific tests, if necessary. Dental x-rays and dental periodontal probing are very helpful in assessing the degree of periodontal involvement.

Gingival Pigmentation

Amalgam tattoo is a very common condition in which dental amalgam is implanted into mucous membrane or alveolar bone at the time of amalgam removal or placement, endodontic filling, or tooth extraction. Although these tattoos can occur on other mucosa, the gingiva is by far the most common area involved. Dental amalgam that enters a socket area, an ulcer, or a cut in the gingiva is relatively inert and thereby discolors or tattoos the tissue without causing other signs or symptoms.

Signs and Symptoms

The gingiva appears focally blue-black to brown. The pigmented area is usually well demarcated. No symptoms of pain, growth, or lumps or bumps are present.

Diagnosis

The diagnosis of amalgam tattoo is best based on the clinical appearance and lack of other symptoms. Freckles, moles, and **malignant** melanomas of the gingiva are rare and may appear similar to an amalgam tattoo; however, these lesions usually manifest other signs and symptoms. Dental x-rays of the area will demonstrate radiopaque amalgam about half the time. Biopsy is sometimes necessary.

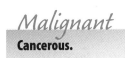

Malignant

Cancerous.

Treatment and Intervention

The amalgam tattoo is common, benign, and usually left untreated unless esthetics is a consideration. The dental team needs to distinguish tattoos from melanomas by the above criteria.

Gingival Fibrous Hyperplasia

Fibrous overgrowth of the gingiva can be caused by certain drugs and medications (dilantin, cyclosporin), hereditary overgrowth, or as a sequelae of chronic gingivitis with resultant scarring.

Signs and Symptoms

The gingiva appears enlarged and pale, is relatively firm to touch, and is not usually painful. The gingiva may overgrow and actually submerge the crowns of the teeth. It may cause movement, malocclusion, and malalignment of teeth. In edentulous patients the growth of the alveolar mucosa is frequently molded by the denture and conforms to the shape of the internal surface of the denture.

Diagnosis

The diagnosis of gingival hyperplasia is usually based on clinical signs and symptoms. A history of dilantin therapy or familial history helps distinguish types. Presence of a loose-fitting, removable dental appliance helps determine the irritation type of gingiva hyperplasia. Localized lesions may have to be biopsied to distinguish them histopathologically from other gingival growths.

Treatment and Intervention

Gingival overgrowth interferes with dental or dental prosthesis function. Dilantin-induced overgrowth can be somewhat controlled by strict hygienic intervention. Surgical removal of gingival hyperplasia is the treatment that provides the best cure, but the overgrowth will probably recur unless the stimulus is removed.

DISEASES OF THE MUCOSA: SOFT LUMPS AND BUMPS

Because touch and palpation are very useful as parameters of assessment, certain changes of the mucosa are detected as lumps and bumps. Some of the most common ones can be subclassified as soft, firm, or bony hard.

Fordyce Granules

These are small (1 to 2 mm), soft, multiple, yellow-white submucosal nodules seen bilaterally in the buccal mucosa and upper labial mucosa and lips of about 80% of the patients (Figure 11.4). They are developmental sebaceous glands and should be considered "normal" for that patient.

Signs and Symptoms

Patients are seldom aware of their existence because they are not painful or of significant size to elicit symptoms. They are usually noted by medical or dental personnel at oral examination.

Diagnosis

The diagnosis is almost always based on size, location, color, and texture as described.

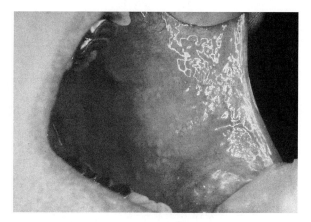

FIGURE 11.4
When Fordyce granules are present, the buccal mucosa shows bilateral nodules.

Treatment and Intervention

No treatment is necessary. Dental personnel need to familiarize themselves with the existence of Fordyce granules so that they will not confuse them with other lumps.

Papillomas and Verrucae

Squamous papillomas and verruca vulgaris are benign growths that appear clinically similar. Papillomas are considered as benign neoplasms, whereas verruca vulgaris is a virus-induced growth (wart). These lesions are rather common findings and have been noted on almost every mucosal surface.

Signs and Symptoms

These lesions are most frequently white or pale pink in color and raised. The surface shows numerous pointed or blunted finger-like extensions raised from the mucosa either on a single stalk or as multiple projections.

Diagnosis

Diagnosis is based on the appearance, a history of slow or no growth, and the color. Occasional papillomas may be less white or more firm; however, most feel quite soft. Patients who have clinical papillomas should be questioned and examined for warts of the hands and the habit of chewing on warts. Occasionally warts are venereal in origin.

Treatment and Intervention

Although theoretically infective, spread to other people is very uncommon. A rare verrucous cancer may clinically resemble these papillary growths. Papillomas and verrucae should therefore be documented and pointed out to the attending dentist. Excisional surgery is recommended.

Mucoceles

These are lesions caused by rupture of the minor salivary gland ducts with resultant spillage of mucin into the tissue. Trauma is the most common cause, although occasionally lesions are caused by ductal obstruction. A ranula is a large mucocele involving the floor of the mouth.

Signs and Symptoms

These lesions usually appear as blue to blue-white, raised submucosal swellings that are very soft. Superficial lesions resemble blisters. A history of short duration with rapid growth and collapse is common.

Diagnosis

Although these lesions are frequently caused by minor trauma and therefore occur most frequently on the lower labial mucosa, a history of trauma is frequently not available. Diagnosis is based on signs and symptoms and histopathologic examination. Rare malignant salivary gland cancers clinically resemble these common mucoceles.

Treatment and Intervention

Manipulation of the oral mucosa (trauma) can cause these lesions. The lesions usually need to be excised. Puncture of the mucocele results in collapse of the lesion, but it will probably reoccur. These lesions occasionally become enlarged. Any observed mucocele should be recorded and reported for definitive therapy.

Fibrous Hyperplasia (Fibromas) and Pyogenic Granulomas

These lesions result from chronic irritation to an area with reactive proliferation of collagen and fibroblasts (fibroma) or capillaries and fibroblasts (pyogenic granuloma). A long-standing pyogenic granuloma will ultimately mature into a fibroma.

Signs and Symptoms

Fibromas tend to be pink and soft (Figure 11.5, *A*), whereas pyogenic granulomas tend to be red, blue or black (Figure 11.5, *B*), and are frequently ulcerated. Both can occur on any mucosal surface, including the gingiva. Fibromas are seldom painful but may become very large (5 cm), whereas pyogenic granulomas tend to be irritating and bleed readily. Fibromas are often present for years, pyogenic granulomas for months. Note that the pregnancy tumors discussed as a component of pregnancy gingivitis are really pyogenic granulomas.

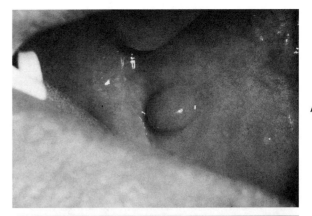

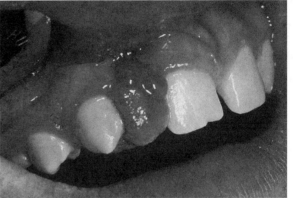

FIGURE 11.5

A, Fibroma. This soft, painless pink growth of the buccal mucosa was present for 4 years. **B,** Pyogenic granuloma. This gingival growth occurred over a 4-month period in a pregnant woman.

Diagnosis

Because these lesions are caused by chronic low-grade irritation, the source of irritation may be ascertained and contribute to the diagnosis. Common sources include sharp or broken teeth, dental calculus, habitual sucking of buccal or labial mucosa through the space of a missing tooth, loose-fitting dentures, and chronic lip biting. A linear, white, slightly raised fibrous hyperplasia located bilaterally on the buccal mucosa at the line of occlusion is called the linea alba and should be considered "normal" for most individuals.

Treatment and Intervention

Occasional salivary and connective tissue tumors may appear as fibromas or pyogenic granulomas. If the irritant remains, a fibroma or pyogenic granuloma may reoccur. Fibromas about a dental prosthesis must be removed, because the fibrous hyperplasia can both cause and be caused by poor fitting dentures.

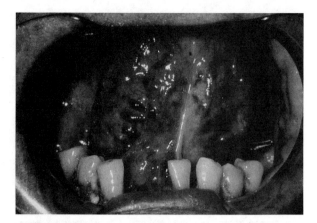

FIGURE 11.6

Lingual varices. The ventral tongue is involved in this older male.

Hemangioma and Varix

Hemangiomas are benign overgrowths of blood vessels within mucosa, whereas a varix is a dilated or **varicose vein**. Varices are so common they can be considered normal for adults over age 60 (Figure 11.6). Hemangiomas are a less common finding.

Varicose vein

A dilated, tortuous vein that appears swollen and blue.

Signs and symptoms

Hemangiomas are soft, may be raised or flat, and are usually red or blue-red in color. Size ranges from very small (1 mm) to involvement of the total mucosa or skin (birthmark). They can be located on any mucosal surface. Varices are usually soft, blue to blue-black, slightly raised, and vary in size from 1 to 5 mm. They are frequently multiple and are most often located on the ventral tongue, floor of the mouth, lateral tongue, and buccal mucosa.

Diagnosis

The diagnosis is usually based on color, location, palpation, and a history of little or very slow growth. Many of these lesions blanch if pressure is applied; this phenomenon aids in diagnosis.

Treatment and Intervention

Mucosal hemangiomas are sometimes excised, whereas varices are usually recognized and left alone. Lesions are sometimes removed to confirm diagnosis or for esthetic purposes. Neither entity causes any real sequelae. Rare large hemangiomas may be associated with certain syndromes. Therefore it is advised that they be removed for histopathologic diagnosis.

DISEASES OF THE MUCOSA: FIRM LUMPS AND BUMPS

The fibromas previously discussed may range from soft to firm. Other firm lumps of the mucosa include benign and malignant tumors of nerve, muscle, connective tissue, and salivary glands. Chronic inflammation and infection of the submucosa may also result in firm lumps of tissue.

Signs and Symptoms

Benign lumps tend to be of long duration, slow growing, painless, and are freely movable. The mucosa is usually stretched but intact. Malignant lesions tend to be attached or bound to adjacent tissue, fast growing, ulcerated, and may cause pain or numbness. Chronically inflamed areas are slow growing and somewhat painful.

Diagnosis

Differentiation of the above is usually based on histopathologic study of excised tissue.

Treatment Intervention

Immediate referral is important for any firm lump with the above mentioned malignant characteristics.

Palatal Tori and Mandibular Tori

These are developmental bony lesions that grow with the young patient and usually cease growth in adulthood. Palatal tori are found in about 25% of the population, whereas mandibular tori have been noted in 8% of patients.

Signs and Symptoms

Tori are bony hard, painless, attached to the jaws, and frequently lobulated. The palatal torus is located at the midline of the hard palate, whereas the mandibular tori are usually bilateral and attached to the mandible, lingual to the bicuspid roots (Figure 11.7). Tori are covered with mucosa, which can be stretched and occasionally ulcerated.

Diagnosis

The location and appearance are diagnostic. Adult patients are frequently unaware of their existence. Adults usually do not give a history of growth.

Treatment and Intervention

Recognition is the most important consideration, because no treatment is necessary. The only danger would be failure to diagnose and inappropriate treatment. Patients with large tori should be encouraged to maintain their teeth in good condition, because such tori can present a problem with prosthetic design and may have to be removed before denture construction. Bony growths in other areas should be

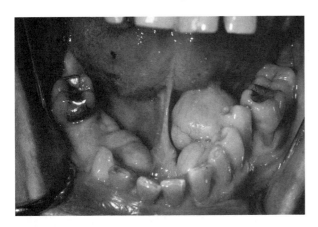

FIGURE 11.7

The mandibular tori on this patient has been present for many years.

pointed out to the dentist, because they may represent other more serious conditions.

Bony Cysts, Tumors, and Inflammatory Processes

Infections of the bone secondary to dental infection, **cysts** of the bone secondary to dental infection or tooth formation, and tumors of the bone- or tooth-forming apparatus usually are benign. All can cause lumps that are bony hard, usually asymmetric, and as a group are rather common. Common odontogenic cysts include inflammatory cysts, which form in the apical bone of an infected tooth, and dentigerous cysts, which form about the crown of impacted teeth. These cysts are slow growing, often expand the bony plates, and are well demarcated on radiograph. They are usually not painful and are often detected incidentally. Chronic infection (periapical granuloma) of the apical bone is also common and may cause circumscribed radiolucency with minimal bone expansion. The offending tooth is usually easily identified by an obvious carious lesion, vitality testing (negative), or percussion sensitivity.

Cyst

An epithelial-lined, fluid-filled cavity.

Cysts and granulomas are usually not very painful. Periapical abscesses are extremely painful, causing toothache and marked percussion sensitivity. The abscessed area may not be visualized with x-ray. Although cysts, granulomas, and abscesses are benign, they can cause considerable bone destruction and increase the risk of fracture. Malignant neoplasms, on the other hand, both originate in and metastasize to the jaws. Therefore any unexplainable bony lump or swelling should be brought to the attention of the dental team.

Treatment and Intervention

Periapical abscess, granulomas, and cysts usually resolve when the infected pulpitis is treated by root canal therapy or extraction. Sometimes apical surgery is necessary. Dentigerous cysts are treated by surgical excision and extraction of the impacted tooth. Because other less-common, morbid bony and odontogenic cysts and tumors may clinically present similar to the above, it is advisable to 1) submit excised tissue for histopathologic diagnosis and 2) initiate posttreatment follow up to ensure lesion resolution.

ULCERS

Ulcers are defined as breaks in the oral mucosa and may represent the clinical presentation of a number of diseases. Upon discovery of oral ulcers, it is important to carefully note pain, recurrence, number of lesions, location, duration, and coexisting lesions of the mouth and other areas of the body (Table 11-1). All of these features help distinguish ulcers of similar clinical presentation.

Aphthous Ulcers

These common ulcers affect more than 20% of the population and are frequently called "canker sores" or "stomach ulcers." These recurrent ulcers are caused by an immune hypersensitivity against the oral mucous membranes. Factors such as minor local trauma, stress, certain foods, gastrointestinal diseases, and mucosal manipulations usually cause predisposed patients to develop these acute ulcers. When trauma causes these ulcers, the size of the ulcer exceeds the amount of trauma; that is, a 1-cm ulcer may develop from a toothbrush abrasion to the mucosa. Ulcers last from 7 to 14 days and do not scar. Most patients give a family history of canker sores.

Signs and Symptoms

Aphthous ulcers appear on mucosa, which contains minor salivary glands. These ulcers are usually singular, round, punched-out, or crater-like. They have yellow-white membranous coatings and a red inflamed border (Figure 11.8). Aphthous ulcers are extremely painful.

Diagnosis

Aphthae can be diagnosed clinically by the crateriform appearance, location (aphthae are seldom, if ever, located on the gingiva or hard palate), history of recurrence, and other features. Lymphadenopathy

Aphthae

Canker sores.

frequently accompanies aphthae but fever is rare. Culture of the ulcers is nonspecific.

Table 11.1

Acute Oral Ulcers

Type	Prevalence	Location	Morphology	Cause	Treatment

Recurrent aphthous	20%–30% recurrent	Labial and buccal mucosa
		Tongue
		Soft palate
			Singular
			Round crater
			  3–10 mm
				Immune hypersensitivity
				Predisposing factors:
				  Trauma
				  Foods
				  Stress
				  GI disease
				Familial
					Corticosteroids
					Anesthetics

Primary herpetic gingivostomatitis	<1%	Gingiva All other mucous membranes Vermilion	Small multiple ulcers Fever Malaise	Herpes simplex I Immune suppression	Acyclovir and nutrient fluid

Herpes labialis	30%–40% recurrent	Lips
		Vermilion
		Skin
			Multiple
			  Blisters 1 × 1 mm
			  Ulcers coalesce
			  Crust
				Herpes simplex I
				Predisposing factors:
				  Fever/Cold
				  Sun
				  Trauma
					Acyclovir and topical preparations

Intraoral recurrent herpes	<1% recurrent	Hard palate
		Gingiva
			Multiple
			  Small ulcers
			    1 × 1 mm
				Herpes simplex I
				Predisposing factors:
				  Trauma
				  Fever/cold
					Topical anesthesia

Vesiculobullous skin disorder	Rarely recurrent	All mucous membranes	Multiple
			Large blisters
			  Large ragged ulcers
			  Skin, eye, genital lesions
				Skin Disorders
				Allergy
					Usually corticosteroids

Traumatic	Isolated singular	Area of acute or chronic trauma	Variable	Trauma:
				  Biting
				  Denture
				  Chemical
					Remove cause

FOM, Facial oral mucosa.

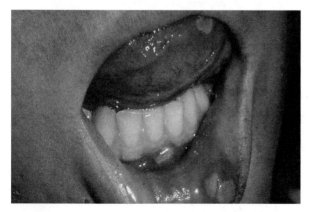

FIGURE 11.8

This patient developed multiple recurrent apthous ulcers several days after dental treatment.

Treatment and Intervention

These ulcers cause considerable discomfort. Susceptible individuals develop ulcers in stressful situations and ulcers can be further induced or aggravated by oral manipulation or minor trauma. Therefore it is necessary to be especially careful with dental manipulations, packs, or gauze and other minor traumatic oral events such as suctioning in susceptible patients.

Treatment of small and individual ulcers is usually restricted to a protective oral bandage (orabase), perhaps with a topical anesthetic. More severe and multiple lesions are treated with topical corticosteroids, systemic steroids, and topical anesthetic. The dentist should be alerted to the presence of these ulcers, because they can interfere with patient comfort and mastication. Severe frequent and multiple aphthae-like ulcers may actually indicate more severe disorders such as leukopenia, leukemia, allergic manifestations,

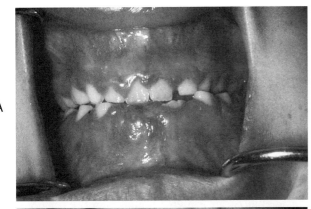

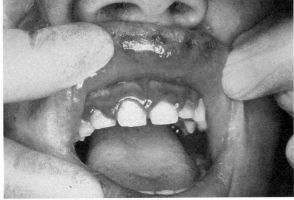

FIGURE 11.9

Primary herpetic gingivostomatitis. **A,** This young child has multiple ulcers and gingivitis. **B,** Note the lip ulcers and necrotitis gingivitis in this adult with primary herpes.

Crohn's disease and others; therefore further testing of these cases may be indicated.

Primary Herpetic Gingivostomatitis

This condition is caused by herpes simplex type I virus and affects less than 1% of the population. Children are most frequently infected, and a history of exposure to a patient with recurrent herpes labialis (cold sore, fever blister) is common. This condition is caused by the same virus, which causes recurrent herpes of the lips.

Occasional adult patients with recurrent herpes labialis who are immune deficient will also develop primary gingivostomatitis.

Signs and Symptoms

The patient with a primary infection usually demonstrates fever, malaise, and irritability. The lips, oral mucosa, gingiva, and pharynx develop multiple blisters (vesicles), which rapidly ulcerate to form yellow-white ulcers (Figure 11.9, A). The gingiva is edematous, red, painful to minor stimulation, and bleeds freely. Frequently the gingiva becomes vesicular or ulcerated and may resemble trench mouth (Figure 11.9, B).

Diagnosis

The diagnosis is based on the total clinical presentation. Cytology (smear) of a vesicle will reveal viral infected cells microscopically, which help identify the cause. Although children are most commonly infected and patient age therefore becomes a diagnostic parameter, occasional cases occur in adults (see Table 11.1). The disease must be distinguished from erythema multiforme, pemphigus, and other uncommon more morbid dermatologic conditions in adult patients.

Treatment and Intervention

Recognition is extremely important, because the vesicular lesions are contagious to all personnel. Gloves, meticulous hygiene, use of disposable instruments, careful viral sterilization techniques, and barrier techniques are necessary. Rare complications of viremia, including herpes encephalitis, can be devastating to patients. Bed rest is usually mandatory. Patients must be closely observed for fluid (dehydration) and nutrient intake, which is difficult because of the pain of the oral ulcers. Intravenous (IV) fluids and hospitalization are sometimes necessary. Oral lesions are treated with peroxide rinses and antibiotic mouthwash for secondary infection and viscous xylocaine for pain relief. A cold, bland diet is best tolerated. The disease usually subsides spontaneously in about 14 days. Many patients develop recurrent herpes lesions later.

Recurrent Herpetic Ulcers

Herpes simplex is a common contagious virus. It causes ulcerations called cold sores, fever blisters, or sun ulcers of the lips or oral cavity. The following three clinical forms of ulcers are quite easily recognizable:

1 Recurrent herpes labialis
2 Recurrent intraoral herpes
3 Primary herpes gingivostomatitis.

Upon initial contact with herpes simplex type I virus, most patients (80% of the adult population have antibodies) develop subclinical infections with less than 1% developing primary gingivostomatitis. Half of those infected (40% of the population) develop recurrent labial or intraoral lesions, whereas the other half infected never develop clinical disease. Recurrent lesions are usually initiated by exogenous or endogenous factors such as fever, upper respiratory infection, minor trauma, sunlight, or stress.

Signs or Symptoms

Lesions of the vermilion area of upper and lower lip (herpes labialis) account for the vast majority of incidence (see Table 11.1). The rare intraoral recurrent lesions are confined to the free and attached gingiva and the palatal mucosa (see Table 11.1). Clinically, recurrent herpetic lesions are usually multiple or clustered and are preceded by a burning or a tingling prodrome, closely followed by formation of fluid-filled blisters. Individual blisters are usually very small (13 mm) but tend to coalesce with adjacent blisters. The blisters rapidly ulcerate

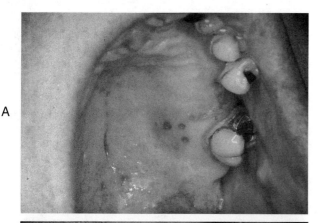

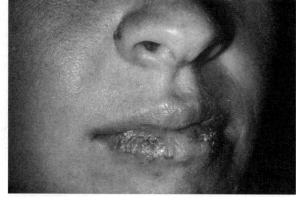

FIGURE 11.10

A, Ulcer stage of intraoral recurrent herpes. **B,** Crust stage of herpes labialis.

intraorally (Figure 11.10, *A*) or dry and crust on the lips, leaving the patient with irritating and somewhat unsightly crusted ulcers (Figure 11.10, *B*). In 7 to 14 days the ulcers heal without scarring. Recurrence may occur at unspecified rates but usually occurs in the same general area of the lips or mouth. Intraoral and extraoral lesions seldom occur simultaneously.

Diagnosis

Intraoral lesions can be diagnosed because of their specific location, vesicle stage, multiple small ulcerations and recurrence. Lip lesions have characteristic prodrome, vesicle stages, and crusting appearance. Cytology of vesicular fluid content demonstrates virally infected cells. Associated lymphadenopathy can occur. Lesions must be distinguished from rare vesiculobullous diseases of the oral cavity.

Treatment and Intervention

Severity of lesions can supposedly be reduced by application of ice pencils or lipid solvents (ethyl chloride) at the prodrome stage. Most therapy, such as commercial preparations containing phenol, xylocaine and silver nitrate, is palliative. Antiviral drugs (acyclovir) are effective in reducing lesion duration and in prevention of lesions when administered at an early stage.

Patients who have a history of recurrent lesions are susceptible to exogenous factors such as trauma or drying. This necessitates identification of such patients and care during oral manipulations to not initiate lesion formation. Lip balms and oral lubricants may give the patient additional protection. The prodromal and vesicular stages are infectious; therefore it is extremely important to recognize these lesions and to practice preventive procedures to protect staff and other patients from contagion.

Acute Ulcers of Chemotherapy

Acute oral ulcers are expected complications of chemotherapy or direct therapeutic irradiation. Chemotherapeutics can cause or predispose the patient to such ulcers by causing myelosuppression or immunosuppression, by directly damaging the oral mucosa, by inhibiting mucosa cell renewal, by causing xerostomia (dry mouth), by promoting overgrowth of opportunistic virus, fungi, and bacteria, and by combinations of these.

Signs and Symptoms

The signs and symptoms vary. The mucosa usually appears reddened, and multiple aphthous-like ulcers can develop on almost any mucosal surface. Gingival lesions resemble acute necrotizing gingivitis (see previous discussion). Patchy milky white plaques of candidiasis, which scrape off and leave a raw bleeding base, are common. The mucositis and ulcerations are usually very painful and may preclude the patient from chewing, swallowing, or drinking. Occasionally primary herpes gingivostomatitis accompanies other lesions or even predominates.

Diagnosis

These lesions should be anticipated in chemotherapeutically treated cancer patients. Certain drugs cause specific lesions. In general, lesions should be cultured for specific organisms even if these organisms represent secondary infective agents. The presence of vesicles preceding ulcerations suggests herpes virus is involved.

Treatment and Intervention

Anticipation is the key to prevention and treatment. Specific side effects can be predicted before therapy begins or lesions develop. Good dental hygiene using a soft bristle brush helps prevent ulcerative gingivitis. Dryness of the mouth can be treated with petrolatum (lips) and artificial saliva for the oral mucosa. Hydrogen peroxide rinses or glycerin peroxide lubricants can provide both an antiseptic and cleansing effect. Prophylactic administration of nystatin rinses and tetracycline suspension mouthwashes may prevent or abort bacterial or fungal ulcerations. Any traumatic or irritating procedures to the patient's oral cavity should be minimized, and irritating dental condition or prosthesis should be corrected or removed before chemotherapy. If lesions develop, culture and sensitivity tests are helpful.

The patient's food and fluid intake should be monitored and the diet adjusted to include foods the patient can tolerate. Liquid breakfast preparations, milk shakes and bland, cold, soft foods are best tolerated; coarse and acidic foods should be avoided. Rinses of xylocaine and benadryl give some topical symptomatic relief, and antibiotic, antiviral, and nystatin therapy can be started when indicated. Hydrocortisone preparations are helpful in reducing the inflammatory sequelae if herpes is ruled out. Specific antibiotics can be administered as per culture and sensitivity (see Chapter 10).

Other Ulcers

Acute oral ulcers are encountered from such conditions as trauma, burns, chemicals, loose-fitting dental prostheses, or as an end stage of several of the vesiculobullous diseases, such as pemphigus, pemphigoid, erythema multiforme, and drug reactions.

Signs and Symptoms

Most of these lesions appear as nonspecific ulcerations of any mucosal surface and can be easily confused with severe aphthae or primary herpes. The ulcers of the vesiculobullous diseases are preceded by blisters and are frequently multiple in number and area of location (Figure 11.11, *A*). Blisters of the oral mucous membrane, however, are usually short lived, because the tissue is readily sloughed after the simplest oral function. Therefore the absence of blisters does not preclude the possibility of a vesicular disease. Traumatic, chemical, or thermal injuries are usually found in specific locations, such as pizza burn of incisive papilla, cheek biting of buccal mucosa, or medicine burn of the gingiva next to an aching tooth (Figure 11.11, *B*).

Diagnosis

An accurate patient history is important. Most vesiculobullous diseases are associated with blisters and ulcers of the skin, eyes, genitalia, or anus and are recurrent. An associated history of medication preceding oral lesion development provides a clue to allergic or drug idiosyncracy as a cause of the ulcers. If questioned, the patient may admit to trauma, use of over-the-counter drugs and chemicals, topical use of aspirin (see Figure 11.11, *B*) on the mucosa, and factitial (self-inflicted) injury.

Treatment and Intervention

If vesiculobullous or allergic conditions are suspected, immediate medical consultation is necessary. If injury is suspect, the offending agent should be removed. If local ulcerations exist, topical application of an oral bandage, steroid, or benzocaine ointments may be necessary to enhance healing. Severe or numerous oral ulcers may be treated

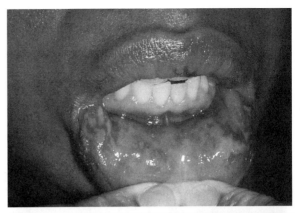

A

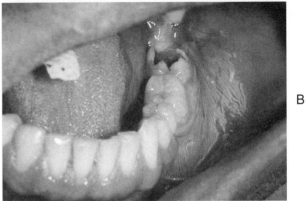

B

FIGURE 11.11

A, Erythema multiforme. This vesiculobullous disease resembles primary herpetic gingivostomatitis. **B,** Aspirin burn.

nonspecifically with the regimen used for chemotherapy patients and specifically with the therapeutic drugs for the causative disease.

ULCERATED ORAL CANCER

Oral cancer effects approximately 30,000 people annually and often presents clinically as a chronic ulcer. The most common type of oral cancer is the epidermoid (squamous cell) carcinoma. The epidermoid carcinoma is most common in older males who smoke, consume above-average quantities of alcohol, and practice poor oral hygiene.

Excessive sun exposure is an important carcinogen for squamous cell carcinoma of the lips. Such cancer, however, has been reported in adults of both sexes, almost any age, and any degree of habituation. Most premalignant and early cancers do not present as ulcers but rather as changes in mucosal color.

Signs and Symptoms

Cancerous ulcers are relatively nonpainful and of long duration. Usually the ulcer margins are raised, firm, and fixed

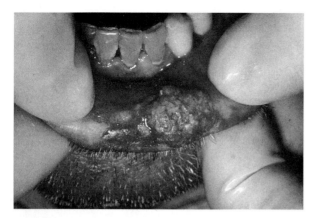

FIGURE 11.12

Ulcer stage of squamous cell carcinoma.

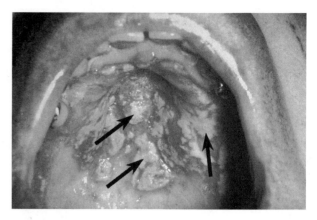

FIGURE 11.13

Subject with candidiasis (*arrows*). These white areas scrape off.

(Figure 11.12). Because the lesion is not painful, often the patient is not aware of its presence or is unconcerned. Very large lesions can cause fixation or destruction of adjacent tissues with loss of muscular function, tooth mobility, or displacement of structures. Firm, painless nodal enlargement in the neck signals metastasis. Oral cancer most frequently is located on the lip (one third of cases), floor of mouth, posterior lateral tongue, and retromolar-pillar areas. These are considered high-risk locations.

Diagnosis

All chronic ulcers should be held suspect, especially in high-incidence oral locations and in high-risk patients. Because the intraoral locations are difficult to examine and because lesions are asymptomatic in early stages, a thorough oral examination is mandatory in any high-risk patient. Biopsy of the suspicious lesion is usually necessary.

Treatment and Intervention

The dentist should be alerted to suspected lesions. Treatment varies according to type of cancer, histopathologic grade, and surgical stage. A person who has or who has had an oral cancer has up to 10 times the chance of developing a second primary cancer compared with a noncancer patient. Therefore upon examining an oral cancer, an oral assessment should be completed with special attention to changes suggestive of a secondary primary lesion.

WHITE LESIONS OF THE ORAL MUCOSA

Candidiasis (Moniliasis)

This superficial fungus is found in most oral cavities but grows in pathologic numbers secondary to such conditional stages as the following:

1 Antibiotic or steroid therapy

2 HIV and AIDS
3 Chemotherapy
4 Poorly controlled diabetes mellitus
5 Leukemia or leukopenia
6 Poor denture hygiene
7 Neonatal infection and certain hormonal diseases

Signs and Symptoms

Lesions can arise on almost any mucosal surface and consists of milky white curdlike membranous areas that partially scrape off with a gauze sponge (Figure 11.13). Frequently the area beneath the removed curd is red, raw, irritated, and bleeds. Frequently the lesions are not entirely white, but appear as red, inflamed, sore mucosa with only rare white patches. The infection is very superficial and the mucous membrane is usually intact.

Diagnosis

The white curd represents colonies of fungus, which can be demonstrated by cytologic smear or culture. Materia alba and denture powders can accumulate about teeth and beneath dental appliances and clinically resemble candidiasis. Aspirin burns of the mucosa create white lesions that scrape off and are easily confused with candidiasis. History of predisposing factors is often important to help include candidiasis and exclude aspirin burn and foreign material.

Treatment and Intervention

The fungal infection is to be treated with topical or systemic antifungal medicines such as nystatin. It is important that the precondition be identified along with the fungus, because the precondition may cause the more serious sequelae. If the infected patient wears dentures or partial dentures, the appliance should also be periodically treated with nystatin cream or soaked in antiseptic so that it will not reinfect the patient. Denture hygiene is necessary to prevent candidal organisms from growing beneath the denture.

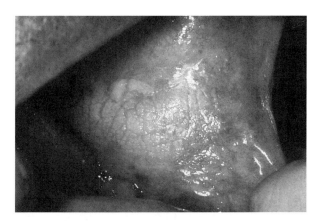

FIGURE 11.14
Hyperkeratosis.

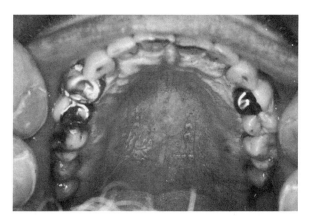

FIGURE 11.15
Nicotine stomatitis. These white and red lesions occurred in a pipe smoker.

Dentures should be cleaned routinely and left out at night if possible, especially in patients taking antibiotics. Careful sterilization of infant pacifiers and nipples should also be practiced in infected children.

Keratosis

When the oral mucosa accumulates layers of keratin or parakeratin, it will appear white (Figure 11.14). (The term "leukoplakia" is sometimes used to describe a white mucosal patch. This term should be avoided, because it implies precancerous change to some dentists and physicians.) Oral keratosis is a very common condition found in most mouths and is usually caused by a chronic low-grade physical irritation. It is a callous within the mouth.

Signs and Symptoms

Keratosis can be found on any surface but is usually noted on areas subjected to low-grade stimulus such as an edentulous ridge in a patient who does not have dentures, an area of the cheek adjacent to a pipe stem, or an area of the cheek that is sucked between the teeth because of habit. The white area usually appears flat and at times may be rough, cracked, or corrugated. Margins of the lesion can vary from well demarcated to diffuse.

Diagnosis

Although the term "keratosis" is a histopathologic term, diagnosis is frequently made on clinical location, evidence of chronic stimulation, or disappearance of the lesion after the stimulant is withdrawn. If the lesion is in an area of high cancer incidence or if it persists after the stimulus is removed, biopsy becomes necessary.

Treatment and Intervention

A white patch in the oral mucosa that is not readily explainable has a 16% chance of being cancerous or malignant. This chance increases from white patches of the floor

of the mouth, ventral lateral tongue, or retromolar area. All such lesions should be charted and reported to the dentist.

Nicotinic Stomatitis

This is a common, benign lesion of the hard and soft palate caused by chronic thermal irritation secondary to pipe or cigar smoking. This lesion is rare in cigarette smokers. The palate becomes white and hyperkeratotic, and the orifices of the palatal minor salivary glands become inflamed and red.

Signs and Symptoms

The unprotected palate (a denture gives protection) appears white and dry and is often cracked to give a dry river-bottom appearance. Multiple, red, 1-mm, round areas appear within the white area and are usually located within the center of raised, white, pebbly papules (Figure 11.15).

Diagnosis

The area, classical appearance and history of smoking cigars or a pipe are diagnostic. Biopsy is seldom necessary.

Treatment and Intervention

The condition is benign, not premalignant, and therefore no therapy is necessary. Other areas of high cancer incidence should be examined thoroughly, because the nicotinic stomatitis lesion indicates that the patient is a heavy smoker and thereby cancer prone.

Dysplasia and Early Oral Cancer

Dysplasia is a premalignant condition that may ultimately develop into epidermoid carcinoma. Dysplastic mucosa and early carcinomas of the oral cavity are related to incidence of

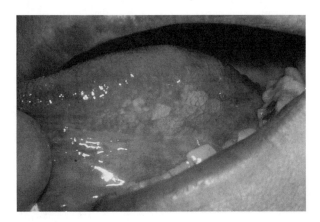

FIGURE 11.16

Epithelial dysplasia. Biopsy shows precancerous changes.

tobacco usage (including smokeless tobacco) and alcoholism, whereas lip cancer is related to smoking and sunlight exposure. Cancer and dysplasia can have clinical manifestations such as white lesions, ulceration, swelling, and erythroplakia. These manifestations are discussed elsewhere.

Signs and Symptoms

These lesions are often difficult or impossible to distinguish clinically from keratosis on the basis of clinical appearance alone. Like keratosis, these lesions are white, demarcation varies, surface texture varies from smooth to rough, and size is extremely variable (Figure 11.16). Dysplasia has been noted in lesions as small as 3 mm in diameter. The white surface does not scrape away with a gauze sponge.

Diagnosis

Location and history of chronic irritation are important features in distinguishing dysplasia from keratosis. Any persistent white plaques in areas of high cancer incidence should be biopsied. Cytology of white oral lesions has not proven useful in cancer detection. White lesions of non–cancer-prone oral areas are much less suspect, especially if a chronic irritant is identifiable. These areas should nevertheless be followed up by the dental team. If the lesion is diagnosed as dysplasia, local excisional surgery is the best treatment. If the lesion is diagnosed as cancer, a therapy of surgery, radiation and chemotherapy is dictated by grade, stage, and location of the tumor.

Leukoedema

This common developmental condition is noted most often in African Americans and is present in up to 40% of the population.

Signs and Symptoms

The buccal mucosa bilaterally appears filmy, opalescent, blue-white, folded, and often lacy. These areas feel soft and smooth.

If the mucosa is stretched, the linear striations disappear and the mucosa appears a normal pink color and consistency. The patient is seldom aware of the presence of this condition.

Diagnosis

This condition is always bilateral and of buccal mucosa only. Extreme examples might be confused with such dermatologic conditions as lichen planus or white sponge nevus.

Treatment and Intervention

The condition is "normal" for the affected patient.

Other White Lesions of the Oral Mucosa

Numerous uncommon hereditary and dermatologic conditions may cause white lesions of varying patterns and locations. These conditions include lichen planus, lupus erythematous, white sponge nevus, pachyonychia congenita, and others. Most of these lesions are associated with other oral or dermatologic manifestations detectable by history or physical examination. If the presence of white oral lesions cannot be readily justified, other considerations must be made by the dentist and appropriate tests should be ordered.

RED LESIONS OF THE ORAL MUCOSA

An inflamed oral mucosa appears red and is usually swollen and painful. In addition, chronically dried mucosa also becomes readily inflamed. Nonspecific infection and xerostomia should be considered when assessing painful, reddened oral mucosa.

Radiation Mucositis

Direct therapeutic radiation of oral mucosa causes mucositis secondary to direct tissue damage, xerostomia and opportunistic infection.

Carcinoma in Situ, Dysplasia, and Oral Cancer

The term erythroplakia is frequently used to describe clinical red mucosal lesions that are not inflammatory and that cannot be otherwise diagnosed clinically by location, specific morphology, or history. Most erythroplakias are premalignant carcinoma in situ, dysplasia, or malignant carcinomas. Again, smoking, alcoholism, and oral sepsis play an important (but not exclusive) causative role.

Signs and Symptoms

These lesions are red, nonpainful, and often appear velvety. They are usually smooth and soft (Figure 11.17). The patient is

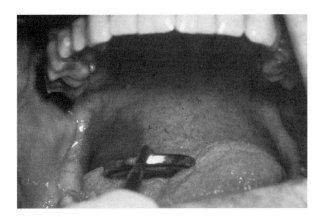

FIGURE 11.17

Erythroplakia. The red spot is carcinoma in situ.

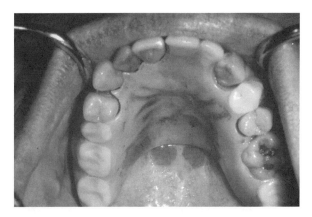

FIGURE 11.18

Papillary hyperplasia. This patient wears a poorly fitting retainer.

seldom aware of their presence, so historical data is usually absent. The intraoral areas involved most frequently are similar to those previously noted for premalignant and malignant white lesions and ulcers. Not uncommonly erythroplakias are associated with adjacent speckled white areas and chronic ulcers.

Diagnosis

The location, lack of signs of inflammation, association of risk habits, history of previous oral cancer, and elimination of other conditions are important considerations. Cytology may be helpful as a screening technique, but biopsy is the definite diagnostic technique.

Treatment and Intervention

Carcinoma in situ and dysplasia are premalignant lesions that may progress to cancer. In general, surgical excision and withdrawal of tobacco and alcohol are the best treatment. Some of these lesions regress after removal of tobacco and alcohol alone. Epidermoid carcinoma is treated with surgery, radiation, and chemotherapy, depending on the size, spread, stage, grade, and location of the growth and the patient's health status. Early recognition is the key to good prognosis. At-risk patients must be thoroughly examined for oral cancer regularly using the suggested technique for oral assessment.

Denture Sore Mouth and Papillary Hyperplasia

These conditions are related to and are caused by one of the following: 1) ill-fitting dentures, 2) improper denture hygiene with resultant sepsis, 3) candidal infections of denture covered mucosa, 4) denture material (acrylic) intolerance, or 5) acrylic allergy.

Signs and Symptoms

Denture sore mouth is characterized by the appearance of bright red mucosa beneath a denture in such a fashion that when the denture is removed, the red "image" of the denture is easily visualized on the mucosa. Often the tissues are slightly irritated and painful; however, painless lesions are most common. Frequently the mucosal texture becomes roughened or pebbly, especially when the hard palate is involved. Papillary hyperplasia results when contact with the above-mentioned causal factors is long standing and usually involves the palatal areas beneath a maxillary denture. The palate acquires numerous pink to red papillary or cobblestone projections that are firm and fibrotic (Figure 11.18). Pain and ulceration of the area rarely occur.

Diagnosis

The location, characteristic denture demarcation, and peculiar clinical appearance are diagnostic. Diagnostic smears or culture for candida is helpful in determining the role of these organisms in lesion presentation. Occasionally patients must be tested for acrylic allergy (rare) after the other etiologic factors have been eliminated.

Treatment and Intervention

Preventing lesions in long-term patients is possible by reinforcing principles of denture hygiene, either through patient education or personal service. When lesions exist, the cause must be identified before treatment commences. Often proper hygiene and nystatin therapy solve the problem. If the dentures are poor fitting, they should be evaluated, conditioned, relined, or remade. Usually the fibrotic papillary lesions of papillary hyperplasia must be surgically removed before dentures can be refitted. If acrylic intolerance or allergy is identified as the cause, dentures have to be fabricated or lined with nonacrylic materials.

DISEASES OF THE TONGUE

The pointed filiform papillae of the dorsal tongue are especially sensitive to environmental insult and intrinsic disease;

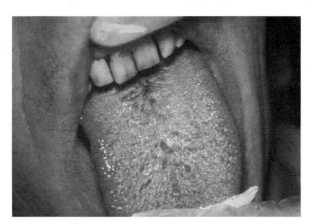

FIGURE 11.19

Brown hairy tongue. This patient is a heavy smoker.

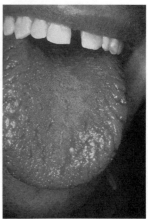

FIGURE 11.20

Fissured tongue.

therefore specific changes of the dorsal tongue commonly indicate such conditions. The tongue mucosa is susceptible to most of the other mucosal diseases that cause ulcers, lumps and bumps, and color changes and have been discussed previously.

Hairy Tongue

This condition is a manifestation of hyperkeratinization of filiform papillae and may be caused by such factors as bacterial overgrowth secondary to antibiotics or drugs, low-grade stimulation by heat or stomach acid, heavy smoking, xerostomia, and loss of normal tongue function. The color of the hyperplastic "hairy" papillae is dictated by chromogenic bacteria (black hairy tongue), the presence of tobacco pigments or coffee (brown hairy tongue), or the presence of keratin (white hairy tongue).

Signs and Symptoms

These conditions are painless and the signs vary according to cause:
1 Black hairy tongue: The filiform papillae of the dorsal tongue are very elongated and black in color. The tongue appears unsightly and may gag the patient if the elongated papillae tickle the soft palate. The condition is usually secondary to systemic antibiotic administration with resultant overgrowth of chromogenic bacteria with the hyperkeratosis.
2 Brown hairy tongue: The filiform papillae are elongated and brown (Figure 11.19). This condition is frequently secondary to combinations of smoking, drinking hot coffee or tea, or chronically using lozenges.
3 White coated tongue: The dorsal tongue appears coated with a thick, white plaque that does not scrape off. This condition is usually secondary to inactivity (coma, mouth ulcers), gastric hyperacidity and use of antacids.

Treatment and Intervention

Because the condition is asymptomatic and nonthreatening, treatment is usually initiated for esthetic reasons. The causative agent must be identified and removed if possible. Tongue brushing will promote desquamation and reduce the severity of the discoloration and gagging. Prophylactic tongue brushing may be necessary in susceptible patients.

Fissured Tongue

This condition affects 5% of the population and tends to increase in incidence with age. The etiology is unknown.

Signs and Symptoms

The dorsal tongue appears cracked or fissured with multiple cracks radiating toward the lateral margins (Figure 11.20). Some patients complain of mild to moderate burning pain. Almost half the patients with fissured tongue also have geographic tongue.

Diagnosis

A clinical diagnosis is based on the characteristic appearance.

Treatment and Intervention

Treatment is unnecessary. Sometimes the fissured tongue should be cleansed with a toothbrush or peroxide rinse to avoid burning or superficial bacterial entrapment with subsequent infection.

Atrophic Glossitis

This condition usually effects the entire dorsal tongue surface and may be a manifestation of pernicious anemia, folic acid deficiency, pellagra, chronic anemias, gluten intoler-

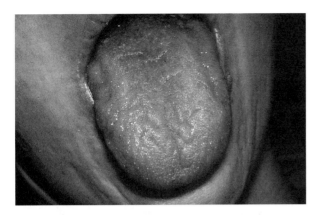

FIGURE 11.21
Atrophic glossitis. This patient has dry mouth.

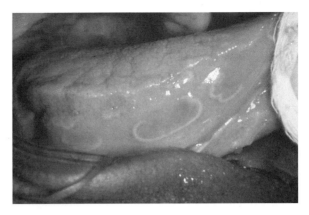

FIGURE 11.22
Benign migratory glossitis. The location and pattern change frequently.

ance, or allergy. Xerostomia and chronic atrophic candidiasis can also cause a similar condition.

Signs and Symptoms

The entire dorsal tongue appears reddened, flat, and smooth with atrophy of filiform and fungiform papillae (Figure 11.21). The patient often complains of a scalding or burning and intolerance of hot or spicy foods. Taste is sometimes altered. The duration of symptoms is almost always chronic.

Diagnosis

Careful attention should be paid to a presentation or history of malaise, dermatitis, neuropathy, dementia, gastritis or stomach surgery, anemia, or steatorrhea. An assessment of chronic dry mouth or evidence of candidiasis frequently yields diagnostic information. Hemoglobin tests, RBC morphology examination, and serum cobalamin (vitamin B_2) may be necessary if anemia or pernicious anemia is suspected. An allergic history and food diary may help identify an allergen.

Treatment and Intervention

If systemic disease is suspected, this condition and other associated signs should be brought to the attention of a physician. Topical anesthetics give temporary symptomatic relief but are too often used without regard for causality. Saliva substitutes and vitamin supplementation is occasionally helpful. Candidiasis can be treated by the dentist.

Benign Migratory Glossitis

This is a specific condition of the dorsal tongue that affects 2% of the general population. Such etiologic agents as psychosomatic predisposition, nonspecific vitamin B

deficiency, and allergy have been suggested but not proven.

Signs and Symptoms

Lesions seem to occur most frequently at times of stress. The dorsal and lateral tongue shows patchy atrophy of filiform papillae and the lesions appear reddened and inflamed. The lesion periphery frequently demonstrates whitened C-shaped, slightly raised rings of hyperkeratotic papillae. Multiple lesions at one time are usual. The pattern of atrophy with hyperkeratosis changes rapidly and the lesions frequently appear as continents of a world map, hence the term migratory glossitis or geographic tongue (Figure 11.22). At times the tongue will return to normal but recurrent lesions can be expected. The lesions infrequently cause a burning sensation but are usually asymptomatic; therefore the patient may not be aware of recurrence or chronicity.

Diagnosis

This condition is clinically recognizable by its location, migratory pattern, recurrent history, and characteristic morphology. Rarely, lateral tongue lesions must be distinguished from white lesions or erythroplakia. This condition infrequently manifests as a patchy manifestation of atrophic glossitis.

Treatment and Intervention

Recognition and diagnosis is important so that this condition is not be confused with erythroplakia and inappropriately biopsied. Erythroplakia (carcinoma in situ, dysplasia and epidermoid carcinoma) almost never occurs on the dorsal tongue. Patients should be checked for dermatologic diseases and other associations with atrophic glossitis. Some patients respond to vitamin supplementation perhaps as a psychosomatic placebo.

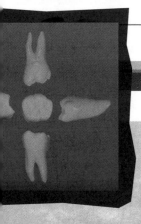

Points for Review

- Dental assistants' role in an oral examination
- Identification of the signs and symptoms of common oral disease, their diagnosis, treatment, and intervention
- Definitions of related terms

Self-Study Questions

1. Which of the following statements is TRUE about aphthous stomatitis ulcers?
   a. Usually occur on the hard palate
   b. Frequently associated with a family history of recurrent mouth ulcers
   c. Caused by the herpes virus
   d. Seldom painful
   e. Lasting immunity developing after the first infection

2. What are the usual initial symptoms immediately after infection with herpes simplex I virus?
   a. Blisters of palate
   b. Blisters of lips
   c. Ulcers of gingiva and oral mucous membranes
   d. Ulcers of the eyes
   e. Subclinical (no) lesions

3. All of the following are symptoms of primary oral herpes EXCEPT which one?
   a. Dry mouth
   b. Fever
   c. Oral ulcers
   d. Gingivitis
   e. Pharyngitis

4. Which conditions predispose to oral candidiasis?
   a. Antibiotic therapy
   b. Immune suppression
   c. Diabetes mellitus
   d. Cortisone medications
   e. All of the above

5. Which oral growth is most often associated with pregnancy?
   a. Pyogenic granuloma
   b. Hemangioma
   c. Varices
   d. Fibromas
   e. All of the above

6. Why should oral dysplasia be diagnosed and distinguished from other oral white lesions?
   a. Dysplasia is a skin disease
   b. Dysplasia will become painful
   c. Dysplasia often develops into oral cancer
   d. All metal fillings must be removed next to the dysplasia
   e. Two of the above

7. All of the following are associated with the development of oral squamous cell (epidermoid) carcinoma EXCEPT which one?
   a. Smoking tobacco
   b. Alcohol
   c. Poor oral hygiene
   d. Smokeless (spit) tobacco
   e. Hairy tongue

8. What is the most likely cause of papillary hyperplasia of the palate?
   a. Pipe smoking
   b. Wearing the upper denture at night
   c. Candidiasis
   d. Antibiotic administration
   e. B and C only

9. What are the usual causes of fissured and geographic tongue?
   a. Developmental
   b. Bacterial infection
   c. Vitamin deficiency
   d. Unknown
   e. A, B, and C

10. What do patients with oral erythroplakia most likely have?
    a. Pizza burn
    b. Premalignant or malignant disease
    c. Candidiasis
    d. Geographic tongue
    e. Leukoedema

11. Leukoedema is best characterized as which of the following?

   a. White thickening of the buccal mucosa

   b. Malignant bone marrow disease

   c. Chronic cheek biting

   d. Sunburn

   e. An oral manifestation of a skin rash

12. Enamel hypoplasia is usually caused by which environmental agent?

   a. Caries

   b. Fever and childhood infection

   c. Pregnancy

   d. Smoking

   e. Fluoride

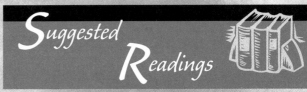

Suggested Readings

Antoon JW, Miller RL: Aphthous ulcers: a review of the literature on etiology, pathogenesis, diagnosis and treatment, *JADA* 101:803, 1980.

Banoczy J, Szaba L, Csiba A.: Migratory glossitis: a clinical histologic review of seventy cases, *Oral Surg Oral Med Oral Pathol* 39:113, 1975.

Barrett AP: Gingival lesions in leukemia: a classification, *J Periodontol* 55:585-588, 1984.

Dreizen S: Oral candidiasis, *Am J Med* 77:28-33, 1984.

Lynch DP: Oral candidiasis: history, classification and clinical presentation, *Oral Surg Oral Med Oral Pathol* 78:189, 1994.

Miller RL et al: *General and oral pathology*, St Louis 1995, Mosby.

Neville BW et al: *Oral and maxillofacial pathology*, Philadelphia, 1995, WB Saunders.

Regezi JA, Sciubba J: *Oral pathology: clinical-pathologic correlations*, ed 3, Philadelphia, 1999, WB Saunders, pp 77-88, 98-129.

Scully C: Orofacial herpes simplex infections:current concepts in the epidemiology, pathogenesis and treatment, *Oral Surg Oral Med Oral Pathol* 68:701, 1989.

Spruance S et al: The natural history of recurrent herpes simplex labialis, *N Engl J Med* 297:69, 1977.

Waldron CA, Shafer WG: Leukoplakia revisited: a clinicopathologic study of 3256 oral leukoplakias, *Cancer* 36:386, 1975.

Chapter 12

Radiology and Radiation Safety

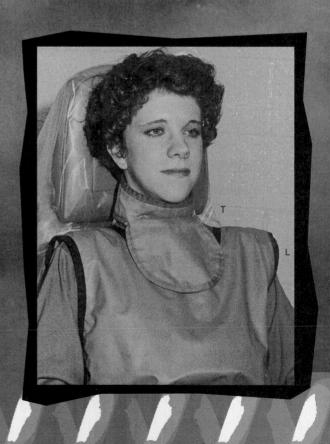

Chapter Outline

Learning Objectives

On completion of Chapter 12, the student should be able to do the following:

- Define key terms.
- Describe atomic structure as it relates to production of x-radiation.
- Describe the basic components of an x-ray unit and how they affect the x-ray beam.
- Explain the production of x-radiation.
- Discuss the ways in which x-radiation interacts with matter.
- Describe the process by which the latent image is produced and converted to a visible image.
- Discuss image quality using the following terms: density, contrast, resolution, distortion, unsharpness, and magnification.
- Identify the principal chemical components of processing solutions and describe the functions of each.
- Discuss the cause of and remedy for major film exposure and processing errors.
- Discuss the biologic effects of radiation.
- List the basic principles of radiation safety and explain how each affects occupational exposure to radiation.
- List and describe methods by which patient exposure to x-radiation can be reduced.

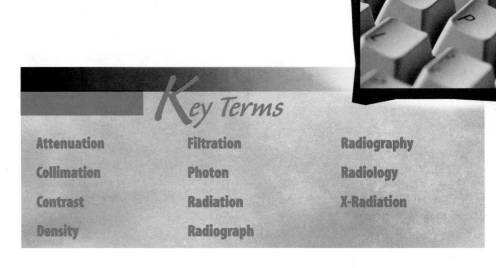

Key Terms

Attenuation	Filtration	Radiography
Collimation	Photon	Radiology
Contrast	Radiation	X-Radiation
Density	Radiograph	

RADIATION PHYSICS

To understand the physics of **radiation,** one must first understand the atom. Atoms are the smallest indivisible units of matter. They consist of a nucleus and an electron cloud. The nucleus is composed of variable numbers of subatomic particles, called *protons* and *neutrons.* Protons have a positive charge; neutrons have no charge and are said to be neutral. Together, protons and neutrons are referred to as *nucleons* because they make up the nucleus of the atom. The electron cloud that surrounds the nucleus is called a cloud because subatomic particles, called *electrons,* orbit the nucleus at high speed. An electron has a negative charge equal in magnitude to the positive charge of a proton, but an electron weighs much less than a proton (1840 times less).

> **Radiation**
>
> The transmission of energy by waves through space.

An atom is considered neutral when the number of positive charges in the nucleus (protons) equals the number of negative charges (electrons). When the number of positively and negatively charged particles is unequal, the atom is *ionized* (changed into an ion). A substance made up of only one kind of atom is called an *element.* Elements have unique atomic numbers (symbolized by Z, which stands for the number of protons) and atomic mass (symbolized by A, the number of nucleons). The atomic number and atomic mass of several elements commonly used in **radiography** are listed in Table 12.1.

The electrons orbit the nucleus at different distances. For simplicity, these distances are grouped into electron shells, which are labeled with letters from the inside out, starting with K. The electrons in each shell have specific binding energies; *binding energy* is the force needed to remove an electron from its shell. The closer an electron is to the nucleus, the harder it is to remove it from its shell and therefore the higher is its binding energy (Table 12.2).

> **Radiography**
>
> The making of radiographs by passing radiation through an object of interest and capturing the resultant energy on an image receptor.

Radiation is defined as the transmission of energy. Two types of radiation are necessary for radiography: particulate or corpuscular energy and electromagnetic energy. Corpuscular (particulate) radiation transmits energy in the form of charged particles that have mass. Alpha particles (such as the nucleus of a helium atom, which has a positive charge of 2 [2] and an atomic mass of 4) and beta particles (high-speed electrons) are examples of corpuscular radiation. Beta particles are essential for the production of x-rays.

X-rays are an example of electromagnetic radiation. Electromagnetic radiation transmits energy in a wavelike pattern. The shape of the wave pattern is determined by an electric and a magnetic field (hence the name electromagnetic). The energy of electromagnetic radiation is de-

Table 12.1

Atomic Number and Mass of Elements Commonly Used in Radiography

Element and symbol	Atomic number (Z)	Atomic mass (A)*
Aluminum (Al)	13	27
Copper (Cu)	29	63
Gadolinium (Gd)	64	157
Lanthanum (La)	57	139
Lead (Pb)	82	208
Niobium (Nb)	41	93
Tungsten (W)	74	184

*Rounded to the nearest whole number.

Table 12.2

Binding Energies of Tungsten Electron Shells

Electron shell	Binding energy (keV)*
K	68.4
L	12.1
M	2.8
N	0.59
O	0.08
P	Approximately 0

*keV, Kiloeletron volt.

scribed as a small packet, or *quantum*. These packets have no electric charge and are weightless. Electromagnetic radiation is separated by different wave patterns, or frequencies. *Frequency* is the number of waves per unit of time (for example, cycles per second). This arrangement is called a *spectrum.*

Photon

A weightless packet of pure energy.

X-radiation

A type of electromagnetic radiation that moves in divergent straight lines from the source at the speed of light, with a wavelength measured in angstroms (Å).

Radiograph

The visual image produced by exposing and processing radiographic film.

An x-ray is a weightless packet of pure energy with no electrical charge that moves through space with a specific frequency (less than 5 angstroms) at the speed of light. This packet of energy is also called a **photon** of **x-radiation.**

The phenomenon of x-rays was discovered by Wilhelm C. Roentgen in 1895. He found that a fluorescent plate glowed when placed near a cathode ray tube. He surmised that the fluorescence was caused by radiation, which he called "x-radiation" ("x" was for unknown). News of Roentgen's discovery spread rapidly. Otto Walkoff, a German dental surgeon, exposed the first dental **radiograph** just 2 weeks after Roentgen's discovery. James Morton, C. Edmund Kells, and William Rollins all have been credited with the exposure of the first dental radiograph in the United States. The equipment used by these pioneers was slow and inefficient and not without danger. Clarence Dally, one of Thomas Edison's assistants, died of the effects of x-radiation in 1904. Although he claimed to be resistant to the effects of radiation, C. Edmund Kells endured numerous operations as a result of exposure to x-radiation and ultimately took his own life.

The exposure time for Roentgen's first radiograph was 15 minutes; modern exposure times are measured in fractions of seconds. This dramatic reduction in exposure time is the result of improved image receptor sensitivity (discussed later) and the design of the x-ray unit. The typical x-ray unit is shown in Figure 12.1.

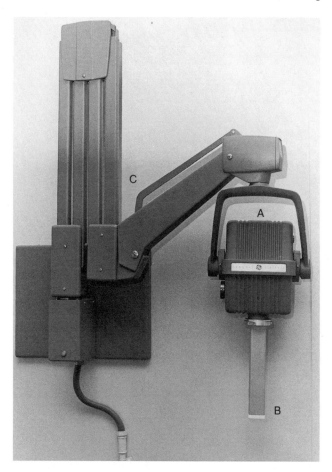

FIGURE 12.1

X-ray unit. **A,** Tube head. **B,** Rectangular collimator. **C,** Control arm.

X-Ray Equipment
Coolidge Tube

The Coolidge tube, or hot cathode ray tube, is a leaded glass receptacle that contains a cathode and an anode within a vacuum. The cathode is negatively charged and consists of a tungsten filament seated in a molybdenum focusing cup. A low voltage current is used to heat the filament immediately before exposure. The anode is positively charged and is made up of a tungsten target (1 × 4 mm) imbedded in a copper heat sink. The heat sink draws heat away from the tungsten target, reducing thermal damage to the target. The target is sloped to reduce its effective size. A smaller target (sometimes called the source) produces a more geometrically suitable beam of x-radiation. The angling of the target allows for better heat dissipation and extends the life of the target by allowing a larger focal spot but maintaining a small effective size. The sloping of the target to reduce the effective size and the relationship of the cathode and anode are shown in Figure 12.2; the choice of this shape is based on the Benson line focus principle.

Tube Head

The tube head is a heavy metal casing that holds the Coolidge tube immersed in oil. The oil acts as an additional heat sink. An opening in the tube head produces an exit for the useful beam. The tube head casing helps prevent the escape of useless (leakage) radiation from the tube head.

Control Arm

The control arm supports the weight of the tube head and is balanced to permit precise positioning with fingertip control.

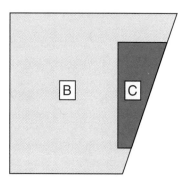
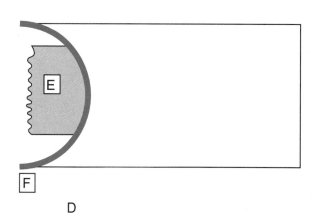

FIGURE 12.2

Components of the x-ray (or cathode ray) tube. **A,** Anode. **B,** Copper heat sink. **C,** Tungsten target. **D,** Cathode. **E,** Tungsten filament. **F,** Molybdenum focusing cup.

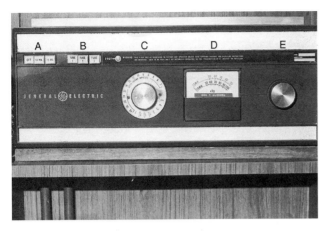

FIGURE 12.3

Control panel. **A,** Milliamperage control. **B,** Tube head selector (used only if several tube heads are operated from the same control panel). **C,** Exposure time selector. **D,** Kilovoltage meter. **E,** Kilovoltage control, which indicates the kilovolt peak selected by the operator.

Control Panel

The control panel allows manipulation of exposure factors: time, kilovoltage peak, and milliamperage. The kilovoltage peak (kVp) is a measure of electric force; kVp describes the potential difference between the cathode and the anode. As kVp increases, the quality of the x-ray beam changes, with the energy being increased. For diagnostic dental radiographs, the kilovoltage ranges from 60 to 90 kV. Line voltage (usually 110 or 220 V) is increased to kilovoltage with a step-up transformer. A step-down transformer reduces line voltage to 8 to 12 volts. The mean energy of the x-ray beam determines the quality of the beam. Beam quality is a function of kVp.

Milliamperage (mA) is the measurement of electric current that passes through the filament. The milliamperage controls the number of electrons "boiled off" the tungsten filament in the cathode. Increasing the milliamperage increases x-ray photon production. Beam quantity is a function both of kVp and mA. In diagnostic dental radiography, the milliamperage usually ranges from 7 to 15 mA. Figure 12.3 shows a typical control panel.

In the context of radiography, time measures the period during which x-ray photons are produced. Electronic timers record time in fractions of seconds. The accuracy of these timers is derived from the use of 60-cycle electrical current. Impulse timers also use 60-cycle electrical current for accuracy; one impulse is equivalent to $^1/_{60}$ of a second. For example:

6 Impulses = $^6/_{60}$ seconds = $^1/_{10}$ of a second

Rectification of the electrical current is a mechanism for protecting the tungsten filament in the cathode and can affect the sensitivity by which exposure time is measured. A half-wave rectified current uses only half of the available input current. A half-wave rectified unit can measure time in $^1/_{60}$ of a second. Full-wave rectification allows the use of all the input current. Consequently, exposure time can be measured in $^1/_{120}$ of a second. A three-phase generator produces a current with essentially a constant potential or no fluctuations in the beam energy. A three-phase, fully rectified generator can produce exposure times measured in $^1/_{360}$ of a second.

Timer Switch

The timer switch is also called a deadman switch. Activation of the timer switch sets the production of x-radiation into motion. When the timer switch is pushed, there is a very short delay before x-rays are produced. This delay allows the Coolidge tube to heat up. It is important to keep the timer switch depressed until the indicator sound stops and the indicator light goes out.

X-Ray Generation
Filtration

Filtration is the process by which lower wavelength photons (less energetic photons) are removed from the beam of radiation. In dental radiography, Aluminum is the most common filter material used. Different thicknesses of Aluminum are placed across the opening of the tube head (Figure 12.4). The thickness of the Aluminum depends on the kVp used. For kVp of 70 or greater, 2.5 mm Aluminum total filtration is required by law. The requirement for kV below 70 is 1.5 mm Aluminum. Long wavelength (low energy) photons would not reach the image receptor and can harm the patient; therefore they are best filtered.

> *Filtration*
> **The selective removal of lower energy photons from a beam of radiation. Aluminum is the material most commonly used as a filter in dental radiography.**

Total filtration is the sum of inherent and added filtration in mm of Aluminum equivalence. Inherent filtration results from the glass of the Coolidge tube and oil in the tube head. Generally, inherent filtration is equivalent to 0.5 mm of Aluminum. Added filtration is placed at the opening of the tube head (see Figure 12.6). Several other filter materials can also be used, which include nonrare earth materials such as Copper and Niobium, and band pass or K-edge filters such as Gadolinium, Ytterbium, Yttrium, and Samarium).

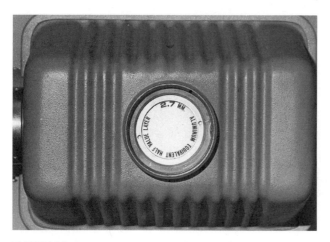

FIGURE 12.4

Filter in place; 2.7 mm of aluminum-equivalent added filtration has been placed over the exit portal in the tube head.

Collimation

Collimation is the reduction of beam spread or area and is achieved in two ways. The primary collimator is a lead diaphragm (see Figure 12.1, *B*) with a central opening in the shape of the desired beam (round or rectangular). Secondary collimation further reduces the dimensions of the x-ray beam. A lead-lined position indicating device (PID) is the most common secondary collimator. The PID is sometimes referred to as a *cone*. The American Dental Association (ADA) Council on Dental Materials, Instruments, and Equipment recommends the use of a secondary collimator that reduces the size of the x-ray beam to that of the image receptor (1 inch x 1$\frac{1}{2}$ inch). This recommendation is largely ignored. A 2.75 inch diameter round beam is much more common and has been the federal requirement for more than 20 years. The 2.75-inch dimension allows almost 4 square inches of the patient's skin to be needlessly exposed to x-radiation.

> *Collimation*
>
> **The reduction of the dimension of a beam of radiation. The dimensions produced with rectangular collimation are 1$\frac{1}{2}$ inches by 2 inches. Round collimation produces a circle 2.75 inches in diameter.**

Generation of X-Rays

Pushing the button on a timer switch sets into motion a chain of events that culminate in production of x-radiation. The instant the timer switch is depressed, the filament in the cathode is heated and a large number of electrons are boiled off of the filament. This process is called *thermionic emission.* Immediately after the cloud of excited electrons is formed, kilovoltage is applied between the cathode and anode and the electrons are attracted to the anode at a high rate of speed. The production of heat is the end result of over 99% of the electron-target interaction. As these electrons strike the tungsten target in the anode, the following four interactions can occur:

1 The high-speed electron can completely miss the target atom.

2 The high-speed electron can dislodge an electron and create an ion. The ion is quickly returned to ground state on neutral.

3 The path of the high-speed electron can be bent or slowed by a close encounter with another shell electron. The radiation produced by this interaction is called *breaking* or *Bremsstrahlung radiation*. Bremsstrahlung radiation accounts for between 80% and 90% of the radiation produced in the x-ray tube head. Bremsstrahlung radiation is referred to as a *polyenergetic beam* because individual photons can have different enemies.

4 If the high-speed electron dislodges an inner-shell electron in the target atom, the radiation produced is called *characteristic radiation* because the energy of the photon is characteristic for the electron shell and target atom. For example, the characteristic radiation produced by dislodging an electron from the K-shell of Tungsten has an energy of 68.4 kV. Because the energy of each photon is the same (for each atom and electron shell) the resultant beam is considered monoenergetic. Characteristic radiation accounts for approximately 10% to 20% of x-radiation produced in the tube head. Most characteristic radiation is generated at kilovoltages greater than 70.

Regardless of the type, the radiation that leaves the opening in the tube head is called the *primary* or *useful beam*. The geometric center of the primary beam is referred to as the *central ray*. The importance of the central ray will become apparent when technique is discussed. Radiation that leaves the tube head by other than the prescribed opening is called *leakage radiation*. If leakage radiation is detected, the x-ray unit should not be used until repaired or replaced.

The generation of x-radiation is a complex process but it occurs in a fraction of a second. X-rays are produced only when the timer is activated.

X-Ray Interaction with Matter

When a photon is produced and directed towards the object of interest, the following four interactions can occur:

1 Absorption

2 Penetration

3 Scatter

4 Generation of secondary radiation

The result of these interactions depends on the energy of the x-ray beam and the **density,** thickness, and shape of the object being

> *Density*
>
> **The overall darkness of a processed radiograph. Density is affected by kVp, mA, exposure time, TFD, and processing.**

imaged. Objects that are bulky, dense, or the use of a low energy beam can result in absorption of the emitted photon. Because the photon is absorbed, the x-ray film is not affected or exposed, and the radiographic image is white. Structures that appear light or white on x-ray film are termed *radiopaque*. An object that has low density, is thin, or the use of a high-energy beam can allow the emitted photon to penetrate the objects and interact with the radiographic film. This allows more emitted protons to interact with the film emulsion, resulting in a dark image on the processed film. Structures that appear dark are described as radiolucent. Some structures appear grey on the processed film. This radiographic appearance is the result of differential absorption of x-radiation by the different structures and tissues.

As x-ray photons traverse the patient's tissues, their path can be deflected and their energy attenuated or reduced. This phenomenon is referred to as *scatter*. Three types of scatter are recognized in dental radiography. When the photon is deflected, **attenuation** of the beam occurs, Thompson or coherent scatter results. Compton or incoherent scatter occurs when the photon is deflected and the beam energy is attenuated. Photoelectric absorption takes place when the incident photon is absorbed and a photon of characteristic radiation from the tissue atom concerned is produced.

> ## Attenuation
> **The reduction of the energy of a beam of radiation as it passes through tissue or structures.**

Scattered radiation degrades the quality of the radiographic image and must also be a consideration in the radiation protection of the patient and operator.

Secondary radiation is produced when the interaction between the photon from the primary beam and the structure of interest produces a photon of x-radiation. Secondary radiation has a lower photon energy than primary radiation. Secondary radiation also adds to the effects of scattered radiation.

The differential absorption of x-rays by matter produces a pattern of exposure on the radiographic film. This pattern is generated by that part of the useful beam that traverses the object of interest (remnant radiation) and is called the *latent image*. The latent image is a chemical change within the film emulsion and is invisible. Processing the latent image produces a silver or visible image.

Radiographic Film

Radiographic film is similar to photographic film with regard to composition and light sensitivity. Both types of film consist of an emulsion of Silver Halide crystals in gelatin. The emulsion coats both sides of a plastic base. Silver Halide crystals (for example, Silver Bromide [AgBr] and Silver Iodide [AgI]) undergo a chemical change when exposed to

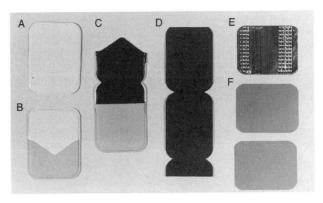

FIGURE 12.5

Contents of a film pack. **A,** Plastic outer covering (front). **B,** Plastic outer covering (back). **C,** Opened film packet. **D,** Black cardboard inner covering. **E,** Lead backing. **F,** Film (two pieces).

light or x-radiation (the latent image). Either one or two pieces of film are wrapped in black paper, along with a lead foil backing, and sealed in either a paper or plastic film packet (Figure 12.5). Many clinicians and patients feel that the paper film packet is more comfortable for the patient. Unfortunately, the paper packets leak if soaked in disinfectant as an infection control procedure.

Dental x-ray film comes in many sizes. Sizes 0-3 are used in the mouth (intraorally), and size 4 can be used either intraorally or extraorally (outside the mouth). Larger films are used extraorally. Film contained in packets is referred to as *direct exposure film* because the film is sensitive to exposure by x-radiation. Larger films must be used in a cassette with intensifying screens to capture an image. This type of film is called *screen film* and is sensitive to the light emitted by the intensifying screens. Intensifying screens convert x-radiation to light. This conversion increases the efficiency of the receptor (speed with which an image is captured) and decreases patient dose. Screens can emit different colors of light depending on their composition. Traditional screens are composed of Calcium Tungstate (Ca_2WO_4) and emit violet light when exposed to radiation. Newer screens are composed of salts of rare earth elements such as Gadolinium and Lanthanum. The Oxybromide screens emit green light and the Oxysulfide screens emit blue light. Film that is sensitive to the light emitted by the particular screen and safe-light filter that is matched to the film should be used.

Film Speed

Film speed is a measure of the film's sensitivity to x-radiation. A fast film type is more sensitive to radiation than a slow film type. Fast film requires less radiation to produce an acceptable radiograph. Use of fast film decreases the patient's exposure to radiation. There are two film speeds available commercially at this time—D speed and E-speed. E-speed film is said to be twice as fast as D-speed film and consequently decreases the patient's dose by half. In clinical practice E-speed actually reduces patient exposure by approximately 40%.

Extraoral screen-film combinations are also rated by speed. A conventional or par speed screen-film combination is arbitrarily assigned a speed of 100. Rare earth screen-film combinations are rated up to 400 speed or four times as fast as par screens. The speed of an intensifying screen is determined by the screen material, screen thickness, and shape and thickness of the phosphor crystal in the screen.

Nonfilm Image Receptors

For a number of years, images have been captured electronically in medical radiography. Images generated in computed tomography (CT) and magnetic resonance imaging (MRI) are stored electronically, processed by a computer, and displayed on a video screen or film. Within the past 5 years, dentistry has achieved the capability of electronic image capture and storage. Intraoral units that use electronic image capture are now commercially available, and several extraoral units are available in prototype for panoramics, plain film, and linear tomography. The image receptor for these units is called a *charge-coupled device* (CCD) or a *linear array*. Most CCD devices require a phosphor layer (much like an intensifying screen) that converts x-radiation to light. The CCD that acts as a camera detects the light. It is converted to a grey scale by a computer. The image is displayed on a video screen and can be printed on paper. CCD-based systems are extremely sensitive to radiation and can record an image with an exposure time of $^2/_{100}$ of a second.

Film Processing

The process by which the latent image is converted to a visible image is called *film processing*. One of the easiest and unfortunately the most common way to produce a nondiagnostic x-ray film is to incorrectly process the radiograph. Every dental office has its own processing method and most of them are wrong. Proper methods for manual and automatic processing will be presented in this section. Methods for maintaining the quality of processing will be discussed later in this chapter. Development and fixation are the two major steps in film processing.

Development

X-ray developer contains several components that act together to convert the exposed Silver Halide crystals to black metallic silver. Sodium Carbonate softens and swells the gelatin in the emulsion to allow the reducing agents to contact the Silver Bromide crystals. Potassium Bromide controls the reaction between the Silver Halide crystals and the reducing agents so that unexposed crystals are not converted to metallic Silver. These chemicals are dissolved in water and preserved with Sodium Sulfite. For proper processing, the

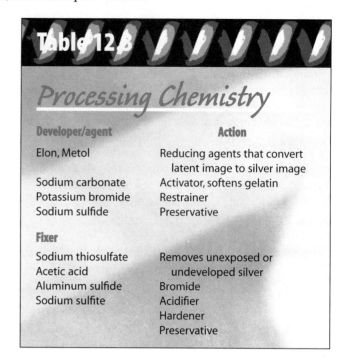

Table 12.3

Processing Chemistry

Developer/agent	Action
Elon, Metol	Reducing agents that convert latent image to silver image
Sodium carbonate	Activator, softens gelatin
Potassium bromide	Restrainer
Sodium sulfide	Preservative
Fixer	
Sodium thiosulfate	Removes unexposed or undeveloped silver
Acetic acid	
Aluminum sulfide	Bromide
Sodium sulfite	Acidifier
	Hardener
	Preservative

developing time *must* be determined by the temperature of the developer. The time-temperature method is the only acceptable process by which to manually process radiographic film. Optimum conditions for manual processing are generally $4^1/_2$ minutes of developing time at 68° F. When the film has been in developer for the correct time, it should be rinsed in clean, running water for 30 seconds, shaken to remove excess water, and placed in fixer. Always remember to follow the time-temperature recommendations of the manufacturer of the processing solutions.

Fixation

The chemical components of radiographic fixer halt the process of development, wash away unexposed Silver Halide crystals, and preserve the resultant metallic silver image. Acetic acid stops development by neutralizing the developing solution. Ammonium Thiosulfate clears the film by washing away the unexposed crystals. The gelatin is hardened to preserve the metallic Silver on the film by Aluminum Sulfide. As with developer, water is the solvent and Sodium Thiosulfate is the preservative in fixer. Fixing time should be twice the developing time. When fixation is complete, film should be rinsed for 20 minutes in clean, running water and then dried.

The processing chemistry for manual and automatic processing is quite similar. However, automatic processing takes less time and therefore must be performed at a higher temperature than manual processing techniques. The chemicals for automatic processing have been modified so that they will last longer in a high-temperature environment. Table 12.3 lists the common components of processing chemistry, and Box 12.1 presents the equipment and steps used in manual processing.

Box 12.1

Procedure

Equipment and Steps for Manual Processing

Darkroom setup

Radiographs must be processed in a room that allows no white light because exposure of the film to white light before developing results in a fog on the film that degrades the quality of the radiographic image. The darkroom should be equipped with the following items:

A room that completely excludes white light; the door should have a lock, and the walls of the room should be a light color

An adequate work surface

An appropriately filtered safelight placed 4 feet or farther from the work surface

Manual processing tanks

A sink with hot and cold running water

A thermometer (although not a mercurial thermometer)

An accurate timer

A film drying rack

Storage space

A source of white light

Steps in manual processing

1. Stir the developer and fixer with different mixing paddles.
2. Check the solution levels and replenish when necessary.
3. Check the temperature of the solutions; remember that the temperature of the developer dictates the processing time. *Note:* Do not use a mercurial thermometer to check solution temperature; if the thermometer breaks, the finish of the tanks will be ruined.
4. Label the film hanger with the patient's name and date.
5. Exclude white light and turn on the safelight.
6. Put gloves on to handle contaminated film packets.
7. Remove all films from their packets, allowing the film to fall untouched onto a paper towel.
8. Discard gloves and securely attach the films to the film hanger, taking care to handle the film by its edges.
9. Using the loaded film holder, gently agitate the developer and then immerse the film in the developer.
10. Cover the tanks and set the timer for the correct developing time.
11. Remove the films from developing tank and rinse them for 20 seconds in clear, running water.
12. Lightly agitate the fixing tank with the loaded film hanger and immerse the films in the fixer.
13. Cover the tanks and set the timer for double the developing time. Films can be viewed wet after 3 minutes of fixation but must be final fixed immediately.
14. Wash the films in clear running water for 20 minutes. Water should be added to the master tank at a rate that circulates the tank contents every 6 minutes.
15. Allow the films to dry.
16. Place the films in appropriate film mount.

Dark Room

Radiographs must be processed in a room that allows no white light. White light will produce fog that degrades the quality of the radiographic image. Some offices will have an automatic processor. However, maintain manual processing tanks in case the automatic processor breaks down (see Box 12.1).

Automatic Processors

Automatic processors consist of a series of rollers that propel a radiograph through developer, fixer, water rinse, and drying cycle (Figure 12.6). Most automatic processors operate at higher temperatures than manual processing. The chemistry is modified to last longer in a warmer operating temperature. Perform quality assurance procedures with automatic

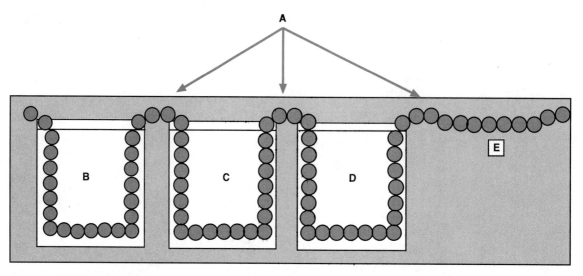

FIGURE 12.6

Automatic processor. **A,** Roller assembly. **B,** Developer tank. **C,** Fixer tank. **D,** Rinse tank. **E,** Dryer.

processing because the solutions can become exhausted between films.

Daylight Loaders

Some dental offices are not equipped with a darkroom. Instead, an automatic processor with a daylight loader is used. A daylight loader is attached over the entry port of the processor. It consists of a box with two hand holes with sleeves and a hinged door. The hinged door has a filtered window through which to place exposed but unprocessed films. The following two major limitations of daylight loaders must be considered:

1 The filter on the hinged door is designed for D-speed film but not necessarily for E-speed film. If E-speed film is used (and it should be) the filter should be augmented or processing should take place in an area with subdued lighting.

2 Aseptic technique is all but impossible to maintain in a daylight loader. Suggested corrections for this problem include the use of a film barrier, soaking the films in a disinfectant for 15 to 20 minutes or changing gloves while your hands are inside the loader. If the dental office uses a daylight loader in lieu of a darkroom, what happens when the processor breaks down must be addressed.

Safelights

The importance of safe lighting can not be minimized. Faster film is more sensitive to light and x-radiation. The safelight should be placed at least 4 feet from the working surface. The purpose of the safelight is to provide enough light to see what you are doing without fogging the image. Maximum brightness for safe lights is 15 watts for direct lighting (light pointed at the working surface) and 25 watts

for indirect safe lighting (light pointed away from the working surface). The safe light filter must match the sensitivity of the radiographic film in use. The Kodak GBX (red) filter can be used for both direct and screen film processing. The Kodak Morlite (orange) filter can be used for direct but not for screen film processing.

All safelight filters wear out eventually. The safety of the filter can be checked with the coin test. Turn off both the white and safelights in the darkroom. Unwrap an unexposed film. Place the film on the working surface with a coin on top of the film. Expose the film to the safelight for 5 minutes then process. If the outline of the coin is visible on the processed film, the safelight filter is defective (or a white light leak may exist). Perform the coin test with the fastest film used in the office. A safelight that is effective for D-speed film may be ineffective if used with E-speed film. White light leaks can also be detected with the coin test. Repeat the process without turning on the safelight.

EXPOSURE AND PROCESSING PITFALLS

The dental radiographer must be able to detect exposure and processing errors to prevent unnecessary patient exposure and wasted time. Use Table 12.4 as a guide to the many possible errors.

Labeling and Film Mounting

Mounted radiographs should be labeled with the patients name, date of exposure, and radiographer. Film mounts are made of cardboard or plastic. Film mounts should be opaque to mask out excess light when the films are viewed.

Table 12-A

Exposure and Processing Pitfalls

Problem	Exposure error	Processing error	Appropriate corrections
Light image	Short exposure time Low kVp Low mA Long TFD Too much filtration Film in backwards	Short processing time Low processing temperature Exhausted processing chemistry	Always check exposure factors before exposing film. Daily quality assurance procedures should minimize the number of thin images caused by inadequate processing.
Distinct pattern on a light image (Figure 12.7, A)	Film packet exposed on wrong side		Appearance of a herringbone, tire track, orange peel, or other embossed pattern across half the film indicates that the film was loaded on the wrong side; always position the lead backing so that the radiation traverses the film *first*.
Dark image	Long exposure time High kVp High mA Short TFD Use of faster film Double exposure	Long processing time High processing temperature Light leaks	Be sure to use the correct target to film distance (TFD). Don't leave the film in the developer too long. When processing film at high temperatures, adjust the developing time accordingly.
Partial image (Figure 12.7, B)	Incorrect film placement Poor position-indicating device (PID) alignment Poor cone-film alignment	Incomplete immersion in processing solutions	Attention to detail is a must; poor PID film alignment (cone cuts) is a common error for the novice and even happens to the experienced radiographer.
Distorted image (Elongation and foreshortening)	Incorrect film placement Bad PID alignment	Excessive bending of film	Double-checking film placement and PID alignment will minimize image distortion.
Brown image		Exhausted developer Insufficient washing	Use developing agents properly and replace them promptly when they become weak.
Green image		Exhausted fixer Possible uneven developing because film is stuck together	Use developing agents properly and replace them promptly when they become weak.
Gray image		White light or safelight leak Inadequate processing Inadequate film washing time	Follow timing guidelines and periodically inspect equipment.
Dark spots (Figure 12.7, C)	Static electricity	Film splashed with developer before processing Dirty rollers (automatic processor) Localized light leak Powder from rubber gloves	Practice safe handling of all items used in the radiographic process and ensure proper servicing, repair, and replacement of automatic processing equipment.
Black lines (Figure 12.7, D and E)	Discharge of static electricity when handling film Creased film	Dripping of fixer on film	Static electricity is more common in the winter months, and wearing rubber gloves for processing the film can aggravate the problem. Rubber gloves are recommended for the processing procedure, but static discharge can be reduced by touching a fabric softener sheet.
Stained images (Figure 12.7, F)	Soaking of film in disinfectant Fluoride in patient's mouth	Localized light leak Chemical splash	Use Polysoft packet and expose the radiographs before applying fluoride.

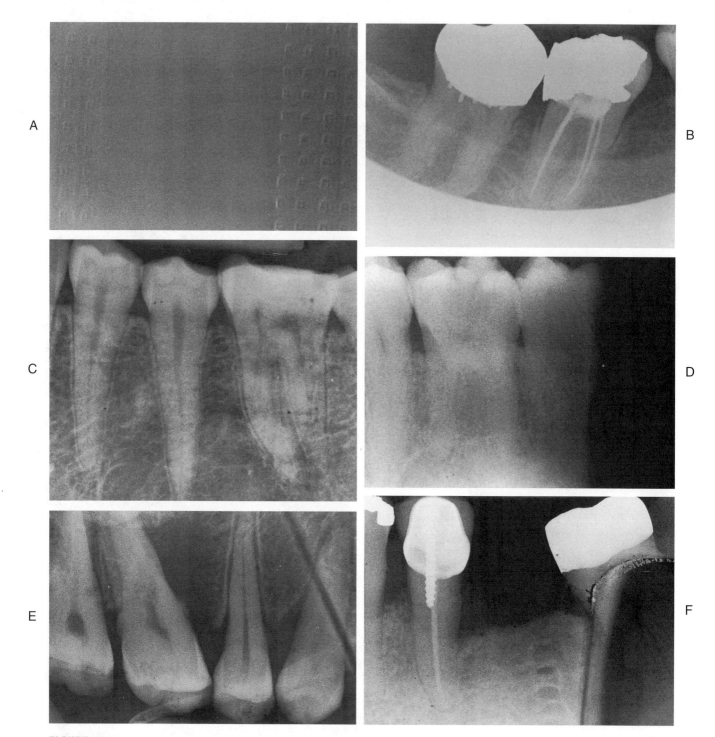

FIGURE 12.7

Exposure and processing pitfalls. **A,** Distinct pattern on a light image. This radiograph was exposed with the back of the packet toward the source of radiation. The fine print on the back of the film packet was embossed with "opposite side toward tube." Two sets of square patterns are visible at the lateral edges of the film. When the film is exposed backward in the patient's mouth, the resultant image displays this pattern and has low density and contrast. **B,** Partial image. Associated with round collimation. Note that the apical regions of all teeth have been cut off. Partial images also can result from incomplete immersion of the film in the processing solutions. **C,** Dark spots. An automatic processor with dirty rollers caused the dark spots on this radiograph. Dark spots also can be caused by powder from rubber gloves and fixer splash. A discharge of static electricity can produce black spots, but these usually appear as black artifacts that look like trees with no leaves. **D,** Black lines. Opening of the exposed but unprocessed film in white light caused the thick black line on this radiograph. Other causes of black lines included a discharge of static electricity and dripping fixer. **E,** Diagonal lines. Creasing of the film causes the black diagonal line that traverses the maxillary first premolar; the black line is the result of disrupted emulsion. This artifact could result in a misdiagnosis, such as root fracture. **F,** Stained image. Overlapping of unexposed films in the processor caused the dark area that covers the apical region of the mandibular second molar. Black scratches can be seen at the periphery of the overlapped region. A fingerprint also can been seen in the region of overlap. Other causes of stained images are light and chemical fog and incomplete processing.

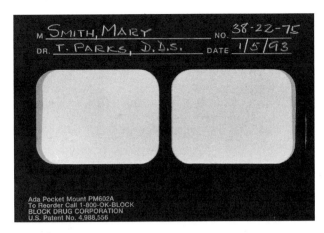

FIGURE 12.8

Labeled radiographic mount. The mount should always be labeled with the patient's name, chart number (if applicable), date, and operator's name.

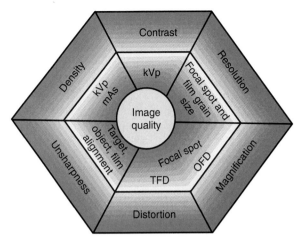

FIGURE 12.9

Visual and geometric factors that determine image quality.

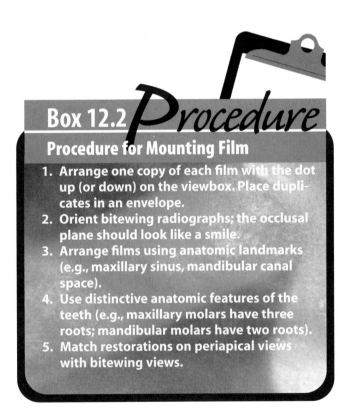

Box 12.2 *Procedure*

Procedure for Mounting Film

1. **Arrange one copy of each film with the dot up (or down) on the viewbox. Place duplicates in an envelope.**
2. **Orient bitewing radiographs; the occlusal plane should look like a smile.**
3. **Arrange films using anatomic landmarks (e.g., maxillary sinus, mandibular canal space).**
4. **Use distinctive anatomic features of the teeth (e.g., maxillary molars have three roots; mandibular molars have two roots).**
5. **Match restorations on periapical views with bitewing views.**

Each intraoral film has an embossed dot. Some practitioners prefer the dot to extend away from the front of the mount (a dimple) and others prefer the dot be oriented towards the operator (a pimple) (Figure 12.8). Everyone in the office should mount films in the same way to avoid confusion. If the dot is a pimple, the right side of the mount corresponds to the left side of the patient. If the dot is a dimple, the right side of the mount corresponds to the patient's right side (Box 12.2).

Film Duplication

With the increased need for multiple copies of radiographs, the properly equipped dental office should have a film duplicator. Duplication must be performed in the darkroom. The duplicating film that is coated with emulsion on only one side is sensitive to visible and ultraviolet light and would be ruined if not used under safe light conditions. Films to be duplicated need to be removed from their mounts, correctly oriented on a film organizer, and covered with duplicating film. The film duplicator is then closed carefully to not disturb the arranged films and activated. The duplicator emits ultraviolet light. Duplicating film responds oppositely from x-ray film. X-ray film becomes darker with increased exposure. Duplicating film becomes lighter with increased exposure. Once exposed, duplicating film should be processed and immediately labeled with the patient's name, date of exposure, and right and left orientation.

CHARACTERISTICS OF THE RADIOGRAPHIC IMAGE

Image quality is dependent upon several image characteristics. These characteristics can be separated into visual and geometric characteristics (Figure 12.9).

Density

Radiographic density is the degree of darkness or blackness of a radiograph. A film that is too dark (high density) or too light (low density) cannot be interpreted. Density can be manipulated by a variety of exposure and processing factors. (Processing factors will be discussed later in the chapter). Kilovoltage, milliamperage, target to film distance (TFD), and time all affect density.

Kilovoltage

Density increases with higher kilovoltage. An increase of 15 kilovolts will double the amount of radiation produced by the x-ray tube and produce an image twice as dark as the original image. To produce equivalent densities when kVp is increased by 15, time must be decreased by half.

For example, current exposure factors are 60 kVp and 1 s. In the equation below, figure out what exposure time should be used for 90 kVp technique while maintaining the same density. Remember that output and density doubles for every 15 kVp increase.

$$60 \text{ kVp} \rightarrow 75 \text{ kVp} \rightarrow 90 \text{kVp}$$
$$1 \text{ s} \rightarrow 0.5 \text{ s} \rightarrow 0.25 \text{ s}$$

Milliamperage and Time

An increase in time or mA will produce a denser film. With some x-ray units, mA and time can be manipulated separately. In units with fixed MA, only time can be manipulated. Often, time and mA are combined into a single unit called *mas* or *milliamperage* times time in seconds. The following formula will allow you to maintain density when manipulating either time or mA:

$$mAs\ 1 = mAS2$$

For example, current exposure factors are 10 mA and 0.6 s. You want to use a 15 mA technique. Figure out what exposure time should be used to maintain the same density.

$$mAs1 = mAs2$$
$$10 \times 0.6 = 15 \times ?$$
$$6 = 15 \times ?$$
$$\frac{6}{15} = ?$$
$$\frac{2}{5} = 0.4 \text{ s} = ?$$
$$0.4 \text{ s} = \text{New time}$$

Target-Film Distance

The distance between the Tungsten target in the anode and the image receptor has been referred to by many names in the literature. TFD is the descriptor used in this text. Other terms include *focal spot to film distance* (FFD) and *source to film distance* (SFD). As the distance between the film and the target increases, the density of the processed radiograph decreases. Another way to describe this interaction is that density (or intensity) varies inversely with the square of the distance from the target to the film. Ms relationship is referred to as the *inverse square law*. The formula is as follows:

$$I \text{ (Intensity, Density)} = \frac{I}{(TFD)^2}$$

The formula is great if you are a physicist, but must be modified to be useful to the dental radiographer. Exposure time is the most easily manipulated variable and is included in the equation that follows:

$$\frac{t_1}{(TFD_1)2} = I = \frac{t_2}{(TFD_2)2}$$

$$t_1 = \text{Old exposure time}$$
$$t_2 = \text{New exposure time}$$
$$TFD_1 = \text{Old TFD}$$
$$TFD_2 = \text{New TFD}$$

For example, current exposure factors are 8 inches TFD and 0.5 s. Your office is converting to a 16 inch TFD to maintain density. Figure out what the new exposure time will be.

$$\frac{t_1}{(TFD_1)^2} = I = \frac{t_2}{(TFD_2)^2} \qquad \frac{0.5 \text{ s}}{(8'')^2} = \frac{?s}{(16'')^2}$$

$$\frac{0.5s}{64} = \frac{?}{256} \qquad \frac{256 \times 0.5}{64} = ? \qquad \frac{128}{64} = \frac{2}{1} = 2s$$

For a short cut, 16 inches is double 8 inches. You can substitute 1 for 8 inches TFD and 2 for 16 inches TFD.

$$\frac{0.5}{(1)^2} = \frac{?}{(2)^2} \qquad 0.5 = \frac{?}{4} \qquad 4(0.5) = 2 = ?$$

Radiographic Contrast

Contrast is defined as the difference in densities viewed on a radiograph. Contrast on radiographic images allows the viewer to detect changes in bone, tooth structure, and sometimes soft tissue. Radiographic contrast is the product of subject and film contrast. Subject contrast is determined by the density, thickness, and atomic weight of the elements that make up the subject. To manipulate subject contrast, kilovoltage has to be varied. kV is the only exposure factor that directly affects contrast. A low kV technique produces high contrast. High contrast images are predominately black and white with only a few intermediate shapes of gray. High contrast images can be described as displaying a short scale of contrast. Conversely, a high kV technique produces low contrast. Low contrast images display a wide range of grays and is also called *long scale contrast*.

High contrast images are useful for detecting dental caries. Low contrast images are used for monitoring periodontal disease.

Contrast

The difference in densities as visualized on a radiograph. High-contrast (short scale) images are produced using low kVp techniques (60 to 70 kVp). Low-contrast (long scale) images are produced using high kVp techniques (90 to 120 kVp).

Film Contrast

Film contrast is determined by the film type and film processing. The film type is selected by operator preference and is more of a factor with extraoral techniques. See p 278-280 for processing information.

Resolution

Resolution is the ability to detect small objects that are very close together. *Detail* is another name for resolution. Film detail depends on the size of the focal spot, proper image geometry, and radiographic contrast. Resolution is enhanced by use of a small effective focal spot. Most dental x-ray units are manufactured with a fixed focal spot size, and medical x-ray generators often employ a variable focal spot size. Adequate radiographic contrast is essential for the operator to be able to differentiate between objects that are close together. Image geometry will be discussed in the next section.

GEOMETRIC CHARACTERISTICS

Image unsharpness, distortion, and magnification are geographic characteristics that influence image quality. The effects of these factors can be demonstrated using the principles of shadow casting.

Image Unsharpness

Image unsharpness is inherent in dental radiography because a radiograph is a two-dimensional representation of a three-dimensional structure. Unsharpness can result from image geometry, patient or film movement, or a large penumbra or secondary shadow. Secondary shadow is the fuzzy indistinct portion of the shadow beyond the primary shadow or umbra. Penumbra is produced by using a short TFD or a large object film distance (OFD).

Image Distortion

Distortion is an alteration of the true shape of an object as visualized on a radiograph. For example, the way people appear in a hall of mirrors in an amusement park is not a true image. Distortion is the product of misalignment of the central ray, film, and long axis of the tooth. The two most common forms of distortion are foreshortening and elongation. They occur with the use of the bisecting angle technique. An image is foreshortened when the object appears shorter on the radiograph than the actual object, and foreshortening is produced when the central ray is directed perpendicular to the film rather than the bisector (Figure 12.10, *A*). The recorded object appears to be longer than the true object when elongation is produced. Elongation occurs when the central ray is directed perpendicular to the long axis of the tooth rather than the bisector (Figure 12.10, *B*). The bisector is an imaginary angle that is calculated by dividing in half (bisecting) the angle created by the film and long axis of the tooth. Correct alignment of the film, tooth, and central ray will minimize image distortion.

Magnification

Magnification is the uniform enlargement of the recorded object and differs from distortion in that the recorded image is uniformly enlarged in magnification whereas the recorded image is selectively enlarged or shortened in image distortion. Magnification can be avoided by using a long TFD and a short OFD (Figure 12.9).

RADIATION BIOLOGY

Radiation biology is the study of the effects of radiation on living organisms. Radiation can adversely affect living tissues. Consequently the radiographer must understand these effects to be able to adequately weigh the risk versus benefits of using x-radiation. Ionizing radiation first exerts its effect at the molecular level. These changes are produced by the absorption of energy by the irradiated tissues. The two mechanisms that are recognized are direct and indirect effects.

Direct Effects

Direct effects are the product of a direct interaction between radiation and living tissue. Direct effects include disruption of molecular bonds by breaking or adding new bonds and destruction of molecules. Direct effects of radiation are less common than indirect effects.

Indirect Effects

Indirect effects occur as a result of radiation contacting water (H_2O) and oxygen (O_2) molecules. This interaction occurs more frequently than direct effects because living tissue is composed predominantly of water. Ionizing radiation and water and oxygen react to form free radicals such as hydrogen peroxide (H_2O_2) and hydroxyl radical (OH-). Free radicals in turn damage surrounding tissues by releasing oxygen or binding to hydrogen. The release of oxygen can disrupt cell and organelle membranes. Binding of free radicals to hydrogen can cause deformation of many important molecules that may inhibit the activity of these molecules.

Cellular Effects

Molecular changes in a biologic system lead to cellular changes. Cellular changes can manifest as somatic effects or genetic effects. A somatic effect can occur in all cell types with the exception of reproductive cells. Somatic effects include destruction of organelles and cell membranes and alteration of cellular proteins. Somatic effects ultimately result

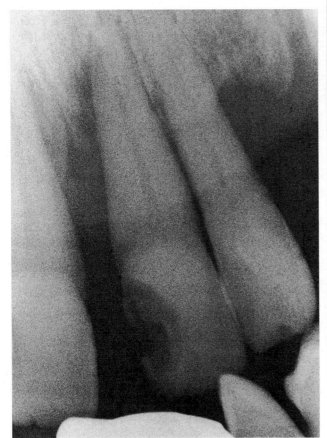

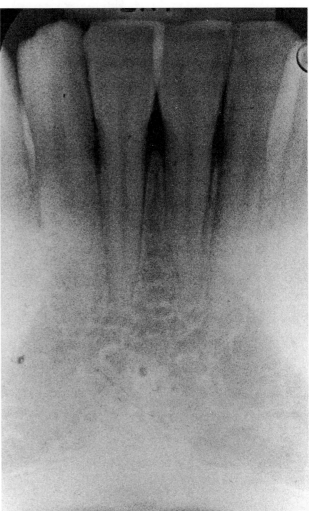

A

B

FIGURE 12.10

Image distortion. **A,** Elongation. Anatomically, these anterior teeth extend beyond the border of the radiograph; that is, the image of the teeth is longer than the actual teeth. **B,** Foreshortening. The image of the teeth is shorter than the actual teeth. Another anatomic landmark that suggests that the object has been shortened on the recorded image is the presence of the inferior border of the mandible.

in cell death. If enough cells die, the tissue and sometimes even the patient can die.

Genetic effects occur in reproductive cells (sperm cells and ova). These effects are produced when radiation damages genetic material such as deoxyribonucleic acid (DNA). In most situations, the damage can be repaired. Unrepaired damage to DNA can generate mutations, which are changes that are passed on to future cell generations and potentially to offspring.

Radiosensitivity

Some tissues are more sensitive to radiation effects than other tissues. Tissues made up of cells with a high rate of cell division or a low degree of differentiation are more ra-

diosensitive. The Law of Bergonié and Tribondeau states this relationship. Radiosensitivity is directly proportional to the mitotic rate and inversely proportional to the degree of differentiation of a particular cell type.

$$\text{Radiosensitivity} = \frac{\text{Mitotic rate}}{\text{Degree of differentiation}}$$

An important exception to this generalization is the small lymphocyte. The small lymphocyte displays a high degree of differentiation and undergoes no cell division once it matures. The small lymphocyte exhibits the highest radiosensitivity of human cells. Other tissues and cells that are highly radiosensitive are reproductive cells, bone marrow and lining mucosa of the gastrointestinal and genitourinary tract. Tissues such as

Relative Radiosensitivity of Human Tissues

Highly radiosensitive

Small lymphocytes
Gonadal tissues
Bone marrow

Moderately radiosensitive

Oral and other gastrointestinal mucosa
Skin
Salivary glands
Small blood vessels

Radioresistant

Muscle
Mature cartilage and bone
Nerve
Brain

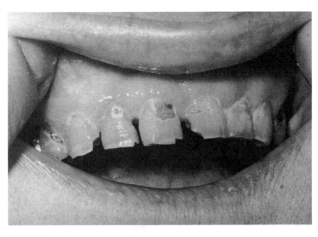

FIGURE 12.11

Radiation caries. The distinctive pattern of hard-tissue destruction is apparent in the oral cavity of this patient who underwent therapeutic irradiation of the head and neck. (Courtesy Department of Dental Diagnostic Sciences, Indiana University School of Dentistry.)

muscle, nerve, and mature bone and cartilage are not sensitive to radiation and are said to be radioresistant. Box 12.3 catalogs the radiosensitivity of representative human tissues.

Radiosensitivity is not always bad. Certain tumors are highly radiosensitive and treated with high doses of ionizing radiation. The treatment regimen for many head and neck cancers (for example, squamous cell carcinoma, nasopharyngeal carcinoma) includes therapeutic radiation.

COMPLICATIONS OF THERAPEUTIC HEAD AND NECK IRRADIATION

Although radiation helps to destroy the tumor, it also damages oral mucosa, blood supply of the bone, taste buds, and salivary gland tissue. Oral mucosa becomes inflamed during radiation therapy of the head and neck and may ulcerate or even slough. Inflammation of oral mucosa is called *oral mucositis*. Oral mucositis is very painful and hard to treat. Luckily it resolves after radiation therapy is completed.

Destruction of the blood supply to the bone by radiation decreases the amount of oxygen and nutrients that reach the bone. Irradiated bone is likely to become infected if traumatized. Pieces of the bone then die and may slough, called *osteoradionecrosis*. Osteo means bone; radio indicates radiation; and necrosis means death. Osteoradionecrosis is exceedingly difficult to treat. Treatment is usually protracted, and cures are rare.

Taste alterations often occur during the course of radiation therapy, which are difficult to manage. In many instances, patients will not like the way their favorite food tastes and may like foods they used not to like. These changes in taste perception usually disappear within 2 to 4 months after completion of radiation therapy.

Salivary glands are also affected by radiation. Salivary flow decreases significantly through the course of radiation therapy and may never return to normal levels. Lack of saliva produces dry mouth or xerostomia. Xerostomia can lead to the development of radiation caries. This is a misnomer because the radiation does not affect the tooth but rather the oral fluids that help to keep the tooth surface clean. The distribution of these carious lesions is quite distinctive (Figure 12.11).

Although radiation is used to treat some cancers, it can also cause cancer. The thyroid gland, breast, and bone marrow are susceptible to radiation-induced cancers. Spindle cell carcinoma is much more likely to occur in a site that has been previously irradiated for the treatment of squamous cell carcinoma.

Effects of Total Body Irradiation

The effects of total body irradiation are determined by dose and dose rate. For example, the $LD_{50/30}$ (lethal dose for 50% of a population 30 days after radiation exposure) is $4^{1}/_{2}$ to 6 Grays in a single exposure, and the total dose in a 6-week fractionated course of radiation therapy can exceed 75 Grays.

The time between exposure to radiation and manifestation of effects is called the *latent period*. The latent period can range from hours to years depending on the dose. The length of the latent period is inversely proportional to the dose; the higher the dose, the shorter the latent period.

Table 12.5

Units of Radiation Measurement

Parameter	Traditional units	S.I.	Conversion
Exposure	Roentgen (R)	Couloumb/kilogram (C/kg)	$1R = 2.58 \times 10 - 4$ (C/kg)
Absorbed dose	Rad	Gray (Gy)	1 rad = 0.01 Gy
Dose equivalence	Rem	Sievert (Sv)	1 rem = 0.01 Sv

Another important concept of radiation biology is that the effects of radiation exposure are cumulative. This does not mean that radiation remains in the body after exposure. It simply means that as the number of radiation exposures increases, so does the amount of damage, albeit nonlinearly. The human body is efficient at repairing radiation damage. However, the body can not be returned to its preirradiation condition. A simplified example is that for every exposure to radiation, 100 cells are damaged and 99 of them are repaired. Obviously if the body is repeatedly exposed to radiation, the damage induced by radiation adds up. Ultimately, failure of a tissue (for example, the lens of the eye) or induction of a cancer (for example, salivary gland tumor or leukemia) can result.

No direct methods of determining the effects of small effects of radiation on humans exist. Therefore any amount of radiation is potentially damaging and must be analyzed when deciding if the benefit of exposing the patient to radiation (sometimes called *diagnostic yield*) outweighs the risk. The purpose of this statement is not to needlessly frighten anyone, but rather to illustrate the point that unnecessary radiographs place the patient at an unacceptable radiation risk.

Radiation Measurements

Radiation is measured in several different units (Table 12.5). Currently, the United States is the only country in which the older traditional units for radiation measurement are still occasionally used. Therefore traditional and Systeme Internationale (SI) units will be presented in this chapter.

Exposure

Exposure is measured in coulombs per kilogram (c/kg) or Roentgens (R). A coulomb/kilogram is equivalent to 3880 Roentgens. Exposure tells how much radiation the patient has been exposed to. Dose tells the amount of radiation absorbed by the patient.

Dose

Dose is measured in Grays (Gy) or radiation absorbed dose (rads). Rads or Grays measure the amount of energy transferred to the patient. One rad equals 0.01 Grays or one centigray. Conversely, one Gray equals 100 rads.

Dose Equivalence

Dose equivalence allows comparison of various types of radiation with x-radiation. Dose equivalence is measured in Sieverts (Sv) or Roentgen Equivalent Man (rems). One Sievert equals 100 rems. For the purpose of dental radiography, the practitioner can assume that 1 R = 1 rad = 1 rem or 1 Gy = 1 Sv. This generalization would not be valid if different forms of radiation were being used or if animals other than humans were being exposed to radiation.

Background Radiation

Although a lot of time has been spent presenting the effects of diagnostic and therapeutic radiation, the contribution of background radiation can not be ignored. Background radiation comes from naturally occurring sources such as cosmic radiation and radioactive elements (Radon gas, Uranium) and from fallout from nuclear testing and radioactive waste. The average yearly dose from natural background radiation (in the United States) is approximately 3 milli-Sieverts or 300 millirems (BEIR V). Any radiographic procedure adds to the amount of radiation absorbed by the patient. Because the amount of background radiation can not be altered, the radiographer is responsible for minimizing the amount of radiation the patient is subjected to during radiographic procedures. The radiographer and others in the office must also be protected from exposure to ionizing radiation. The principles and methods for radiation protection are discussed in the following section.

Table 12.6

Criteria for Selection of Patient Radiographs

Patient type	Child (Primary/mixed dentition; transitional)	Patient type (Before eruption of third molar)	Adult
New patient			
Inspection for dental disease and assessment of growth and development	*Primary:* Bitewing views (BWs) if proximals are closed *Mixed:* BWs and selected periapical views (PAs), or panoramic views and BWs	BWs and selected PAs or full mouth series (FMS), depending on disease state and treatment history	*Dentulous:* BWs or selected PAs, or FMS, depending on disease state and treatment history *Edentulous:* FMS or panoramic survey
Recalled patient			
Clinical caries or high risk of caries	BWs at 6-month intervals until no caries are seen	BWs at 6- to 12-month intervals until no caries are present	BWs at 12- to 18-month intervals
No clinical caries or low risk of caries	BWs at 12- to 24-month intervals	BWs at 18- to 36-month intervals	BWs at 24- to 36-month intervals
Periodontal diseas			
Clinical signs or history of disease	Horizontal or vertical BWs or selected PAs (or both)		
Growth and development			
	Mixed: Selected PAs or panoramic survey	PAs or panoramic survey to assess development of third molar	

Modified from Williamson GF: *Radiographic assessment* In Woodall IR: *Comprehensive dental hygiene care,* ed 4, St Louis, 1993, Mosby.

RADIATION SAFETY

The dental radiographer is responsible for limiting radiation exposure to the patient and eliminating exposure to all office personnel (including the radiographer). Many options exist to minimize radiation exposure, making the process sometimes overwhelming. The development of a philosophy regarding radiation safety is often helpful. The ALARA (as low as reasonably achievable) principle is an excellent basis for developing a radiation safety philosophy. In other words, the amount of radiation exposure to the patient and dental office personnel should be as low as reasonably achievable.

Selection Criteria

The best way to minimize patient exposure to x-radiation is to avoid exposing unnecessary radiographs. Radiographs should be exposed only for the purpose of diagnosis. Administrative radiographs are unnecessary and unacceptable. The use of a film duplicator or double film packets will eliminate the need to expose multiple copies of the same radi-

ographic image. Selection criteria have been developed that assist the clinician in deciding the number of films and time span between radiographic examinations. Some selection criteria allow the clinician to individualize radiographic examinations by using patient history, the current oral condition, and past dental treatment as determinants. Judicious use of selection criteria can reduce the radiation dose to the patient by 100% simply by not exposing unnecessary radiographs (Table 12.6).

Reducing Patient Exposure

When exposure of radiographs is indicated, the radiation exposure to the patient can be reduced in several ways.

Film Speed

Use of E-speed film instead of D-speed film effectively reduces patient exposure by 40% to 50%. This dose reduction has been well documented; unfortunately, the majority of dental practitioners still use D-speed film. One of the reasons that D-speed film is more popular than E-speed film is that D-speed film is less sensitive to technique and processing errors. In addition to being twice as sensitive to x-radiation, E-speed film is also twice as sensitive to exposure and processing errors when compared with D-speed film. Unless proper technique and processing is performed, the image on E-speed film will be of poorer quality than that of D-speed film. The use of E-speed film mandates proper exposure factors, safelighting, processing, and rigorous quality assurance.

Collimation

Two types of collimation can be used when exposing radiographic film: round and rectangular. Patient dose can be reduced by 50% or more by implementing rectangular collimation. Use of rectangular collimation can actually improve the image quality of E-speed film by decreasing the amount or scattered radiation that degrades film quality. Unfortunately, even fewer dental practitioners use rectangular coll-imation techniques than use E-speed film despite the recommendations of the ADA. Several methods occur in which rectangular collimation can be achieved. The rectangular position indicating device (PID) is the most efficient method for implementing rectangular collimation technique. The Rinn Snap-on collimator is attached to the positioning ring of extension Cone Paralleling (XCP) instruments. Rectangular collimation is incorporated into Precision Instruments. Use of rectangular collimation is technically more demanding than round collimation. However, mastery of rectangular collimation techniques is easily achieved after some practice.

Target to Film Distance

A long TFD reduces patient exposure by decreasing the spread of the x-ray beam. The long TFD (14 to 16 inches) is used in the paralleling technique. The paralleling technique additionally reduces exposure to the thyroid gland when compared with the bisecting angle technique.

Kilovolt Peak

High kVp techniques produce a more energetic beam, consequently, fewer low energy photons are generated. Low energy photons are usually absorbed by the patient and have no effect on the resultant image.

Filtration

Filtration selectively removes low energy photons from the x-ray beam. As with use of high kVp techniques, removal of low-energy photons reduces the amount of x-radiation absorbed by the patient. Aluminum is the most common filter material. At least 2.5 mm of aluminum equivalence is required for techniques using kVp between 70 and 90 kilovolts. Besides aluminum, other materials are being investigated with regard to their beam filtering efficiency (for example, Copper, Niobium, and Gadolinium). Box 12.4 displays various dose reduction methods.

Box 12.4

Factors That Help Reduce Patient Radiation Dose

Proper selection criteria
Fastest available radiographic film and screens
Rectangular collimation
Lead apron and thyroid collar
High kVp technique
Adequate filtration
Proper film placement to reduce the number of retakes
Quality assurance procedures in processing
Electronic imaging devices

Patient Shielding

The patient must be covered with a lead apron and thyroid collar for all intraoral and most extraoral dental radiographic examinations. The thyroid collar should not be used for panoramic radiography because it would obscure several important structures. The lead apron virtually eliminates radiation exposure to the gonads, breast, and bone marrow of the sternum, which are three highly radiosensitive tissues. As the name implies, the thyroid collar shields the thyroid gland from radiation exposure. The thyroid collar must be snugly fitted to be effective (Figure 12.12).

Retakes

If a radiograph must be repeated, the exposure to the patient is doubled. Proper film placement, beam alignment, and patient monitoring during exposure will decrease the number of retakes. Occasional retakes are unavoidable because of patient anatomy and management. However, most retakes are caused by poor technique. Keep a record of retakes in the dental office and review the retake log periodically to help identify consistent errors and allow the operators to correct their technique.

Darkroom Procedures

A perfectly placed and exposed radiograph will still need to be repeated if it is not properly processed. Poor processing techniques account for the majority of radiographs that need to be repeated. The darkroom must be "white light tight" and the safelights of correct wattage must be properly placed. The processing chemistry must be monitored continuously to produce radiographs of high quality on a consistent basis. Poor processing can result in an unnecessary retake or a missed diagnosis, neither of which are acceptable.

Radiation Protection for the Operator

A great deal of this section has been devoted to protecting the patient from the effects of ionizing radiation. A radiog-

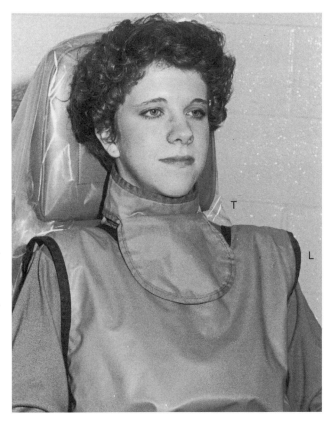

FIGURE 12.12

This patient has been draped with a thyroid collar *(T)* and a lead apron *(L)*.

rapher is potentially exposed to ionizing radiation on a daily basis. The following three principles of radiation protection should guide the radiographic procedures of the office:

1 Time
2 Distance
3 Shielding

Time

Clearly you want to limit the time you are exposed to radiation. Use of the shortest exposure time possible (while still maintaining film quality) is desirable from the patient's and operator's point of view.

Distance

The operator should be at least 6 feet away from the source of x-radiation at the time of exposure. Under no circumstances should you hold the film or the tube head during exposure. If the film (or the patient) needs to be stabilized, let the parent or other adult family member assist with the exposure. Be sure to provide the helper with protective shielding. If the tube head is not stable, the unit should not be used until it is repaired.

Shielding

Shielding is the placement of a radiodense material between the source of radiation and all other people in the dental office. The workload, maximum kVp, location, and proximity to others within the office determine the amount of shielding. For example, shielding should be incorporated into the walls separating the front office and the reception area if the walls are shared with operators equipped with an x-ray generator. Shielding is measured in lead equivalence. Cinder block and dry wall are effective materials for shielding if they are of sufficient thickness. Plywood or thin paneling are not effective shielding materials.

Radiation Monitoring

The goal of radiation safety is to eliminate operator exposure to ionizing radiation. Wearing monitoring devices is an effective way of determining if the operator has been exposed to ionizing radiation in the office. Several types of devices are available. The film badge is the least expensive personal radiation monitoring device. It contains a special type of film sandwiched between small blocks of different types of metal. At monthly intervals, the company processes the film and a report of any exposure is returned to the dental office. The film badge is only effective if it is worn at work. Other radiation monitoring devices use thermoluminescent dosimeters (TLDs) or ionization chambers. These types of devices are more sensitive to radiation exposure but are more expensive.

Radiation Exposure

Maximum occupational exposure values have been set and enacted by OSHA. The maximum permissible dose (MPD) is 0.05 Sv per year. The lifetime permissible dose is calculated using the following formula:

$$\text{Lifetime MPD} = 0.05 \text{ Sv (N- 18)}$$

N indicates the operator's age in years. The current ICRP recommendation is for an MPD limit of 0.02 Sv (N- 18).

From these equations one can determine that operators should be at least 18 years old. For operators under 18 years of age, the MPD has been set to be 0.001 Sv, assuming the individual is in a supervised educational program. The MPD for the operator who is pregnant is 0.005 Sv for the entire pregnancy.

Remember that the effects of radiation are cumulative. Do not feel secure because you cannot see or feel the effects of radiation at the time you are exposed. Further information pertaining to radiation safety and protection can be found in publication no. 35 of the National Commission on Radiation Protection (and Measurement) (NCRP).

The information contained in this chapter has provided an overview of image production, processing, and characteristics and radiation biology and safety. This chapter is by no means all you need to know about dental radiography. Rather, it should be viewed as a framework on which to build a more complete understanding of **radiology** and radiography and to prepare you to take the next step of exposing radiographs on a live patient.

Radiology

The branch of health sciences that deals with the diagnostic and therapeutic uses of radiation.

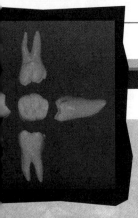

Points for Review

- The definitions of the terms *radiography, radiology, electromagnetic radiation, x-radiation,* and *photon*
- The way in which x-radiation is produced, beginning with turning on the x-ray generator
- The process by which the latent image is produced and converted to a visible image
- The definitions of the terms *exposure time, kVp, mA, film speed, TFD image processing,* and the ways in which these parameters relate to image density and contrast
- The component parts of an intraoral x-ray film packet and an extraoral film cassette
- The difference between Bremsstrahlung and characteristic radiation
- The cause of and remedy for major film exposure and processing errors
- The direct and indirect effects of radiation on living tissue
- The effects of therapeutic radiation on oral structures and the reasons tissues such as teeth and mucosa are differentially affected by radiation
- The maximum permissible dose (MPD)
- The as low as reasonably achievable (ALARA) principle
- The use of selection criteria to reduce patient exposure to radiation

Self-Study Questions

1. What are the type and frequency of a radiographic series determined by?
   a. Selection criteria
   b. Insurance benefits
   c. Patient's age
   d. None of the above
2. Which of the following is *not* considered an image receptor?
   a. Direct exposure film
   b. Panoramic film
   c. CCD
   d. Computer screen

3. What is the consequence of incorrect horizontal angulation?
   a. Elongation of the teeth in the image
   b. Foreshortening of the teeth in the image
   c. Overlapping of the teeth in the image
   d. Magnification of the teeth in the image
4. What is the effect of the increased target-receptor distance used in the paralleling technique?
   a. It prevents overlap
   b. It minimizes shadows
   c. It compensates for increased object-receptor distance
   d. It increases image density
5. Why is a radiographic examination not needed for edentulous patients?
   a. They have no teeth
   b. They cannot stabilize a film holder
   c. Insurance will not pay for the examination
   d. Edentulous patients should receive a radiographic examination
6. Radiolucent structures have which property or properties?
   (1) They absorb most of the x-ray beam
   (2) They absorb little or none of the x-ray beam
   (3) They appear light or white on the film image
   (4) They appear dark or black on the film image
   a. 1, 3
   b. 2, 4
   c. 2
   d. 3
   e. All of the above
7. Radiopaque structures have which property or properties?
   (1) They absorb most of the x-ray beam
   (2) They absorb little or none of the x-ray beam
   (3) They appear light or white on the film image
   (4) They appear dark or black on the film image
   a. 1, 3
   b. 2, 4
   c. 2
   d. 3
   e. All of the above
8. What is the force called that is needed to remove an electron from its shell?
   a. Ionizing
   b. Electromagnetic
   c. Binding energy

d. X-radiation

9. What X-ray equipment contains a cathode and an anode within a vacuum?
   a. Tube head
   b. Coolidge tube
   c. Control arm
   d. Collimator

10. What material is most commonly used as a filter in dental radiography?
   a. Aluminum
   b. Potassium bromide
   c. Silver halide
   d. Silver

Suggested Readings

Barr JH, Stephens RG: *Dental radiology: pertinent basic concepts and their applications in clinical practice,* Philadelphia, 1980, WB Saunders.

Bushong S: *Radiologic science for technologists,* ed 6, St Louis, 1997, Mosby.

Frommer HH: *Radiology for dental auxiliaries,* ed 5, St Louis, Mosby (in press).

Council on dental materials, instruments, and equipment: Recommendations in radiographic practice: an update, *J ADA* 1989: 115-117, 1988.

Miles DA et al: *Radiographic imaging for dental auxiliaries,* ed 3, Philadelphia, 1999, WB Saunders.

Recommendations in radiographic practices: an update: 1988, *J Am Dent Assoc* 118:115-117, 1989.

White SC: *Oral radiology: principles and interpretation,* St Louis, 1999, Mosby.

Wuehrmann AH, Manson-Hing LR: *Dental radiology,* ed 5, St Louis, 1981, Mosby.

*O*ral and *Maxillofacial Radiography*

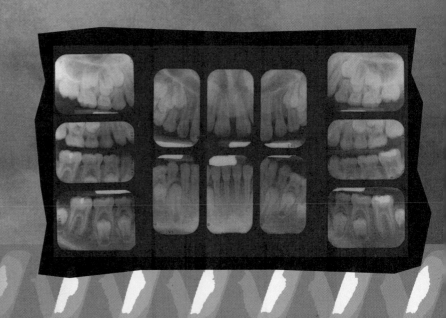

Chapter Outline

Producing Acceptable Dental Radiographs
   The purpose and content of radiographs
Professional Responsibility
Contemporary Equipment and Techniques
   Bisecting angle
   Paralleling technique
   Holding devices
Radiographic Surveys
   Extraoral techniques
   Radiographic needs of children

Radiology for the edentulous patient
Endodontic radiography
Asepsis in Dental Radiography
Patient Procedures
   Bisecting angle technique
   Periapical examination
   Paralleling technique
   Bitewing projections
   Radiographic anatomy
   Mounting radiographs

Learning Objectives

On completion of Chapter 13, the student should be able to do the following:

◼ Define key terms.

◼ List the criteria for selecting radiographs.

◼ Describe the uses of panoramic, cephalometric, tomographic, and direct digital imaging.

◼ List the basic steps needed to expose a full mouth survey of radiographs using the paralleling technique.

◼ List the methods used to modify imaging for pediatric, endodontic, and edentulous patients.

◼ Identify the anatomic landmarks seen in a full mouth series of dental radiographs.

◼ Correctly mount dental radiographs.

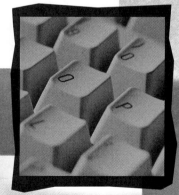

Key Terms

PRODUCING ACCEPTABLE DENTAL RADIOGRAPHS

With a basic understanding of the principles of x-ray photon production, radiation safety, and exposure factors, it is essential to learn how to produce acceptable dental radiographs. Gaining skill in dental radiography involves not only mastery of technique but also problem solving and patient management skills.

The Purpose and Content of Radiographs

Radiographs (x-rays) provide vital diagnostic information to be used when formulating the future treatment of the dental patient. When produced in an accurate and safe manner, radiographs enable the dentist to examine underlying, surrounding, and supporting structures of the head and neck while not significantly adding to health risks to the patient. (In other words, the benefits derived from the radiographs outweigh the risks of radiation exposure.) Many times these structures are not visible in the clinical examination. Therefore a complete diagnosis is not possible without use of radiographs.

However, x-rays are not without risk, and every precaution must be taken by the dental professional to reduce radiation exposure to the patient. Using the least amount of exposure possible should be the rule for diagnostic radiography.

ALARA principle

The philosophy that radiation exposure to the patient must be As Low As Reasonably Achievable.

This philosophy is summarized in the **ALARA principle**: the radiation exposure to the patient must be *As Low As Reasonably Achievable*. The benefits as well as the potential dangers of x-radiation should be clearly discussed with the patient. Demonstrating concern for the patient's health in this manner will assist in establishing rapport with the patient. The patient needs to know that the safest techniques and equipment available are used.

If, after a thorough explanation of the procedure, the patient chooses not to have radiographs, a refusal of consent should be signed by the patient and dentist. This refusal of consent should state that the dentist will be unable to render a complete diagnosis, and consequently, is unable to deliver proper treatment. Although the patient accepts the responsibility for refusal of radiographs, the standard of care is compromised and the dentist may be the target of possible legal action. One of the more common reasons for litigation in dentistry is "failure to diagnose." For this reason the importance of a complete dental data base (including radiographs) cannot be understated.

Many patients refuse radiographs because of the cost. They feel the costs are increased for administrative reasons rather than for appropriate dental care. Another frequent concern is recent exposure to x-radiation for medical purposes. Dental assistants must take the opportunity to educate the patient regarding the critical need for radiographs. For example, if patients have received radiation to the head and neck for the treatment of cancer, they are more susceptible to dental decay and periodontal disease. Consequently, they need radiographic examinations more frequently than the nonirradiated patient. The early treatment of dental conditions is critical to the overall health of these patients.

Radiographs provide information about the status of past dental conditions as well as present treatment needs. It is important to evaluate diseases such as periodontitis over long periods of time. This is one of the reasons radiographs are considered the property of the dentist. Radiographs should be preserved and archived to permit future review of ongoing conditions. The quality of an image is partially dependent on the processing. It is very difficult to compare today's image with a brown blob that used to be a radiographic image.

Government agencies and most dental insurance companies often request radiographs before authorizing payment for treatment. Occasionally, the patient requests that the original radiographs be sent to another dentist. Use of duplicate radiographs or duplicate copies should be kept as a part of the patient record in this instance. The patient should never be reexposed to x-radiation for administrative purposes. The original radiographs should never be given to the patient but forwarded to another health care provider.

As was stated earlier, radiographs are considered the property of the dentist. However, the information contained within the radiograph is the property of the patient. This is an important distinction, which often causes misunderstandings between the patient and office personnel if not adequately explained. The patient can not be denied access to the information contained in the radiograph. An office policy should be made by the dentist for third-party release. This policy must be adhered to at all times.

PROFESSIONAL RESPONSIBILITY

The dentist, who prescribes the necessary survey of radiographs, uses radiographic information combined with the clinical examination and the history to formulate a correct diagnosis. In prescribing radiographs, the dentist has a responsibility to the patient and operator to follow state and federal installation and maintenance radiation safety guidelines to provide safe and efficient radiographic equipment. The patient will then be exposed to the least amount of radiation for the dentist to provide the best dental treatment.

A panel of representatives from the Academy of General Dentistry, Academy of Dental Radiology, American Academy of Oral Medicine, American Academy of Pediatric

Dentistry, American Academy of Periodontology, and the American Dental Association under FDA sponsorship have developed recommendations for selection criteria of dental radiographic examinations. These criteria are displayed in Table 12.6. Many factors are considered and are based on individual patient history and clinical judgment. Patient selection criteria are guidelines for determination of the appropriate radiographic examinations. The dentist will give or imply the authority to expose, process, and mount the x-rays based on these guidelines. The auxiliary will carry out the prescription under the supervision of the dentist. The radiographic diagnosis is the responsibility of the dentist. The dental auxiliary does not have the authority to make a radiographic diagnosis.

Dental professionals must be thoroughly trained in the theory of x-ray production, radiation biology, hygiene, the safe use of radiographic equipment, and various techniques used to expose and process radiographs. Training of allied dental professionals in radiation safety procedures and quality control is also critical to proper patient care. Radiographs of diagnostic value are the result of education and practice of the above-mentioned skills. The use of good technique produces fewer mistakes and retakes. Anytime a radiograph is retaken, the radiation exposure to the patient is doubled for that particular view.

CONTEMPORARY EQUIPMENT AND TECHNIQUES

More powerful and accurate x-ray equipment is allowing the dentist to produce better radiographs with increased definition using less exposure. Faster film speeds, requiring less time, have also contributed to reduced exposures. Minimizing the size of the beam to reduce unnecessary radiation to the areas surrounding the area of interest was a primary concern in early dental radiography. This is easily achieved by collimating the beam to the dimensions of the image receptor. Minimizing distortion and magnification and showing true anatomic relationships and size was probably the second greatest concern of the early radiographer.

Bisecting angle

The concept of directing the central x-ray perpendicular to the line that equally divides the angle formed by the image receptor and the long axis of the tooth.

Bisecting Angle

The **bisecting angle**, or short-cone, technique was one of the earliest techniques used to expose dental radiographs. The concept of bisecting was derived by application of the rule of **isometry**. This theory, known as the Cieszynski's rule of

isometry, states that two triangles having equal angles and a common side are equal triangles. In practice the central ray is directed perpendicular to the line that bisects or equally divides the angle formed by the image receptor and the long axis of the tooth illustrates this relationship. The bisecting angle technique was originated by Dr. W.A. Price in 1904. Because of the distortion inherent in this technique, early dental radiographers continued to search for more simple and consistent techniques.

Isometry

Theory used in bisecting techniques recognizing that two triangles having equal angles and a common side are equal triangles.

Paralleling Technique

Franklin McCormack's development of the right angle, or **paralleling**, technique in 1920 was the initial means of solving many of the problems inherent in the bisecting angle technique. The right angle or paralleling technique was simplified by Drs. G.M. Fitzgerald and William J. Updegrave. Their refinement of this technique, film-positioning devices, and basic instructions are used in most of today's dental practices.

Parallel

Side by side or an equal distance apart.

The paralleling technique requires that the film be placed as parallel as possible to the long axis of the teeth. The central ray is then directed at right angles to the teeth and film. A film holding device is used to maintain the film packet in position and provide an extraoral guide for directing the source of radiation through the region of interest. The paralleling technique provides more consistent radiographic images and is easier to learn and implement than the bisecting angle technique.

Holding Devices

Several holding devices are used for paralleling and bisecting techniques. The "Snap-a-ray" (Figure 13.1) or "Eezee-grip" is one film-holding device that is used with the bisecting angle technique. Other aligning instruments were developed by Dr. William Updegrave. Dr. Updegrave's XCP, extension cone paralleling (XCP), and bisecting angle instruments (BAI) automatically indicate the correct horizontal and vertical angulation for the radiation source. Tubehead angulation settings are no longer necessary when using XCP and BA instruments. The angle of the bite block differs from 90 degrees with the XCP to 105 degrees for the BAI system. Usually a 16-inch target-receptor distance (TRD) is used with XCP and an 8-inch TRD with the BAI system. Both systems include bite blocks for anterior, posterior, and bitewing use. Disposable

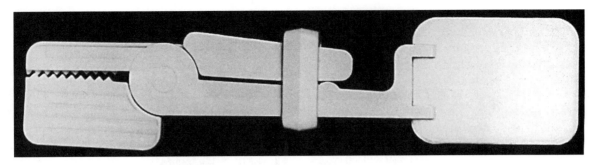

FIGURE 13.1

Snap-a-ray with size 2 film packet attached to anterior portion

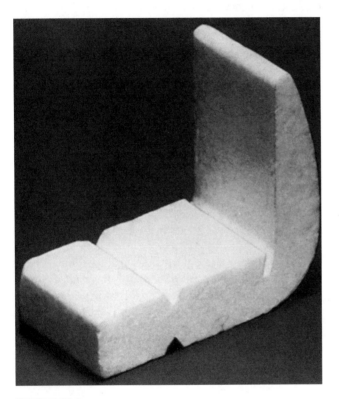

FIGURE 13.2

A styrofoam biteblock can be used for either bisecting angle or paralleling techniques.

bite blocks, made of styrofoam, are also available (Figure 13.2). In addition to the bite blocks, the systems include indicator rods and rings for correct alignment. Figure 13.3 displays the components of the XCP system.

RADIOGRAPHIC SURVEYS

The full mouth survey, or FMS, portrays the teeth and supporting structures with a minimum of 14 single films. These radiographs vary in size according to the individual patient's age, arch shape, range of mandibular motion, technique and holders used, and patient's tolerance.

The FMS usually includes bitewing radiographs for caries detection and evaluation of periodontal support. Periapicals, bitewings, and occlusal projections are taken with intraoral x-ray generators or machines. Occlusal techniques are discussed later in the chapter.

Extraoral Techniques
Panoramic Radiography

Panoramic radiography enables the dentist to see the entire dentition on a single film. The pedodontist and orthodontist use the panoramic projection to predict growth and dental eruption patterns. Oral and maxillofacial surgeons are dependent on the panoramic view for detection of jaw fractures, tumors, impactions, and foreign objects.

Panoramic radiograph

An x-ray that shows the entire dentition on a single film.

Although the ease of imaging is a distinct advantage, the panoramic radiograph has some disadvantages. The most important disadvantage is the loss of **resolution** or detail. Because of the use of intensifying screens for image capture, the resolution of a panoramic image is approximately 10 line pairs per millimeter (lp/mm) as compared with 20 lp/mm with direct exposure radiographic film. Additionally, if the patient is positioned incorrectly, the whole image must be remade.

Resolution

The ability to discern two objects that are very close together.

Tomography

Panoramic radiography is a form of **tomography**. Tomography is a radiographic technique in which a selected segment

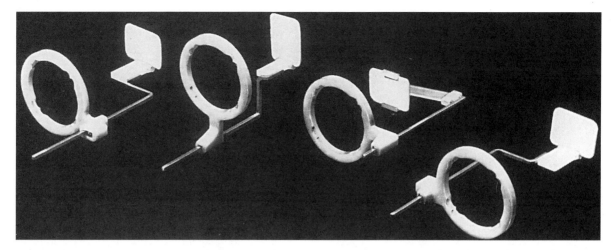

FIGURE 13.3

Extension cone paralleling instruments (XCP).

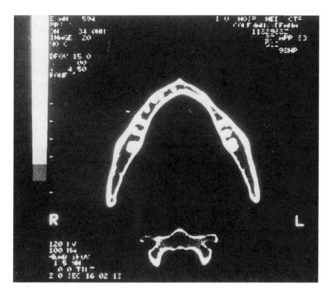

FIGURE 13.4

Computed tomography (CT) of a proposed mandibular implant site.

Tomography

Making an x-ray of a given plane by blurring out the images of other planes.

of the head and neck is imaged for detailed review. Simple tomography is used to evaluate the temporomandibular joint or proposed implant sites displays an image produced with computed tomography (CT) (Figure 13.4). The resolution with CT is measured in line pairs per centimeter rather than lp/mm.

The basic principle of tomography is that the image receptor and radiation source rotate about a fulcrum in opposite directions. Structures located at the fulcrum (or zone of focus) are imaged in focus; areas outside the zone are blurred. Several patterns of movement of the source and receptor exist. Generally, the more complex the movement of the source and receptor, the more in focus the structure appears.

Cephalometric Radiography

Cephalometric radiography is used by orthodontists, oral and maxillofacial surgeons, and prosthodontists to measure the bony structures, teeth, and soft tissues of the head and neck to determine the relationships among them. With the aid of computers, clinicians are able to view the progressive movement of the teeth and jaws and predict the probable result. Figure 13.5 shows an example of a lateral cephalometric projection.

Digital Subtraction

Dentists are utilizing the technique of digital subtraction radiography in the diagnosis and management of periodontal disease. Digital subtraction radiography is a technique in which changes in bone between two images are calculated using a computer. Using this technique, the amount of bone loss or gain can be determined. Figure 13.6 displays an image created using the digital subtraction technique. These images are flat, because only the changes between the radiographs should be evident. ("Flat" in this context means that the images have only a few shades of gray and are monotonous.)

Direct Digital Imaging

Direct digital imaging using a charge-coupled device (CCD) is the latest technologic advance utilizing radiographic

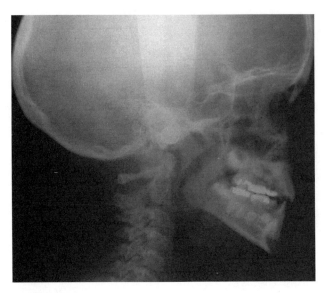

FIGURE 13.5

Lateral cephalometric projection is used to study bone-to-bone relationships and to identify growth patterns.

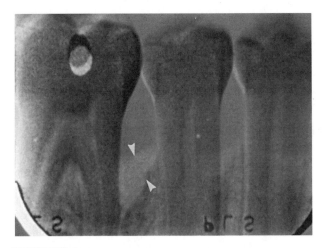

FIGURE 13.6

Digital subtraction radiography is the result of a computer comparing two radiographs taken 6 months apart. The light area (*arrows*) depicts new bone deposition after a periodontal surgical procedure called guided tissue regeneration.

techniques and further reduces exposure to the patient. The CCD is activated by radiation to produce a radiographic image that can be enhanced by computer means. Radiation exposure is significantly decreased with exposure times measured in hundredths of seconds. Density and contrast are enhanced by the manipulation of the gray scale. Because no film is exposed, processing time is saved. The image is displayed instantly on a video monitor and a hard copy is generated on heat sensitive paper. Computer storage of the

image is possible for long term storage. CCD imaging is popular for in-process treatment evaluation and time efficiency.

As computer programmers and dental researchers continue to study the diagnostic needs of practicing dentists and their desire to provide optimum care, developments for producing a more accurate diagnosis continue to evolve.

Radiographic Needs of Children

Education of parents is a prerequisite to proper treatment of the dental needs of children. Many parents are unaware of the importance of maintaining the primary dentition. The parent must be made aware of the important role the deciduous dentition plays in the development and maintenance of healthy permanent teeth. Prevention is key to the long-term health of the child's teeth. The use of radiography allows for evaluation of potential infections, caries, and orientation of the permanent dentition. Accurate treatment planning and eruption problems can be corrected early and therefore have less effect on the child.

Children are prone to develop dental caries. Systematic clinical and radiographic examination allows the dentist to identify early carious lesions and provide conservative treatment. Dental caries are only one indication for radiographs in children. Panoramic radiographs are used to identify developmental disturbances such as supernumerary teeth (extra teeth), anodontia (absence of teeth), and conditions such as amelogenesis imperfecta, the failure of the enamel to fully develop.

Radiation Safety for Children

Radiation safety is most important in children. Developing cells are most affected by radiation. The factors to be considered in how often a child should be exposed to x-radiation include the existing dental needs, previous radiographs, and arch size. The child's emotional state, attitude, and cooperation must also be considered.

The first radiographic survey is usually taken at 3 years of age. By the age of 3 the primary dentition is usually fully erupted. Patient selection criteria recommend that radiographs be ordered only for the benefit of the patient. Radiographs should be periodically exposed depending upon the caries experience, periodontal status, and dentofacial development of the child.

A lead apron and thyroid collar should be used every time radiation is in use. Because the bone density in children is much less than adults, the exposure time can usually be reduced by one third that of the recommended adult dosage.

Children are very curious and should be given a full explanation during each appointment when radiographs are exposed. This explanation may need to be repeated, considering the short attention span of children. It is usually best to take the child to the operatory alone. The child can then view the operator as the authority and not be distracted by the parents' explanation and authority. It is

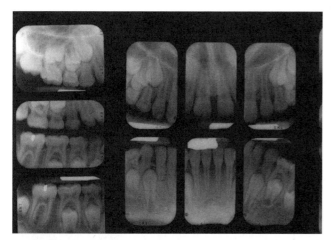

FIGURE 13.7

Full mouth radiograph survey displaying mixed dentition.

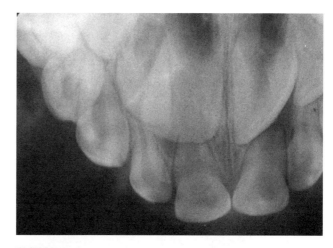

FIGURE 13.8

Occlusal projection detecting supernumerary teeth.

helpful to show the child the equipment used and the radiographs of other children to make them comfortable. Most often, children react favorably to a confident and thorough operator. An emergency should be the only time a child is forced to cooperate in the taking of radiographs. Many times a frightened, uncooperative child can be transformed into a cooperative dental patient with a thorough explanation of the procedure.

Extraoral films should be taken first to gain the confidence of the child. Extraoral films provide much of the growth information needed in children. The paralleling technique should be used when possible for the intraoral radiographs. The use of the paralleling technique decreases radiation exposure to the child's thyroid gland. The flatness of the palate in children often requires radiographic technique modification. The XCP bite block can be trimmed with scissors to accommodate size 0 film. When film holders need to be stabilized, it may be necessary to use cotton rolls to assist in stabilization. In the bisecting angle technique, the vertical angulation must be increased in the maxilla to compensate for the flatness of the children's palates.

Pediatric Surveys

The number of films in a pedodontic or child's survey, varies greatly. For the child with primary dentition, the FMX would consist of four size 0 posterior periapical radiographs, two size 2 occlusal projections of the anterior teeth, and two size 0 bitewing radiographs. For the child with mixed dentition, a FMX would consist of 10 size 2 periapical projections (six anterior, four posterior) and two size 2 bitewing projections (Figure 13.7) combined with any needed extraoral projections. Bitewing surveys are ordered for recall exami-nations according to selection criteria. Combinations of intraoral, periapical, bitewing, occlusal, extraoral panoramic, and cephalmet-

ric films are among the choices of radiographic surveys for the child dental patient.

Occlusal projections can be used to capture a complete arch on one film (Figure 13.8). Occlusal projections most often are used for a rapid survey of one arch to detect supernumerary or impacted teeth, fractures, cysts, tumors, and malignancies. Foreign bodies, such as salivary stones, or sialoliths, can also be detected. For children, the size 2 packet is used for occlusal projections. Larger (size 4) occlusal film is used for some of the same purposes in adult radiography. The film is placed flat on the occlusal plane with the teeth of the opposing arch stabilizing the film packet for the occlusal exposure.

Panoramic projections display the entire midface in a single view (Figure 13.9, *A* and *B*). However, because of the lower resolution of the panoramic radiograph, it should be used as an adjunct rather than a replacement for intraoral radiographs. Another difficulty experienced when attempting to produce an acceptable panoramic projection of a child is matching the arch size to the zone of focus. Some panoramic units allow the operator to manipulate the size of the focal trough as well as collimator size to more accurately image the child patient.

Radiography for the Edentulous Patient

A diagnostic review precedes any prosthetic replacement of the teeth. A radiographic examination is necessary even if patients say they have no teeth. Many times root tips remain years after the teeth have been extracted. Residual infection can also be seen long after the extractions have been performed. Pathology such as cysts and malignant tumors are also detected by radiographs of the edentulous patient. Many other pathology

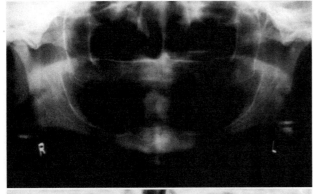

A

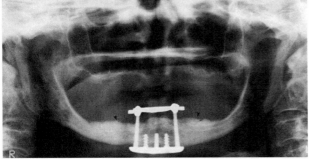

B

FIGURE 13.9

Panoramic radiographs of edentulous patients. **A,** Note how thin this mandible appears. Compare this mandible with the mandible in *B.* **B,** Note the implant and the hydroxylapatite augmentation (*black arrows*).

conditions may also exist and may never be detected if the appropriate diagnostic radiographs are omitted.

To view the dental arches or ridges, many combinations of intraoral, extraoral, and occlusal films are used. Most often the panoramic film is used to show both dental arches on one film. Figure 13.9, *A* and *B* shows the relationship of the mandibular and maxillary arches in the edentulous patient. If the patient is partially edentulous, the remaining teeth should be imaged using intraoral radiographs. For example, if a patient is edentulous in the maxilla but has a full complement of mandibular teeth, panoramic radiograph and periapical views of the remaining teeth are necessary.

Endodontic Radiography

Endodontics is the specialty of dentistry that deals with the diagnosis and treatment of diseases of the dental pulp. The perfection of the technique of root canal therapy (RCT) has saved more teeth than ever in this century. RCT involves removal of the diseased pulp, sterilization and shaping of the pulp canals, and filling of the pulpal cavity with a filling material (e.g., gutta percha).

High-quality radiographs are necessary to view the stages of endodontic treatment. The root length is determined in the initial radiograph. As treatment progresses, the positions

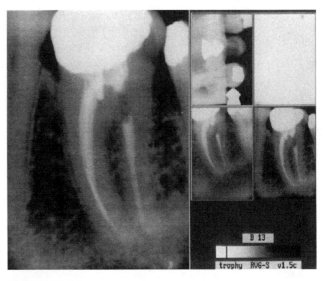

FIGURE 13.10

This charge-coupled device (CCD) image was captured with a CCD sensor rather than with radiographic film.

of the files need to be radiographically evaluated, while the instruments are left in place. Exposure of the radiograph is made difficult by the restricted access caused by use of the rubber dam and the presence of files. To avoid distortion of the root during radiographic procedures during RCT, the paralleling technique is recommended.

Again, because of restricted access during treatment, modifications in technique may be necessary. Many dentists use hemostats and visually parallel the film to the long axis of the root. Several other film-holding devices have been developed exclusively for endodontic radiography. Direct digital imaging using a CCD as the image receptor is especially well suited for endodontic radiography. Figure 13.10 displays an image of completed endodontic therapy in a molar using CCD imaging.

Once the pulpal cavity is cleaned and points placed, a postoperative radiograph is then needed before sealing the canal or canals. Some teeth have more than one canal. With multi-rooted teeth, such as the maxillary molars, modification of technique is necessary because of superimposition of the buccal and palatal roots.

Clark's rule (also known as the *SLOB* rule, *Same Lingual Opposite Buccal*) is a localization technique used to separate the buccal and lingual roots. Two radiographs are taken of the target image with the exact same vertical angulation. The first image is a standard periapical projection. The tubehead and position indicating device (PID) angulation are adjusted to the mesial in the second radiograph so that the lingual root then appears mesial and the buccal root appears distal. In other words, if the structure moves in the same direction as the radiation source from the first radiograph to the second, the structure is located towards the lingual surface. If the structure moves in the opposite direction from the source, it is located toward the buccal surface. This method allows greater visualization during treatment.

ASEPSIS IN DENTAL RADIOGRAPHY

As with any other dental procedure, universal precautions are mandated in dental radiography. The operator should wear gloves, mask, and protective eyewear and clothing. All surfaces in the operatory (including the tubehead, control panel, and timer switch) should be covered with plastic. Surfaces that cannot be covered must be sprayed with an appropriate disinfectant. The American Academy of Oral and Maxillofacial Radiology has developed guidelines for infection control in dental radiography.*

The weakest link in asepsis in dental radiography is the darkroom. Particular care must be taken when removing radiographic film from its protective packet. The packet is contaminated but its contents are not. The film packet must be opened in a way that allows the contents to drop onto a clean surface without contamination. If more than one film is being processed, all packets should be opened and emptied at the same time. Then the contaminated gloves should be discarded, hands washed, and the radiographic film processed. Although the processing chemistry is harsh, it does not sterilize radiographic film. The solutions can become contaminated with microorganisms just as easily as any other material used in dentistry.

Because of the potential for contamination, use of daylight loaders is not recommended unless the film packets have been disinfected (by immersion in an appropriate agent), or have a protective outer coating. Radiographic film can be obtained with the outer coating in place or the protective coating can be applied to traditional film packets. It is virtually impossible to take off a pair of contaminated gloves within the confines of a daylight loader.

PATIENT PROCEDURES

A great deal of patient preparation is required before making the first radiographic exposure. First, appropriately drape the operatory. Then explain the procedure to the patient. The patient should be instructed to remove all jewelry, eyeglasses, and oral prostheses. Provide a denture cup containing water for storage of any prosthesis during the procedure. Place the lead apron and thyroid collar on the patient, make the exposure settings, and assemble the armamentarium. Now exposure of radiographs may begin.

Two techniques have evolved for the exposure of intraoral radiographs: the bisecting angle and the paralleling techniques. The theory behind these techniques is explained earlier in the chapter. The bisecting angle technique is based upon distortion of image geometry and should be used only if the paralleling technique cannot. A short description of the bisecting angle technique follows the discussion of the paralleling technique.

*Information regarding these guidelines can be obtained by contacting the American Academy of Oral and Maxillofacial Radiology; c/o Dr. Kevin O. Carroll, Executive Secretary; PO Box 55722; Jackson Mississippi 39296.

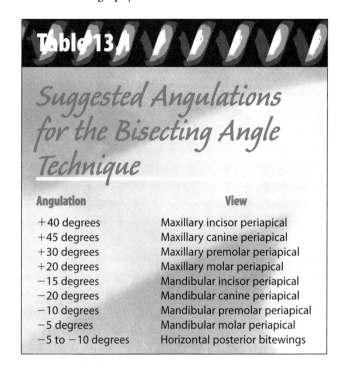

Table 13.1

Suggested Angulations for the Bisecting Angle Technique

Angulation	View
+40 degrees	Maxillary incisor periapical
+45 degrees	Maxillary canine periapical
+30 degrees	Maxillary premolar periapical
+20 degrees	Maxillary molar periapical
−15 degrees	Mandibular incisor periapical
−20 degrees	Mandibular canine periapical
−10 degrees	Mandibular premolar periapical
−5 degrees	Mandibular molar periapical
−5 to −10 degrees	Horizontal posterior bitewings

The paralleling technique is based upon aligning the film packet and the long axis of the tooth of interest parallel to one another. The central ray is then directed perpendicularly to the image receptor. The image receptor must be placed as far away from the tooth of interest as possible. This arrangement (increased object film distance [OFD]) produces magnification and image unsharpness. To compensate for these distortions, a long target receptor distance must be used. One of the advantages of the paralleling technique is that the patient can be placed in any position as long as the relationship between the tooth, image receptor, and central ray are maintained. A diagram showing packet placement, a photograph and radiographic example are displayed for each periapical and bitewing projection used in the paralleling technique.

Bisecting Angle Technique

Although the same structures are captured on periapical films using the bisecting angle technique and the paralleling technique, the relationship between the image receptor and the tooth of interest is different in each technique. The image receptor is placed as close as possible to the tooth of interest. The angle formed between the image receptor and the tooth of interest is calculated, and the central ray is projected perpendicularly to the bisector of the angle just calculated. Each patient is different; therefore each angle will be different. The angulations listed in Table 13.1 should be considered as approximations rather than absolute values.

The vertical angulation of the tubehead and PID is zero when they are positioned parallel to the floor. When the PID's

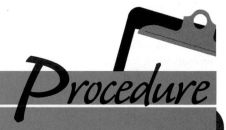

Box 13.1

Paralleling Technique

Mandibular incisor region

The mandibular central and lateral incisors are captured in this projection (Figure 13.11, *A*).

1. Insert the film packet vertically on the bite block of the anterior film-holding instrument. Be sure the film is secure in the slot on the bite block. Size 1 film is recommended.
2. Align the center of the film packet with the midline of the mandibular incisors (Figure 13.11, *B*). Place the packet as far away from the teeth of interest as possible. Doing so allows the film packet to be oriented parallel to the long axis of the teeth. If the patient has a short lingual frenum, the packet may have to be placed on the dorsal surface of the tongue.
3. Ask patient to close carefully on the bite block to retain film position.
4. Slide the aiming ring down the indicating rod as close as possible to the patient's face. Center the PID with the aiming rings (Figure 13.11, *C*).
5. Make the exposure. Figure 13.11, *D,* shows an example of a well-placed mandibular incisor periapical projection.

Mandibular canine region

The mandibular canine is centered on the film packet in this projection. Make sure to include the distal of the lateral incisor in this view (Figure 13.12, A).

1. Insert the film onto the bite block of the anterior film-holding instrument. Size 1 film is recommended. Be sure the film is secure in the slot of the bite block.
2. Center the film packet on the canine (Figure 13.12, B).
3. Have the patient bite on the bite block to stabilize the film and holder.
4. Slide the aiming ring down the aiming rod as close as possible to the patient's face. Align and center the PID of the x-ray with the aiming ring.
5. Make the exposure.

Mandibular premolar region

The mandibular premolars, distal of the canine and mesial of the first molar, are captured in this projection (Figure 13.13, A).

1. Place the film packet horizontally, in the bite block of the posterior film holding device. Use size 2 film and be sure the film is secure in the slot of the bite block.
2. Make sure the film packet is centered on the center of the second premolar. Be sure to include the distal of the canine in the premolar projection. It is important that the bite block rest on the occlusal surface of teeth of interest. Placing the film packet at the center of the arch maximizes room to allow for maintaining a parallel orientation between the teeth and the central ray (Figure 13.13, B).
3. Patient should close the mouth slowly and firmly to stabilize the position of the film.
4. Slide the aiming ring down the indicator rod as close as possible to the face. Align and center the PID with aiming ring (Figure 13.13, C).
5. Make the exposure.

Figure 13.13, D shows an example of a mandibular premolar periapical projection. Capturing the distal of the canine is not as easy as it looks. In most instances, the mesial portion of the film packet will have to be placed at the midline of the mandible. This packet location is also much more comfortable for the patient.

Mandibular molar region

The mandibular molar periapical projection should contain the first, second, and third molars (Figure 13.14, A).

1. Place the film horizontally in the bite block of the posterior film holder. Size 2 film is recommended. Be sure the film is secure in the slot of the bite block.
2. Center the film packet on the second molar. The bite block should rest 0 the occlusal surfaces of the mandibular molars (Figure 13.14, B). If the film packet is centered on the

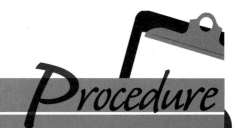

Box 13.1

Procedure

Paralleling Technique—cont'd

second molar and the third molar is incompletely captured, consider a panoramic or lateral oblique projection. Many times the third molar can be imaged on a periapical film, but the view is distorted to the extent that it is useless from a diagnostic standpoint.

3. The patient should close the teeth to stabilize the film in position.
4. Slide the aiming ring down the indicator rod as close as possible to the patient's face. Align and center the PID of the x-ray with the aiming ring (Figure 13.14, C).
5. Make the exposure.

Maxillary central incisor region

Center the maxillary central incisor periapical projection on the maxillary midline and capture the central incisors and the mesial of the lateral incisors (Figure 13.15, A). Remember that the maxillary incisors are wider in a mesiodistal direction than their mandibular counterparts.

1. Insert the film vertically in the anterior bite block of the anterior film-holding instrument. Make sure the film is secure in the bite block slot. Size 1 film is recommended.
2. Center film packet with the midline of the central incisors. Remember to place the film packet as far as possible from the teeth of interest. This arrangement allows the operator to take advantage of the palatal vault for this projection (Figure 13.15, B).
3. Patient should close the teeth to stabilize the film by resting the incisal edges on the bite block.
4. Slide the aiming ring down the indicator rod, as close to the patient's face as possible. Align and center the PID of the x-ray unit with the aiming ring (Figure 13.15, C).
5. Make the exposure.

Maxillary lateral incisor region

The maxillary lateral incisor periapical projection should be centered on the lateral incisor and capture the distal of the central incisor and the mesial of the canine (Figure 13-16, A). This projection is not mirrored in the mandibular arch because of the difference in widths between maxillary and mandibular incisors.

1. Insert the film vertically in the anterior bite block of the anterior film-holding instrument. Make sure the film is secure in bite block slot. Size 1 film is recommended.
2. Center film packet with the lateral incisor. Remember to place the film packet as far as possible from the teeth of interest. This arrangement allows the operator to take advantage of the palatal vault for this projection (Figure 13.16, B).
3. Patient should close the teeth to stabilize the film by resting the incisal edges on the bite block.
4. Slide the aiming ring down the indicator rod, as close to the patient's face as possible. Align and center PID of the x-ray unit with the aiming ring (Figure 13.16, C).
5. Make the exposure.

Maxillary canine region

The maxillary canine has a split personality. The mesial half of the tooth acts like an anterior tooth, the distal half like a posterior tooth. Because of this, it is important to concern yourself with capturing the mesial interproximal portion of the maxillary canine in this projection and capturing the distal interproximal portion in the premolar projection (Figure 13.17, A).

1. Place the film vertically on the anterior bite block of the film-holding instrument. Size 1 film is recommended. Make sure the film is secure in the slot of the bite block.
2. Center the film packet on the canine far from the palatal surface as possible (Figure 13.17, B). Remember that the maxillary canine is the longest of the permanent teeth.
3. Patient should close the teeth firmly to stabilize the film with the maxillary teeth.

Continued

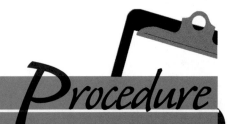

Box 13.1

Procedure

Paralleling Technique—cont'd

4. Slide the aiming ring down the indicator rod to the patient's face. Align and center the PID of the x-ray unit with the aiming ring (Figure 13.17, *C*).
5. Make the exposure.

Maxillary premolar region

This projection captures the maxillary premolars, distal of the canine, and mesial of the first molar (Figure 13.18, *A*).

1. Insert film packet horizontally into the bite block of the posterior film-holding instrument. Size 2 film is recommended. Be sure the film is secure in the slot of the bite block.
2. Center the film packet with the second bicuspid. The packet should be placed as close to the midline of the palate as possible (Figure 13.18, *B*). The mesial corner of the film packet may need to be bent down (not creased) for patient comfort.
3. Patient should close the teeth slowly and firmly to stabilize the film against the occlusal surfaces of the mandibular teeth.
4. Slide the aiming ring down the indicator rod to the patient's face. Align and center the PID of the x-ray unit with the aiming ring (Figure 13.18, *C*).
5. Make the exposure.

An example of a well-placed maxillary premolar periapical projection is shown in Figure 13.18, *D*.

Maxillary molar region

This projection captures the maxillary first, second, third molars and maxillary tuberosity (Figure 13.19, *A*).

1. Insert the film packet horizontally on the posterior bite block of the film-holding instrument. Size 2 film is recommended. Be sure the film is secure in the slot of the bite block.
2. Center the film packet on the second molar. The packet should be placed at the midline of the palate (Figure 13.19, *B*). Beginning radiographers tend to produce a gag reflex in the hardiest of patients, because they wiggle the film packet against the soft palate. It is essential to place the packet where you want it with a minimum of adjustment. The longer this film stays in the mouth, the more likely the patient is to vomit.
3. Patient should close the teeth firmly to stabilize the film against the occlusal surfaces of the mandibular teeth.
4. Slide the aiming ring down the indicator rod to the patient's face. Align and center the PID of the x-ray unit close to the aiming ring (Figure 13.19, *C*).
5. Make the exposure.

It is sometimes impossible to capture both the entire first molar and the tuberosity. When in doubt, capture the tuberosity. In most instances the first molar will be captured in its entirety in the premolar periapical projection.

---

angulation is directed downward toward the floor, the angulation is positive and upward toward the ceiling is negative.

For the bisecting angle technique, facial landmarks are used to orient the central ray and the bisector. For maxillary projections, the line from the tragus of the ear to the ala of the nose is used. The occlusal plane should then be horizontal. For radiography of the mandibular regions, the line from the tragus of the ear to the corner of the mouth should be horizontal. Patient cooperation should be stressed during the procedure. Patient movement compromises the quality of the exposed image and therefore lack of patient motion is essential. The operator should be sure the tubehead is also completely motionless before exposing the radiograph.

Periapical Examination

Film size selection is made according to the size of the dental arch. Most often size 2 packets are used for adult examinations and size 0 and 1 film are used for children's examinations. Adults with narrow dental arches may require use of size 1 films in the anterior regions. Review the selection criteria for the recommended number of exposures for the individual patient.

Paralleling Technique

The paralleling technique records the long axis of the teeth in specific areas of the oral cavity. The procedures described uses the RINN film holding device to secure the packet (Box 13.1 and Table 13.2).

Table 13.2

Evaluation For Exposing, Processing, and Mounting Radiographs

Procedure

	4	3	2	0	X
Exposing radiographs					
1. Select and position equipment.					
2. Select correct film.					
3. Wash hands.					
4. Put on gloves.					
5. Place protective covering on patient.					
6. Explain procedure to patient.					
7. Center oral cavity region in projection.					
8. Insert film packet securely in bite block.					
9. Align center of film.					
10. Place film packet parallel to long axis of teeth.					
11. Patient close carefully with film in position.					
12. Position aiming ring.					
13. Center PID with aiming ring.					
14. Make exposure.					
15. Remove film from patient's mouth.					
16. Secure film for developing.					
17. Remove gloves.					
18. Wash hands.					
Processing radiographs					
1. Check developer, water, and fixture levels.					
2. Stir both solutions.					
3. Check temperatures.					
4. Label film hanger.					
5. Use safe light.					
6. Put on gloves.					
7. Remove film onto towel.					
8. Remove gloves.					
9. Attach film to hanger.					
10. Immerse film in developer.					
11. Cover tank.					
12. Set timer					
13. Remove film from developer.					
14. Rinse for 20 seconds.					
15. Immerse film in fixer.					
16. Cover tank.					
17. Set timer.					
18. Remove film from fixer.					
19. Rinse 20 seconds in running water.					
20. Hang film to dry.					
Mounting radiographs					
1. Label mount.					
2. Identify embossed dot on film.					
3. Sort and arrange exposed film for mounting.					
4. Place film in mounts.					

Materials needed: Film packets; Bite block; Aiming ring with indicating rod; Container for exposed film.

The numeric criteria: 4 Excellent; 3 Good but some improvement needed; 2 Below average, usable, and improvement needed; 0 Unsatisfactory; X Not able to evaluate.

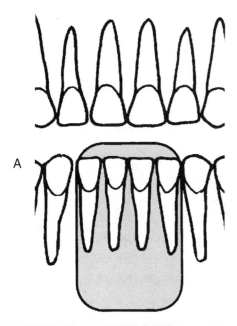

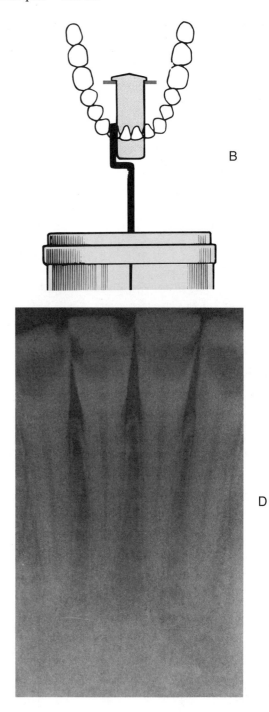

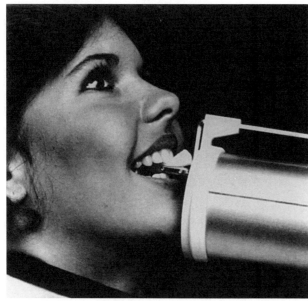

FIGURE 13.11

Mandibular incisor periapical projection. **A,** Diagram of teeth to be included in projection. **B,** Relationship of positioning instrument to the teeth. **C,** Proper orientation of positioning instruments and the PID. **D,** Beginning radiographers often have difficulty with this projection because they try to place the film packet too close to the teeth. Note the facial and proximal caries. (*A, B,* and *C,* Courtesy the Rinn Corporation.)

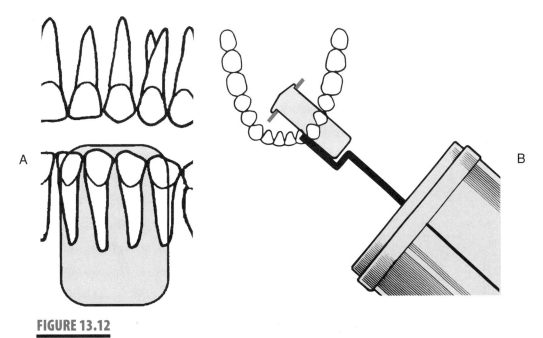

FIGURE 13.12

Mandibular canine periapical projection. **A,** Diagram of teeth to be included in projection. **B,** Relationship of positioning instruments to the teeth. (Courtesy the Rinn Corporation.)

Bitewing Projections

The bitewing projection captures the crowns of the maxillary and mandibular teeth in equal proportions. Bitewings are used to evaluate interproximal carious lesions and crestal bone status. Because of these uses, it is essential that the interproximal contacts be open so that these areas can be appropriately evaluated. Attention must be directed towards achieving the correct horizontal angulation for each bitewing projection. Bitewing projections can be taken of the anterior teeth with the film packet oriented with the long axis of the packet parallel with the long axis of the teeth. These projections are called vertical bitewings. Vertical bitewings can also be taken of the posterior teeth. These projections are often used in patients with moderate to severe periodontitis. Posterior horizontal bitewing projections are generally used for the evaluation of dental caries. Bitewing surveys are the most commonly ordered radiographic surveys in dentistry (Box 13.2).

Radiographic Anatomy

Knowledge of normal radiographic anatomy is essential to the radiographer. The mounting of radiographs requires the mastery of certain radiographic landmarks to prevent improper mounting, which can result in treating the wrong tooth. Two terms that need to be defined before a study of normal radiographic landmarks takes place are **radiopaque** and **radiolucent.**

Structures that are radiopaque appear light or white on a processed radiograph because most or all of the photons are blocked or absorbed by the object of interest. If no photons reach the receptor, a white or light image will result. Enamel, dentin, bone, and metallic restorations are representative examples of radiopaque structures. A radiolucent structure appears black or dark on the processed radiograph. X-ray photons easily pass through these structures or are only slightly attenuated. Soft tissues, the pulp, and the periodontal ligament space are examples of radiolucent structures.

Problems arise when several structures are seen on a radiograph with varying radiodensity. Suppose that one structure is very radiopaque and one is very radiolucent. The structure in the middle can be described as a relative radiopacity or relative radiolucency depending on which end of the spectrum it is closest. The structure in the middle can also be described as radiopaque or radiolucent when compared with an adjacent structure.

Radiopaque
Not allowing penetration of radiation.

Radiolucent
Permeable to radiation; luminous.

Text continued on p. 317

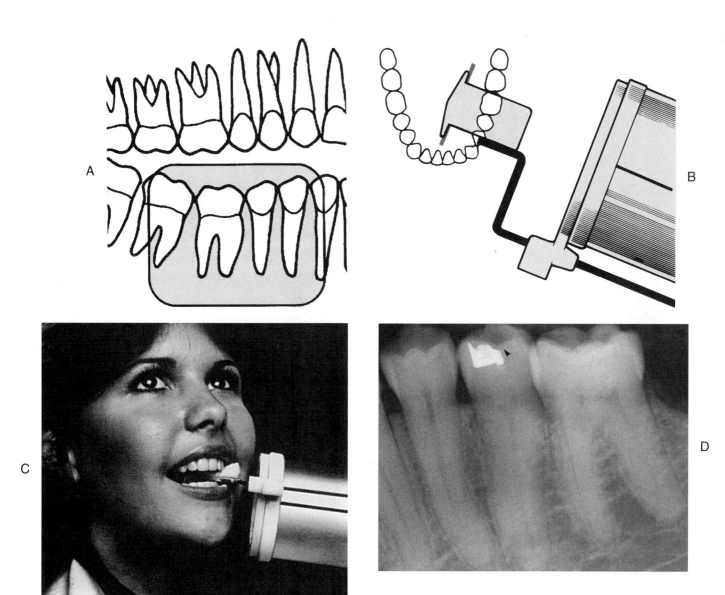

FIGURE 13.13

Mandibular premolar periapical projection. **A,** Diagram of teeth to be included in projection. **B,** Relationship of positioning instrument to the teeth. **C,** Proper orientation of positioning instruments and the PID. **D,** Calculus is evident on the canine and first molar. A defective occlusal amalgam restoration is present on the second molar (*arrow*). If you look closely, you will see two mesial roots on the first premolar. (*A, B,* and *C,* Courtesy the Rinn Corporation.)

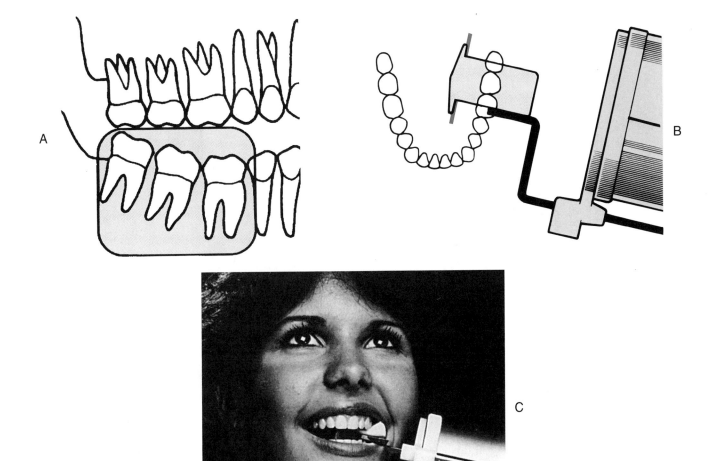

FIGURE 13.14

Mandibular molar periapical projection. **A,** Diagram of teeth to be included in projection. **B,** Relationship of positioning instrument to the teeth. **C,** Proper orientation of positioning instruments and the PID. (Courtesy the Rinn Corporation.)

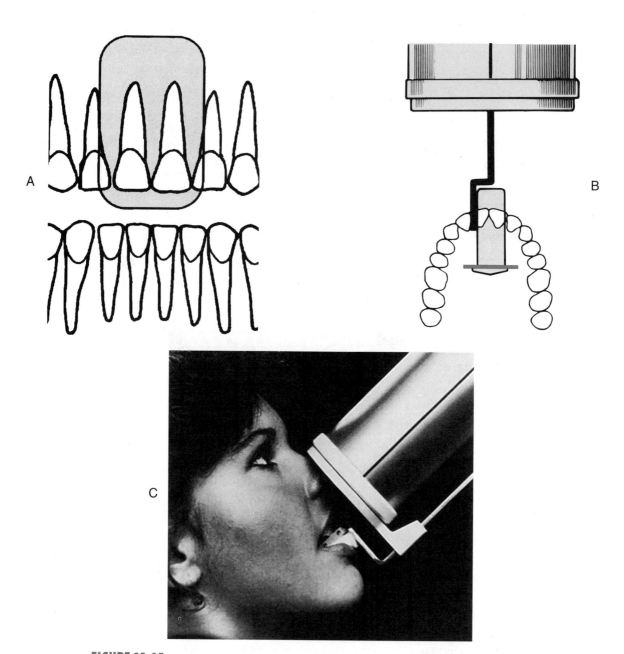

FIGURE 13.15

Maxillary central incisor periapical projection. **A,** Diagram of teeth to be included in projection.
B, Relationship of positioning instrument to the teeth. **C,** Proper orientation of positioning instruments and the PID. (Courtesy the Rinn Corporation.)

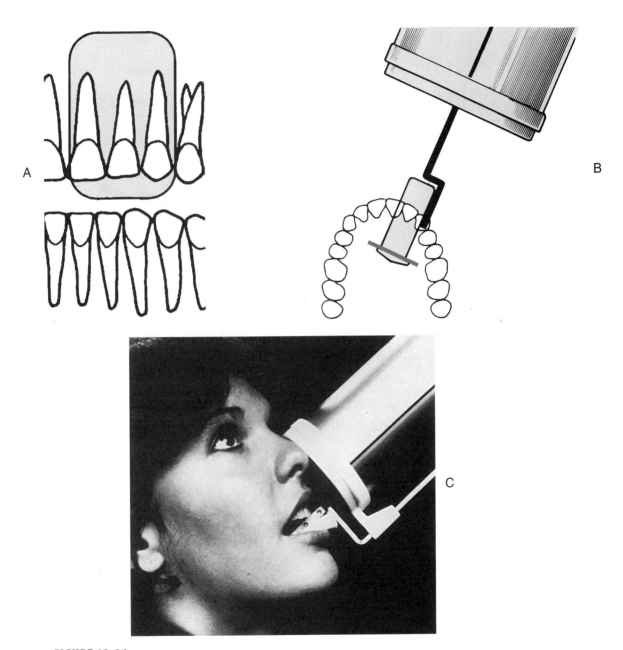

FIGURE 13.16

Maxillary lateral incisor periapical projection. **A,** Diagram of teeth to be included in projection. **B,** Relationship of positioning instrument to the teeth. (Courtesy the Rinn Corporation.)

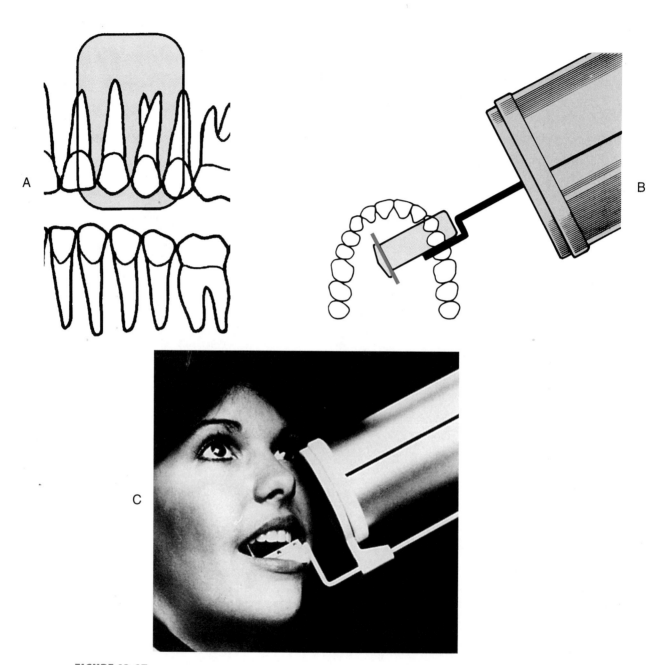

FIGURE 13.17

Maxillary canine periapical projection. **A,** Diagram of teeth to be included in projection. **B,** Relationship of positioning instrument to the teeth. **C,** Proper orientation of positioning instruments and the PID. Note: The distal interproximal contact of the maxillary canine is usually obscured by the palatal cusp of the maxillary first premolar. This is *not* a positioning error. (Courtesy the Rinn Corporation.)

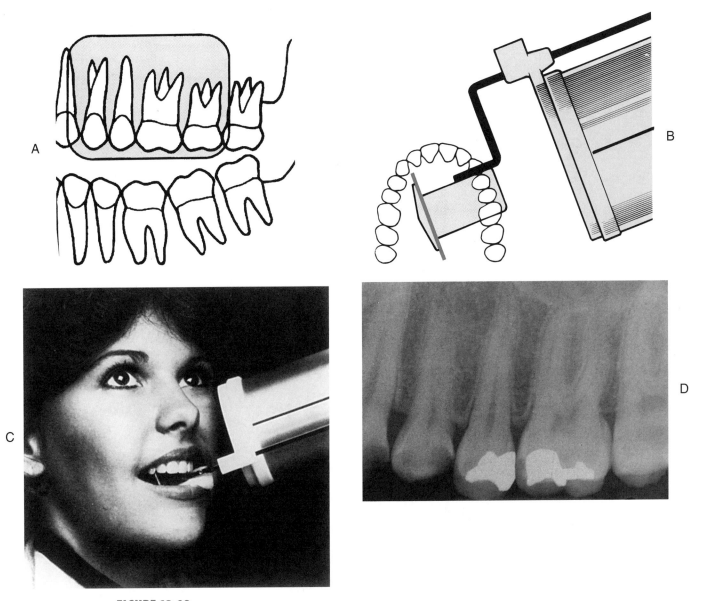

FIGURE 13.18

Maxillary premolar periapical projection. **A,** Diagram of teeth to be included in projection. **B,** Relationship of positioning instrument to the teeth. **C,** It is essential to include the distal interproximal contact area of the canine in this projection, because it is usually overlapped in the canine view. (*A* and *B,* Courtesy the Rinn Corporation.)

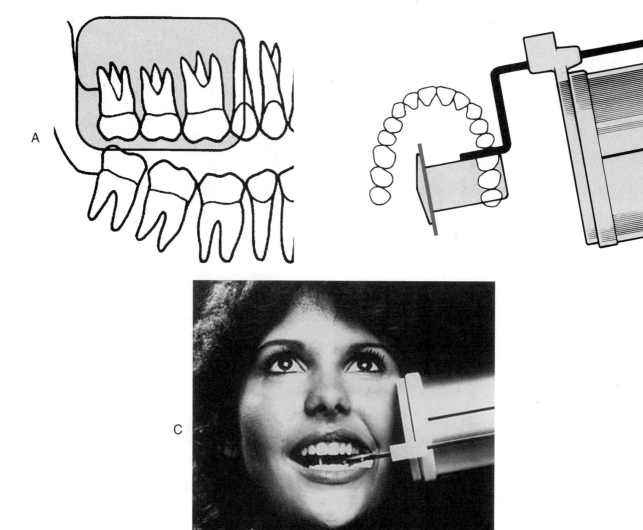

FIGURE 13.19

Maxillary molar periapical projection. **A,** Diagram of teeth to be included in projection. **B,** Relationship of positioning instrument to the teeth. **C,** Note: Centering the second molar on the biteblock produces an excellent image of the third molar and maxillary tuberosity. (Courtesy the Rinn Corporation.)

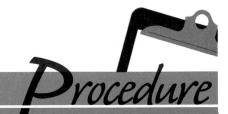

Box 13.2

Procedure

Procedure for Premolar and Molar Bitewing Projections

Premolar Bitewing Projection

The horizontal premolar bitewing captures the maxillary and mandibular premolars, the distal view of the maxillary and mandibular canines, and the mesial view of the maxillary and mandibular first molars (Figure 13.20, *A*).

1. Insert film packet horizontally into the bite block of the bitewing-holding instrument. Size 2 film is recommended. Be sure the film is secure in the slot of the bite block.
2. Center the film packet with the second bicuspid. The packet should be placed as close to the midline of the palate as possible (Figure 13.20, *B*). The mesial corner of the film packet may need to be bent down for patient comfort (bent not creased). Make sure that the distal surfaces of the maxillary and mandibular canines are captured.
3. Patient should close the teeth slowly and firmly to stabilize the film against the occlusal surfaces of the mandibular teeth.
4. Slide the aiming ring down the indicator rod to the patient's face. Align and center the PID of the x-ray unit with the aiming ring (Figure 13.20, *C*).
5. Make the exposure.

An example of a well-placed horizontal premolar bitewing projection is shown in (Figure 13.20, *D*).

Molar bitewing projections

This projection captures the crowns of the maxillary and mandibular first, second, and third molars (Figure 13.21, *A*).

1. Insert the film packet horizontally on the bitewing bite block of the film-holding instrument. Size 2 film is recommended. Be sure the film is secure in the slot of the bite block.
2. Center the film packet on the second molar. The packet should be placed at the midline of the palate (Figure 13.21, *B*).
3. Patient should close the teeth firmly to stabilize the film against the occlusal surfaces of the mandibular teeth.
4. Slide the aiming ring down the indicator rod to the patient's face. Align and center the PID of the x-ray unit close to the aiming ring.
5. Make the exposure.

Figure 13.21, *C*, displays an example of a horizontal molar bitewing projection. The interproximal contact between the maxillary first and second molars is difficult to open in the molar projection. In most instances, this contact is opened in the premolar bitewing projection. Do not worry about unerupted third molars. Remember why the bitewing is being exposed.

The teeth are complex structures made up of tissues of varying radiodensity (Figure 13.23). The pulp consists of blood vessels, nerves, and other soft tissues needed for the development and maintenance of the teeth. The pulp is radiolucent and usually described as a pulp chamber because the outline of the pulp is evident but the components are not. Enamel is the hardest tissue in the body, is the most radiopaque, and covers dentin, which is also radiopaque but not as much as enamel. Dentin and bone have comparable radiodensities. The junction between enamel and dentin is called the *dentinoenamel junction* or *DEJ*. The decision whether to treat carious lesions is based in part on the location of the lesion relative to the DEJ.

Cementum has a radiodensity similar to dentin and covers the dentin of the root of the tooth. The cementoenamel junction of CEJ is a landmark used to determine the loss of bony attachment around a tooth. Bone loss is measured from the height of the bone to the CEJ. Radiographs only show that periodontal disease has been present but give no information about disease activity and should be used as an adjunct to the diagnosis of periodontal disease. They are no substitute for the clinical examination.

The cementum is surrounded by a radiolucent space, referred to as the *periodontal ligament space.* The periodontal ligament consists of several tissues that are radiolucent.

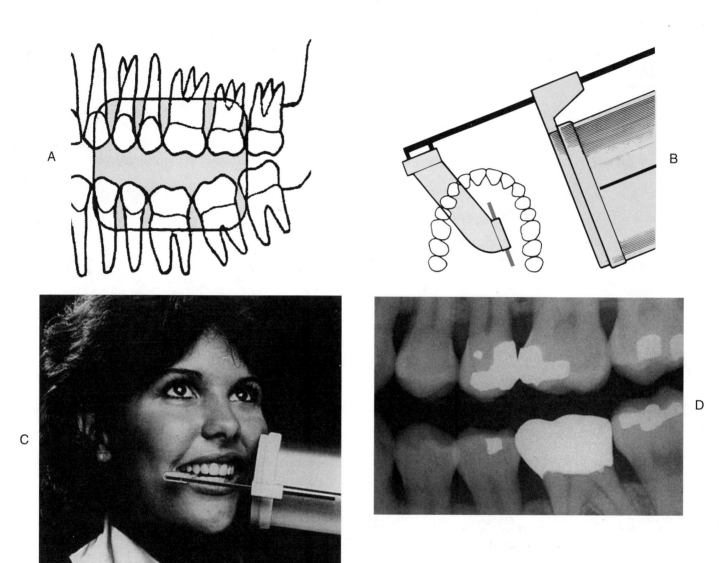

FIGURE 13.20

Premolar bitewing projection. **A,** Diagram of teeth to be included in projection. **B,** Relationship of positioning instrument to the teeth. **C,** Proper orientation of positioning instruments and the PID. **D,** The distal of both maxillary and mandibular canines are included in this projection. Note how the teeth of both arches are equally displayed. (*A, B,* and *C,* Courtesy the Rinn Corporation.)

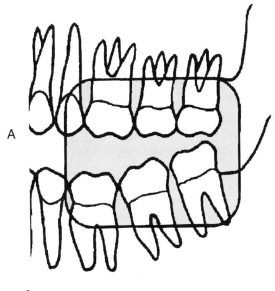

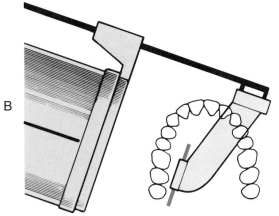

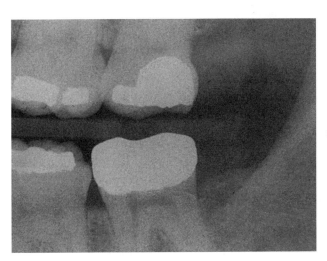

FIGURE 13.21

Molar bitewing projection. **A,** Diagram of teeth to be included in projection. **B,** Relationship of positioning instrument to the teeth. **C,** The contact between the maxillary first and second molar is often overlapped in a properly placed molar bitewing projection. (*A* and *B,* Courtesy the Rinn Corporation.)

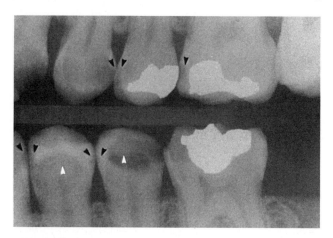

FIGURE 13.22

Dental caries on premolar bitewing projection. *Black arrows* indicate proximal carious lesions. *White arrows* indicate facial carious lesions.

Immediately adjacent to the periodontal ligament space is a rim of dense bone, called the *lamina dura.* The lamina dura can become thickened or even disappear in certain pathologic conditions. The bone that surrounds the lamina dura is called *cancellous bone,* is not as radiodense as the lamina dura, and contains irregularly shaped opacities called *trabeculae.* The relative lucencies around the trabeculae are made up of bone marrow and are called *bone marrow spaces.* Bone without marrow spaces is called *cortical bone* and can be found at the inferior border of the mandible and at the crest of the alveolar bone (bone that surrounds and supports the teeth).

Mounting Radiographs

Looking at a jumble of 20 images can sometimes seem overwhelming. The confusion can be doubled by us-

ing two film packets and not processing them as separate entities. Remember that the correct mounting (Box 13.3) of radiographic images is essential for accurate diagnosis.

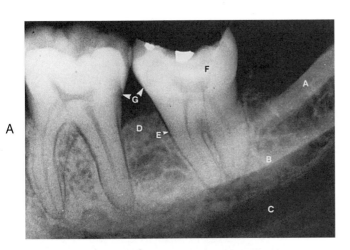

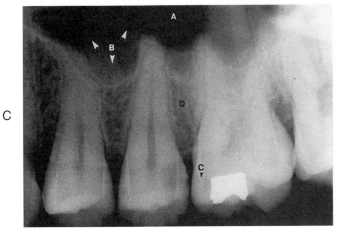

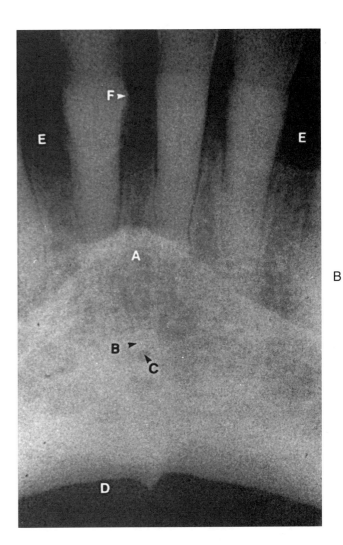

FIGURE 13.23

A, Mandibular molar periapical. *A,* External oblique ridge. *B,* Internal oblique ridge. *C,* Mandibular canal space. *D,* Horizontal bone loss. *E,* Periodontal ligament space. *F,* Dental caries. *G,* Cementum enamel junction. **B,** Mandibular incisor periapical. *A,* Mental Ridge. *B,* Genial tubercle. *C,* Lingual foramen. *D,* Inferior border of mandible. *E,* Horizontal bone loss. *F,* Calculus. **C,** Maxillary premolar periapical. *A,* Soft tissue shadow of nasolabial fold. *B,* Soft tissue shadow of gingiva.*C,* Proximal caries. *D,* Widened periodontal ligament space.

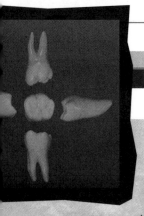

Points for Review

- Radiation safety techniques
- Asepsis in dental radiography
- Patient procedures, including bisecting angle techniques, periapical examinations, paralleling techniques, bitewing projections, and special radiographic needs
- Radiographic anatomy
- Mounting techniques

Self-Study Questions

1. What is (are) involved in taking x-rays?
   a. Mastery of technique
   b. Problem solving
   c. Patient management
   d. All of the above

2. What principle(s) emphasize the philosophy that the least amount of exposure possible should be the rule for diagnostic radiography?
   a. DAU principles
   b. Ethics principles
   c. ALARA principle
   d. All of the above

3. What organization(s) has (have) developed recommendations for selection criteria of dental radiographic examinations?
   a. Academy of Dental Radiology
   b. Academy of General Dentistry
   c. Academy of Pediatric Dentistry
   d. All of the above

4. Training of allied dental professionals in radiation safety procedures and quality control is critical to proper patient care.
   a. True
   b. False

5. Why can operators now produce better radiographs than in the past?
   a. Radiographic equipment is less expensive
   b. Larger and more powerful x-ray equipment exists
   c. Accuracy of equipment provides increased definition with less exposure.
   d. All of the above

6. What technique was one of the earliest techniques used to expose dental radiographs?
   a. Long-cone technique
   b. Short-cone (bisecting angle) technique
   c. Right angle (paralleling) technique
   d. Extension cone (paralleling) technique

7. How many x-ray films are usually included in a full mouth survey?
   a. Minimum of 14
   b. Minimum of 4 bitewing radiographs
   c. Maximum of 24
   d. None of the above

8. What film can be used to enable the operator to see the entire dentition on a single film?
   a. Tomograph
   b. Cephalometric projection
   c. Panoramic
   d. Digital

9. At what age should the first x-ray of a child be taken?
   a. At least by 2 years
   b. Usually at 3 years
   c. Not before 4 years
   d. None of the above

10. How can film holders be stabilized when taking pedo x-rays?
    a. Assistant hold the film
    b. Use of cotton rolls
    c. Use of XCP bite block
    d. None of the above

11. The American Academy of Oral and Maxillofacial Radiology has developed guidelines for infection control in dental radiography.
    a. True
    b. False

12. What is the weakest link in asepsis in dental radiography?
    a. Content of the film
    b. Operatory procedures

c. Darkroom procedures

d. None of the above

13. The bisecting technique should be used only if the paralleling technique cannot.
   a. True
   b. False

14. For what anatomic guide is the line from the tragus of the ear to the ala of the nose used?
   a. Mandibular projections
   b. Maxillary projections
   c. Anterior projections
   d. Occlusal projections

15. What sequence is followed to expose periapical x-rays using the paralleling technique?
   a. Slide aiming ring down to the patient's face, insert film into bite block, center film packet, have patient bite on block
   b. Insert film into bite block, have patient bite on block, center film packet, slide aiming ring down to patient's face
   c. Insert film into bite block, center film packet, have patient bite on block, and slide aiming ring down to the patient's face.
   d. None of the above

16. The premolar bitewing includes the maxillary and mandibular premolars, the distal view of the maxillary and mandibular canines, and the mesial view of the maxillary and mandibular first molars.
   a. True
   b. False

17. How does a radiolucent structure appear on a processed radiograph?
   a. Black
   b. Light
   c. White
   d. Pale gray

18. What anatomic landmark is used to determine the loss of bony attachment around a tooth?
   a. CEJ
   b. Apex of the root
   c. Occlusal and incisal surface of the teeth
   d. All of the above

19. When mounting radiographs, how should the x-rays be placed?
   a. Dimple up
   b. Pimple up
   c. Occlusal plane curved down
   d. Most posterior image on the film toward the center of the mount

20. What region of the dentition would be represented by a x-ray film showing a radiolucent midline?
   a. Maxillary molar region
   b. Cuspid region
   c. Mandibular premolar region
   d. Maxillary incisors

Suggested Readings

Barr JH, Stephens RG: *Dental radiology: pertinent basic concepts and their applications in clinical practice,* Philadelphia, 1980, WB Saunders.

Bushong S: *Radiologic science for technologists,* ed 6, St Louis, 1997, Mosby.

Council on Dental Materials, Instruments, and Equipment: Recommendations in radiographic practices: an update, 1988, *J Am Dent Assoc* 118:115-117, 1989.

Goaz PW, White SC: *Oral radiology: principles and interpretation,* ed 2, St Louis, 1987, Mosby.

Miles DA et al: *Radiographic imagine for dental auxiliaries,* ed 3, Philadelphia, 1999, WB Saunders.

White SC: *Oral radiology: principles and interpretation,* ed 4, St Louis, 1999, Mosby.

Wuehermann AH, Manson-Hing LR: *Dental radiology,* ed 5, St Louis, 1981, Mosby.

Chapter 14

General Pharmacology and Pain Control

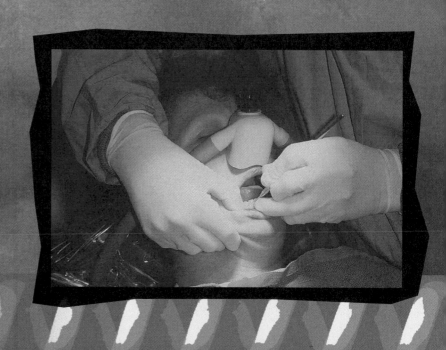

Chapter Outline

Learning Objectives

On completion of Chapter 14, the student should be able to do the following:

■ Identify key terms.

■ Discern the difference between brand names and generic names of drugs.

■ Define the Controlled Substances Act and its classifications.

■ Describe drug effects and drugs associated with abuse.

■ Describe the drugs and armamentarium for use in pain control in dentistry including nitrous oxide.

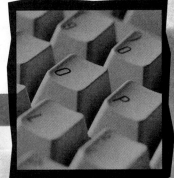

Key Terms

Analgesia	Antiinflammatory	Hypersensitivity
Anesthesia	Depressants	Sedative
Antagonism	Drug Interaction	Vasodilator
Antibiotic		

PHARMACOLOGY

Pharmacology is the study of chemical agents and their affects on living processes. Chemicals with therapeutically useful actions are called drugs. This chapter is about the use of drugs such as antibiotics, anesthetics, analgesics, and **sedatives** as they relate to dentistry and their reactions and general properties of these drugs. The drugs used today are obtained from plants (including microorganisms), minerals or chemicals, animals, or through synthetic development.

Sedative
A drug that causes a calming or unaroused effect.

The scope of pharmacology is expansive. Clinical dentistry is primarily concerned with the usefulness or medicinal use of drugs to treat disease and eliminate or minimize pain with the fewest side effects. Two basic areas of pharmacology exist, which allow comparison and evaluation of drugs. Pharmacokinetics and pharmacodynamics deal with the relationship between the dose of a drug given and the physiologic effect of that drug in treating the patient.

Pharmacokinetics describes the relationship between the rate absorption, distribution, biotransformation, and excretion of drugs and can be thought of as what the body does to a drug when it is administered. Pharmacodynamics is the study of the mechanism of action and physiologic effects of drugs and can be described as the study of what the drug does to the body. Some drugs may stimulate, depress, or block biochemical or physiologic processes to provide relief of symptoms such as in pain control, and others may favorably alter the course of disease by modifying the body's response. Conversely, some drugs are useful only because they have minimal effects on the body but can destroy harmful organisms such as bacteria or eliminate pathogenic cells such as cancer. From a clinical standpoint, one of the most important properties of a drug is its selectivity or ability to produce its desired effects with minimal side effects.

Certain conditions occur such as exposure of the drug to air, temperature changes, and exposure to light that will modify the effectiveness of drugs. Age and weight, allergy, and cumulative use of a drug can also affect its usefulness.

1 Age and weight: The greater the weight of the patient the larger the dosage or strength of the drug.
2 Allergy: Some patients are allergic or sensitive to specific drugs and will be given a substitute.
3 Tolerance and accumulative effects: The body can build up a tolerance to a drug used over a prolonged period. Although some drugs are destroyed or eliminated by the body, a continued and faster intake of the drug can result in an excessive amount of the drug if not eliminated fast enough.
4 Administrative channel: A drug injected has faster results than one given by mouth, for instance, drugs that must be absorbed through tissue must often be given in larger doses.
5 Pathologic condition: The type of infection or pathologic agent will determine the type of drug to be used; the amount; and the route of administration.

DRUG INTERACTIONS

Drug interaction can occur when two or more drugs cause a side effect of negative response. For instance, when tranquilizers are taken with an antihistamine, a significant increase exists in the analgesic effects of the narcotic. This interaction is called *synergism* because the action of drugs together, their combined effect, is greater than the effect of either drug alone. Acetaminophen (Tylenol) plus hydrocodone bitartrate taken together, can be more effective than either drug by itself. If the action of the drugs together create an undesirable effect the condition is called **antagonism**.

Drug interaction
When two or more drugs, given concurrently, produce an altered pharmacologic response.

Antagonism
When the action of drugs together produce an undesirable effect.

When a drug is used repeatedly, greater dosages may be required to produce the same effect over a period. This is called *drug tolerance* because the body becomes accustomed to the drug. Side effects such as drug dependency can also occur. Some individuals have **hypersensitivity** to specific drugs and can have allergic reactions. In addition, some drugs can cause unexpected results or idiosyncrasy. For instance, some **depressants** will cause an individual to become very anxious or excited. Excessive amounts or overdose of drugs can cause poisoning (toxic dose) or death (lethal dose).

Hypersensitivity
A reaction or altered response of an individual to a drug.

Depressants
Drug used to reduce anxiety.

Dental assistants should obtain a complete list of the patient's current medications because of the potential for drug interactions, bleeding (for example, Coumadin or even aspirin therapy), and various cardiac conditions. Several reference books may be available in a dental office such as *Patient Drug Facts, Facts and Comparisons*, the *Physician's Desk Reference, Mosby's Dental Drug Reference*, and *Mosby's GenRx*.

ROUTES OF ADMINISTRATION

Drugs can be administered through several pathways or routes of administration, including the following:

- Inhalation: Breathing a gaseous substance (e.g., nitrous oxide sedation)
- Topical: Application on the surface of the mucosa or skin (e.g., topical anesthetic solutions)
- Transdermal: Through the skin (e.g., nicotine patches)
- Rectal: Suppositories or enemas
- Oral: Tablets, capsules, or liquids
- Sublingual: Under the tongue (e.g., nitroglycerin)
- Parenteral: Injection through a hypodermic syringe
- Subcutaneous: Injection under the skin
- Intramuscular: Injection within the muscle tissue
- Intravenous: Injection directly into a vein

PRESCRIPTIONS

A prescription is a written order authorizing a pharmacist to provide a certain drug to a patient. Only the dentist can prescribe medication. Prescription pads should be kept in a secure place and only be given to patients under authorization and direct supervision of the dentist. A copy of the prescription should be kept in the patient's record for future reference and medical-legal considerations. A record of all drugs dispensed must be kept. Remember that a prescription is dispensed only with the direct order of the dentist.

Drugs may be identified by their brand or generic names. Brand names are registered drug names or trademarks given by the drug company and are always capitalized. Generic names are generally the chemical name of the specific drug that any company may use. These names are not capitalized. Zylocaine, for example, is a brand name for the generic drug lidocaine. Drugs are also classified legally based on their availability to the public. Prescription drugs are controlled by federal and state law and are only available on orders of a doctor. All other drugs that may be purchased without prescription are called *over-the-counter* (OTC) *drugs*.

Prescription Writing

A prescription is the written instruction by a dentist or physician for the preparation and administration of a drug or medicine. A controlled drug is legally available only by the order of the doctor's prescription. Some prescriptions are not refillable and will be stated as such on the prescription and container. A dental assistant must never write a prescription, sign the prescription, or dispense a drug. Any instruction for drug use must be made by the doctor and should include written instructions as prescribed by the doctor. All drugs administered should be documented on the patient's records and should include the following:

Table 14.1

Latin Abbreviations Used in Prescription Writing

Abbreviation	Latin	English Meaning
a.c.	Ante cibum	Before meals
b.i.d.	His in die	Twice a day
c.	Cum	With
caps.	Capsula	Capsule
d.	Dies	Day
gt(t)	Gutta	Drop(s)
h.	Hora	Hour
h.s.	Hora somni	At bedtime
o.h.	Omni hora	Every hour
P.C.	Post cibum	After meals
P.O.	Per os	By mouth
p.r.n.	Pro re nata	As needed
q.	Quaque	Each, every
q.h.	Quaque hora	Every hour
q.i.d.	Quater in die	Four times a day
s.	Sine	Without
Sig.	Signa	Label
Sol.	Solutio	Solution
tab.	Tabella	Tablet
t.i.d.	Ter in die	Three times a day
ung.	Unguentum	Ointment
ut dict.	Ut dictum	As directed

- Dose and route of administration
- A file copy of prescription
- Drug prescribed
- Date and time

Table 14.1 lists the Latin abbreviations used in prescription writing. A written prescription should include the following information:

Demographic data
- Prescriber's name, address, and telephone number
- Patient's name and date of prescription

Superscription
- Rx the abbreviation for "recipe" meaning to take

Inscription
- Name and strength of the drug

Subscription
- Quantity of the drug

Signature

Directions for use
- Amount of drug in a single dose
- Route of administration
- Frequency of administration

Prescriber's signature
- Doctor's name with degree printed and signature

DEA number
- Drug Enforcement Agency (DEA) number if the drug is for a controlled substance

If prescriptions are called into the pharmacy, the prescription should be recorded on the patient's chart.

Some states may require further information such as the following:
- Patient's address and age
- If a generic brand can be substituted by the pharmacist
- If refills are permitted

DRUG ABUSE

Substance abuse of prescription medications is becoming more prevalent in contemporary dental practice. A drug is a chemical substance used to treat diseases but some are addictive, causing compulsive use of the drug. Narcotic drug use can cause physical dependence, an altered physiologic state produced by chronic exposure to a drug, which necessitates continued administration to prevent withdrawal illness. Withdrawal is the physical or psychologic distressed condition caused by the discontinued use of a chemical agent such as codeine or nicotine. Drug use can also cause psychologic dependence or habitual, compulsive use of the drug that differs from physical addiction because it does not result in withdrawal illness.

Controlled Substances Act

The Controlled Substances Act is a federal mandate that is divided into five schedules of drugs based primarily on the drug's potential for abuse. Under these laws, a doctor is authorized to prescribe these medications and is issued a Federal Drug Enforcement Agency (DEA) identification number.

Schedule I

Schedule I drugs have no accepted medical use, a high potential for abuse, or are used for research purposes. Examples include heroin, LSD, and marijuana.

Schedule II

Schedule II drugs have a high potential for abuse and accepted medical uses. Prescriptions for this class may be issued only pursuant to a written prescription (no telephone prescriptions) and may not be refilled: meperidine (Demerol), oxycodone (Percodan), and codeine.

Schedule III

Schedule III drugs have less abuse potential than I and II and accepted medical uses. This class may be called in by telephone or issued pursuant to a written prescription and may be refilled up to five times or within 6 months from date of issue. Examples include acetaminophen with codeine (Tylenol #3), hydrocodone (Lortab 7.5), and other similar products.

Schedule IV

Schedule IV drugs have low abuse potential and accepted medical uses. The prescribing information is the same as for Schedule III drugs. Examples include benzodiazepines (Valium) and propoxyphene (Darvon).

Schedule V

Schedule V drugs have low abuse potential and accepted medical uses. These drugs do not require a prescription under federal law but are always controlled by a pharmacist; however, some states place these drugs in a higher schedule and therefore must be prescribed. Practitioners should keep a supply of drugs, especially narcotics, in the office because of their potential for abuse and theft. Dentists may legally dispense drugs in some states.

Dental Personnel's Responsibility in Controlled Substance Abuse

Any patient suspected of altered behavior because of any influence of drugs should be brought to the attention of the dentist immediately. Otherwise benign treatment may be dramatically altered in the presence of abuse. Also, many of these patients have "shopped" many other offices for drugs. Prescription blanks should not be accessible to patient areas where the possibility of theft may occur.

Commonly Abused Drugs

Alcohol

Alcohol is a depressant and commonly abused drug that may cause impaired judgment, slurred speech, drowsiness, confusion, and aggressive behavior. Although alcohol has wide social acceptance, its status as a potent drug is often overlooked. Antianxiety drugs coupled with alcohol can produce a deadly cocktail.

Narcotic Analgesics

Narcotics are often abused for their euphoric effect. These drugs depress the central nervous system and produce pinpoint pupils, drowsiness, respiratory depression, nausea, or stupor. Overdose will cause slow and shallow breathing, clammy skin, convulsions, coma, and possible death. Narcotics include opium, morphine, codeine, heroin, meperidine, and methadone.

Depressants and Antianxiety Agents

Depressants and antianxiety agents may produce drowsiness, fatigue, paranoia, staggering, slurred speech, confusion, and aggressive behavior. Benzodiazepines are stimulants that may produce similar states. Overdose will cause shallow, dilated pupils, weak and rapid pulse, coma, and possible death. Depressants include choloral hydrate, barbiturates, glutethimide, methaqualone, and tranquilizers. Cannabis agents include marijuana, hashish, and hashish oil.

Stimulants and Hallucinogens

Stimulants and hallucinogens may produce excitement, illusions, increased wakefulness, talkativeness, and hallucinations. These agents may also cause bizarre behavior, psychotic symptoms, poor perception of time and distance, violent reactions and possible death. Stimulants include cocaine amphetamines, phenmetrazine, and methylphenidate. Hallucinogens include LSD, Mescaline, Psilocybin-Psilocyin, NDA and PCP.

DRUGS COMMONLY USED IN DENTISTRY

Antibiotics

Antibiotic

Drug to kill or inhibit the growth of bacteria.

Antibiotics are chemical substances that inhibit or destroy bacteria and other microorganisms. The use of an **antibiotic** should be based on the following criteria:

1 An established need for the drug (antibiotics are not effective against viral infections)
2 Knowledge that the particular antibiotic is effective for the causative bacteria or microorganism
3 No allergies to the drug
4 Awareness of possible side effects of the drug

Prophylactic antibiotic use is recommended for all dental procedures that are likely to cause bleeding for high-risk patients. These patients may have had open-heart surgery, various forms of heart disease, rheumatic fever, or valve or joint replacement. Although this treatment is controversial, the antibiotic Keflex, Amoxicillin, or Ampicillin, may be administered before dental treatment and continued for a short time after treatment.

All antibiotics disrupt the normal microbial balance of the skin, mucous membranes, and gastrointestinal tract. This may permit drug resistant bacteria or fungi to proliferate. A new infection, called a *superinfection*, may occur at the original site or elsewhere in the body. For example, during antibiotic therapy, an overgrowth of *Candida albicans* may occur in the mouth. Females, prone to genital yeast infections, may be particularly susceptible to antibiotics.

In warm climates with sunny seasons some antibiotics can cause photosensitivity or sensitivity to the ultraviolet rays. Tanning beds should not be used when taking these drugs.

Types of Antibiotics

Penicillins

Penicillin is a generic term for a group of antibiotics similar in chemical structure but differing in spectrum and absorption rate. The primary use of penicillin in dentistry is to reduce inflammation (**antiinflammatory**) and combat infections caused by gram-positive bacteria such as strepto-cocci and is not useful in gram-negative bacteria, viruses, or fungi. Penicillin is available in a variety of formulations such as penicillin V and penicillin G. Amoxicillin and ampicillin are known as extended spectrum penicillins, which are used to treat staphylococci infections and other infections resistant to other forms of penicillin. As with most antibiotics, the effectiveness of penicillins has become somewhat diminished because of newer resistant bacteria. Injudicious prescribing of antibiotics has added to this problem. Hives, swelling, shock, and death are acute reactions that can be caused by the administration of penicillin (see Chapter 22).

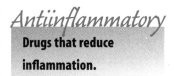

Antiinflammatory

Drugs that reduce inflammation.

Cephalosporins

This group of antibiotics is chemically related to penicillin. However, they are broad-spectrum antibiotics because they are active against gram-positive and gram-negative organisms. Their use in dentistry is primarily for susceptible organisms or when other drugs are ineffective.

Erythromycin

Erythromycin resembles penicillin and may be used in patients who are allergic to penicillin or when organisms have become penicillin resistant. Erythromycin may upset the stomach and should be taken with food or milk.

Tetracyclines

Tetracycline antibiotics affect a wide range of microorganisms. The administration of tetracyclines from the second trimester of pregnancy to approximately 8 years of age may produce permanent discoloration of the teeth. The extent of the staining is related to the time, dosage, and duration of the involved drug. Staining may vary from slight yellow or gray discoloration to dark gray or purple banding of the teeth. This type of discoloration is often a dental problem, requiring cosmetic correction by the dentist.

Antifungal Agents

These drugs are used for fungal infections such as those caused by *Candida albicans*. Nystatin and ketoconazole are two such agents in dentistry.

Antiviral Agents

These agents are used in dentistry for treating herpetic lesions associated with the oral cavity. Acyclovir (Zovirax) is an example of this type of drug.

Epinephrine

Epinephrine is sometimes called *adrenaline* and acts as a vasoconstrictor to narrow the blood vessels, stimulate the heart, and increase the blood pressure. It is also

Vasodilator

Drug used to cause blood vessels to expand.

a **vasodilator** causing the blood vessels to expand, thereby increasing circulation, pulse rate, and potential bleeding. Epinephrine causes the dilation, or opening, of the bronchioles to the lungs and is used in local anesthetics and gingival retraction cords to increase the duration of the anesthetic effect and control bleeding. It causes a reversal of the skin and mucus reactions and is also used as an emergency drug for medical emergencies such as anaphylactic shock because it acts very rapidly to counteract and reverse the most severe effects of the histamine response. The percentage of epinephrine added to the anesthetic solution is called the *epinephrine ratio*. For routine dental treatment, the most widely used epinephrine ratio is 1:100,000. This means that one part epinephrine per 100,000 parts of anesthetic solution is used. When longer duration of anesthetic is needed, a ratio of 1:50,000 is used. The vasoconstrictive property of the epinephrine is maximized at a ratio of 1:200,000; therefore increasing the epinephrine dose does not add to vasoconstriction. Epinephrine degenerates in the body very rapidly so it is very short acting, possibly making a second dose of epinephrine necessary. Epinephrine is administered either intermuscularly (IM) in the arm muscle or subcutaneously (SC) beneath the skin. All anesthetic cartridges are labeled and usually color-coded by the manufacturer as to epinephrine content.

Corticosteroids

Corticosteroids such as hydrocortisone, 100 mg IM or intravenously (IV), will also reduce swelling and capillary dilation. However, their onset of action is slow. The main function of corticosteroids is to prevent a relapse of the crisis after epinephrine has had its initial effect.

Hemostatics

Hemostatics are used to stop bleeding where a slow flow of blood exists. They are not used effectively for a profuse flow of blood from large vessels and cannot be absorbed or injected into the blood stream. They are used near an incised vessel to rapidly coagulate (clot) the slow flow of blood and stop bleeding.

Gelfoam is an absorbable hemostatic, gelatin sponge cut into small pieces and used in a surgical site (such as removal of a tooth) to stop bleeding. It is usually absorbed within 4 to 6 weeks. Oxidized regenerated cellulose and oxidized cellulose (Novacell, Oxycel) are chemically modified surgical gauze used to control bleeding from an extraction. Astringents are used on the tissue around the bleeding area to cause the tissue to contract thus stopping the bleeding. A styptic is a concentrated form of astringent used to stop bleeding in a small area.

Tranquilizers

Tranquilizers are used to treat emotional stress and anxiety. These etiologic factors cause and exacerbate (increase) chronic pain. Tranquilizers treat this chronic pain, decrease anxiety and stress, and relax the muscles. Examples include Valium and Elavil.

Antihistamines

Antihistamines are used to treat mild-to-moderate allergic reactions and also for sedation. Benadryl (diphenhydramine) is an example of this type of drug. Diphenhydramine, 5.0 mg, or chlorpheniramine, 10 mg, may be administered IM for a long-term histamine response. Antihistamines are most effective in controlling edema (swelling) and pruritus (itching). They have little effect on blood pressure or bronchodilation. Although antihistamines are helpful in treating mild allergic reactions, they are of little value in treating severe or anaphylactic reactions.

Oxygen

The most useful single agent for resuscitation is oxygen. Oxygen should be readily available with appropriate accessories for its use. Every person in the dental office should be familiar with its use in an emergency situation including the operation of the equipment (See Chapter 22).

Other Miscellaneous Drugs

- Calcium hydroxide: Used for pulp capping, pulpotomy, or a cavity liner.
- Euginol: An active ingredient of oil of cloves is used with zinc oxide as a sedative and analgesic agent in dental cements and liners.
- Alum: An astringent, styptic, and hemostatic topical agent.
- Aromatic spirits of ammonia: A respiratory stimulant used to prevent fainting or shock.
- Atropine: Decreases the secretion of saliva and mucus thus drying the mouth and throat. May be administered 2 hours before dental surgery.
- Hydrogen peroxide: Diluted and used as a mouthwash or irrigating solution.
- Cresol: Used topically to treat root canals and as an antiseptic.
- Tannic acid: Found in tea and may be used to stop bleeding.

PAIN CONTROL IN DENTISTRY

Reducing anxiety and controlling pain are essential in the dental practice. Anxiety and depression can increase a patient's tolerance to analgesics. Horace Wells, who discovered the use of nitrous oxide in 1844, introduced pain control.

In 1904, an ester type of local anesthetic was introduced followed in 1948 by an amine type of local anesthetic, which was hypoallergenic. Electronic anesthesia, introduced in the 1990s, is the most recent form of pain control. Injectable local anesthetics are an effective and frequently used method of pain control. However, many patients are anxious about the injection process, postoperative numbness, and possible allergic responses. Therefore hypnosis and electronic anesthesia are alternatives to anesthetic injection. When discussing pain control, several terms are important to remember.

Analgesia

A reduction in pain without producing unconsciousness.

Anesthesia

Total or partial loss of physical sensation.

The term **analgesia** refers to a reduction in a reflex reaction caused by a painful stimulus (nociception). The reaction can be relative or absolute in its intensity. **Anesthesia** relates to the loss of sensory perception that can be accomplished on a local or peripheral basis by local anesthetic drugs that do not significantly alter consciousness with conventional dosage or on a general or central basis by general anesthetics that also produce an unconscious state.

The two principle classes of analgesic agents are narcotics and nonnarcotics. Consciousness can be altered through use of electronic anesthesia, analgesics, anxiolysis, sedation, or hypnosis. Electronic anesthesia provides nerve stimulation to control pain. Analgesic drugs dull the perception of pain and can be nonnarcotic or narcotic. Anxiolysis provides noticeable reduction of anxiety with little or no apparent drowsiness. Sedation causes noticeable change in awareness often characterized by drooping eyelids or slurred speech. Hypnosis produces a state of sleep.

Electronic Anesthesia

Today, an estimated 300 million local anesthetic injections are administered annually in the United States. Approximately 47 million people are considered dentally anxious. Some of their fears may be relieved by electronic anesthesia. Electric nerve stimulators have been developed, which can control pain. These units, called *transcutaneous electrical nerve stimulators* (TENS), have been used in medical fields to control acute, chronic, and postsurgical pain for several years. The unit provides a signal that intercepts pain sensation.

This system provides an anesthetic alternative for cavity and crown and bridge preparation and cementation procedures. Electronic nerve stimulators provide dental assistants and dental hygienists with a safe and easy-to-use anesthetic

system for restorative and preventive procedures, saving time for the dentist (Box 14.1).

Because electronic anesthesia is new to most patients, patients should know that it is operated by a 9-volt battery and is perfectly safe to use. The electrodes that are placed on the face would be referred to as *pads* or *patches*. Let the patient know that a tingling feeling will occur as the anesthesia begins and a quivering in the muscle will take place when anesthesia has reached the needed level. The patient should know that the dial can be turned up to remove any discomfort during the procedure and another anesthesia can be administered if needed.

Analgesics

Analgesics reduce or abolish pain without producing unconsciousness. Analgesics can be strong, moderate, or mild. These drugs act by blocking transmission of pain senses or they can increase a patient's pain threshold and reduce the ability to feel the pain sensation.

Mild Analgesics

Mild analgesics are used for the relief of low intensity pain, such as headaches and most common dental procedures. Mild analgesics are not addictive and have minimal side effects in healthy patients and are available without prescription. Examples of these drugs are the acetylsalicylic acids (aspirin), such as Bayer aspirin, Bufferin, Empirin, Ibuprofen (Motrin), and acetaminophen (Tylenol). The class of drugs known as *nonsteriod antiinflammatory drugs (NSAIDS)*, to which ibuprofen belongs, includes many of the newer brand names such as Ansaid, Aleve, Anaprox, Naprosyn, and Toradol.

Moderate-to-Strong Analgesics

Moderate-to-strong pain is often controlled by a combination of a mild analgesic and a narcotic such as codeine. These drugs are called *opioids* or *opium derivatives*. A brand name example is Tylenol with codeine, Fiorinol with codeine, Empirin with codeine, Anaprox, Nasprosyn, Darvon, Darvocet, Advil, Motrin, and Nuprin. Narcotic drugs used as strong analgesics are capable of producing physical and psychologic dependence and their continued long-term use should be prescribed with caution. However, appropriate medication for adequate pain relief should not preclude the proper use of available drugs. Unrelieved pain should not be a requisite of clinical dental practice.

Codeine is often used when an analgesic stronger than aspirin or a similar drug is required. Codeine is generally used in combination with aspirin or acetaminophen. This combination increases the pain-relieving effects of both drugs and permits the use of smaller qualities of both drugs. Oxycodone (Percodan) and hydrocodone (Lortab) are codeine

Box 14.1

Procedure

Procedure for Using Electronic Anesthesia

1. Explain the use of electronic anesthesia to new patients (Figure 14.1, *A*).
2. Wipe the pad placement site with alcohol to remove facial oils and makeup and dry the skin.
3. Open the foil pouch and insert the slide-lock connectors into the electrode pad. Make sure the pouch is folded closed to prevent dehydration of the pads and maintain adhesion and conductivity.
4. To eliminate surprising the patient, make sure the amplitude knobs are turned off and the light is not glowing.
5. Have the patient's mouth open to adjust facial tissue changes to attached pad and place negative (green) electrode pad on treatment side of the face for greater stimulation (at least $^1/_2$ inch between the pads) and plug lead wire into output jack.
6. Place the pads at the apices of the upper bicuspids just below the zygoma for treatment on mandibular teeth (Figure 14.1, *B*).
7. Place the pads at the apices of the upper bicuspids just below the zygoma for treatment on maxillary teeth (Figure 14.1, *C*).
8. The patient or operator will gradually increase the amplitude until the patient feels significant tingling. Pause for 20 to 30 seconds between increases of amplitude for the body to accommodate the stimulation. Minimum therapeutic level is reached when the operator can visually observe muscle contractions, approximately 2 to 5 minutes. Stimulation can be increased as necessary to "dial out discomfort."
9. Always turn the unit off when removing or relocating the pads or storing the stimulator.
10. When completed, you should gently pull the pads while supporting the skin tissue and dispose them. Clean the outer case with rubbing alcohol and do not immerse in water; clean the leads with mild soap and water (Figure 14.1, *D*).

derivatives often used for moderate-to-severe pain. Meperidine (Demerol) is also widely used in dentistry. Strong analgesics include Demerol, Percocet, Percodan, Tylax, Vicodin, and Dalophine.

Anxiolytics and Sedatives

The major classes of the drugs differ in mechanism of action but the sedative effects are similar and dose-dependent. Sedatives are used routinely in dentistry to produce a calming-to-unarrousable affect for the relief of apprehension. However, they may produce paradoxical excitation (arousal or opposite effect). Sedation depresses the central nervous system (CNS). This group of drugs is comprised of the barbiturates, benzodiazepines, and antihistamines. Benzodiazepines have unsurpassed sedative and anxiolytic efficacy and a higher therapeutic index than barbiturates. An example of a benzodiazepine is diazepam (Valium). Midazolam (Versed) is another useful benzodiazepine often employed in intravenous sedation. Because the barbiturates have no advantage over the benzodiazepines, their

use has diminished in modern practice. Chloral hydrate, an antihistamine previously used for sedation in pediatric dentistry, is irritating to the gastrointestinal tract and often exhibits paradoxical responses similar to the barbiturates. The primary use of a barbiturate in dentistry is to produce drowsiness or sleep and to calm an excitable patient during treatment (Box 14.2).

Intravenous Sedation

IV sedation involves the use of drugs administered directly into the vein to produce light conscious or deep sedation for achieving preoperative sedation. IV sedation requires advanced training for the doctor administering this technique and usually requires a specific license or permit in most states. Midazolam (Versed) is a popular drug for this use. In addition to controlling anxiety, this drug also produces amnesia so that the patient does not remember much of what occurred during treatment. The onset of sedation with this drug is usually within 30 seconds. Much of the safety associated with IV sedation is that the patient remains conscious and will respond verbally to instructions

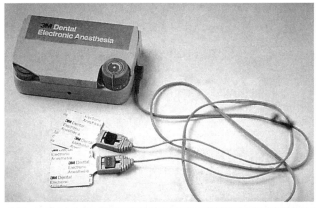

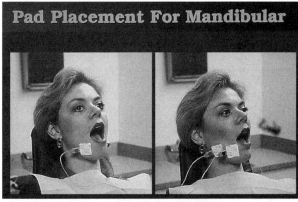

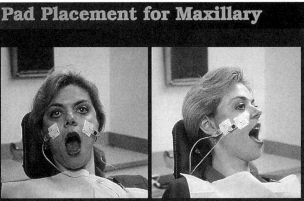

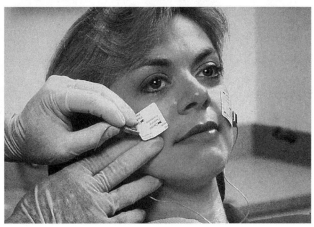

FIGURE 14.1

A, Electronic anesthesia. **B**, Mandibular pad placement. **C**, Maxillary pad placement. **D**, To remove, gently pull the pads while supporting the skin tissue. (Courtesy 3M)

Box 14.2

Sedation Levels

Level I
Awake and calm (no evidence of drowsiness)

Level II
Awake but sedated (slowed or slurred speech)

Level III
Asleep but easily aroused (verbally)

Level IV
Asleep but difficult to arouse (shake/shout)

Level V
Asleep and unarousable (except by surgical stimulus)

Light sedation would describe Levels I and II, with occasional drifting to Level III.
Deep sedation would describe Levels IV and V.
General anesthesia is described in Chapter 27.

given by the doctor. These patients require proper monitoring of their vital signs, including pulse oximetry, and the dental team must be prepared to act quickly and appropriately in the event of an emergency. Because intravenous sedation necessitates adequate perfusion, ventilation, and oxygenation, adequate local anesthesia is preferred whenever possible.

Nitrous Oxide Sedation

A combination of nitrous oxide and oxygen gases is used to achieve conscious sedation and analgesia. Nitrous oxide will reduce sensations of pain, discomfort, or gagging that the patient may experience during dental treatment. Nitrous oxide sedation acts to relieve psychologic stresses and apprehension and relaxes the patient, but pain control still depends on the effective use of local anesthesia. The nitrous oxide and oxygen mixture will increase the percentage of oxygen that the patient is breathing. This will increase the oxygen supply to the heart. As with all types of sedation, adequate pain control should rely on adequate, effective local anesthesia.

Box 14.3 — *Procedure*

Procedure for Assisting the Dentist in Nitrous Oxide Administration

Materials needed
Full nitrous oxide and oxygen tanks
Mask and proper tubing
Informed consent form
Patient record

1 Check the tanks of nitrous oxide and oxygen to ensure that the tanks are sufficiently full and operational (Figure 14.2, *A*).
2 Choose the proper mask and attach it to the unit tubing.
3 Recline the patient in the dental chair and describe the effects and sensations of nitrous oxide sedation.
4 Secure informed consent.
5 Instruct the patient to breathe normally during the procedure.
6 Start the flow of oxygen and place the mask comfortably over the patient's nose (Figure 14.2, *B*).
7 Adjust the flow of 100% oxygen to 5 to 8 L for approximately 1 minute.
8 Observe the rubber bag on the gas unit that indicates the patient's breathing volume.
9 Increase the nitrous oxide at the rate of 1 L per minute while the oxygen flow is decreased at a similar rate.
10 Determine how the patient feels.
11 When the desired level of sedation is achieved, administer the local anesthetic and begin dental procedure (Figure 14.2, *C*).
12 Return the nitrous oxide control to 0 and the oxygen flow to 5 to 8 L for 5 to 10 minutes to stabilize the patient.
13 Remove the patient's mask and confirm how the patient feels.
14 Record the levels of gases in the patient's chart (important for medical-legal purposes).

Under the Dental Practice Act in some states, the assistant is allowed to aid in the administration of nitrous oxide under the direct supervision of the dentist. Although nitrous oxide sedation has a good safety record, proper technique is necessary. Nitrous oxide sedation can be a pleasant experience for most patients, but nitrous oxide is a drug and not intended for recreational purposes or chronic use by dental personnel. Significant side effects and spontaneous abortions have been reported by continued exposure to nitrous oxide. All equipment should meet current safety standards including the use of a scavenging system to remove gases. The patient's mask should fit snugly, and high volume evacuation should be employed during treatment to reduce ambient levels of nitrous oxide exhaled by the patient.

Nitrous Oxide Equipment

The office may be equipped with built-in or mobile equipment in the treatment rooms. Both types of equipment are the same except for the size of the tanks of gas. In addition to the tanks in use a reserve tank of oxygen should be available. In most states, nitrous oxide has to be ordered by the doctor. It is also necessary to comply with OSHA and state requirements for safe installation and storage of these supplies.

Nitrous oxide is supplied in blue tanks and oxygen is supplied in green tanks. The gases are dispensed through controls and gauges attached to the unit. The flow of gases is measured in liters per minute. During the procedure, the patient is maintained at a maximum of 6 to 7 L of combined gases. The equipment also includes a rubber bag, which is partially inflated during the administration of the gases.

The gases are administered through a scavenging mask that fits snugly over the patient's nose. Masks are available in different sizes to accommodate adults and children. The mask may be either disposable or sanitized before reuse and should fit snugly on the patient's face to prevent gaps around the edges (Box 14.3 and Table 14.2).

ANESTHESIA

Several methods are used in dentistry to achieve anesthesia and pain control. This one aspect of dentistry is important in all dental procedures. Depending on the patients and their needs, the dentist may perform one of the following methods of anesthesia to achieve pain control.

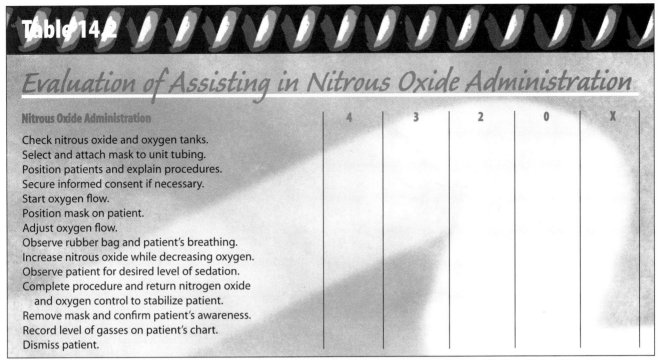

Table 14.2

Evaluation of Assisting in Nitrous Oxide Administration

Nitrous Oxide Administration	4	3	2	0	X
Check nitrous oxide and oxygen tanks.					
Select and attach mask to unit tubing.					
Position patients and explain procedures.					
Secure informed consent if necessary.					
Start oxygen flow.					
Position mask on patient.					
Adjust oxygen flow.					
Observe rubber bag and patient's breathing.					
Increase nitrous oxide while decreasing oxygen.					
Observe patient for desired level of sedation.					
Complete procedure and return nitrogen oxide and oxygen control to stabilize patient.					
Remove mask and confirm patient's awareness.					
Record level of gasses on patient's chart.					
Dismiss patient.					

The numeric criteria: 4 Excellent; 3 Good but some improvement can be made; 2 Below average, usable, needs to improve skill; 0 Unsatisfactory; X Not able to evaluate.

General Anesthesia

General anesthesia is the most desirable in terms of control and reaction from the patient and it carries the greatest risks to the patient's health and safety. A qualified anesthesiologist specially trained in anesthesia most often, safety, administers this method in a hospital setting. Emergency life-support equipment is immediately available if ever the need arises. Most procedures in dentistry also require the use of a local anesthetic in addition to the general anesthetic given. This is done to help control local bleeding and immediate postoperative pain. The patient requires less general anesthesia when local anesthesia is used in conjunction (see Chapter 27).

Local Anesthesia Combined with Oral Sedation or Injection Medication

Oral sedation medication acts to lessen the anxiety and fear that accompanies a patient on the trip to the dentist and the procedures performed. The oral sedation, which is also combined with a local anesthesia, helps the patient to relax and feel drowsy and pain free. The patient is issued a prescription for the premedication, which is usually taken before the dental procedure. It can also be administered at the time of the procedure but takes time to achieve the same desired effects. Oral sedation is unpredictable in effect and should therefore be administered in advance of the scheduled procedures to achieve reasonable predictability. Oral sedation is usually in the form of a tablet, capsule, powder, or liquid. Sedation may be achieved by intramuscular or intravenous injection, which requires advanced training. Whenever patients receive sedation, they should not be left alone or allowed to travel until the effects have decreased.

Local Anesthesia

Local anesthetic agents are the most frequently used form of pain control in dentistry. These agents provide safe, effective, and dependable anesthesia of suitable duration for virtually all forms of dental surgery. Local anesthesia that anesthetizes only the area being treated is relatively easily administered and has an excellent safety record. Several local anesthetic agents commonly used for dental treatment include the following:

- Zylocaine (with epinephrine)
- Zylocaine (without epinephrine)
- Carbocaine
- Octocaine
- Procaine
- Oracaine

Some patients are hypersensitive to these drugs. Therefore another anesthetic may be administered. For instance, zylocaine and Carbocaine are both amide types of local anesthetic. Neither drug can be used for a patient hypersensitive to amide-types of local anesthetics. The two most frequently used forms of local anesthesia administration

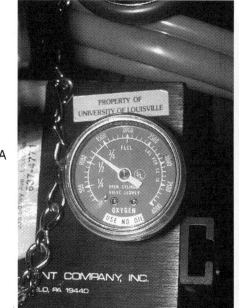
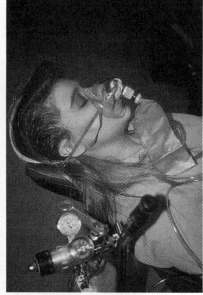
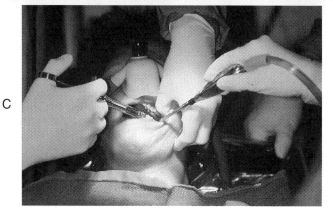

FIGURE 14.2

Assisting in the administration of nitrous oxide. **A,** The gauge indicates the level of gas remaining in the tanks. **B,** When the oxygen is started, the mask should be placed comfortably over the patient's nose. **C,** When the desired level of sedation is achieved, local anesthesia can be applied and the dental procedure can proceed.

are infiltration anesthesia and block anesthesia. General armamentarium used with local anesthesia include the following:
- Aspirating syringe
- Two capules of topical anesthesia
- Disposable needle
- Two cotton tip applicators
- Three 2x2 gauze
- Needle guard

The procedure for administering local anesthetics will be discussed later in this chapter (Box 14.6).

Topical Anesthetics

Topical anesthetics are used directly on the tissues to provide temporary anesthesia. The topical anesthetic ointment is the most popular method to provide mucosa anesthesia or temporary numbness of the gingiva tissue before introducing the needle or for temporary relief from the pain of oral injuries. Topical anesthetic ointment is placed with a cotton tip applicator directly on the injection site to anesthetize or numb the tissue. Approximately 2 to 5 minutes are required for optimum effectiveness because the rate of onset of topical anesthesia is slow.

Box 14.4

Supraperiosteal Injection Sites*

Posterior superior alveolar injection (Figure 14.3, A)
Middle superior alveolar injection (Figure 14.3, B)
Anterior superior alveolar injection (Figure 14.3, C)
Maxillary central incisor (Figure 14.3, D)
Maxillary lateral incisor (Figure 14.3, E)
Maxillary cuspid (Figure 14.3, F)
Maxillary first bicuspid (Figure 14.3, G)
Maxillary second bicuspid and mesiobuccal first molar
   (Figure 14.3, H)
Mandibular incisor (Figure 14.3, I)

*Dark indicator pinpoints injection site.

Liquid topical anesthetics are thick liquids containing flavoring agents. They are also available in flavored spray aerosols. The liquid can be placed directly into the patient's mouth to swish or if the patient has a gag reflex, the spray can be applied to a single area to the intraoral tissues before taking impressions or radiographs. Liquid topical anesthetics (Diclone) that have low viscosity and are tasteless, odorless, and are significantly effective can also be used.

Infiltration of Anesthesia or Supraperiosteal Injections

To obtain anesthesia, using this method, the medication is placed directly into the soft tissues at the site of the dental procedure and near the involved tooth with a short needle. Infiltration is achievable and is primarily used in the maxillary teeth because of the porous nature of the alveolus cancellous bone. This bone, which supports the teeth in this region, has many tiny openings that allow the solution to spread through the bone towards the apices of the tooth where the nerve fibers enters the teeth. This method may also be used secondarily to block gingival tissues surrounding the mandibular teeth.

When an infiltration injection is needed in the anterior maxillary area, the upper lip is reflected upward and the bevel of the needle is inserted at the height of the gingiva at the mucobuccal fold, toward the bone. The medication is discharged slowly at the site where the needle enters the tissue. Anesthesia occurs rapidly after deposition of the solution, usually in 5 to 10 minutes (Box 14.4 and Figure 14.3).

Mandibular Block Anesthesia

As opposed to the maxillary cancellous bone, the mandibular bone is dense and compact and called *cortical* bone. Because this type of bone does not have many tiny openings that allow diffusion of anesthetic solution, profound anesthesia is impossible for the mandibular teeth and is con-traindicated; therefore block anesthesia is used for these teeth. However, the injection can be given to children under the age of 7 years. When this action is needed, the anesthetic solution is deposited in the region superior and medial (area of the lingual) to where the nerve vascular supply enters the mandibular canal. In this area, the blood supply enters and exits the mandible. This anesthetizes the teeth in the quadrant where injected plus half of the tongue and lower lip.

Because the inferior alveolar nerve is so close to the blood vessels, the dentist cautiously makes this injection so that the medication is not deposited directly into the blood stream, which could have serious adverse effects for the patient. To keep the medication from going into the blood stream, the dentist aspirates, which means to draw back, up, and in. If the needle is in a blood vessel when the dentist aspirates, blood can be seen entering the anesthetic cartridge. If this happens, the dentist repositions the needle before any more anesthetic is deposited. The operator may use a long or short needle. In general, depending on the anesthetic agent used, achieving profound anesthesia may take longer when locking a nerve than to obtain the same result when infiltrating. The patient may feel pins and needles or a warmth or tingling sensation in the lip moving from the corner of the mouth as it spreads to the middle of the lower lip. Half the tongue may also feel similar sensations. The patient may state that the lip feels large and swollen. Block injections are administered in the sites illustrated in Figure 14.4.

Periodontal Ligament Injection

The periodontal ligament injection is an alternative type of infiltration injection. The anesthetic solution is injected in a special syringe under pressure directly into the periodontal ligament and surrounding tissues (Box 14.5 and Figure 14.5). The onset of anesthesia is quick and the duration of action is relatively short. This type of injection is sometimes used as the primary method of anesthesia but more often is used as an adjunct to conventional techniques.

Intraseptal Technique

An intraseptal injection is used when ordinary injections fail to provide profound anesthesia to the pulp of a tooth. This technique allows the anesthetic to be injected into the cancellous bone between the teeth, directly contacting the nerve fibers where they enter into the apical foramen and periodontal membrane. This procedure is initiated by piercing the hard cortical plate of bone with a bur and entering into the cancellous bone. When proper depth is reached, the bur is removed, and the dentist injects the needle and anesthetic directly into this opening. Anesthesia should be immediate.

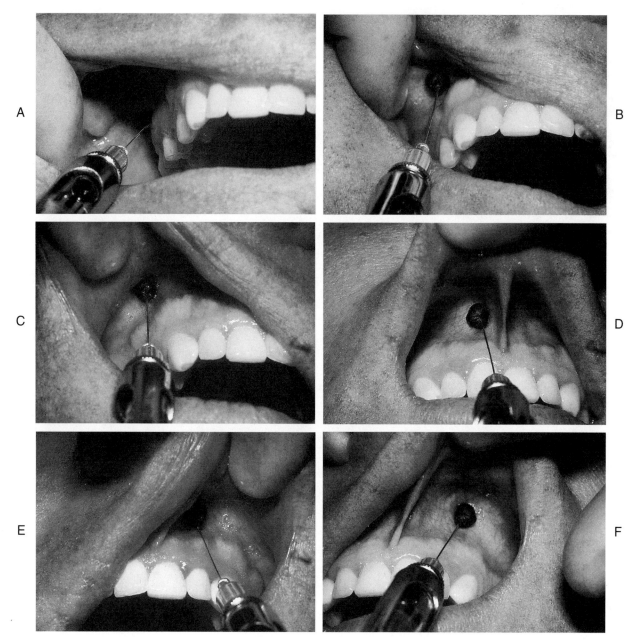

FIGURE 14.3

Supraperiosteal injection sites. **A**, Posterior superior alveolar injection. **B**, Middle superior alveolar injection. **C**, Anterior superior alveolar injection. **D**, Maxillary central incisor. **E**, Maxillary lateral incisor. **F**, Maxillary cuspid.

Intraosseous Injection

Intraosseous injection is sometimes used when other types of injections were unsatisfactory. It has the advantage of localized action as opposed to a block injection, which anesthetizes a larger area. Some patients prefer this one tooth numbness as opposed to the fat lip sensation. The anes-

thetic solution is injected though the gingival and cortical plate directly into the spongy portion of the bone. The needle fits on a standard syringe and has a sliding sleeve over the needle, which retracts into the needle body as the needle penetrates the tissues. The injection site is anterior to the tooth to be anesthetized and takes advantage of the thin interproximal bone.

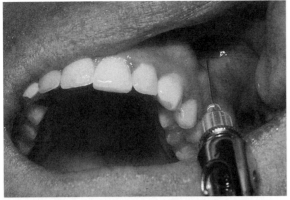

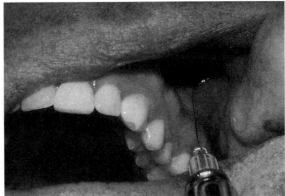

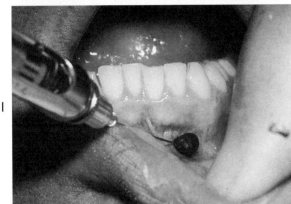

FIGURE 14.3, cont'd

Supraperiosteal injection sites. **G**, Maxillary first bicuspid. **H**, Maxillary second bicuspid and mesiobuccal first molar, I, mandibular incisor.

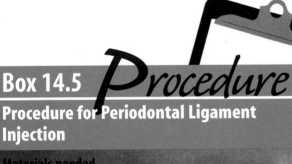

Box 14.5 *Procedure*

Procedure for Periodontal Ligament Injection

Materials needed
Topical anesthetic
Cotton tip applicator
2x2 gauze
Syringe
Anesthetic cartridge

1 Place topical anesthetic on the injection site.
2 Use sterile 2x2 gauze to grasp and hold the upper lip securely when giving the injection.
3 Remove the cap from the syrijet (Mark II by Mizzy, Inc) syringe.
4 Activate the lever.
5 Insert the cartridge (Figure 14.5, *A*).
6 Set the dial.
7 Place the syringe tip against the injection site and activate (Figure 14.5, *B*).

PARTS OF A SYRINGE

An anesthetic syringe used in dentistry may look somewhat different than a conventional syringe and is designed to work with cartridges (Figure 14.6). These same syringes are not designed to draw medications from a multidose vial of medication, as are conventional syringes

Syringe

The thumb ring, finger grip, and finger bar help the dentist have far greater control by using only one hand to aspirate on the needle entering the site of injection. The barrel of the syringe allows the cartridge to be loaded into the syringe and also holds the syringe in place. One side of the barrel is larger than the other for loading, and the opposite side has a window, which allows the operator to aspirate and view any blood cells entering the syringe. The piston rod pushes down the rubber stopper inside of the cartridge, which forces the solution out through the needle. To load the cartridge, a spring mechanism is provided inside the finger grip area allowing the piston rod to be pulled back thus loading the cartridge. The two types of local anesthetic syringes generally used in dentistry are the aspirating and self-aspirating syringes.

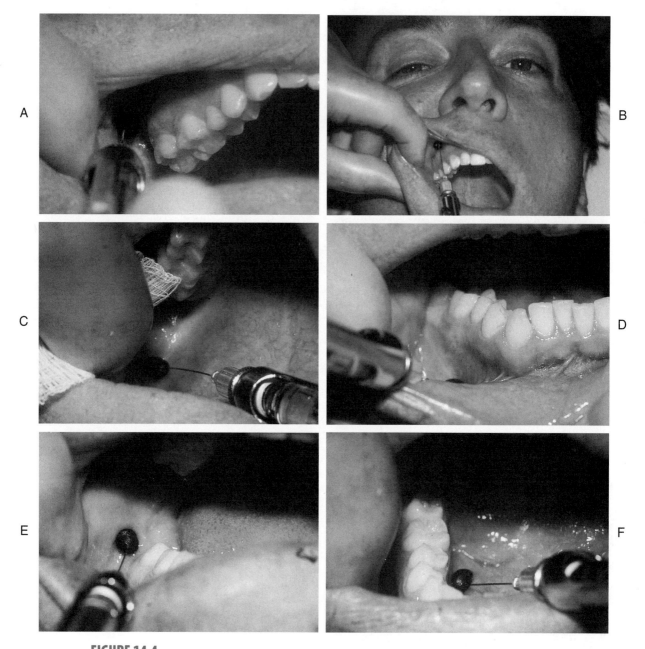

FIGURE 14.4

Block injection sites. **A**, Zygomatic. **B**, Infraorbital. **C**, Mandibular. **D**, Mental. **E**, Long buccal. **F**, Lingual.

Aspirating Syringe

The aspirating syringe has a small hook harpoon that attaches into the rubber stopper enabling the dentist to aspirate. This is accomplished by first loading the cartridge into the syringe and then tapping on the thumb ring with the heel of the hand forcefully, engaging the rubber stopper. The threaded tip allows the hub of the needle to be at-tached to the syringe. The shorter cartridge end of the needle passes through the small opening in the center of the threaded tip and punctures the rubber diaphragm on one end of the anesthetic cartridge. The syringe must be sterilized between patients, following guidelines for infection control.

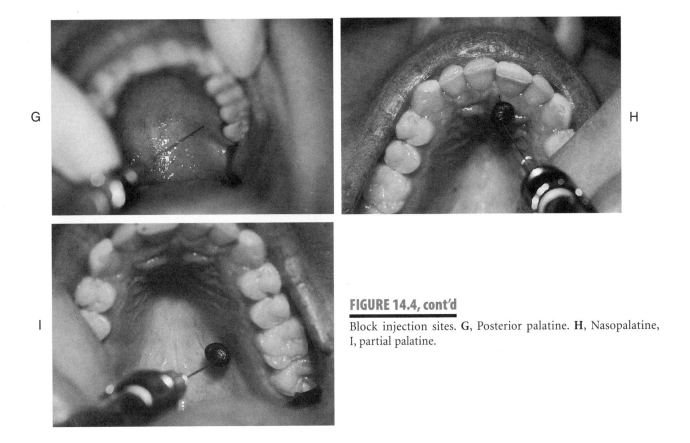

FIGURE 14.4, cont'd

Block injection sites. **G**, Posterior palatine. **H**, Nasopalatine, I, partial palatine.

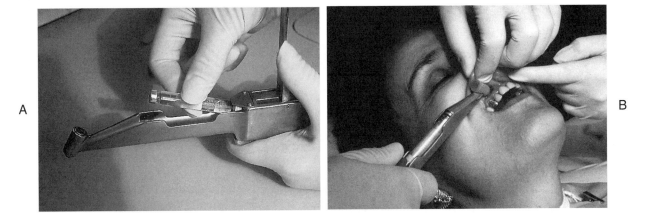

FIGURE 14.5

Periodontal ligament injection. **A**, Insertion of cartridge. **B**, Placement of syringe tip against the injection site and activation.

Self-Aspirating Syringe

Self-aspirating syringes do not have a harpoon to engage the rubber stopper. The syringe is designed to eliminate the procedures described earlier. This type of syringe has a barrel-shaped end on the piston rod instead of the harpoon (Figure 14.7). A small amount of anesthetic is released through the needle to eliminate air.

Cartridge

The cartridge has a rubber stopper on one end of the glass tube and a cap with a rubber diaphragm at the other end. The glass is encased in a clear plastic coating in case of breakage, preventing mishaps for the patient and dentist.

Needle

The needle consists of a short or cartridge ends and long or injection ends with the needle hub in the center. The needle itself is hollow through which the anesthetic solution flows. Two lengths are commonly used in dentistry, a

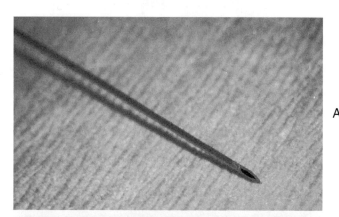

A

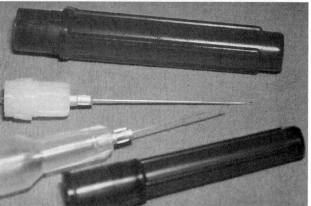

B

FIGURE 14-8

A, Close-up illustration of a beveled needle. **B,** Short and long needles with sheaths removed.

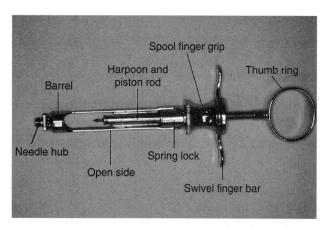

FIGURE 14.6

Parts of the aspirating anesthetic syringe used in dentistry.

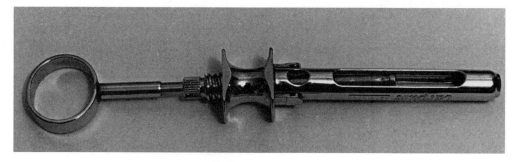

FIGURE 14.7

Self-aspirating syringe.

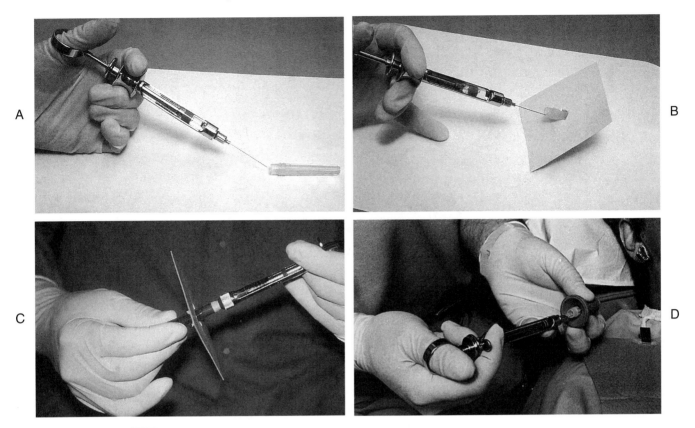

FIGURE 14.9

The needle cap should be replaced cautiously. **A,** One-handed technique with cap laying on a tabletop. **B,** One-handed technique using a safety shield. **C,** Two-handed technique using a safety shield. **D,** Safety cap holder.

1-inch or short needle for infiltration anesthesia, primarily in the maxilla, and a $1^5/_8$-inch or long needle for block anesthesia, primarily in the mandible. Short, $^5/_8$-inch and ultrashort, $^3/_8$-inch needles also exist. The needles are encased in a protective covering and are disposable. The protective plastic cap is sealed and is tamper-proof to ensure sterility. It consists of a plastic cap encasing the capsule and a needle guard that covers the needle itself. Needles are gaged, which refers to the thickness (lumen or bore) of the needle.

Gages are numbered so that the larger the gage number, the smaller and thinner the bore of the needle. The gage numbers range from 14 to 30. Gage numbers 25, 27, and 30 are the most commonly used. Figure 14.8 is a close-up illustration of a beveled needle.

Recapping Needle

Extreme care should be taken to avoid a needle stick, which most often occurs when recapping the needle. Self-capping syringe and needle designs are available to eliminate this risk. This is the time the health care providers are most likely to be stuck with a needle. Although a variety of techniques and devices for recapping can be used, the technique recommended by most safety and health agencies is the *scoop technique.* This is accomplished by making a scooping motion with the uncapped needle, sliding it into the needle sheath lying on a flat surface (Figure 14.9). If a needle stick should occur, the injury must be reported to the dentist immediately (Box 14.6). See Chapters 18 and 22 for more information on handling sharps.

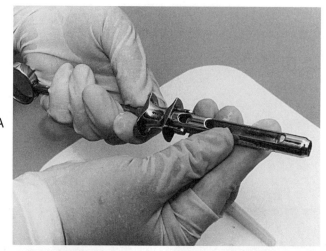

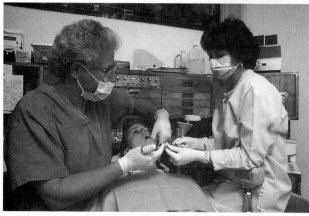

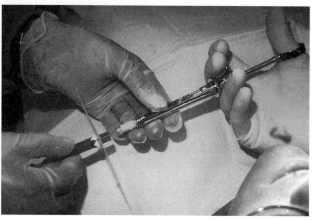

FIGURE 14.10

Procedures for administering local anesthetic. **A,** Unwrap the sterile syringe, hold the syringe in hand, and use the thumb ring or finger bar to pull the plunger (top-loading syringe). **B,** When passing the syringe to the dentist, the assistant places the thumb ring over the dentist's thumb and then the syringe is laid into the dentist's open hand. **C,** The assistant removes the needle guard.

CONSIDERATIONS WHEN ADMINISTERING ANESTHETICS

The success or effectiveness of providing anesthesia can depend on the condition of the surrounding tooth tissue (Table 14.3).

Paresthesia

When the effects of the anesthesia do not go away within a reasonable time after the patient receives dental care, pares-

thesia, or persistent anesthesia, has occurred. Although this happens infrequently it is a serious complication when it does occur. It is most often the result of damage to the nerve or surrounding tissues. Paresthesia usually resolves by itself without treatment in a matter of weeks. However, if the damage to the structures is severe enough, it may be permanent. The usual complaint is continued numbness several hours after receiving dental treatment. This can be a serious adverse effect, and the dentist should respond directly to the patient's questions concerning this occurrence. These conditions are often described on the postop instructions and may

Box 14.6

Procedure for Administering Local Anesthetics

Materials needed

Aspirating syringe
Two capules of topical anesthesia
Disposable needle
Two cotton tip applicators
Three 2×2 gauze
Needle guard

Application of topical anesthetic

1 Place the ointment or other medication on a sterile cotton-tipped applicator.
2 Dry the injection site with a dry gauze sponge.
3 Apply the ointment to the site.
4 Leave the applicator in place for 1 to 3 minutes before proceding with the injection.

Preparing the anesthetic syringe

5 Choose the syringe, needle, and type of anesthetic directed by the dentist.
6 Unwrap the sterile syringe. Hold the syringe in your hand and use the thumb ring to pull back the plunger (Figure 14.10, *A*).
7 With your other hand, load the anesthetic cartridge into the syringe. The rubber stopper end goes in first, toward the syringe.
8 Securely grasp the syringe in one hand. If using an aspirating syringe, use the other hand to apply firm pressure until the harpoon is engaged into the rubber stopper. (This step is not necessary when using a self-aspirating syringe.)

9 Remove the protective cap from the needle but do not remove the needle guard.
10 Screw the needle into position on the syringe.
11 Remove the needle guard and express a small amount to clear any air bubbles from the cartridge and needle.
12 Place the syringe on the tray ready for use and out of the patient's sight.

Passing the syringe

13 Loosen the needle guard but do not remove it.
14 The assistant receives the topical anesthetic applicator with one hand and passes the syringe with the other. The exchange should be made just under the patient's chin and out of the patient's line of vision.
15 When passing the syringe to the dentist, the assistant places the thumb ring over the dentist's thumb and then the syringe is laid into the dentist's open hand (Figure 14.10, *B*).
16 The assistant removes the needle guard (Figure 14.10, *C*).
17 When the injection is complete, the assistant receives the syringe and carefully replaces the needle cover. The one-handed capping technique is the most safe. Always use a safety shield when using the two-handed cap technique. A two-person capping technique can expose the assistant to unnecessary risk of possible injury and infection.

be included in the overall treatment informed consent (see Chapter 21).

Infected Areas

Infections generally make most anesthetics ineffective. The infection itself changes the environment of the surrounding tissues, rendering anesthesia difficult at best. This usually can be overcome by increasing the amount given or switching to different anesthetics. The dentist can also use a more central nerve block technique. The dentist needs to be aware of this and will usually discover this during the health history, which should be updated often.

Table 14-3

Evaluation of Assisting with Administration of Local Anesthetic

Administration of Local Anesthetic	4	3	2	0	X
Place topical on applicator.					
Dry injection site.					
Apply topical to site.					
Secure syringe and load anesthetic cartridge.					
Engage plunger into stopper.					
Remove protective cap from needle and place into syringe.					
Remove needle guard and express air bubbles.					
Place on tray.					
Loosen needle guard.					
Place syringe in operators hand and remove needle guard.					
Receive syringe and replace needle cover.					
Secure syringe on working area.					

The numeric criteria: 4 Excellent; 3 Good but some improvement can be made; 2 Below average, usable, needs to improve skill; 0 Unsatisfactory; X Not able to evaluate.

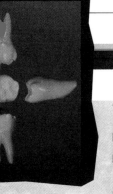

Points for Review

- Drug classifications
- Drug abuse and understanding law enforcement
- Routes of drug administration and the role of the dental assistant
- Methods of pain control and use of materials and equipment
- Considerations of anesthetic administration

Self-Study Questions

1. What is a generic drug?
   a. Chemical name of a specific drug
   b. Name of a registered drug given by the drug company
   c. A general name given to all drugs
   d. A and b
2. What is the name of the Act under which drugs are regulated?
   a. Drug Enforcement Act
   b. Schedule of Drugs Act
   c. Controlled Substances Act
   d. Dental Practice Act
3. What type of drug is recommended for dental procedures that may cause bleeding in high-risk patients?
   a. Antiviral agent
   b. Prophylactic antibiotic
   c. Epinephrine
   d. Antihistamine
4. What is a primary reason for combining two drugs such as codeine and acetaminophen?
   a. Increases pain relief
   b. Reduces drug dependency
   c. Reduces stomach upset
   d. None of the above
5. What color is the nitrous oxide tank?
   a. Green
   b. Red
   c. Blue
   d. Black

6. What are the two most frequently used forms of local anesthesia for dental treatment?
   a. Infiltration
   b. Block
   c. Nitrous
   d. A and b
7. What is the reason the operator aspirates before injecting local anesthetic?
   a. To prevent injecting anesthetic directly into the blood stream
   b. To remove air from the cartridge
   c. To prevent bleeding in high-risk patients
   d. None of the above
8. How can an accidental needle stick be prevented?
   a. Do not recap
   b. Use the one-handed scoop technique
   c. Use a needle shield
   d. All of the above
9. What is the major contraindication for use of tetracycline during pregnancy?
   a. Discoloration of mother's teeth
   b. Discoloration of newborn's teeth
   c. Miscarriage
   d. All of the above
10. What route of sedation administration can determine the exact dose needed?
    a. Oral
    b. Subcutaneous
    c. Intravenous
    d. Sublingual

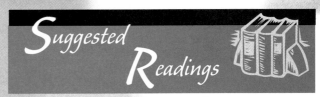

Suggested Readings

2000 Mosby's GenRx, ed 10, St Louis, 1999, Mosby.

Anderson JA: Reversal agents in sedation and anesthesia, *Anesth Prog* 35:43-47, 1988.

Becker DE: The respiratory effects of drugs used for conscious sedation and general anesthesia, *JADA* 119:153-156, 1989.

Becker DE: Pharmacological considerations for conscious sedation: clinical applications of receptor function, *Anesth Prog* 38:33-38, 1991.

Clark MS, Brunick AL: *Handbook of nitrous oxide and oxygen sedation*, St Louis, 1998, Mosby.

Cook-Waite Laboratories: *Manual of local anesthesia in dentistry*, New York, 1990, Waite Laboratories, Inc.

Drug Facts and Comparisons: *Facts and comparisons*, St Louis, 2000, Mosby.

Malamed SF: *Handbook of local anesthesia*, ed 4, St Louis, 1997, Mosby.

Malamed SF: *Sedation: a guide to patient management*, ed 4, St Louis, Mosby (in press).

Unit IV

Clinical Principles and Techniques

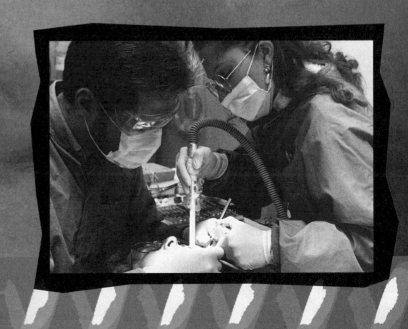

Chapter 15

Dental Materials and Clinical Application

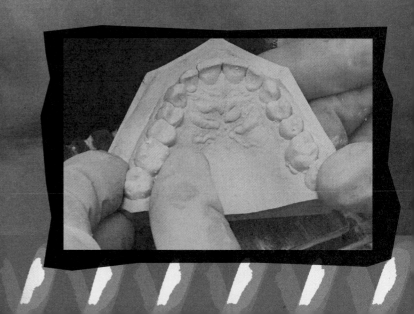

Chapter Outline

Dental Materials
Properties of Dental Materials
Dental Cements
   Zinc phosphate cement
   Polycarboxylate cement
   Zinc oxide-eugenol cement
   Calcium hydroxide
   Dental varnishes
   Glass-ionomer cements
   Resin cements
   Bonding agents
Dental Amalgam
   Mercury

Resin-Based Restorative Materials
   Polymerization shrinkage
   Adhesion to tooth structure
Impression Materials
   Impression trays
   Boxing impressions
   Custom trays
   Elastomeric impression materials
   Hydrocolloid impression materials
   Irreversible hydrocolloid-alginate
   Reversible hydrocolloids
   Waxes
   Gypsum

Learning Objectives

On completion of Chapter 15, the student should be able to do the following:

- Define key terms.
- List the factors that contribute to adhesion.
- List the major types of cements and important properties of each.
- Describe the types of amalgam alloy available and their advantages and disadvantages.
- Describe the types of composite resin available and their differences.
- Describe the nature of reversible and irreversible hydrocolloids.
- List and describe the categories of elastomeric impression materials.
- Describe the various dental gypsum products and their properties.

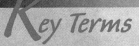

Key Terms

Activator or Catalyst	Corrosion	Retarder
Adherent	Dew Point	Sealer
Alloys	Exothermic	Sedative or Obtundent
Base	Expansion	Solution
Buffer	Initiator	
Contraction	Liner	

Box 15.1

Procedure

Procedures and General Safety Instructions for Working in the Dental Laboratory

Precautions when using gas

1. Make sure the rubber tubing is properly attached before opening gas outlets.
2. Always light the match before opening the gas jet.
3. Close the jet at once if flame should go out.
4. Do not place flame near any inflammable object.
5. Keep face away from Bunsen burner when lighting.
6. Do not smoke.

Precautions when using equipment and tools

1. Keep instruments out of pockets. Do not allow pockets to become "tool chests."
2. Turn off all power equipment before leaving it.
3. Change wheels and brushes at low speeds or when the machine is in the "off" position. Automatic chucks can be used on lathes.
4. Do not allow long hair to be caught in running equipment.
5. Grasp electric plugs not the cord when inserting and removing the plugs.

6. Use safety glasses when using a handpiece, lathe, model trimmer, or other similar equipment.
7. Keep floors clean and wipe any liquids immediately. Powders will track throughout laboratory and clinic and may be slippery.
8. Report any injuries such as hands, fingers, or arms becoming irritated to dentist or office manager.

Precautions when using acids

1. Keep acid pickling jars covered at all times when not in use.
2. Do not lean over the jars and avoid breathing fumes.
3. Do not remove any object with fingers; use only special forceps designed for that purpose.
4. Immediately wash with copious amount of water if acid should splash on face or hands and report such an accident immediately. Sodium bicarbonate (baking soda) will neutralize acid.

DENTAL MATERIALS

Dental materials are the bonding agents, cements, amalgam, metals, plastics, porcelain, impression materials, stones, polishing agents, and waxes used by the dentist or other dental personnel in treating patients. These materials generally fall into the following two categories:

1 Those that are placed in the mouth
2 Those that are used in the laboratory during the fabrication of intraoral appliances (dentures, bridges, crowns, and removable partial dentures)

Certain safety precautions should be followed when working in the laboratory (Box 15.1).

PROPERTIES OF DENTAL MATERIALS

The American Dental Association (ADA) has developed standard tests to measure the properties of dental materials.

A specification list refers to the standardized test methods and required minimum results essential for successful performance of a material. The specifications ensure the quality of the material, and if the material complies, it receives the seal of acceptance or certification that can be displayed on the label as certified by the ADA. However, the operator will determine which material to use for the procedure according to the physical, mechanical, chemical, and biological properties.

Physical properties refer to thermal conductivity and expansion, optical qualities, and electrical conductivity. For example, metals conduct heat and cold quickly through a material and may produce sensitivity, whereas plastic and porcelain are poor thermal conductors. Therefore insulating cement may be used in deep cavities to protect the pulp. Also heat will cause expansion of materials and cooling will produce contraction. Waxes and plastics have high coefficients of expansion and porcelain has a relatively low expansion. Optical factors such as color, shade, translucency, opacity, and lighting conditions affect the appearance of a restoration.

This is why tooth-colored materials such as composites are preferred over metal restorations in the anterior teeth. Electrical currents may be produced by the presence of two different metals in the acidic saliva, such as gold and amalgam restorations in the mouth. The electrical flow from one material to the other through the tooth can cause a shocking pain (galvanism) to the patient. Corrosion from this phenomenon may affect the material by causing discoloration or tarnish.

Mechanical properties involve the internal reaction (response or strength) of a material to outside (external) forces that cause the material to deform or break. Materials must have high compressive strength or hardness to withstand biting forces and high tensile strength to resist stretching, permanent indentation, and fracture under pressure. Therefore the operator usually uses amalgam, gold, or a high-strength composite material in posterior restorations.

Chemical properties concern corrosion and absorption of fluids. Ideally, dental materials should not adversely react with other materials they touch. For instance, some mouth rinses contain alcohol, which may dissolve some resin restorations, and some resins may absorb water or other fluids leading to discoloration, swelling, or bacteria contamination.

Dental materials also have biological properties because they are placed in the mouth and should be compatible with mouth fluids and other conditions to not adversely affect oral tissues. Because materials are composed of a wide variety of chemicals such as metals and resins, they may have allergic or systemic effects on the patient. Dental personnel should be aware of the potential adverse affects on the patient to minimize any risk to the patient and also be prepared if an allergic reaction does occur.

DENTAL CEMENTS

Cement has been used in dentistry to describe a number of materials that are used as luting agents to bond restorations to the tooth. Cavity **liners** and bases are placed in cavities to

Liner

A material used to line or seal a cavity preparation to protect the pulp.

protect the pulp; periodontal dressings are used to cover surgical sites; and restorative materials are used. No one cement has been developed that can meet the requirements of all of these uses. Cements should generally possess high strength, biocompatibility, and low solubility. Most cements can be mixed to varying consistencies depending on their intended use. In general, the strength of a cement can be controlled by the amount of powder that is added to the liquid. For instance, a cement is stronger as more powder is added into the liquid. The amount of powder added to the liquid also controls the cement's hardness, solubility, setting time, and dimensional change. The setting time is controlled in the following ways:

Table 15.1

Uses of Dental Cements

Type	Use	Name
Luting	Cement crowns or orthodontic appliances	Zinc oxide-eugenol
		Zinc oxide-no eugenol
		Zinc phosphate
		Zinc polycarboxylate
		Glass-ionomer
Bases	Insulators	Zinc oxide-eugenol
		Zinc oxide-no eugenol
		Zinc polycarboxylate
		Glass-ionomer
Liners	Sealers	Zinc oxide-eugenol
		Calcium hydroxide
		Glass-ionomer
	Varnishes	Copalite
		Copal
		Copanol
Temporary	Fillings	Zinc oxide-eugenol
		Zinc oxide-no eugenol
Pulp capping	Endodontic treatment	Zinc oxide-eugenol
		Zinc oxide-no eugenol
Tissue dress	Periodontal treatment	Zinc oxide-eugenol
		Zinc oxide-no eugenol

- Temperature of the slab
- Moisture contamination
- Particle size of the powder
- Rate of incorporation of the powder into the liquid
- Amount of **retarder** used

If the material is to be used for luting a restoration, it is mixed to a thin fluid consistency that will adapt to the restoration and the tooth. Materials used as a **base** or restoration are normally mixed to a stiff, putty-like consistency. See Tables 15.1 and 15.2 for a reference of the type, use, and name of dental cements.

Retarder

A chemical that slows the rate of a reaction.

Base

The main ingredient of a material or a type of cement placed on the pulpal floor of a cavity prep to form a base or bulk of material.

Zinc Phosphate Cement

Zinc phosphate cement has been used for many years in dentistry and still remains popular with many practitioners. It is

Table 15.2

Dental Materials

Material	Composition	Use	Proportions	Mixing Utensil	Spatula	Working (W), Setting (S) Times	Division	Manipulation	Consistency	Placement
Gypsum products										
Plaster	$CaSO_4 \times \frac{1}{2} H_2O$	Study models	Water: 45-50 ml Powder: 100 gm	Flexible bowl	Stiff	W:60 sec S:8-16 min	Add powder to liquid	Vigorous stirring	Putty-like	Place in impression with spatula
Dental stone	$CaSO_4 \times \frac{1}{2} H_2O$	Casts	Water: 30-32 ml Powder: 100 gm	Vacuum mixer		W:60 sec S:8-16 min	Same	Same	Same	Same
High-strength dental stone	$CaSO_4 \times \frac{1}{2} H_2O$	Dies	Water: 19-24 ml Powder: 100 gm	Vacuum mixer		Same	Same	Same	Same	Same
Composites										
Composite resin (self-cured)	Two pastes: bis-GMA or UDMA + fillers + amine. Bis-GMA or UDMA + fillers + peroxide	Esthetic filling	Equal volumes of both pastes	Paper pad	Stiff plastic	W:60 sec S:2-4 min	Mix two pastes	Vigorous spatulation	Thick	Small placement instrument or directly injected into cavity
Composite resin (light-cured)	One paste: bis-GMA or UDMA + fillers + diketone	Esthetic filling	None	Paper pad	None	W:Extended S:20 sec	None	None	Thick	Same as above
Impressions										
Alginate	Sodium alginate + $CaSO_4 \times \frac{1}{2} H_2O$ + sodium phosphate	Impression for study models, some casts	Powder: one scoop Water: one vial	Flexible bowl	Stiff	W:2-5 min S:3-5 min	Add powder to water	Vigorous spatulation	Creamy	Place in tray with spatula
Polysulfide	Two pastes: polysulfide + filler Lead dioxide + filler	Final impression	Equal lengths of pastes	Large paper pad	Stiff	W:5-7 min S:8-12 min		Vigorous spatulation	Varies	Same as above
Addition silicone	Two pastes: vinyl siloxane Silane + chloroplatinic acid	Final impression	Equal lengths of pastes	Large paper pad or automix	Stiff	W:2-4.5 min S:3-7 min		Vigorous spatulation	Varies	Same as above

Material	Composition	Use	Ratio	Mixing surface	Consistency	Time	Technique	Mix	Placement
Consensation silicone	Two pastes or paste and liquid: polydimethyl siloxane + fillers Tin octoate	Final impression	See directions	Large paper pad or automix	Stiff	W:2-5 min S:3-7 min	Vigorous spatulation	Varies	Same as above
Polyether	Two pastes: polyether + fillers Sulfonic ester + thickener	Final impression	Equal lengths of pastes	Large paper pad	Stiff	W:2-3 min S:6-7 min	Vigorous spatulation	Varies	Same as above
Cements									
Dycal (calcium hydroxide)	Two pastes	Liner, pulp protection, direct cap (Stimulates secondary dentin)	Equal lengths of pastes	Treated paper pad	Stiff	W:60 sec S:1-2 min	Stirring motion for 10 sec	Creamy	Thin layer placed in cavity with small placement instrument
Zinc-oxide Eugenol	Paste:zinc oxide Liquid:eugenol, oil of cloves	Linner, pulp protection obtundent base, temporary, root canal, perio dressing	1:1 See directions	Treated paper pad	Stiff	W:30-60 sec S:7-9 min	Mix half portion of powder into liquid, then smaller portions / Divide powder in three portions	Creamy to putty-like	Varies with use
Zinc phosphate	Paste:zinc oxide Liquid:phosphoric acid	Luting base	See directions	Cool glass slab (above dew point)	Stiff	W:90 sec S:5-9 min	Mix increments from small to large over large area of the slab / Divide powder into several portions	Base: thick Luting:creamy	See directions
Zinc polycarboxylate	Paste:zinc oxide Liquid:polyacrylic acid	Luting	See directions	Paper pad	Stiff	W:2-3 min S:7-9 min	Mix all powder into liquid at one time; mix for 30 sec	Creamy	See directions
Glass-ionomer	Paste:fluorosilicate glass Liquid:polyacrylic acid	Pulp protection, luting, restoration	Varies by use	Chilled glass slab or paper pad	Stiff	W:2 min S:6-8 min	Mix half of powder into liquid at a time / Divide powder in two portions	Base:thick Luting:creamy	See directions
Alloys									
Amalgam	Paste:Ag-Sn and Ag-Cu Liquid:Mercury	Restoration	1:1	Capsule		W:2-4 min	Mechanical trituration	Semisolid mass	See directions

Box 15.2

Procedure

Procedure for Mixing Zinc Phosphate Cement

Equipment needed

Zinc phosphate powder
Zinc phosphate liquid
Cement spatula
Glass slab
Powder scoop

1. Be sure that all surfaces of the cavity preparation are clean and dry immediately before placing the cement. When a casting is to be luted, it must be cleaned ultrasonically and wiped with alcohol to remove traces of polishing agents.
2. Isolate the area in the mouth with a rubber dam or cotton roll.
3. Provide pulp protection as needed.
4. Cool the glass slab under running water to about 65° F.
5. Dry the glass slab thoroughly.
6. Dispense the proper amount of powder.
7. Pat the powder into a flat rectangular shape with the spatula.

8. Divide the mass into sixths.
9. Divide one of the sixths into halves (the portion that is divided into halves should be the portion nearest to the liquid to be mixed first).
10. Dispense the appropriate amount of liquid near the center of the glass slab.
11. Mix one of the half portions into the liquid and spatulate for 15 seconds.
12. Spatulate over at least half of the surface of the slab using a rotary and back and forth motion and make sure all liquid from edges is continually brought back into the mass.
13. Add the second half portion and spatulate for 15 seconds.
14. Add each of the six portions and spatulate for 15 seconds each.
15. Add powder until the mix consistency is appropriate for luting or a base.
16. Complete the mix in 90 seconds to 2 minutes.

Solution

A single phase containing more than one component (for example, sugar dissolved in water).

Buffer

An ingredient that neutralizes acid.

used as a luting agent or a base and is supplied as a powder and liquid (Box 15.2). A baking soda and water **solution** will help dissolve cement from the glass slab and spatula and the ultrasonic cleaner.

The powder is mainly zinc oxide with other modifiers and pigmenting agents. The ingredients are mixed, fused together under high heat (calcination), and ground into a powder. The liquid is primarily phosphoric acid in water. Other agents such as zinc or aluminum are added to **buffer** or slow the rate at which the cement sets. Zinc phosphate is also available with a tannin fluoride and radiopaque additive. The liquid bottle should be kept tightly sealed at all times because the liquid will gain or lose water, depending on the humidity, which affects the setting time and properties of the cement.

As the powder and liquid are mixed, heat is given off in an **exothermic** reaction. This heat must be removed or the cement will set too fast and have reduced strength. To dissipate the heat, a glass slab is used, which can be cooled by holding it under cold water. It must be cooled above the **dew point** to avoid moisture on the slab. *Moisture will cause the cement to set too fast.* The powder is added to the liquid in small portions (increments) and mixed over a large area of the slab for 90 to 120 seconds. The correct powder-to-liquid ratio is critical to ensure that the cement has optimum strength and low acidity and solubility. The cement is mixed to a thin, stringy

Exothermic

Any reaction that produces heat.

Dew point

The point of coolness at which moisture will form.

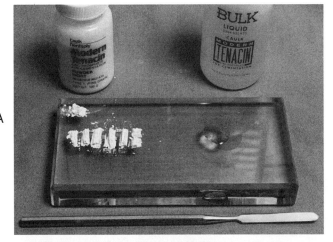

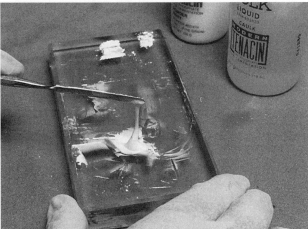

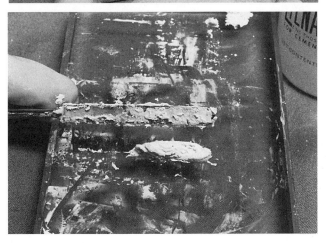

FIGURE 15.1

Mixing zinc phosphate cement. **A,** Dispense zinc phosphate powder and liquid according to manufacturer's directions. **B,** Mix to a stringy consistency for luting. **C,** Mix to a thick, putty-like consistency for a base. Always read the manufacturer's directions.

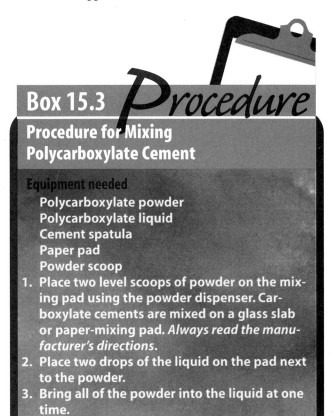

Box 15.3 *Procedure*

Procedure for Mixing Polycarboxylate Cement

Equipment needed
   Polycarboxylate powder
   Polycarboxylate liquid
   Cement spatula
   Paper pad
   Powder scoop
1. **Place two level scoops of powder on the mixing pad using the powder dispenser. Carboxylate cements are mixed on a glass slab or paper-mixing pad.** *Always read the manufacturer's directions.*
2. **Place two drops of the liquid on the pad next to the powder.**
3. **Bring all of the powder into the liquid at one time.**
4. **Spatulate for about 30 seconds.**

consistency for luting and to a thick, putty-like mass for use as a base.

Luting consistency should be a creamy mass that lifts off the slab with the spatula to a length of about $^3/_4$ inch before snapping back onto the slab. Apply a thin coat to the interior of the casting (Figure 15.1).

Base consistency should be stiff and putty-like. Continue adding powder until appropriate stiffness is obtained. Insert into a dried cavity.

Polycarboxylate Cement

Polycarboxylate cements are powder-liquid formulations. The primary advantage to this group of cements is their ability to chemically bond to tooth structure and some metals.

The powder is primarily zinc oxide with small amounts of magnesium oxide. The liquid is a solution of polyacrylic acid and water. Other polymers may be added to reduce the viscosity (thickness) of the liquid to permit easier mixing (Box 15.3).

The manufacturer usually supplies devices to properly proportion the powder and liquid. The mixing should

Box 15.4

Procedure for Mixing Zinc Oxide-Eugenol Cement

Procedure

Equipment needed
- Zinc oxide powder
- Zinc oxide liquid
- Cement spatula
- Liquid dropper
- Powder scoop
- Treated mixing pad

1. Shake the bottle and place a level scoop of powder on the treated mixing pad.
2. Dispense one drop of liquid for each level scoop of powder.
3. Mix one-half of the powder into the liquid (Figure 15.2).
4. Spatulate with a firm, steady, and back-and-forth motion.
5. Bring the remaining powder into the mix and spatulate thoroughly (the consistency for a lining or luting mix should be creamy and smooth. A mix for a base should be putty-like so it can be rolled into a ball or rope shape).
6. Mix for 30 seconds or less.
7. Place the luting mix into the crown and pass it to the operator, or the pad can be held out to the operator.
8. Roll the base mix into a rope or ball shape and pass it to the operator on the spatula or pad.

be rapid and ideally completed in no more that 30 to 60 seconds. The cement should be used while it exhibits a shiny surface. Once the shine disappears, the cement becomes stringy, difficult to manipulate, and should be discarded.

Zinc Oxide-Eugenol Cement

The zinc oxide-eugenol (ZOE) cements are used as temporary restorative materials, liners, temporary luting agents, root canal fillings, periodontal dressings, impression materials, and cavity bases. The eugenol is a **sedative or obtundent** that reduces pain sensitivity when the cement is used as a base in deep cavity preparations. Zinc oxide-eugenol cement should not be used under composite resins because it will retard the setting reaction of the composite resin material. It is also available with tannin fluoride and radiopaque additives (Shofu).

Sedative or obtundent

A medicated material that has soothing properties and decreases sensitivity.

The powder is primarily zinc oxide (Box 15.4). Various additives may be incorporated to improve the strength, reduce brittleness, and accelerate the setting reaction. The liquid is mainly eugenol but other oils may be added to modify

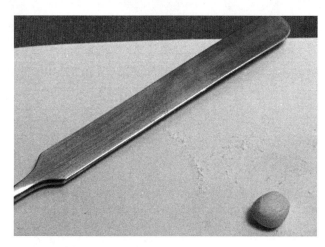

FIGURE 15.2

Mixing zinc oxide-eugenol cement. Mix one half of the powder into the liquid and spatulate with a firm, steady, back-and-forth motion. Add powder as needed for luting or base consistency.

the viscosity. Accelerators may also be added to increase the rate of reaction. Tannin fluoride and radiopaque additives have also been added (Shofu).

The appropriate amount of liquid and powder are placed on a paper-mixing pad. Shake the powder to fluff it because it will settle as it sets and cause the measurement to be more compact. The powder is divided into two equal portions that are incorporated into the liquid over a period of 30 seconds. Further mixing for another 30 to 60 seconds produces a suitable consistency.

Modified Zinc Oxide-Eugenol Cements

Modifications of the powder or liquid by the addition of other ingredients have been attempted to improve the properties of ZOE cement. Resin (polymethyl methacrylate) has been added to the powder to increase the compressive and tensile strength of the cement. A second type of modification adds quartz or alumina particles and rosin to the powder and ethoxybenzoic acid (EBA) to the liquid. The resulting cement is less brittle and stronger but some products exhibit increased solubility in oral fluids. Mixing procedures are the same as for zinc oxide-eugenol.

Other Zinc Oxide-Based Cements

Zinc oxide is used with or without a eugenol base as a periodontal dressing. These materials are available as powder and liquids or as a two-paste system. Zinc oxide eugenol is used in endodontics as an antiseptic temporary cement and a bulk liner for deep cavities and is also provided in a two-paste system to be used as a liner.

Calcium Hydroxide

Calcium hydroxide has been used to line deep cavities that closely approximate the pulp. It has the ability to stimulate secondary dentin formation. However, with the growing popularity and clinical success of glass-ionomer cements and dentin bonding agents, the use of calcium hydroxide is declining. Many clinicians still advocate its use as a direct pulp-capping agent. Most products are two-paste systems that are easy to mix and place (Box 15.5). It is also available in a premixed syringe system and light cure system. Calcium hydroxide sets rapidly in a moist, warm atmosphere and must be placed quickly. These cements are weak and brittle and should be placed in thin layers (not greater that 0.5 mm).

Dental Varnishes

Dental varnishes are used to line the cavity to protect the pulp from dental materials that irritate the pulp. Cement bases with phosphoric acid components such as zinc phosphate will irritate the pulp, and a varnish will be used as a **sealer** for the dentinal tubules from the irritant. In this case the varnish is placed under the zinc phosphate base. Varnish is also placed over a prepared vital tooth before luting an inlay or crown. Varnish is placed

Sealer

A material used to seal the dentinal tubules to protect the pulp.

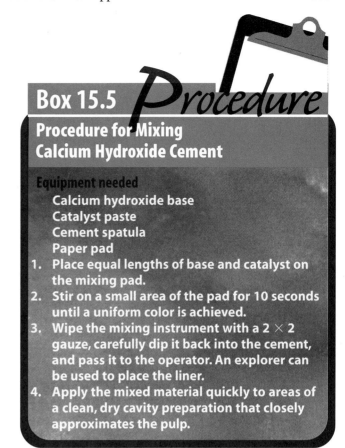

Box 15.5 *Procedure*

Procedure for Mixing Calcium Hydroxide Cement

Equipment needed
- **Calcium hydroxide base**
- **Catalyst paste**
- **Cement spatula**
- **Paper pad**

1. **Place equal lengths of base and catalyst on the mixing pad.**
2. **Stir on a small area of the pad for 10 seconds until a uniform color is achieved.**
3. **Wipe the mixing instrument with a 2 × 2 gauze, carefully dip it back into the cement, and pass it to the operator. An explorer can be used to place the liner.**
4. **Apply the mixed material quickly to areas of a clean, dry cavity preparation that closely approximates the pulp.**

in thin layers (usually two) on the pulpal floor, cavity walls, and cavo surface margins. Varnishes cannot be used under acrylic resin because of the adverse effects they have on the setting reaction of acrylic resin materials. Glass-ionomer cements are replacing these materials.

Glass-Ionomer Cements

These cements and their modified derivatives offer a promising array of advantages. They are adhesive materials and can form a chemical bond to enamel and dentin. They release fluoride, exhibit translucency, and are biocompatible. Their various formulations may be used as luting agents, bases, liners, and restorative materials. Dentin conditioners are available to enhance the bonding strength of glass ionomer cements by removing the protein or smear layer from the dentin. The conditioner is placed for approximately 10 seconds and then rinsed before placement of the glass ionomer cement (Box 15.6). Glass ionomer cement is available in blendable shades for esthetic considerations. The light-cured versions are an exciting addition to the armamentarium of the dental team (Figure 15.3).

The traditional glass-ionomer cements consist of a powder of aluminosilicate glass that is fluoride-rich. The liquid is a solution of polyacrylic acid in water. In some products,

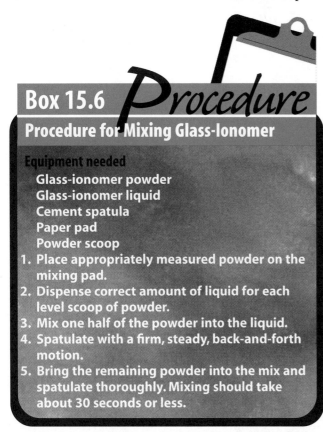

Box 15.6 *Procedure*

Procedure for Mixing Glass-Ionomer

Equipment needed
 Glass-ionomer powder
 Glass-ionomer liquid
 Cement spatula
 Paper pad
 Powder scoop
1. **Place appropriately measured powder on the mixing pad.**
2. **Dispense correct amount of liquid for each level scoop of powder.**
3. **Mix one half of the powder into the liquid.**
4. **Spatulate with a firm, steady, back-and-forth motion.**
5. **Bring the remaining powder into the mix and spatulate thoroughly. Mixing should take about 30 seconds or less.**

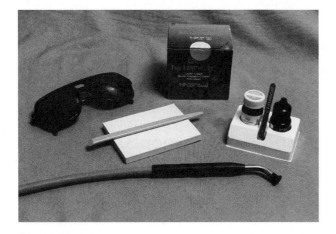

FIGURE 15.3

Setup for using light-cured glass ionomer cements.

itaconic acid has been added to reduce the viscosity of the liquid, and tartaric acid is used to modify the setting reaction by extending the working time and reducing the setting time.

The proper amount of liquid and powder are dispensed on a paper pad. The powder is divided into two portions and mixed into the liquid within 30 seconds. The cement must be used while the surface has a shiny appearance to achieve bonding with the tooth.

Resin Cements

Resin cements are self-cured, light-cured, or dual cured and may be powder-liquid or paste-paste formulations. On mixing, a hard, rigid polymer is formed that provides adhesion to tooth structure in some cases. These cements set very quickly if they are self-cured, have low solubility, and have high compressive strength. Removing excess set cement can be a tedious procedure.

Bonding Agents

The success of a restoration can be determined by the seal between two structures. This can be accomplished by adhesion for retention of dentures to the patient's mouth or bonding amalgam and composite restorations to enamel and dentin. Bonding may be produced mechanically or chemically. Mechanical attachment such as retentive pots and slots in a tooth prepared for restoration locks the material into irregularities on the surface of the **adherent,** whereas chemical bonding is achieved through a chemical interaction between the atoms and molecules in the two surfaces.

Adherent
The material on which the adhesive is placed.

The surface of the adherent should be perfectly clean and free of debris and oil. The liquid must be thin enough to flow into small irregularities on the surface of a material. The stronger the chemical attraction of two materials, the stronger the bond. If the liquid exhibits considerable shrinkage as it sets, it may pull away from the adherent and break the bond. If the adhesive and the adherent possess different coefficients of thermal expansion, changes in temperature will produce different rates of expansion and contraction, producing stress in the bond and failure.

DENTAL AMALGAM

Amalgam results when mercury (a liquid metal at room temperature) is combined with one or more solid metals. Dental amalgam has been used as a restorative material for almost 150 years and provides proven clinical performance at minimal costs (Box 15.7).

Dental amalgams may be classified according to their composition and specifically by the amount of copper that is present. Conventional, low-copper amalgam **alloys** contain less than 6% copper along with silver (67% to 74%), tin (25% to 28%), and sometimes zinc (less than 2%). High-copper alloys contain 12% to 30% copper

Alloys
A mixture of two or more metals.

Box 15.7

Procedure

Procedure for Mixing Amalgam

Equipment needed

- Amalgam alloy pellets
- Mercury in dispenser
- Amalgamator
- Capsule and pestle
- Cotton pliers
- Gauze sponge or squeeze cloth
- Amalgam well
- Amalgam set-up

1. Set up the amalgamator, precapsulated amalgam, cotton pliers, and amalgam well.
2. Consult the recommendations of the manufacturer of the amalgam alloy regarding the proper time and speed settings for your particular amalgamator. Set the amalgamator to the suggested settings.
3. Break the seal in the capsule.
4. Place the capsule into the arms of the amalgamator and close the protective cover (if applicable) (Figure 15.4, *A*).
5. Turn the amalgamator on; it will stop after the set amount of time has elapsed.
6. Remove the capsule and dispense the amalgam mass into the amalgam well (Figure 15.4, *B*).
7. Secure the amalgam in the amalgam carrier and pass it to the operator.

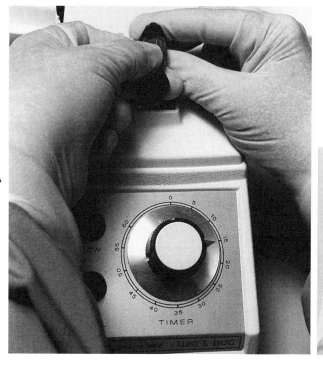

A

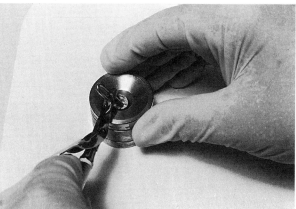

B

FIGURE 15.4

Amalgam alloy procedures. **A,** Activate the preproportional capsule and place it into the amalgamator. **B,** Dispense the amalgam mass into the amalgam well to place it into the carrier.

that is added at the expense of silver. These alloys are a major improvement over low-copper alloys.

Although amalgam alloys corrode, high copper alloys corrode less than conventional alloy. Some corrosion in the space between restorative material and tooth is beneficial because it tends to seal out saliva, bacteria, and other substances that may seep into the crevice. The particle shape of amalgam alloy may be lathe-cut or spherical-shaped conventional alloy. Lathe-cut particles are irregular-shaped and composed primarily of silver and tin. The small particle size produces a stronger amalgam that polishes easily. Spherical-shaped alloys are also primarily composed of silver and tin but are produced under high pressure, causing varied particle sizes that produce an amalgam that can easily be compressed.

Three important steps need to be considered in the preparation of dental amalgam restoration. These steps are critical to the handling and mechanical properties of the amalgam.

Proportioning

An amount of mercury must be available to thoroughly wet all of the alloy particles to ensure a uniform reaction and optimal properties in the set amalgam. In general, a mixture of 1:1 or equal volumes of mercury and alloy particles produces a workable mass. Less mercury is needed when mixing spheric alloys because the smooth, round particles are more easily wetted than the irregularly shaped lathe-cut particles.

Dispensing the Mercury and Alloy

Two common methods for dispensing the correct amounts of mercury and alloy include the following:

1 Separate proportions of mercury and amalgam alloy
2 Preproportioned capsules

Most manufacturers supply pellets of alloy made by compressing the powder particles together. The mercury is dispensed by volume from a specially designed, adjustable bottle. The advantage to this system is that the mercury and alloy ratio can be adjusted to suit the practitioner.

Preproportioned capsules are also available, which contain specific amounts of alloy and mercury ready for trituration. This delivery system has the advantages of convenience and less risk of spilling the mercury. The disadvantages include the inability to alter the mercury and alloy ratio and slightly higher cost. Pressing the capsule between the thumb and fingers may activate some capsules to release the mercury and others are placed in a press to break the seal between the alloy and mercury. Other systems contain a "pillow" that holds the mercury and ruptures on trituration. Twisting the two halves of the capsule activates other systems.

Trituration

The alloy particles should be thoroughly coated by the mercury. Mixing is typically done by placing the capsule containing the mercury, alloy, and pestle in a mechanical amalgamator. Amalgamators operate at different speeds. Make sure to follow the manufacturer's suggestions concerning the recommended time for trituration.

Condensation

After trituration, the amalgam is placed in the prepared tooth in small increments. The cavity must be totally dry because any moisture contamination of the amalgam will weaken the amalgam and cause a delayed **expansion** of alloys containing zinc. Instruments called *condensers* are used to force the amalgam into the cavity to adapt the mix to the cavity, remove excess mercury, and pack the particles of the alloy close together. The amalgam should be packed firmly to ensure that each increment is completely condensed. However, spheric particles will require lighter forces because of their round shape offering less frictional resistance to the condenser. As the cavity is packed with amalgam, the condensation forces bring excess mercury to the surface. The cavity should be overfilled with amalgam so that the mercury-rich layer can be removed during the carving procedure (see Chapter 36).

Expansion
An increase in the dimensions of an object.

Carving

The condensed mass of amalgam should be allowed to partially set before beginning to carve the amalgam to anatomic form. The carved restoration may be lightly burnished or smoothed with a burnisher, which will further adapt the amalgam to the cavity.

Polishing

Even properly carved and burnished amalgam restorations have a rough surface. This surface is more subject to tarnish and plaque accumulation. Polishing will produce a smooth surface, help reduce tarnish and **corrosion**, and will look and feel better to the patient. The best polish can be achieved by using a series of abrasives at a later appointment (at least 24 hours after placing the amalgam).

Corrosion
Chemical attack on a material causing deterioration.

Mercury
Biocompatibility

Concerns are expressed about the biocompatibility of amalgam, especially regarding its mercury content. Two perspectives of the issue involve the patient and the dental team.

The Patient

Amalgam has been used in dentistry for almost 150 years. However, no published evidence exists in the scientific literature that amalgam causes any adverse biologic reactions to patients other than extremely rare allergies that are localized to the adjacent oral tissues.

Mercury Hazards

The greatest hazard to dental personnel is long-term exposure to mercury vapor generated from spills. Care should be taken in the following ways when dispensing mercury:

Preproportioned capsules should be used to limit the possibility of a mercury spill.

Mercury should be stored away from sources of heat such as autoclaves.

Scrap amalgam should be stored in a sealed container, preferably filled with used x-ray fixer solution.

RESIN-BASED RESTORATIVE MATERIALS

Resin-based materials have been widely used for restoring cavities in anterior teeth and are increasingly used in posterior restorations (Figure 15.5). Because these materials are tooth-colored, they provide an esthetic alternative to amalgam.

The first acrylic resins, based on polymethyl methacrylate, were especially subject to the following problems that are common to all polymers (plastics or resins):

- Polymerization shrinkage
- Low strength
- High coefficient of thermal expansion
- Low modulus of elasticity.

This led to failure because of leakage at the margin of the cavity, recurrent caries, and lost restorations. The properties of the acrylic resins could be improved by adding fillers (small particles) of quartz or various glasses to resin, which results in a composite material that exhibits less polymerization shrinkage. Resins are available as two-paste or single-paste systems. The two-paste system has an **activator or catalyst** that when combined, initiates the setting reaction (polymerization). The single-paste system uses light-cured materials to initiate setting, allowing more time for placement. These pastes are available in syringes or capsules. Irreversible eye damage can occur when using the ultraviolet (UV) light; therefore light shields or glasses should be used for protection.

Activator or catalyst

A chemical that reacts with a chemical initiator to start a reaction.

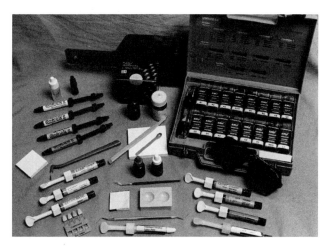

FIGURE 15.5

Syringe and self-curing composite resin systems and light cured-composite resin systems. Use caution when using the visible light-curing unit because light of this wavelength can cause irreversible eye damage. Light shields or special glasses should be used to protect the eyes of patients and personnel.

Polymerization Shrinkage

Regardless of the method used as an **initiator** to the setting reaction, all composite resins exhibit **contraction** or shrinkage when polymerized. To minimize this pulling away or contraction, the operator can first hold the light source next to the tooth structure on the opposite side of the filling. Composite resin materials will flow slightly toward the light source, pulling the composite material toward the tooth structure. Special bonding agents can also be used to adhere the composite to the tooth structure, helping to eliminate gaps, staining, and recurrent caries at the cavomarginal surfaces.

Initiator

Source of energy (chemical, light, or heat) that starts a reaction.

Contraction

A shortening or reduction in size of an object.

Adhesion to Tooth Structure

The acid etch technique was developed to adhere or bond the resin to the tooth and prevent leakage. When an etching acid is placed on enamel, some of the mineral structure is removed creating an irregular, porous surface. Various acids may be used such as citric, maleic, and nitric, but the most common acid used is phosphoric. A liquid bonding resin is then flowed into the irregularities and polymerized thus

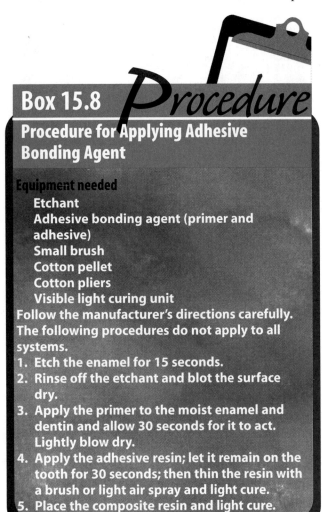

Box 15.8 *Procedure*

Procedure for Applying Adhesive Bonding Agent

Equipment needed
- Etchant
- Adhesive bonding agent (primer and adhesive)
- Small brush
- Cotton pellet
- Cotton pliers
- Visible light curing unit

Follow the manufacturer's directions carefully. The following procedures do not apply to all systems.

1. Etch the enamel for 15 seconds.
2. Rinse off the etchant and blot the surface dry.
3. Apply the primer to the moist enamel and dentin and allow 30 seconds for it to act. Lightly blow dry.
4. Apply the adhesive resin; let it remain on the tooth for 30 seconds; then thin the resin with a brush or light air spray and light cure.
5. Place the composite resin and light cure.

mechanically locking the resin into the porous surface. When the composite resin is placed over the bonding resin, the two resins chemically unite, creating a strong and durable bond.

Bonding to dentin has proven to be much more difficult because of its varying composition and moisture content. Early bonding agents for dentin were modified enamel bonding agents that produced a weak and unstable bond. Modern dentin bonding agents (or universal bonding agents) interact with the dentin to produce a chemical and mechanical bond that approaches the strength of the enamel bond. Most dentin bonding systems use a primer that is a hydrophilic wetting agent that can soften and penetrate the superficial layer of dentin. The primer is followed by a liquid adhesive that is cured before placing the composite resin.

Bonding Amalgam

Some of the dentin bonding agents are now being used in an attempt to bond amalgam to tooth structure (Box 15.8). This would serve to reduce microleakage and sensitivity, help retain the amalgam in the preparation, and reinforce weakened tooth structure.

IMPRESSION MATERIALS

Many dental procedures require the use of a model or replica of the patient's mouth. Material that is inserted into the mouth as a semisolid and allowed to harden can be used to make an impression of the mouth. This is called *impression material*. The impression is removed and another material such as plaster is poured into the impression to produce the model. These models are used for diagnosis and treatment planning, legal records, fabrication of orthodontic appliances, and for various laboratory procedures during the construction of dentures and cast restorations.

To produce an accurate replica, impression materials should possess certain properties. The material should have adequate working time for mixing, placing in a tray, and inserting into the mouth. After it is placed in the mouth it should harden quickly. Impression materials should be biocompatible with the oral tissues. The material must be able to flow and wet the teeth and other oral structures to record them accurately. Different impression materials have different abilities to record this detail, and the material should be chosen based on the amount of detail that is required. The impression should be flexible enough to be removed from undercut areas but should return to its original shape. The impression should not change dimensions after removal from the mouth until the impression can be poured. Ideally, the material should not be expensive but should be easy to use not deteriorate when stored for long periods.

Impression Trays

Impression materials are placed in various types of trays designed for particular procedures and placement positions (Figure 15.6). Wax, preformed into a rope-shape, may be placed around the rim or periphery of the tray to provide length or cover rough edges of the tray. The following types of trays are used for taking impressions:
- Solid metal, rimmed, or rimless
- Water-cooled
- Perforated
- Stock plastic, solid or perforated
- Custom acrylic resin

Boxing Impressions

Boxing an impression means placing a thin wax strip around the prepared impression to confine the gypsum material, usually plaster (Box 15.9). The boxing will form the base of the model and eliminate trimming oversized models. Rubber base formers can also be used for boxing.

Custom Trays

Elastomeric impression materials are placed in custom trays that are fabricated from acrylic resin materials (Box 15.10).

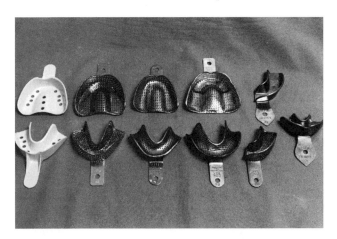

FIGURE 15.6

Examples of preformed impression trays. From left to right: plastic stock trays, perforated metal rimlock (with dentition), edentulous, partial dentition, and solid metal quadrant trays.

These trays may be constructed with self-cured or light cured materials or they can be constructed by using vacuum form equipment.

Classifications

Impression materials fall into two general categories: nonelastic or rigid and elastic. The nonelastic materials (plaster, wax, ZOE, and impression compound) have limited use. The elastic materials may be further divided into two groups: hydrocolloids, which use water as their major ingredient and elastomers, which are based on rubbery materials.

Elastomeric Impression Materials

The four major types of elastomeric impression materials are polysulfides, condensation silicones, addition silicones, and polyethers. Each of the four types has advantages and disadvantages, and a selection of which material to use is based on these factors. The procedures for mixing these materials are similar.

Polysulfides

Polysulfides, often called *rubber base*, are the oldest elastomeric impression materials. They flow well and are capable of good reproduction of detail. Polysulfide is available in a heavy, regular, and light-bodied impression material. The heavy-bodied polysulfide is used in the tray to help get a good final impression. Because of the stiff, heavy body consistency of this tray material, the dentist can firmly press the light-bodied impression material over the teeth and into the cavity prep. Some dentists may use the regular-bodied material for this same purpose. However, the light-bodied material is placed in a syringe because it is the correct consistency to flow into the detailed cavity preparation and surrounding structures.

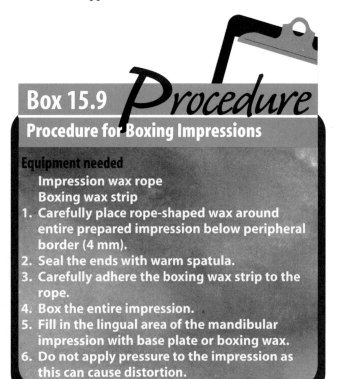

Box 15.9 *Procedure*

Procedure for Boxing Impressions

Equipment needed
   Impression wax rope
   Boxing wax strip
1. **Carefully place rope-shaped wax around entire prepared impression below peripheral border (4 mm).**
2. **Seal the ends with warm spatula.**
3. **Carefully adhere the boxing wax strip to the rope.**
4. **Box the entire impression.**
5. **Fill in the lingual area of the mandibular impression with base plate or boxing wax.**
6. **Do not apply pressure to the impression as this can cause distortion.**

Mixing

To mix the impression material, dispense equal lengths of the heavy-bodied base and catalyst onto a large, paper mixing pad (Box 15.11). The lengths will vary depending on the size of the custom tray. Two to three 6-inch lengths of each paste may be adequate for an average size tray. Do not allow the pastes to touch each other before mixing.

After the heavy-bodied material is placed on the pad, dispense $1^1/_2$ to 2 inch lengths of light-bodied base and catalyst onto the smaller paper pad. Mix the light-bodied material first, allowing about 60 seconds, by picking up the catalyst (brown paste) on the spatula and combining it with the base material. At the beginning of the mixing procedure, the spatula is held in a near vertical position and a stirring action is used to blend the two pastes together. After the material is mixed, wipe the spatula with a clean paper towel to remove excess material on spatula. This helps to provide a homogenous mix. Continue mixing with a back and forth motion with the spatula held in a horizontal position until all streaks are eliminated and a homogeneous mix is attained.

Preparing the Heavy-Bodied Tray Material

Before placing the heavy-bodied material into a tray, the tray is coated with a thin layer of rubber base adhesive and allowed to dry. The heavy-bodied material is then mixed and placed into the prepared impression tray before placing the light-bodied material into the syringe.

Box 15.10

Procedure

Procedure for Fabricating Quadrant Custom Impression Trays

Equipment needed

- Wax
- Plaster models
- Spatula
- Acrylic powder (polymer) or liquid (monomer)
- Paper cup
- Vaseline

1. Set out and prepare the equipment (Figure 15.7, *A*).
2. Cut stops in spacing material.
3. Form spacing material over working arch (Figure 15.7, *B*).
4. Measure powder.
5. Measure liquid and add to powder.
6. Mix powder and liquid together.
7. Always wear a mask when mixing acrylic resin materials.
8. Roll acrylic resin into a rope shape (Figure 15.7, *C*).
9. Place acrylic resin over arch.
10. Shape acrylic resin to form a handle (Figure 15.7, *D*).
11. Check stops.
12. Trim excess material and smooth rough edges with handpiece or trim excess material with laboratory lathe (Figure 15.7, *D*).

Preparing the Light-Bodied Syringe Material

The syringe is also prepared before beginning tooth preparation. Inserting the plastic, disposable tip into the retainer cap and screwing the cap onto the barrel of the syringe assembles it. The O-ring on the plunger should be lubricated with petroleum jelly to allow the plunger to move smoothly through the barrel of the syringe. The syringe is loaded by holding the barrel in a near vertical position and pushing it through the mix several times. When the syringe is loaded, insert the plunger into the syringe and pass it to the dentist.

Placing the Light-Bodied Material

Placing the light-bodied material must be executed quickly and precisely to provide sufficient time for the dental assistant to remove the retraction cord from around the tooth, gently dry the teeth with compressed air, and allow the dentist to immediately inject the impression material into the sulcus surrounding the tooth.

During the initial application of syringe material, the dentist will watch for any potential distortion of the impression material caused from saliva or blood. The dentist will inject the light-bodied material into the sulcus and gradually cover the prepared tooth with the impression material. The injection process should be slow and continuous to minimize air entrapment. The tip of the syringe should be moved so that it follows the impression material rather than moving ahead of it. The dentist will continue to inject the light-

bodied material onto the occlusal surfaces of the posterior teeth and lingual surfaces of the anterior teeth. Remaining syringe material will quickly be placed in the impression tray over the heavy-bodied material.

Placing the Heavy-Bodied Material

The dentist will immediately seat the tray with firm pressure and hold it steady for 10 to 12 minutes while the impression material polymerizes to avoid distorting the material. The impression will be removed and allowed to set for about 20 minutes to permit time for elastic recovery to occur.

Removing the Impression from the Mouth

When the dentist can leave a fingernail print in the impression material, it is sufficiently set. When this occurs, the impression will be carefully removed from the mouth and an impression will be taken of the opposing arch along with a bite registration. The dental assistant should make sure that the patient is cleaned before dismissal.

These materials exhibit some shrinkage soon after the impression is removed from the mouth because of the evaporation of water, a by-product of the setting reaction, from the impression. Ideally, the impression should be poured with dental stone within 1 hour. The impression should be prepared for the dental laboratory following infection control measures.

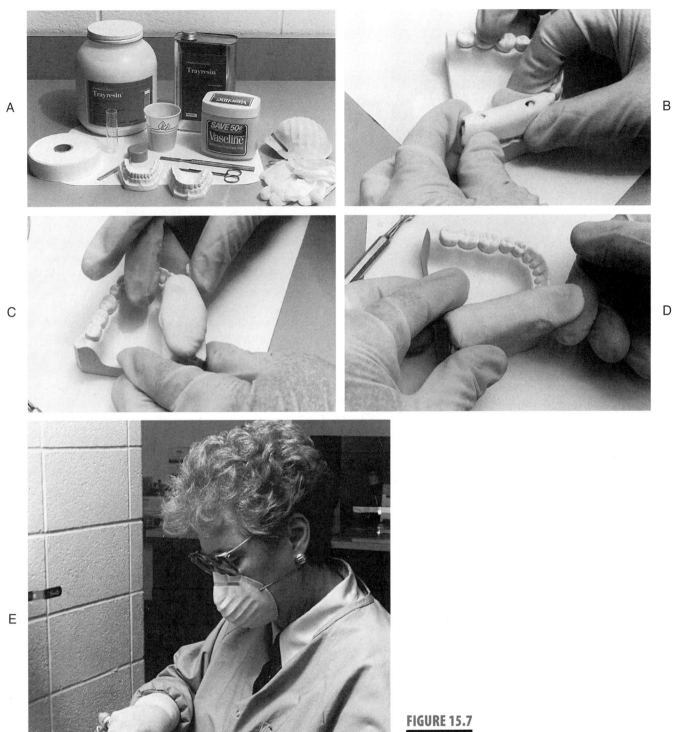

FIGURE 15.7

Fabricating custom trays. **A,** Prepare the equipment needed. **B,** Form spacing material over the working arch. **C,** Roll acrylic into a rope and place over arch. **D,** Shape the acrylic resin to form a handle. **E,** Trim excess material and smooth rough edges with handpiece.

Box 15.11

Procedure

Procedure for Mixing Elastemeric Impression Materials

Equipment needed
- Light-bodied impression material
- Heavy-bodied impression material
- Large and small paper pads
- Two spatulas
- Assembled impression syringe
- Vaseline
- Cleaning brush for the syringe
- Custom tray lined with adhesive
- Tray adhesive (retraction cord should be in place)

An assistant is essential during the impression procedure.

1. Assemble material (Figure 15.8, *A*).
2. Assemble the syringe for the impression material.
3. Dispense equal lengths of heavy-bodied base and catalyst onto a large, paper mixing pad.
4. Dispense $1\frac{1}{2}$--to 2-inch lengths of light-bodied base and catalyst onto a smaller paper pad.

5. Mix the light-bodied material first by placing the catalyst (brown) into the base (white) and mix until it is a uniform color, allowing about 60 seconds (Figure 15.8, *B*).
6. Mix the heavy-bodied material and load the prepared tray (Figure 15.8, *C*).
7. Load the syringe, insert the plunger into the syringe, and hand to the dentist (Figure 15.8, *D*).
8. Remove the retraction cord and gently dry the teeth.
9. Assist the dentist while injecting the light-bodied impression material.
10. Hand the dentist the filled tray and assist while the impression material polymerizes—about 20 minutes.
11. Remove the impression material and clean the patient.
12. Pour the impression within 1 hour.
13. Follow infection control procedures in preparing the impression for the dental laboratory.

Polysulfides are the most flexible elastomeric material and are easy to remove from the mouth. Recovery from deformation is somewhat slow and the impression should be allowed to set for about 20 minutes before pouring. They have a long working time and setting time (8 to 10 minutes). Polysulfides are biocompatible, the least costly, and relatively easy to use.

New Delivery Systems

Most of the elastomers are available as two-paste systems. Usually equal lengths of the pastes are dispensed on a paper pad and thoroughly mixed with a spatula. The catalyst for condensation silicones is often in liquid form. Various consistencies are available depending on the amount of fillers that the manufacturer has added.

Many of the products are available as automix systems. Both pastes are contained in a cartridge. The cartridge is placed in an extruder "gun" and the pastes are ejected as the trigger is pulled. The pastes are ejected directly into a mixing tube. This system is easier to use, results in less wasted material, more uniform mixes, and saves time (Box 15.12).

Condensation Silicones

Condensation silicones have good flow but because of their ability to absorb moisture (hydrophobic), they must be used in a dry, clean field. They have the highest shrinkage of all of the elastomeric materials because of the release of ethyl alcohol as a by-product of the setting reaction and are not as flexible as polysulfides but recover rapidly from deformation. Condensation silicones have medium working and setting times (5 to 7 minutes), are biocompatible, have moderate cost, and mix easily.

Addition Silicones (Polyvinyl Siloxanes)

Conventional polyvinyl siloxane materials flow relatively well and should also be used in a dry field. They have better dimensional stability and more accuracy than polysulfide impression materials. Some products release hydrogen during the setting reaction; this does not affect the dimensions of the impression but may cause bubbles on the surface of the model and may be avoided by waiting for 1 hour before pouring. Other products contain a hydrogen-absorber (palladium) to prevent the release of

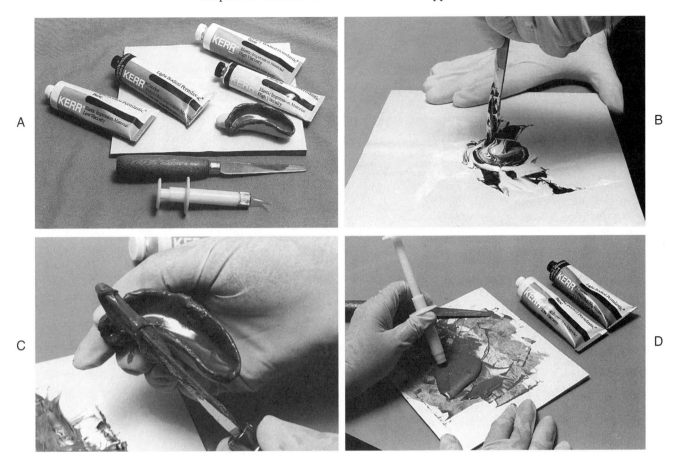

FIGURE 15.8

Mixing polysulfide impression materials. **A,** Assemble all equipment and supplies needed. **B,** Begin mixing the heavy-bodied (brown) catalyst into the base (white) and then continue mixing until it is uniform in color. **C,** Using the spatula, place the uniform mix into the tray. **D,** Mix the light body base thoroughly and place in syringe. (Courtesy Kerr Manufacturing and Dr. Alan Boghosian.)

the gas. They have medium flexibility and readily recover from deformation. Working and setting times are in the medium range (5 to 7 minutes). These materials are biocompatible, are somewhat more expensive, but are easy to mix and use. Newer formulations are more hydrophilic and will wet the oral tissues more easily resulting in fewer voids.

Polyethers

Polyethers possess low flow but will flow onto the oral tissues well because of their hydrophilic (water-loving) nature. They have good dimensional stability unless stored in a humid atmosphere. Under moist conditions, the material will absorb water and swell. Polyethers are stiff, may be difficult to remove from the mouth, and exhibit good recovery. Both the working and setting times are short, which can be a problem when taking an impression of several prepared teeth. Biocompatibility is usually good; however, some patients may become sensitive to the catalyst and experience a burning sensation in the oral tissues and ulceration. These materials are more expensive than other elastomeric materials.

Tissue Management

A tissue management system can be used to provide a dry working area, free of debris. Retraction cord and astringent solutions are used to reduce the flow of blood in the working area. A plastic syringe can be used to place the astringent solution. A small amount of blood can distort the impression and make it unusable.

Hydrocolloid Impression Materials

Hydrocolloid impression materials are based on water and therefore possess several unique properties. They exist in two forms known as *sol* and *gel*. A sol acts and appears as a thick liquid. A gel is a semisolid that has a jelly-like consistency. The gel is produced from the sol (a combination of water and dispersed molecules of a solid material) during the setting process that is called *gelation*. During gelation, part of the sol is converted to fibrils (fiber-like aggregates of molecules) that become interlocked. Most of the water is captured between the fibrils.

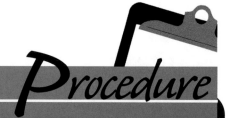

Box 15.12

Procedure for Automix Cartridge System

Equipment needed

Tray with adhesive
Cartridge or gun
Free-flo syringe
Retraction cord

1. Assemble extrude cartridge gun (Figure 15.9, *A*).
2. Apply adhesive to tray and allow 10 minutes to air dry before teeth are prepared, isolated, and retraction cord is placed.
3. Remove cap from extrude extra cartridge and discard. Extrude $1/2$ inch of material and attach new (green) medium mixing tip to cartridge.
4. Load impression tray with extrude extra material (Figure 15.9, *B*).
5. Remove cap from wash material cartridge and discard. Extrude $1/2$ inch of material and attach new mixing tip to cartridge.
6. Extrude wash material into front of Kerr Free-Flo syringe, while the assistant is loading the impression tray.
7. Snap extrude disposable syringe tip onto mixing tip for direct-to-mouth delivery.
8. Remove retraction cord and syringe from prepared teeth using a scrubbing action in interproximal areas, margins, and occlusal surfaces.
9. Insert filled tray over teeth and hold motionless in patient's mouth for approximately 4 more minutes until material is set (Figure 15.9, *C*).
10. Remove tray with snap motion. Rinse with water and blow dry. Impression may be disinfected with cold, sterilizing solution.

Figure 15.9, *D* shows the final impression.

Hydrocolloids are subject to dimensional changes resulting from gaining or losing water. If water is lost by evaporation, the hydrocolloid shrinks and the impression loses its accuracy. Hydrocolloids are capable of absorbing or imbibing water, which will not accurately correct the dimensional change caused by evaporation. Moisture is also lost through a process called *syneresis*. As gelation occurs, the fibrils interlock and squeeze some of the liquid and other constituents to the surface of the hydrocolloid. Syneresis occurs regardless of the humidity of the atmosphere.

Hydrocolloids may gel either by a reduction in temperature or a chemical reaction. Lowering the temperature slows the movement of the molecules of the solid phase and allows them to join to form fibrils. Raising the temperature may reverse this process, and the gel is converted by the heat to the sol state. The temperature at which the gel is converted to sol is much higher than the temperature at which the sol undergoes gelation. This temperature difference is called *hysteresis*.

Gelation may also occur through a chemical reaction involving the dispersed solid phase. This cannot be reversed and an irreversible impression material is formed. Hydrocolloids used in dentistry may be reversible or irreversible with the latter being the most popular.

Irreversible Hydrocolloid-Alginate

Alginates are supplied as a powder that is mixed with water to produce the sol (Box 15.13). The sol is placed in a tray and inserted into the mouth to make the impression. After gelation, the impression is removed.

The advantages of alginate impression materials are their ease of manipulation, low cost, minimum equipment, and flexibility. Alginate impressions are used to fabricate study models and for models used in the construction of complete and partial dentures. Alginate, however, lacks the stability and necessary detail reproduction for use in the fabrication of crowns and fixed partial dentures.

The powder is sodium or potassium salts of alginic acid that is derived from seaweed. It reacts chemically with calcium sulfate hemihydrate (plaster of paris) to produce the gel, *calcium alginate.*

The rate of setting is retarded by the addition of trisodium phosphate. Varying the temperature of the water used in mixing can also control the setting rate.

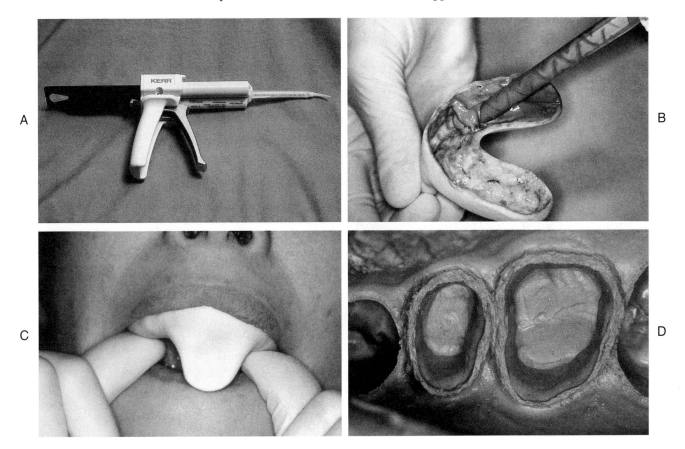

FIGURE 15.9

Extrude extra cartridge dispensing system. **A,** Kerr extrude dispenser. **B,** Place impression material into a custom tray. **C,** Seat tray securely over teeth. **D,** Remove tray and check impression for detail.

Cooler water slows the reaction and warm water causes acceleration.

Selection of Impression Tray

Usually perforated, rimlock, stock trays are used to secure the alginate impression. The perforations and rimlock help to hold in the alginate impression material in the tray. The maxillary and mandibular trays are available in many sizes. The dentist or dental assistant will try several trays and select the tray that best fits the patient's oral cavity (Box 15.14). The following procedures should be followed:

- Select perforated rimlock tray.
- Place tray making sure the tray covers all teeth and the alveolar process causing no pressure on teeth or gingiva tissue. Leave $1/4$-inch clearance between occlusal surface, soft tissue, and tray. The tray must cover the maxillary tuberosities and mandibular retromolar pad.
- Adjust the tray with wax to allow for extra length.

Manipulation

The recommended amount of water is placed in a rubber mixing bowl, with the appropriate amount of powder is sifted in. The powder and water are spatulated for about 60 seconds, the mix is placed in a perforated tray, and the tray is seated in the patient's mouth. Initial set of the alginate is indicated by a loss of tackiness. After 2 or 3 additional minutes, the tray is removed and the impression is rinsed with water and poured immediately. The impression may be stored for 1 hour if it is wrapped in a wet paper towel.

Evaluation of Impressions

Dental assistants should learn to self-evaluate their work until they are able to successfully accomplish each task with minimum correction (Table 15.3). Refer to the procedures for manipulating and taking alginate impressions.

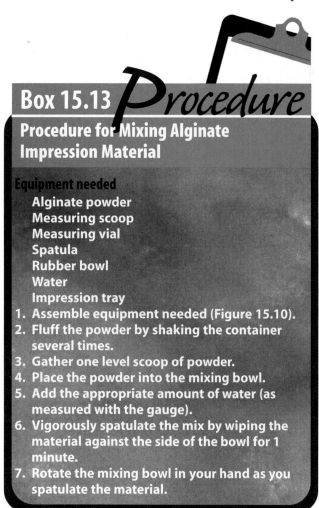

Box 15.13 *Procedure*

Procedure for Mixing Alginate Impression Material

Equipment needed
- Alginate powder
- Measuring scoop
- Measuring vial
- Spatula
- Rubber bowl
- Water
- Impression tray

1. Assemble equipment needed (Figure 15.10).
2. Fluff the powder by shaking the container several times.
3. Gather one level scoop of powder.
4. Place the powder into the mixing bowl.
5. Add the appropriate amount of water (as measured with the gauge).
6. Vigorously spatulate the mix by wiping the material against the side of the bowl for 1 minute.
7. Rotate the mixing bowl in your hand as you spatulate the material.

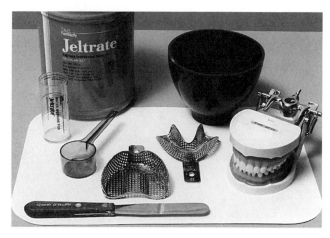

FIGURE 15.10

Equipment and material needed for taking an alginate impression on a dentoform.

Reversible Hydrocolloids

These hydrocolloids are supplied as a gel that is heated to convert it to a sol, placed in a special tray, and seated in the patient's mouth. Cooled water is circulated through the tray, and the reversible hydrocolloid undergoes gelation with the reduction in temperature.

Reversible hydrocolloids are based on water (80%) and agar (10% to 15%), which is derived from seaweed and other additives. The properties of reversible hydrocolloid are similar to alginate impression materials. However, they reproduce surface detail more accurately and may be used in making impressions for crown and bridge construction. Reversible hydrocolloids have largely been replaced by the more dimensionally stable and easily handled elastomers.

Waxes

Waxes have a wide variety of applications in dentistry. They have been used as impression materials, in the construction of crowns, bridges, partial denture frameworks, dentures, and other laboratory procedures (Figure 15.12). This variety of uses requires waxes with different properties and compositions. Many waxes are derived from natural sources such as insects, plants, and petroleum. Paraffin is a by-product of petroleum distillation. Plants provide waxes such as carnauba and candilla. Synthetic waxes are also used because of their consistent composition and properties.

Waxes possess the highest coefficients of thermal expansion of any dental material. Therefore their dimensional stability depends on maintaining a constant temperature during the storage of a wax pattern. Because waxes are blends of different waxes, they do not possess any constant properties such as melting points.

Types of Dental Wax

Inlay Wax
Inlay wax is used to construct wax patterns that are used in the construction of crowns and bridges. It is composed primarily of paraffin with carnauba, beeswax, and other ingredients used to modify its handling characteristics.

Sticky Wax
Sticky wax has a composition of beeswax and resins and is used to temporarily attach parts of appliances during the construction of the final product.

Carding Wax
Carding wax is used to box impressions to contain the stone during the pouring process.

Base Plate Wax
Base plate wax is used during the construction of removable partial dentures and full dentures to set the teeth in position.

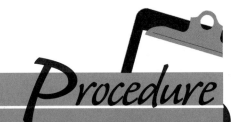

Box 15.14

Procedure for Taking Alginate Impression

Equipment needed

Alginate powder
Measuring scoop
Measuring vial
Spatula
Rubber bowl
Water
Impression tray

1. Make sure any unnecessary appliances are removed from the patient's mouth and try in tray for proper size (Figure 15.11, *A*).
2. Gather the material together with spatula and insert into tray when it is smooth and lump-free. Do not overload tray.
3. Maxillary tray procedure:
   - Insert material into tray from posterior of tray, flowing forward with spatula.
   - Do not overfill posterior portion of palate area of tray.
   - Dip fingers into water and smooth over alginate.
   - Spread a small amount of alginate over occlusal surfaces of teeth and into vault of palate, if necessary.
   - Rotate corner of tray first over maxillary arch, making sure handle is in line with nose and then gently bring tray forward over anterior teeth.
   - Flex lip over tray to force impression material into vestibule for complete impression (Figure 15.11, *B*).
   - Do not move or pull tray forward after it is in place or air voids will occur.
   - Remove excess material from mouth with dental mirror.
   - Hold tray securely in mouth for 3 to 5 minutes.
   - Remove tray and check impression for accuracy.
   - Spray impression with antiseptic solution for infection control and remove excessive moisture. Place a wax extension on the tray for additional length if necessary and for patient comfort.
4. Mandibular tray procedure:
   - Insert material into mandibular tray from lingual side of tray using only half of material at a time.
   - Place other half of material into side of tray, flowing material into anterior area. Load tray in 30 seconds.
   - Insert tray by rotating the corner over the arch using the side of the tray to push cheek out and allow tray to slide into position (Figure 15.11, *C*).
   - Place posterior of tray over teeth and lower the anterior portion of the tray into place.
   - Center handle and make sure tray is in place (Figure 15.11, *D*).
   - Remove the tray when material is firm by pulling upward with a quick snap, being careful not to hit the tray on the maxillary teeth.
   - Check impressions for accuracy (Figure 15.11, *E*).
   - Carefully rinse impressions with disinfectant and remove excessive moisture.
5. Use wax to obtain a bite registration.
6. Have patient rinse mouth and clean patient's face before dismissing.

Because of this use, they are usually pink and supplied in sheets. The main component is paraffin plus beeswax and carnauba.

Bite Registration Paste

Wax is used for securing a bite registration. In addition, bite registration paste is available and used to secure an occlusal registration or relationship. The composition of these registration pastes is zinc oxide. Bite registration paste is a two-paste system used with bite occlusal frames to hold the material and is primarily used for securing an accurate occlusal registration for inlays, crowns, and fixed partials. The base and accelerator are mixed together until their consistency is uniform (Figure 15.13). A small amount is then placed on both sides of the frame and placed in the mouth with the teeth properly occluded until the material is set.

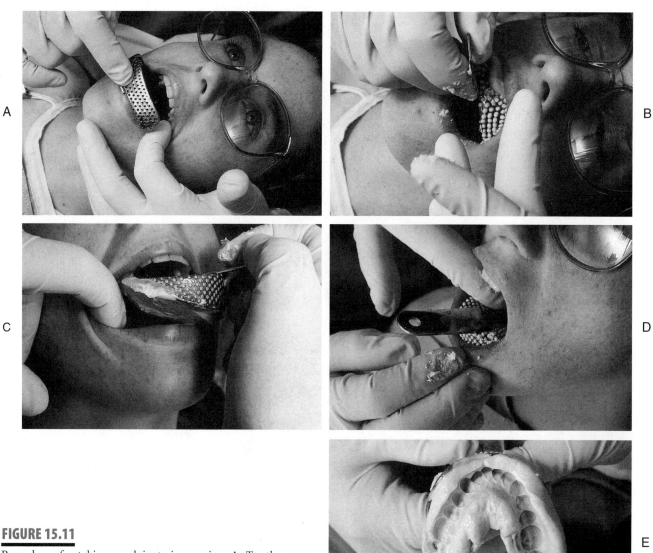

FIGURE 15.11

Procedures for taking an alginate impression. **A,** Try the upper and lower trays for proper size. **B,** Flex lip over the maxillary tray to force impression material into the vestibule for complete impression. **C,** To properly place the mandibular tray, use the side of the tray to push the cheek out. **D,** Make sure the handle is centered and the tray is in place. **E,** Always be sure to check the impression for accuracy and spray for infection control.

Gypsum

Many procedures in dentistry require the use of a model of the patient's mouth. These models are most readily constructed by obtaining an impression and pouring it up with a dental plaster or stone. Several forms of gypsum are available. Although the chemical composition of each product is identical, a difference in the shape and density of the powder particles exists.

Gypsum has been commonly called *plaster of Paris*. It is calcium sulfate dihydrate ($CaSO_4 \times 2\ H_2O$), which is a nat-

urally occurring mineral. The production of the various forms of gypsum requires heating the dihydrate to get rid of most of the water to form calcium sulfate hemihydrate ($CaSO_4 \times 2\ H_2O$). If the dihydrate is heated in air, a large, porous, irregular particle is formed. Heating under pressure produces particles that are smaller, denser, and more regular in shape. Adding water to the hemihydrate powder reverses the procedure and results in the following setting reaction:

$$CaSO_4 \times 1/2\ H_2O + 1\,1/2\ H_2O\ CaSO_4 \times 2\ H_2O$$
(calcium sulfate dihydrate)

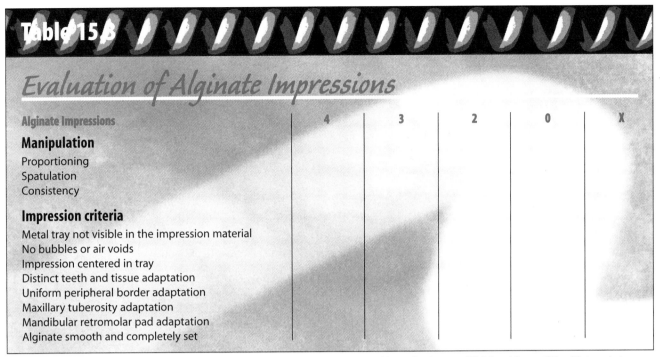

Table 15.3

Evaluation of Alginate Impressions

Alginate Impressions	4	3	2	0	X
Manipulation					
Proportioning					
Spatulation					
Consistency					
Impression criteria					
Metal tray not visible in the impression material					
No bubbles or air voids					
Impression centered in tray					
Distinct teeth and tissue adaptation					
Uniform peripheral border adaptation					
Maxillary tuberosity adaptation					
Mandibular retromolar pad adaptation					
Alginate smooth and completely set					

The numeric criteria: 4 Excellent; 3 Good, but some improvement can be made; 2 Below average, usable, needs to improve skill; 0 Unsatisfactory; X Not able to evaluate.

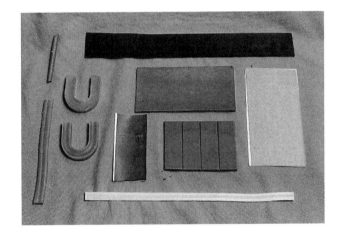

FIGURE 15.12

Types of dental waxes include wax rope, occusal wax rims, boxing wax, baseplate wax, carding wax, bite registration wax, and various utility wax.

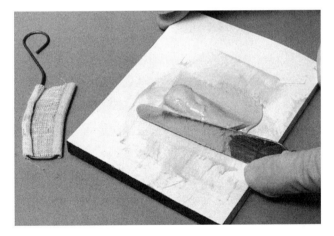

FIGURE 15.13

Bite registration paste system.

Heat is produced during this reaction and as an expansion of the gypsum. Dihydrate also forms as crystals. As the material sets, the crystals eventually contact and push against each other to produce the expansion. The different forms of hemihydrate produce different amounts of expansion with the porous form exhibiting the most expansion.

Types of Gypsum
Dental Plaster
Dental plaster is a porous hemihydrate used to pour up study models. Because of dental plaster's porous nature, more water is needed to mix plaster. The proper powder and water ratio is *50 cc water to 100 g powder*. This excess water will eventually produce larger voids in the set material and a reduction in its strength. Extended mixing time will also

Box 15.15

Suggestions for Working with Hemihydrate Materials

Powder-to-water ratio

Increasing the amount of water produces a thin mix that slows the reaction rate and results in a weaker set material.

Mixing time

A proper mix can usually be obtained in about 90 seconds. Excessive mixing will break the forming crystals. The net effect is the production of more crystals that contact sooner, thus increasing the setting rate of the mix and producing added expansion.

Mixing temperature

Within normal temperature ranges encountered in the dental office, the effect on the setting rate will not be significant when mixed.

Setting time

The setting time can be changed by altering the amount of powder to water, use of slurry water, addition of salt (accelerator) or vinegar (retarder), use of warm, cold or room temperature water, rate of spatulation, length of spatulation.
- Shorten setting time by use of warm water, use of more powder, rapid spatulation, or use of an accelerator.
- Lengthen setting time by use of cold water, slow spatulation, or use of retarder.

Rules

1 Read manufacturer's directions.
2 Keep material away from drains.
3 Keep material free from moisture.
4 Keep in airtight containers.
5 Order as needed.
6 Measure powder and water.
7 Put water in bowl first.
8 Wash equipment immediately after use.
9 Rinse bowl first.
10 Let power soak into water slowly.
11 Spatulate against side of bowl.
12 Mix well.
13 Place on vibrator.
14 Never add powder or water to mix.
15 Use good equipment.

weaken the material. Once mixing has begun, the consistency of the mix should not be altered by the addition of more powder or water.

Dental Model Stone

The hemihydrate particles of dental stones are smaller, denser, and more regular in shape. Less water is required during mixing, resulting in a final product that is denser, stronger, and harder. The proper powder and water ratio is *30 cc water to 100 g powder*. It also exhibits less setting expansion. The recommended powder and water ratio should be carefully maintained or a weaker mix will result. Dental stone is used to pour up working casts and to construct orthodontic appliances rather than plaster because it is stronger.

Class II Die Stone

Class II die stone is a denser and stronger stone that is used to produce working models and dies for crown and

bridge construction. The proper powder and water ratio is *24 cc water to 100 g powder*. Less water is needed for this mixture.

Manipulation

The manner in which the hemihydrate is mixed with water will affect the rate of reaction and the properties of the final gypsum material. Dental assistants can change the setting reaction time of gypsum materials by regulating the amount of water to powder used and controlling the temperature of the water (Boxes 15.15 and 15.17).

Measuring Devices

Many measuring devices are used in dentistry for measuring gypsum powder, water, impression materials, and cements. Height and width of materials, teeth, and periodontal pocket depths are also measured. The dental assistant should learn what these measuring devices are, what they are used for, and how to use them (Figure 15.14). The gram

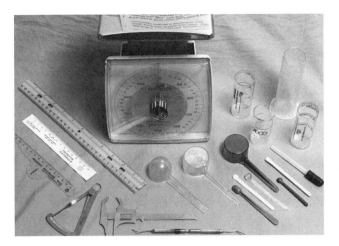

FIGURE 15.14

Measuring devices routinely used for dental procedures are the standard rule, millimeter rulers, caliper gauge, boley gauge, periodontal probe, gram scale, manufacturer graduated cylinders, premeasured scoops, milliliter graduated cylinder, and pipet.

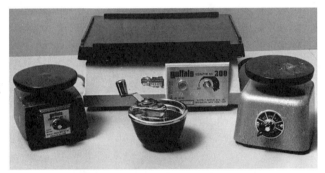

A

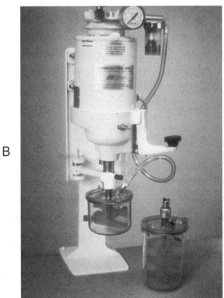

B

FIGURE 15.15

Mixing devices. **A,** Mechanical mixer (center) and three types of vibrators. **B,** Whip mix vacuum power mixer system. (Courtesy Whip Mix Corporation, Louisville, Ky)

Box 15.16 *Procedure*

Procedure for Using Vacuum Mixer

Equipment needed
   Vacumixer with attachments
   Gypsum in vacumixer bowl
1. **Place gypsum in vacumixer bowl.**
2. **Attach lid to bowl and insert cap into hole on lid.**
3. **Position drive nut into chuck and mix.**
4. **Hold bowl with both hands and mix on slow for 20 to 30 seconds or on high for 10 to 15 seconds.**
5. **While the vacuum is engaged, remove mixer from chuck and vibrate material from sides to bottom of bowl.**
6. **Remove tube from mixing bowl.**
7. **Separate lid and paddle from bowl and rinse thoroughly.**
8. **Carry bowl to vibrator and pour impressions.**

scale or dietetic spring scale is used to measure gypsum materials and other solids. The milliliter-graduated cylinder and cubic centimeter graduated cylinder are also used to measure liquid.

The gypsum manufacturer will usually include a premeasured scoop and graduate to use with impression materials. Gypsum materials are measured using the rubber mixing bowl, scoop and scale for the powder, and a graduate for measuring water.

Other types of measuring devices are rulers and boley gauges, which measure length, width and circumference. Periodontal probes measure the depth of periodontal pockets.

Mixing Devices

Gypsum can be mixed by hand with a spatula and rubber bowl, with a hand mechanical mixer or a vacuum power mixer (Figure 15.15, *A* and *B* and Box 15.16). Vacuum systems can be used to remove air from the mixture and produce a smooth, bubble-free mix. Once the machine is turned on, check the pressure gauge; it should read 10 lb; mixing pressure should read 25 lb; and should be mixed for 20 seconds.

Box 15.17

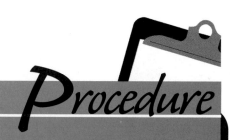

Procedure for Mixing Gypsum and Pouring Impressions

Equipment needed

- Dental plaster or stone
- Alginate impressions of dental arches
- Vibrator
- Rubber bowl
- Graduated cylinder
- Scales for weighing powder
- Cement spatula
- Large spatula
- Water

1. Assemble the equipment needed (Figure 15.16, *A*).
2. Rinse the impression in running water and remove excess water from the impression.
3. Trim away excess alginate that may extend beyond the palatal area or lingual and facial flange of tray.
4. Prepare a mix of gypsum material:
   - Plaster: 50 cc water to 100 g powder
   - Model stone: 30 cc water to 100 g powder
   - Die stone: 24 cc water to 100 g powder
5. Place room temperature water into the rubber bowl.
6. Slowly add the measured amount of gypsum into the water, letting the powder soak into the water slowly.
7. Use a stiff spatula to stir the mixture, scraping the sides of the bowl to ensure that all of the powder has been incorporated into the water. Never add additional powder or water to mix after mix has been vibrated.
8. Use the vacuum mixer to produce a smooth, bubble-free mix (see Box 15.16).
9. Use a vibrator to reduce any remaining bubbles but do not overvibrate (Figure 15.16, *B*).
10. Hold the impression tray on the vibrator at a slight angle and turn on the vibrator.
11. Place a small amount of gypsum at one posterior aspect of the impression with the cement spatula and allow it to flow slowly into each tooth imprint to minimize bubble entrapment (Figure 15.16, *C*). Do not overvibrate, which might cause bubble formation. Begin on one side of the impression and let the gypsum flow around to the opposite surface.
12. Completely fill the impression.
13. Remove the impression from the vibrator.
14. Add two or three small amounts of gypsum to produce a rough, undercut surface.
15. Prepare a second mix of gypsum as before but use 26 cc of water to produce a thicker mix. Place this mass in a pile on the working surface and use the spatula to shape the stone so that it is about $3/_4$ inches thick and covers a large enough area to receive the original pour.
16. Use the spatula to shape the second pour to the first. You may use a double mix of gypsum instead of two separate mixes. Place the additional mass in a pile on the working surface and use the spatula to shape the stone so that it is about $3/_4$ inch thick. Place the impression tray with gypsum onto the mass and shape the gypsum around the impression-filled material, being careful not to cover the tray (this would lock the tray into the material and make it difficult to separate) (Figure. 15.16, *D*).
17. Make sure the tray handle is parallel to working surface.
18. Allow the gypsum to set (approximately 1 hour or until heat dissipates). If the material sets too long the impression material will harden, making it difficult to separate.
19. Separate impression material from gypsum with a careful up-and-down motion to not to break teeth.

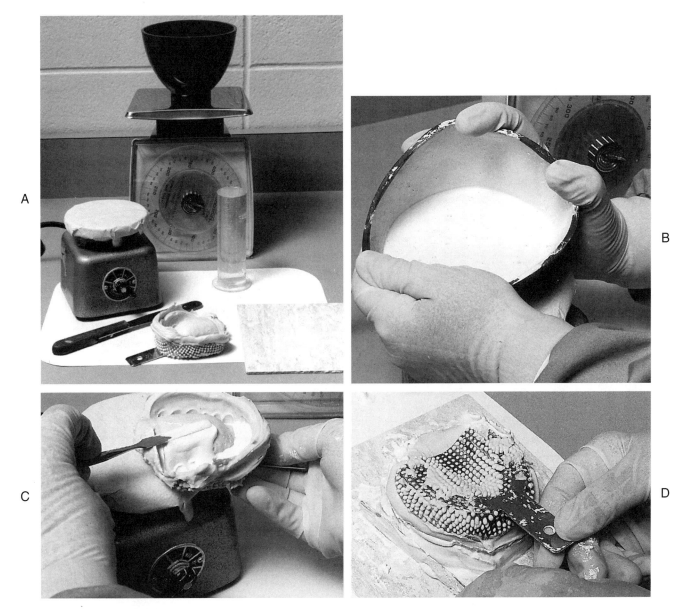

FIGURE 15.16

Procedure for mixing gypsum and pouring impressions. **A,** The equipment necessary for preparing a gypsum model include the gram scale to measure the gypsum, milliliter graduate for measuring water, rubber bowl, spatula, vibrator, and impression. **B,** Use a vibrator to reduce any remaining bubbles but do not overvibrate. **C,** Add small increments of gypsum materials with the cement spatula. Be sure to cover all the occlusal and coronal surfaces before filling the impression. **D,** After filling the impression, form a base with the remaining gypsum (rubber base former may be used to contain the gypsum for the base). Place the impression on the gypsum mass and form the sides of the base. Be sure to keep the handle parallel with the table top.

Trimming Study Models

Present well-trimmed and finished study models to the patient when treatment planning. These models can indicate the care the office staff takes when they perform various dental proce- dures. The laboratory area and equipment should be kept clean and in good working order. The trimmer blade should be sharp to allow for quick and smooth trimming, and the plaster trap should be kept clean (Box 15.18 and Tables 15.4 and 15.5).

Box 15.18

Procedure

Procedure for Trimming Study Models

Equipment needed

Model trimmer
Gypsum models
Ruler
Pencil
Sheet wax
Sharp knife
Fine sandpaper

1. Prepare the model trimmer:
   - Make sure that the table on the trimmer is perpendicular to the grinding wheel (Figure 15.17, A).
   - Turn on the water valve to produce a flow of water that will prevent the grinding wheel from becoming clogged. The model trimmer is never used without water flowing through it, and the water is never stopped until the discharged water is clear and free of stone.
2. The base of the model should make up approximately $1/3$ of the total height of the model. The anatomic portion of the model containing the teeth and gingival tissues will make up the other $2/3$ of the model (Figure 15.17, B).
3. Before trimming, soak the model in water for 2 to 3 minutes and use slurry water if more time used.
4. Remove all bubbles from the occlusal surfaces of the teeth to prevent interference when the models are occluded.
5. Preparing the maxillary model:
   - Place the model with the teeth facing down on a flat surface. The anterior teeth and premolars should be touching the flat surface.
   - Draw a line parallel to the flat surface around the base portion of the model, approximately $2 1/2$ inches up from the flat surface.
   - Trim the base to this line on the model trimmer.
   - Carefully trim the heal so that the model can be set flat on the trimmer table and gently move the base evenly against the trimming wheel making sure that the model base is parallel to the wheel.
   - The base should be about $1/2$ inch thick at its thinnest part (palate).
   - The sides of the maxillary model are trimmed parallel to an imaginary line running through the buccal cusps of the posterior teeth. The sides of the trimmed cast

   should be about $3/8$ inches from the buccal surfaces of the teeth.
   - Trim the anterior portion of the model to form a V, aligning the point of the V with the midline of the arch (Figure 15.17, C).
   - The V will intersect the previously trimmed sides in the canine area.
6. Preparing the mandibular model:
   - Trim the sides of the mandibular model like the maxillary model, with an imaginary line running parallel to the buccal cusps of the posterior teeth. The sides of the trimmed cast should be about $3/8$ inches from the buccal surfaces of the teeth.
   - The anterior portion of the model should be trimmed in a smooth arch from canine to canine. Maintain the $3/8$-inch distance from the buccal surfaces of the teeth.
7. Trimming both models:
   - Place the maxillary model on the trimmer and trim the back of the model to within $3/8$ inches of the most posterior tooth. This cut should be perpendicular to the midline of the model.
   - Occlude the maxillary and mandibular models. Place a wax bit between the models to protect the cusps (Figure 15.17, D).
   - Place the occluded models on the trimmer with the maxillary model on top of the mandibular model and trim the back (heel) of the mandibular model until it is even with the back (heel) of the maxillary model.
   - Place the occluded models on their heels on the trimmer table and trim the base of the mandibular model so that it is parallel with the base of the maxillary model. The base should be approximately $1 1/4$ inches thick. Both bases should be $1/2$ inches thick at their thinnest part. Total height should be about $2 1/2$ inches.
8. Finishing the models:
   - Smooth all trimmed areas and the lingual area of the mandibular model with a sharp knife and fine sandpaper.
   - Fill in any small holes with additional stone while the models are wet.
   - Allow the models to completely dry.
   - Place the models in hot soap solution (supersaturated Ivory flakes) for 15 minutes.
   - Rinse; remove excess soap; dry; and polish with a damp cloth.

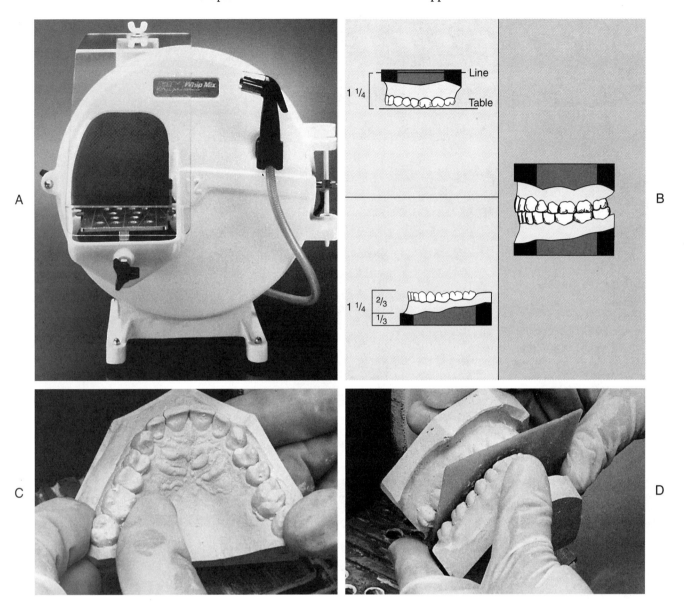

FIGURE 15.17

Trimming study models. **A,** Make sure the table is perpendicular to the wheel and the water is on to keep the wheel clear. **B,** Measure the base and sides of the gypsum models. **C,** Trim the sides of the maxillary model and form a V to parallel the sides of the model with the central groove alignment of posterior teeth and incisal alignment of anterior teeth. When trimming the mandibular model, trim a smooth, rounded arch from cuspid to cuspid. **D,** Trim the models together with a wax bite to protect cusps. (Photos for *A, C,* and *D* courtesy of Whip Mix Corporation, Louisville, Ky)

Table 15-4

Evaluation of Pretrimmed Study Models

Pretrimmed Study Models	4	3	2	0	X
Manipulation					
Proportioning					
Spatulation					
Consistency					
Pouring					
Base					
Neatness					
Removal					
Pretrimmed models					
No bubbles or air voids					
No fractured teeth					
Anatomic reproduction of teeth and tissue					
Reproduction of maxillary tuberosity					
Reproduction of mandibular retromolar pad					
Uniform vestibule					
Adequate base (approximately $^3/_8$ inch)					

The numeric criteria: 4 Excellent; 3 Good but some improvement can be made; 2 Below average, usable, needs to improve skill; 0 Unsatisfactory; X Not able to evaluate.

Table 15-5

Evaluation of Trimmed Study Models

Trimmed Study Models	4	3	2	0	X
Total height ($2^1/_2$ in)					
Height parallel					
Maxillary-anatomic detail					
Mandibular-anatomic detail					
Base accuracy-art					
Maxillary angles					
Mandibular angles					
Porous-free					
Total esthetics					

The numeric criteria: 4 Excellent; 3 Good but some improvement can be made; 2 Below average, usable, needs to improve skill; 0 Unsatisfactory; X Not able to evaluate.

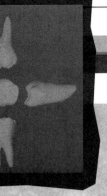

Points for Review

- Properties, characteristics, and manipulation procedures for dental cements, impression materials, gypsum, amalgam, and resin-based restorative materials.
- Types and uses of dental wax.
- Occlusal registration procedures.
- Powder-to-water ratio, mixing time, mixing temperature, setting time, and manipulation of dental materials.
- Procedures for model trimming.
- Precautions and infection control methods for the dental laboratory.

Self-Study Questions

1. Thermal conductivity and expansion refer to what property?
   a. Chemical
   b. Physical
   c. Biological
   d. Mechanical
2. What is the chemical name for dental stone?
   a. Calcium hydroxide
   b. Bis-GMA
   c. Calcium sulfate dihydrate
   d. Potassium sulfate
3. How will the water-to-powder ratio being too high effect the strength of dental stone?
   a. Stronger mix
   b. Weaker mix
   c. No difference
4. Which type of gypsum has the smallest and most dense crystal structure?
   a. Plaster
   b. Class I stone
   c. Class II stone

5. Which is the best method for slowing the reaction rate of an alginate impression material?
   a. Use warm water
   b. Use cold water
   c. Add alginic acid
   d. Mix slow
6. Which type of cement is anticariogenic?
   a. Zinc oxide eugenol
   b. Zinc phosphate
   c. Glass-ionomer
   d. Dycal
7. Which cement serves as an obtundent?
   a. Zinc oxide eugenol
   b. Zinc phosphate
   c. Glass-ionomer
   d. Calcium hydroxide
8. What is the name of a mixture of two or more metals?
   a. Activator
   b. Alumina
   c. Alloy
   d. Cross-linking
9. The dental assistant can control the strength of cement through what process?
   a. Cooling the glass slab
   b. Use of retarders
   c. Controlling the amount of powder-to-liquid ratio
   d. A and c
10. What property can moisture contamination affect the mixing of zinc phosphate?
    a. Setting time
    b. Strength
    c. Hardness
    d. Shading

Suggested Readings

Craig RG: *Restorative dental materials*, ed 10, St Louis, 1997, Mosby.
Craig RG, Powers JM, Wataha JC: *Dental materials: property and manipulation*, ed 7, St Louis, 2000, Mosby.
O'Brien WJ: *Dental materials*, Chicago, 1989, Quintessence.
Phillips RW, Moore BK: *Elements of dental materials*, ed 5, Philadelphia, 1994, WB Saunders.

Chapter 16

Nutrition and Dietary Counseling

Key Points

- Review of basic nutritional concepts
- Influence of nutrition on general and oral health
- Process of modifying the food habits of patients

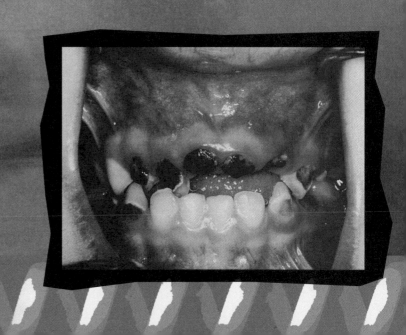

Chapter Outline

Nutrition and Dietary Counseling
Review of basic nutritional concepts
Nutrition and Oral Health and Disease
**Nutritional influences during tooth
development**
**Postnatal nutrition and dental
development**

Role of the dental assistant
Nutrition and dental caries
Nutrition and Periodontal Disease
Systemic factors
Local factors
Dietary Interview
Dietary Management

Learning Objectives

On completion of Chapter 16, the student should be able to do the following:

■ Define key terms.

■ Discuss the food guide pyramid's purpose and limitations and the contributions to nutrition made by each food group.

■ Categorize the nutrients required by the body into six broad areas and discuss classification, function, and food sources.

■ State what nutrients have the most influence on tooth development.

■ Discuss the problem of nursing-bottle caries and prevention.

■ Discuss the role of the dental assistant in providing dietary guidance through the life cycle, including pregnancy, infancy, and adulthood.

■ Explain the role of carbohydrates in the etiology of dental caries.

■ Explain the nutritional influences on periodontal disease.

■ Summarize the dietary goals for the United States.

■ State the indications for and the guidelines and steps followed in dietary counseling.

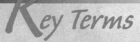

Key Terms

Adequate Diet	Diet	RDA
Balanced Diet	Fat	Sugar
Calories	Minerals	USRDA
Cholesterol	Nutrient	Vitamins

NUTRITION AND DIETARY COUNSELING

Dental professionals are in a unique position to supply the health service of nutrition and dietary counseling because about one-half of the U.S. population seeks regular dental care. Dental care provides a mechanism for ongoing examination, evaluation, and recommendation.

Nutrients

A substance required by the body for health and function and categorized into proteins, carbohydrates, fats, vitamins, minerals, and water.

The term *nutritional* refers to the **nutrients** in foods and their systemic effects, or their general influence on the body following digestion, absorption, and use. In contrast, the term *dietary* refers to the local, as opposed to the systemic or general, effects of foods on the teeth and other structures in the mouth.

Review of Basic Nutritional Concepts

Diet

The pattern or regimen of food intake.

Adequate diet

An eating pattern that includes a variety of foods and provides all the nutrients essential for good health.

The **diet** refers to the pattern of food intake. The diet recommended for general health should provide virtually all of the nutrients normally required for the development and maintenance of healthy oral tissues. The general requirements for an **adequate diet** are discussed in the next section.

Recommended Dietary Allowances

The recommended dietary allowances (**RDA**) are suggested levels of intake of certain key nutrients designed to maintain good nutrition in healthy persons. The allowances are broad to allow for the variations of requirements that occur in the general population; they are set higher than the minimal requirements to provide for nutritional needs during periods of

RDA

Recommended dietary allowances of the levels of nutrient intake based on age, sex, and activity of the U.S. population.

stress and permit adequate growth and development. The recommended nutritional levels can be readily obtained by choosing a diet that provides adequate variety and quantity of foods.

Food Guides

Based on the RDA, the following two similar guides have been prepared to simplify the composition of an adequate diet:

1 The *Food Guide Pyramid* (the U.S. Department of Agriculture and the U.S. Department of Health and Human Services)
2 The *Guide to Good Eating* (National Dairy Council) (Figure 16.1)

These food guides provide an outline of what to eat each day and are general plans that let you choose a healthful diet that is right for you.

Foods are classified into five basic groups according to their contribution of several key nutrients, with emphasis placed on key foods in each group as important sources of certain nutrients. These daily food plans give a basis for an adequate diet and encourage a wide choice in food selection. The purpose of the guides is to provide a practical method of planning food selection.

Milk Group

The milk group includes all kinds of milk and cheeses, including cottage cheese, yogurt, ice cream, and milk. Foods in this group supply most of the calcium and significant amounts of riboflavin (B_2) and protein in our food supply, in addition to some of almost all essential nutrients. The recommended servings of milk (or its equivalent) are in Table 16.1.

Meat Group

The meat group includes meat (beef, veal, pork, lamb, and wild game); fish and shellfish; poultry, eggs, legumes (such as dry beans), peas, lentils, and peanuts; and nuts. These foods provide the major supply of protein, iron, niacin, thiamin (B_1), and other members of the Vitamin B complex and of the mineral nutrients. Two-to-three servings from the meat group are recommended daily. Three servings are recommended for pregnant women. One serving equals 2 to 3 oz of boneless, lean cooked meat; poultry or fish; two eggs or one cup of cooked, dry beans or peas.

Vegetable sources of proteins such as cooked dry beans or peas, soy extenders, and nuts by themselves supply protein lacking in essential amino acids (incomplete protein). The consumption of animal protein (complete protein) such as meat, fish, poultry, eggs, milk, or cheese at the same time complements the incomplete protein so that complete protein necessary for body building and maintenance is available. Examples of complementary protein feeding in this manner are chile con carne with beans, split

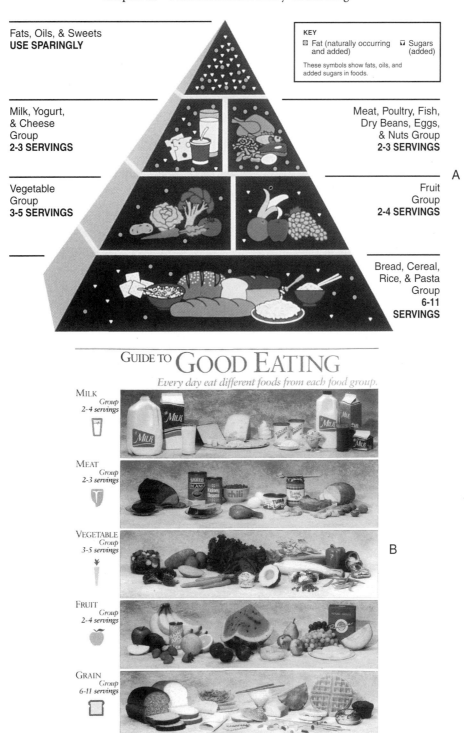

FIGURE 16.1

A, *Food Guide Pyramid.* **B,** *Guide to Good Eating.* (National Dairy Council.)

pea soup with milk, and tuna chow mein with cashew nuts. Foods containing dry beans and peas and nuts can also be combined with grain to enhance protein use (for example, baked beans and brown bread, beans and rice, peanut butter sandwich).

Fruit and Vegetable Group

The fruit and vegetable group is actually two separate groups but is discussed here as one group. It includes all fresh, canned, frozen, and dried fruits and vegetables, except dried beans and peas. The latter are placed in the meat group because of their high protein content. Fruit and vegetables supply most of the vitamin C in our diet and are abundant sources of vitamin A and numerous other **vitamins** and **minerals** such as iron.

Two-to-four servings of fruits and three-to-five servings of vegetables are recommended daily. Citrus fruit (such as oranges, grapefruit, and tomatoes) is recommended daily for vitamin C. Dark green, leafy or orange vegetables and fruits are recommended three or four times weekly for vitamin A. A serving of cooked fruit or vegetables or juice is $1/2$ cup (4 oz), or a portion ordinarily served, such as a medium apple, banana or potato, or one half of a medium grapefruit.

Vitamins

A class of nutrients that are essential components of the body's enzyme systems, usually required by the body in small amounts and present in minute quantities in foods.

Minerals

Certain inorganic elements essential in human nutrition.

Grain Group

The grain group includes all grains such as barley, buckwheat, corn, oats, rice, rye, wheat, and the breads. The breads recommended are breakfast cereals, grits, and noodle and pasta products made from them (see Figure 16.1). The grain group is a significant source of the thiamin (B_1), iron, niacin, and other essential nutrients in our food supply. Grain is an important, economic source of carbohydrate.

Approximately 6-to-11 servings of enriched, fortified, or whole grain foods is recommended daily. A serving is one tortilla, slice of bread, pancake, or small waffle; half of an English muffin, hamburger bun, or bagel; 1 cup of ready-to-eat cereal; and $1/2$ cup of cooked cereal, rice, grits, pasta, or noodles. Milk combined with cereal improves the use of grain proteins for body building and repair. Examples of grains combined with products for high-quality protein include cheese pizza, macaroni casserole, and beans and rice.

Others

Foods that contain mostly fats, sweets, and alcohol are placed in the "others" category. They are often referred to as *empty calorie* foods because they contain **calories**, **fat**, and little else. They do not (or should not) take the place of foods from the five major food groups described earlier in supplying nutrients. Specific amounts or servings are not recommended but, rather, should be determined by individual caloric needs. Fats and oils, sweets, desserts, chips and related products, condiments, and beverages such as coffee, tea, fruit drinks, alcoholic products, and soft drinks are included in this category.

Using the Dietary Guide

A diet based on the guide discussed earlier supplies most or all of the caloric needs of the average adult, and provides the major portion of the recommended allowance of all other essential nutrients. Additional calories and nutrients are supplied by eating some foods from the "others" food group as needed or desired. Fluoride may need to be supplemented for infants and children who are breast-fed only or live in areas where fluoride is not in the water.

These guides can be useful for the dental auxiliary who seeks to advise patients regarding their choice of desirable foods under normal conditions. Ordinarily, consumed food, and not synthetic supplements used instead, should be the main source of providing dietary requirements.

USRDA and the Food Label

The **USRDA** (U.S. recommended daily allowances or "daily value") is another guide that was prepared for use in nutrition labeling of foods. The objective is to list on food labels those nutrients judged most important and necessary to maintain a positive state of health and to include an excess to allow for individual variations (Figure 16.2). The USRDA (daily value) will generally be higher than the RDA. The percentages of nutrients listed at the top of the

Calories

A measure of energy in foods. They are obtained from the protein, carbohydrate, and fat in the diet.

Fat

Several compounds that are insoluble in water but soluble in fat solvents such as ether and chloroform.

USRDA

U.S. recommended daily allowances. A guide developed by the food and drug administration (FDA) for use in nutrition labeling of foods. Also called *daily value*.

Table 16.1

The Guide to Daily Food Choices—A Summary

Food Group	Servings	Major Contributions	Foods and Serving Sizes*
Bread, cereals, rice, pasta	6-11	Starch Thiamin Riboflavin[†] Iron Niacin Folate Magnesium[‡] Fiber[‡] Zinc	1 slice of bread 1 oz ready-to-eat cereal $1/2$-$3/4$ cup cooked cereal, rice, pasta
Vegetables	3-5	Vitamin A Vitamin C Folate Magnesium Fiber	$1/2$ cup raw or cooked vegetables 1 cup raw leafy vegetables
Fruits	2-4	Vitamin C Fiber	$1/4$ cup dried fruit $1/2$ cup cooked fruit $3/4$ cup juice 1 whole piece of fruit 1 melon wedge

Milk, yogurt, cheese	2 (adults[§])
	3 (children, teens, young
	   adults, pregnant or
	   lactating women)
		Calcium
		Riboflavin
		Protein
		Potassium
		Zinc
			1 cup milk
			$1^1/2$ oz cheese
			2 oz processed cheese
			1 cup yogurt
			2 cups cottage cheese
			1 cup custard/pudding
			$1^1/2$ cups ice cream

Meat, poultry, fish, dry beans, eggs, nuts	2-3	Protein Niacin Iron Vitamin B$_6$ Zinc Thiamin Vitamin B$_{12}$[‖]	2-3 oz cooked meat, poultry, fish 1-$1^1/2$ cups cooked dry beans 4 T peanut butter 2 eggs $1/2$-1 cup nuts
Fats, oils, sweets	Foods from this group should not replace any from the other groups. Amounts consumed should be determined by individual energy needs.		

Adapted from the US Department of Agriculture, revised edition of former *Basic Four Food Groups Guide,* 1985.
*May be reduced for child servings.
[†]If enriched.
[‡]Whole grains especially.
[§]≥25 years of age.
[‖]Only in animal food choices.

Nutrition Facts

Serving Size 1/2 cup (114g)
Servings Per Container 4

Amount Per Serving

Calories 90   Calories from Fat 30

% Daily Value*

Total Fat 3g	5%
Saturated Fat 0g	0%
Cholesterol 0mg	0%
Sodium 300mg	13%
Total Carbohydrate 13g	4%
Dietary Fiber 3g	12%
Sugars 3g	
Protein 3g	

Vitamin A	80%	Vitamin C	60%
Calcium	4%	Iron	4%

* Percent Daily Values are based on a 2,000 calorie diet. Your diet values may be higher or lower depending on your calorie needs:

	Calories	2,000	2,500
Total Fat	Less than	65g	80g
Sat Fat	Less than	20g	25g
Cholesterol	Less than	300mg	300mg
Sodium	Less than	2,400mg	2,400mg
Total Carbohydrate		300g	375g
Fiber		25g	30g

Calories per gram:

Fat 9   •   Carbohydrates 4 •   Protein 4

This label is only a sample.

FIGURE 16.2

Sample of the revised FDA labeling format.

food label (% daily value) are based on the USRDA for an "average" 2000 calorie diet.

Nutrients

Approximately 50 nutrients are required by the body for health and function. These nutrients are classified into the following six broad categories:

1 Proteins
2 Carbohydrates
3 Fats
4 Vitamins
5 Minerals
6 Water

Most foods contain several nutrients and calories. No one food is a complete source of all nutrients, even though some have specific nutrients added. All essential nutrients (those that must be eaten because the body cannot make them) are available in common foods; therefore, supplements are an unnecessary expense for most healthy people who eat a varied, well-selected diet. Many different combinations of foods furnish essential nutrients for optimal health. Eating a variety of fresh and minimally processed foods helps ensure obtaining virtually all needed nutrients.

Energy and Calories

Energy is required for growth and all body functions, such as breathing and digestion, maintaining normal body temperature, and physical activity. Calories are a measurement of energy. The more active people are, the more calories they use.

Calories are obtained from the protein, carbohydrate, and fat in the foods eaten. Protein and carbohydrate each supply about 4 calories per gram of food (28 g 1 oz). Fat supplies 9 calories per gram.

Carbohydrates

The major function of carbohydrates is to provide energy for the body. Carbohydrates also prevent the use of protein as a source of energy, allowing protein to be available for its primary purpose: tissue-building and cell replacement. Furthermore, carbohydrates provide the all-important fiber, or roughage, that the body needs. Although humans cannot digest dietary fiber, it is an important part of a well-**balanced diet**. The **sugars**, however, contribute little more than energy in the diet, hence the term *empty calories* (junk food). In contrast, the complex

Balanced diet

An eating regimen that incorporates meals consisting of foods from several of the food groups at each meal.

Sugar

Carbohydrates classified as either monosaccharides or disaccharides, all having a sweet taste and being cariogenic.

carbohydrates often contribute many other nutrients such as vitamins, minerals, water, protein, and fiber.

Proteins

Protein in the diet supplies the amino acids and nitrogen needed to make body protein that is essential for growth and body repair. Only dietary proteins can perform this unique function. However, proteins can also be used to supply energy and when the diet does not provide sufficient energy from carbohydrate and fats, proteins may be "wasted" for energy needs even at the expense of body protein. Generally, vegetable sources of protein such as grains, nuts, and fruits are incomplete, whereas proteins from animal sources such as eggs or milk are complete.

Fats

Fat is part of the structure of the body's cells. Stored body fat provides insulation and protects vital organs by forming a cushion around them. Fats are our most concentrated source of energy, providing 9 calories per gram, considerably greater than the 4 calories per gram provided by carbohydrates and proteins. In addition, fats are the carriers of the fat-soluble vitamins A, D, E, and K, aid in their absorption, and provide for their storage in the adipose tissue. Dietary fats also provide an essential fatty acid necessary for proper growth and healthy skin. Finally, fats add to our enjoyment of foods because of their flavor, contribution to desirable food texture, and provide for a feeling of fullness (satiety). Frequently the amount of fat in the diet is underestimated because many people think only about visible fats such as butter, margarine, lard, cooking and salad oils. However, foods also contain "invisible" fat, such as the fatty streaks in marbled beef, the fats contained in nuts, other meats and dairy products, and that present in many processed foods, such as potato chips.

Some of the major sources of fat include dairy products, eggs, meat products, and cooking fats and oils of both animal and vegetable origin. In general, vegetable fats have a low degree of saturation (they are high in polyunsaturated fatty acids), whereas animal fats have a high degree of saturation (high in saturated fatty acids). However, all naturally occurring fats are actually mixtures of saturated, monosaturated, and polyunsaturated fatty acids.

Presently, about 40% of the total calories in the American diet are derived from fats. This excess intake at the expense of other nutrients may contribute to such serious diseases as diabetes, obesity, and atherosclerosis. *An association exists between elevated levels of cholesterol in the blood, a high saturated fat diet, and heart disease.*

In general, the ingestion of saturated fats increases

Cholesterol

A fat-soluble substance that is manufactured only by animals, including humans, and therefore only present in animal-source foods.

blood **cholesterol** levels, and polyunsaturated fats and monosaturated fats decrease the cholesterol level. Because of this, the following dietary changes to reduce serum cholesterol have been advocated and are likely to reduce the risk of heart disease:

- Reduce saturated fat by increasing the consumption of vegetable-source foods and fish and fowl and decreasing the consumption of animal-source foods, especially dairy products made from whole-milk, pork, and beef.
- Increase polyunsaturated fat and monosaturated fat by using salad and cooking oils and margarine and shortenings made from vegetable oils.
- Reduce dietary cholesterol by eating fewer animal-origin foods, especially organ meats, whole milk, and egg yolks.

Vitamins

The vitamins are a group of substances that are present in small amounts in foods and are necessary for the normal functioning of the body. They are essential components of the body's enzyme systems and also function as hormones. The human body cannot manufacture most of the vitamins it needs and therefore must obtain them from the diet. However, vitamin D can be formed in the skin, and the intestinal bacteria can make vitamin K and certain B vitamins.

B-Complex Vitamins

At least eight different essential vitamins are part of the B-complex vitamins and primarily involved in the following:

- Release of energy from food (thiamin, niacin, riboflavin, pantothenic acid, and biotin)
- Formation of red blood cells (folic acid and vitamin B_{12})
- Release of energy from foods (as well as its role as an antianemic coenzyme B_6)

Vitamin-B complex is often considered as one entity because its component vitamins frequently occur together in the same foods. Table 16.2 summarizes the major points of interest concerning the function, food sources, requirements, and deficiencies of the eight essential B vitamins.

Vitamin C (Ascorbic Acid)

Vitamin C is essential in the manufacture of collagen, the protein that serves as the "cement" holding connective tissues together, including the periodontal ligament. Ascorbic acid is present almost exclusively in the vegetable and fruit food groups. Citrus fruits and green, leafy vegetables are popular sources. The RDA is about 50 mg.

The dietary deficiency of ascorbic acid is scurvy, a severe disease rarely encountered in the developed countries. The oral changes associated with this disease may include severe gingivitis with heavy bleeding and swelling, although plaque is most important in the initiation of gingivitis.

Vitamin A

Vitamin A is essential for the formation of visual purple, a substance related to the maintenance of normal vision in

Table 16.2

Functions, Dietary Sources, Requirements, and Deficiencies of B-Complex Vitamins

Vitamin	Function	Major Dietary Sources	Adult Daily Requirement	Deficiency Manifestation
B₁-thiamine	Coenzyme in carbohydrate and protein metabolism	Pork, whole and enriched cereal grains, legumes, meats	1.0 - 1.5 mg	Beriberi; possible oral manifestations
B₂-riboflavin	Coenzyme in carbohydrate and protein metabolism	Milk, green vegetables, meat, fish, and eggs	1.5 - 1.7 mg	Lesions of the lips mouth, eyes, and skin
Niacin - (nicotinic acid)	Coenzyme in carbohydrate and protein metabolism	Meat, legumes, enriched or whole grain cereals	13 - 18 mg	Pellagra
B₆-(pyridoxal, pyridoxamine, pyridoxine)	Amino acid metabolism	Whole grain cereals, milk, meat, and vegetables	2 mg	Rare, possible oral manifestations
Panthothenic acid	Active in coenzyme A	Widely distributed in many foods	Not yet established	Unlikely
B₁₂-cyanocobalamine	Nucleic acid metabolism (red blood cell formation)	Animal foods; meat and dairy products	Not yet established	Unlikely but not dietary in origin
Folic acid (folacin)	Purine metabolism (red blood cell formation)	Green leafy vegetables organ meats	0.4 mg	Macrocytic anemia
Biotin	Essential for activity of enzyme systems	Widely distributed in many foods	Not yet established	Unlikely

dim light (Table 16.3). In addition, this vitamin contributes to the maintenance of the skin and the membranes that line the eyes, mouth, respiratory, genitourinary, and gastrointestinal tract. Vitamin A is also essential for normal growth and development of the skeletal system and dentition. The main sources of vitamin A are butter, eggs, milk, liver, and some fish. Plant foods, particularly those having an intense green or yellow color, are excellent sources of carotene, which the body can convert into vitamin A.

The early signs of vitamin A deficiency are night blindness (inability to adapt to the dark) and the development of rough, sandpaper-like skin.

Vitamin D

Vitamin D promotes the absorption of calcium and phosphorus and is essential for the formation of sound bones and teeth (see Table 16.3). Because exposure to sunlight converts a compound present in the skin to vitamin D, humans probably derive a major portion of this vitamin from sun exposure of the skin. The best dietary source is fortified milk.

The RDA of vitamin D is 400 international units (IU). A deficiency of this vitamin in childhood leads to rickets, characterized by a severely defective skeletal system. In adult life, the deficiency disease is osteomalacia, which results in a softening of the bones. Like vitamin A, excess levels of vitamin D tend to accumulate in the body.

Vitamin E

Vitamin E functions as an antioxidant, helps in the formation of red blood cells, and promotes the stability of biologic membranes (see Table 16.3). The richest sources of vitamin E are the various seed or vegetable oils, but vitamin E is widely distributed in many other foods. No natural deficiencies of vitamin E have been observed in humans. Food faddists have claimed the vitamin has almost supernatural powers but these claims have little scientific foundation. The cosmetic benefits from applying vitamin E to the skin are exaggerated. However, vitamin E supplements may be beneficial for those who suffer from a circulatory disease in the legs that causes pain and difficulty in walking (intermittent claudication).

Table 16.8

Fat-Soluble Vitamins

	A	D	E	K
Active chemical forms	Retinol	Cholecalciferol	Tocopherols	Vitamin K_1 phylloquinone and K2 menaquinone
	3-dehydroretinol Retinal Retinoic acid Carotenoids	Ergocalciferol	α, β, γ, etc. Tocotrieols	

Important food sources	Liver
	Egg yolk
	Butter, cream
	Margarine
	Green and yellow
	  vegetables
	Apricots
	Cantaloupe
		Irradiated foods
		Small amounts in:
		  Butter
		  Egg yolk
		  Liver
		  Salmon
		  Sardines
		  Tuna fish
			Wheat germ
			Leafy vegetables
			Vegetable oils
			Egg yolk
			Legumes
			Peanuts
			Margarine
				Cabbage
				Cauliflower
				Spinach
				Other leafy
				  vegetables
				Pork liver
				Soybean oil and other
				  vegetables oils

Solubility to cooking, drying, etc.	Gradual destruction
	  by exposure to air,
	  heat, and drying;
	  more rapid at high
	  temperatures
		Stable to heating,
		  aging, and storage
		Destroyed by excess
		  ultraviolet irradiation
			Stable to methods
			  of food processing
			Destroyed by rancidity
			  and ultraviolet
			  irradiation
				Stable to heat, light,
				  and exposure to air
				Destroyed by strong
				  acids, alkalis, and
				  oxidizing agents

Functions	Maintains function of
	  epithelial cells, mucous
	  membranes, skin, bone;
	  constituent of visual pigments
		Calcium and phos-
		  phorus absorption
		  and use in
		  bone growth
			Protects cell
			  structures
				Necessary in formation
				  of four factors
				  essential for clotting
				  of blood

Deficiency signs and symptoms	Night blindness
	Glare blindness
	Rough, dry skin
	Dry mucous
	  membranes
	Xerophthalmia
		Rickets
		Soft bones
		Bowed legs
		Poor teeth
		Skeletal deformities
			Increased hemolysis
			  of red blood cells
				Slow clotting time of
				  blood
				Some hemorrhagic
				  disease of newborn
				Lack of prothrombin

Adult human requirement	Male 1000 RE
	  (5000 IU);
	Female 800 RE
	  (4000 IU)
		Children and
		  adolescents 400 IU
			Male 15 IU
			Female 12 IU
				Unknown

Table 16.4

Some Minerals Essential to Health

Mineral	Best Source	Important Functions	Deficiency Symptoms

Calcium	Milk
	Cheese
	Sardines and other
	   whole canned fish
	Vegetable greens
		Normal development
		  and maintenance
		  of bones and teeth
		Clotting of the blood
		Normal heart action
		Normal muscle activity
		Iron use
			Retarded growth
			Poor tooth formation
			Rickets
			Slow clotting time of blood
			Porous bones

Phosphorus	Meat, poultry, fish
	Milk
	Cheese
	Dried beans and peas
	Whole grain products
		Formation of normal bones
		  and teeth
		Cell structure
		Maintenance of normal blood
		  tissue
		Normal muscle activity
			Retarded growth
			Poor tooth formation
			Rickets
			Porous bones

Magnesium	Whole grains Nuts Soybeans Green, leafy vegetables	Production of energy Protein synthesis Bone-building Acid base balance	Hyperexcitability Weakness Depression Tremors Convulsions
Iodine	Seafoods Iodized salt	Formation of thyroxine, a hormone that controls metabolic rate	Goiter Slow metabolism

Iron	Liver, organ meat
	Oysters
	Vegetable greens
	Dried beans and peas
	Dried fruits
	Egg yolk
	Whole grain or
	  enriched products
		Formation of hemoglobin of the
		  red blood cells
		Carrying oxygen to body tissues
			Anemia characterized by:
			  Weakness
			  Dizziness
			  Loss of weight
			  Gastric disturbances
			  Pallor

Copper	Liver Dried beans and peas Meat Nuts Cereals	Formation of hemoglobin	Anemia (see iron)

Vitamin K

In addition to being widely distributed in foods, vitamin K is manufactured by the human intestinal bacteria and is necessary for the formation of several factors in blood that are responsible for blood clotting. No RDA has been established. A deficiency is rare, however, vitamin K injections are commonly given to infants immediately after delivery because an inadequate reserve of this vitamin occurs in the newborn.

Minerals

Twenty one minerals are considered essential in human nutrition and have many functions in the body (Table 16.4). For example, calcium, phosphorus, magnesium, and fluorine are important parts of bones; sodium, potassium and chlorine are electrolytes that function in the maintenance of acid-base balance and body fluids; iron, copper, and cobalt are essential in red blood cell formation; other minerals including magnesium, manganese, zinc, and molybdenum function as components of various enzyme systems.

Minerals are divided into two broad categories. The macrominerals (calcium, phosphorus and magnesium) are those elements required by the body in relatively large quantities (300 to 800 mg), whereas microminerals, or trace elements, are those required in very small amounts (less than 100 mg).

Macrominerals

Calcium and Phosphorus Calcium and phosphorus are the most abundant minerals in the body. They occur together as the major components of both the skeletal and dental tissues, providing rigidity to the bones and teeth. In addition, calcium in the blood functions in muscular contraction, blood clotting, nerve function, and enzyme activation. Phosphorus regulates acid-base balance and assists in energy release.

Magnesium Magnesium is an essential part of bone and soft tissues and is also involved in energy production. Major sources are whole grain cereals, nuts, legumes, cocoa, and some dark green, leafy vegetables.

Microminerals (Trace Elements)

Iron Most of the body's iron is present in the blood as hemoglobin, which carries oxygen from the lungs to the tissues and returns carbon dioxide from the tissues to the lungs. An inadequate intake of iron will lead to iron-deficiency anemia, which occurs most frequently in infants, children, and pregnant and lactating women. For this reason, iron supplements are often recommended for these groups, especially pregnant women.

Iodine Iodine is primarily found in the thyroid gland, where it is a component of the thyroid hormone, which controls energy production.

Potassium and Sodium Potassium and sodium function prominently in the maintenance of water and electrolyte balance.

Water

Water is second only to oxygen among life's basic requirements. One can exist several weeks without food but only a few days without water. Water is the universal solvent or medium in which all metabolic reactions occur; for example, taste, digestion, absorption, circulation, and excretion.

As the major transport fluid, water (in blood or other body fluids) is responsible for delivery of all other nutrients required for growth and maintenance of life. At the same time, water carries off byproducts of metabolic reactions, whether they are to be used elsewhere in the body or to be eliminated as waste.

The constant presence of water between cells and tissues lubricates and cushions tissues against friction and shock. So much water exists within and around the cells, tissues, and organs (approximately 50% to 60% of our body weight is water) that it contributes substantially to body structure; water is the most abundant nutrient in our bodies.

A suitable allowance for water for most adults is 2 L daily. Much of this quantity is contained in prepared foods. Some water is contained in almost all foods.

NUTRITION AND ORAL HEALTH AND DISEASE

The nutritional needs for maintaining the health of the oral structures are similar to those for the remainder of the body. Optimal maternal nutrition is required for the best calcification of the primary dentition, and proper nutrition during infancy and childhood is particularly important for the maintenance of excellent dental structures in the permanent dentition. Furthermore, dietary intake and plaque control following the eruption of the teeth have profound influences on the health or disease status of the teeth and their supporting structures. The need for nutrients (especially iron) and energy also increases during pregnancy.

Nutritional Influences During Tooth Development

Vitamin A, C, and D deficiencies along with deficiency and imbalanced ratios of calcium and phosphorus cause malformations in the structure of the developing tooth.

Vitamin A is required for the promotion of the health of the oral structures such as the teeth, periodontium, and oral mucous membranes. Inadequate vitamin A intake affects the development of the enamel. Vitamin C deficiency during tooth development results in impaired dentin formation. Inadequate amounts of vitamin D or calcium, phosphorus, or imbalanced ratios of calcium and phosphorus result in imperfect calcification of the teeth. Vitamin D deficiency during tooth development may result in an increased susceptibility of caries. Fluoride is essential in the mineralization of teeth and bones, playing the most important role in the formation of teeth with caries resistance.

Postnatal Nutrition and Dental Development

Nutrients needed once the teeth have erupted into the mouth are found in an adequate, balanced diet. With the exception of fluoride, no special nutrient requirements exist for the teeth. Furthermore, ingesting nutrients in excess of

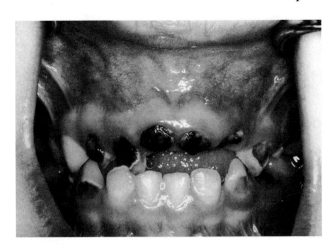

FIGURE 16.3

An infant with nursing bottle caries. (Courtesy Dr. Guy Furnish, Louisville, Ky.)

the RDA in an attempt to increase the resistance of the oral structures to disease is not always necessary.

Nursing Bottle Caries

Excessive decay with extensive destruction of the teeth is occasionally seen in 2-to 4-year old children. This condition may be associated with misuse of the nursing bottle, pacifier, or foods and liquids eaten by the infant at nap or bedtime. Because of reduced salivary flow during sleep, all foods or liquids, except water, should be avoided within 1 hour of nap or bedtime. This includes milk, fruit juices, formulas, and soft drinks.

Use of these liquids may lead to the pattern of excessive caries commonly referred to as *nursing bottle decay* (Figure 16.3), a rampant caries with extensive and rapid carious destruction of the maxillary incisors and primary first molars. In advanced cases, the entire dentition may be affected. Sugar-dipped pacifiers should also be avoided. Frequent breast-feeding can also cause severe or rampant caries of the primary dentition in infants.

Role of the Dental Assistant

The dental assistant can be helpful to those patients who are about to become parents by inquiring about their nutritional beliefs and practices. For example, expectant mothers should be cautioned against highly restrictive dieting for weight control. If the pregnant patient is not consuming a varied, balanced diet and limiting sweet intake, now is an ideal time to try to correct problem habits. New parents may need to be cautioned about adding sugar to a baby bottle and dipping the pacifier in honey. Patients should make sure their teenagers do not skip meals or snack on "junk" food. Iron-deficiency anemia may be a problem for some infants and children. Cereals that have added iron are useful for avoiding this problem. Adults can be advised to reduce calories or increase exercise to avoid weight gain. The elderly should be advised in the need for a balanced diet.

In general, dietary goals should include eating less fat and more carbohydrate (with almost twice the current intake of complex carbohydrate). Alterations in the current diet to achieve this recommended change include increased consumption of whole grains, fruits and vegetables, and decreased intake of foods high in refined and processed sugars, salt, cholesterol, and saturated and total fat. Diets low in fiber are associated with increased colon cancer, diabetes, and heart disease. Dental health should improve if more grains, fruits and vegetables, unsaturated fats, monosaturated fats, and whole grain cereals are eaten with a corresponding decrease in refined and processed sugars.

Nutrition and Dental Caries

Dental caries results from the interplay of the following three important factors (Figure 16.4):

1 Bacteria
2 Host
3 Diet

Role of Bacteria

Bacteria are essential for the initiation of dental caries. Certain bacteria, particularly *Streptococcus mutans*, can manufacture glucan, a sticky substance, from dietary sucrose. The glucan aids bacteria in adhering to the tooth and therefore is important in the build up of bacterial plaque. The result of plaque build up and sugar is production of acid. Frequent use of sugars and some starches leads to continuous acid production.

Role of the Host: Individual Susceptibility

Each person varies in the susceptibility to dental caries. This may be because of the interaction between plaque bacteria, diet, and host. With average host susceptibility and mechanical cleansing, the intake of sugars will be the major factor. If plaque control and diet are good, the major determinant of

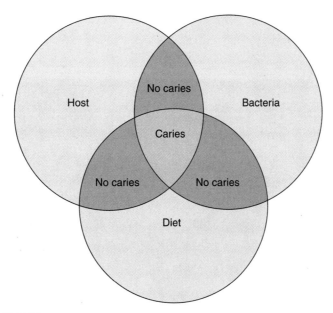

FIGURE 16.4

Critical factors in caries etiology include the host, bacteria, and diet.

caries is the susceptibility or resistance of the tooth surface (influenced largely by fluoride) and the protective qualities of saliva.

Role of Diet

In the absence of dietary sugars acting locally in the mouth, caries will not occur. The various sugars have differing abilities to produce carious lesions. Sucrose has a greater cariogenic potential than other sugars, but maltose, lactose, glucose, fructose, and their mixtures do have high caries-producing abilities in rodents. Flour and starches are usually not cariogenic, but when starch is used in conjunction with sugar, the potential cariogenicity increases.

Sugar Substitutes

Substitute sweeteners are potentially attractive alternatives to sucrose. The principal sugar substitutes available are saccharine, aspartame ("Nutrasweet"), sorbitol, and mannitol. Saccharine is currently used in cosmetics, drugs, dentifrices, mouthwashes, and "Sweet and Low," although it is not recommended for most children, pregnant or young women of child-bearing age, or for excessive use, because it causes tumors in animals. Aspartame is a much safer product and is used in a wide range of food products. It is the principal ingredient in "Equal." Sorbitol and mannitol are used in a wide variety of food products, including toothpaste, candies, and other snack products, but excessive intake can have a laxative effect.

NUTRITION AND PERIODONTAL DISEASE

Systemic Factors

The nutritional status of the individual obviously has some bearing on the development and health of the periodontal tissues. Nutritional factors do not cause periodontal disease by themselves, but they can alter host susceptibility to periodontal disease or modify its progress. Many specific nutrients influence the periodontal structures. For example, a protein deficiency increases susceptibility to periodontal infection and suppresses repair. Folic acid deficiency lowers the host defense mechanisms in the gingiva. Vitamin C deficiency increases the inflammatory gingival response to plaque bacteria, and altered dietary calcium:phosphate ratios may cause alveolar bone resorption in edentulous ridge areas.

Although nutrition can alter the host response to bacterial plaque, nutritional therapy alone has not cured periodontal disease. Similarly, good nutritional practices alone will not prevent periodontal disease.

Local Factors

Local irritation from plaque and calculus play the major role in the initiation of periodontal disease. Deficiencies of specific vitamins or other nutrients, in the absence of local factors, will not produce periodontal destruction.

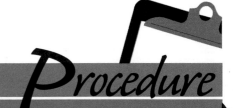

Box 16.1

Procedure for Conducting a Dietary Interview

Step 1

Ascertain everything consumed on an ordinary weekday, including snacks, supplements, gum, and fluoridated water.

Note the time when meals and snacks are eaten, how much of each was ingested in household measures, how the food was prepared, and if any sugar was added to any of the foods or beverages or gum.

Be sure the food diary described by the patient represents the typical intake pattern.

Step 2

Note the foods that have been sweetened with added sugar, including soft drinks (all carbonated beverages and beer should be circled, diet or not, because of their acidity), sugar added to coffee, cookies, cakes, pastry, jam, candy, cough drops, cough syrup, fruits canned in syrup, and other foods that have an overtly sweet taste. Dried fruits such as figs, dates, prunes, apricots, and raisins should be circled because they are highly concentrated sweets. However, fresh fruits with their high water and fiber content, such as apples, oranges or pears, are not.

Step 3

Classify the remaining foods into one or more of the appropriate food groups. Circle the 5 food groups and place a check mark for each serving of food eaten in a particular category.

Classify all of the sweets in Step 2 in the "others" food category.

Step 4

Evaluate the adequacy of the diet by comparing the servings from each food group with the servings recommended in the dietary guide.

Determine the frequency and consistency (sticky or nonretentive) of presweetened foods and assess their potential in contributing to the patient's problem.

From the information collected and analyzed, determine the need of the patient for dietary counseling. For example, a patient with rampant decay problems and considerably faulty food intake obviously has a high need for major counseling, probably with considerable reinforcement from you and the dentist on subsequent visits. Conversely, a patient with a slight caries problem and minor dietary problem would likely need only minimal (brief) counseling.

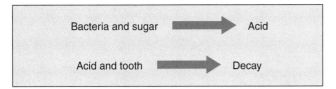

FIGURE 16.5

Key events leading to dental decay.

Therefore dietary management should receive secondary emphasis in periodontal treatment unless definite evidence of nutritional inadequacy occurs. Treatment in the dental office and oral hygiene procedures practiced by the patient are of first importance. Improvement of nutritional status can usually only supplement those measures in preventing or treating periodontal disease. The addition of vitamins to an already adequate diet is of doubtful value in either the prevention or treatment of periodontal disease.

DIETARY INTERVIEW

The dietary interview is a screening device to determine the patient's current food intake pattern and assess the need for dietary counseling. It is conducted by listing the patient's responses on paper concerning their current dietary regiment. It is a quick and easy procedure that can disclose the probability of a dietary problem arising in the near future that is likely to adversely affect the patient's oral health. If no problems are uncovered in the interview, the patient is experiencing no oral problems that may be related to the diet and is not likely to in the future, counseling is usually not needed. However, if potential problems are encountered or if the patient is experiencing dietary related oral problems, some form of diet counseling is probably indicated (Box 6.1).

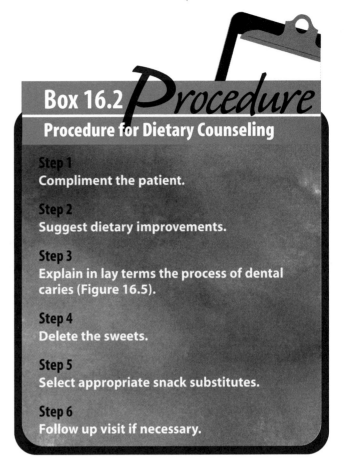

Box 16.2 Procedure

Procedure for Dietary Counseling

Step 1
Compliment the patient.

Step 2
Suggest dietary improvements.

Step 3
Explain in lay terms the process of dental caries (Figure 16.5).

Step 4
Delete the sweets.

Step 5
Select appropriate snack substitutes.

Step 6
Follow up visit if necessary.

DIETARY MANAGEMENT

After the patient has the dietary interview and its evaluation, the last step in a dietary counseling session is to help the patient select an adequate, balanced, noncariogenic diet. The following steps are recommended for this process (Box 6.2).

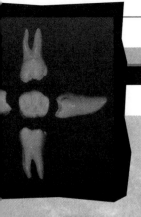

Points for Review

- The basic nutritional guidelines as presented in the food pyramid
- Nutrients including carbohydrates, proteins, fats, vitamins, and minerals
- The influences of nutrition on oral health and disease during various stages of life
- The relationship of nutrition to dental caries and periodontal disease
- The role of the dental assistant in dietary management
- The procedure for dietary interviewing and counseling

Self-Study Questions

1. What is the practical government plan for daily food selection that diagramatically illustrates the makeup of an adequate diet called?
   a. RDA
   b. USRDA
   c. *Guide to Good Eating*
   d. *Food Guide Pyramid*
2. Foods from which food group provide the major daily supply of protein, iron, niacin, and thiamin in the diet?
   a. Meat
   b. Milk
   c. Vegetable
   d. Grain
3. Which two vitamins do most fruits and vegetables abundantly supply?
   a. A and B-complex
   b. B-complex and C
   c. C and D
   d. A and C

4. How many daily calories are considered "average" for food labeling purposes?
   a. 1500
   b. 1700
   c. 2000
   d. 2400
5. According to the nutrition label that now appears on most packaged foods, what is the maximum daily intake of fat?
   a. 25 g
   b. 45 g
   c. 65 g
   d. 85 g
6. Which nutrient has the major function of supplying energy to the body?
   a. Carbohydrate
   b. Fat
   c. Protein
   d. Vitamins
7. Which food group contributes to fiber?
   a. Fructose
   b. Glucose
   c. Sucrose
   d. Lactose
8. Which of the following dietary changes would most likely improve cardiac health?
   a. Increased saturated fats relative to polyunsaturated
   b. Decrease saturated fats relative to polyunsaturated
   c. Decrease dietary cholesterol
   d. B and d
9. Which of the following minerals is an essential component of hemoglobin?
   a. Iron
   b. Iodine
   c. Potassium
   d. Sodium
10. The three critical factors involved in caries etiology are bacteria, host and which of the following?
    a. Acid
    b. Plaque
    c. Diet
    d. Saliva

11. Which sugar has the greatest cariogenic potential?

    a. Sucrose

    b. Glucose

    c. Fructose

    d. Maltose

12. Which of the following sugar substitutes is the safest product?

    a. Amount consumed

    b. Frequency of consumption

    c. Timing of ingestion

    d. Type of sugar

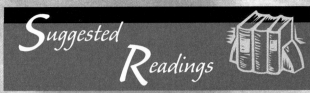

Suggested Readings

National Dairy Council: *Calcium: a summary of current research for the health professional*, Rosemont, Ill, 1984, NDC.

National Dairy Council: *Calcium currents*, vol 1, Rosemont, Ill, 1985, NDC.

National Dairy Council, Dairy Council Digest: *The food group approach to eating in the 1990s*, 64 (1), Rosemont, Ill, 1993, NDC.

National Dairy Council, *Guide to good eating*, Rosemont, Ill, 1989, NDC.

Nizel AE, Papas AS: *Nutrition in clinical dentistry*, ed 3, Philadelphia, 1989, Saunders.

Pollack RL, Kravitz E: *Nutrition in oral health and disease*, Philadelphia, 1985, Lea and Febiger.

Rugg-Gunn AJ: *Nutrition and dental health*, New York, 1993, Oxford University Press.

United States Department of Agriculture, U.S.D.H.H.S: *Dietary guidelines for Americans*, Washington, DC, 1985, USDA.

United States Senate Hearings: *Select committee on human needs*, Washington, DC, 1977.

Preventive Dentistry and Advanced Oral Health Procedures

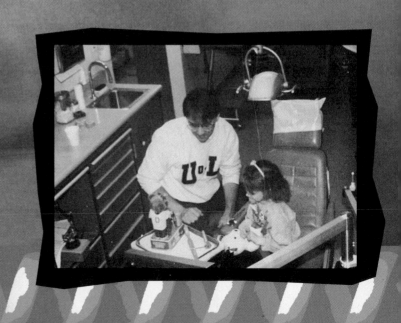

Chapter Outline

Learning Objectives

On completion of Chapter 17, the student should be able to do the following:

- Define key terms.
- Explain the role of plaque in the causes and prevention of periodontal disease.
- Discuss the causes and prevention of dental caries.
- Explain the role of the dental assistant in a patient education program.
- Discuss the various oral hygiene aids used in a patient education program.
- Explain the rationale, methodology, and instrumentation used in dental prophylaxis and coronal polishing.
- Discuss the advantages of and the steps used in applying pit and fissure sealants.
- Explain the rationale and value of water fluoridation and the use of fluoride supplements.
- Discuss the use of topical fluorides in dentistry and the steps used in their application.
- Explain the rationale and procedures employed in a maintenance recall program.

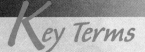

Key Terms

Calculus	Dental Prophylaxis	Plaque
Coronal Polishing	Edentulous	Preventive Dentistry
Demineralization	Gingivitis	Sealants
Dental Caries	Health	

WHAT IS PREVENTIVE DENTISTRY?

Preventive dentistry

Procedures in the practice of dentistry and community health programs that prevent the occurrence of oral diseases and abnormalities.

Preventive dentistry is the procedure in the practice of dentistry and community **health** programs that prevents the occurrence of oral diseases and abnormalities. It differs from other dental procedures in that its achievement requires the combined efforts of the dental team, patient, and community.

Dental Caries

Even with the benefits of fluoridated community water for most people in the United States, **dental caries** continues to affect at least 80% of the population. Fortunately, a significant decline in caries has occurred since 1975. Tooth decay has been reduced by about one third in school children, largely because of the widespread use of fluorides. Unfortunately, about 20% of children continue to have a relatively high caries experience. Young adults are also experiencing a decline in caries. Older adults, however, have not yet attained appreciable reductions in caries.

Health

A state of complete physical, mental, and social well-being, not merely the absence of disease or infirmity.

Dental caries

A bacterial disease of the teeth involving decay, disintegration, and destruction of the structure.

Periodontal Disease

Periodontal disease affects about 70% of the adult population. Most of those afflicted have **gingivitis**, a reversible, preventable condition affecting primarily the gingiva. Periodontitis, a more serious form of the disease affecting the supporting structures of the teeth (the periodontium), affects about 22% of American adults. Deterioration occurs slowly, episodically, and infrequently in most cases. A significant improvement has occurred in oral hygiene, with a corresponding improvement in gingival health in the American population in recent years.

Gingivitis

A reversible, preventable, inflammatory periodontal condition affecting the gingiva, caused primarily by dental plaque.

Tooth Loss and Edentulism

In the 1940s, tooth loss was common, increased rapidly with age, and was more prevalent among lower income groups. These basic patterns have not really changed, although the severity of tooth loss has diminished. The percent of the entire **edentulous** population declined from 13% to less than 5% between the 1950s and 1980s.

Edentulous

Without teeth; loss of all of the natural teeth.

PLAQUE AND PERIODONTAL DISEASE

The various diseases that affect the periodontium are collectively known as *periodontal (gum) disease*. Gingivitis is an early, inflammatory condition limited to the gingival tissues. Periodontitis is a more advanced problem in which the supporting structures of the teeth (the alveolar bone, cementum, and periodontal ligament) are affected.

Some of the signs of gingivitis are redness of the gingiva and swelling or bleeding when the gums are probed. Untreated gingivitis may continue to progress from limited or extensive inflammation of the gingiva to periodontitis, involving bone loss and pocketing around the tooth.

Oral Hygiene

Inadequate oral hygiene is the main problem leading to periodontal disease. Control of the disease depends on regular professional maintenance care and meticulous personal oral hygiene. Regular professional cleaning, up to four times per year in advanced cases, along with reinforcement of oral hygiene instruction, is essential for the maintenance of periodontal health.

The Role of Plaque

Plaque is a soft, sticky mass of bacteria organized on the tooth surface and other oral structures. The greatest growth of bacteria occurs at the gingival margin, where plaque tends to provoke inflammation (redness, bleeding, and gingivitis). Toxic products manufactured by the plaque bacteria may

Plaque

A collection of organized bacteria growing in a deposit of soft material on the surface of a tooth.

Calculus

> **Plaque that has mineralized (hardened) from calcium salts in the saliva.**

eventually do enough damage to the soft tissues so that bone loss, pocket formation and periodontitis results. In addition, hard deposits (**calculus**, or mineralized plaque) may be found attached to tooth surfaces if the soft plaque is not removed.

DENTAL CARIES

Dental caries, or cavities, is a bacterial disease of the teeth involving decay and a progressive disintegration and destruction process. Dental visits should begin between the age of 6 months and 1 year, preferably by the time the first tooth appears. Caries is associated with the use of sugars in the diet. The following simplified diagram summarizes the most important factors necessary for caries to occur:

Sugar + Bacteria = Acid
Acid + Tooth + Time = Caries

Calcium salts from saliva get into tooth structures following its eruption, resulting in maturation or greater calcification, which protects the tooth from caries. Saliva also protects against dental caries because of its washing action, buffering capacity (ability to counter the effects of acidity), and antibacterial activity.

Dietary Factors

Dietary factors that contribute to the development of dental caries include the type of sugar consumed, its concentration, frequency and timing of ingestion, and physical nature. Of the various sugars, sucrose (ordinary table sugar) is the most cariogenic (caries-causing) sugar, but other sugars (such as fructose and lactose) can also cause caries, but less so. Retentive foods cause greater damage to the tooth than nonsticky liquids that clear the mouth faster. The most cariogenic foods are those containing high concentrations of sucrose in a retentive form consumed frequently, especially between meals.

Bacterial Factors

Specific bacteria are necessary for caries to occur. Numerous organisms exist in the plaque, but the ones of special interest in caries development are the streptococci, lactobacilli, and actinomyces organisms. The one factor that all these bacteria have in common is that they all release acids in the presence of sugars. This acid is responsible for the **demineralization** of the enamel, initiating the caries process.

Demineralization

> **A breakdown of the tooth structure with a loss of mineral content.**

Prevention of Dental Caries

Dental caries can be prevented or at least controlled through the use of the following preventive measures:

1 Mechanical removal (brushing and flossing)
2 Pit and fissure sealants
3 Dietary measures
4 Fluorides

PREVENTIVE PROGRAM OUTLINE

A typical sequence of preventive services that may be used in a dental office includes the following (these procedures would be offered depending on individual patient needs):

1 Oral hygiene instructions and dietary counseling (see Chapter 16)
2 **Dental prophylaxis**
3 Sealants
4 Fluorides
5 Maintenance recall

Dental prophylaxis

> **A professional cleaning (scaling and polishing) of the teeth, consisting of complete mechanical removal of all hard and soft deposits.**

The Preventive Dental Assistant

Working under the supervision of a dentist, dental assistants can provide most preventive services directly to patients, depending on state dental practice acts. These include oral hygiene instruction, dietary counseling, **coronal polishing** of teeth, supragingival scaling, pit and fissure **sealants**, and topical fluoride applications. In addition, the dental assistant can take and develop radiographs, secure and pour study casts for treatment planning, and perform blood pressure monitoring. Skills in communication and interpersonal relations make the difference between success and failure in practice and are indispensable in preventive dentistry. Patients must be intimately involved in the learning

Coronal polishing

> **A cleansing and polishing of the coronal surfaces of the teeth by the use of motor-driven rubber cups, bristle brushes, and paste.**

Sealants

> **A plastic material (polymer) that bonds to the enamel tooth surface through mechanical locking, creating an effective barrier that prevents occlusal caries.**

Box 17.1

Procedure

Procedure for Oral Hygiene Patient Evaluation

Materials needed
Mouth mirror
Explorer
Cotton forceps
Probe
Air and water syringe
Disclosing material
Large mirror
Toothbrush
Toothpaste
Floss
Disposable mouth mirror
This procedure helps the patient understand the need for patient education.

1. Ask the patients questions concerning their preventive program, such as whether they have received oral hygiene instructions, are having any problems, and what hygiene aids they use and how often.
2. Examine the patient's teeth and gingiva to get a general impression of mouth cleanliness and gingival health. Check for food debris and calculus and to see if the gingival tissues are firm and healthy pink or swollen and enlarged.
3. Relate the state of health and disease present to the plaque in the patient's mouth and explain what plaque is in terms the patient can understand and how it is relates to the patient's oral condition.
4. Use disclosing materials to identify any plaque.
5. Have the patient chew the tablet until dissolved, then forcefully swish with saliva throughout the mouth. Tell the patient to rub the saliva on all outside surfaces of the teeth with the tongue before expectorating. Swish for 15 to 30 seconds.
6. Have the patient rinse mouth with water to remove excess disclosing film (a disclosing solution may be painted on with a cotton swab or a small amount may be placed under the tongue and then swished around).
7. Have the patient hold a large mirror to view the stained areas in the mouth after the disclosure {Figure 17.1).
8. Use a small mirror for the lingual surfaces.
9. Tell the patient to disclose daily, before and after plaque removal.
10. After about 2 weeks, the effectiveness of the patient's program should be reviewed on a follow-up visit.

process, and the information must relate to their specific problems.

ORAL HYGIENE INSTRUCTION AND PATIENT EVALUATION

Chairside instructions in proper home care procedures can yield daily dividends in oral health when followed by the patient. Patient instruction is preceded by oral hygiene evaluation follow up and the disclosing of plaque (Box 17.1 and Table 17.1).

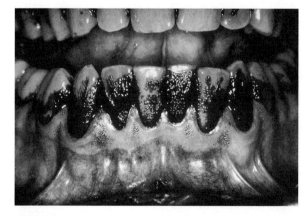

FIGURE 17.1

Disclosed mouth showing the amount and distribution of plaque on the facial surfaces of the lower teeth.

Table 17.1

Evaluation of Oral Hygiene Patient Evaluation

Patient Education	4	3	2	0	X
Secure materials and equipment.					
Seat and prepare patient.					
Discuss patient's oral hygiene knowledge.					
Ask about existing dental problems.					
Wear protective eye wear, gloves, and mask.					
Examine teeth and gingival tissue.					
Relate findings and discuss plaque.					
Use disclosing materials for 15 to 30 seconds.					
Ask patient to rinse and view with mirror.					
Discuss findings.					
Discuss at home disclosing and brushing.					
Set a follow up appointment.					

The numeric criteria: 4 Excellent; 3 Good but some improvement can be made; 2 Below average, usable, needs to improve skill; 0 Unsatisfactory; X Not able to evaluate.

STEP-BY-STEP GUIDE FOR PATIENT EDUCATION

Effective patient education is different from other areas of dentistry. With most dental procedures, the immediate outcome rests directly with the clinician, whereas patient education requires active participation of the patient in a teacher-learner relationship. The objective of patient education, establishment of desirable health practices, is difficult because it often requires many hours of exposure, training, and reinforcement. For some patients, desired health practices may not be possible at certain times. In offering suggestions regarding patient procedures, the dental assistant should emphasize that each person is different. Therefore the following information will need to be personalized and altered for each patient according to individual needs.

If a preventive program is to be effective, patient education efforts should be periodically repeated and reinforced. Few people will be able to master a new skill after just one lesson and be motivated to continue their efforts indefinitely. After questioning patients regarding their new oral health practices, the dental assistant should perform another oral hygiene evaluation by discussing intraoral observations and then by using disclosing tablets. Do not be surprised if little progress occurs and do not say anything to discourage the patient. Help patient make any necessary improvements in their technique, introducing any other additional aids needed, such as interproximal cleaners or floss holders.

Schedule subsequent instructional visits, lengthening the interval between them, until the patient achieves the desired level of proficiency and health. Continue to reinforce home care during the maintenance recall phase of the patient's treatment program. Help sustain the patient's motivation by commenting positively on the patient's efforts and pointing out any healthy benefits achieved. When appropriate, oral hygiene practices need to be watched so that, through feedback, improvements can be made. People tend to regress in their efforts to achieve proficiency at a skill. Expect periodic setbacks and when they occur, help patients achieve desired goals by working with them in a helpful manner (Box 17.2 and Table 17.2).

ORAL HYGIENE AIDS AND METHODS

The Toothbrush

The two basic types of toothbrushes are *manual* and *automatic*.

Manual Toothbrushes

Dental professionals generally prefer straight handles for maximum efficiency. The bristles may be nylon or natural. Nylon is preferred because the ends are rounded and polished, which make it safer. Soft bristles are safer because they tend to remove plaque without doing harm to the tooth enamel.

Automatic Toothbrushes

Automatic toothbrushes use one or several motions such as back and forth, up and down, or circular and are powered by

Box 17.2

Procedure

Procedure for Patient Education

Materials needed

Mouth mirror
Explorer
Cotton forceps
Probe
Air and water syringe
Floss
Mouth rinse
Toothbrush
Toothpaste
Disposable mouth mirror
Disclosing material
Large mirror
Other patient aides as needed
Educational materials

A combination of regular professional tooth cleaning, reinforcement, or oral hygiene instructions and successful daily plaque removal by the patient is necessary to preserve periodontal health.

1. Initial preventive session
- Operator should be wearing protective eyewear, gloves, and a mask.
- Explain purposes of visit.
- Explain plaque and diet control.
- Have patient rinse with antimicrobial mouth rinse.
- Review any plaque-related oral problems.
- Explain value of preventive measures.
- Explain patient responsibility for oral health.
- Complete an oral hygiene evaluation
- Demonstrate clean, healthy areas in the mouth.
- Show any plaque and related problems.
- Demonstrate disclosing materials.

2. Emphasize need to remove plaque every day
- Advise patient to use disclosing materials daily.
- Explain purpose of aids recommended.
- Demonstrate method of brushing and flossing.
- Have patients show you their procedure.
- Provide positive reinforcement of proper technique.
- Help patient remove all plaque from the mouth.
- Reemphasize the need to disclose regularly.
- Stress the importance of daily plaque removal.
- Underscore the need for proper toothpaste.
- Put hygiene aids in a sealable plastic bag.
- Ask patient to bring the hygiene aides for the next visit.
- Schedule follow-up appointment in one or 2 weeks.

3. Second and subsequent instruction visits
- Question patient about new oral health practice.
- Perform another oral hygiene evaluation.
- Do not say anything to discourage the patient.
- Help patient make necessary technique improvements.
- Introduce any other additional aids needed.
- Schedule subsequent instructional visits.
- Lengthen intervals between visits.
- Continue to reinforce home care.
- Comment positively on the patient's efforts.
- Point out any healthy benefits achieved.
- Expect periodic setbacks.
- Help patients achieve desired goals.

batteries or ordinary house current. They may be especially useful for physically and mentally handicapped people and may have some motivational value for young children.

A sonic toothbrush is also available. It consists of a manual toothbrush combined with an electric ultrasonic emitter in the brush head (Figure 17.2, *A*).

Toothbrushing Methods

The objectives of toothbrushing are to remove plaque, food debris, and stains from the teeth. Toothbrushing also stimulates the gingiva and, with toothpaste, polishes the teeth and applies therapeutic agents such as fluoride and desensitizing

Table 17.2

Evaluation of Patient Education Program

Initial Preventive Session	4	3	2	0	X
Secure materials and equipment.					
Seat and prepare patient.					
Wear protective eye wear, gloves, and mask.					
Give oral hygiene and diet instruction.					
Have patient rinse.					
Examine teeth and gingival tissue.					
Discuss findings and any problems.					
Discuss prevention and patient's role in oral health care.					
Have patient demonstration of cleaning method.					
Reinforcement of proper procedure.					
Demonstrate disclosing materials and dental aides.					
Demonstrate brushing and flossing methods.					
Patient show interpretation of demonstration with help to remove plaque if necessary.					
Reemphasize regular disclosing and need for proper toothpaste, brush, and aides.					
Provide hygiene aides with instructions and follow up appointment.					
Second and subsequent instruction visits					
Secure materials and equipment.					
Seat and prepare patient.					
Wear protective eye wear, gloves, and mask.					
Discuss new health practice.					
Examine teeth and gingival tissue and evaluate conditions.					
Encourage patient positively and help to improve.					
Introduce other aids if necessary.					
Schedule subsequent visit.					
Reinforce home care and point out achievements.					

The numeric criteria: 4 Excellent; 3 Good but some improvement can be made; 2 Below average, usable, needs to improve skill; 0 Unsatisfactory; X Not able to evaluate.

additives. Various toothbrushing methods have been devised to accomplish this task.

Bass Method

The Bass method is also called the *modified bass* or *sulcular*. This method places the bristle ends directly into the gingival sulcus at a 45-degree angle and then vibrates the brush in a small back-and-forth or circular motion, using several strokes in each area (Figure 17.2, *B*). People should work in a systematic pattern, starting preferably on the rearmost tooth of one side of the mouth and then work slowly to-wards the other side of the mouth until all of the facial areas of the teeth in one arch are cleaned.

Scrub-Brush Method

The scrub-brush method is also called the *horizontal* or *circular method*. It places the head of the brush horizontal to the teeth and vibrates the bristles in a small horizontal or circular motion as in scrubbing a floor (Figure 17.2, *C*). This method is best for small children because the horizontal motion is much easier for them to use.

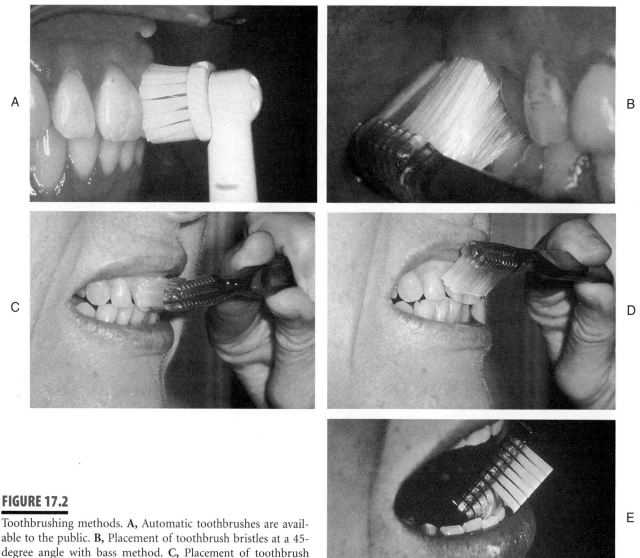

FIGURE 17.2

Toothbrushing methods. **A,** Automatic toothbrushes are available to the public. **B,** Placement of toothbrush bristles at a 45-degree angle with bass method. **C,** Placement of toothbrush bristles horizontally with scrub-brush method. **D,** Placement of toothbrush bristles coronally with charter's method. **E,** Placement of the brush head in the anterior lingual mandibular area with all methods.

Charter's Method

The charter method places the bristles of the brush on the gingiva, tilting coronally (away from the gingiva) at about a 45-degree angle, with the sides of the bristle half on the teeth and half on the gingiva. The bristles are gently manipulated into the interproximal space in a manner that does not damage the soft tissues (Figure 17.2, *D*). A vibratory action is used. This method may be useful in cleaning under the pontics of fixed bridges and around orthodontic appliances.

Cleaning the Occlusal Surfaces

The occlusal surfaces may be cleaned by using short, vibratory strokes, with pressure being maintained to accomplish as deep a penetration of the pits and fissures as possible. Long, sweeping horizontal strokes should be avoided.

Cleaning the Lingual Areas

With all methods, the posterior lingual areas are brushed with a small horizontal or circular motion, holding the brush in a horizontal, diagonal, or vertical position (Figure 17.2, *E*).

Box 17.3

Procedure

Procedure for Flossing

Materials needed
Mouth mirror
Explorer
Cotton forceps
Probe
Air and water syringe
Floss
Large mirror
To begin flossing, do the following:
1. Remove 2 to 3 feet of floss.
2. Wind the bulk of floss lightly around the middle finger, leaving space between wraps to avoid cutting off circulation to the fingers.
3. The rest of the floss is similarly wound around the same finger of the opposite hand. This finger can wind or take up the floss as it becomes soiled or frayed to permit access to an unused portion.
4. The floss is kept taut with about 1 inch of floss between the guiding fingers.
5. The thumb and index finger are used as guides for the upper teeth and the two index fingers are used for the lower teeth.
6. The floss is worked between the teeth in a sawing, back-and-forth motion (Figure 17.3). To avoid injury to the interdental papilla, avoid snapping the floss through the contacts.
7. Once through the contact, slide it under the free gingiva as far as it will go, keeping it taught around the tooth and work it up and down several times. Repeat the process for the adjacent tooth.
8. When the floss becomes frayed or soiled, it is unwound and moved to a clean section.

Toothbrushing Damage

Toothbrushing damage can occur to both the soft tissue (gingival recession) or the tooth surface (toothbrush abrasion).

Frequency of Brushing

Patients should be encouraged to remove plaque thoroughly at least once per day. Disclosing materials should be used daily for about 2 weeks.

Denture Patients

Patients with full dentures will need to use a denture brush to clean all areas of the denture. A nonabrasive cleaner such as a denture cream, mild soap, dishwashing liquid or mild toothpaste should be used on the brush, using short strokes. The denture should always be left out of the mouth when sleeping and kept in water to prevent distortion.

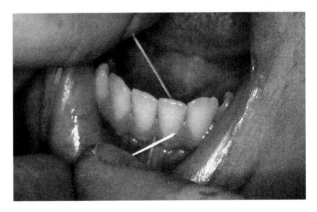

FIGURE 17.3

Patient dental flossing. The floss is wrapped around each tooth in the interproximal area and used with up-and-down strokes.

Dental Floss

Dental floss is an effective means of removing plaque and debris from contact and interproximal areas and some accessible areas of the gingival sulcus that the toothbrush cannot reach (Box 17.3 and Table 17.3).

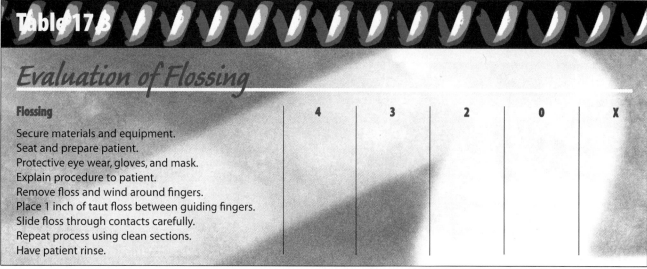

Table 17.3

Evaluation of Flossing

Flossing	4	3	2	0	X
Secure materials and equipment.					
Seat and prepare patient.					
Protective eye wear, gloves, and mask.					
Explain procedure to patient.					
Remove floss and wind around fingers.					
Place 1 inch of taut floss between guiding fingers.					
Slide floss through contacts carefully.					
Repeat process using clean sections.					
Have patient rinse.					

The numeric criteria: 4 Excellent; 3 Good but some improvement can be made; 2 Below average, usable, needs to improve skill; 0 Unsatisfactory; X Not able to evaluate.

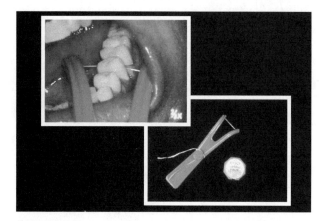

FIGURE 17.4

The FlossMate floss holder. (Courtesy John O. Butler Company, Chicago, Ill.)

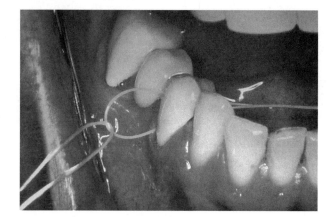

FIGURE 17.5

Using an Eez-Thru floss threader to guide floss under a fixed bridge. (Courtesy John O. Butler Company, Chicago, Ill.)

Floss Holder

The floss holder eliminates the need to use both hands while flossing and makes it unnecessary to place the fingers in the mouth (Figure 17.4).

Floss Threader

A floss threader is a needle or loop device that has an opening at one end through which the dental floss is threaded (Figure 17.5). Dental floss can usually be slipped through an open embrasure space, but when an open contact area is not present, the patient can use either Super Floss or floss threader. This stiff yet flexible device can carry the limp floss under an appliance through a splinted interdental embrasure or very tight contact area, or under pontics, space maintainers, or orthodontic appliances.

Perio-Aid

A perio-aid is a toothpick holder that allows the patient to use an ordinary, round toothpick as a cleaning device in various areas of the mouth (Figure 17.6). It is useful in cleaning the depression in teeth where dental floss cannot reach; for example, interproximally in areas of gingival recession, or following periodontal surgery. It can also be used to trace along the gumline, removing plaque.

In using a perio-aid, a firm, round toothpick is inserted into an opening at either end of the device, breaking off the excess toothpick length. The end of the toothpick is then carried to the area to be cleaned by merely holding the device with one hand.

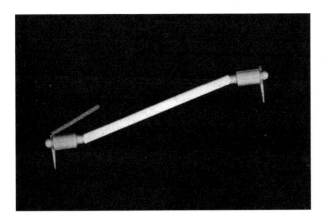

FIGURE 17.6

The perio-aid enables the patient to use an ordinary toothpick as a cleaning device.

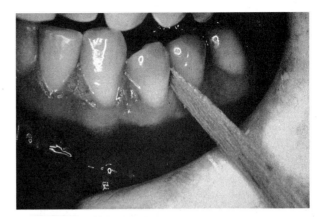

FIGURE 17.8

Using a Stim-U-Dent wedge-stimulator.

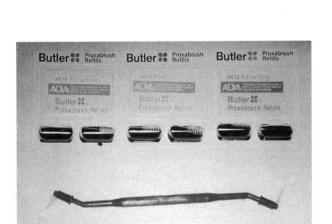

FIGURE 17.7

An interdental brush with replacement refills.

Interdental Brushes

Interdental brushes are small cone-shaped or cylindrical-shaped bristle brushes or a single tuft of brushes attached to a handle (Figure 17.7). They are especially useful for cleaning and removing plaque in interdental areas when the interdental papilla is missing or reduced in height or when sufficient space exists in the interproximal embrasure. This space permits insertion of the aid without injuring the soft tissue.

Interdental Tip Stimulator

The interdental tip stimulator is used primarily for stimulating the periodontal tissues, when necessary. These aids are generally not used in clinically healthy areas with intact interdental papilla, where interdental devices are usually unnecessary and can be harmful. The tip is inserted interdentally and slightly coronally. A gentle rotary motion, which provides intermittent pressure against the gingival tissue, should be applied to a slow count of ten.

Wedge Stimulator

Wedge stimulators are made of wood or plastic and most are triangular in cross section (Figure 17.8). The majority of wood wedges are available in birch or balsa. They can be used to massage the interdental gingiva in areas where the gingival papilla is missing and, to a lesser extent, for cleaning in these areas.

Dentifrice

Toothpaste contains detergent agents that help dislodge food residues. Abrasives such as pumice help remove stain. Because abrasives tend to dull the tooth luster, polishing agents are added. A highly polished tooth surface will stain less readily and remain cleaner longer. Flavoring agents that provide acceptable taste to the dentifrice, may promote more frequent brushing by imparting a feeling of cleanliness. Some toothpastes now incorporate a compound that reduces calculus formation, especially when used regularly following a dental prophylaxis. These tartar-control dentifrices may be helpful for those individuals who tend to accumulate excessive calculus between professional cleaning intervals.

Mouth Rinsing

The use of a toothbrush and supplemental cleaning aids will disperse and loosen food particles, plaque, and food debris. Their further removal will be aided by vigorous rinsing of the mouth using fluids such as water, fluoride mouth rinses, salt solutions, or commercial mouthwashes. Rinsing is also recommended after meals and snacks when toothbrushing and interdental cleaning is not possible.

Plaque-Control Kits

Commercially prepared kits are available that commonly contain a plastic dental mirror, toothbrush, dental floss, disclosing materials, and a printed sheet of oral hygiene instructions prepackaged in a plastic bag.

Mouth Rinses (Nonfluoride)

Cosmetic mouth rinses remove oral debris and temporarily do the following:
- Provide a pleasant taste and good feeling to the mouth
- Lower the bacterial count of the oral cavity and reduce halitosis.

Therapeutic mouth rinses have an active agent that prevents, arrests, or helps reverse an oral disease process, such as gingivitis or caries.

Irrigation Devices

Oral irrigators direct a high-pressure stream of water through a nozzle to the teeth and gingiva. Most use a receptacle for water that is propelled by a motor driven pump. These irrigators clean nonadherent bacteria and debris from the oral cavity, especially from inaccessible areas around orthodontic appliances and fixed prostheses.

DENTAL PROPHYLAXIS

Scaling

Calculus provides a highly retentive surface for bacteria and thus promotes the accumulation of dental plaque. Because of its rough surface and location, adequate removal of plaque from calculus is often difficult or impossible. Therefore calculus must be eliminated to facilitate adequate plaque removal. Calculus is removed by scaling the teeth, using instruments such as ultrasonic and sonic scalers, hand scalers, and curettes. Dental assistants can legally perform coronal or supragingival scaling in several states.

Supragingival scaling consists of the removal of calculus and plaque from the coronal (crown) tooth surface. Calculus that is coronal to the margin of the gingiva is termed *supragingival*; subgingival calculus is apical to the gingival margin, inside the gingival sulcus or pocket and is therefore not visible. Scaling is usually performed with a pull motion by engaging the apical border of the calculus with the selected instrument and dislodging it with a firm movement in the direction of the crown. It is accomplished by powerful, short-working strokes.

Supragingival Calculus Removal

Supragingival (supramarginal) calculus is located coronal to the gingival margin and is not normally generalized to a particular area of the tooth. It is most commonly found on the following:
1 Lingual surface of mandibular anterior teeth
2 Buccal of maxillary molars apical to the height of contour
3 Teeth out of alignment or occlusion

In addition, if recession of the gingival tissues has taken place, subgingival calculus can be seen as supragingival calculus.

Supragingival calculus is usually irregular and bulky. Large calculus deposits may fill in the interproximal spaces between adjacent teeth or extend over the free gingival margin if left unattended. The shape of supragingival calculus will vary according to the anatomy of the tooth and contour of the gingival margin. The presence of the tongue, lips, and cheeks will also control the shape of the calculus deposit.

Calculus may be attached by acquired pellicle, irregularities in the tooth surface, or direct attachment of the calcified calculus matrix to the surface of the teeth. Calculus attached by the thin, acellular pellicle layer on all exposed smooth tooth surfaces is easily removed because it has not penetrated into the enamel. Calculus in minute irregularities such as enamel cracks, carious lesions, or cementum spaces caused by resorption, toothbrush abrasion, or scaling grooves may be difficult to detect and completely remove because of the inability of the instrument to catch the slight irregularities. Calcified calculus may also be difficult to identify because of the lack of distinction between calculus and cementum (Box 17.4 and Table 17.4).

Identification

Examination and identification of supragingival calculus can be accomplished by direct observation using proper lighting, retracting tissue, and slightly drying the area with the air syringe. Compressed air flow will dry the wet calculus and increase visibility, and the mouth mirror will provide indirect vision when needed. The intraoral camera can also increase vision for these observations. The explorer helps detect calculus in proximal areas not directly observable. Furthermore, transillumination by reflecting light through teeth may reveal calculus as a dark shadow on the tooth.

Instrumentation

Effective instrumentation for scaling, as with other dental procedures, is accomplished by the following:
1 The principles of positioning
2 Visibility through lighting, tissue retraction, and a clean, dry field

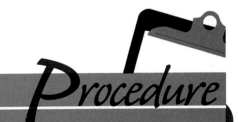

Box 17.4

Procedure for Supragingival Calculus Removal

Materials needed

Mouth mirror
Explorer
Cotton forceps
Probe
Scaler selection
Air and water syringe

1. Prepare operatory, patient, and infection barriers.
2. Examine the oral cavity.
3. Retract tissue.
4. Grasp instrument using modified grasp.
5. Position instrument with light grasp.
6. Apply finger rest near site (third finger and little finger together will provide a firm fulcrum when scaling).
7. Apply lateral pressure and begin strokes using a tight grasp.
8. Use thumb to roll instrument as the instrument is adapted to the tooth form.
9. Control instrument movement by using hand and arm together.
10. Limit stroke length to height of calculus.
11. Position blade at correct angulation to begin working stroke, approximately 70 degrees, when using the placement stroke.
12. Grasp instrument securely and apply appropriate lateral pressure when using the working stroke.

13. Use activation strokes to remove calculus:
    • Vertical and oblique strokes are used most and horizontal strokes can be used for inaccessible areas.
    • Use pull strokes in coronal direction to prevent calculus from damaging the soft tissue.
    • Use short, smooth, even strokes to remove calculus and longer, lighter strokes for finishing and smoothing the surfaces.
    • Overlap each stroke to ensure complete scaling.
14. Use a hand-wrist-forearm unit action for increased strength and control of instrument and pressure.
15. As the stroke is completed, the grasp is lightened and the blade is positioned for further strokes.
16. Calculus is removed incrementally around the tooth during circumferential instrumentation.
17. Check frequently with explorer for complete scaling and progress.
18. Rinse oral cavity.
19. Provide any further oral hygiene instructions.
20. Provide postoperative instructions if necessary.

3 Stability of instrument grasp and finger rest
4 Knowledge of tooth form and function
5 Instrument use

When removing calculus, the dental assistant should correctly adapt the scaling instrument to the tooth surface and soft tissue. The working end of the scaler must be positioned to conform with individual tooth morphology (shape). After the instrument is secured and the proper fulcrum is acquired, the blade of the scaler or curette is adapted to the tooth surface, pressure is applied, and stroke or movement application begins.

Instrument Pressure

The fulcrum pressure should provide an even balance with sufficient amount of pressure to remove the calculus. Proper instrument grasp and finger rest will control the pressure and length of each stroke while preventing laceration of the soft tissue. The thumb and index finger are placed near the junction of the handle and shank with the second finger on the shank and ring finger in the rest position (Figure 17.9). The instrument handle is rolled between the fingers to maintain correct tooth adaptation as the tooth is cleaned (Figure 17.10). Angling the face of the blade approximately between 70 and 80 degrees from the tooth surface forms the working angle of scalers and curettes. The blade of the instrument is placed against the tooth with light, moderate or heavy pressure, called *lateral pressure*. Place the scaler or curette with light pressure until the instrument is positioned and vary the pressure according to the hardness and attachment of the calculus deposit.

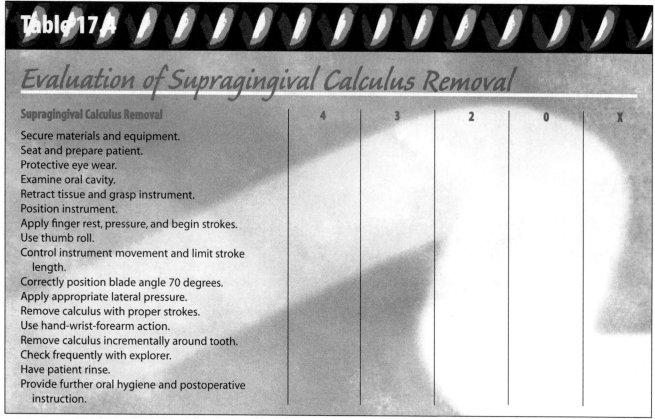

Evaluation of Supragingival Calculus Removal

Supragingival Calculus Removal	4	3	2	0	X
Secure materials and equipment.					
Seat and prepare patient.					
Protective eye wear.					
Examine oral cavity.					
Retract tissue and grasp instrument.					
Position instrument.					
Apply finger rest, pressure, and begin strokes.					
Use thumb roll.					
Control instrument movement and limit stroke length.					
Correctly position blade angle 70 degrees.					
Apply appropriate lateral pressure.					
Remove calculus with proper strokes.					
Use hand-wrist-forearm action.					
Remove calculus incrementally around tooth.					
Check frequently with explorer.					
Have patient rinse.					
Provide further oral hygiene and postoperative instruction.					

The numeric criteria: 4 Excellent; 3 Good but some improvement can be made; 2 Below average, usable, needs to improve skill; 0 Unsatisfactory; X Not able to evaluate.

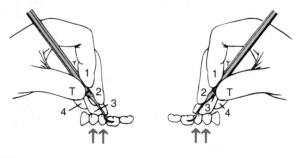

FIGURE 17.9

The thumb and index finger are placed near the junction of the handle and shank with the second finger on the shank and ring finger in the rest position. (Courtesy Darby ML: *Mosby's comprehensive review of dental hygiene,* St Louis, 1998, Mosby.)

Instrument Stroke (Movement)

Positioning the instrument is called the *placement stroke* and applying pressure and scaling is called the *working stroke*. Pressure that is too light may only burnish the calculus and make it more difficult to detect. In addition to lateral pressure, various types of instrument movements or strokes exist that will aid in effective removal of calculus deposits. These movements are referred to as the *action, function,* and *direction strokes.* Action strokes are the pulling, pushing,

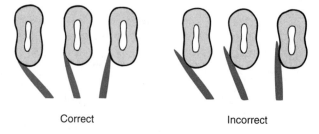

Correct   Incorrect

FIGURE 17.10

The instrument handle is rolled between the fingers to maintain correct tooth adaptation as the tooth is cleaned. (Courtesy Darby ML: *Mosby's comprehensive review of dental hygiene,* St Louis, 1998, Mosby.)

push-pull, and walking motions. Each stroke is identified by the following actions:

1. Pull: Coronal movement as instrument pulls calculus loose
2. Push: Insertion of curette into subgingival space and positioning it for pushing function
3. Push-pull: The up-and-down movement of the explorer tip on the side of the tooth
4. Walking stroke: The movement of the probe to the bottom of the sulcus or pocket and up in a circular direction

Function strokes are used for exploratory or assessment when examining a tooth surface or working strokes used, or to remove calculus from a tooth surface. The following directions of the instrument movement identify the other types of stroke:

1 Vertical: Parallel to the long axis of the tooth
2 Horizontal: Perpendicular to the long axis of the tooth
3 Diagonal (oblique): Diagonal to the long axis of the tooth
4 Circular: 1 to 2 mm diameter strokes used with a porte polisher to apply polishing paste or desensitizing agent
5 Circumferential: Vertical or diagonal strokes around the tooth

Root Planing

Scaling usually leaves the tooth with a rough and scratched surface that favors rapid re-establishment of plaque and calculus. To help prevent this, the tooth surface must be planed with suitable scalers or curettes and then polished with abrasive paste on a rotary rubber cup or brush. Smooth, polished tooth surfaces resist calculus formation and are more conducive to effective plaque control measures.

Hand Instruments used in Scaling and Root Planing

The names given to the basic instruments used in performing scaling and root planing describe the shape and design of the blades or the way the instrument is used. The following instruments are designed for a specific use:

• Explorers
• Scalers curettes, which include sickles, chisels, hoes, and files

Sickle Scalers

The sickle scaler has a curved or straight blade with a triangular cross section, two cutting edges, and a pointed tip, designed to remove gross supragingival calculus from the anatomic crown of the tooth. The two basic types of scalers are anterior and posterior. The anterior sickle scalers may be straight or hooked (Figure 17.11). Posterior sickle scalers have an angled shank to make for easier access to posterior interproximal areas (Figure 17.12). Small sickle blades are useful beneath the contact area of anterior teeth when a curette is not available (Figure 17.13). The sickle scaler is used with a vertical or oblique pulling stroke.

Chisels, Hoes, and Files

Chisels and hoes are designed for gross supragingival calculus removal but are infrequently used today because of the refinement of curettes and the advent of ultrasonic devices.

If selected, the hoe is used on the facial and lingual surfaces or proximal surfaces of teeth adjacent to edentulous areas. The blade is placed under the calculus deposit making a two-point contact. The side of the shank is held against the crown of the tooth at a 90-degree angle and a pull vertical stroke is made.

The chisel scaler is used to remove gross supragingival calculus from exposed proximal surfaces of anterior teeth. A horizontal push stroke is used. Do no push calculus toward the sulcus or pocket.

Files are a series of miniature hoes lined up on a round or rectangular base. They are rarely used today because they tend to gouge and roughen root surfaces. However, fine files are useful in narrow, deep pockets and are sometimes used for removing rough amalgam and overhanging margins of dental restorations. Use the file with a pull stroke and do not use excessive pressure because of gouging potential.

Curettes

Curettes are used for supragingival and subgingival scaling and root planing. It is the most commonly used instrument for these purposes. The shape of the instrument allows for easy entry into a pocket because its shank and blade design enables it to conform to the curvatures of the root more readily than any other instrument. The sickle scaler has a pointed tip, whereas the curette has a spoon-shaped blade with two curved cutting edges united by a rounded toe (Figure 17.14). Both instruments have two cutting edges (**C**). The sickle has a **V**-shaped back when viewed in cross section, and the back of a curette is rounded.

Curettes are usually used as double-ended instruments, with blades that are mirror images of each other. The length and angulation of the shank and the dimensions of the blade differ between brands of the instrument. Curettes are usually identified by the name of the designer and are numbered in sets. For example, the Gracey $^3/_4$ curette is a double-ended instrument with blades that are mirror images.

Rigid curettes are used to remove moderate calculus whereas finishing curettes are used to remove light calculus deposits. The curette is recommended for fine supragingival calculus near the free gingival margin because it will not irritate or cause trauma to the soft tissue if used properly. The blade is positioned with the face angled approximately 70 degrees to the tooth surface. Use only strokes in a vertical or oblique direction.

Ultrasonic and Sonic Instruments

Ultrasonic instruments are used for scaling, root planing and stain removal. These units consist of an electric power generator that delivers high vibrations to a handpiece, and a foot or hand control (Figure 17.15).

Removable ultrasonic tips of different shapes are placed into the handpiece and used for scaling, root planing, and other periodontal procedures. Electrical energy generated by the power unit is carried to numerous metal strips that encircle the handpiece. The tips convert the electrical energy into mechanical energy in the form of rapid vibrations. These vary from 20,000 to 29,000 vibrations per second, causing the tip of the insert to move $^1/_{1000}$ of an inch in

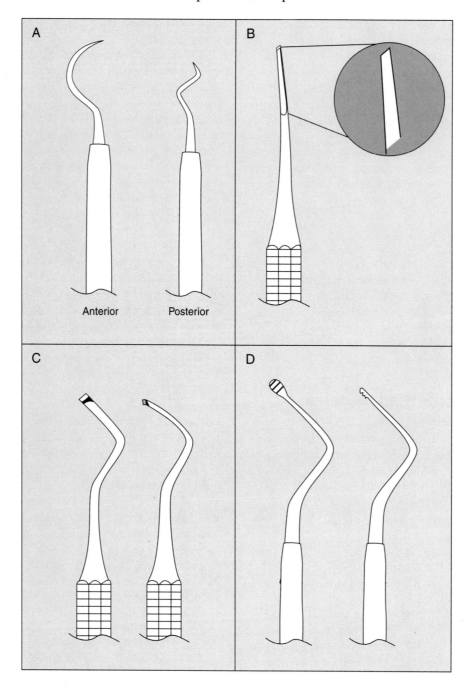

FIGURE 17.11

Various types of scalers. **A,** Anterior and posterior and sickle scaler. **B,** Chisel scaler. **C,** Hoe scaler. **D,** Files.

various directions. The vibration of the tip and the spraying and cavitation effect of the fluid coolant accomplish the removal of plaque, calculus, and stain. All tips are designed to operate in a wet field and have attached water outlets. The spray is directed at the end of the tip to dissipate the heat generated by the ultrasonic vibrations.

After the desired tip is inserted into the handpiece, the instrument must be adjusted with regard to the power and water spray. Usually, the lowest power setting consistent with effectiveness is used. After adjustment, the handpiece is held between the fingers before use to guard against excessive vibration heat production.

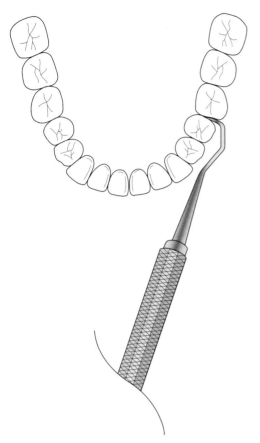

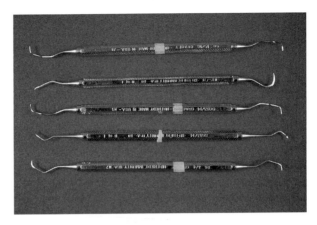

FIGURE 17.13

Set of curettes and scaler.

FIGURE 17.12

Posterior sickle scalers have an angled shank to make for easier access to posterior interproximal areas.

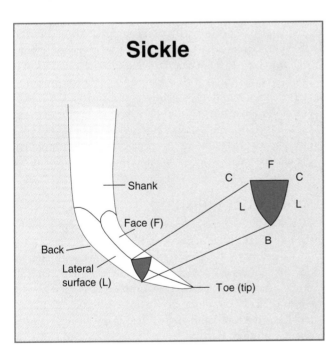

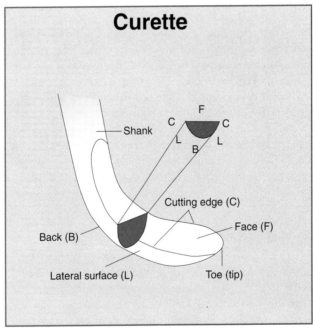

FIGURE 17.14

The parts of a sickle scaler and a curette are illustrated side-by-side for comparison. The pointed tip of the sickle. The rounded tip of the curette. In the cross-section adjoining each figure, the following parts are labeled: *F,* Face. *C,* Cutting edges. *L,* Lateral surface. *B,* Back.

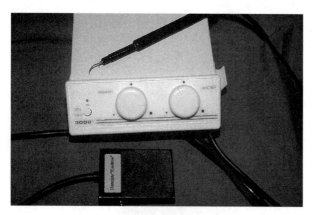

FIGURE 17.15

Ultrasonic unit.

A new type of instrument for scaling is the sonic scaler, which is air driven, producing vibrations in sonic range of 2,300 to 6,300.

Coronal Polishing

Up until recently, dental procedures were typically performed by the dentist and dental hygienist. However, in 25 states (1996) coronal polishing to the level of the gingival crown can be delegated under certain circumstances to the expanded function dental assistant who has been trained in the technique. Several states permit coronal scaling by trained dental assistants. Scaling and polishing the teeth removes stain, plaque, and other debris; polishes dental restorations; and may constitute the final step of a professional prophylaxis. It may be accomplished as the final step of other procedures, such as following the taking of impressions or inserting crowns or fixed prostheses to ensure the mouth is free of debris. It may also be used as the initial step of some procedures, such as the application of the rubber dam, pit, and fissure sealants or the taking of impressions. In many of these circumstances, depending on state dental practice acts, the dental assistant may be the person delegated to perform these procedures (Box 17.5, Table 17.5, and Figures 17.16 and 17.17).

Dental Stains

Stains are pigmented deposits within or on the surface of the teeth, tooth coatings (pellicle, plaque, and calculus), dental restorations, and prostheses. Although thick stains can be rough and therefore harbor plaque deposits, they are considered primarily a cosmetic problem. As such they are relatively harmless and do not directly cause disease, but when they are apparent to the patient, they can be quite objectionable. Stains result from carious enamel, dentin and cementum, and from discoloration by bacteria, blood, foods, metals, chemicals, tobacco, tea, coffee, drugs, and disturbances.

Devices for Polishing

Polishing can be adequately performed with a rubber cup or brush inserted into a special prophylaxis angle that is attached to a handpiece (Figure 17.18, A). The prophy angle may be made of metal (autoclavable) or plastic (disposable) (Figure 17.18, B). The assistant will select a small or large prophy tray depending on the need.

Pumice Cup

Pumice cups or glass dappen dishes are used to hold the pumice or other polishing pastes and disclosing solutions during a prophylaxis. The finger handle allows the operator to work close to the mouth without spilling or dripping the solutions. The metal cups are used more routinely than the glass dappen dishes because of the ability to autoclave the metal cups (Figure 17.18, C).

The rubber cup, consisting of a rubber shell with or without web-shaped configurations in the hallow interior, works well on the facial and lingual tooth surfaces (Figure 17.18, D). Bristle brushes, available in wheel and cup-shapes, can be used on the occlusal surfaces of the teeth to clean in the grooves and fissures, thereby cleaning and polishing the tooth and any restorations in this area (Figure 17.18, E).

The cups and brushes are used with different types of cleaning and polishing pastes. A popular polishing paste consists of flour of pumice of various grits (from fine to coarse), glycerine, flavoring and color additives, and a fluoride compound to minimize sensitivity. The handpiece is operated at the slowest rotation speed consistent with effectiveness to lessen heat and possible tissue trauma.

Dental tape or floss with polishing paste is used for polishing the proximal surfaces. It is gently passed through each contact area, kept at a right angle to the long axis of the tooth, and activated with a firm up-and-down motion. In this manner, the floss is gently passed below the gingival margin to loosen debris that may have lodged in the gingival sulcus. The dental assistant should be careful not to injure the gingiva while performing this procedure. Finally, the area is rinsed with warm water to remove all remnants of paste.

Air-Powder Polishing

Developed in the early 1980s, air-powder polishing involves the use of an instrument called the *Prophy-Jet*. This special device delivers a slurry of water and sodium bicarbonate under air and water pressure. A specially designed handpiece propels the mixture against the tooth on activation of a foot control. The nozzle in the handpiece is held several millimeters from the tooth and angled diagonally, using a constant circular motion. Care must be employed to aim the stream at the tooth and to avoid the soft tissues. An application of the spray should be limited to 3 to 5 seconds on any specific spot of the tooth surface. This device effectively removes extrinsic stains and soft deposits by mechanical abrasion and at the same time provides warm water for rinsing.

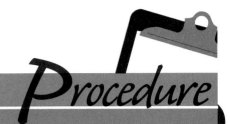

Box 17.5

Procedure for Coronal Polishing

Materials needed

Mouth mirror
Explorer
Cotton forceps
Probe
Selection of scalers
Antiseptic mouth rinse
Prophy angle
Handpiece
Rubber dam
Prophy rubber cups
Prophy brushes
Dappen dish
Paste
Saliva ejector
Air and water syringe
Dental floss
Disclosing material

Precautions

Power-driven instruments such as the prophylaxis angle can cause patient discomfort, trauma to the gingival tissues, and abrasion to the coronal tooth surfaces. To minimize these problems, use the minimal pressure, application of the rubber cup or brush, and hand piece speed consistent with procedure objectives.

1. Have patient rinse with antiseptic mouth rinse before the procedure to minimize risk of bacterial infection to the operator.
2. Patient and operator should be wearing appropriate protective eyewear and the operator should also be wearing a facemask and gloves.
3. Position the patient in a supine position in the dental chair, with the head comfortably supported by the headrest.

Use of prophylaxis angle

4. Attach prophylaxis angle to handpiece.
5. Insert rubber cup or brush into prophy angle.
6. Place small amount of moist paste into cup or brush.

7. Distribute paste over surfaces of a few teeth to be polished. Replenish paste on cup or brush as needed, keeping it moist.
8. Use a modified pen grasp to hold the handpiece and prophy angle. Establish a finger rest (fulcrum) with the third finger and activate the power.
9. Operate handpiece at slow speed; use a minimal application force and short, intermittent application intervals to minimize heat.

Use of rubber cup

10. Beginning with the distal surface of the most posterior tooth in a quadrant, adapt cup to fit each surface of the tooth.
11. Use light pressure to allow edge of cup to flare slightly and enter gingival sulcus without harm to this delicate area.
12. Use sweeping or patting motion, keeping cup in contact with tooth for a few seconds at a time.
13. Proceed from the posterior to the anterior and from the gingival to the incisal or occlusal area of each tooth.
14. Have patient turn left and open the mouth slightly to give operator good access to the facial surfaces of the upper and lower right quadrants and lingual surfaces of the upper and lower left quadrants.
15. Polish posterior teeth in these quadrants, maintaining the 9 o'clock position. Retract patient's cheek with mouth mirror, using lower anterior area for finger rest.
16. Use water spray and saliva ejector or vacuum periodically to remove polishing debris and excess saliva.
17. Have patient face center and close the mouth slightly. Retract patient's lips with mouth mirror or your fingers. Polish facial surfaces of all anterior teeth, using fingers for retraction and lower anterior teeth for fulcrum.

Continued

Box 17.5-Cont'd

Procedure

Procedure for Coronal Polishing

18. Have patient turn right to give good access to the facial surfaces of the upper and lower left quadrants and lingual surfaces of the upper and lower right quadrants.
19. Shifting to the 11 o'clock position, have the patient's head centered and mouth opened wide to obtain good access to the lingual surfaces of the maxillary anterior teeth.
20. Approach from behind the patient's head. Use mirror to reflect light and gain indirect vision. The occlusal surfaces may be polished in this position, using the adjacent teeth as a fulcrum.

Use of bristle brush

21. This device can be used on occlusal surfaces if necessary to remove stain and plaque. Avoid placing revolving brush near any soft tissue (gingiva, lips, cheek, and tongue) to prevent harm.
22. Use a firm finger rest, fulcrum, and a slow handpiece speed.
23. Apply polishing paste to brush and then to occlusal surfaces of a few teeth to be polished.
24. Bring brush close to tooth, activate power, apply revolving brush slowly, lightly, and intermittently to occlusal surfaces.
25. Use a short, brushing motion and follow inclined planes.
26. Replenish paste periodically as needed. Keep it moist.

27. Be systematic. For example, start with the maxillary right posterior quadrant and continue around the maxillary arch to the most posterior left tooth.
28. Drop down to the most posterior left tooth, following the same procedures and continuing around to the most posterior right tooth. The operator will be in the same position for polishing the surfaces of right posterior teeth using a dental mirror for retraction and lower anterior teeth for fulcrum.

Use of dental floss

29. Use dental floss with polishing paste to polish all proximal surfaces following the same routines described earlier.
30. Gently pass floss through each contact area at right angle to the long axis of the tooth.
31. Activate with a firm up-and-down motion to allow the floss to gently pass below the gingival margin and loosen any debris that may have lodged in the gingival sulcus.
32. Be careful not to injure the gingiva during this procedure.
33. When finished, have the patient rinse mouth with water, dry and inspect for any remaining stain, plaque, or other soft debris. A disclosing tablet may be used to be sure all plaque has been removed.

PIT AND FISSURE SEALANTS

About half of all decay occurs in the pit and fissure areas of the tooth. The unusual shape of these pits and fissures makes them especially vulnerable to caries. Occlusal fissures, seen in cross-section, have a wide variety of forms. Narrow pits and fissures are difficult to clean because the toothbrush bristles may be too large to penetrate the constricted opening (Figure 17.19). This sheltered environment harbors bacteria, plaque, and food debris, enabling the caries process to begin and advance quickly.

Although fluorides are effective agents for combating caries, they are least effective on the occlusal surfaces compared with the smooth (proximal, facial, and lingual) surfaces. The use of pit and fissure sealants provides a means of protecting these vulnerable occlusal areas. Presently, the application of a pit and fissure sealant is the only established method of preventing occlusal decay.

All commercial sealant systems are supplied with a phosphoric acid etchant to condition the enamel. Etching produces microscopic porosities (small surface irregularities) in the enamel surface, increasing the retention of the

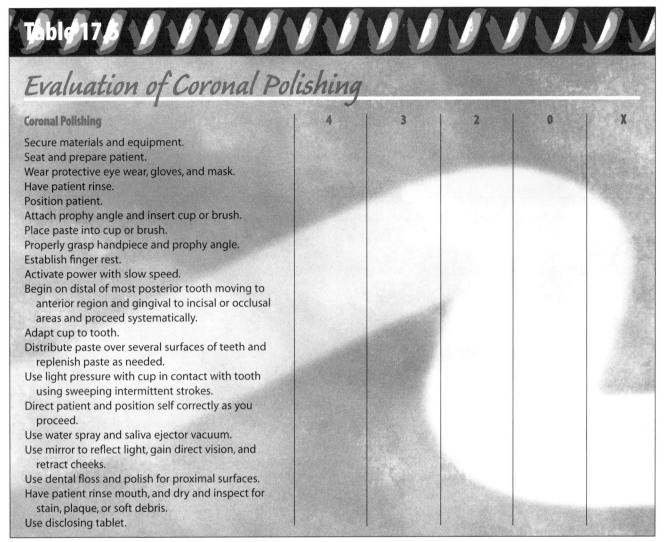

Table 17.5

Evaluation of Coronal Polishing

Coronal Polishing	4	3	2	0	X
Secure materials and equipment.					
Seat and prepare patient.					
Wear protective eye wear, gloves, and mask.					
Have patient rinse.					
Position patient.					
Attach prophy angle and insert cup or brush.					
Place paste into cup or brush.					
Properly grasp handpiece and prophy angle.					
Establish finger rest.					
Activate power with slow speed.					
Begin on distal of most posterior tooth moving to anterior region and gingival to incisal or occlusal areas and proceed systematically.					
Adapt cup to tooth.					
Distribute paste over several surfaces of teeth and replenish paste as needed.					
Use light pressure with cup in contact with tooth using sweeping intermittent strokes.					
Direct patient and position self correctly as you proceed.					
Use water spray and saliva ejector vacuum.					
Use mirror to reflect light, gain direct vision, and retract cheeks.					
Use dental floss and polish for proximal surfaces.					
Have patient rinse mouth, and dry and inspect for stain, plaque, or soft debris.					
Use disclosing tablet.					

The numeric criteria: 4 Excellent; 3 Good but some improvement can be made; 2 Below average, usable, needs to improve skill; 0 Unsatisfactory; X Not able to evaluate.

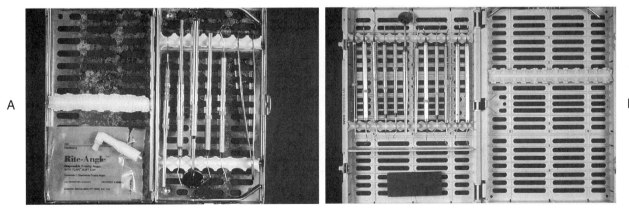

A   B

FIGURE 17.16

Prophy set-ups. **A,** Small prophy set up includes a mirror, explorer, sickle scaler, universal curette, pumice cup, prophy angle, and suction tip. **B,** Large prophy set up includes a mirror, explorer, probe, sickle scaler, universal curette, area specific curettes, sealant brush handle, dressing pliers, sharpening stones, pumice cup, prophy angle, suction tip, aspirating syringe, and A/W syringe tip. (Courtesy Hu-Friedy.)

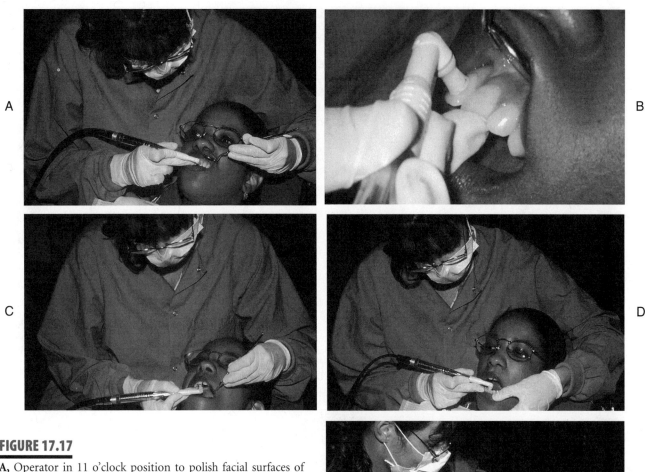

FIGURE 17.17

A, Operator in 11 o'clock position to polish facial surfaces of maxillary anterior quadrant. Mirror is used for retraction; fulcrum is on adjacent tooth. **B,** Close-up view of polishing technique. **C,** Operator in 11 o'clock position to polish lingual surfaces of upper anterior teeth. Indirect vision and mirror are used; fulcrum is on adjacent tooth. **D,** Operator in same position for polishing lingual surfaces of lower anterior teeth. Direct vision is used; fulcrum is on adjacent tooth. **E,** Operator in 10 o'clock position to polish mandibular right posterior teeth. Direct vision is used and mirror helps to retract teeth.

resin to the enamel (Box 17.6, Table 17.6, and Figure 17.20).

TOPICAL FLUORIDE THERAPY

The use of fluorides topically is an effective means of reducing caries. The term *topical fluoride therapy* refers to the use of systems containing relatively large concentrations of fluoride that are applied directly (topically) to erupted tooth surfaces to help prevent dental caries. Thus the term includes the use of fluoride rinses, dentifrices, pastes, gels, foams, and solutions that are applied in various manners to erupted teeth by the patient and dental professional in the dental office. Systemic fluoride exerts

its beneficial effect on the teeth before they erupt, whereas topical fluorides work after the teeth erupt.

The following two procedures for administering topical fluoride treatments involves:

1 Using a solution
2 Applying fluoride gel or foam using a disposable tray

The second procedure is currently more common. With either technique, the teeth should be exposed to the fluoride for 4 minutes (Box 17.7 and Table 17.7).

Special Note

Whether solutions, gels or foams are used, care should be taken to minimize the amount of fluoride inadvertently

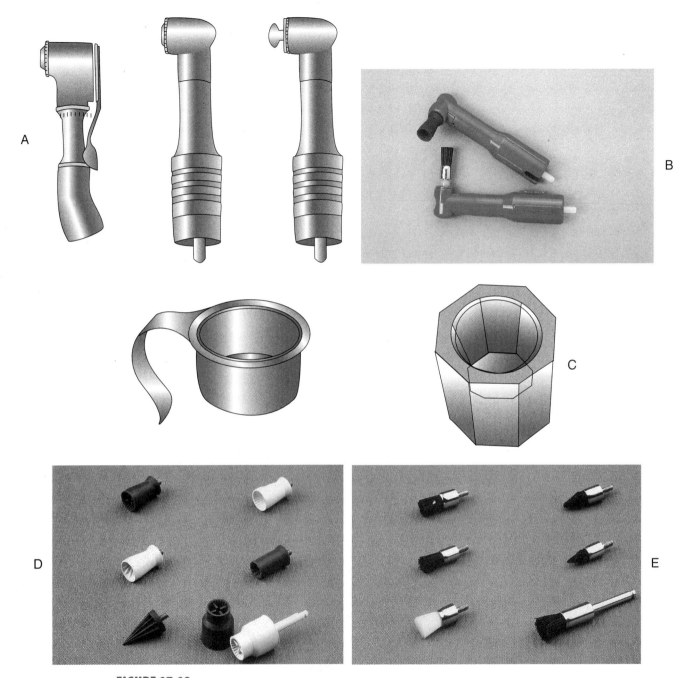

FIGURE 17.18

Devices used for polishing. **A,** Autoclavable prophy angles (from left to right) latch, screw type, snap on. **B,** Disposable prophy angles. **C,** Pumice cup and dappen dish. **D,** Rubber prophylaxis cups. **E,** Bristle brushes for prophylaxis.

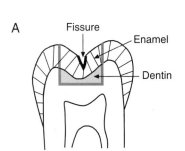
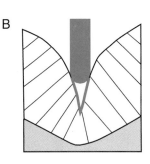
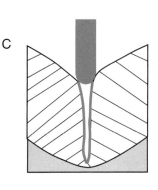
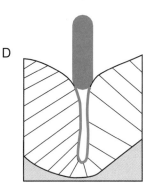

FIGURE 17.19

Cross section of variously shaped fissures. **A,** Tooth showing fissure enlarged. **B,** The toothbrush bristle, superimposed is larger than the opening to the wide V-shaped fissure. **C,** Long, narrow fissure. **D,** Long, constricted fissure with bulbous bottom.

Box 17.6

Procedure

Procedure for Application of Sealants

Materials needed

Mouth mirror
Explorer
Cotton forceps
Probe
Prophy angle
Handpiece
Prophy rubber cups
Dappen dish
Paste
Saliva ejector
Cotton rolls
Air and water syringe
Sealant material
Activator light
Always wear protective eyewear, mask, and gloves.
Patient should wear protective eyewear and rinse with antimicrobial mouth wash.
Follow manufacturer's directions.

1. Prophylaxis coronal surface of the teeth with pumice and rinse well with water. Avoid using pumice on occlusional surface.
2. Isolate quadrant with rubber dam or cotton rolls and air-dry teeth for at least 30 seconds with air syringe (Figure 17.20, *A*).
3. Apply etchant over occlusal surface with brush or cotton pellet for 60 seconds.
4. Rinse each tooth thoroughly for 30 seconds and suction.

5. Dry well for 15 to 30 seconds per tooth with air syringe.
Inspect etched surface for frosty, dull, chalky-white appearance. Reetch for additional 20 seconds if necessary. *Do not allow saliva to contaminate etched surface.* Maintain a dry field by replacing cotton rolls if they become saturated with saliva. The quadrant must be absolutely dry.
6. Insert disposable cartridge into applicator handle and adjust tip for either arch (Figure 17.20, *B*).
7. Remove cap.
8. Apply sealant (45 seconds) by depressing lever and slowly moving cartridge tip along fissures while dispensing sealant (Figure 17.20, *C*). If more than one tooth is to be sealed, seal the most posterior tooth first using only two teeth per mix.
9. Cure by holding light source about 1 to 2 mm from tooth surface and exposing all coated surfaces for 20 seconds (Figure 17.20, *D*). *Wear protective amber eyewear to protect eyes.*
10. Check margins with explorer.
11. Dry teeth, place articulating paper between teeth, have patient bring teeth together, and adjust occlusal discrepancies, if necessary.
12. Reevaluate sealants during recall visits.

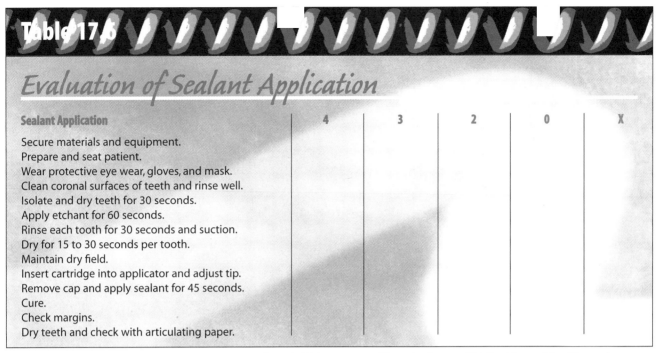

Table 17.6

Evaluation of Sealant Application

Sealant Application	4	3	2	0	X
Secure materials and equipment.					
Prepare and seat patient.					
Wear protective eye wear, gloves, and mask.					
Clean coronal surfaces of teeth and rinse well.					
Isolate and dry teeth for 30 seconds.					
Apply etchant for 60 seconds.					
Rinse each tooth for 30 seconds and suction.					
Dry for 15 to 30 seconds per tooth.					
Maintain dry field.					
Insert cartridge into applicator and adjust tip.					
Remove cap and apply sealant for 45 seconds.					
Cure.					
Check margins.					
Dry teeth and check with articulating paper.					

The numeric criteria: 4 Excellent; 3 Good but some improvement can be made; 2 Below average, usable, needs to improve skill; 0 Unsatisfactory; X Not able to evaluate.

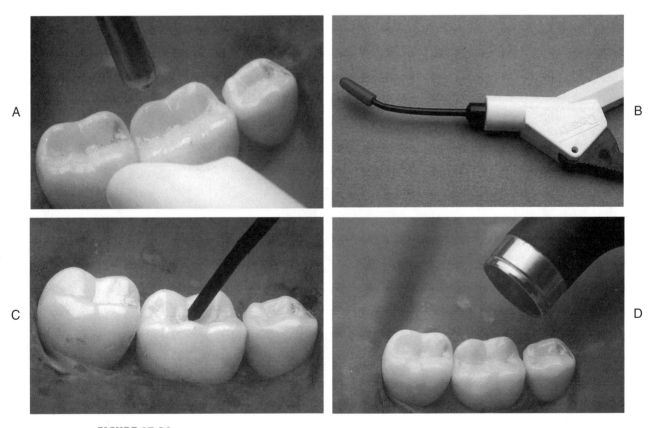

FIGURE 17.20

Procedure for application of sealants. **A,** Isolate quadrant with rubber dam or cotton rolls and air dry teeth. **B,** Disposable cartridge is inserted into applicator. Be sure to adjust the tip for either arch. **C,** Apply the sealant by slowly moving the cartridge tip along the fissure. **D,** Cure by holding light source 1 to 2 mm from tooth surface and exposing all coated surfaces for 20 seconds. Be sure to wear protective amber eyewear.

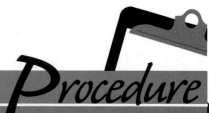

Box 17.7

Procedure for Topical Fluoride Application

Materials needed

Mouth mirror
Explorer
Cotton forceps
Probe
Selection of scalers
Mouth rinse
Prophy angle
Handpiece
Rubber dam
Prophy rubber cups
Prophy brushes
Dappen dish
Paste
Saliva ejector
Air and water syringe
Floss
Suction
Cotton applications
Cotton rolls and holder
Fluoride solution, gel, or foam
Trays

Preparation

Operator should wear mask and protective
    eye-wear.
Have patient rinse with antimicrobial
    solution.
Have patient wear protective eye wear.
Polish coronal surfaces of the teeth if
    indicated.
Have patient rinse thoroughly.
Place patient in upright position.
Have high velocity suction ready.

Procedure for applying topical solution

1. Isolate quadrant or quadrants to be treated with cotton rolls and holders.
2. Dry teeth with compressed air.
3. Wet teeth continuously with fluoride solution on cotton-tipped applicators for 4 minutes.
4. Use frequent loading of cotton-tipped applicators to keep teeth moist.
5. Remove cotton rolls and holders and suction excess saliva from patient's mouth.
6. Repeat process for each area of the mouth.
7. When finished, have patient expectorate all excess fluoride from mouth.
8. Advise patient not to eat, drink, or rinse for 30 minutes.

Procedure for applying gels and foams

1. Select appropriate sized trays for patient (Figure 17.21, *A*).
2. Try unloaded trays in the mouth for fit.
3. Dry tray with compressed air.
4. Insert 3mm of gel/foam in tray ($^1/_3$ full) (Figure 17.21, *B*).
5. Dry teeth with compressed air.
6. Insert trays into mouth.
7. Place saliva ejector between trays or have patient drool over sink.
8. Instruct patient to bite gently against trays and move lips and cheeks for 4 minutes (Figure 17.21, *C*).
9. Remove trays after 4 minutes.
10. Use high vacuum evacuator to remove remaining fluoride or have patient expectorate.
11. Advise patient not to eat, drink, or rinse for 30 minutes.

Table 17

Evaluation of Topical Fluoride Application

Topical Fluoride Solution	4	3	2	0	X
Secure materials and equipment.					
Seat and drape patient.					
Provide protective eye wear for patient.					
Wear protective eye wear, gloves, and mask.					
Have patient rinse with mouthwash.					
Polish coronal surfaces of teeth.					
Have patient rinse.					
Isolate quadrant.					
Dry teeth.					
Place fluoride solution continuously for 4 minutes.					
Remove cotton rolls and suction saliva.					
Repeat process.					
Have patient expectorate excess fluoride.					
Advise patient not to eat, drink, or rinse for 30 minutes.					
Topical Fluoride Gel and Foams					
Secure materials and equipment.					
Seat and drape patient.					
Provide protective eye wear for patient.					
Wear protective eye wear, gloves, and mask.					
Select tray and try in mouth.					
Dry tray.					
Insert 3 mm ($\frac{1}{3}$ full) foam in tray.					
Dry teeth.					
Insert trays into mouth.					
Place saliva ejector.					
Instruct patient to bite against trays.					
Use suction to remove fluoride.					
Advise patient to not eat, drink, or rinse for 30 minutes.					

The numeric criteria: 4 Excellent; 3 Good but some improvement can be made; 2 Below average, usable, needs to improve skill; 0 Unsatisfactory; X Not able to evaluate.

swallowed by the patient during the application. Using only the required amount of fluoride to adequately perform the procedure facilitates this. The dental assistant should keep the patient in an upright position, using high-velocity suctioning apparatus, and have the patient expectorate thoroughly for 1 minute after treatment is completed. When the procedure is completed, the patient is usually told not to rinse, drink, or eat for 30 minutes.

The most comprehensive approach to caries prevention combines multiple fluoride therapy with pit and fissure sealants, oral hygiene instruction, and dietary counseling.

MAINTENANCE RECALL

An important aspect of a recall program is to periodically review the patient's efforts at disease control to ensure

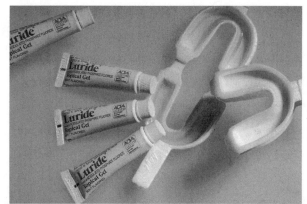

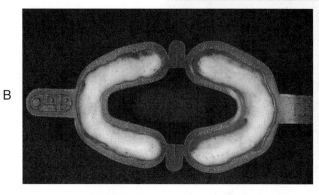

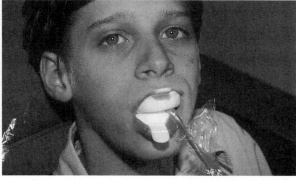

FIGURE 17.21

Procedure for applying gels and foam. Select appropriate-sized tray. **A,** Using no more than the recommended amount of fluoride will help minimize the amount of fluoride inadvertently swallowed by the patient. **B,** Insert 3 mm of gel into tray. **C,** After the trays are inserted, place the saliva ejector between trays and instruct patient to bite gently against trays while moving lips and cheeks for 4 minutes.

their program is effective. Most patients need periodic reinstruction and positive reinforcement to have a successful outcome. Dental assistants' enthusiasm and empathy for the patient, coupled with effective teaching skills, can make a difference in whether the preventative goals for the patient are maintained. Recall appointments should be scheduled initially at 3 months, then at 6 months, according to the needs of the patient.

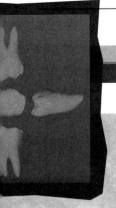

Points for Review

- Importance of preventive dentistry programs
- General oral health status in the United States
- Role of the dental assistant in preventive dental care
- Importance of attitude in dental health care
- Definition of plaque, caries, and periodontal diseases
- Oral hygiene instruction and patient education program
- Instrument identification and use
- Application techniques for pit and fissure sealants, fluoride therapy, and coronal polish

Self-Study Questions

1. Who controls the major efforts for following preventive measures?
   a. Patient
   b. Dental assistant
   c. Dentist
   d. Hygienist
   e. Community

2. What is the most efficient, effective, reliable, and inexpensive method of reducing caries in a community?
   a. Fluoridation of the community water supply
   b. Fluoridation of the school water supply
   c. Distributing fluoride supplements to schoolchildren
   d. Weekly fluoride mouth rinse programs in schools
   e. School-based topical fluoride programs

3. What are the signs of gingival inflammation?
   a. Redness
   b. Swelling
   c. Bleeding
   d. A and b
   e. All of the above

4. What causes inflammatory periodontal disease?
   a. Dental neglect
   b. Plaque
   c. Calculus
   d. Poor nutrition
   e. C and d

5. What causes dental caries?
   a. Sugar
   b. Bacteria
   c. Acid
   d. Time
   e. All of the above

6. What is the best method of preventing occlusal decay?
   a. Plaque control
   b. Dental sealants
   c. Dietary counseling
   d. Water fluoridation
   e. Multiple fluoride therapy

7. What kind of bristles does the preferred type of toothbrush have?
   a. Natural bristles
   b. Nylon bristles
   c. Hard bristles
   d. Soft bristles
   e. B and d

8. Who mainly benefits from using a floss holder?
   a. Patients lacking manual dexterity
   b. Nursing personnel assisting debilitated patients
   c. Parents flossing the teeth of their young children
   d. Patients with a strong gag reflex
   e. All of the above

9. Which useful aid is used for reshaping the interdental gingiva that has been destroyed by periodontal disease?
   a. Interdental tip
   b. Interdental brush
   c. Dental floss
   d. Soft toothbrush
   e. All of the above

10. Which of the following mouth rinses does the ADA accept for controlling plaque and gingivitis?
    a. Scope
    b. Cepacol
    c. Listerine
    d. Plax
    e. Lavoris

11. For a preventive program is to be effective, how should patient education efforts be approached?
    a. Initiated by the dentist
    b. Initiated by the dental auxiliary
    c. Repeated and reinforced
    d. Taught using study models and radiographs
    e. Taught in a separate appointment

12. How can the dental assistant help patients preserve periodontal health?
    a. Provide a regular dental prophylaxis
    b. Provide instruction in oral hygiene
    c. Reinforce the patients' oral hygiene efforts
    d. Establish an appropriate recall schedule
    e. All of the above

13. What is a hand instrument often used to remove gross supragingival calculus from the crown of the tooth called?
    a. Sickle scaler
    b. Hoe
    c. File
    d. Curette
    e. Ultrasonic scaler

14. What is the procedure sometimes delegated to a dental assistant that involves removing stain and plaque and polishing dental restorations called?
    a. Scaling
    b. Coronal reshaping
    c. Coronal polishing
    d. Dental prophylaxis
    e. Tooth cleaning

15. Fluorides are *least* effective on which tooth surfaces?
    a. Proximal
    b. Facial
    c. Lingual
    d. Occlusal

16. In applying dental sealants, acid conditioning is accomplished by using which of the following?
    a. Phosphoric acid
    b. Sulfuric acid
    c. Acetic acid
    d. Hydrofluoric acid
    e. Carbonic acid

17. Which of the following steps in the dental sealant procedure, if indicated, is performed *first*?
    a. Washing the teeth
    b. Isolation
    c. Prophylaxis
    d. Acid conditioning
    e. Applying the rubber dam to maintain dryness

18. One part per million of fluoride in the water will reduce caries in a population by about which percentage?
    a. 20%
    b. 40%
    c. 60%
    d. 80%

19. What does the term *topical fluoride therapy* refer to?
    a. Home-use fluoride rinses and gels
    b. Fluoride-containing toothpastes
    c. Professionally applied fluoride solutions and gels
    d. Fluoride-containing prophy pastes
    e. All of the above

20. Which of the following fluoride systems has the ADA accepted for professionally applied topical fluoride applications?
    a. 8% stannous fluoride
    b. Acidulated phosphate fluoride 1.23%
    c. 2% sodium fluoride
    d. A and b
    e. All of the above

21. The ADA accepts all of the following toothpastes as effective decay-preventive dentifrices *except* which one?
    a. Pepsodent
    b. Crest
    c. Colgate
    d. Aim
    e. Aquafresh

22. How often should recall appointments be scheduled?
    a. About every 3 months
    b. About every 6 months
    c. Initially at 3 months, then 6 months
    d. About every year
    e. According to the needs of the patient

23. What is the most efficient way to identify supragingival calculus?
    a. Disclosing solution
    b. Use of an explorer
    c. Visual observation and compressed air
    d. Transillumination

24. What is the approximate angulation degree established between the tooth surface and instrument before initiating a stroke?
    a. 10 to 20
    b. 30 to 50
    c. 70 to 80
    d. 90 to 100

Burt BA, Eklund SA: *Dentistry, dental practice, and the community*, ed 5, Philadelphia, 1999, WB Saunders.

Carranza Jr FA, Newman MG: *Clinical periodontology*, ed 9, Philadelphia, WB Saunders (in press).

Genco RJ: *Contemporary periodontics*, ed 2, St Louis, Mosby (in press).

Grant DA, Stern IB, Listgarden MA: *Periodontics*, ed 6, St Louis, 1988, Mosby.

Harris NO, Christen AG: *Primary preventive dentistry*, ed 5, Stamford, Conn, 1999, Appleton & Lange.

Kentucky Cabinet for Human Resources: *The Kentucky oral health survey*, Frankfort, Ky, 1987, 1989.

Lindhe J: *Textbook of clinical periodontology*, ed 2, Copenhagen, 1989, Munksgaard.

Mandel ID, editor: Symposium on current and future uses of antimicrobial mouthrinses, *J Am Dent Assoc* 125 (suppl 2), 1994.

McDonald RE, Avery DR: *Dentistry for the child and adolescent*, ed 7, St Louis, 2000, Mosby.

Newbrun E: *Cariology*, ed 3, Chicago, 1989, Quintessence.

Nikiforuk G: *Understanding dental caries*, Basel, Switzerland, 1985, Karger.

Wilkins EM: *Clinical practice of the dental hygienist*, ed 8, Baltimore, Md, 1999, Williams & Wilkins.

Woodall IR: *Comprehensive dental hygiene care*, ed 4, St Louis, 1993, Mosby.

Meskin LH: Caries diagnosis and risk assessment: a review of preventive strategies and management, *J Am Dent Assoc* 126 (special suppl), 1995.

Meskin LH: Dental sealants, *J Am Dent Assoc* 128:485-488, 1997.

Chapter *18*

*B*arriers to Disease Transmission

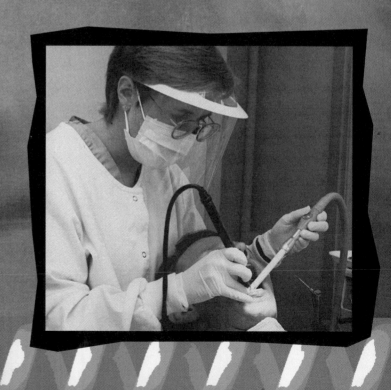

Chapter Outline

Ethical Issues
Legal Issues
Principles of Infection Control
    Sterilization processes
    Disinfection process

Recycling the dental operatory
Asepsis of dental support areas
Asepsis in radiology
**Removal of personal protective
    equipment**

Learning Objectives

On completion of Chapter 18, the student should be able to do the following:

■ Define key terms.

■ Describe the operation of an autoclave, dry heat sterilizer, and chemical vapor sterilizer.

■ Characterize an ideal disinfectant and the subjective levels of applications.

■ Give the major properties including beneficial aspects and disadvantages of the following disinfectant groups: alcohols, detergents, iodine compounds, chlorine-containing compounds, phenol derivatives, and aldehydes.

■ Describe the barrier technique.

■ Describe the process of recycling the dental operatory.

■ Categorize dental instruments relative to the level of infection control needed.

■ Describe adequate infection control procedures for dental laboratory and radiology support areas.

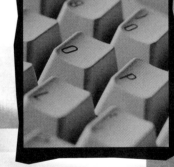

Key Terms

ETHICAL ISSUES

Infection control is the prevention of the spread of infectious diseases to healthy people. This is accomplished by using **aseptic** techniques. The infection control guidelines issued for dentists by the Center for Disease Control (CDC) is the policy recommendation of the American Dental Association (ADA).

Aseptic

Free of viable micro-organisms

The prevention of diseases spreading to patients is a major priority of all dental practices. The onset of HIV and AIDS initially created some ethical problems for health professions. Because of initial fear about the spread of the disease, questions arose concerning whom, how, where, and who would treat these patients. Fears concerning the reputation of a practice from healthy patients could occur that might result in a practice losing income. As a result, health professions, including dentistry, often were reluctant to treat these patients. However, while these problems may still exist, they are no longer ethical questions for the following reasons:

1 Our current knowledge of the disease and its method of transmission
2 The now standard practice of using universal precautions in providing health care services such as dentistry
3 The ADA's official position on the treatment of these patients
4 The 1990 enactment of the Americans with Disabilities Act

Since the late 1980s, knowledge of this disease has greatly increased. The disease is not transmissible in the course of most normal social interaction and seems to be spread only through direct body fluid-to-body fluid contact. As a result of this knowledge, the use of universal precautions effective enough to protect against the much more contagious Hepatitis B virus has become the professional standard of care.

Numerous studies have proved that proper use of universal precautions protects the provider from the patient, the patient from the provider, and one patient from another. The effectiveness of universal precautions has made the discrimination of patients in their health care treatment unjustified.

The 1990 Americans with Disabilities Act made it illegal to discriminate against a person just because they are HIV positive. In a similar manner, in 1991 the American Dental Association updated its code of ethics regarding patient selection. The official position of the dental profession is that dentists have an ethical obligation to treat those in need, and to decline care *solely* on the basis of a patient's HIV status is unethical.

Thus, treatment of HIV or AIDS patients is no longer an option; it is an ethical obligation if the dentist has the technical expertise to accomplish the treatment needed and appropriate universal precautions are maintained.

These ethical and legal standards regarding the treatment of patients apply not only to the dentist but also to everyone on staff, including the dental assistant. Treatment of patients with diseases is now a normal part of dental practice. If anyone, including the physician, nurse, dentist, or assistant, is unable to comply with these ethical and legal standards, they will need to find another occupation. They cannot stay in the health professions and refuse to treat these patients.

LEGAL ISSUES

The Occupational Safety and Health Administration (OSHA) regulates prevention of disease transmission to employees of dental health care offices. The entire intent of infection control is to stop infectious disease transmission. This is generally accomplished by either destroying the pathogenic potential of infectious organisms or by preventing transfer of disease-producing organisms from contaminated surfaces to the human host.

PRINCIPLES OF INFECTION CONTROL

Bacteria, viruses, and some fungi cause infectious diseases. **Sterilization** is the process that destroys all biologic material capable of reproduction. In other words, an item that has no living bacteria, viruses, yeast, or other biologically active material in or on its surfaces is sterile. An object is either sterile, with no life forms, or is nonsterile, with no contamination. In contrast, disinfection means the reduction or elimination of disease-causing microorganisms from surfaces. A **disinfectant** will kill pathogens but many living microbes could remain.

Sterilization

The process that eliminates all living micro-organisms

Disinfectant

A substance that destroys vegetative state microbial pathogens

Sterilization Processes

Numerous ways to sterilize equipment exist; however, the following have ready application in the dental office for sterilization of reusable instruments:

1 **Autoclave**
2 Dry heat
3 Unsaturated chemical vapor (Table 18.1)

Autoclave

Chamber containing saturated steam generally at 121°C used for sterilization

Table 18.1

Dental Sterilizer Operating Characteristics

Sterilizer Type	Operating Temperature (IC)	Time at Temperature
Autoclave	121	15 min
Autoclave (high)	132	4-8 min
Dry heat	160	120 min
Dry heat	170	60 min
Chemical vapor	132	20 min

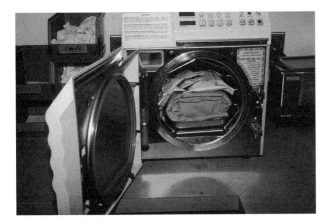

FIGURE 18.1

Midmark M9 ultra clave. Loading techniques provided by the manufacturer should be followed to achieve complete sterilization.

Autoclave

Autoclaves use saturated steam at a temperature of 121° C (250° F) to create sterile conditions. The microbes are killed when their proteins are denatured. The 121° C temperature is higher than what can be achieved by boiling a pan of water on the stove. The laws of physics dictate that water at 100° C (212° F) at sea level will produce steam. The only way to raise the temperature of steam is to allow the steam to build pressure. The chamber of an autoclave is strong and allows the steam to build pressure inside to about 16 lb per square inch. As a result of the pressure, the temperature increases to 121° C. Once this temperature is reached, most manufacturers of autoclaves recommend a 15-minute exposure of instruments. The time should be extended to 20 or more minutes if the autoclave contains a large mass of instruments.

The autoclave has proved to be a very effective and rapid means of sterilizing medical equipment (Figure 18.1). A drawback to the use of the autoclave is that the steam may react with metal instrument surfaces causing discoloration and dulling of cutting surfaces. Autoclaved items may also retain water from condensation of the steam. In addition to the traditional autoclave, effective high-temperature autoclaves are sold that operate at 132° C (270° F). Because of the increased temperature, the recommended cycle time is reduced to between 4 and 8 minutes.

Although this method is much quicker than the conventional autoclave, the dentist may find greater rates of instrument corrosion and the assistant must be attentive to the amount of material sterilized per load. The times given are for the sterilization portion of a cycle only. Do not include the time to heat the unit to the desired temperature or the time for the unit to reduce the internal temperatures to a safe level at the end of a run as part of the sterilizing time. Instrument packages and cassettes should be dried before removing them from the sterilizer.

Dry Heat

Sterilization can also be achieved by placing instruments into a dry heat sterilizer that is heated to 150° C to 170° C. This oxidizes microbes. The simplest dry heat sterilizer is nothing more than a typical kitchen oven. The heating in these gravity convection ovens is not uniform and they are not recommended for dental office sterilization procedures. The accepted dry heat sterilizers use forced air circulation within the sterilizer. In these systems, a load of instruments will be sterilized after 1 hour at 170° C (340° F).

Unsaturated Chemical Vapor

The unsaturated chemical vapor sterilizer was developed to reduce the instrument corrosion caused by the saturated steam of an autoclave. It is physically similar to an autoclave, but operationally, the chemical vapor sterilizer uses a mixture of alcohol, water, formaldehyde, and other trace chemicals to create a nonsaturated vapor inside the chamber (Figure 18.2).

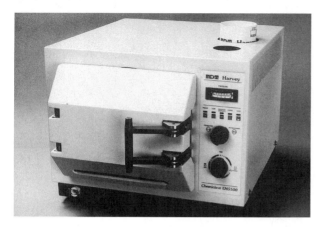

FIGURE 18.2

Unsaturated chemical vapor sterilizer operating at 132° C.

Microbial killing occurs by protein denatentation and reaction with the formaldehyde. The operating temperature of the unsaturated chemical vapor sterilizer is 132° C (270° F) and the recommended exposure time is 20 minutes. The manufacturer's instructions to use porous instrument wraps and careful loading techniques must be observed for effective sterilization to occur. Fabrics and plastics absorb the vapors and should not be used for 24 hours after sterilization to avoid skin irritations.

Disinfection Process

Categories of Effectiveness

Sterilization is an absolute but disinfection may not kill *all* living material. Some disinfectants may be more effective than others; therefore comparisons are often made between the different types of disinfecting agents. In the health care industry, the following accepted categories of effectiveness include:

1 Sterilants and disinfectants: Chemicals that kill all bacteria, including bacterial endospores, viruses, and fungi on prolonged contact (10 hours).
2 Intermediate disinfectants: Hospital disinfectant that will kill *Mycobacterium tuberculosis* var. bovis cells but may not inactivate endospores. The label will also include a claim for virucidal and fungicidal activity.
3 Low-level disinfectants: Chemicals that kill many normal bacteria and viruses may not have an effect on fungi or endospores.

Caution When Using Disinfectants

Regardless of the product selected, be certain to follow exactly all of the manufacturer's directions for mixing and diluting; proper application shelf-life, activated use-life, and reuse-life; and all safety warnings.

Disinfectant Types

Choosing the best disinfectant for a particular task is difficult for dental health care workers, especially because of exaggerated or distorted claims made by some manufacturers. General properties of an ideal disinfectant are described in Box 18.1. All available disinfectants are not ideal; therefore dental health care workers must compare and decide which product will best serve the specific needs of the practice (Table 18.2).

Microbial destruction by disinfectants typically involves chemical reactions between the disinfectant and vital contents of the cell. The usual targets for bacterial cells include the cell wall, nuclear material such as DNA, and the enzymes found in the cytoplasm. Because these chemical reactions are not highly specific or selective, the disinfections will also react with heat tissue products, such as proteins found in blood serum and saliva. Thus, high levels of contaminating tissues, sometimes referred to as *bioburden*, can quickly reduce or eliminate the effectiveness of chemical disinfectants. When a disinfectant actually kills an organism, they are called **bactericide**, **fungicide**, or **germicide** agents. If the chemical inhibits the growth of microbes but does not kill them, the agent is considered to be a **bacteriostatic** agent.

Bactericide
An agent that kills bacteria

Fungicide
An agent capable of destroying fungi

Germicide
An agent that destroys pathogenic micro-organisms

Bacteriostatic
An agent that inhibits bacterial growth

Table 18.2

Disinfectants Used in Dental Infection Control Programs

Disinfectant Type	Recommended by ADA	Tuberculocidal	Surface Use	Comments
Alcohols Isopropyl & ethyl	No	Yes	No	Useful as an antiseptic.
Detergents Quaternary Ammonium Compounds	No	No	Yes	Found in some mouthwashes and floor-care products.
Iodine compounds	Yes	Yes	Yes	Will stain surfaces; used in surgical scrubs.
Chlorine compounds Hypochlorite (bleach)	Yes	Yes	Yes	Make fresh daily.
Chlorine dioxide	Yes	Yes	Yes	Make fresh daily; reduce odor.
Phenolics	Yes	Yes	Yes	May irritate tissues.
Aldehydes Glutaraldehyde	Yes	Yes	Yes	Good for immersion; not a cold sterilant; 2-4 wk life.

Alcohols

Ethyl and isopropyl alcohols have been used for years as disinfectants. They cause rapid **denaturation** of proteins and dissolve many fat or lipid molecules. The alcohols work over a large spectrum of microbes, including most viruses and hardy bacterial cells such as *M. tuberculosis*. The most effective concentration of alcohol is 70%. Unfortunately, alcohols have little, if any, effect on endospores, are not effective cleansing agents, and do not leave a antimicrobial residue. Because of these shortcomings, the ADA and CDC do not accept these alcohols for use as a surface disinfectant in the dental office.

Denaturation

A process in which proteins lose their configuration and biologic activity

Detergents

Detergents are chemicals that form bridges between water-loving solutions and water-insoluble molecules, such as fats. Because fats are necessary for the cell to function, altering cells with detergents usually results in death of the cell. The most common group of disinfecting detergents are the quaternary ammonium compounds.

Detergents

Synthetic cleansing agents with soap characteristics

Quaternary ammonium compounds work well on gram-positive bacteria. In contrast, substantial evidence exists that quaternary ammonium compounds have little effect on gram-negative bacteria, *M. tuberculosis*, Hepatitis B virus, and selected yeast and fungi. The ADA once accepted these compounds for use in the dental office, but because of their limited scope of effectiveness, the ADA no longer lists them as an acceptable group of disinfectants. However, the quaternary ammonium compounds exhibit low toxicity for human tissues and can be found in germicidal soaps and some mouthwashes.

Iodine and Iodophores

For years iodine has been used for minor scrapes. It also has antimicrobial properties. Because pure iodine is not water soluble, salts of iodine, such as potassium iodide, are dissolved in alcohol. This is referred to as **tincture** of iodine. In this form, iodine will inactivate virtually all pathogenic bacterial, including spores, viruses, and fungi. Although iodine is ideal as an antimicrobial, it has several negative properties, including

Tincture

An alcoholic solution of a particular substance, such as tincture of iodine

irritation and staining of skin and corrosion of metal instruments. Some of these problems are overcome by combining iodine with a carrier molecule that forms an iodophor. The ADA accepts iodophor-containing products as surface disinfectants based on their abilities to kill many microorganisms and to remain on environmental surfaces as an active residue. Solutions of iodophores do not store well after dilution and must be prepared daily.

Iodophor solutions have minimal toxicity for human tissues and are often used as **antiseptics**. They are often the active agent in surgical scrubs and can be used on skin and mucosal surfaces. After the surfaces are scrubbed, the iodophores residual antimicrobial activity remains strong even when rinsed with water.

Antiseptics

A chemical compound that inhibits bacterial growth and can be used on the surface of living tissue

Chlorine-Containing Compounds

Chlorine mixed with water causes **oxidation** of biologic molecules and is an effective antimicrobial compound. Hypochlorite solutions are simply household bleaches diluted 1:10 for sporicidal activity or 1:00 for general use, including inactivating the Hepatitis B virus. The bleach-based disinfectants must be made fresh daily. They often degrade metal and plastic instruments and some people consider the odor offensive. A newer group of chloride-containing compounds is known as *chlorine dioxide preparations*. These are also effective antimicrobials but with reduced odor and only limited corrosiveness for instruments. Both types of chlorine-based disinfectants can be irritating to the skin.

Oxidation

Loss of electrons by an atom or compound

Phenol-Based Antimicrobials

In the mid 1800s, Joseph Lister used carbolic acid (phenol) as a spray in his first attempts to perform aseptic surgery. His findings demonstrated that phenol was a powerful agent for killing infectious disease-producing microbes. However, phenol is not in general use today because of its high level of toxicity.

Phenol can be chemically modified to form molecules that are less irritating to tissues and in some cases have greater antibacterial properties than phenol. These derivatives of phenol are termed *phenolics*. A frequently used phenolic is the natural-occurring cresols obtained from coal tar. Cresols are good surface disinfectants. The synthetic phenols can also cause skin and eye irritations. Soaps or scrubs of hexachlorophene, a synthetic phenolic, often control infections of the skin. A prescription is required to purchase hexachlorophene-containing soaps.

Glutaraldehydes

Glutaraldehydes are the most widely used disinfectants in the dental profession. They have a wide antimicrobial range including Hepatitis viruses and *M. tuberculosis* cells. Bacterial spores are also killed in 6 to 10 hours of exposure. In addition, glutaraldehydes have good cleaning characteristics because of their ability to penetrate biological materials, such as blood.

Some accept the fact that because glutaraldehydes kill spores, they can be used to sterilize equipment. But the ADA no longer accepts these cold sterilants based on a number of reasons, including the compound's inability to inactivate occluded or embedded microbes and the variabilities encountered when the reuse life is considered.

Glutaraldehydes are generally usable for 2 to 4 weeks after dispensing to the clinic; however, the effects bioburden, dilution with rinse water, and contamination by other agents, such as detergents, must be taken into account to determine the actual time when glutaraldehyde solutions must be changed.

One of the first uses of glutaraldehyde was as a tissue fixative for electron microscopy. The concentration as a fixative is usually 2.0%, whereas, the disinfecting solutions range from 2.0% to 3.2%. Thus, glutaraldehydes are obviously damaging to human tissues and should be handled only with gloved hands. Glutaraldehyde-treated instruments should never be used on patients without completely rinsing them with water. Prolonged exposure of selected instruments to glutaraldehyde solutions can lead to discoloration and corrosion of the instrument surfaces, including the cutting edges.

Alternatives to Sterilization or Disinfection

Aseptic techniques are required to eliminate the spread of infectious diseases in the dental operatory. Asepsis in the operatory requires physical tasks and an understanding of universal precautions, which mean that all patients must be thought of as potentially infectious. Therefore the infection control procedures used for patients who are known to harbor infectious diseases must be the same procedures applied universally for all patients seeking treatment. Proper application of universal precautions is not just a checklist of things to do but also is an attitude generated in the dental professional's mind (Boxes 18.2 and 18.3 and Table 18.3).

Personal Protection

The dental healthcare worker is at risk of infection by pathogenic microbes from the patient. Several experiments have been performed using colored or dyed saliva and looking for the dye after a procedure. In virtually all cases, the dentist and assistant were contaminated with patient saliva from the waist up, including their hair. For the dental staff, obviously, sterilization is not possible and most high- and intermediate-

Box 18.2

Universal Precautions

All patients must be presumed infectious.

All treatment personnel must wear gloves, masks, and eye-protection during treatment.

A heat process must sterilize all critical and semicritical instruments and items; liquid sterilants are not acceptable.

All touch and splash surfaces must be disinfected with an EPA-registered, hospital-grade disinfectant.

All contaminated waste must be disposed of carefully and properly.

level disinfectants are not compatible with human tissues. The best approach is to wash the exposed skin with soap, followed by a suitable barrier.

The OSHA regulations indicate that long-sleeved gowns, gloves, and a face shield or mask and protective eyewear are required as the minimal level of barrier protection (Figure 18.3). Masks and gloves should be changed after each patient or when saturated with liquid or punctured. Washing gloved hands between patients is not acceptable. Gloves need not be sterile, but should fit well and be comfortable. Similarly, masks must be comfortable and fit well, especially around the nose. Protective eyewear must shield against spatter from the sides and front. For routine dentistry, gowns need not be changed between patients only when visibly soiled. No protective clothing or equipment should be worn outside of the treatment area.

Handwashing

Handwashing is one of the most important actions taken to prevent transfer of microorganisms from one person to another. Washing for 15 seconds with plain soaps or detergents is effective in lifting and removing many contaminating microorganisms and normal flora microorganisms from the top layers of skin. Germicidal soaps will inhibit many of the microorganisms that remain buried in the sweat glands and hairshafts of the skin. Every dental team member should begin the day with two consecutive 15-second handwashes with soap and water followed by adequate rinsing. The thumbs, fingertips, and areas between and around the fingernails should receive particular attention (see Chapter 27).

During the typical workday, your hands should be washed before gloving and after gloves are removed. Also,

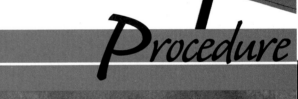

Box 18.3

Procedure for Operatory Asepsis

Procedure

Before seating the patient

1 Remove all unnecessary items from the operatory.

2 Preplan the materials needed during treatment. Unit dose dispensing.

3 Use individualized, sterilized bur blocks for each procedure.

4 Identify fixed equipment and methods of infection control.

5 Place radiographs on the view box and review patient records before initiating treatment.

Chairside infection control

1. Use care when receiving, handling, or passing sharp instruments.

2 Take special precautions with syringes and needles.

3 Avoid touching unprotected switches, handles, and other equipment once gloves have become contaminated.

4 Avoid entering drawers or cabinets once gloves have become contaminated.

5 Treat used or contaminated instruments.

Posttreatment infection control

1 Continue to wear personal protective clothing during clean up.

2 Remove all disposable barriers.

3 Clean and disinfect all items not protected by barriers.

4 Remove the tray with all instruments to the sterilization and clean-up area.

5 Sterilize handpieces between patients.

6 Place contaminated waste and soft goods soiled with blood or saliva in sturdy, leak-proof bags.

7 Handle sharp items carefully.

8 Remove personal protective clothing.

Table 18.3

Evaluation for Operatory Asepsis

Operatory Asepsis	4	3	2	0	X
Before seating the patient					
Remove all unnecessary items.					
Prepare materials and equipment.					
Prepare operatory infection barriers.					
Prepare radiographs.					
Review patient records.					
Chairside infection control					
Take precautions for handling sharps.					
Avoid touching unprotected areas and equipment.					
Wear protective glasses, gloves, and mask.					
Avoid entering drawer after gloved.					
Secure contaminated instruments.					
Posttreatment infection control					
Wear protective clothing.					
Remove disposable barriers.					
Clean and disinfect area.					
Remove tray with instruments.					
Sterilize handpieces and instruments.					
Secure contaminated waste and sharps.					
Remove protective clothing.					

The numeric criteria: 4 Excellent; 3 Good but some improvement can be made; 2 Below average, usable, needs to improve skill; 0 Unsatisfactory; X Not able to evaluate.

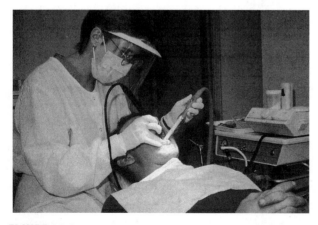

FIGURE 18.3

A properly protected dental assistant, wearing gloves, mask, eyewear, and gown.

wash before and after going to lunch, taking a break, using the restroom, or any other time they become contaminated. Dry your hands with disposable or single-use towels. When washing times are too short or technique is poor, the opportunity for disease transmission may occur for the following reasons:

- Fingertips, thumbs, and the areas between the fingers are washed poorly or may be skipped entirely.
- The dominant hand is generally washed less thoroughly than the nondominant hand.
- Microbe counts under the fingernails may remain high.

Because soap containers and sink equipment will become contaminated, the handwashing product should be a liquid and kept in a foot-operated dispenser. Ideally, the sink should be equipped with foot- or elbow-operated faucets, or use a paper towel as a barrier when turning off the water with your hands.

Whether antimicrobial handwashes should be used instead of plain soaps or detergents has not been established because of the lack of well-controlled studies comparing infection rates with different products. For most routine nonsurgical activities, handwashing for 15 seconds with plain soaps is sufficient because most of the transient or contaminating microorganisms on the skin will be washed off.

If you have problems with skin irritation because of the effects of soap or frequent handwashing, try another handwashing product. Finally, hand lotions are helpful to prevent hands from chapping caused by frequent handwashing.

Gloves

Significant risks exist for dental health care personnel and patients when gloves are not used. Ungloved hands are the mechanism by which dental personnel have acquired HBV infections from their patients. Transmission of infectious agents including Herpes virus from ungloved provider to patient has also been documented. Gloves must be worn whenever you anticipate contact with blood, saliva, mucous membranes, or blood-contaminated objects or surfaces. Two categories of gloves routinely used in the dental clinic include (1) thin latex or vinyl exam gloves used during patient treatment and (2) heavy-duty or utility gloves used for cleaning operations.

Many types of exam gloves are on the commercial market. Factors to consider when choosing gloves include the type of procedure, tactical sensitivity required for the procedure, and comfort of the wearer. The following are categories of exam gloves:

1 Latex gloves (sterile and nonsterile)
2 Vinyl gloves (sterile and nonsterile)

No data currently exist to indicate differences in barrier effectiveness between vinyl and latex gloves. Sterile gloves (often marketed as sterile surgical gloves) are recommended specifically for surgical procedures, such as oral and periodontal surgery involving contact with penetrated or injured tissues. Nonsterile gloves (often marketed as examination gloves) provide an adequate level of protection for operative or general dentistry procedures. Gloves must be changed between patients, whether they are worn for treatment or examination. Exam or surgical gloves used in patient care should not be washed. Hands should always be washed after removing gloves because the potential for damage to a glove during dental procedures is high.

Allergic reactions to gloves or glove powder may be corrected by trying a different brand of gloves or by using hypoallergenic gloves.

General-purpose utility gloves are thicker gloves that are only appropriate for use during cleanup and disinfection procedures. Whereas, the typical dishwashing glove is acceptable, gloves made of rubber are more puncture- and disinfectant-resistant and are strongly recommended. Unlike gloves used during patient care, utility gloves can be washed and reused; however, be sure to replace them if they become cracked, worn, or show other evidence of deterioration.

Masks

Spatter containing blood and saliva is generated during dental procedures from equipment such as the handpiece, air-water syringe, or ultrasonic scaler. A mask must be worn to protect the mucous membranes of the nose and mouth from exposure to the airborne blood and saliva. Several guidelines for the use of masks includes the following:

- Choose a style that can be adjusted to fit your face comfortably and tightly.
- Keep your beard and mustache groomed so that the mask fits well and can be worn effectively.
- Always change the mask between patients and if it gets wet.
- Remove the mask when treatment is over. Do not leave it dangling around your neck; either wear it properly or take it off.
- Never leave the operatory with a mask in place or around your neck.
- When removing a mask, handle it only by the elastic or cloth tie string; never touch the mask.

Protective Eyewear

Protective eyewear must be worn to protect the mucous membranes of the eyes from projectiles and spatter of blood and saliva. The risk of exposing the tissues of the eyes to blood and body fluids is well documented. Viruses such as Hepatitis B and Herpes simplex have been transmitted to dental staff whose eyes were spattered with saliva or blood.

Choice of eyewear depends on the nature of the procedures that are being performed; however, prescription or safety glasses equipped with side shields are considered to be the minimal acceptable protective eyewear. Goggles afford the greatest eye protection. As an alternative to protective glasses or goggles and a mask, a face shield may be worn by the clinician. Because many dental procedures produce flying objects from materials such as amalgam restorations or crowns, protective eyewear for the patient should also be considered.

Clinic Uniforms

Coats and gowns provide additional protection from possible exposure to blood and other body fluids. When selecting a gown, consider those with the greatest coverage for your body. The isolation gown is ideal and recommended because it fits closely around the neck and the long sleeves cover the arms. Gloves should overlap the sleeves of the clinic coat.

Gowns should be changed whenever they have been sprayed with saliva or blood or are visibly soiled.

Like masks and gloves, clinic coats should only be worn in clinics and support areas. They should not be worn in nonclinical settings such as staff lounges, office or record supply rooms, or outside of the building.

Vaccinations

Additional protection of the dental health care worker is provided through immunizations. By OSHA mandate, all persons with patient exposure in either clinical or laboratory settings must be given the opportunity by the employer to receive the vaccine to prevent Hepatitis B. Hepatitis B is a major health hazard for members of virtually all health occupations and is of particular concern to dental health care personnel. Any person may decline to receive the vaccine and remain at risk. Until recently, about 18,000 health care workers became infected with HBV each year, and approximately 1000 of these became chronic carries of the virus.

Clinic scrubs and uniforms should be kept clean and laundered daily. Many dental practices provide uniforms for all office personnel and contract with a commercial laundry to maintain the uniforms or provide a uniform rental service on a weekly basis.

Two types of HBV vaccines available are made from plasma and recombinant DNA technology. Both are considered safe and effective in producing immunity to HBV. Vaccines are available for other infectious diseases and are generally given during childhood. A notable exception is the influenza virus vaccine. The viruses causing the seasonal flu tend to vary significantly and human immunity to these viruses is not long-lived; thus, annual reimmunization against the prevalent viral form is recommended for all health care workers. Because many pathogens exist that presently have no vaccine, including HIV, non-A and non-B Hepatitis and Hepatitis C, no vaccine can replace adherence to universal precautions, which is mandatory for all health care workers.

Dental health care personnel are likely to come into contact with many different infectious agents; therefore, vaccinations for measles, mumps, rubella, tetanus, and poliomyelitis should be considered if you have not already had these diseases or have not been immunized against them. Most people receive these as children but verification is always in order. In addition, yearly influenza vaccinations should be considered.

Recycling the Dental Operatory

Every dental health care worker should ensure that each patient is protected against risk of infection from contamination. To accomplish this, the dental operatory and adjacent support areas must be processed for infection control between each patient. Three major steps regarding infection control in the dental operatory include the following:

1 Aseptic preparation of the operatory
2 Control of contamination generated during treatment
3 Disposal of consumable products and sterilization and disinfection of reusable materials

Between Patient Operatory Preparation

To efficiently prepare an operatory, it should be arranged to facilitate thorough cleaning following each patient. To achieve this, the operatory must be kept as uncluttered as possible to reduced the number of items that could become contaminated. This includes reducing the number of items on tables and counter tops. Seldom-used equipment and materials should be removed from the operatory. For the best infection control results, only supplies essential to the scheduled procedure should be on the counters.

Individual Tray Set-Ups

The clinical staff must organize the materials for treatment in advance. The individualized tray system for each procedure has all instruments and items normally used for categorical clinical procedures. The dental assistant should carefully preplan for any unique procedure to ensure that everything needed for that treatment session is available to the dentist. This will eliminate the need to enter cabinets or drawers wearing contaminated gloves.

The tray system not only includes instruments but also contains sufficient consumable supplies to complete a given procedure. The consumables are dispensed by unit dose, which means that each tray contains enough supplies for that procedure only. Typical consumable items include gauze squares, cotton pellets, cotton rolls, applicator sticks, and rubber dams. Having the tray set up eliminates cross-contamination of the general supply stock because the clinician does not reach into a supply container while working on a patient. This also reduces unnecessary resterilization of consumable supplies.

The unit dose concept is extended to instruments; for example, the dental team may use individual, sterilized bur blocks for each procedure. Using individualized blocks containing only the burs required for a given procedure eliminates the contamination of other, unneeded burs, and additional clean up is not required.

Perhaps the most overlooked part of preplanning infection control in the operatory is the patient chart. The temptation is great to have the chart readily available next to the dentist, to write notes with a gloved hand during a procedure, or to place an x-ray on the view box. When this happens, the chart is contaminated either by spatter or direct contact with contaminated hands. Therefore preplan the chart location away from the patient's head, place the x-rays on the viewer before treatment, and if notes must be made, record them temporarily on paper that can be discarded when the operatory is cleaned.

Control of Operatory Surface Contamination

A quick look at the front of a protective face shield or eyeglasses worn during routine work in the operatory will reveal significant spatter following most dental procedures. The generation of sprays containing potentially infectious microorganisms is virtually impossible to eliminate from the dental operatory; therefore all surfaces in an operatory must be considered contaminated. In addition, continual handling of air and water syringe lines, saliva ejectors, and light handles with gloved hands inadvertently leaves these pieces of equipment contaminated. Because the equipment and fixtures are not removable, sterilization is not an option and disinfection of these surfaces must be accomplished.

Table 18.4

Typical Barrier Products and Their Use

	Plastic Bag	Sheet Plastic	Paper	Aluminum Foil	Deli Gloves
Chair headrest	+*	+			
Chair control buttons	+	+			
Light handles	+	+		+	
Handpiece hoses	+*				
Air and water	+*				
Syringe and lines	+*				
Bracket table	+	+	+*		
Countertops		+	+*		
X-ray head	+	+			
X-ray controls		+			+
Wall light switches					+

*Strong preference for use by most dental offices.

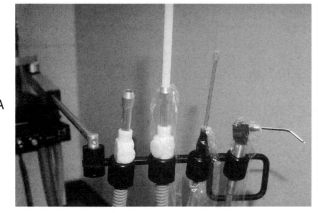
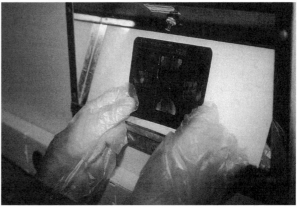

A   B

FIGURE 18.4

A, Air and water lines are covered with plastic sleeves to protect them from splatter. **B,** Disposable deli gloves are quick and effective barriers that keep charts and x-rays from coming in contact with contaminated surfaces.

Two general methods to protect these surfaces exist. The first is to wipe or scrub all surfaces with hospital-level (tuberculocidal) or better disinfectants between each patient. From a practical standpoint, to clean every surface is a time-consuming task, plus most disinfectant solutions recommend a 10-minute waiting period before the disinfected surfaces are dried or used. An alternate approach to disinfection of the operatory surfaces is to shield the surfaces with barriers or protective coverings. Today, most dental offices use a combination of surface disinfection and barrier protection of the surface to reduce the potential of disease. Table 18.4 shows typical barrier products that will greatly reduce the need for surface disinfection following common dental procedures.

Use of Infection Control Barriers

Before applying surface barriers, rub the surface with an intermediate disinfectant. Once the area is dry, place the cover over the entire surface and secure it. For countertops, water-impervious covers such as butcher paper held in place with a few pieces of tape is usually sufficient. Dental chair backs can be covered with plastic bags and, if the bag is long enough, the chair buttons will also be protected.

Air and water lines are continually being exposed to spatter and general chairside contamination. The best way to protect these lines to cover them with a plastic sleeve up to the point where the functional tip is attached (Figure 18.4). This includes handpieces, air and water syringes, and saliva

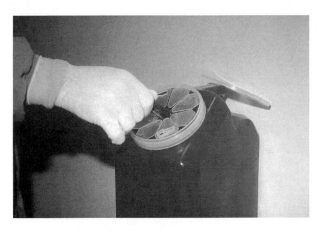

FIGURE 18.5

A typical OSHA-approved sharps container.

ejectors. Some dental supply houses now stock long, thin, plastic sleeves that can be cut to length to cover the hoses. Plastic covers or aluminum foil can be used to protect light handles.

The most difficult area to manage infection control while in the dental operatory is the patient chart. Remember that everything that is touched by a gloved hand after patient contact is contaminated. Thus, when information must be recorded in a chart, do not pick up a pen and write until either a barrier such as disposable deli gloves further protects the gloved (contaminated) hands or the exam gloves are removed and the hands are washed (Figure 18.4, *B*).

Discarding of Contaminated Materials

Recycling a barrier-protected operatory requires removal of all surface protective covers and disinfection of the area where the barrier joined the equipment. New barriers are applied. The used material should be discarded as indicated by individual state regulations. For most localities, this means the public trash system for lightly contaminated barriers. If visible blood or excessive moisture are involved, many communities require disposal as a biohazard waste. Check with local authorities for exact procedures and details.

In most dental offices contaminated waste, soft goods soiled with blood or saliva, should be placed in sturdy, leak-proof bags. Ideally, these bags will be attached to the back of the chair convenient to the clinician, but out of sight of the patient. Sharp instruments such as needles and scalpel blades should be placed intact into OSHA-approved, puncture-resistant containers (Figure 18.5). *Never* remove sharps with anything other than forceps. All bags and containers should be disposed of at the clinical receptacle.

Handle sharp items carefully. Appropriate procedures for handling sharp instruments during operatory recycling include the following:

- Wear sturdy utility gloves when cleaning contaminated instruments or other sharp items.
- Avoid picking up sharp instruments by the handful.
- Keep a log of injuries that should include the date of injury, person injured, cause of injury, patients name (if involved), description of situation, witness, action taken, outcome, and follow-up if necessary.

Infection Control During Patient Treatment

The use or clinical treatment step is obvious and the primary source of contamination. From the perspective of the dental health care worker, caution and good judgment must be continually exercised to avoid personal contamination.

Handling Sharps

The most common incident for the dental professional is the parenteral wound such as cuts on the hands by sharp instruments and needle sticks. The OSHA guidelines cover these areas but two aspects of the guidelines need reinforcement for the dental profession. OSHA prefers that all injection needles be discarded after a single use; however, most dentists retain the anesthesia syringe at the chairside throughout a procedure. If this is done, the needle must be resheathed using either a one-handed scoop technique or mechanical manipulation of the sheath. Both systems remove the hand and fingers from the proximity of the exposed needle.

Another problem is the safe placement of handpieces following use on patients. Often contaminated burs are left in the handpiece chuck and in some operatory settings workers are in danger of being scrapped or punctured by these burs as they move around the operatory. Common sense suggests that burs be removed from handpieces at the completion of a procedure and that brackets for holding handpieces be positioned away from normal movement patterns in the operatory. A major problem during patient treatment is that the level of mental concentration on the procedure by the clinical staff is quite high and the proximity of potentially dangerous sharps is forgotten. Therefore observe the following:

- Keep hands away from rotating instruments.
- Dispose of needles and other sharp items promptly and appropriately.
- Avoid any quick motions that would bring one hand toward the other or the instrument across the plane of any part of your body when handling sharp instruments.
- Point sharps away from yourself.
- Use the proper technique at all times when passing sharp instruments. The point should be held away from everyone, including yourself.

Instrument Cleaning

Once a procedure is completed, the operatory must be prepared for the next patient. Instruments must be gathered and prepared for sterilization. The dental health care worker must wear proper personal protective equipment including utility gloves during this operation. The instruments may be washed directly at this point; although some prefer placing instruments into a holding tank containing an intermediate (hospital-level) or better disinfectant. The benefits of this step include reduction of viable microbes before contact by the office staff and prevention of drying or crusting of debris on instruments at the beginning of the cleaning cycle. Soaking instruments for hours may lead to corrosion of the surfaces.

After the instruments are removed from the operatory, they are considered clean. The hand method of cleaning using a brush to remove all biologic debris and cements from instruments is acceptable, assuming that the cleaning solution has the properties of an intermediate disinfectant and that splashing is kept to a minimum.

Using ultrasonic cleaners is the preferred method of cleaning. These are effective and greatly reduce the potential for cuts and punctures to the operatory staff. A wide variety of ultrasonic cleaners are available. Refer to the specific manufacturer's recommendations regarding the type of cleaning solutions to use and the length of time needed to clean a typical load.

After cleaning, rinse the instruments with generous amounts of tap water. Remember that these cleaned instruments may still harbor infectious microorganisms. Personal protective equipment must therefore be used. The rinsed instruments are dried and are then ready for packaging.

A major concern of most patients is the passage of diseases from previous patients through the use of contaminated instruments. Although not all instruments have to be sterilized, the great majority of them will need to be sterilized. According to the classification of hospital items proposed by Spaulding, the three levels for preparation of instruments for reuse include the following:

1 Critical

Sterilization is required for all items that penetrate skin, mucous membranes, or bone. Instruments include all surgical devices, explorers, scalers, and burs.

2 Semicritical

Sterilization or high-level disinfection is required for all items that may touch saliva or intact mucosal tissues. Typically, items included in this category are handpieces, mirrors, amalgam condensers, x-ray holders, and reusable impression trays. If at all possible, these instruments should be sterilized following use.

3 Noncritical items

Intermediate-level disinfection is required for operatory surfaces such as light handles, counter tops, x-ray heads, and dental chairs. Noncritical items come in contact with only intact skin surfaces.

Cleaning and Lubricating Handpieces

The CDC guidelines state that all handpieces should be treated with a heating process capable of sterilization between each patient use (Figure 18.6). In use, handpieces

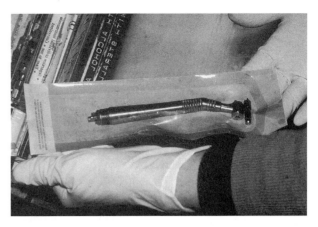

FIGURE 18.6

Handpiece packaged and ready for sterilization in an autoclave or unsaturated chemical vapor sterilizer.

rarely contact open wounds and should be considered semicritical; however, the spray generated readily covers the handpiece and because of its construction and inner workings, the inside of the handpiece is often contaminated. Surface disinfection cannot eliminate this contamination. Therefore sterilization that will penetrate to the internal parts of the handpiece is recommended.

Dental handpieces are precision instruments that will give many years of trouble-free service if they are installed, operated, and maintained according to the manufacturer's directions. The dental assistant should read, understand, and follow the instructions for the handpieces. These instructions are usually well-illustrated and quite easy to follow. In a short period, the dental assistant will become familiar with the maintenance and cleaning procedures for the equipment used in many professional settings.

Instrument Sterilization

Many different ways of packaging instruments for sterilization exist; however, certain principles must be applied to the process. First of all, use only bags, pouches, or wraps that have been designed for the sterilizer you are using. For example, paper bags work well in an autoclave but char and disinfect in dry heat sterilizers. Specially designed sealing plastic tubes work well in autoclaves and dry heat sterilizers but are not recommended for unsaturated chemical vapor units because the vapor cannot readily penetrate through the plastic.

When using metal or plastic cassette systems, the dental assistant should place the cleaned instruments into the cassette and keep it closed. Wrap the entire unit with paper or cloth and secure the edges with tape (Figure 18.7). This will provide excellent protection against contamination once the cassette is removed from the sterilizer and placed on the shelf.

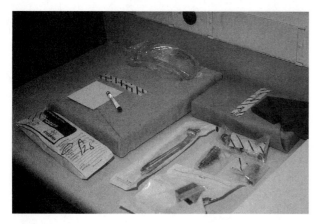

FIGURE 18.7

A wrapped cassette system and other supplies ready for use. The marker tape indicates that the cassette has been through the sterilizer.

Secondly, tightly capped containers should never be used because steam and chemical vapors cannot penetrate into the interior of the container. Similarly, biohazard bags should not be tightly closed when sterilizing the contents.

A third consideration in any sterilization cycle is verification that the sterilizer worked properly. Only using biologic monitors can do this. The CDC and ADA recommend weekly monitoring of sterilizers using biological indicators. This can be done in the office; however, several university-based sterilizer monitoring services are available (Figure 18.8).

Many sterilizer bags and tapes have chemical markers that change colors following sterilization. These should be checked daily to confirm that the packages were subjected to sterilizing conditions. Only the weekly biologic monitor is sufficient to verify that the conditions were maintained sufficiently to achieve sterility. Chemical indicators cannot be used as substitutes for biologic indicators. Because of the open space within cassettes, stacking them flat in the sterilizer is acceptable.

When loading the sterilizer, follow the manufacturer's recommendations. In general, placing individual packages on edge rather than flat is best. But be careful not to overload the unit and make sure the minimum exposure times are achieved. Wrapped cassettes may be placed flat in the sterilizer.

The Cassette System to Manage Instruments

An increasing need occurs in dental offices to develop more effective ways to organize, clean, sterilize, and store dental instruments. Manufacturers have developed cassette systems that provide efficiency and methods of infectious disease control. Cassettes are designed to hold complete procedural set ups (Figure 18.9). A number of accessory-perforated, stainless steel boxes also exist, which can provide easy orga-

nization for smaller items (Figure 18.10). This allows the dental assistant to have organized and sterile set ups ready for immediate use.

A cassette can be opened and set directly on the prepared working area, with the instruments removed directly from the cassette and replaced into the cassette as the procedure is completed. This reduces cross-contamination from handling the instruments and also reduces the processing time. Too much handling of the instruments can cause workers to drop or damage them or stick themselves with the sharp objects.

After debris are removed from the instruments, they are positioned in a cassette or on a tray according to the sequence in which they were used. The cassette is kept together during cleaning and sterilization as the instruments can be washed and sterilized in the cassette. Following proper sterilization techniques, the dental assistants can store the cassettes in a readily accessible area. Using cassettes allows for easier training of new staff (see Chapter 21).

Asepsis of Dental Support Areas
Storage Areas

Determine the amount of storage space available. Although dental offices often have a limited amount of space for storage, all supplies should be stored in an organized manner providing quick and easy retrieval. Supplies should also be organized so new materials are placed toward the back and older materials brought forward. This keeps materials rotating so that older supplies can be used first.

Too many bulky supplies should not be ordered at one time unless plenty of storage space exists. Special attention should be given to supplies such as x-ray film that must be refrigerated or gypsum that should be stored in a dark, cool, or dry area. The storage space should have sufficient light to help in finding smaller items quickly. Supply shelves and bins should be clearly labeled to make it easier to find the items.

Personnel responsible for handling storage of supplies should have knowledge of OSHA, the federal guidelines regarding the use and storage of materials handled in the dental office. Dental offices are required to have material safety data sheets on file that contain the following product information:

1 Name, address, and emergency telephone number of the manufacturer who makes the chemical or material
2 Hazardous ingredient data such as permissible exposure limits
3 Physical and chemical data that includes boiling and melting points, evaporation rate, vapor pressure, and water solubility
4 Fire and explosion hazard data such as flash point, flammable limits, and extinguishing media
5 Reactivity data that includes stability and conditions to avoid, incompatibility, and any hazardous by-products

UNIVERSITY OF LOUISVILLE
SCHOOL OF DENTISTRY
ROBERT STAAT, PhD
PROFESSOR OF MICROBIOLOGY

Call toll-free 1-800-000-0000 for new supply of samples
Local 000-0000

Acct. number: 1828

Clinic: W...
Dentist: Dr. ...
Address:
City: P...   State: OH   ZIP:

Telephone: 614-.........   Clinical contact person: Sherri

Type of sterilizer: Autoclave   Payment: #3734   5/16/95
Number of samples required: 1
Date started: 3/1/92   Renewal date: 2/28/96   #: 1828

For samples received through 05/18/95

Results

Month			Week beginning*		
June 1994	6: S	13: S	20: N	27: S	
July	4: S	11: S	18: S	25: S	
August	1: S	8: S	15: S	22: S	29: S
September	5: S	12: S	19: S	26: S	
October	3: S	10: S	17: S	24: S	31: S
November	7: S	14: S	21: S	28: S	
December	5: S	12:	19: S	26:	
January 1995	2:	9: S	16: S	23:	30: S
February	6: S	13: S	20: S	27:	
March	6: S	13:	20: S	27: S S	
April	3: S	10: S	17:	24: S	
May	1: S	8: S	15: S	22: S	29: S
June 1995	5: S	12: S	19: S	26:	

S or DS = Sterile; N = Nonsterile; Blank = No sample received; B = Broken in mail.
*Date is most often determined by postmark on return envelope.

Samples sent:	7/1/93	Lot #:	J3GKHH
	12/9/93		C4GKSJ
	6/2/94		G4GLGB
	9/21/94		K4GLJI
	3/21/95		J4GLID

FIGURE 18.8

Sterilizer monitoring report.

6 Health hazard data such as eye, skin, and respiratory protection, routes of entry, carcinogenicity, signs and symptoms of exposure, and emergency and first aid procedures

7 Precautions for safe handling and work practices such as handling and storing precautions, waste disposal method, normal clean up, and waste disposal methods

8 Control measures such as respiratory protection, ventilation needs, protective clothing or equipment, and safe work practices

OSHA makes the ultimate decision when disposing hazardous materials. However, local and state laws also govern the disposal of medical waste. Dental workers should understand

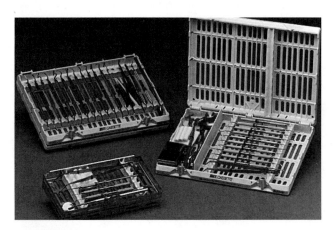

FIGURE 18.9

An instrument management system provides efficiency in instrument standardization and sterilization and time management. (Courtesy Hu Friedy)

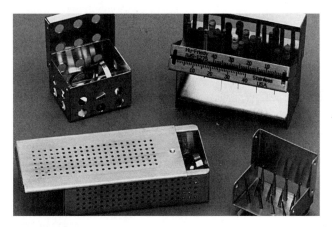

FIGURE 18.10

Accessory boxes are available to provide convenient methods for organizing smaller items. (Courtesy Hu Friedy)

the regulations identified by OSHA regarding medical waste or biohazards. See Figure 18.11 for an example of material safety data sheets.

For More Information, You Can Contact The Following:

Business and Legal Reports
64 Wall Street
Madison, Connecticut 06443-1513
Telephone: (203) 245-7448

Controlled substances must also be handled carefully and locked as soon as they are received. Because first-aid kits often contain drugs, they must also be secured in a safe place out of the patient's sight and reach. Many dentists have all drugs locked in an office safe with a limited number of staff able to unlock it. This protects the patient, dental personnel, and dentist.

Expiration Limits

Identify the expiration limits of dental material, shelf-life, or length of time material is usable, and storage requirements. Some materials must be refrigerated.

Delivery Time

Define the delivery time needed, making sure to allow extra time for items that may often be more difficult to get during a normal delivery time.

Infection control within the dental laboratory equipment requires extra attention. Because most work is done on models, it is easy to forget that the models were made from impressions taken of the patient's mouth. Thus, with no infection control efforts, the patients potentially infectious saliva and blood is readily transferred to the impression and then to the model. In addition to impressions, models, fixed and removable prostheses, and bite registration records should be disinfected to protect the patient and health care team.

Impressions

Ideally, a dental impression should be rinsed with tap water after removal from the mouth and then disinfected. Several different disinfectants can be used (Table 18.5). The rinsed impressions are placed in a closable container with an appropriate disinfecting solution. Zip-lock plastic bags work well in this application. Some manufacturers suggest that a saturating spray of disinfectant is suitable but some professionals suggest the immersion approach to reduce generation of potentially irradiating aerosols and mist.

Polyether-based impressions do not perform well when immersed in most disinfectants. For polyether impressions, the only recommended procedure is to spray them with disinfectant and keep them moist with disinfectant treated towels. Care must be taken to not generate excessive aerosols of disinfectant in the laboratory. Following a 15-minute exposure to the disinfectant, the impressions are rinsed with water and ready to be poured with stone.

Dental Stone Casts

Poured gypsum casts may be sprayed with an iodophor disinfectant after they have been separated from the impression. The cast can also be soaked for 10 minutes in an iodophor solution (not applicable to master casts because of the potential for surface damage). This is required *only* if the impression was not disinfected before pouring the cast.

Wax Registration Records

Disinfect wax registration records by soaking them in an iodophor or dilute (1:100) household bleach for 10 minutes.

Fixed and Removable Prostheses

Before sending fixed and removable prostheses to the dental laboratory for repair, adjustment, or delivery to the

Material safety data sheet
May be used to comply with
OSHA's Hazard Communication Standard,
29 CFR 1910.1200. Standard must be
consulted for specific requirements.

U.S. Department of Labor
Occupational Safety and Health Administration
(Nonmandatory form)
Form approved
OMB No. 1218-0072

Identity *(as used on label and list)*

Note: Blank spaces are not permitted. If any item is not applicable, or no information is available, the space must be marked to indicate that.

Section I

Manufacturer's name

Emergency telephone number

Address *(number, street, city, state, and ZIP code)*

Telephone number for information

Date prepared

Signature of preparer *(optional)*

Section II — Hazardous ingredients and identity information

Hazardous components (specific chemical identity; common names [or names])	OSHA PEL	ACGIH TLV	Other limits recommended	% *(optional)*

Section III — Physical and chemical characteristics

Boiling point	Specific gravity (H_2O = 1)	
Vapor pressure (mm Hg)	Melting point	
Vapor density (AIR = 1)	Evaporation rate (Butyl Acetate = 1)	

Solubility in water

Appearance and odor

Section IV — Fire and explosion hazard data

Flash point (method used)	Flammable limits	LEL	UEL

Extinguishing media

Special firefighting procedures

Unusual fire and explosion hazards

(Reproduce locally)

OSHA 174, Sept. 1985

Continued

FIGURE 18.11

Material safety data sheet.

Section V — Reactivity data

Stability	Unstable		Conditions to avoid	
	Stable			

Incompatibility *(materials to avoid)*

Hazardous decomposition or byproducts

Hazardous polymerization	May occur		Conditions to avoid	
	Will not occur			

Section VI — Health hazard data

Route (or routes) of entry: Inhalation?   Skin?   Ingestion?

Health hazards *(acute and chronic)*

Carcinogenicity: NTP?   IARC monographs?   OSHA regulated?

Signs and symptoms of exposure

Medical conditions
generally aggravated by exposure

Emergency and first aid procedures

Section VII — Precautions for safe handling and use

Steps to be taken in case material is released or spilled

Waste disposal method

Precautions to be taken in handling and storing

Other precautions

Section VIII — Control measures

Respiratory protection *(specify type)*

Ventilation	Local exhaust	Special
	Mechanical *(general)*	Other

Protective gloves	Eye protection

Other protective clothing or equipment

Work and hygienic practices

FIGURE 18.11, cont'd

Material safety data sheet.

Table 18.5

Appropriate Disinfectants for Use on Impression Materials*

Impression material	Disinfectants†			
	Glutaraldehydes	Iodophors	Sodium Hypochlorite	Phenolics
Alginate	No	Yes	Yes	No
Polysulfides	Yes	Yes	Yes	Yes
Polyethers (spray appl.)	No	Yes	Yes	Yes
Silicones	Yes	Yes	Yes	Yes
Hydrocolloids	No	Yes	Yes	Insufficient data

*Adapted from Miller CH, Palenik CJ: *Infection control and management of hazardous materials for the dental team,* St Louis, 1998, Mosby.
†Proposed according to manufacturer's recommendation.

patient, wash the appliance thoroughly in an antimicrobial detergent. Resin dentures and appliances of noble alloys (containing precious metals) should be disinfected in a 1:100 solution of household bleach for 10 minutes. Fixed and removable prostheses of nonnoble alloys should be disinfected using an iodophor or phenol compound.

Laboratory Area

Routine procedures such as adjusting and polishing removable dental appliances require a laboratory area where infection control must be practiced. The major rule in this situation is that the appliance should be disinfected before it gets to the laboratory bench. Virtually no infection control problem exists with rag wheels, and brushes if the prostheses are disinfected before laboratory work. In practice, this is not always feasible.

Actual work on the appliance should be done with unused supplies such as fresh pumice (50 to 60 g per unit dose) for each new case and sterilized material including reusable rag wheels. The work area must have a vacuum exhaust system capable of containing any aerosol generated during the grinding or polishing steps. After completion of the appliance, the pumice will be discarded into a contaminated waste bag and the wheel disinfected will be cleaned and sterilized. The pumice tray and splashguard will be disinfected with an intermediate-level disinfectant.

Asepsis in Radiology

Infection control principles should also be observed when dental assistants take radiographs because the equipment and film can be contaminated, which could result in the transmission of infectious agents. Barriers best protect radiographic equipment as chemical disinfection is difficult. In preparation for exposing periapical radiographs, place a polyethylene bag or plastic wrap over the tube head and hand holds so that they will be protected from contamination when the head is positioned for various exposures. The exposure control switch should be protected with a disposable plastic covering if a foot-activated switch is not available. Remember that a gloved hand is contaminated. However, another simple approach to contamination control of the control panel is the use of deli gloves to cover contaminated examination gloves.

Proper handling of contaminated films is important for effective infection control. After the films are exposed, place them on a paper towel or in a disposable cup. Cover or replace the contaminated gloves when you get to the film processing area to not contaminate surfaces within the darkroom. Most plastic-covered films and film pouches in use today can be disinfected without harming the film. Refer to the manufacturer's instructions for disinfection of films.

In the darkroom, the technician who is wearing fresh gloves or still wearing the deli gloves should peel open each film and spill it out of its wrapping onto a flat surface. After doing this with all exposed film, remove and dispose of wrapping then remove and dispose of contaminated gloves and place the film into the processor slot or film holder for developing. Once the films are loaded into the processor, infection-control problems are at a minimum because neither developer nor fixer promote microbial survival or growth. Discard all contaminated materials including gloves, cups, and film covers. Films, holders, and other items placed in the mouth must be disinfected or preferably sterilized after each use.

When an automatic film processor with daylight loader is used, contamination of the fabric light shield is likely to be a problem. See Boxes 18.4 for suggestions to prevent contamination and Table 18.6 for evaluation for handling contamination.

The bite holder required on some panoramic x-ray units should be autoclaved if possible.

If heat sterilization is not possible, clean it thoroughly with soap and water and use an EPA-registered disinfectant and sterilant chemical according to the manufacturer's directions (Box 18.5). Rinse thoroughly after disinfection. When replacing bite holder, order autoclavable units.

Removal of Personal Protective Equipment

After the instruments have been scrubbed and packaged for sterilization and other clean-up tasks have been completed, personal protective equipment may be removed. The proper method of removing a mask is to grasp it only by the cloth or elastic strings, not by the mask itself. Protective eyewear and face shields should be cleaned with soap and water and then disinfected or prepared for sterilization. Do not touch the eyewear with ungloved hands because it is likely to be contaminated with spatter of blood and saliva.

After removing your gown, immediately place it in the soiled linen container. Gowns must be washed according to the OSHA guidelines (that is, in the office using a normal laundry cycle or by a professional laundry equipped to handle the items). Employees are not allowed to take clinic gowns home to be washed with the household laundry. Utility gloves should be washed with soap before removal. Lastly, thoroughly wash your hands (Box 18.6 and Table 18.7).

Box 18.4 *Procedure*

Procedure for Handling Contaminated Film

1. Place the exposed film in a paper cup previously set aside for this purpose.
2. Remove soiled gloves and put on a pair of clean gloves.
3. Place the cup inside the daylight loader and close the lid.
4. Place the gloved hands through the light shield, unwrap the film packet, and drop the film onto the surface inside the loader.
5. Place the film wrapping into the cup. Remove the gloves, turn them inside out, and place them in a paper cup.
6. Drop the film in the chute for developing.
7. Remove hands from the loader, lift the lid, and dispose of paper cup and waste.
8. Wash hands thoroughly.

Table 18.6

Evaluation for Handling Contaminated Film

Handling Contaminated Film	4	3	2	0	X
Secure material and equipment.					
Place exposed film in paper cup.					
Remove soiled gloves and put on clean gloves.					
Place cup inside daylight loader.					
Unwrap film packet.					
Place film wrapping into cup.					
Remove gloves and place in cup.					
Place film in developing chute.					
Dispose of paper cup.					
Wash hands.					

The numeric criteria: 4 Excellent; 3 Good but some improvement can be made; 2 Below average, usable, needs to improve skill; 0 Unsatisfactory; X Not able to evaluate.

Box 18.5

EPA Regulations

1. Separate regulated medical waste into separate containers.
   - Sharps (used and unused needles, scalpel blades, burs, etc.); fluids in quantities over 20 cc; other regulated medical waste
2. Determine the quantity to be disposed (weigh).
3. Package waste containers so they are the following:
   - Rigid; leak-resistant; impervious to moisture; puncture-resistant (for sharps); sealed for shipping
4. Label outer containers with a water-resistant label indicating, "medical waste," "infectious waste," or the universal biohazard symbol (insert drawing).
5. Store containers in a protected areas to maintain their integrity and prevent odor. Refrigerate as necessary.
6. Mark inner containers with a water-resistant tag or write the following with indelible ink:
   - Your name; address or permit number
7. When shipping the outermost container in indelible ink, mark it as follows:
   - Your name; your state permit or ID number or your address if you have no ID number; transporter's name and permit or ID number or address; if shipping instruction is given by the service you use, follow their instructions
8. Several disposal methods are available; choices may vary according to your state and local area.
   - If allowed in your area, you may transport via your own vehicle to a health care facility or a destination with

which you have a written agreement to accept your regulated medical waste; use a transporter with EPA notification (in the seven affected EPA jurisdictions); use a service that will receive your waste via registered mail with return receipt or UPS, if allowed; use a pick-up service approved by your state

9. Recordkeeping
   - Maintain a log for 3 years (in the seven affected EPA jurisdictions)

   If you use a transporter, log the following information:
   - Transporter's name and address; transporter's state permit or identification name, if required by the state; quantity of medical waste transported (by treated and untreated category); date of shipment; signature of the transporter's representative

   If you transport waste by your own vehicle to a disposal facility, log the following information:
   - Name and address of the disposal facility; quantity of medical waste transported (by treated and untreated category); date of shipment

   If you use registered mail log the following:
   - Request return receipt and keep the originator's receipt and the returned receipt for 3 years; quantity of medical waste shipped (by treated and untreated category); name and address of the facility to which the waste is shipped

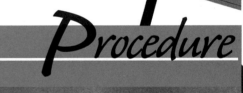

Box 18.6

Procedure

Procedure for Infection Control

Before seating patient, wash hands and use new mask and gloves; check cleanliness of eye protection and clinic gown.

Ready patient protection materials including bib and glasses.

Verify patient schedule outside the operatory.

Remove all unnecessary items from operatory.

At the beginning of a regular clinic session, disinfect counters, light handles, headrest, control buttons, and all other working areas.

Place barrier covers on air and water syringe lines, handpiece lines, light handles, headrest, chair backs and control buttons, counter tops, and other appropriate equipment.

Flush water lines.

Do not touch unprotected surfaces such as records, drawer handles, and x-ray controls with contaminated gloves; use disposable deli gloves as quick protection.

Always check that the chemical indicators have changed on packages containing sterilized instruments; monitor sterilization cycles weekly using biologic indicators.

Use disposable materials when possible.

Use either mechanical barriers or the one-handed

scoop technique when recapping syringe needles.

Use rubber dams whenever possible.

Place all contaminated instruments into cassette at conclusion of procedures.

Dispose of contaminated soft goods in leak-proof containers or bags.

Dispose of used sharps in OSHA-approved containers.

After seeing each patient, recycle the operatory by replacing barrier covers and disinfecting exposed surfaces.

Clean instruments wearing heavy (nitrile) utility gloves.

Verify that all instruments are in proper working order and that no instruments or burs are missing from tray set ups.

Disinfect all impressions and appliances before transferring to the laboratory.

Use sterilized acrylic burs, rag wheels, and fresh pumice when making adjustments to removable appliances.

At the conclusion of a clinic session, never wear gown, masks, or gloves outside clinical area.

Table 18.1

Evaluation for Infection Control

Infection Control	4	3	2	0	X
Wear gloves.					
Remove unnecessary items from operatory.					
Disinfect operatory.					
• Counters					
• Light handles					
• Headrest					
• Control buttons					
Place barrier covers.					
• Air and water syringe lines					
• Handpiece lines					
• Light handles					
• Headrest					
• Chair backs					
• Control buttons					
• Counter tops					
Flush water lines.					
Do not touch unprotected surfaces.					
Check chemical indicators on packages.					
Monitor sterilization cycles.					
Verify patient schedule.					
Wash hands.					
Protective eye wear, gloves, and mask.					
Seat, drape, and provide glasses for patient.					
Place rubber dam.					
Use one-handed scoop technique.					
Secure contaminated instruments.					
Dispose of contaminated materials.					
Dispose of sharps.					
Recycle operatory.					
Clean instruments.					
Verify instruments presence.					
Disinfect impressions and appliances.					
Remove protective clothing.					

The numeric criteria: 4 Excellent; 3 Good but some improvement can be made; 2 Below average, usable, needs to improve skill; 0 Unsatisfactory; X Not able to evaluate.

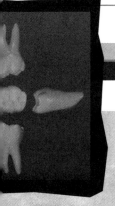

Points for Review

■ The methods of operation for different dental sterilizers must be understood

■ The different types of disinfectants and appropriate uses for each

■ Means other than sterilization and disinfection must be used to avoid occupational hazards

■ The correct method to recycle an operatory between patients

■ Microbial contamination control exercised in the operatory and other dental support areas

Self-Study Questions

1. Which term does the statement, "the absence of all living organisms define?"
   a. Antiseptic
   b. Disinfectant
   c. Sterilization

2. In which sterilizer is saturated steam used?
   a. Autoclave
   b. Chemiclave
   c. Dry heat oven

3. What is the purpose of intermediate-level disinfectants?
   a. Kill pathogens, including the tubercle bacillus but not spores
   b. Kill pathogens, including the tubercle bacillus and spores.
   c. Kill bacterial and viral pathogens but not the tubercle bacillus.

4. Which disinfectant is best suited for immersion of contaminated instruments?
   a. Chlorine-based compounds
   b. Iodophores
   c. Glutaraldehydes

5. Light handles and chair switches are best kept free of infectious microbes using which technique?
   a. Disinfectants
   b. Barrier techniques
   c. Dry heat sterilization

6. According to the CDC, what must be done to current handpieces?
   a. Disinfected with alcohol
   b. Exposed to sterilizing conditions
   c. Disinfected with a high level disinfectant

7. How often should a dental sterilizer be tested using biologic monitors?
   a. Daily
   b. Weekly
   c. Monthly

8. For ideal infection control how often should a laboratory rag wheel be sterilized?
   a. Never, disinfection is sufficient
   b. Daily
   c. Between each patient

9. What must the assistant wear when cleaning used instruments?
   a. Clinic or latex gloves
   b. Nitrile based utility gloves
   c. Gloves are not needed to handle disinfected instruments

10. Which instrument is considered critical and must be sterilized?
    a. Dental explorers
    b. Amalgam condensers
    c. X-ray heads or cones

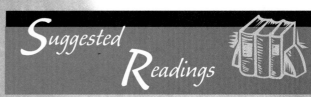

Suggested Readings

Cottone JA, Terezhalmy GT, Molinari IA: *Practical infection control in dentistry*, Philadelphia, 1991, Lea and Febiger.

Miller CH, Palenik CJ: *Infection control and management of hazardous materials for the dental team*, ed 2, St Louis, 1998, Mosby.

Tortora GJ, Funke BR, Case CL: *Microbiology: an introduction*, Redwood, Calif, 1995, Benjamin/Cummings.

Centers for Disease Control and Prevention: Recommended infection-control practices for dentistry, Morbidity, Mortality Weekly Reports RR-8 (42):1-12, 1993.

Chapter 19

Dental Instruments and Equipment

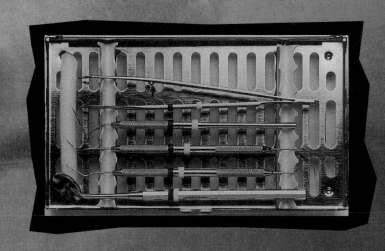

Learning Objectives

On completion of Chapter 19, the student should be able to do the following:

■ Define key terms.

■ Identify described instruments and explain their use.

■ Explain GV Black's instrument formula.

■ Identify handpieces and the attachments.

■ Demonstrate instrument sharpening.

■ Identify, label, and define the functions of rotary cutting instruments.

■ Be able to clean and lubricate dental handpieces and attachments correctly.

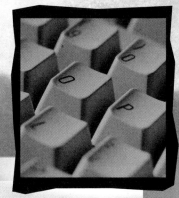

Key Terms

Bevel	Cylindrical	Retract
Cassettes	Hone	Rotary Instruments
Conical	Laser	Tactile

DENTAL INSTRUMENTS

Dental instruments include a variety of large and small hand instruments that are used for specific purposes or multiple procedures. The term *armamentarium* describes all of the materials, equipment, and supplies that dental personnel need to complete a specific procedure. Some instruments are used in the patient's mouth and others are used in dental procedures performed outside the mouth. Dental instruments come in an assortment of numbered sizes and are grouped in categories such as explorers, probes, and scalers. They can also be grouped according to their use such as basic, operative, periodontic, or surgical.

Dental instruments are also defined as *hand-cutting* or *rotary-cutting*. A hand-cutting instrument can cut hard or soft tissue by the pressure applied with the hand, whereas the rotary-cutting instrument is an electrical handpiece and drill (bur, stone, point, diamond, wheel, or disc). Today, **laser** handpieces are used in dentistry for intra-oral procedures.

Many dental instruments look alike, therefore it may take time to learn the identity and use of each type. This is important to assist the dentist during a busy procedure. Instrument coding and procedural trays or **cassettes** help to organize and sterilize instruments.

Laser
The handpiece that converts electromagnetic radiation to frequencies of highly amplified and coherent visible radiation to cut hard and soft tissues

Cassettes
Specially designed set-up tray used for organizing instruments and accessories for dental procedures and sterilization

HAND INSTRUMENTS

Instrument Identification

Dental hand instruments are identified and described by their name, basic design, number, and function. For example, *amalgam condenser* or *plugger* describes the name and function of this instrument. An amalgam condenser is used to condense or compact amalgam alloy into a cavity preparation. Amalgam condensers, like other hand instruments, have a common basic design. The selection of an amalgam condenser for use in a procedure is determined by the size of the preparation and the shape of the functional end of the instrument. Smaller instrument tips may be used for smaller areas, whereas larger sizes may be used for larger preparations.

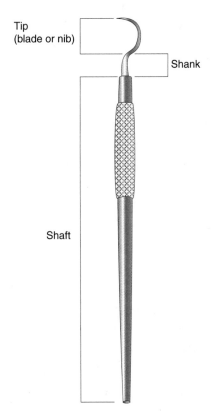

FIGURE 19.1
Dental hand instruments have three parts: tip, shank, and shaft.

Dr. GV Black's textbook, *Operative dentistry* (1908), established the first classifications and categories for dental instruments by describing the instruments by their design and using mathematical formulas

Design

Dental hand instruments may be single- or double-ended and may vary in shape and appearance. However, the length of these instruments is fairly uniform among manufacturers. They are made of carbon steel or surgical stainless steel and some are plastic. Although instrument tip designs have changed with the introduction of new dental materials, the basic hand instrument style remains the same.

Shaft

The shaft is the handle portion of the instrument that the operator holds (Figure 19.1). Manufacturers of dental instruments offer a variety of handle selections that include solid, or lighter, hollow handles. The shape may be octagon, round, or have a **tactile** balance variance. They may be serrated, smooth, stippled, or a combination of textures. The diameter may

Tactile
The sense of touch

vary in size from standard to large, and the tips and handles are swedged or permanently combined and are usually available only in the standard complete handle and tip combination. They are not sold separately but special combinations of handles and tips can be ordered from the manufacturer. Expanded function dental assistants or hygienists are often able to order their own instruments and should try several styles to get a sense for grasp and tactile sensitivity preference. The larger, hollow handle provides a lighter instrument that may allow for a firmer grasp without finger cramping and tension.

Shank

The shank is the portion of the instrument located between the handle and the tip. It may be straight or angled to provide the operator with increased accessibility for the instrument tip to reach interproximal tooth surfaces. The shank may be straight-, single- (monangle), double- (binangled), or triple-angled. The direction of thrust and amount of pressure applied determines the angle and flexibility of the shank. The angulation of the shank also allows the patient to be more relaxed by not having to open the mouth as wide.

Shanks may be more flexible or rigid to allow the operator to put more pressure on the instrument without breaking it. This is determined by how the instrument is used. The finger rest also helps the operator provide appropriate forces when packing or scaling (see Chapter 20).

Tip

The tip of the instrument is also called the *blade* or *nib* and is referred to as the working, functional, placement, or condensing ends and cutting edge of the hand instrument. The tip can be used to cut hard and soft tissue; condense restorative materials; remove calculus; place cements and restorative materials; or detect imperfections of the tooth. Tips are angulated to conform to cavity preparation configurations, interproximal tooth shapes, and reach subgingival areas.

Bevel

The angle or slope of the sharp or working ends of a dental cutting instrument

Thin, flexible, and sharp knife-like blade tips allow the operator to reach tight interproximal areas to contour restorative materials.

The term **bevel** refers to the angle of the cutting edge of the blade. The tips of instruments, such as the explorer, need to be thin for the operator to have greater tactile sensitivity in detecting imperfections but they must be firm enough to prevent breakage of the tip.

Dental assistants and hygienists need to know how to sharpen the working ends of dental hand-cutting instruments correctly to damage the sharp surface. Sharpening stones are available for this purpose (see p. 471). Various manufacturers of instruments offer variations in instrument tips. Probes, for example, are available with color-coded tips to more easily identify the measurement increments.

Formula Description

GV Black developed a numbering system that describes the handle, shank, and tip. These numbers are especially important for identifying and ordering instruments. If three numbers appear on the handle, those numbers provide the following information:

1 The first number on the left refers to the width of the blade in tenths of a millimeter.
2 The second number refers to the length of the blade in millimeters.
3 The third number refers to the angle of the blade in relationship to the long axis of the handle in centigrade (circle with l00-degree measurements).

If a fourth number appears on the instrument, the cutting edge of the tip is at an angle. The first number remains the same, referring to the width of the blade. However, the second number refers to the angle of the cutting edge, the third number refers to the length of the blade, and the fourth number refers to the angle of the blade in relationship to the long axis of the handle.

Instruments are identified by right (R) and left (L), depending on which side of the cavity they are to be used. These instruments look alike except that the working ends are reversed.

Instrument Description

Some dental instruments have specific uses and others have several uses and can be used in different procedures. Also, plastic rather than metal dental instruments are essential for use with certain dental materials. The following instrument descriptions are identified by procedural cassette set up. Specialty instruments will be listed and described in later chapters.

Examination Instruments

The dentist may use several different tray set ups for examination procedures. The exam set up is often referred to as the *basic set up* and includes the mirror, explorer, and dressing pliers. An exam cassette will often also contain a probe and suction tip. Color-coded rings added to the instrument's shaft can help to identify the procedural code and also the instrument's position in the cassette (Figure 19.2). These instruments are found on most tray set ups but are also part of the exam set up, which is generally arranged for emergency appointments and basic examinations. The examination or preventive set up may include either the small or large prophy, pedodontic prophy and sealant, or root planing set up, depending on patient dental needs and procedure used.

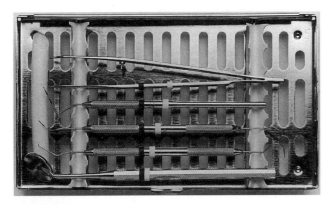

FIGURE 19.2

Exam set up: mirror, explorer, probe, dressing pliers, and suction tip. (Courtesy Hu-Friedy.)

Mouth Mirror

The mouth mirror is used to magnify and reflect the operating area, illuminate the mouth, **retract** the tongue and soft tissue, and to protect tissue from injury during tooth preparation. These mirrors are distortion-free and may be plain or magnifying. They range in a variety of sizes averaging from $^3/_4$ to 2 inches. Some mouth mirrors are double-sided or hinged for angle adjustment. The cone socket mirrors are detachable from the handle so that they can be replaced if broken or marred. Hand mirrors for patients and mirrors for aiding in taking intraoral photographs are also available.

Retract

To draw or pull back as in holding back the cheek, lip, tongue, or intraoral tissues as part of a dental procedure

Explorer

Explorers are used to examine the tooth surface and detect imperfections in the pit and fissures and interproximal areas around restorations. They also are used to detect calculus and explore pockets around the neck of the tooth. Explorers are single- or double-ended; straight or curved; and they have sharp, flexible tips (Figure 19.3). These tips must be thin and flexible for the operator to feel any defect and get into interproximal areas but firm enough to withstand pressure without bending or breaking.

Probe

A probe looks similar to the explorer. The tip is marked in millimeters to measure the depth of the periodontal pockets (Figure 19.4). They are single- or double-ended, and the working ends are straight, curved, or at right angles. They may be combined with explorers and are available with color-coded surfaces.

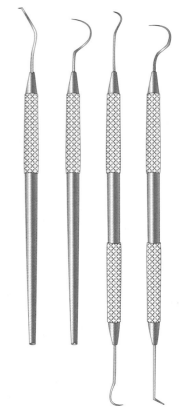

FIGURE 19.3

Explorers are single- or double-ended; straight or curved, with sharp flexible tips.

Dressing Pliers

Dressing pliers are also called *cotton pliers* or *forceps*. They are used to pick up, hold, or carry materials to and from the mouth (Figure 19.5). Therefore these pliers have the ability to lock. Tips may be straight or angled and are available with plain or serrated tips for better grip.

Saliva Ejector

Saliva ejectors are used to reduce the amount of water and fluid in the mouth during a dental procedure. They are available in plastic or metal and are tubular in form (Figure 19.6). The plastic saliva ejector is disposable and can be shaped to fit in the mouth where needed. Some ejectors are not flexible and others have tongue retractors attached.

Suction Tip

The suction tip is used to remove fluid and debris from the mouth during a dental procedure. Suction tips may be plastic (disposable) or metal (reusable) and are available in various sizes, lengths, and shapes. They are tubular in shape and may be straight, curved, or angled. Plastic and metal suction tips can be autoclaved.

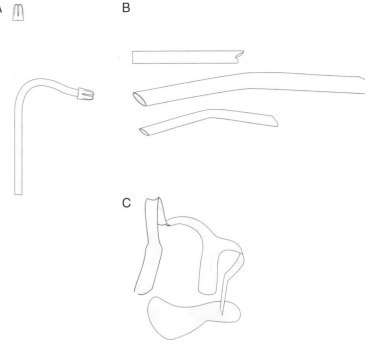

FIGURE 19.6

Moisture control. **A**, Saliva ejector. **B**, Suction tips. **C**, Cotton roll holder.

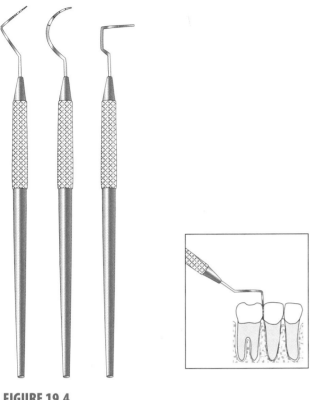

FIGURE 19.4

Probes are marked in millimeters to measure the depth of periodontal pockets.

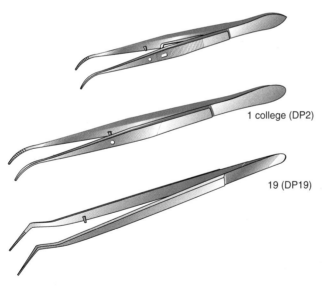

1 college (DP2)

19 (DP19)

FIGURE 19.5

Dressing pliers are used to pick up, hold, or carry materials to and from the mouth.

Cotton Roll Holders

Cotton roll holders are metal devices that hold cotton rolls in place on the buccal and lingual surfaces of the mandibular teeth. They aid in isolation from moisture and help reflect or hold back the cheek and tongue while providing treatment.

Aspirating Syringe Tip

Aspirating syringes are small, **cylindrical**, and slightly curved metal tips that are used on the high-power aspirating unit to remove blood and debris from the cervix of the tooth during root planing or from the tooth socket and tissue areas during a surgical procedure (Figure 19.7, *A*). These tips can be autoclaved before use.

Cylindrical
A cylinder or tube shape

Air and Water (A/W) Syringe Tip

Air and water syringe tips are small, cylindrical, and slightly curved metal tips used on the air and water syringes (Figure 19.7, *B*). These tips can be autoclaved before use.

Hand-cutting Instruments

The cutting edges of the hand-cutting instruments remove decay and form the various angles by cutting and shaping the internal cavity angles. These instruments come in pairs and may be single- or double-ended. They are marked right- or left-handed by indented rings. They may also be identified with commonly used tools such as the hatchet, chisel, or hoe.

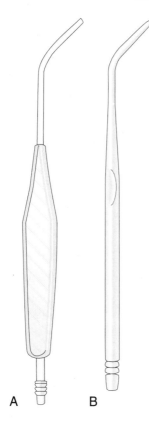

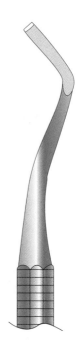

FIGURE 19.8

The hatchet's cutting edge is parallel to the angle of the handle.

FIGURE 19.7

Syringe tips. **A,** Aspirating syringe tip. **B,** Air and water syringe tip.

Hatchet

The hatchet is used to remove hard caries, prepare retentive areas, and sharpen internal line angles. The cutting edge is parallel to the angle of the handle (Figure 19.8). If the bevel is on the right side of the blade when the dental assistant is holding the instrument in the working position, it is the left cutting edge. If the bevel is on the left side of the blade in this position, it is the right cutting edge. These instruments come in large and small pairs.

Chisel

The chisel is used for planing and breaking away the enamel and carious material of the tooth. The cutting edge forms a right angle to the long axis of the handle (Figure 19.9). This angle is called a bevel. If the bevel is toward the handle it is called a standard bevel and if it is away from the handle it is called a reverse bevel. An indented ring around the shaft designates the reverse bevel end. Chisels are available in several shapes and sizes and are commonly called a straight, Wedelstaedt, or binangle chisel. The straight and Wedelstaedt chisels are used primarily in the maxillary arch. The binangle chisel has two shank angles which provides the ability to reach into the cavity floor and push.

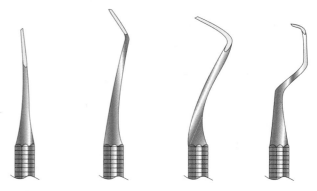

FIGURE 19.9

The chisel's cutting edge forms a right angle to the long axis of the handle.

Hoe

The hoe is used for removal of hard caries and forming the line angles on anterior teeth. The cutting edge forms a right angle to the long axis of the handle and is used with a pulling force (Figure 19.10).

Angle Former

Angle formers are used for defining line angles, defining retentive form in the dentin, and placing bevels on enamel margins of anterior teeth. The blade is beveled on three sides (Figure 19.11).

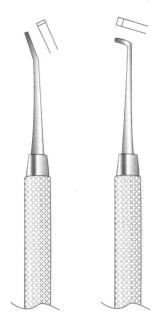

FIGURE 19.10
The hoe's cutting edge forms a right angle to the long axis of the handle.

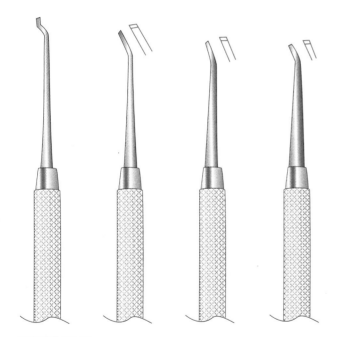

FIGURE 19.11
The blade of the angle former is beveled on three sides.

Gingival Margin Trimmers

The margin trimmer is considered a modified hatchet and is used primarily to develop a bevel on the gingival enamel margins and remove enamel from the floor of the cavity. The

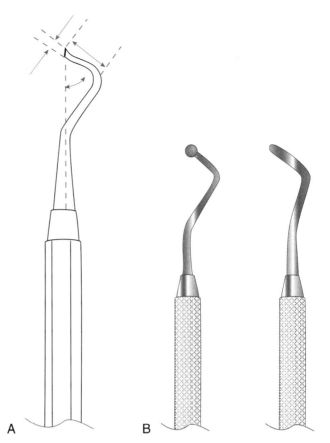

A   B

FIGURE 19.12
A, The blade of the margin trimmer is curved and the cutting edge is at an angle to the long axis of the handle. **B,** Excavators are spoon-shaped with the edge of the spoon tapered to a sharp cutting edge.

blade is curved and the cutting edge is at an angle to the blade (Figure 19.12, *A*).

Excavators

Excavators are used to remove soft caries and are often used in carving amalgam and direct wax patterns. They are spoon-shaped with the edge of the spoon tapered to a sharp cutting edge. It has a binangle shank with the spoons' cutting edge parallel to the angle of the handle (Figure 19.12, *B*).

Discoid-Cleoid

The discoid shape is similar to the shape of the spoon excavator and is also used to remove the soft caries material. They are also used to carve, shape, and finish an amalgam alloy restoration. The cleoid shape looks similar to the discoid shape, except it has a nib or claw to form a groove or corner. The discoid and cleoid spoon shapes are sharpened for carving. These instruments are usually double-ended to form a discoid-cleoid excavator and are available from small to large sizes.

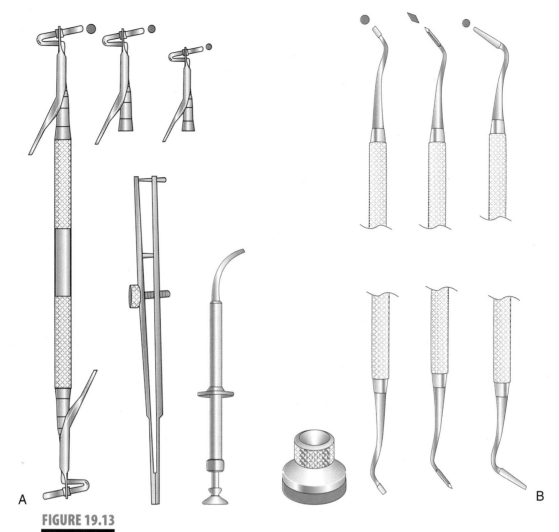

A

B

FIGURE 19.13

A, Amalgam carriers and amalgam well. **B,** Amalgam condenser tip is available in many shapes and sizes.

Amalgam Operative Instruments

Amalgam Carrier

The amalgam carrier is a hollow-tip instrument that has a lever-action handle for picking up, carrying, and placing amalgam alloy into the cavity preparation (Figure 19.13, *A*). The instrument is single- and double-ended and may be angled. The hollow carrier tip comes in various sizes from mini to jumbo.

Amalgam Condenser

The amalgam condenser is also called a *plugger* and is used to pack and condense amalgam material into a cavity preparation. Pluggers are available in a number of sizes and shapes and may have flat, smooth, or serrated tips. The double-ended type usually has different sized tips to place small increments of material and build to larger amounts of material. Some dentists prefer to use an automatic condenser,

which works with a condensing contraangle and latched points of varying sizes and shapes. It condenses by vibration when the dental assistant applies pressure to the alloy filling material (Figure 19.13, *B*).

Carver

The carver is used to carve and form the preset amalgam alloy into the anatomic shape of the tooth. They come in various shapes, and selection is determined by the operator's preference (Figure 19.14).

Burnisher

Burnishers are designed to condense, smooth, and polish amalgam at the preset stage. They come in a number of shapes and are selected according to the operator's preference (Figure 19.15, *A*).

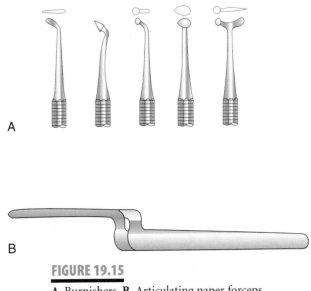

FIGURE 19.15

A, Burnishers. **B**, Articulating paper forceps.

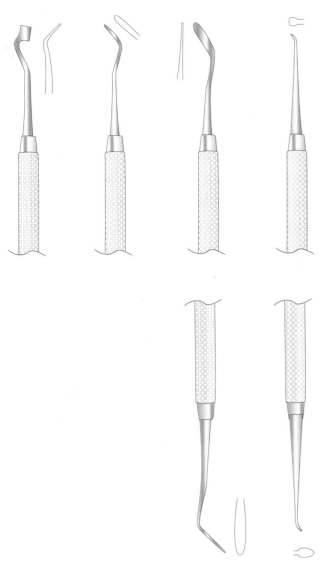

FIGURE 19.14

Carvers are selected by operator preference.

Articulating Paper Forcep

Articulating paper forceps are metal or plastic forceps used to hold the articulating paper in place to check the occlusion of the teeth following placement of an amalgam restoration (Figure 19.15, *B*).

Amalgam Well

The amalgam well is a small stainless steel-weighted container that is designed to handle amalgam easier (see Figure 19.13, *A*). The amalgam alloy is placed in the well after it has been mixed and ready to place in the cavity preparation. This helps hold the mass in place for securing it into the amalgam carrier.

Bur Stand

The bur stand is a small metal box that is used to hold and secure the burs during the procedure and sterilization.

Matrix Retainer

The matrix retainer is a stainless steel device used to hold the matrix band in place while the dental assistant condenses the amalgam alloy into the cavity preparation. It has two threading devices used to hold the matrix band in place and to tighten the matrix band around the tooth. Three common types of retainers include the following:

1 The Toffelmier retainer, available in straight and contraangle (Figure 19.16, *A*)
2 The ivory retainer (Figure 19.16, *B*)
3 The automatic retainer

Matrix

Matrices are used to form a wall where the proximal surface of the tooth is missing, allowing for the amalgam alloy to be condensed in place. They are various thicknesses of stainless or carbon steel strips, designed to fit a designated matrix retainer (Figure 19.16, *C*).

Separate separators are used to spread adjacent teeth apart slightly to place a restoration in a proximal preparation when space is needed to place the filling (Figure 19.16, *D*).

Composite Operative Instruments

The composite or plastic instruments are used for applying all types of composites, to trim away excess composite material, or for cosmetic contouring (Figure 19.17, *A*). They are available in various sizes and shapes.

A gold knife or scalpel is often used to smooth the proximal surfaces of a composite restoration. Much practice and

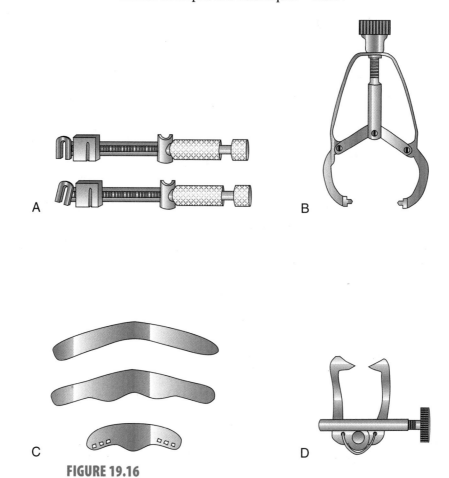

FIGURE 19.16

A, Toffelmier retainers. **B**, Ivory retainer. **C**, Matrices. **D**, Separator.

caution must be used if these instruments are used for finishing composites.

Composite Brush Handle

The composite brush handle is the same handle that is used with the sealant brush. It is made from stainless steel and is designed to hold the composite brush insert (Figure 19.17, *B*).

Cord Packer

The cord packer or *gingival* cord packers are used for inserting the hemostatic cord into the gingival sulcus around the neck of the tooth (Figure 19.17, *C*). They may have a spoon- or disc-shape and may be smooth or serrated.

Composite Placement Instrument

Usually a plastic placement instrument is used to place composite restorations. One end of the instrument may be shaped like a beaver tail, the other one like a condenser tip without serration, or both ends may be the same or some variation of these shapes.

Composite Mixing Instrument

These composite mixing instruments are usually made of plastic in varying shapes. Often the manufacturer provides composite mixing sticks.

Composite Matrix

Plastic strips are used as matrices for composite restorations. They may be precut in various lengths or on a roll to cut to desired length.

Composite Matrix Clip

The matrices may be hand-held, or a metal or plastic clip can be used to hold the matrix in place.

Miscellaneous Mixing Instruments

Cement Spatula and Mixing Pads

Cement mixing instruments, also called *cement spatulas*, are used to mix dental cements (Figure 19.18, *A*). Cement spatulas are made of plastic or stainless steel and are usually flat-, single-, or double-ended instruments. The double-

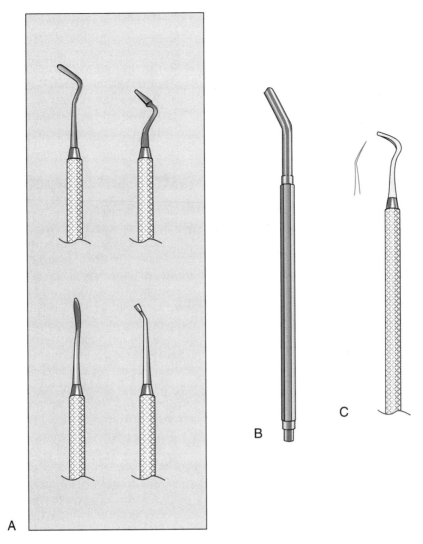

FIGURE 19.17

A, Composite and plastic instruments. **B**, Composite brush holder. **C**, Cord packer.

ended instrument may be combined with a spatula on one end and a loading instrument on the other end to scoop up and place mixed cement into a crown or inlay preparation or smooth and shape temporary restorations. These instruments are also available with extra-large handles to fit more comfortably in the palm of the hand and are available in several lengths. The blade has a rounded working end that may be flexible or rigid according to use. The cement spatulas are used with glass slabs or paper pads of varying sizes and shapes. Some manufacturers provide small double-ended spatulas with their dental materials (Figure 19.18, *B*).

Cement Placement Instrument

Cement placement instruments are single- and double-ended and used to place dental cement (Figure 19.18, *C*).

Some placement instruments have small, round ball tips that are used to place calcium hydroxide or other cement liners and can be used as small burnishers. Other placement instruments may have a flat-ended plugger to place and contour the cement base in undercut areas and flat surfaces of the pulpal floor, and the other end may have a hoe-shaped removal instrument for carving a smooth pulpal-axial floor. These instruments may also have a flat-end ball on one end combined with a flat-end plugger on the other.

Cement Removal Instrument

Cement removal instruments have as harp cutting blade to remove dried cement. Scalers are often used for this purpose (Figure 19.18, *D*).

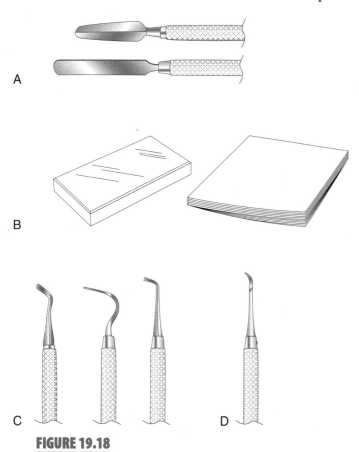

FIGURE 19.18

Cement instruments. **A**, Cement spatulas. **B**, Mixing surfaces. **C**, Cement placement. **D**, Cement removal.

Plaster/Impression Spatulas

In addition to the cement spatulas, a variety of spatulas are designed to mix plaster and impression materials. These spatulas may be made of plastic, stainless steel, or a cobalt-chromium alloy. These instruments vary in size and are usually single-ended and available with a flexible, firm, or extra rigid blade. The blade varies in flexibility, size, and shape according to the material that will be used.

Knives, Gauges, and Calipers

The laboratory knife has a sharp and rigid blade with a wooden handle. It is used for cutting and trimming various dental materials in both. The boley gauge is also used in clinical and laboratory procedures for such applications as endodontic, prosthetic, and operatory techniques. It is calibrated in millimeters and $1/10$ millimeter scales. The Iwanson spring caliper is used to measure thickness of crowns before and after casting. It is also calibrated in $1/10$ millimeter scales. The caliper with sharp points is used to measure porcelain and metal, and the caliper with rounded points is used for measuring wax and plastic.

Waxing Instruments

Various waxing instruments are available that may be used in the dental office laboratory and operatory. Wax spatulas, carvers, and brushes are used to place, carve, and smooth wax during such procedures as preparing base plate and wax rims. Waxing instruments such as the PKT (Peter K. Thomas) instruments are used to flow molten wax, remove excessive wax, contour, carve, and perfect tooth form for fabrication of a crown or bridge.

Instrument Sharpening

Professional dental assistants are a valuable member of the dental team and perform many procedures to better serve the needs of the patient, increase office productivity, and decrease stress to the operator. The dental assistant sharpening the hand-cutting instruments is one way to help the practice. Some instruments, however, must be sent back to the manufacturer for sharpening. Sharp hand-cutting instruments are necessary to remove dental caries, properly form the angles of the cavity preparation, finish the alloy and composite restoration, scale during prophylaxis, and cut hard and soft tissue during surgical procedures. Dull instruments do not cut hard tooth structure efficiently, increasing the amount of time the dental assistant has to complete the preparation and lowering the quality of the preparation. Dull instruments require additional pressure to be applied to the tooth, causing patient discomfort and trauma to hard and soft tissue. This additional strain causes unnecessary stress and fatigue to the operator. *Dental assistants should only sharpen instruments that have been sterilized.*

The dental assistant can test the blade by placing the cutting edge of the instrument on the thumbnail. If it catches or does not slide smoothly when the assistant draws it lightly across the nail, it is sharp. The dental assistant can also tell when the instrument is dull by looking at it in direct light or under a magnifying glass. A sharp instrument has little nicks or flat spots on the angle of the cutting edge and the intersecting blade surface.

Types of Sharpening Devices

Many types of sharpening devices are available. They can be categorized as hand-sharpening stones, handpiece mandrel-mounted stones, and mechanical-sharpener. Because the purpose of sharpening is to provide a smooth, sharp cutting edge, the device to use is the one that produces the best result. Check the sharpness of instruments routinely. The small cutting surfaces can be viewed with a magnifying glass. The dental assistant should also know the angle of the cutting surface of the blade to maintain the same angle (Figure 19.19, *A*).

Hand-Sharpening Stone Technique

Hand-sharpening stones, also called *unmounted stones*, are made of natural and artificial abrasive materials that are hard enough to grind, recontour, and smooth the metal cutting edge of the dental instrument. The India and Arkansas

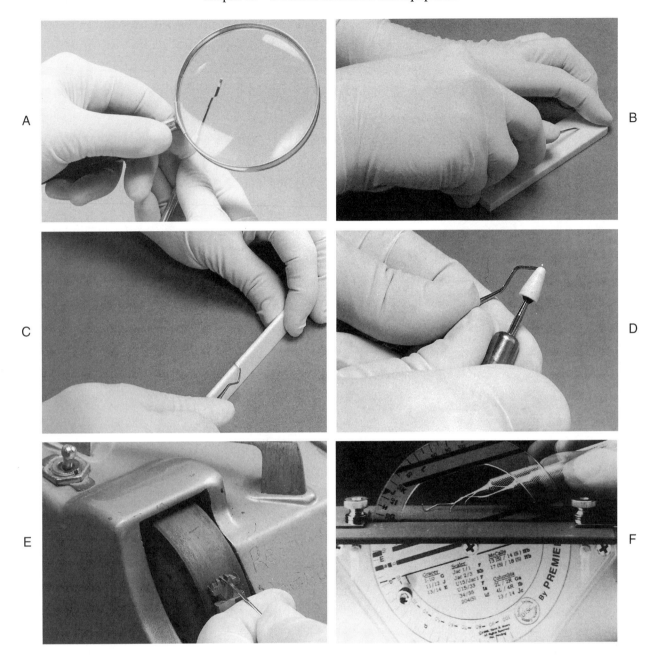

FIGURE 19.19

Techniques used to show dental instruments. **A,** Check blade of instrument with magnifying glass. **B,** Flat Arkansas stone. **C,** Tapered stone. **D,** Handpiece mandrel mounted stone. **E,** Mechanical sharpening. **F,** Disk simplified sharpening. (Courtesy Premier Dental Products Co.)

stones are natural, and the Arkansas stone is available in a hardwood box for convenience. The grit determines the coarseness of the stone. Stones are available in super-fine, fine, medium, and hard grit. Coarser grit provides greater sharpening and recontouring capacity for extremely dull instruments. The ceramic stone provides fine grit and is lubricated with water when sharpening. The sharpening stone size, thickness, and shape varies. Sharpening stones may be rectangular with a flat or grooved surface for all-purpose

use. They may also be wedge-, **conical**-, or cylindrical-shaped for use with specific instrument shapes.

Sharpening oil is available to lubricate the stone during sharpening. This helps to prevent damage to the instrument tips from heat build-up during the grinding process and helps to float away metal particles. The manual sharpening technique is

Conical

A cone shape

excellent if instruments are inspected routinely and properly maintained. The dental assistant should know cutting-edge designs to properly sharpen the instrument.

Flat Arkansas Stones The flat Arkansas stone provides a good basic method for sharpening hand-cutting instruments. After you the dental assistant inspects and evaluates the angle of the cutting instruments to be sharpened, they are laid aside while the assistant prepares the armamentarium (Figure 19.19, *B*).

Tapered, Conical, or Cylindrical Stones The tapered stone is thicker on one side and tapers to a thinner side. Both sides are rounded for use in sharpening instruments with curved blades such as curettes and spoon excavators. The flat surface can be used for general sharpening purposes. The conical or cylindrical stones are sold in various diameters and are also used to sharpen instruments with curved blades.

The dental assistant should make sure the stone is lubricated with oil. The curvature of the blade to be sharpened determines which stone to use. The stone is held between the thumb, index finger, and middle finger with the remaining two fingers resting on the stone to securely hold it. Place the bevel edge of the blade on the stone surface. The instrument is then firmly drawn around surface of the stone, turning the stone in the opposite direction and repeat if necessary. Carefully smooth off, or **hone** any roughness on the opposite, noncutting surface of the instrument (Figure 19.19, *C*).

Hone

To sharpen or smooth a cutting edge

Handpiece Mandrel-Mounted Stone Technique

Mandrel-mounted stones and unmounted abrasive wheels are composition stones that are not as hard as the Arkansas stones. They are available in varying sizes, shapes, and grits to be used with a motor-driven handpiece. The unmounted wheels are used with screw-type mandrels. These mandrel-mounted stones are also available in flat- (wheel), conical- and cylindrical- shapes and are used primarily the same as the flat- and rounded-shaped hand stones. The advantage of the motor-driven stones is the speed at which an instrument can be sharpened. This can also be a disadvantage if the person sharpening the instrument is not properly trained in using the handpiece. Excess metal can be removed quickly, changing the cutting edge of the blade and even making it nonfunctionable.

The dental assistant should grasp the instrument firmly to stabilize it during the procedure. The operator must have adequate control of the rotational speed of the stone and grasp of the handpiece. Hold the handpiece firmly with a strong palm grasp, using the thumb of the hand holding the handpiece as a support (fulcrum) for the index finger of the hand holding the instrument. The fingers, hand, wrist, and elbow should remain fixed to help stabilize the instrument while the cutting edge is moved over the stone in firm inter-

mittent strokes. Properly place the bevel of the blade over the stone surface. Carefully smooth off any roughness on the noncutting surface (Figure 19.19, *D*).

Mechanical Sharpening Technique

The mechanical sharpener provides a faster method of sharpening instruments but must also be used with a great deal of care to not remove too much metal or change the design of the instrument. The lathe-type sharpener has a large Arkansas stone wheel with three smaller attached wheels. The large wheel has an instrument guide with three slots to hold the instrument in place. The center slot is for instruments such as the chisel and hoe, which have cutting edges perpendicular to the long axis of the blade. The right and left slots are for instruments such as gingival margin trimmers, which have right- and left-angle bevels that are not perpendicular to the long axis of the blade. The smaller size wheels are for sharpening instruments such as scalers, which have right- and left-angle beveled, curved-blades.

Another mechanical sharpener is the suter-fine sharpener. The instructions for use are similar for all lathe-type mechanical devices. Lubricate the wheel surface by following the manufacturer's directions. This reduces overheating of the instrument. Grasp the instrument firmly and carefully guide the cutting edge of the blade to the wheel with gentle pressure so that the blade touches the wheel evenly. Hold the blade evenly on the wheel, check the instrument, and repeat if necessary. Metal burs on the cutting edge can be smoothed and removed, or honed by using the felt buffing wheel (Figure 19.19, *E*, Box 19.1, and Table 19.1).

Other Sharpening Techniques

One of the new instrument sharpening methods is the disk simplified sharpening system. The dental assistant should always follow the manufacturer's directions (Figure 19.19, *F*).

ROTARY INSTRUMENTS

Hand-cutting instruments were used exclusively for dental procedures until the introduction of the first rotary cutting instruments in 1846. These instruments were adapted from an earlier invention called the *spinning wheel*. In 1871, Morrison introduced the first handpiece, which was belt-driven by a foot-controlled engine and was similar to the earlier spinning wheel. In 1880, the first electric belt-driven dental engine began replacing the foot-controlled engine. These dental engines used slow-speed handpieces that were gear-driven. The electric belt-driven handpieces were later supplemented by the introduction of the high-speed, gear-driven handpieces and later the air-driven, turbine handpieces.

The heat produced from the increased cutting speed of these instruments caused the need for a coolant system to be used during operative procedures. Initially, the dental assistant would spray water and air over the tooth while the dentist prepared the restoration, which led to the addition of an

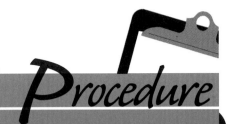

Box 19.1

Procedure

Procedure for Sharpening Instruments

Flat Arkansas stone
1. Lubricate the stone.
2. Place the stone on a hard, flat surface and grasp instrument firmly.
3. Place bevel of blade on stone and with stiff action draw instrument over surface of stone toward operator.
4. Smooth off (hone) any roughness on the opposite noncutting surface.

Tapered Arkansas stone
1. Lubricate the stone.
2. The curvature of the blade is sharpened by grasping the instrument and firmly drawing the blade over the round edge of the stone.
3. Finish by smoothing off any roughness on noncutting surface.

Handpiece mandrel mounted stone
1. Lubricate the mounted stone, grasp the instrument firmly, and use the palm grasp with thumb and index finger for support.
2. Carefully pass the bevel of the blade over the stone surface.
3. Smooth off any roughness on the noncutting surface.

Mechanical device
1. Lubricate the stone wheel.
2. Guide the cutting edge to the wheel evenly.
3. Smooth off any roughness.

Disk simplified sharpening system*
1. Identify cutting surface. Hold the instrument so the tip is toward you and the last section of the shank, which is closest to the cutting surface, is perpendicular to the floor. The lower edge of the blade is the cutting surface.
2. Select appropriate angle setting from instrument reference guide. Loosen screw. Rotate protractor dial until red line matches setting; tighten screw. No oil or water is required.
3. Rest blade on sharpening platform with instrument handle held parallel to black guide lines. Establish finger rest on platform.
4. Pull arm toward you while keeping wrist rigid. At all times instrument handle should remain parallel to guide lines. Repeat short strokes until desired sharpness is obtained.
5. For instruments with a curved cutting surface (curettes), rotate fingers slightly as you draw instrument toward you. Start at the heel of the cutting surface and finish stroke at the tip.

Courtesy Premier Dental Products Co.

Table 19.1

Evaluation of Sharpening Instruments

Techniques	4	3	2	0	X
Secure materials and equipment.					
Wear eye protection.					
Lubricate stone.					
Place bevel of blade on stone surface.					
Grasp instrument.					
Draw instrument over stone.					
Smooth off roughness.					

The numeric criteria: 4 Excellent; 3 Good but some improvement can be made; 2 Below average, usable, needs to improve skill; 0 Unsatisfactory; X Not able to evaluate.

air and water coolant and debriment system to be added to the handpiece.

Later a light system was added to provide more visibility while working in the oral cavity. More recent developments include the addition of minute television receptacles that magnify the tooth to allow high visibility for the operator. The laser handpiece has been introduced to dentistry, which will further increase efficiency for the dental practice and comfort for the patient.

Dental Handpieces and Attachments

The dental handpiece and rotary attachments such as burs, stones, and discs are the basic instruments used by the dentist and dental personnel for restorative and preventive dentistry. Without the use of the handpiece and attachments, if they become inoperable, the dentist is unable to perform the majority of the dental procedures (see Chapter 18). Therefore the dental assistant should be able to identify the handpieces and attachments and understand how they are used and maintained. Manufacturers provide the instructions for equipment use and maintenance. The dental assistant must be able to maintain these handpieces to keep them operable, and the expanded duty dental assistant, in most instances, needs to have the skills to operate the handpiece to perform various restorative and polishing procedures. The operational use of these handpieces by the dental assistant is determined by state regulations.

Conventional Handpieces and New Innovations

Dental handpieces have changed tremendously over the last 40 years as they have progressed from slow speed, belt driven, to medium-speed, electrotorque, and ultra-speed, air driven. Air and water was incorporated into the handpiece, and technology has introduced fiber-optic halogen lighting, digital image magnification, and laser to dental handpieces recently. The dental assistant should be familiar with all handpieces used in dental practice. Therefore the following information provides an overview of these various handpieces:

> The dental assistant should be knowledgeable of the handpieces used in the office, ask to read the manufacturer's directions for the use and maintenance of those handpieces, and feel free to ask the dentist any questions about their use and care.

Low-Speed Handpiece

The low-speed handpiece is a conventional electric, motor-driven, gear-driven instrument. It operates at speeds of 5000 to 10,000 revolutions per minute (rpm). With modification, the low-speed handpiece can reach 50,000 rpm. The handpiece is used with a contraangle or prophylaxis angle and is used primarily for finishing, polishing, and laboratory procedures.

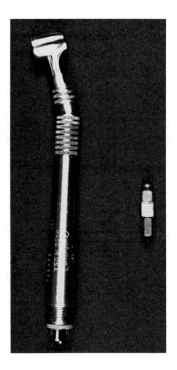

FIGURE 19.20

The high-speed handpiece is also called the *ultra-speed* or *air-driven handpiece.*

High-Speed Handpiece

The conventional high-speed handpiece, which is often referred to as an *electrotorque handpiece*, is also gear-driven (Figure 19.20). Since the introduction of the ultraspeed handpiece, this handpiece is considered a medium-speed handpiece operating between 100,000 to 800,000 rpm. It is used primarily for restorative dentistry where the operator wants greater control of the contact or touch between the instrument and the tooth or restoration surface. It is also used for laboratory procedures where greater speed or higher torque is needed.

The ultra-speed or air-driven handpiece is a high-speed handpiece that uses compressed air rather than being gear-driven. The air is forced into the head of the handpiece, against small turbines that rotate the bur or other attachments. These attachments, such as burs and stones, are held in place by friction grip rather than the latch-type. The air-driven handpiece operates with speeds from 100,000 to 600,000 rpm. Although these instruments have high speed they also have low torque and stall with moderate pressure.

The advantage of this handpiece is the time in which the dental procedure can be completed, the low vibrations placed on the tooth, and the reduced trauma to the tooth. This provides greater efficiency and comfort for the patient. The disadvantage is the high-speed frictional heat that is produced during cavity preparation, which is avoided by spraying air or water on the instrument tip while completing the procedure. This condition is improved by the addition of an air and water coupler system attached to the air-driven handpiece. The inclusion of the coolant within the air-turbine handpiece is an added feature of the ultraspeed handpiece. Cooling systems have been developed that are equipped with selectors. The selector allows the operator to control the air, water, or a combination of air and water through the foot rheostat.

Fiber Optic Light Handpiece

The high-speed torque handpiece was improved with the addition of a fiber optic, intraoral light. The fiber optic light is enclosed in the handpiece to provide direct light on the working area, improving vision in the oral cavity during various procedures (Figure 19.21). The fiber optic handpiece is attached to a control box, which contains the light source.

Portable Handpiece

Light weight, miniature electric handpiece motors and handpiece units have been developed for portable and alternative use. These are portable handpieces and units that can be used outside the dental operatory (see Chapter 20).

Dental Lasers

Dental lasers are making a dramatic change in dentistry today and have the potential to change how dentistry is performed in the future. Several types of lasers have been adapted for dental treatment. A variety of hard- and soft-tissue applications are currently being identified. Because of lasers, a reduced need for anesthesia exists. The dentist can perform surgical procedures without hemorrhage, and less edema and postoperative discomfort that facilitates operator use and increases patients acceptance exists. The laser also ablates or removes bacteria through the cutting process thus providing a new concept for periodontal treatment. Studies in progress suggest promising applications for decay removal, root canal treatment, preparation of tooth structure, and bonding. The adaptation introduced with dental lasers is flexible delivery systems and handpiece arrangements, facilitating intraoral placements (Figure 19.22).

Laboratory Turbine Handpiece

Manufacturers provide an air turbine handpiece for laboratory procedures such as carving porcelain or gold. The handpiece weighs less than 2 oz and performs quietly at speeds in excess of 250,000 rpm.

Intraoral Video Camera

Fully integrated intraoral video cameras with fiber-optic light sources have been developed. These miniature cameras provide color and full-face focus to a single tooth focus with

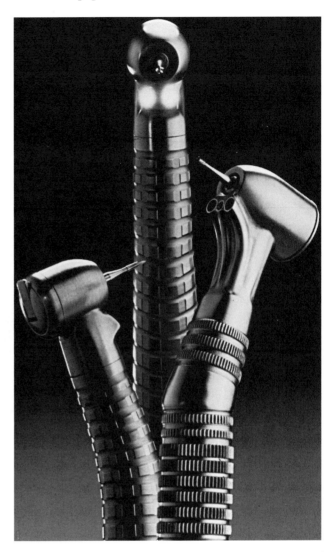

FIGURE 19.21

The fiber optic light system adds direct light to the oral cavity, improving vision. The fiber optic light system also includes air and water spray. (Courtesy Midwest Dental Division)

a clear illumination and 30x magnification. The camera image is exactly as seen by the eye. These systems include a 13 inch color monitor, a color printer, and a mobile cart that can be moved from one operatory to the next or as a remote unit linking up to five operatories (Figure 19.23). They also include a disposable sleeve to cover the entire handpiece for asepsis and a cover for the camera lens, which can be cold sterilized or thrown away.

Handpiece Attachments

Straight, contraangle, and right angle handpiece attachments are available for use with the low- and high-speed handpieces. The attachments are used to hold the rotary cutting instruments such as burs, stones, and discs.

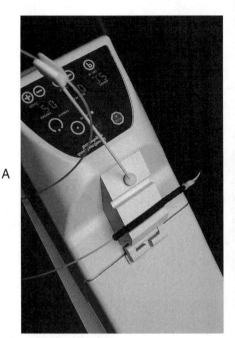

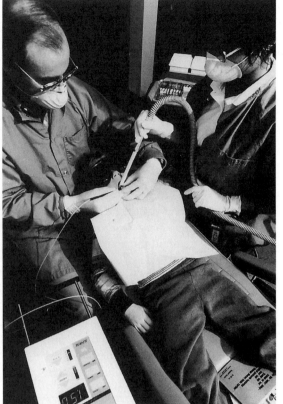

B

A

FIGURE 19.22

The dental laser is adding another dimension to dental equipment. **A**, Laser system. **B**, Laser procedure with operator and dental assistant. (Courtesy Dr. Frederick Parkins, University of Louisville School of Dentistry, Louisville, Ky.)

Straight Handpiece

The straight handpiece varies in diameter and length and is tubular (Figure 19.24). It is used primarily for laboratory work or procedures in which the rotary cutting instrument (bur) works in alignment with the handpiece.

Contraangle Handpiece Attachment

The contraangle handpiece is tubular and attached to the straight handpiece to hold rotary cutting instruments, which work at right angle to the long axis of the handpiece, in place. The contraangle may have a latch-type or friction-grip head.

Latch-Type Head The latch-type head has a latch device that locks the rotary instrument in place (see Figure 19.24). The latch is opened, the bur is placed in position, and the latch is closed around the instrument to lock it into place.

Friction-Grip Head The friction-grip head holds the rotary cutting instrument in place by friction against a chuck inside the head (see Figure 19.24). The friction-grip heads require specific tools to place and remove burs.

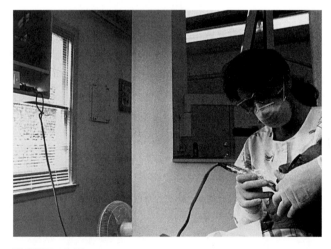

FIGURE 19.23

Intraoral video cameras with a fiber optic light source provide clear illumination and magnification. The dental assistant in this photograph is using the video camera as an educational aid.

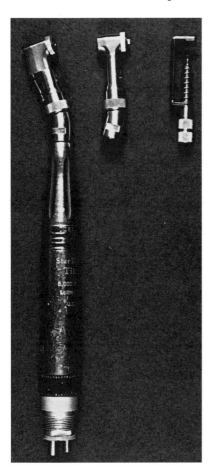

FIGURE 19.24
Low-speed straight handpiece with adapter and latch contraangle. Friction grip attachment and bur changer are to the right.

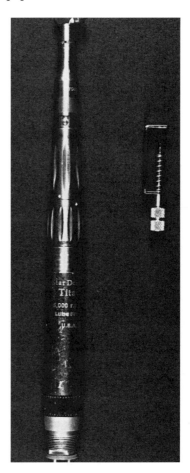

FIGURE 19.25
The low-speed straight handpiece is shown with a right angle friction-grip attachment.

Right Angle Handpiece Attachment

The right angle handpiece attachment is used for prophylaxis procedures and has a snap-on or screw head (Figure 19.25). Although the contra-angle can be used, the prophylaxis right angle attachment is designed to prevent wear from the abrasive paste materials.

ROTARY CUTTING ATTACHMENTS

The term *rotary cutting attachments* refers to dental burs, diamond points, stones, discs, and wheels. They are designed to meet specific dental needs for removing caries, cutting the hard tooth structure, and polishing the teeth. They are also used for grinding, finishing, and polishing various restorative materials. They may fit directly into the straight handpiece or into the contraangle handpiece, determined by the design of the shank. Those that fit into the straight handpiece have a long shank and those that fit into the contraangle have a shorter latch or

friction-grip shank. Some rotary cutting instruments are mounted and others are unmounted and must snap or screw onto a mandrel before inserting into the handpiece.

Cavity Preparation Burs

Burs are the rotary cutting instruments that are attached to the handpiece and used to cut hard tooth tissue and trim and finish dental restorative materials. The parts of the bur are the shank, neck, and head (Figure 19.26).

The neck is the portion of the bur that narrows to connect the shank with the head. The blade is the fine head or cutting portion of the bur. The blade configuration of the bur and the size and shape will vary according to the procedure in which it will be used. Burs must meet quality testing standards; therefore some manufacturers will plastic coat the bur head to protect the blades from damage until they are ready for use. Burs will last longer when they are used with a light touch to cut dentin, amalgam, or

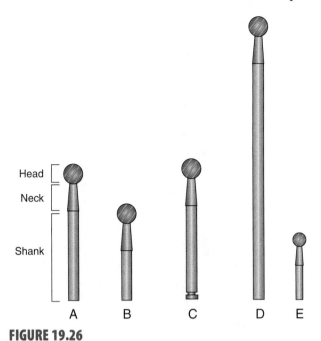

FIGURE 19.26

Bur shank designs. **A**, Friction grip (FG). **B**, Friction grip short shank (FGSS). **C**, Latch-type (LA). **D**, Straight handpiece (HP). **E**, Miniature (mini).

gold. They wear faster when used to cut porcelain or composite materials. Also, some cold sterilization solutions tend to dull the burs by affecting their carbide bonding materials if they are left in the solution too long. Dull burs should be replaced as soon as possible because they take more time to complete a given procedure.

Debris should be gently removed from the bur with a stiff bristle brass or nylon brush. A nongum, soft pink rubber eraser can be used for removing debris from the bur blades by pushing the bur into the eraser two or three times. Most burs can be ultrasonically cleaned but they need to be placed into a holder or bur block to keep the blades from rubbing against other metal surfaces while being cleaned. Most burs can be processed through common sterilizing equipment, but the dental assistant must follow the manufacturer's directions for sterilizing procedures.

The shank is the part of the bur that fits into the handpiece. Burs are made from regular steel and tungsten carbide. The carbide burs will often have nickel-plated shanks to protect against corrosion and provide a more secure grip by the handpiece chuck. Others have gold-plated shanks, groove, or marks on the neck for easy identification in the bur block and also to distinguish the manufacturer's brand.

The length and shape of the shank depends on how the bur will be used. The straight, long shank is used with the straight, low-speed handpiece and is used primarily for laboratory work. The latch-type shank is used with the latch-type contra-angle handpiece, which locks into the shank

groove. The friction-grip shank is used with the gear-driven, friction-grip contra-angle handpiece. The high-speed turbin handpieces also use a friction grip shank that is more slender. Burs are available with the following shank types:

1　FG-friction grip
2　FGSS-friction grip short shank
3　LA-latch type
4　HP-straight handpiece
5　CA-contra-angle
6　Miniminiature

Several basic bur shapes are used primarily for cavity preparation. These regular carbide burs are usually defined as six-bladed burs and categorized by their shapes and use. Each bur shape has a different series of numbers that indicates the size of the bur. The low number indicates a small bur head size, and the larger the number, the larger the bur head size (Figure 19.27).

Round (#$^1/_4$-8)

Round burs can be applied to various dental procedures depending on their size. The smallest round bur, #$^1/_4$ and $^1/_2$, is used for making retention grooves. The medium sizes are used to remove interproximal caries in incisors and opening up teeth for endodontic procedures. The largest round burs are used at low speed to remove caries on the cavity floor (Figures 19.27 and 19.28, *A*, *B*, and *C*).

Inverted Cone (#33 $^1/_2$-39)

The inverted cone bur is used for producing undercuts for retention of filling materials at the junction of cavity walls and floor (Figures 19.27 and 19.28, *D* and *E*).

Straight Fissure Plain (#56-57-L) and Straight Fissure Crosscut (#556-558-L)

The straight fissure plain and straight fissure crosscut burs are used to produce a flat floor and parallel sided cavity preparation. They are used to remove enamel to access caries of the dentin, to produce retentive locks and for gross reduction for crown preparations. They are available in long for better access (Figures 19.27 and 19.28, *F*, *G*, and *H*).

Tapered Fissure Plain (#168-171-L) and Taper Fissure Crosscut (#699-703-L)

Taper fissure plain and taper fissure crosscut burs are used to produce flat floor and wall cavity preparations that taper slightly. They are particularly useful to avoid undercuts such as for inlay and crown preparations and for making retentive locks. The are available in long versions (Figures 19.27 and 19.28, *I* and *J*).

Taper Dome (#1169-1170-L)

The taper dome bur appears the same as the taper fissure except that it has a rounded top that allows it to penetrate enamel and is excellent for drilling pin holes.

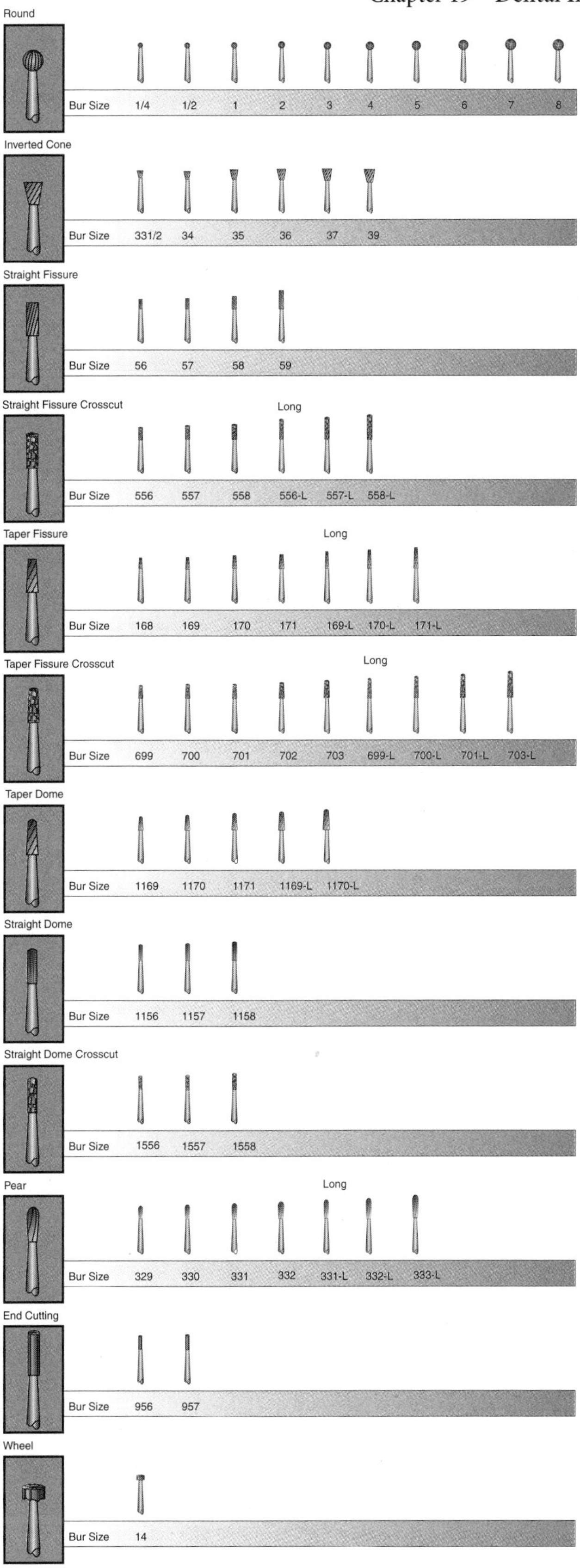

FIGURE 19.27

This bur graph identifies the regular carbide burs by shape and size.

Straight Dome (#1156-1158) and Straight Dome Crosscut (#1556-1558)

The straight dome plain and straight dome crosscut combines the benefits of the round bur and fissure burs by allowing enamel penetration and side-cutting without changing the bur.

Pear-Shaped (#329-333-L)

The pear-shaped burs combine the functions of several burs. They are used to produce an occlusal cavity preparation in which a rounded cavity floor is needed. They can make the initial entry cut in the enamel, remove caries, and produce rounded undercuts in a cavity preparation (Figures 19.27 and 19.28, *K*, *L*, and *M*).

End Cutting (#956-957)

The end cutting bur is used for cutting a smooth flat shoulder on crown preparations. The sides of the bur are smooth so that they do not undercut the tooth or cause laceration of the tissue (Figures 19.27 and 19.28, *N*).

Wheel (#14)

The wheel bur is used for trenching and preparing retentive grooves and ledges (Figure 19.27). A variety of mounted and unmounted **rotary instruments** are used in handpieces to trim and finish amalgam alloy, gold, composites, enamel, and other materials. The grit determines how and when they are used in the finishing process. They are classified as trimming and finishing burs, diamond points, stones, discs, wheels, and rubber points (Figures 19.27 and 19.28, *O*).

> *Rotary instruments*
>
> **Power-driven instruments, often called *dental drills*, which are used to cut hard and soft oral tissue and other materials**

Trimming and Finishing Instruments

Burs

The trimming and finishing burs are used for shaping and smoothing composites, amalgams, gold and enamel, dentin, and other materials (Figure 19.29). They have 12- and 40-blades that remove less material as they revolve than regular cutting burs. This produces a smoother finish that is less likely to discolor or stain and a better fit and seal because of the smooth finish. The trimming and finishing burs remove material at a slower rate and therefore are better for equilibration. These burs are also excellent to remove the striations and grooves often left by diamond burs. The 40-blade trimming and finishing burs produce an ultrafine finish because they have more than

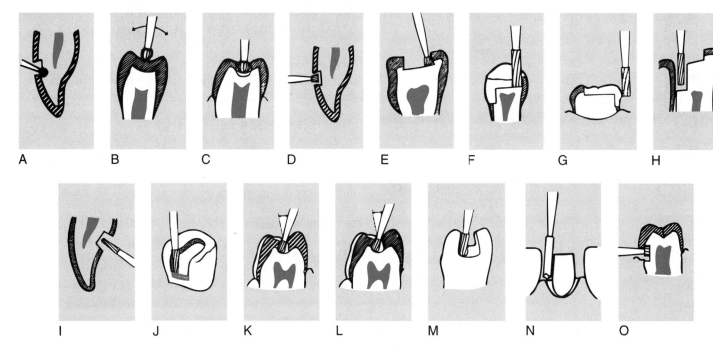

FIGURE 19.28

Cavity Preparation Bur Types. Round burs are used to: **A,** Produce retention points. **B,** Make occlusal adjustments. **C,** Remove caries. Inverted cone burs are used to produce undercuts for retention of restorative materials such as: **D,** Labial surface. **E,** Occlusal surfaces. Straight fissure and straight fissure crosscut burs are used for: **F,** Gross reduction (plain fissure). **G,** Gross reduction (straight crosscut fissure). **H,** Better access (long plain fissure). Taper fissure plain and taper fissure crosscut burs are used for: **I,** Prepare preparation. **J,** To prepare retentive locks. Pear shape burs are used for: **K,** Making entry cuts. **L,** Shaping cavity preparations. **M,** Additional penetrations. Long end-cutting burs are used for: **N,** Cutting smooth flat shoulders on crown preparations. The smooth, safe sides of this bur ensure that no laceration of tissue or undercutting of the tooth occurs. Wheel burs are useful for: **O,** Trenching and preparation of retentive grooves and ledges.

6 times the number of blades a regular carbide bur has, producing an extremely smooth finish (Figure 19.30).

The expanded function dental assistants in designated states use these burs to trim and finish amalgam and composite restorations; therefore the expanded function dental assistant should understand their use and application.

Diamond Points

Diamond points are friction grip abrasives designed in a variety of sizes and shapes and are mounted on regular and short shanks. Unmounted diamond disks are available to use on handpiece mandrels. The shapes are similar to the carbide burs. Diamond abrasives are round, inverted cone, cylinder, cone, straight dome, taper dome, pear, flame, pointed, and wheel shaped. They are considered equivalent

to the 6- and 12-fluted burs. The diamond points are designed to perform the same functions as the carbide burs. Diamond instruments such as the Shofu GingiCurettage FG points are also used to remove soft tissue around the neck of the tooth.

The benefit of diamond points is their abrasive qualities to cut quickly and cause less patient trauma than carbide burs. Diamond points are manufactured through an electroplating bonding process that produces microfine grit diamond instruments. They are available in coarse grit diamond points for removing large bulks of hard tooth structure. The fine and ultrafine points are used for trimming and finishing procedures using light strokes. Diamond points can be purchased individually or in kits. Dressing stones are available to remove glazed or clogged surfaces of diamond points.

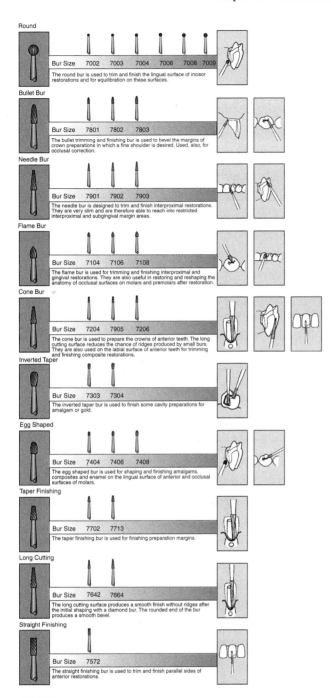

FIGURE 19.29

12-Blade trimming and finishing burs are designed for trimming, shaping, and finishing restorative materials.

Stones

Stones are fast-cutting instruments used to finish enamel, porcelain, composites, and gold and silver alloys. They are mounted and unmounted and are available in a wide range of shapes and sizes (Figure 19.31). The mounted stones come in friction grip (FG), straight handpiece (HP), and contraangle (CA) shanks.

The green stones are used to remove the bulk of material during the finishing process and for occlusal adjustment. The green stones come in various grits and are made of silicon carbide abrasives. The white stones are made from micrograined aluminum oxide grits, which produce a finer texture to provide a smoother surface when finishing enamel, composites, and porcelain. Mounted and unmounted lab stones made of pure aluminum oxide grits are also available. The pink stones are for finishing precious ceramic metals; the white stones are for finishing semiprecious and nonprecious ceramic metals; and the coral stones are for finishing chrome-cobalt and nickel alloys. The unmounted stone wheels fit onto straight handpiece mandrels and are available in several sizes and grits.

Discs

Discs are used for creating interproximal separation, contouring embrasures, shaping, and finishing cavity preparations and restorations (Figure 19.32). They are single- or double-sided and vary in thickness, size, and shape. The shape varies from flat to concave or convex and may be plain or perforated. Discs are molded or they have plastic, paper, or metal backings coated with a variety of abrasive grits such as diamond, silicon carbide, quartz, sand, and garnet. Grits are extrafine, fine, medium, coarse, and extracoarse. Plastic and paper discs are excellent for contouring tooth and restorative materials because of their flexibility. They can be mounted on either the snap-on or screw-on mandrel. Thin-flexible diamond discs with crystals around the edges of the disc are available. A popular molded disc is the Damascus disc often called the *JoDandy disc.*

Rubber Cups, Discs, Wheels, and Points

Rubber cups, discs, wheels, points, and minipoints are used for finishing and polishing composite, amalgam, gold, and cast alloys (Figure 19.33). They can be used on subgingival and interproximal surfaces and are impregnated with polishing ingredients to provide fast, smooth results without pumice, tin oxide, or fuss. The ingredients or grits used in these abrasives provide different levels of polish without the use of pumice or tin oxide. For instance, the Shofu brownies give a smooth to satin finish; the greenies give a lustrously polish; and the supergreenies give a superpolish. The manufacturer designates abrasiveness and identifies coloring. The abrasive instruments are used with straight, contraangle, and friction grip handpieces. These instruments are available in amalgam, composite, enamel, gold, porcelain adjustment, and polishing kits.

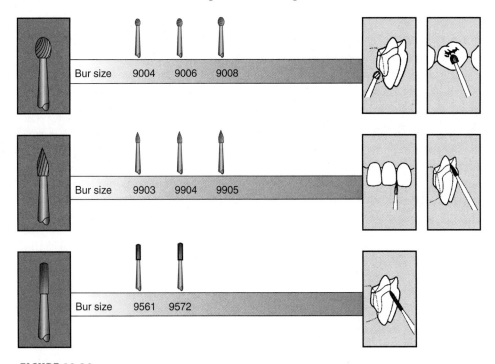

FIGURE 19.30

40-Blade trimming and finishing burs produce an ultrafine finish on composite, gold, and natural tooth material.

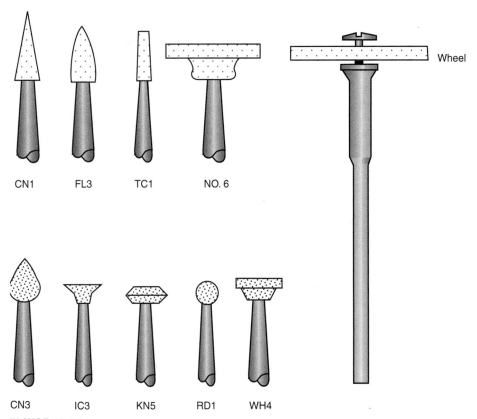

FIGURE 19.31

Stones are fast-cutting abrasive instruments used to finish enamel, porcelain, composites, gold, and silver alloys.

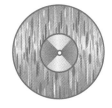
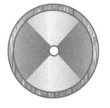
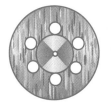
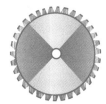

	911H-220	940-220	918PB-220	365-220
Straight handpiece	911H-220			
(RA latch)	911H-220			
Unmounted	911H-220			

FIGURE 19.32

Diamond discs, like sandpaper discs, vary in shape, size, and flexibility.

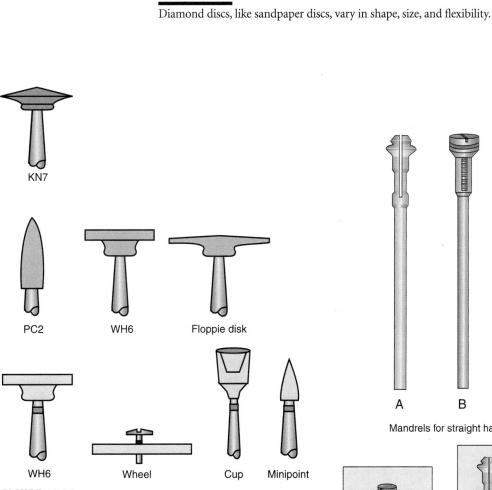

KN7

PC2   WH6   Floppie disk

WH6   Wheel   Cup   Minipoint

FIGURE 19.33

Rubber abrasive instruments are available in varying size, color, and shape.

Mandrels

Mandrels are heavy-duty, stainless steel shanks used to hold discs and wheels in the straight, contraangle, or friction-grip handpieces. They are available with a snap-on, regular screw, or pin screw head (Figure 19.34).

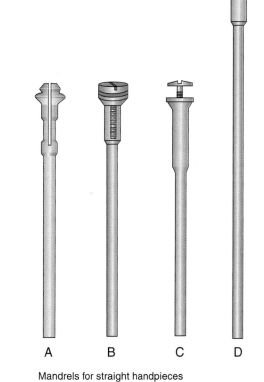

A   B   C   D

Mandrels for straight handpieces

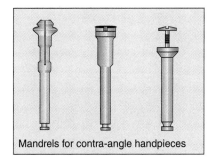

Mandrels for contra-angle handpieces

Mandrels for friction grip handpieces

FIGURE 19.34

Mandrels are used to hold discs and wheels in the straight handpiece, contraangle attachment, or friction grip handpiece. **A**, Snap-on. **B**, Screw-on. **C**, Pin-head screw. **D**, Long screw-on.

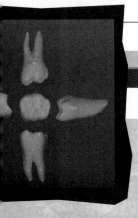

Points for Review

- Intraoral video cameras
- Dental lasers
- Laboratory turbine handpiece
- Instrument management and infection control of instruments
- Identification of examination instruments and hand-cutting
- Clinical instruments, laboratory instruments, hand-pieces, and contraangles
- Handpiece attachments and conventional handpieces
- Sharpening instruments
- Types of burs and trimming and finishing instruments

Self-Study Questions

1. The three numbers on a dental hand instrument refer to the width of the blade, length of the handle, and angle of the blade.
   a. True
   b. False

2. The basic set up includes the mouth mirror, explorer, cotton forceps, and probe.
   a. True
   b. False

3. What are the five basic hand-cutting instruments used often in dental procedures?
   a. Hatchet, hoe, chisel, scaler, and excavator
   b. Hatchet, hoe, chisel, angle former, and gingival margin trimmer
   c. Hatchet, hoe, chisel, discoid and cleoid, and explorer
   d. None of the above

4. What is the name of the cutting instrument with the edge parallel to the angle of the handle and used to prepare retentive groove and sharpen internal line angles?
   a. Hatchet
   b. Hoe
   c. Chisel
   d. Gingival margin trimmer

5. What is the name of the instrument with a curved blade, the cutting edge at an angle to the blade, and used to develop a bevel on cavosurface margin?
   a. Hatchet
   b. Hoe
   c. Excavator
   d. Gingival margin trimmer

6. What is the name of the instrument that is spoon-shaped and used to remove the soft caries from a tooth?
   a. Hatchet
   b. Hoe
   c. Excavator
   d. Gingival margin trimmer

7. Before sharpening a dental instrument by hand, the dental assistant should lubricate the stone with water.
   a. True
   b. False

8. The dental assistant should only sharpen instruments that have been sterilized.
   a. True
   b. False

9. What type of handpiece attachment is most often used for prophylaxis procedures?
   a. Contraangle attachment
   b. Latch-type attachment
   c. Right angle attachment
   d. All of the above

10. What bur does the series #56-57 represent?
    a. Round
    b. Taper
    c. Straight fissure plain
    d. Inverted cone

11. What bur does the series #$1/_4$-8 represent?
    a. Round
    b. Taper
    c. Straight fissure plain
    d. Inverted cone

12. What bur does the series #956-957 represent?
    a. Straight dome
    b. Straight dome crosscut
    c. Pear-shaped
    d. End-cutting

13. What devices are used to shape and smooth composites, amalgams, gold, enamel, and dentin?
    a. #14 wheel bur
    b. Rubber cup and pumice
    c. Finishing bur
    d. Sandpaper disc

14. Green stones are used to remove the bulk of material during the finishing process and for occlusal adjustment.
    a. True
    b. False

15. Mandrels are available in what shapes?
    a. Snap-on
    b. Regular screw
    c. Pin screw head
    d. All of the above

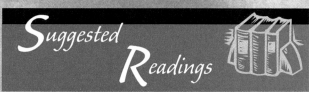

Suggested Readings

Finkbeiner BL, Johnson CS: *Mosby's comprehensive dental assisting: a clinical approach*, St Louis, 1995, Mosby.

Miyasaki-Ching C: *Chasteen's essentials of clinical dental assisting*, ed 5, St Louis, 1997, Mosby.

Roberson TM, Heymann HO: *Sturdevant's art and science of operative dentistry*, ed 4, St Louis, Mosby (in press).

Woodall IR: *Comprehensive dental hygiene care*, ed 4, St Louis, 1993, Mosby.

Chapter 20

Current Concepts of Dental Chairside Assisting

Key Points

- Dental auxiliary utilization (DAU)
- Four-handed sit-down dentistry
- Principles of work simplification
- Practice efficiency methods

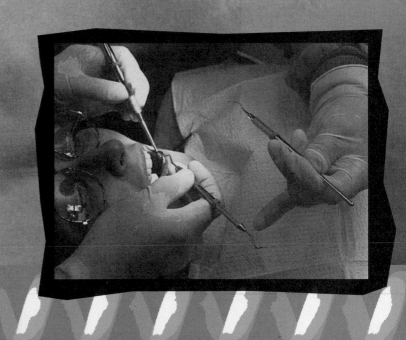

Chapter Outline

Concepts of Chairside Assisting
   Dental auxiliary utilization
Selection and Use of Dental Equipment
   Dental chair
   Operator's clinical chair
   Assistant's clinical chair
   Operator's unit
   Assistant's unit
   Dental light
   Room lighting
   Dental cabinets
   Waste receptacles
Four-Handed Sit-Down Dentistry
   Principles of work simplification
   Principles of motion economy

Classification of motions
Assistant, patient, and operator
   positioning
Principles of Material and Instrument
   Handling
Storage of materials chairside
Manipulation of materials chairside
Standardized tray setups and procedures
Assembly, delivery, and return of
   instruments
Practice Efficiency Methods and Instrument
   Application
Managing instrumentation techniques
General Guidelines for Visibility and Access
   to the Oral Cavity

Learning Objectives

On completion of Chapter 20, the student should be able to do the following:

▪ Define key terms.

▪ Define the roles and operating zones for the operator, assistant, and patient.

▪ State the principles of dental auxiliary utilization.

▪ Discuss the type and operation of equipment most suitable for dental auxiliary use.

▪ State the general objectives of four-handed sit-down dentistry.

▪ Describe the basic principles of work simplification.

▪ Identify the concepts for motion economy.

▪ Describe the practice efficiency methods.

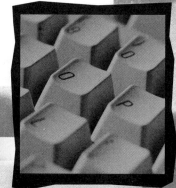

Key Terms

Dental Assistant (DA)

Dental Auxiliary
   Utilization (DAU)

Expanded Duty Dental
   Assistant (EDDA)

Four-Handed
   Dentistry

Motion Economy

Operator

Personnel

Sit-Down Dentistry

Work Simplification

CONCEPTS OF CHAIRSIDE ASSISTING

Dental assistant (DA)

A general term that refers to the chairside assistant, office assistant, office manager, laboratory assistant, expanded duty assistant, and any specialty assistant, such as an orthodontic or oral surgery assistant

The chairside **dental assistant (DA)** plays a major role in creating a relaxed, pleasant environment in which to provide quality dental health care. The chairside assistant works under the direction and supervision of the dentist; this arrangement is called direct supervision. The dentist and staff work together to build a good employer-employee relationship in order to achieve maximum results. The development of good professional interpersonal relationships and working skills increases the efficiency of the dental office and produces a relaxed working environment.

Personnel

The dental assistant, dental hygienist, laboratory technician, or other employees.

Operator

An individual who provides direct patient care

NOTE: In this chapter the terms **personnel** or *staff* are used when referring to the dental assistant, hygienist, laboratory technician, or other employees working in the dental office. The term **operator** is used to refer to the individual providing direct patient treatment such as the dentist, advanced function dental assistant, or the dental hygienist.

Dental Auxiliary Utilization

Dental auxiliary utilization (DAU)

The performance of dental procedures with the aid of allied dental personnel according to the accepted principles of practice, which have been determined through research

The principles of **dental auxiliary utilization (DAU)** are guidelines that can increase operational efficiency when providing dental services. Research has shown that following these principles can save the dentist and staff time and energy and can enable them to work more comfortably and smoothly as a team. These guidelines promote efficiency, ease of operation, good physiological health, comfort, and proper visibility.

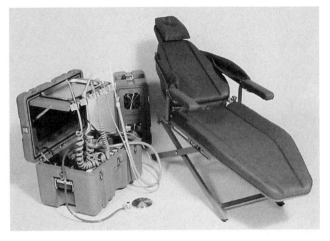

FIGURE 20.1

As dental assistants are delegated advanced functions in preventive dentistry, portable equipment will become essential in providing dental services outside the traditional practice setting.

The principles of DAU help the operator, chairside assistant, and patient to maintain proper posture and position. This positional relationship is called the *triad*. It allows the operator to work smoothly with the chairside assistant to use the assistant's services correctly and efficiently. Proper positioning of the patient and proper selection and positioning of the dental equipment enable the dentist and chairside assistant to interact with ease and comfort.

SELECTION AND USE OF DENTAL EQUIPMENT

The dental assistant often is involved in evaluating and helping to select new operatory equipment when replacement becomes necessary. For this reason, the assistant must understand some of the criteria involved in selecting equipment for dental auxiliary utilization and four-handed sit-down dentistry.

Dental Chair

Over the years dental chairs have been redesigned to meet current styles and needs. Today's dental chairs are both more comfortable and more functional than previous models. Also, because more dental procedures are being performed outside the office setting, new portable equipment has become available (Figure 20.1).

Dental chairs are arranged in the operatory in basically the same way for right- and left-handed operators, regardless of the quadrant being treated. The basic requirements are as follows:

1 *Position adjustability.* The supine, or reclining, position is routinely accepted by most patients for dental procedures. The dental chair should place the patient in the full supine position, which is used unless a heart disorder or some other physical condition must be taken into consideration. For example, some patients with specific heart problems must sleep on two pillows at night; these individuals should be positioned about 22 degrees from horizontal. A pregnant woman may be more comfortable on her side or in a more upright position with a pillow tucked into the side of the chair for support. Some operators prefer to scale or polish the lingual surface of the lower anterior teeth with the patient in a more vertical position. An important rule to remember when placing a patient in the supine position is "toes no higher than the nose." Otherwise, too much blood may accumulate around the head and neck, and the patient may become uncomfortable.

2 *Contouring.* The dental chair should be contoured and padded to give complete and comfortable support to the trunk, head, arms, and legs when the patient is placed in the supine position.

3 *Back adjustability.* The back of the chair should be adjustable from a vertical position to a full horizontal position (90 degrees).

4 *Thin back.* The back should also be thin—$2^1/_2$ inches maximum at a point 6 inches down from the top end of the chair. This allows the back of the chair to rest over the operator's thighs with the operator sitting erect, shoulders relaxed, arms at the sides, and legs comfortably under the back of the chair. A distance of 14 to 16 inches from the patient's mouth to the operator's eyes is the best visual distance for the operator. New types of eyewear have been developed to enhance the operator's vision.

5 *Narrow back.* The back of the dental chair should be narrow (6 inches maximum) to allow the operator and assistant to sit close to the patient's head and mouth when the chair is in the supine position.

6 *Single-piece back.* A single-piece chair back is recommended over a split-back model because the hand control switches that operate the chair are more conveniently located on the single-piece style.

7 *Power controls.* Many dental chairs now are power operated with foot controls. This allows positioning of the dental chair during a procedure without touching the controls.

  Dual controls allow both the operator and the assistant to adjust the chair. Solid, one-piece chair backs have an advantage over the split-back style because they allow hand switches to be placed at the head of the chair for easy access from both the operator and assistant positions.

  The adjustments for the leg portion of the dental chair should be combined with the back adjustment to en-

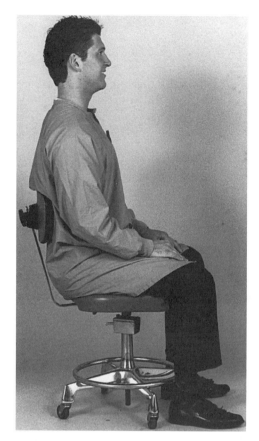

FIGURE 20.2

The operator's chair should have a stable base and adequate back support.

sure patient comfort when the chair is placed in the vertical or supine position. The lower half of the chair should have an independent adjustment to allow for individual patient differences.

  The chair should be able to be lowered to 14 inches above the floor or lower to place the upright patient near eye level with the seated operator or assistant.

8 *Seating and dismissing capability.* Equipment should not be attached to the dental chair, so that patients can be seated and dismissed from either side of the chair. This may be important for access by disabled patients. This capability also allows the chair to be used by either left- or right-handed operators and prevents inefficient traffic patterns from developing around the chair.

Operator's Clinical Chair

The operator's chair or stool should offer maximum comfort and support (Figure 20.2). The basic requirements are as follows:

1 *Independent mobility.* The operator's clinical chair should be completely mobile and independent of the dental

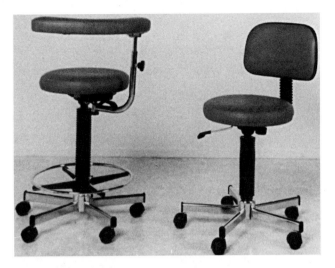

FIGURE 20.3

The assistant's clinical chair should have a stable base, a foot adjustment mechanism, and waist support to prevent tipping when the chairside assistant bends forward. (Courtesy DNTL Corp.)

chair, which allows easy repositioning during procedures performed by either a right- or left-handed operator.

2 *Back support.* The chair back should be stable and padded for comfort and should have vertical and horizontal adjustments in order to apply positive pressure to the small of the operator's back.

3 *Padded, uncontoured seat.* The operator's stool should be padded, but the seat should not be contoured because contours tend to separate the operator's legs or force them into a fixed position.

4 *Vertical adjustability.* The vertical adjustment for the seat of the operator's stool should allow a minimum low of 14 inches so that all operating personnel can sit with the thighs parallel to the floor or the knees slightly raised.

5 *Stable base.* The operator's chair should have a stable base with four large casters placed within the circumference of the seat. This arrangement provides stability for the seated operator, allows easy repositioning, and prevents the operator's heels from hitting the casters and the wheels from catching or binding on floor surfaces.

Assistant's Clinical Chair

The assistant's clinical chair or stool must be comfortable and should have a stable body support component (Figure 20.3).

1 *Independent mobility.* Like the operator's chair, the assistant's stool should be completely mobile and independent of the dental chair.

2 *Stable base.* The chair should have a broad, stable base with five large casters that are located outside the circumference of the seat. This gives the assistant a secure base when leaning forward to view the operating field.

3 *Padded, uncontoured seat.* The stool should be padded sufficiently to provide comfort during lengthy dental procedures, and the seat should not be contoured.

4 *Body support.* The body support component, which extends around the waist, should be convertible for either right- or left-handed assisting positions and should be capable of vertical and horizontal adjustment. These adjustments allow the chairside assistant to lean comfortably toward the patient.

5 *Vertical adjustability.* The assistant's stool should adjust from a low of 17 inches to a maximum height of 21 inches. The height adjustment mechanism should not require the assistant to get off the chair or to contaminate the hands.

Operator's Unit

Equipment for the dental practice is selected to complement the office design, to support the work pattern, and to take maximum advantage of available space. The type of unit chosen must be flexible enough to allow the operator to practice solo (alone) or dual (with an assistant) (Figure 20.4). The basic requirements are as follows:

1 *Flexibility of use.* The location of instruments, such as the air and water syringe, on both the operator's and the assistant's sides allows the operator to work solo or with a team. It also allows the equipment to be used by both right- and left-handed operators if more than one operator is involved.

Mounted styles are attached to the dental chair, wall, or cabinets. A unit mounted to the dental chair has the least amount of flexibility.

The mobile style is often called the split-cart side delivery system. This system offers maximum flexibility because it can be moved to meet the needs of left-handed or right-handed operators without hookup changes. When the procedures are finished, the mobile unit can be moved aside to allow the operator and staff to move freely within the operatory or between operatories.

2 *Work surface.* The operator's unit has a work surface that can support an instrument setup or other portable equipment, such as an ultrasonic scaler. Electrical outlets must be available on the unit or nearby to provide power to portable equipment.

Equipment Design

The design of equipment is changing because of an increased emphasis on infection control. The recommended location of handpieces and holders has been below the work surface of the operator's unit to allow the operator unobstructed access to instruments and portable equipment. However, because handpieces cause a water and saliva vapor or mist that contaminates the working area, new operator

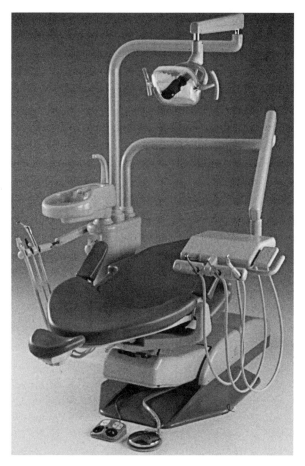

FIGURE 20.4

Operator unit attached to chair with auxiliary attachment and light. (Courtesy A-dec, Inc.)

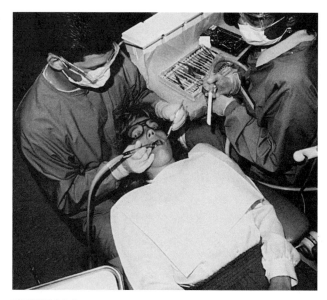

FIGURE 20.5

Operating unit is placed next to the operator's leg.

units are available with handpieces and holders above the work surface.

The operator's unit should be placed with the handpieces adjacent to the operator's right leg and right hand (if the operator is right-handed) when the elbow is down against the side and the forearm is relaxed and extended forward and outward (Figure 20.5). The palm of the hand should face up to lift the handpiece or air and water syringe from the holder.

Unit and Handpiece Operation

Most operator units currently in use in dental offices have at least two high-speed handpieces because of the frequent bur changes necessary when using friction-grip handpieces. One low-speed handpiece with a latch-type attachment usually is adequate because changing the burs is not as difficult or time-consuming. Handpiece holders are equipped with automatic switches that activate the handpiece when it is removed from the holder. Figure 20.6 and Box 20.1 present an overview of the control functions of the operator's unit.

Tri-Flow Syringe

The tri-flow syringe is a three-way combination syringe that supplies air, water, and spray. The syringe has a quick disconnect, autoclavable metal tip. The handpiece is connected to the operator's unit by a free-hanging (30 inches), and coiled cord (18 inches), which provides sufficient length to reach the patient. The syringe is operated by pressing the blue button for water, the orange button for air, and the two buttons together for spray.

Foot Control (Rheostat)

The single foot control rheostat operates all types of handpieces. The handpiece control is located on the floor and is used primarily to control the handpiece drive and to provide an air signal to turn on the water and air for the handpieces. It is activated by turning the base portion of the foot control to the right or left. The air and water are activated by putting foot pressure on the foot control button. The foot control also has an optional chip blower or ultrasonic scaler button and a fiberoptics button (this button allows the operator to turn on the fiberoptic light in the handpiece without operating the handpiece at the same time). The rheostat should be operated with the right foot because the right leg (for right-handed operators) is not under the chair and therefore is free. This also allows proper positioning of the dental chair and operator.

Radiographic Viewbox

All patient records and radiographs should be reviewed outside the clinical area before dental procedures are begun to avoid contamination of the records and other areas of the office. Records should never be handled during patient treatment.

Assistant's Unit

The general purpose of the assistant's unit is to hold instruments, equipment, and supplies for dental procedures. For the unit to meet basic team practice requirements, it must accommodate both solo and dual practice needs. This means that it must conveniently support the chairside assistant's activities during four-handed procedures and must also support the solo operator performing dental procedures without an assistant. The basic requirements are as follows:

1 *Independent mobility.* The most important requirement for the assistant's unit is that it allow both the operator and the assistant to perform dental procedures with a minimum of reaching (class IV) movement and body twisting (class V) movement. As with the operator's unit, the assistant's unit must be free of any attachment to the dental chair so that clinical personnel can move around the head and foot of the patient's chair. This promotes efficient traffic flow in the operatory and allows the patient to be seated and dismissed from either side of the dental chair.

2 *Height adjustability.* The assistant's unit should be height adjustable. It should be adjusted to a level below the chairside assistant's elbow, and when the assistant is working with a right-handed operator, the unit should be placed over the assistant's legs to the left side and behind the patient's head (Figure 20.7). This arrangement is reversed with a left-handed operator.

3 *Work surface.* The assistant's unit should have a work surface that can hold two tray setups; that is, it should measure approximately 14 × 28 inches. This saves the chairside assistant time and energy by providing sufficient space for instruments, materials, and supplies, as well as room to mix and prepare materials.

4 *Storage.* The unit should provide easily accessible storage space for restorative materials and a few support instruments and supplies. Units with a sliding top allow the chairside assistant to reach materials by sliding the top forward to open the back half; this offers access to the amalgamator, restorative materials, and supplies needed for operative procedures. Additional space can be made

Box 20.1

Control Functions of the Operator's Unit

1. *Master on/off toggle switch*: Operates the air-actuated shutoff valves for the air and water supplies. This toggle should be off whenever the unit is not in use.
2. *On/off indicator:* Gives visual proof that the unit is pressurized when the master on/off toggle is turned on.
3. *Air coolant flow control:* Adjusts the flow of air to all handpieces. Turning the knob fully clockwise shuts off the air coolant.
4. *Water coolant on/off toggle:* Used to manually cut off the flow of water to all handpieces.
5. *Water coolant flow controls:* Independently adjust the flow of water to each handpiece.
6. *Automatic handpiece hangers:* Activate the handpiece when it is removed from the holder and shut off the air and water to handpieces when they are hung up and not in use.
7. *Manual lock-out toggles:* Used when two or more handpieces are out of their hangers at the same time. The toggle is flipped to the left to "lock out" the handpiece not in use. For normal automatic operation, the toggles are flipped to the right, toward the red dot.
8. *Arm break valve:* Holds the arm at the selected height. The toggle is moved backward to set the break and forward to release it.
9. *Light intensity button:* Used to adjust the intensity of the fiberoptics. Light intensity is decreased by turning the button clockwise (Figure 20.6).

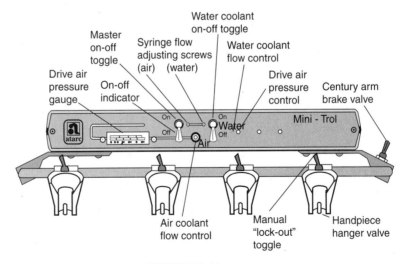

FIGURE 20.6

Operator's control unit.

available by sliding the top back. The sliding top should be closed when high-speed cutting instruments are used, because the unit is close to the patient's head, raising the possibility of air and water spray-mist contamination of exposed materials.

5 *Air and water syringe.* The chairside assistant's unit should have a combination air, water, and spray syringe located at a 45-degree angle to the floor and below the work surface. This allows easy "pick up" by the assistant and a smooth, consistent arm movement during dental treatment. The air and water syringe should be mounted on the left side of the unit so that the assistant can pick up and use the syringe with the left hand when assisting a right-handed operator.

6 *High-velocity evacuation.* The unit should have a high-velocity evacuation (HVE) system with a light, flexible, noncollapsing hose mounted on the right side of the unit.

7 *Electrical outlet.* The assistant's unit should also have an electrical outlet for the amalgamator, endodontic sterilizer, or other portable electrical equipment that may be used during treatment.

8 *Waste receptacle.* Appropriate disposable waste receptacles should be provided so that waste materials can be discarded immediately after use during treatment procedures. This allows the chairside assistant to keep a clean, uncluttered tray setup.

Operation of the Assistant's Unit

The mobile unit can provide storage space and a work area for instruments, equipment, and supplies. It also can provide the tri-flow air and water syringe, saliva ejector, HVE handpiece, and water outlet with a flow control. Figure 20.8 and Box 20.2 present more information on the control functions of the assistant's unit.

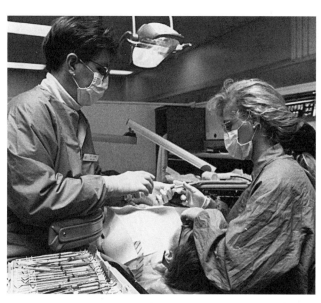

FIGURE 20.7
Placement of assistant's unit with operator in 1 o'clock position.

Box 20.2
Control Functions of the Assistant's Unit

1. *Water outlet:* A standard quick disconnect that supplies cold water for the ultrasonic scaler, jet polisher, hydrocolloid tubing, or other accessories.
2. *Water flow control:* Adjusts the amount of water dispensed from the water outlet.
3. *Master on/off toggle:* Controls the shutoff valve for the air and water supply to the tri-flow syringe, saliva ejector, and high-velocity evacuator. This toggle should be off when not in use. If the assistant's unit is post mounted, the toggle may be connected to the operator's utility center and therefore controlled by the operator's master on/off switch.
4. *On/off indicator:* Shows visually that the unit is pressurized when the master toggle is on.
5. *Optional switch:* A low-voltage outlet that is available for several uses. It may be used as a call switch, for wiring into the office vacuum pump control, or for other low-voltage electrical purposes.
6. *Accessory on/off toggle:* Controls the air and water shutoff valve for accessory equipment (Figure 20.8).

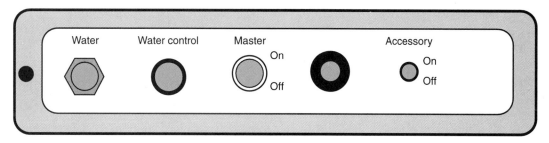

FIGURE 20.8
Controls for assistant's unit.

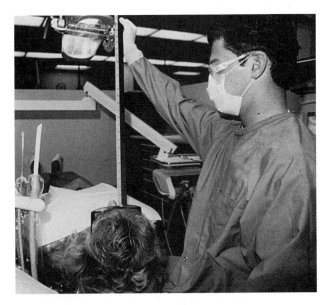

FIGURE 20.9
The best focal distance for the dental light is 24 to 30 inches from the patient's mouth.

Dental Light

The dental light should not interfere with patient or staff traffic patterns or with the seating and dismissing of patients from either side of the dental chair. A ceiling-mounted light is out of the way of the team and patients and is conveniently located for adjustment during procedures. It should be capable of being easily adjusted by the operator or the assistant from either side of the dental chair. This accommodates both right- and left-hand operatory setups, as well as dual and solo operating arrangements.

The assistant or operator projects and confines the beam to the oral cavity. The light should be kept in a downward position when not in use. When needed, it should be turned on and then raised slowly until it is projected on the mouth. The beam should never fall over the patient's eyes. The best focal distance for the dental light is 24 to 30 inches from the patient's mouth (Figure 20.9). This distance prevents the light from obstructing the operator or assistant and also reduces the effects of shadowing created when hands and instruments enter the field of operation.

Room Lighting

Room lighting also is important to patient comfort, because the patient faces the ceiling when placed in the full supine position. High-intensity ceiling lights can cause eye discomfort for patients during treatment, as well as shadows in the operatory. Perimeter, or border, lighting provides sufficient illumination and reduces eye discomfort for patients and staff.

Dental Cabinets

The dental operatory should have a minimum number of cabinets in order to maximize the work or traffic area. Sink cabinets located on both the operator's and the assistant's sides of the operatory increase utilization for both right- and left-handed setups. The cabinets should have the air, water, electricity, and vacuum utility connections for the operator's and assistant's units, and they should be 25 inches high. This is low enough for sit-down utilization, and it allows the operator or assistant to comfortably use the sink as needed. A knee control bar about 20 to 21 inches above the floor on each side of the sink is recommended so that the faucet can be activated without using the hands.

Waste Receptacles

Waste receptacles should be located in convenient areas and should have foot control lids. Sharps should be disposed of in approved containers, and contaminated materials should be disposed of in leak-proof approved bags.

FOUR-HANDED SIT-DOWN DENTISTRY

Four-handed sit-down dentistry and team dentistry increase the productivity of the practice while maintaining a high quality of dental services. These operating procedures minimize operator and staff fatigue and stress during delivery of dental treatment. The term **four-handed dentistry** refers to the procedures provided while an operator works with a dental assistant. During these procedures the dental assistant passes all dental instruments and supplies to the operator. **Sit-down dentistry** refers to procedures provided by the operator and chairside assistant while sitting down in a predetermined position or zone. The term *team* refers to the operator and

Four-handed dentistry
Procedures practiced while the dentist and dental assistant work together

Sit-down dentistry
Procedures provided by operators and chairside assistants while sitting down in a zone

Expanded duty dental assistant (EDDA)

A credential given to a dental assistant who has had additional training and therefore is allowed to perform certain intraoral procedures previously performed only by the dentist

Work simplification

The process of simplifying and standardizing all dental tasks

Motion economy

Involves minimizing body motions to accomplish tasks

staff, who work together to provide dental treatment. The title **expanded duty dental assistant (EDDA)** refers to a dental assistant with additional training to whom certain dental procedures, called advanced functions or expanded duties, are delegated. These procedures are duties that once were performed only by the dentist.

Quality dental care can be delivered efficiently through the use of four-handed sit-down dentistry, which is based on the principles of **work simplification** and **motion economy**. Four-handed dentistry organizes and standardizes every basic constituent of the dental practice in order to take maximum advantage of patient treatment time. For example, through patient diagnosis and treatment planning, a patient's appointments can be sequenced to take advantage of operator and staff time and energy. Because certain procedures are more difficult and time-consuming, it often is advantageous to schedule them in the morning, when the dentist and staff are rested, or to sequence them with less strenuous treatments.

Principles of Work Simplification

Four-handed dentistry supports the principles of work simplification, which involve simplifying and standardizing all dental tasks. For example, a 100% savings can be achieved by eliminating unnecessary equipment, instruments, procedural steps, and movements, and a 50% savings can be realized by combining steps in a procedure or by combining two instruments into one (Campbell, 1996). Equipment, patient schedules, and procedural steps can be rearranged to take greater advantage of time and space. The staff should always be alert for opportunities to simplify procedures and equipment and increase practice efficiency.

The objectives of four-handed dentistry are based on the use of trained allied dental personnel, who function as chairside dental assistants and as expanded function dental auxiliaries. The operator and chairside assistant use basic principles of motion economy to achieve comfort and minimize fatigue and stress during patient treatment. The expanded function dental assistant is trained to perform the highest level of procedures that can legally be delegated. This allows the dentist to concentrate on procedures that require a higher level of professional education, experience, and decision making.

Principles of Motion Economy

The basic principles of motion economy have been developed through time and motion studies. These principles include planning for the usual, not the unusual. They involve the use of body motions that require the least amount of time, thus minimizing the number of body motions needed to accomplish a task. This would include shortening the length of motions (the distance required to reach an object) and using smooth, continuous motions rather than inconsistent or zigzag motions. Motion economy includes treatment sequencing and prepositioning of instruments and materials according to their use in a particular dental procedure. Instruments and materials also should be located as close to the point of use as possible. For this reason, work surfaces, cabinet tops, trays, operating stools, and equipment should be designed and arranged for the greatest comfort and operational efficiency. In addition, good lighting is a primary requirement for enhancing the visual field. All these principles help minimize the number of eye fixations or eye movement.

Classification of Motions

Motions are classified into five categories, ranging from simple to complex.

- Class I motions involve movements of the fingers only.
- Class II motions involve movements of the fingers and wrist.
- Class III motions involve movements of the fingers, wrist, and elbow.
- Class IV motions involve movements of the entire arm from the shoulder.
- Class V motions involve movements of the arm and twisting of the body.

The operator and the chairside assistant should use class I, II, and III motions rather than class IV and V motions, which are the most time-consuming and fatiguing motions because they require gross muscular activity, refocusing, and reaccommodation of the eyes.

Assistant, Patient, and Operator Positioning

The objectives of a proper working position are (1) to ensure the comfort and safety of the patient and the operating team and (2) to obtain good visibility of and access to the operating site. The patient's well-being is most important in the delivery of dental treatment. Good isolation, oral evacuation, and effective operating techniques minimize the risk of the patient swallowing or aspirating dental materials or debris. The use of safety glasses by both the patient and the operating team can prevent eye injuries during dental treatment. In addition, a face mask or face shield provides an infection barrier and protects the dental team from saliva and water spray. Instruments and materials should be transferred only in the operating area. This further reduces the risk of dropping an instrument or dental materials into the patient's eyes or face.

The patient can be made comfortable, and safe access and visibility can be increased through patient, operator, and assistant positioning techniques. These techniques require an understanding and use of activity zones. Activity zones for the operating team are based on the positions of the operating team and equipment in relation to the patient's oral cavity. These zones are stated in terms of clock positions (Figures 20.10 and 20.11).

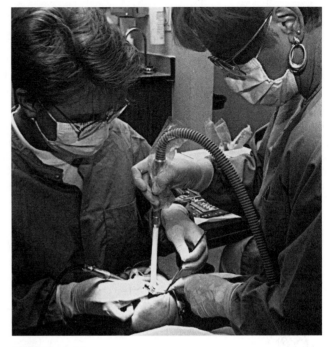

FIGURE 20.10

Four-handed dentistry. The principles of work simplification are applied through the use of allied dental personnel and four-handed sit-down dentistry.

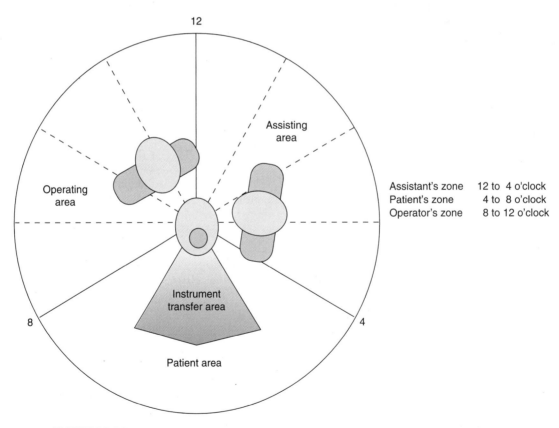

Assistant's zone   12 to 4 o'clock
Patient's zone   4 to 8 o'clock
Operator's zone   8 to 12 o'clock

FIGURE 20.11

Operator, assistant, and patient zones.

Patient's Zone

The patient's zone is located in the 4 to 8 o'clock position. This zone includes the "transfer area" because it is the area in which instrument transfer takes place. Careful use and preservation of this position is important because it keeps the instruments out of the patient's sight and reduces patient apprehension. It also allows the operator's hands and eyes to remain in the treatment area and reduces class V movements for the assistant. This area should be clear of obstructions so that patients can be easily seated and dismissed, and no fixed equipment should be placed over the patient. Teamwork is important, and each team member must be constantly aware of the others' activities in order to make adjustments as necessary and to permit maximum team functioning.

The patient is positioned in the dental chair such that the oral cavity is centered over the operator's lap at the height of the operator's elbow (Table 20.1). The operator's forearms should be parallel to the floor when the hands are in the working position in the oral cavity. The operator should not have to reach up to work in the oral cavity, because this can cause stress and discomfort to the operator's arms, shoulders, neck, and back muscles. Box 20.3 illustrates the procedure for seating patients.

Operator's Zone

The operator's zone is located in the 8 to 12 o'clock position. This zone is the primary area of activity for the dentist. The 8 o'clock position is seldom used when the patient is in the supine position because it places the operator in a long axis position to the patient and forces the operator to reach and lean with the elbow held high. The 9 o'clock position often is used for giving lower right quadrant anesthetic injections and for some prosthetic procedures. The 11 to 12 o'clock position is the primary operating area for most procedures (Figure 20.12).

The principles of four-handed dentistry emphasize work simplification and the adaptation of the work environment to the operator rather than adaptation of the operator to a fixed environment.

The operator should sit comfortably with the thighs parallel to the floor or the knees slightly raised. The back of the dental chair should rest on the operator's thigh with the patient's mouth in line with the operator's elbow and sagittal plane. The operator's shoulders and arms should be parallel to the floor, with the elbows close to the sides. The operator's back and neck should be relatively straight, which may require that the eyes be directed slightly downward. The distance from the operator's eyes to the patient's mouth should be no less than 14 inches. Some operators tend to bend forward during dental treatment. The operator should sit square on the stool, not on the edge, in a vertical position and should lean from the hips. This reduces pressure on the backs of the thighs and muscle fatigue from bending and compressing internal organs; it also allows the back of the

Box 20.3 *Procedure*

Procedure for Seating Patients

1. Before the patient is received, the dental chair should be in a ready position:
   - Place the dental chair seat at a comfortable height for the patient, approximately 17 inches from the floor.
   - Elevate the chair back to a comfortable sitting position.
   - Raise the arm of the chair.
2. Complete the following steps when seating the patient:
   - Indicate where the patient is to sit and assist the patient if necessary.
   - Once the patient has been seated, lower the arm of the chair.
   - Place the napkin and chain.
   - Provide the patient with safety glasses.
   - Elevate the chair base after letting the patient know what you are about to do.
   - Fully tilt the chair seat
   - Lower the backrest slowly to the horizontal position.
   - Adjust the patient's position to the proper location of the patient's head.
   - Lower the operating light so that it is within reach of the properly seated assistant.
   - Make special adjustments as necessary for patients with physical disabilities.

operator's stool to provide support to the small of the operator's back.

Assistant's Zone

The assistant's zone is located in the 12 to 4 o'clock position (see Figures 20.10 and 20.11). This is the primary activity area for the assistant. The central vacuum, air and water syringe, and assistant's cart with instruments, dental materials, and some equipment are located in this area to enable the

Table 20.1

Evaluation of Seating Patients

Seating Patients	4	3	2	0	X
Position dental chair					
Check height.					
Check chair back.					
Raise arm rest.					
Seat Patient					
Greet patient.					
Indicate seating.					
Lower arm rest.					
Place napkin and chain.					
Provide patient safety glasses.					
Elevate chair.					
Recline chair.					
Adjust patient.					
Adjust light.					
Assist patients with disabilities.					

The numeric criteria: 4 Excellent; 3 Good but some improvement can be made; 2 Below average, usable, needs to improve skill; 0 Unsatisfactory; X Not able to evaluate.

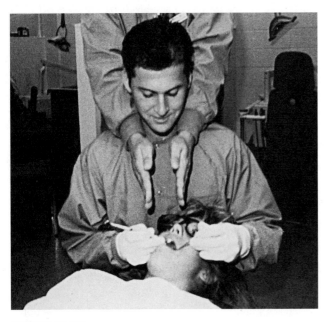

FIGURE 20.12

The operator's back and neck should be kept relatively straight with the eyes directed slightly downward toward the patient's mouth. The head should not be held at an angle.

chairside assistant to transfer instruments, retract, evacuate, and maintain visibility in the working area for the operator. To carry out the various chairside activities, the assistant must maintain a clear zone, must be able to see what opera-

tions are being performed, and must have access to the working area (oral cavity). The primary working position, which allows the chairside assistant access and visibility in all quadrants of the mouth, is the 3 to 4 o'clock position. The assistant's stool is placed as close to the dental chair as possible, with the edge of the stool that is toward the patient's head in line with the patient's oral cavity. The assistant's eye level should be 3 to 4 inches above the operator to enhance access and visibility. The assistant's neck and back should be relaxed but relatively straight, and the assistant should lean from the hips. The assistant's legs should be parallel to the side of the dental chair with the feet resting on the stool's foot support or on the floor.

PRINCIPLES OF MATERIAL AND INSTRUMENT HANDLING

Efficient storage and manipulation of materials and handling of instruments are work simplification principles that can help the chairside assistant eliminate unnecessary activity and improve overall efficiency.

Storage of Materials Chairside

Materials should be stored as close to the working area as possible. However, because of facility space design, most operatories are rather small and compact. This means that only frequently used materials should be stored in the most easily accessible areas of the assistant's cabinet. Containers should be the minimal practical size so that a limited amount of all necessary materials can be kept in the assistant's cabinet. These materials could include precapsulated amalgam and small bottles of cements. Color-coded or labeled trays and tubs for dental materials can be prearranged, set up for specific procedures, and made readily accessible within the operatory. Color coding aids in easy identification. Materials can be premeasured or prepackaged according to the amount needed for particular procedures.

Manipulation of Materials Chairside

Efficiency can also be improved at chairside by anticipating the operator's needs and preparing, delivering, and cleaning up materials in a limited amount of time with a minimum amount of motion. Because dental materials are prepared immediately before use, the assistant must be able to anticipate when the operator will actually need the material. The assistant also can move the tray or tub to the upper right side of the assistant's cabinet so that the material can be prepared and manipulated on the lower left side of the cabinet. This allows the material to be mixed closer to the area of operation and passed a shorter distance. The assistant should hold the prepared material in the right hand and deliver it to the operator within the transfer zone as near to the patient's mouth as practical. By holding the material in the right hand, the assistant keeps the left hand free to transfer instruments, wipe the mirror, or suction if necessary.

Disposable items such as mixing pads, spatulas, cups, and suction tips should be used as often as practical to eliminate cleanup procedures. Disposable items are placed in waste receptacles immediately after use. Nondisposable spatulas and placement instruments, as well as the cutting instruments, should be wiped clean of debris immediately after use and taken immediately to the sterilization area after dismissal of the patient. The assistant's cabinet top and instrument tray should be kept clean and in order throughout the dental procedure.

Standardized Tray Setups and Procedures

Prepared standardized tray systems offer an effective way to increase both office efficiency and staff confidence and morale. They allow the dentist and staff to concentrate on patient care rather than operational procedures. Standardized tray setups provide a disciplined approach to infectious disease control and at the same time promote greater efficiency during dental treatment.

Tray Setups

Standardized tray setups use several different types of trays on which to place the instruments.

> ## Box 20.4
> ### Benefits of Standardized Tray Setups
>
> - Efficiency can be increased and stress decreased during patient treatment by having sterile, organized instrument setups ready for immediate use by the operator and chairside assistant.
> - The time saved and the efficiency of operation afforded by use of an instrument management and infection control system can promote patient satisfaction and confidence.
> - Standardized tray setups are adaptable to any dental procedure and any dental office.
> - Clean up, processing, and preparation of operatory are reduced no matter the number of operatories.
> - Tray setup systems are relatively inexpensive.
> - Income can be increased and more patients can be seen with less effort.
> - The effort, time, and cost involved in training allied dental personnel can be reduced.

- *Open operational or surgical trays* are available in a variety of colored resins and stainless steel. They may be plain, flat trays with raised sides or may have molded instrument holders. Removable rubber or resin instrument holders are available for the plain flat tray. The trays are set up with selected, sterilized loose instruments or packaged instruments and supplies (Box 20.4 and Table 20.2).
- *Cassette trays* (Figure 20.13) are made of lightweight resin or stainless steel. They are designed with removable rails (plastic instrument holders), which can be adapted to small or large setups. Cassettes have locking covers that secure the instruments in place. Instruments are placed in the tray rails according to use and are used directly from the tray (Box 20.5 and Table 20.3).

The cassette trays are prepared by coding or indexing each cassette and selecting the most commonly used instruments for each dental procedure, coding the instruments by procedure, and placing them in the indexed trays. Color coding can be done for instruments, trays, treatment procedures, and operatory rooms.

Tray setups should have all items needed for each dental procedure, and double-ended instruments should be used whenever possible to reduce the number of instruments on the tray.

Assembly, Delivery, and Return of Instruments

Tray setups should be assembled in a central sterilization area in the dental office. Each setup should include the cassette with standardized instrument selection, sterilized handpieces, adapters (if necessary), and angles. A bur brush

Table 20.2

Identifying Instruments and Materials for Tray Setups

Process	Procedure	Instruments and Material
Patient preparation	Examination	Napkin, mirror, explorer, cotton forceps, eye protection
	Topical anesthetic	Cotton applicator, anesthetic spray, disposable needle, syringe
Amalgam procedures	Rubber dam	Instruments, material, clamps, floss, lubricant
	Moisture control	Suction tip, air, water, and syringe tips
	Cutting	Burs, bur block, changing tool, hand-cutting instruments
	Matrix application	Retainer, band, wedges, application burnisher
	Lining/base	Varnish, liner/base, mixing pad or slab, spatula, placement instruments and other items
	Amalgam placement	Amalgamator, alloy, placement mercury, dappen dish, carrier, pluggers
	Carving	Carvers, burnisher
	Occlusal check	Articulating paper, holder
	Oral debris removal	Aspirator tip
	Waste removal	Container for sharps and other materials

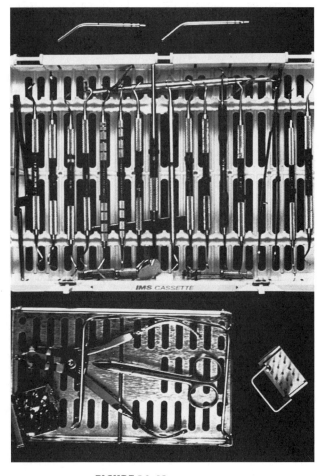

FIGURE 20.13

Cassette instrument system.

Box 20.5

Benefits of the Cassette Tray System

- After completion of the procedure, the instruments are checked for removal of any heavy debris and then secured and sterilized directly in the cassette.
- Cassette trays can be sterilized by steam autoclave, chemical vapor, or gas, and they fit into most dental office sterilizers.
- Cassette systems reduce cross-contamination by the dental assistant handling the instruments; instrument damage resulting from handling and dropping, as well as replacement costs; and instrument processing time.

should be included. The assembled tray setups should be labeled, dated, and stored in an appropriate area away from dirty instruments and trays. The tray should be placed in the operatory just before the start of dental treatment, and the sterilization wrap should not be removed until the operator is ready to begin the procedure. The chairside assistant should do a quick inspection to ensure that all instruments are on the tray. Additional instruments should be packaged, labeled, and available to the operator and chairside assistant in case of unanticipated needs during treatment procedures.

At the end of dental treatment and after the patient has been dismissed, the chairside assistant should inspect the tray setup carefully to make sure that all instruments have been counted and placed on the tray in the standard arrangement. If a cassette is used, the lid must be closed and

Table 20-3

Suggested Standardized Cassette Tray Setups

Cassette Type	Setup	Instruments and Material
Preventative	Examination	Cassette, mirror/handle, explorers, probe, dressing pliers, suction tip
Periodontic	Prophy/sealant	Cassette, mirror/handle, explorer, dressing pliers, sickle scalers, curette, sealant brush/handle, pumice cup, prophy angle, suction tip
	Small prophy	Cassette, mirror/handle, explorer, sickle scalers, curettes, pumice cup, prophy angle, suction tip
	Large prophy	Cassette, mirror/handle, explorers, probe, sickle scalers, curettes, sealant brush handle, dressing pliers, sharpening stones, pumice cup, prophy angle, suction tip, aspirating syringe, A/W syringe tip, cassette clip
	Root planing	Cassette, mirror/handle, explorers, probe, sickle scalers, root planing curettes, curettes, dressing pliers, sharpening stones, pumice cup, prophy angle, suction tip, aspirating syringe, A/W syringe tip, cassette clip
Restorative	Amalgam	Cassette, mirror/handle, explorer, excavator, cavity preparation, placement instruments, amalgam carrier, amalgam plugger, cleoid-discoid, carvers, burnishers, dressing pliers, accessory boxes with clamps, matrix, retainer, and other items, bur stand with burs, rubber dam forceps, articulation forceps, amalgam well, rubber dam punch, suction tip, aspirating syringe, A/W syringe tips, cassette clip
	Composite	Cassette, mirror/handle, explorer, excavator, cavity preparation, placement instruments, composite brush handle, carvers, burnisher, gingival retractor, plastic filling, wax carver, cosmetic contouring, dressing pliers, bur stand with burs, articulation forceps, parts box with clamps, rubber dam forceps, rubber dam punch, gingival cord packer, suction tip, aspirating syringe, A/W syringe tip, cassette clip
	Universal amalgam/composite	Cassette, mirror/handle, explorer, excavator, cavity preparation, placement instruments, composite brush handle, amalgam carrier, amalgam plugger, cleoid-discoid, composite filling, burnishers, dressing pliers, accessory boxes with clamps, matrix, retainer, and other items, bur stand with burs articulation forceps, amalgam well, rubber dam forceps, rubber dam punch, gingival cord packer, suction tip, aspirating syringe, A/W syringe tip, cassette clip

Continued

Table 20-3—Cont'd

Suggested Standardized Cassette Tray Setups

Cassette Type	Setup	Instruments and Material
	Crown and bridge	Cassette, mirror/handle, explorer, probe, excavator, dressing pliers, cord packer, spatula, carver, plastic filling, cement remover, cavity preparation, scissors, bur stand, articulating forceps, crown remover, suction tip, aspirating syringe, A/W syringe tip, cassette clip
	Porcelain veneer placement	Cassette, mirror/handle, explorer, dressing pliers, gingival cord packer, brush handle, spatula, cement remover, articulating forceps, scissors, bur stand and burs, crown remover, suction tip, aspirating syringe, A/W syringe tip, cassette clip
	Endodontic	Cassette, mirror/handle, explorer, probe, endodontic explorer, endodontic pliers, excavator, spreader, root forceps, plastic filling, stainless steel ruler, endodontic pluggers, bur stand and burs, parts box, rubber dam clamps, rubber dam forceps, endodontic box, suction tip, aspirating syringe, A/W syringe tip, cassette clip
Surgical	Peridontal surgery Cassette I	Cassette, mirror/handle, explorer, probe, furcation probe, periodontal chisels, periosteal elevator, periodontal file, periodontal knives, surgical curette, dressing pliers, tissue pliers, aspirator handle/tip, rongeurs, suction tip, aspirating syringes, A/W syringe tip, cassette clip
	Cassette II	Cassette, cheek retractor, scalpel handle, root planing curettes, curettes, hemostat, scissors, needle holders, suture scissors, scalpel blade remover
	Extraction	Cassette, mirror/handle, scalpel handle, periosteal elevator, root tip elevators, surgical curette, bone file, dressing pliers, irrigation syringe, cheek retractor, mouth props and gags, scalpel blade remover, crown remover, suction tip, aspirating syringe, A/W syringe tip, cassette clip
	Suture removal	Cassette, mirror/handle, dressing pliers, scissors, curette, suction tip
	General practice periodontal surgery	Cassette, mirror/handle, explorer, furcation probe, periodontal knives, periosteal elevator, periodontal file, root planing curettes, curettes, chisels, scalpel handle, dressing pliers, tissue pliers, needle holder, scissors, scalpel blade remover, hemostat, rongeurs, suture scissors, suction tip, aspirating syringe, A/W syringe tip, cassette clip

A/W, Air and water.
Courtesy Hu-Friedy.

secured. The lid must not be forced close if the hinges bind, because this reduces their durability and may break the hinges. Burs and the air and water syringe tips also must be placed back on the tray; small instruments and burs often are thrown away by accident. Instruments should be inspected routinely to see if they are dull, bent, or broken. If necessary, they should be sharpened or replaced (see Chapter 19 for sharpening procedures).

Aspirating syringes should be disassembled in the sterilization area. Instruments and handpieces should be washed with soap and water to remove gross debris and cement as soon as possible (heavy utility gloves are used for this purpose). Burs should be brushed under water to remove debris (for further information, see Chapter 19). All disposable materials should be placed in proper containers, not on the cassettes or trays.

PRACTICE EFFICIENCY METHODS AND INSTRUMENT APPLICATION

The dental assistant must understand the terms *efficiency* and *effectiveness* as they relate to the practice of dentistry. Efficiency refers to the output (energy and time) required to produce quality dental care with minimum waste, expense, or unnecessary effort. Effectiveness, on the other hand, refers to the ability to achieve desired results; it is doing the right things. Practicing efficiency methods is important in the dental office.

Managing Instrumentation Techniques

The management of instruments involves reducing or eliminating unnecessary movement of the operator and assistant through standardized instrument transfer and material handling methods. In other words, the chairside dental assistant can save time by not having to reach back and forth to the cabinet for instruments, thus interrupting the flow of treatment procedures. This can be accomplished first by proper positioning of the operator, patient, and assistant and then by using appropriate techniques, such as establishing a secure instrument grasp and finger rest position, developing a hand instrument transfer system, properly using the mouth mirror to retract appropriate intraoral soft tissues, and properly placing the oral evacuation tip.

Instrument Grasp

A stable grasp of the dental instrument is essential for controlling movement and maintaining a firm fulcrum (finger rest). Dental instruments are exchanged and dental materials are prepared so frequently during procedures that the operating team must use efficient methods of instrument transfer to reduce fatigue and stress. The smooth transfer of instruments during dental treatment requires more coordination and communication between the oper-

ator and the assistant than any other facet of clinical practice.

The appropriate grasp for the dental instrument is firm but not tight or rigid, because this would lessen the tactile sensitivity and effectiveness of instrumentation and cause fatigue to the operator's fingers, hand, and arm. A firm grasp increases fingertip tactile sensitivity and allows for good control and flexibility of the dental instrument. The operator must be able to feel any irregularities on the tooth surface with the explorer; a tight or rigid grasp would eliminate this sensitivity. The operator also must have a firm grasp on the instrument to be able to rotate and turn it without dropping it.

The three basic types of instrument grasps are the pen grasp, the palm grasp, and the palm-thumb grasp. Most hand instruments are used with the pen grasp or modified pen grasp. Forceps are used primarily with a palm grasp, and hand-cutting instruments, such as chisels, are used with a palm grasp.

A general rule for using instruments with a pen grasp is to pass the working end of the instrument toward the operator so that it may be grasped and used at the operative site with the same grip. Hand instruments used with the palm grasp (e.g., forceps, scissors, and syringes) should be passed with the handle toward the operator. The operating team should practice instrument transfers until they feel comfortable with them.

Pen Grasp

The conventional pen grasp, the one used for writing, concentrates the point of support of the pen on one location where the fingertips cover the pen tip area. However, because considerable more pressure and force are needed in dentistry, the modified pen grasp provides four points of support to be applied to the instrument. This allows for more control of the dental instrument.

Modified Pen Grasp

The modified pen grasp (Figure 20.14) is the basic instrument grasp. It supplies up to four points of support, allowing good instrument control and providing the ability to apply considerable force to the instrument. The instrument is supported by four control points: the balls of the thumb and the first finger, the end of the second finger, and the side of the third finger. Some have difficulty holding the instrument securely using the four pressure points while maintaining a stable finger rest or fulcrum. In such a case three points of support are satisfactory, which allows the third finger to be used for the fulcrum. The small finger can be used to support the third finger or extended out of the way. The key is to have good support for the instrument and a good, solid finger rest.

Palm Grasp

The palm grasp (Figure 20.15) has limited application and is used primarily as a power grasp. The handle of the instrument is held in the palm of the hand with the fingers in a

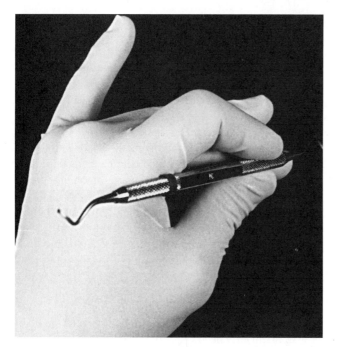

FIGURE 20.14
Modified pen grasp.

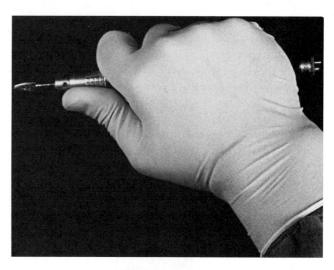

FIGURE 20.16
Palm-thumb grasp.

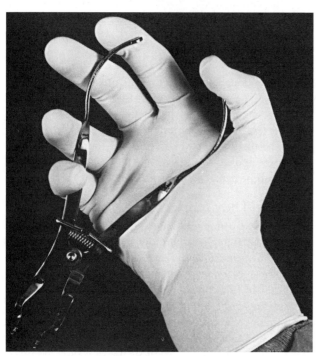

FIGURE 20.15
Palm grasp.

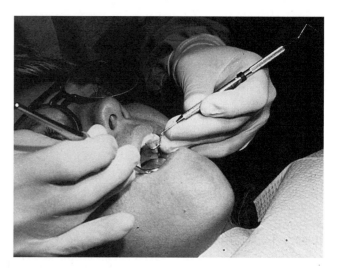

FIGURE 20.17
For dental procedures in the maxillary central incisor area, the operator uses a "mirror" and a finger rest or fulcrum on the right premolar occlusal area and an "explorer" and a finger rest on the left premolar occlusal area.

cupped position. The thumb acts as a pivot or fulcrum point of control.

Palm-Thumb Grasp

The palm-thumb grasp (Figure 20.16) is used with straight instruments, such as the straight chisels, for applying pressure.

Finger Rest Position (Fulcrum)

A finger rest position (Figure 20.17) is also referred to as a *fulcrum*. A fulcrum must always be used when instruments are placed on the teeth with any amount of pressure. The purpose of the fulcrum is to act as a point of support and rest from which to manipulate or rotate the fingers and instrument. It provides stability and helps the operator control the instrument. This stability prevents injury to oral tissues and therefore patient comfort and safety. The operator will feel more secure in manipulating instruments when a good finger rest has been established.

When the three-finger pen grasp is used, the ring finger maintains the fulcrum position. The fingers are slightly curved for relaxation and support. The fulcrum must be maintained on firm, solid tooth structure. The patient's lip, chin, or cheek should not be used for a finger rest because these tissues are too soft and flexible. Whenever possible, the finger rest should be in the same arch (maxillary or mandibular) and the same quadrant (right or left) as the tooth receiving treatment (Table 20.4). The fulcrum finger must maintain a firm hold with moderate pressure to secure the instrument when force is applied. Too much pressure on the finger rest can result in finger fatigue and less control of the instrument. For example, heavy pressure on the movable mandible can cause fatigue to the jaw and discomfort for the patient. The maxillary, on the other hand, is stationary and offers an excellent finger rest. A fulcrum on the maxillary teeth should be used whenever possible for maxillary instrumentation because of this stability and patient comfort.

Instrument Transfer

Instrument transfer takes place in the transfer area, which is below the patient's mouth in the patient's zone. Transferring instruments in this area keeps the instruments out of the patient's sight, provides a system of transfer that prevents instrument collision between the operator and assistant, and serves as a safety measure in case an instrument or medication is dropped. This system of instrument transfer reduces the number and types of motions and allows the operator to maintain finger rest while focusing the eyes only on the work site.

As the operator and assistant develop skills in instrument transfer, the operator must inform the assistant of his or her needs before treatment. As the team becomes more proficient, the assistant comes to anticipate the operator's needs. If the operator decides to use a new material or technique, the assistant must be informed of these changes ahead of time to maintain a high-quality treatment system.

The hand instrument exchange consists of five phases: (1) the signal, (2) the approach, (3) the retrieval, (4) the delivery, and (5) the withdrawal:

The Signal

The operator maintains the finger rest position while holding the instrument with the modified pen grasp and signals readiness to transfer by lifting the instrument from the oral cavity with the fingers only (class I) movement. The instrument is released by the operator as the assistant draws it

away and the new instrument is placed into the working position (Figure 20.18).

The Approach

The assistant selects the instrument to be delivered with the left hand and holds it with a pen grasp (between the thumb and first and second fingers) along the end of the shank opposite the end to be used by the operator. The instrument is held with the working end of the instrument pointed toward the tooth being treated and the cutting end of the instrument pointed up if treating the maxillary or down if treating the mandible. The assistant holds the instrument in a ready position 8 to 10 inches from the oral cavity. When the operator signals, the assistant places the left hand next to the operator's working hand with the new instrument parallel to and about 1 inch above the operator's instrument. The assistant extends the small finger of the left hand in readiness to grasp the used instrument from the operator. This prevents tangling and collision of instruments during transfer (Figure 20.19).

The Retrieval

The assistant firmly grasps the used instrument with the small finger and draws it out of the operator's hand. While the assistant lifts the hand slightly above the operator's hand, the pickup finger is rotated into the palm (Figure 20.20).

The Delivery

After the assistant folds the retrieved instrument into the palm, the new instrument is delivered by lowering it into the operator's fingers and releasing it in the same working position. Once the operator has the new instrument, the assistant (1) holds the used instrument between the little finger and ring finger, (2) tips the palm of the hand parallel to the floor, (3) pushes the instrument into the palm with the working end of the instrument toward the body, (4) places the thumb under the instrument shaft, (5) grasps the instrument between the thumb and index finger, and (6) rotates (baton) it out of the grasp of the little finger onto the top of the hand between the thumb and first two fingers (modified pen grasp position). The instrument is held about 1 inch from its nonworking end in readiness for the next delivery (Figure 20.21).

The Withdrawal

If the procedure has been completed, the assistant withdraws the retrieved instrument and returns it to the standardized sequence on the cassette (Figure 20.22).

Exercises for the Hand

Because dentistry requires frequent, repetitive movements of the wrist, hand, and fingers to grip and use instruments, the dentist and staff are more likely to have numbness or tingling in the fingers and hands, as well as aching or numb fingers, hands, or forearms. Direct pressure over the carpal

Table 20.4

Guidelines for Mirror and Finger Rests

These general guidelines are provided to assist the operator in gaining visibility and access in any area of the mouth while following the principles of four-handed sitdown dentistry.

Area of operation	Visualization	Operator's position	Patient's chair position	Patient's head position	Retraction	Finger rest	Suctioning
Upper right posterior teeth							
Buccal	Direct	10-11	Backrest horizontal	Turned toward assistant, straight, chin elevated slightly	Operator–Left index finger	Handpiece head on left index finger	Lingual
Occlusal	Indirect	11	Backrest horizontal	Straight, chin elevated slightly	Operator–Right third finger	Buccal surface of right posterior teeth	Lingual
Palatal	Indirect	10-11	Backrest horizontal	Turned toward operator, chin elevated	Operator–Left index finger	Buccal surface of posterior teeth	Lingual, posterior
Upper anterior teeth							
Labial	Direct	11	Backrest horizontal	Straight, chin elevated slightly	Operator–Left index finger	Occlusal surface of right bicuspid teeth or incisal surface of anterior teeth	Lingual, opposite
Palatal	Indirect	11	Backrest horizontal	Straight, chin elevated slightly	Assistant retracts with left index finger or mirror with solo operator.	Occlusal surface of right bicuspid teeth or edge of incisal teeth	Labial, opposite
Upper left posterior teeth							
Buccal	Direct	10-11	Backrest horizontal	Turned toward operator, chin elevated lightly	Operator–Left index finger	Anterior incisal edge of anterior teeth	Buccal, posterior
Occlusal	Indirect	9-11	Backrest horizontal	Turned toward operator	Assistant retracts with left index finger or mirror with solo operator	Occlusal surface of right cuspid or bicuspid teeth	Buccal
Palatal	Direct	9-10	Backrest horizontal	Turned toward assistant, chin elevated slightly	Assistant retracts with left index finger or mirror or left index finger with solo operator	Labial surface of lower anterior teeth	Lingual, posterior

Lower left posterior teeth

Surface	Vision	Position	Chair	Head position	Retraction	Illumination	Mirror
Buccal	Direct	11	Backrest horizontal	Turned toward operator	Operator–Left index finger on mirror.	Labial surface of lower anterior teeth	Buccal, posterior
Occlusal	Direct	10-11	Backrest horizontal	Straight, chin elevated	Assistant retracts buccal tissues. *Solo mirror.	Labial surface of lower anterior teeth	Buccal
Lingual	Direct	10-11	Seat and backrest horizontal	Turned slightly toward assistant	Operator retracts dam or tongue with mirror. Assistant retracts buccal tissues.	Labial surface of lower anterior teeth	Buccal

Lower anterior teeth

Surface	Vision	Position	Chair	Head position	Retraction	Illumination	Mirror
Labial	Direct	11	Backrest horizontal	Straight or turned slightly toward operator or assistant	Operator retracts lower lip with thumb and index finger.	Buccal surface of lower right cuspid or bicuspid teeth	Lingual, opposite
Lingual	Direct and indirect	11	Backrest horizontal	Straight or turned slightly toward operator or assistant	Operator retracts tongue with back of mirror.	Buccal surface of lower right cuspid or bicuspid teeth	Lingual, opposite

Lower right posterior teeth

Surface	Vision	Position	Chair	Head position	Retraction	Illumination	Mirror
Buccal	Direct	9-10	Backrest horizontal	Straight or turned slightly toward assistant	Operator–Left index finger	Labial surface of lower anterior teeth	Lingual
Occlusal	Direct	11	Backrest horizontal	Turned slightly toward operator, chin lowered slightly	Operator–Left index finger and assistant retracts tongue with mirror	Buccal surface of lower posterior teeth	Lingual
Lingual	Direct	11-12	Backrest horizontal	Maximally turned toward operator, chin slightly elevated	Operator retracts tongue with mirror.	Buccal surface of lower posterior teeth	Lingual, posterior

*Expressed as positions on a clock face.

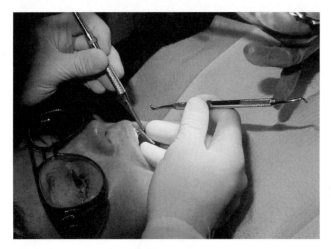

FIGURE 20.18
Signal.

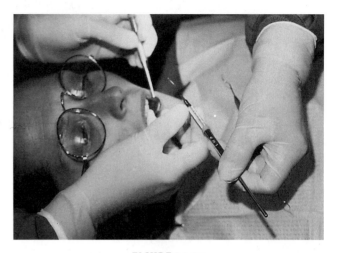

FIGURE 20.21
Delivery.

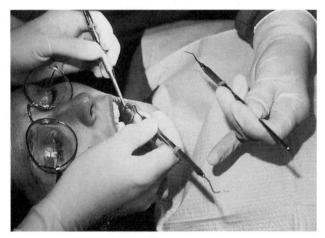

FIGURE 20.19
Approach.

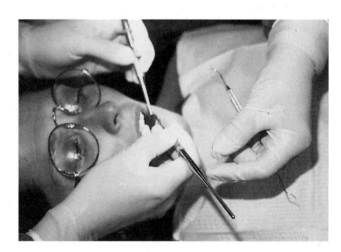

FIGURE 20.22
Withdrawal.

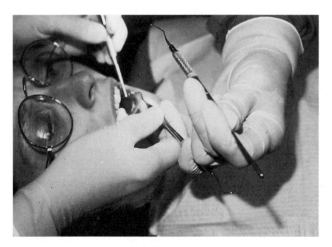

FIGURE 20.20
Retrieval.

tunnel and mechanical stress to the fingers, hands, and wrists can cause carpal tunnel syndrome. The dental assistant should take a few minutes intermittently to reevaluate body positioning techniques and procedures. Stressful tasks should be rotated, and breaks should be taken regularly to relax the fingers and hands (Figure 20.23). Daily warm-up exercises for the hands and fingers, as well as other preventive measures, can help reduce stress and prevent the development of compression neuropathies.

Mouth Mirror Use and Soft Tissue Retraction

The mouth mirror is available in many sizes and has several purposes. It provides indirect vision, such as allowing the operator to view the work area in the maxillary arch without bending or twisting the neck and body (class V

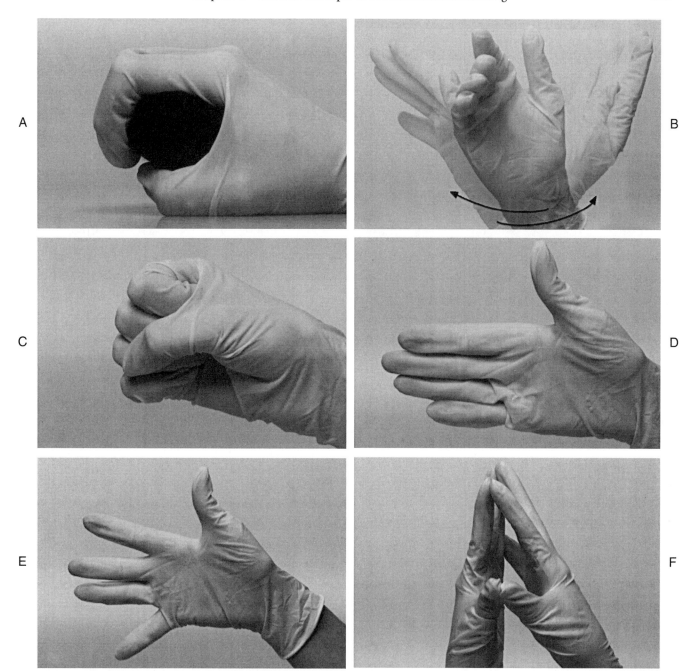

FIGURE 20.23

Exercises for relaxing the hands and fingers. **A,** Hand, finger, and palm muscle massage: Using a flexible exercise handball, gently rotate and massage the ball for approximately 3 to 5 minutes in each hand. **B,** Wrist and arm rotation: First with the right arm raised and then with it lowered along side, rotate the hand at the wrist 15 times clockwise and 15 times counterclockwise. Repeat with the left hand. **C-E,** Hand, thumb, and finger hyperextension: Make a snug fist, with the fingers in the palm of the hand and the thumb extended over the fingers; tighten the grasp. From this position, extend the thumb up and open the fingers, keeping them together; then stretch the fingers as far apart as comfortable. Do this 15 times with the right hand and repeat with the left hand. **F,** Finger and thumb pressure: Place the fingers and thumbs together, with the palms facing each other. Gently press the fingers and thumbs against each other and then release the pressure. Do 15 repetitions.

movements). It also allows the operator to provide indirect illumination by reflecting the light from the overhead dental lamp onto the tooth surface. Because the anterior teeth are translucent, the mouth mirror also is used for transillumination (Figure 20.24). This means that the operator can reflect light through the anterior teeth to check for decay. The mouth mirror is used to retract the cheeks and tongue, which allows better vision into the work area of the mouth. The operator and assistant also use their gloved fingers (usually the index or third finger) to retract the cheek. Table 20.4 presents further information on retraction.

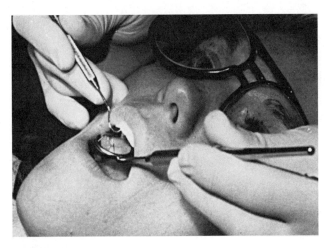

FIGURE 20.24

The mouth mirror is used for indirect vision, indirect illumination, and transillumination and for retraction of the cheeks and tongue.

Oral Evacuation

The operator must have visibility and access in all areas of the mouth during dental treatment. Proper use of a rubber dam aids in achieving greater access to the area of treatment, visibility, and infection control (see Chapter 33 for more details on the use of a rubber dam). An high-velocity evacuator also is used to keep water and debris from accumulating in the field of operation and can be used to retract the cheek and tongue. This evacuation system works on the vacuum principle, which involves suctioning the water and debris from the patient's mouth. The high-velocity suction force and an improperly placed HVE tip (also called the suction or vacuum tip) can "catch" and injure the very delicate soft tissues of the mouth. For this reason, it is essential that the dental assistant understand the use of the suction tip and become proficient in placement techniques.

Placement of the High-Efficiency Evacuation Tip

The most commonly used HVE tip is made of disposable plastic. Metal tips that can be autoclaved are also used. The tips are contoured and have slanted openings at both ends; this slant allows the tip to be adapted to either the maxillary or the mandibular arch and either right or left.

The suction tip is attached to the HVE hose, which is connected to the evacuation system. The assistant must be careful not to touch the soft palate with the suction tip because this could cause the patient to gag. To avoid this, the assistant should always make sure that the tip is held securely and rests with the extended back of the opening on hard tooth structure or is placed firmly against the tongue or other firm tissue. If soft tissue is caught in the suction tip, the assistant carefully rotates the tip while dropping the hose end of the

A 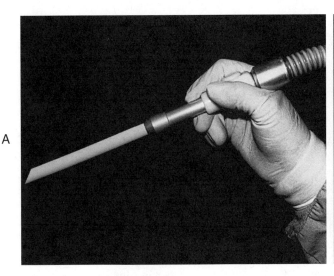 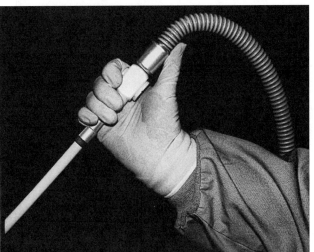 B

FIGURE 20.25

High-velocity evacuator (HVE) grasp. **A,** Modified pen grasp (general grasp). **B,** Palm-thumb grasp, often called the "thumb to nose" grasp.

tube until the suction breaks. The oral evacuator can be turned off if necessary.

The dental assistant holds the vacuum tip in the right hand with a modified pen grasp (Figure 20.25, *A*) or the reverse palm-thumb grasp (Figure 20.25, *B*); the hose is held under the assistant's right arm next to the body. This arrangement gives the assistant maximum control of the HVE tip and hose.

It often is easier for the operator to allow the assistant to enter the mouth with the HVE tip first, to "get into position" (Figure 20.26, *A* and *B*), and then to enter with the handpiece and mouth mirror. The HVE tip is positioned by placing the opening of the tip next to the site of treatment while using the side of the tip to retract the tongue or cheek. The assistant must be careful to keep the tip out of the operator's "visionary area" (see Table 20.4 for suctioning tip placement).

GENERAL GUIDELINES FOR VISIBILITY AND ACCESS TO THE ORAL CAVITY

The area of treatment in the oral cavity determines the operator's position and the positions of the patient's head and the dental chair. The area of treatment also determines whether the operator will have direct or indirect visual access, the manner in which the tissue is retracted, and the finger rest position. In addition, it determines the placement of the oral evacuation tip by the dental assistant.

NOTE: Use of a rubber dam eliminates the need to retract the cheek and tongue.

Table 20.4 presents general guidelines that can help the operator and chairside dental assistant gain visibility and access to any area of the mouth while following the principles of four-handed sit-down dentistry.

A 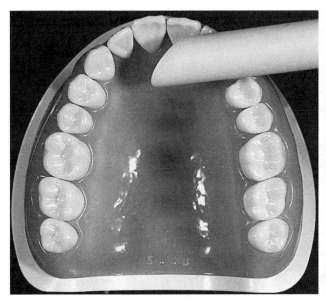 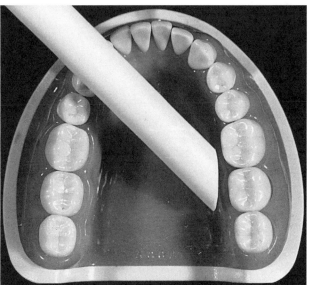 B

FIGURE 20.26

General placement of the high-velocity evacuation (HVE) tip. HVE placement is a critical task for the dental assistant in all restorative procedures. **A,** Upper and lower anterior HVE top placement. The HVE tip is placed opposite the operator's working area; that is, the tip is placed labial to anterior teeth when the working area involves the lingual surface. **B,** Upper and lower posterior HVE tip placement. The HVE tip generally can be placed near the lower buccal or lingual molar area when the working area involves a posterior tooth surface.

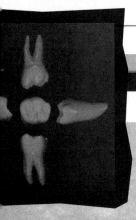

Points for Review

- Criteria for selecting and using dental equipment
- Four-handed sit-down dentistry
- Principles of material and instrument handling
- Standardized tray setups and procedures
- Practice efficiency methods
- Instrument application

Self-Study Questions

1. Identify the criteria that is *not* essential for selecting a chairside assistant's unit.
   a. Can be used by right- or left-handed operators
   b. Provides a work surface that can be placed over the assistant's legs
   c. Has two drawers for storage
   d. Is height adjustable

2. What is the proper operating zones for the assistant?
   a. 8 to 12 o'clock
   b. 12 to 4 o'clock
   c. 4 to 8 o'clock
   d. 12 to 2 o'clock

3. What is the general objective of four-handed sit-down dentistry?
   a. To minimize operator fatigue and stress during delivery of dental services
   b. To enhanced patient safety
   c. To increase patient comfort
   d. To avoid collision of instruments

4. What is the classification of motions that involves movement of the fingers and wrist?
   a. Class I
   b. Class II
   c. Class III
   d. Class IV

5. What is the effect of a proper instrument grasp?
   a. Decreased fingertip tactile sensitivity
   b. Transfer out of the patient's sight
   c. Enhanced patient safety and less postoperative discomfort
   d. Fatigue in the operator's fingers, hand, and arm

6. What type of instrument grasp is used for condensing an amalgam?
   a. Pen grasp
   b. Modified pen grasp
   c. Palm grasp
   d. Palm-thumb grasp

7. What is the purpose of a well-established fulcrum?
   a. Stability for controlled action of the instrument
   b. Oral tissue injury
   c. Minimal operator fatigue and stress
   d. Increased productivity

8. What is the main purpose of a mouth mirror?
   a. Patient safety
   b. Prevention of oral tissue damage
   c. Direct vision
   d. Indirect illumination

9. What is the purpose of proper instrument transfer?
   a. To avoid collision of instruments
   b. Patient comfort
   c. Stability
   d. Increased productivity

10. What instrument transfer involves grasping the used instrument with the small finger and drawing it out of the operator's hand?
    a. Signal
    b. Approach
    c. Retrieval
    d. Delivery

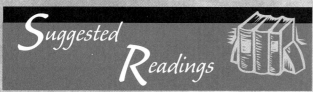

Suggested *Readings*

Barton RE, Matteson SR, Richardson, RE: *The dental assistant,* ed 6, Philadelphia, 1988, Lea & Febiger.

Campbell E et al: *Practice management,* Louisville, Ky, 1996, University of Louisville School of Dentistry.

Castana FA, Alden BA: *Handbook of clinical dental auxiliary practice,* ed 2, Philadelphia, 1980, JB Lippincott.

Charbeneau GT et al: *Principles and practice of operative dentistry,* ed 3, Philadelphia, 1988, Lea & Febiger.

Ciancio SG, editor: Oral irrigation: a current perspective, *Biol Thera Dentistry* 3:33, 1988.

Finkbeiner BL, Johnson CS: *Mosby's comprehensive dental assisting: a clinical approach,* St Louis, 1995, Mosby.

Green EJ, Brown ME: Body mechanics applied to the practice of dentistry, *J Am Dent Assoc* 67:679, 1963.

Kilpatrick HC: *Functional dental assisting,* Philadelphia, 1977, WB Saunders.

Miyasaki-Ching CM: *Chasteen's essentials of clinical dental assisting,* ed 5, St Louis, 1997, Mosby.

Reap CA: *Complete handbook for dental auxiliaries,* Chicago, 1981, Quintessence Publishing.

Robinson GE et al: *Four-handed dentistry manual,* ed 6, Birmingham, 1990, University of Alabama School of Dentistry.

Spohn EE, Halowski WA, Berry TG: *Operative dentistry procedure for dental auxiliaries,* St Louis, 1981, Mosby.

Sturdevant CM et al: *The art and science of operative dentistry,* ed 3, St Louis, 1995, Mosby.

Torres HO, Ehrlich A: *Modern dental assisting,* ed 6, Philadelphia, 1999, WB Saunders.

Waterman GE: Effective use of dental assistants, *Public Health Rep* 67:390, 1952.

Chapter 21

Oral Diagnosis and Treatment Planning

Key Points

- Patient history
- Clinical examination
- Charting oral conditions
- Treatment planning and presentation

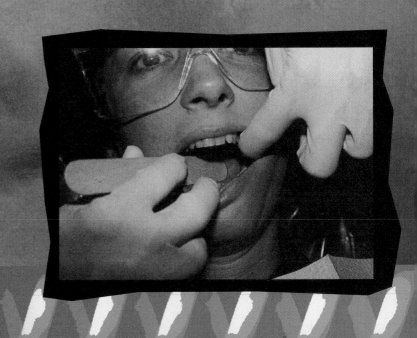

Chapter Outline

Learning Objectives

On completion of Chapter 21, the student should be able to do the following:

- Define key terms.
- Identify the purpose of oral diagnosis and treatment planning.
- List the procedures involved in oral diagnosis.
- Discuss the importance of assessing the patient's general physical condition and taking vital signs.
- Demonstrate the ability to obtain patient vital signs.
- Demonstrate charting techniques.

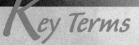

Key Terms

Biopsy	Diastolic	Palpation
Culture	Hypertension	Percussion
Diagnosis	Olfaction	Systolic
Diastema		

\#   _____

Name _____
              Last

Address _____
              Street/P.O. box

Soc. Sec. # _____   _____   _____

Employer _____   _____

Person responsible for account

   Name_____   Relationship to patient _____

   Address_____
              Street/P.O. box   City   State   Zip

   Home phone #_____   Work phone # _____

Insurance   Do you have dental insurance? ☐ Yes ☐ No   Medical ☐ Yes ☐ No

   Name of insurance company _____

Referral: Who referred you to this office? _____

FIGURE 21.1

Sample patient personal history form.

ORAL DIAGNOSIS AND TREATMENT PLANNING

The purpose of oral **diagnosis** and treatment planning is to identify the overall medical and dental health of the patient and to plan dental treatment according to diagnostic findings. In order to secure a comprehensive overview and oral diagnosis of the patient's health, the dental assistant will need to schedule an initial interview and complete a preliminary examination. The preliminary examination usually includes completing the patient's personal, medical, and dental health history as well as completing a physical and oral examination. The dentist will use this data to plan treatment for the patient. Once the treatment plan is completed, the dentist will often have the dental assistant present the plan to the patient.

Diagnosis
An evaluation of existing conditions

Initial Interview

The initial patient interview should be approached in a well-organized professional manner. The quality of the diagnosis and treatment plan depends on the accuracy of the information gathered during the interview process. Before any treatment can be administered the dental assistant should obtain a personal, medical, and dental history. Part of taking the patient's history is recording the vital signs, which include blood pressure, pulse, temperature, and respiration rate. Information obtained from the vital signs directly influences oral diagnosis and treatment planning for the patient. A preliminary examination of the head and neck as well as the hard and soft tissue of the oral cavity is also part of oral diagnosis, and the results will become part of the overall treatment plan. Diagnostic aids such as radiographs and study cast are also needed.

Accurate documentation of all findings must be made. The data gathered will allow the dentist to determine the course of treatment that will assure the best care possible for the patient. It is important that these guidelines be followed because of the possibility of legal questions that could surface in the future. For that same reason, the signature of the patient or the patient's guardian must be obtained before any treatment is attempted (see Chapter 3).

Today's patients are sophisticated about their health care and disease transmission. Infection control is important to both the patient and the dental office. Follow sterile procedures beginning with the initial visit (see Chapter 18).

Personal History

The personal history record may be completed by the patient on a form such as that shown in Figure 21.1. These questions can be completed by the patient and will need little discussion. However, the medical and dental history should be completed by the dental assistant or other office staff. By having a staff member complete the patient medical and dental history, the patient will have an opportunity to communicate and discuss any questions they may have. This allows the apprehensive patient an opportunity to become more comfortable with the office environment. If the patient feels comfortable, they will be less stressful and more manageable as a patient. If the patient has an opportunity to ask questions, the dental assistant will be able to make sure the patient understands. This time with the patient gives the dental assistant an opportunity to evaluate the overall personal physical appearance of the patient. Any abnormality should be recorded on the patient chart and reported to the dentist for further observation. For instance, the dental assistant can observe the following conditions:

Weight: Is the patient under or overweight?

Skin: Does it appear pale or flushed?

Eyes: Are they focused, bloodshot, or dilated?

Face: Is there any swelling or bruises?

Gait: Does the patient limp or show any discomfort in movement?

Speech: Is there any slurring of words?

Accent: Could there be any difficulties in communicating with the patient?

Medical History

The medical history form should include direct and indirect questions. A direct question asks the patient to answer yes or no in response to the presence of a particular medical condition such as, "Are you presently under the medical care of a doctor and taking any medication?" See question #2 (Figure 21.2). An indirect question requires the patient to respond to the presence of symptoms that might suggest a medical condition the patient may not be aware of. For instances, an indirect question could be, "Do you have chest pains on exertion?" See question #13 (Figure 21.2). *The dental assistant should ask about any medication the patient may be taking.* Certain medication will alert the dentist to possible contraindication or circumstances that suggest treatment be delayed. A medical consultation with the patient's physician may be indicated if certain medications are taken or if certain conditions are observed (Figure 21.3). See Chapter 5. A few carefully phrased questions may reveal information that is significant in determining future treatment.

Uses for the Medical History

- Documentation of information that will assist in the diagnosis of oral conditions and treatment planning
- Evaluation of the patient's general health
- Identification of conditions which require precautions, adaptation, or the postponement of treatment

- Establishes the need for referral or consultations with physicians or dental specialist
- Assessment of emotional and psychologic factors or attitudes that might affect treatment
- Prevention of medical emergencies occurring during the course of treatment
- Alerts to the possibility of cross-contamination
- Obtaining baseline information, to be referred to during the course of treatment
- Evidence in legal proceedings

Dental History

Information regarding the patient's past dental experience is a valuable tool in determining the course of any treatment. Statements made by the patient about his or her dental history will allow the dental assistant to evaluate the patient's attitude about dentistry and the value the patient places on dental care. The Dental History form shown in Figure 21.4 is comprehensive.

Dental History Questions

The following questions provide examples of information that may be needed for the patient's dental history:

- Chief complaint: Why is the patient seeking dental treatment at this time?
- Extraction: What was the reason for extractions and were there any complications?
- Restorations: What types of restorations does the patient have and what was the last time they had treatment?
- Orthodontic treatment: What was the nature of the treatment and how long was the patient in treatment?
- Oral hygiene: What type of prevention program was the patient practicing and how often do they brush and floss?
- Prosthetic appliance: What type of appliances, if any, does the patient have and what was the reason for constructing the appliance? Did the patient have any difficulty with the appliance?
- Periodontal treatment: What type of periodontal procedures has the patient received and what was the date of patient's last cleaning?
- Oral habits: What special oral habits does the patient have? Give details.

Each of these questions present a significant amount of information that will influence the practitioner's decisions regarding treatment.

Methods of Examination

There are several methods that the dental assistant can use to examine the patient.

Palpation

The examiner feels and gently presses on the area to be examined. **Palpation**

Palpation

Examination using the sense of touch

Medical history questionnaire

To best treat your dental health needs, we ask that you answer the following questions: Why did you come to the dental clinic today? _____

1. Have you been seen by a physician during the past year?   ☐ Yes ☐ No
2. Are you presently under medical care and/or taking any medication?   ☐ Yes ☐ No
3. Have you ever had a prolonged illness or been hospitalization?   ☐ Yes ☐ No
    If yes, please state details:

_____

4. Check for any of the listed conditions and/or events that you have now or had in the past.

☐ Heart disease or attack	☐ Kidney trouble	☐ Emphysema	☐ AIDS
☐ Angina pectoris	☐ Ulcers	☐ Tuberculosis	☐ HIV-positive
☐ Rheumatic fever	☐ Enlarged glands	☐ Asthma	☐ Nervousness
☐ Heart murmur	☐ Thyroid disease	☐ Hay fever	☐ Sickle cell disease
☐ Heart surgery	☐ Diabetes	☐ Allergies	☐ X-ray treatment
☐ Artificial heart valve	☐ Hemophilia	☐ Hepatitis (type)	☐ Chemotherapy
☐ Heart pacemaker	☐ Persistent diarrhea	☐ Yellow jaundice	☐ Surgery
☐ Congenital heart disease	☐ Arthritis	☐ Venereal disease	☐ Epilepsy or seizures
☐ Stroke	☐ Chronic cough	☐ AIDS-related complex	☐ Hypertension

Others, please specify: _____

5. Have you lost weight without dieting in the last few months?   ☐ Yes ☐ No
6. Have you ever been sick from a shot for dental treatment?   ☐ Yes ☐ No
7. Have you or any relative had a bleeding problem?   ☐ Yes ☐ No
8. Have you ever had serious bleeding after tooth extractions?   ☐ Yes ☐ No
9. Do you have hay fever?   ☐ Yes ☐ No
10. Are you allergic to any foods, clothing, or animals?   ☐ Yes ☐ No
11. Do the following medications make you ill? Aspirin   ☐ Yes ☐ No
     Penicillin or antibiotics?   ☐ Yes ☐ No Sulfa drugs   ☐ Yes ☐ No
     Barbiturates (sleeping pills)   ☐ Yes ☐ No Local anesthetics (novocain)   ☐ Yes ☐ No

     Any other medicines, specify: _____

12. Have you ever had any operations?   ☐ Yes ☐ No

     If yes, specify: _____

13. Do you have chest pains on exertion?   ☐ Yes ☐ No
14. Are you ever short of breath on exertions?   ☐ Yes ☐ No
15. Have you ever had painful or swollen joints?   ☐ Yes ☐ No
16. Do you have any blood disorder such as "thin" or "tired" blood?   ☐ Yes ☐ No
17. Are you on a special diet?   ☐ Yes ☐ No
18. Females: Are you pregnant? If yes, what month? _____   ☐ Yes ☐ No
19. Does any information exist concerning your medical or dental health you feel should be known
     by your dentists?   ☐ Yes ☐ No
20. What is the name and address of your physician (family doctor)? Telephone # _____

_____

To the best of my knowledge, the stated responses are correct and true. If my health history changes, I will inform the dentist at the next appointment.
I understand that patient care in the dental school clinic usually requires at least one 4-hour appointment every 2 weeks or one 2-hour appointment every week. I also understand that the dental school charges for dental treatment, and payment for each procedure is required when it is started unless it is paid for by a third party (insurance company, KY Medical Assistance Program, etc.) or a payment plan is arranged with the school's patient services office.

_____   _____   _____

Patient's signature   Signature of parent or guardian   Date

FIGURE 21.2

Sample patient medical history form.

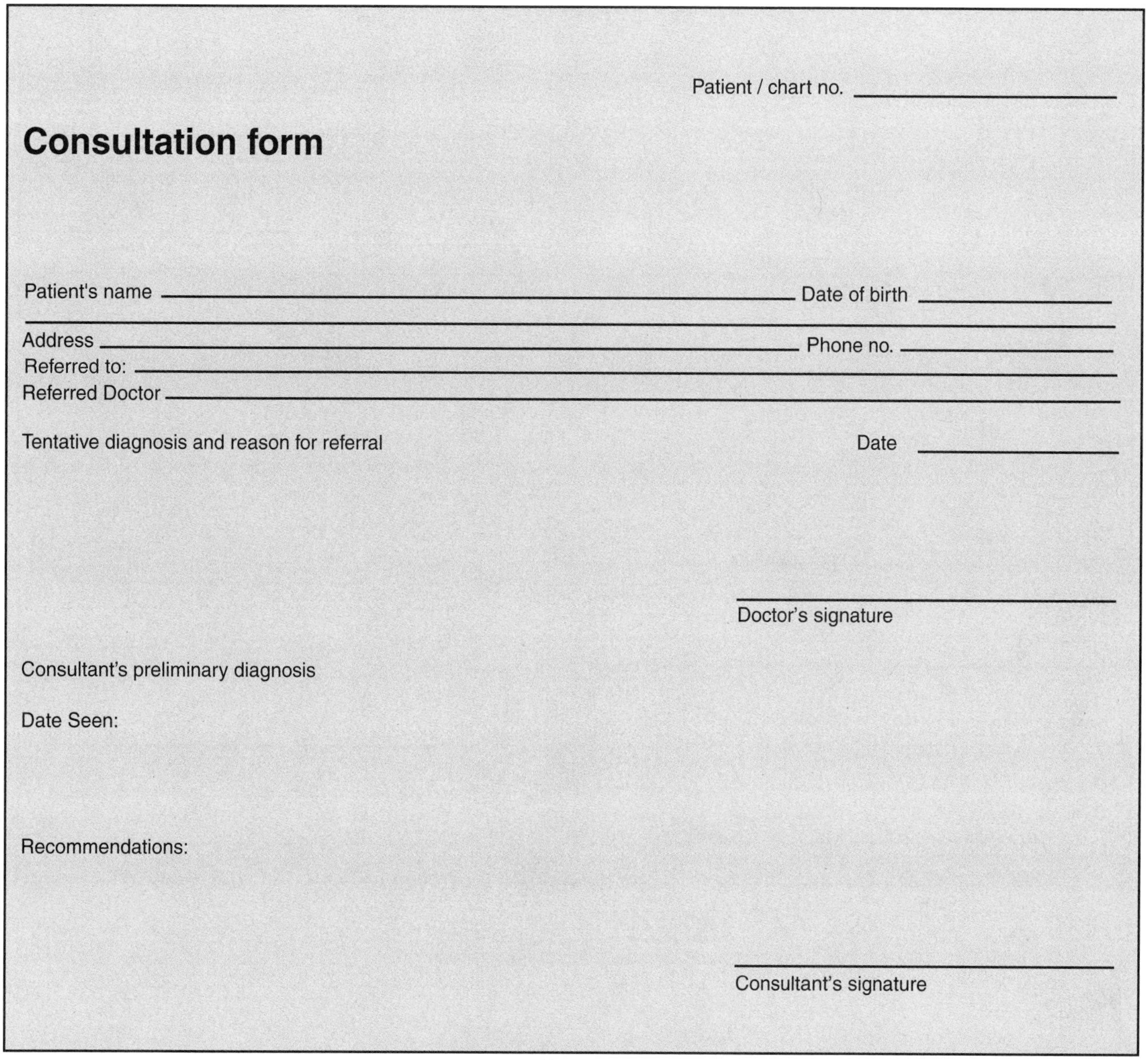

Consultation form

Patient / chart no. _____

Patient's name _____ Date of birth _____

Address _____ Phone no. _____
Referred to: _____
Referred Doctor _____

Tentative diagnosis and reason for referral   Date _____

_____
Doctor's signature

Consultant's preliminary diagnosis

Date Seen:

Recommendations:

_____
Consultant's signature

FIGURE 21.3

Sample medical consult form.

may be accomplished with the use of a single finger or several fingers. The sense of touch is used to identify abnormalities. The change in texture of tissue is frequently the first sign of disease. The tissue will become thicker, larger, or smaller and will be tender when examined.

Auscultation

The sense of hearing is an important tool in the diagnosis of a patient. The operator might listen for abnormal breathing sounds. TMJ disorders produce sounds such as clicking or popping. The blood pressure is obtained with this technique.

Percussion

Tapping (**percussion**) on the tooth or soft tissue will produce sounds of various pitch. The fingers or an instrument may be used. When using an instrument against tooth structure a higher pitched sound will suggest a tooth has normal support. A lower pitched sound will suggest less support, and the patient may express pain.

Percussion
Examination by striking an area and evaluating the sounds and sensations

Dental history

Chief complaint: (see oral diagnosis chart)

History of extractions
Complications: Yes No
Reason for: Caries _____ Malposition_____
Periodontal disease _____ Trauma_____

Restorative: Any restorations: Yes No
Date of last restoration _____
General   Amalgam _____ Silicate _____
type   Gold _____ Resin _____

Orthodontic treatment: Yes No
Duration of treatment
From _____ To _____
Comment: _____
_____
_____
_____

Oral hygiene:
Has patient ever received oral hygiene instructions? Yes No
Has patient ever received disclosing tablets? Yes No
Toothbrush: Hard   Medium Soft
Frequency:
_____ times daily ____ am ____ hs ____ ac ____ pc ____ other

Prosthetic: Any appliances: Yes No
Type
RPD _____ Location _____ Duration _____
FPD _____ Location _____ Duration _____
Is the patient experiencing any difficulty or complaints
with the above appliances?   Yes No
Specify: _____
Reason for not replacing any missing teeth (be brief): ____
_____
Does anyone in the family wear dentures?   Yes No

History of periodontal treatment
    Perio surgery   Yes No
    Occlusal adj   Yes No
    Prophylaxis   Yes No
    Frequency   every _____ month / years

        Months / years since last prophylaxis

Habits:
Mouth breathing   Yes No   Check biting   Yes No
Bruxism   Yes No   Pipe smoking   Yes No
Tongue thrust   Yes No   Other   Yes No
Specify: _____
_____

Dental floss: Yes No
Water irrigation Yes No
  Type _____
Dentifrice   Yes No
  Type _____
Mouthwash   Yes No
  Type _____

FIGURE 21.4

Sample patient dental history form.

Olfaction

An **olfaction** examination using the sense of smell can detect odors that may suggest the presence of certain medical or physical conditions. For instance, kidney or liver conditions may produce specific odors.

Olfaction
Examination using the sense of smell

Observation

During initial interview or observation, allied health personnel can gain a considerable amount of information about the patient, both physical and psychologic, by simply observing the patient.

Vital Signs

Although individual adult vital signs, temperature, pulse, respiration, and blood pressure vary, there is a normal range, which is shown in Table 21.1. The dental assistant can record the patient's vital signs through the following methods.

Blood Pressure

Blood pressure is the measurement of the force of the blood pressing against the walls of the vessels and arteries. This measurement is based on the correlation of blood pressure and sounds. The sounds are known as the *sounds of Korotkoff*, named after the man who first described them,

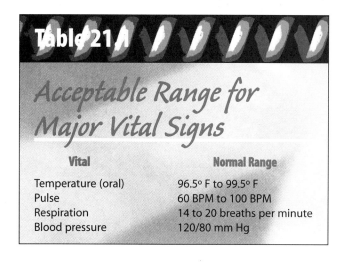

Table 21.1

Acceptable Range for Major Vital Signs

Vital	Normal Range
Temperature (oral)	96.5° F to 99.5° F
Pulse	60 BPM to 100 BPM
Respiration	14 to 20 breaths per minute
Blood pressure	120/80 mm Hg

Box 21.1 Procedure

Procedure for Taking Blood Pressure

1. **Explain the procedure to the patient.**
2. **The patient is seated with forearm resting at heart level, palm facing upward.**
3. **Place deflated cuff 1 inch to 2 inches above the elbow and apply snugly. The cuff should be placed directly against the skin to obtain an accurate reading. Refer to Figure 21.5.**
4. **Locate the brachial artery and palpate with finger tips.**
5. **Place the stethoscope disk firmly, but without pressure, directly against the antecubital fossa, the shallow area inside the elbow. Tighten valve of pump and inflate cuff to at least 20 mm Hg above the point the sound disappears.**
6. **Release the pressure slowly, 2 mm Hg to 3 mm Hg per second, to allow for a gradual drop in pressure.**
7. **Note the pressure at the first sound; this is the systolic pressure. (Figure 21.6, B).**
8. **Continue to release the pressure until the sound completely disappears; this is the diastolic pressure. (Figure 21.6, C).**
9. **Record the measurement with the systolic pressure reading over the diastolic pressure reading. (Table 21.1)**

Nicolai S. Korotkoff (1874-1920). These sounds are heard in the following phases:

- Phase 1: The first appearance of sound, a faint tapping becomes a loud clear tapping.
- Phase 2: As the pressure of the cuff is continually lowered the tapping becomes a murmur or swishing sound.
- Phase 3: A loud thumping sound replaces the murmur.
- Phase 4: A muffling of sound is heard.
- Phase 5: As the pressure is completely released, all sound disappears.

The patient's blood pressure is taken with a sphygmomanometer and a stethoscope (Box 21.1). The sphygmomanometer is a device that consists of an inflatable cuff connected by rubber hoses to a hand pump (bulb) and a pressure gauge; the gauge is called a manometer (Figure 21.5). The cuff is wrapped around the patient's upper arm and inflated. The flow of blood is usually smooth and silent. As the cuff tightens it pinches the artery and causes the blood flow to become rough, and the artery vibrates. The stethoscope allows these sounds to be heard. The cuff is inflated until the flow is completely stopped and becomes silent. In Figure 21.6, *A* the cuff pressure is 160. As the pressure of the cuff is released the flow of blood can be heard once again. The first sound heard is the **systolic** pressure. In Figure 21.6, *B* the systolic pressure equals 140 mm Hg. The cuff pressure at this time is 140. This is the maximum pressure exerted against the arteries as the heart is working to pump blood through the constricted artery. As the pressure decreases and blood begins flowing smoothly and quietly, the point at which the sound disappears is the **diastolic** pressure. In Figure 21.6, *C* the diastolic pressure equals 80 mm Hg. The cuff pressure at this time is 80. This is the minimum pressure against the arteries as the heart is at rest. The pressures are measured and recorded as millimeters of mercury (mm Hg). The systolic reading is always recorded over the diastolic reading which is this case would read 140/80 mm Hg.

Systolic

The maximum pressure exerted against the arteries as the heart is working to pump blood through the constricted artery

Diastolic

The lowest pressure exerted against the arterial walls; the heart is at rest

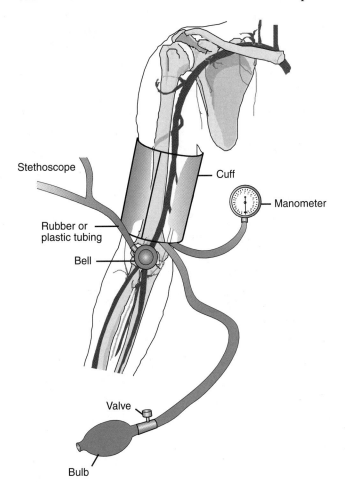

FIGURE 21.5

The parts of a blood pressure monitor are the cuff, control valve, bulb, and mercury gauge (manometer).

There are several considerations in the selection of the size of the cuff to be used. Cuff sizes are child, adult, large adult, and thigh. A thigh cuff is often used for an obese patient. It is the diameter of the patient's arm that determines the size of the cuff to be used, not the patient's age. A cuff that is too narrow will give a reading that is inadvertently high. Choosing a cuff that is too wide gives a reading that is below the actual reading (Box 21.2). The correct size should cover at least two thirds of the upper arm and wrap completely around the arm. If a second reading is indicated, allow time for the circulation of the arm to return to normal.

The sphygmomanometer is available with a mercury manometer (Figure 21.7) or an aneroid manometer (Figure 21.8). The mercury manometer is considered the most reliable for clinic use. The aneroid is calibrated against the mercury manometer to check for accuracy.

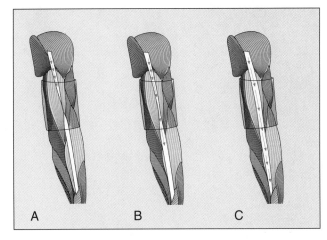

FIGURE 21-6

A, The cuff is inflated, pinching the artery, causing the blood flow to completely stop. **B,** As the cuff pressure is released, the artery enlarges, allowing the blood to begin to flow and the first sound of systolic pressure can be heard. **C,** As the pressure continues to decrease, the blood begins flowing smoothly again and the sound disappears, indicating the diastolic pressure.

Box 21.2 *Take note*

Errors in the Blood Pressure Reading

Improper positioning of the patient: The position of the artery in which the blood pressure is measured must be at the level of the heart.

Improper deflation of the cuff: The pressure should be lowered 2 mm to 3 mm per heartbeat. A slower rate will cause the diastolic reading to be erroneously high. If the cuff is deflated too quickly, the reading will be erroneously low.

Improper positioning of the cuff: A narrow cuff is created when the cuff is applied too loosely, which causes the reading to be excessively high.

Anxiety and apprehension of the patient: The reading will be erroneously high if the patient is not given time to relax before the procedure.

Defective equipment: A defective air release valve or rubber tubing that is too porous will make it difficult to control the inflation and deflation of the cuff. The needle on the dial should indicate *zero* when the cuff is deflated.

Electronic units are available that will automatically inflate and deflate the cuff. A digital readout is given. Automatic blood pressure monitors make it possible to monitor the medically compromised patient during dental treatment.

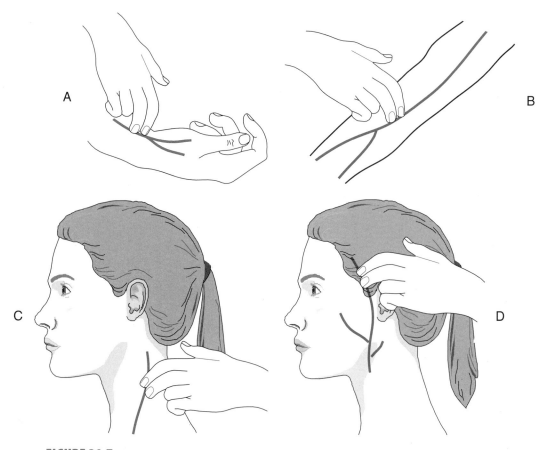

FIGURE 21-7

A, The radial artery pulse position is most often used in dental examination (Courtesy General Medical Corporation). **B**, The brachial artery pulse can be felt on the inside of the arm just above the bend of the elbow (Courtesy GMC). **C,** The carotid artery pulse can be felt along the side of the neck (Courtesy GMC). **D**, The temporal artery pulse can be felt in front of the ear (Courtesy GMC).

Age and the medical history of the patient must be considered before determining if the pressure reading is normal or abnormal. Usually a reading classified as normal would be 120/80 or below. A classification of borderline would be from 130/85 to 140/90. Readings above this would be considered abnormal and **hypertension** is suspect. The dentist may request a physician's consultation before beginning or continuing treatment. A dentist can predict that 10% to 20% of patients will have high blood pressure readings; one third of those will not be aware of this condition. The American Dental Association suggests that every new patient, including children, should have his or her blood pressure checked. All other patients should be checked at least once a year. Since hypertension is an asymptomatic condition (that is, a condi-

Hypertension

An abnormal elevation of the blood pressure

tion without symptoms), this procedure can be an invaluable health service to the patient.

Pulse

The pulse is the throbbing sensation felt when the fingers are pressed lightly against an artery. This sensation is the alternating of the expansion and contraction of the arteries as the blood is pumped into them with each beat of the heart. The pulse rate is the count of the heartbeats. See Box 21.3 and Figure 21.7 for the procedure for taking a pulse.

Pulse rates higher than normal may be due to exercising, stimulants such as coffee or tea, emotions, eating, smoking before the examination, and some heart conditions. A pulse rate higher than 100 for adults is classified as *tachycardia*. Lower rates can be due to sleep, depressants, not eating, or possibly a prolonged illness. Adult pulse rates lower than 60 are classified as *bradycardia*. The pulse should be noted as to strength and rhythm.

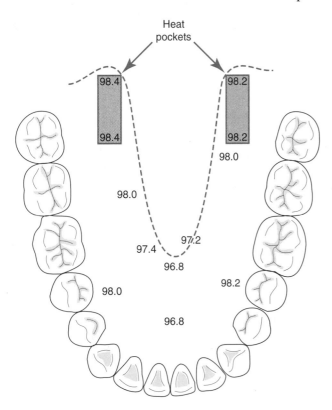

FIGURE 21-8

Place the thermometer under the patient's tongue in a hot spot. (Redrawn from PyMatt Corporation, Somerville, New Jersey.)

Temperature

The body temperature is the difference in the amount of heat the body produces and the amount of heat it loses. If a patient is in good health, his or her temperature should range between 96.5° F to 99.5° F. A reading that is a full degree above the patient's normal reading represents a fever. Taking the patient's temperature orally is the most convenient method (see Box 21.4 and Figure 21.8). If the patient has consumed a hot or cold beverage just before the reading, the accuracy of the reading can be affected. Other conditions can also affect the body temperature, for example, the weather or the patient's emotional state.

Types of Thermometers

There are three types of thermometers used in dental offices, (1) glass mercury, (2) disposable thermometer, and (3) electronic thermometer.

1 Glass mercury thermometers are available in Fahrenheit or centigrade (Celsius) increments. The mercury is heated by body temperature and rises along the column to the temperature of the oral cavity. When using a glass fahrenheit clinical thermometer, follow universal precautions.

2 Disposable thermometers are sterile, single use. They are available and recommended because they reduce the pos-

sibility of cross-contamination, are easier to read, and save steps and valuable clinic time. Disposable thermometers are sterile, accurate, convenient and economical. An additional benefit is the assurance a patient has that every effort is being made to protect his or her health.

3 Electronic thermometers are available. Digital readings are obtained within 5 seconds. Disposable tips are used. Some models have printed readouts.

Fahrenheit to Centigrade Conversion

If necessary, a Fahrenheit scale reading can be converted into a Celsius scale reading by subtracting 32 from the reading and multiplying by 5/9. To convert a Celsius scale reading to a Fahrenheit scale reading, multiply by 9/5 and then add 32. For example 98.6° F is equal to 37° C (or Celsius).

Conditions That Affect Body Temperature

There are many internal and external conditions that affect body temperatures. The body temperature will often in-

---

Box 21.3 *Procedure*

Procedure for Taking a Pulse

1. **Explain the procedure to the patient.**
2. **Seat patient with arm and hand supported, palm down.**
3. **Press index and middle finger on the area between the wrist bone and tendon on the thumb side of the wrist (Figure 21.7, A).**
4. **Note pulsing sensation of the artery, if none, reposition fingers.**
5. **Press on the artery without constricting the flow of blood.**
6. **Count the pulse for 1 minute to ensure the most accurate reading.**
7. **Record reading. Note the rhythm—regular, irregular. The strength—strong, weak.**

The most commonly used artery is the radial artery at the wrist. There are several other pulse points convenient for the dental examination: the brachial artery located on the inside of the arm just above the bend of the elbow (Figure 21.7, B); the carotid artery located along the sides of the neck (Figure 21.7, C) and the temporal artery located in front of the ear (Figure 21.7, D).

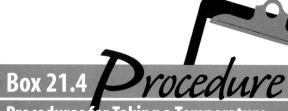

Box 21.4 Procedure

Procedures for Taking a Temperature

1. Explain the procedure to the patient.
2. Place the sterile thermometer in a sterile plastic sleeve.
3. Shake thermometer until it registers below 95° F. Do not hold the thermometer by the tip that is to be placed in the patient's mouth.
4. Place thermometer under patient's tongue in a hot spot. (Figure 21.8). The anterior of the floor of the mouth will give the lowest reading.
5. Instruct patient to close lips around the thermometer and to remain still and quiet. Leave in place for at least 3 minutes.
6. Remove thermometer.
7. Read at eye level. Follow column of mercury.
8. Record temperature.
9. Rinse and sterilize thermometer by soaking in a chemical sterilant according to manufacturer's direction.
10. Store in a dry container.

Using a disposable thermometer

1. Explain procedure to patient.
2. Open package, peel back wrapper to expose handle of thermometer and remove thermometer.
3. Place the thermometer into patient's mouth under the tongue (Figure 21.8). Have patient press tongue down.
4. Leave in place 60 seconds and remove.
5. Wait 10 seconds and read temperature.
6. Discard thermometer.

Box 21.5

Emergency Treatment

There are several common types of emergency treatments encountered in general practice, which will be acknowledged in related chapters:

Pulpotomy: Removal of the dental pulp from the dental chamber.
Pulpectomy: Removal of the dental pulp from the dental chamber and root canal.
Extraction: Removal of a tooth.
Excavation and treatment of a deep carious lesion: Removal of carious material from a cavity and restoration of tooth.

ing. Age and conditions such as menopause cause women to have "hot flashes" and tremendous changes in body temperature. Certain medications and drugs will affect temperatures. Pregnancy is a physical condition that can cause various body sensations including the feeling of warmth or coolness that can change a patient's temperature.

Respiration

Respiration is the inspiration of oxygen and the expiration of carbon dioxide, one complete inhalation and exhalation. A good time to observe the patient's breathing is when the temperature is being taken. Patients have a tendency to control their breathing if they are aware it is being monitored. Observe the rate, rhythm, and depth of respiration. The normal respiration rate for an adult is 14 to 20 breaths per minute. A child's normal rate is 24 to 28 breaths per minute. An adult male's respiration is diaphragmatic, primarily from the abdominal muscles. An adult female's respiration is costal, primarily from the chest. Observe the rise and fall of the chest or upper abdomen; use of other muscles such as the neck or shoulders suggest a possible medical condition.

Classification of Respiration Respiration is classified from normal to abnormal and include the following:

Eupnea: Normal respirations
Hyperventilation: Rapid, deep respirations
Hypoventilation: Slow, shallow respirations
Dyspnea: Difficult respirations
Apnea: Stopped breathing
Respiratory arrest: Failure to resume breathing

Emergency Patients

When a patient makes an appointment because they are in pain, it is important to see them as quickly as possible. Personal and medical histories must be taken if the patient is new or reviewed if the patient is regular; vital signs must be taken before treatment is started. The dentist will complete an emergency examination of the mouth concentrating on the "suspect" area. Radiographs may be indicated (Box 21.5).

crease during illness and people will often complain about being overly hot, cold, or clammy. Exercise can also increase body temperature, often causing sweating. Certain spicy foods, hot coffee, or soup can warm us; and iced tea, ice cream, or cold drinks can cool us. Even emotions can effect body temperatures: fear can cause us to feel cold and anger can cause us to perspire. Of course, hot and cold weather affect us, and a cool swim on a hot day certainly feels refresh-

Clinical Observations

The body's physical appearance offers some indications as to the health of a patient. Some of the general observations can be made by the dental assistant when the patient enters the operatory. The initial clinical examination allows the dental assistant an opportunity to detect any unusual signs or symptoms of potential medical problems.

Physical and Behavioral

The dental assistant should also observe the patient's physical appearance and behavior. For instance, what is the patient's body type; heavy, average, thin? Does the patient move with coordination and smoothness? Does the posture of the patient suggest fatigue or discomfort? The patient's facial expressions may also reveal anxiety or fear. Skin color or "clamminess" may denote a physical problem as well as skin color. A patient's skin color varies according to ethnic background; for instance, the skin may appear a pale ivory or a dark brown when the patient is not feeling well. Any physical or functional abnormalities should be noted and recorded in the patient's chart. Such alertness and concern will help to establish a mutual trust and rapport between the dental assistant and the patient. Just asking the patient how they have felt lately may bring out a potential problem and also indicate a "caring attitude."

While completing the medical and dental history, the dental assistant will be able to evaluate the patient's level of understanding through the inclusion of questions and responses, while at the same time developing a good communication process with the patient. Any speech abnormalities should be noted.

Breath

Breathing is the inhaling and exhaling of air. One's breath can be detected by the vapors, odor, or heat. Through the process of smelling (olfaction), the health care provider or dental assistant can detect "bad breath" or "mouth odors" that may indicate a health problem. The most common odors of the mouth, which can easily be recognized, stem from the buildup of dental plaque. Other odors of the breath may suggest more severe underlying conditions. For instance, the odor of ammonia or alcohol could indicate a kidney problem. Chronic infections of the lungs can also produce bad breath. Liver failure may cause a fishy odor, and dry mouth can cause dead cells to accumulate and decompose, causing bad breath. These odors should be noted so that they can be investigated for origin.

Speech is also a function of the oral cavity as well as respiration and digestion. The teeth, cheeks, tongue, salivary glands, and the tonsils are all part of the process of mastication (the break down of food for digestion) and the digestive system.

Tissues and Organs of the Oral Cavity

Good general health is influenced by the conditions of the oral cavity. The proper function of the oral cavity is essential in sustaining a healthy lifestyle, since chewing, tasting, and swallowing are necessary to our well-being. Anatomy and physiology of the body is discussed in detail in Chapter 8, and Chapter 11 discusses normal and abnormal conditions that are observed during a clinical examination. It is important in the clinical examination to record abnormal findings precisely. For example, if any abnormality is identified, a description and location must be noted.

It is important for the dental assistant to follow a disciplined sequence during a clinical examination of the oral cavity. This means establishing a routine sequence of steps when completing an extraoral and intraoral examination. By following certain steps in order the dental assistant can be efficient in the use of time. As a primary provider of health care services, the dentist and office staff can contribute to the lifelong good health of patients.

Changes in the laws regulating dentistry are providing an opportunity for the dental assistant to perform many procedures that have traditionally been practiced only by dentists. The delegation of providing clinical oral examination to the dental assistants is determined by state regulation.

Oral Habits

The oral habits of patients can contribute to conditions found in the mouth. A mouth breather for instance, will be more likely to have periodontal disease because of the irritation from the continual dryness of the gingival tissue. Bruxism can lead to problematic grinding of the teeth. Bruxism may be diagnosed through temporomandibular joint discomfort, hypersensitivity of teeth, fractures, and erosion or attrition of enamel.

Eating Disorders

There are specific conditions of the oral cavity that can identify patients with an eating disorder. Anorexia nervosa patients have an obsession with weight loss almost to the extent of starvation. Patients with bulimia have excessive appetites. These patient's show certain patterns within the oral cavity that can alert the dental health care worker to the presence of an eating disorder. Self-induced vomiting exposes the patient's teeth to acids found in gastric secretions. These acids will cause a pattern of erosion of enamel and dentin. The patient may have a dry mouth, the palate may be red, and the lips may be chapped and dry. Enlarged parotid and submandibular glands may also indicate an eating disorder. Patients can be instructed in how to minimize the oral health problems caused by these conditions. Topical fluoride treatments may be used in the dental office and the patient may be advised to use fluoride rinses at home. Instruct the patient not to brush immediately after vomiting, this might aid the acids from the stomach in the abrasion of the teeth surfaces, rinsing with a baking soda solution will help naturalize this action. If the patient is a minor, the parents must be made aware of the dental complications that result from an eating disorder.

Oral Cancer Examination

The examiner should inspect the mouth for small lumps or discolored thickenings and discolored patches of tissue. Early detection is vital to the successful treatment of the disease. Almost 25% of patients with cancer of the mouth die because the condition was not diagnosed early. Denture patients should understand the need for a regular oral examination. Teaching self-examination to the patient can save his or her life (Figure 21.9).

Patients with Functional Limitations

A patient with functional limitation has a condition that limits ability to participate in dental treatment in a normal manner. Standard terminology has been developed by the World Health Organization to help aid in communication and treatment of these patients.

A patient with an impairment has limited use or loss of a part of their body or function. A patient with a loss of an arm or vision has an impairment. A patient with a disability has limitations or restrictions that prohibits normal range compared with someone in similar circumstances. A disability may be permanent or only temporary. A patient who cannot climb stairs has a disability. An impairment or disability that results in a patient not being able to do what is normal is considered a handicap.

When treating a patient who is visually impaired, the dental assistant should follow a few simple guidelines to create a helpful atmosphere and allow the patient to feel more comfortable. The assistant should stand close when speaking to the patient. Blind patients need assistance with mobility, therefore allow them to take your arm but do not take their arm. As you pass through a doorway, take a step forward and rotate your arm backward so they know you are going through a door. Give verbal instructions such as "move left," "a chair is right behind you," and "take this in your right or left hand." Use indirect lighting whenever possible to avoid a glare. Appointments or home instructions should be printed in large, bold print.

A patient with hearing loss may be able to understand you if you speak face-to-face. When appropriate, you should use facial expressions or gestures to aid in communication. Never assume that patients cannot hear just because they are older. Certain signs exist that will alert the dental staff to the patient's inability to hear. The dental assistant should ask the following questions:

- Is the patient wearing a hearing aid?
- Does the patient's head or body turn in the direction of the person speaking?
- Does the patient's facial expressions suggest straining to hear?
- Does the patient give inappropriate answers to questions?

Always begin speaking in a normal manner and adjust according to your observations.

If the impairment or disability limits the patient's mobility, an assessment must be made by the healthcare provider as to the amount of assistance a patient may need. If you observe that a patient needs help, ask how you may assist, describe the procedure you are going to perform, and ask if help is needed.

The dental office should be arranged to provide easy access to the operatory for wheelchair patients. Eliminate the need to move other equipment out of the way to make room for a wheelchair. Practice with the office staff using a wheelchair to become familiar with how a patient would receive treatment in your office.

Dental assistants should not treat patients with a disability as if they are helpless. Instead promote their independence by advocating a positive willingness to meet patients' needs.

Pregnancy and Dental Treatment

Special considerations must be made if a patient is pregnant or even suspects pregnancy. The first trimester is the most critical in the development of the fetus. If treatment is necessary, the patient's physician should be consulted. The prescription of drugs should be made only after consultation with the medical doctor. Radiographs should be taken only if absolutely necessary and clearance of the patient's physician is recommended. All necessary treatment should be completed during the second trimester, which is generally the safest time to provide dental treatment.

INTRAORAL AND EXTRAORAL DIAGNOSIS

The dental assistant should record all information received from the clinical examination. In some states dental assistants are delegated with the responsibility to complete the preliminary clinical examination.

Oral Mucosa

The soft tissue lining of the oral cavity is called the *oral mucosa*. The oral mucosa covers all surfaces of the oral cavity except the teeth. Saliva keeps the mucosa moist. The texture of the mucosa varies according to its location in the mouth. There are three types of mucosa in the oral cavity: lining mucosa, masticatory mucosa, and specialized mucosa. The lining mucosa covers the intraoral surface of the cheeks (buccal), lips (labial), soft palate, and sublingual area. Masticatory mucosa covers the attached gingiva and hard palate. Specialized mucosa covers the top surface of the tongue (Figure 21.10).

The three types of oral mucosa have individual appearances or characteristics. A term used to describe these tissues are keratinized and nonkeratinized. Keratinized means that the tissue has a tough fibrous protein substance covering its outer layer. The lining mucosa is nonkeratinized. It is movable and compressible, which means that it should be soft

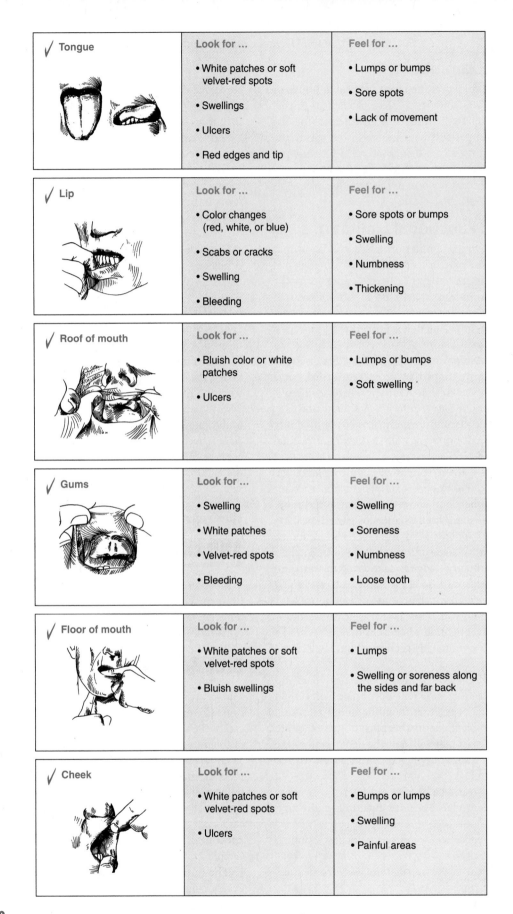

✓ Tongue	Look for …	Feel for …
	• White patches or soft velvet-red spots • Swellings • Ulcers • Red edges and tip	• Lumps or bumps • Sore spots • Lack of movement

✓ Lip	Look for …	Feel for …
	• Color changes (red, white, or blue) • Scabs or cracks • Swelling • Bleeding	• Sore spots or bumps • Swelling • Numbness • Thickening

✓ Roof of mouth	Look for …	Feel for …
	• Bluish color or white patches • Ulcers	• Lumps or bumps • Soft swelling

✓ Gums	Look for …	Feel for …
	• Swelling • White patches • Velvet-red spots • Bleeding	• Swelling • Soreness • Numbness • Loose tooth

✓ Floor of mouth	Look for …	Feel for …
	• White patches or soft velvet-red spots • Bluish swellings	• Lumps • Swelling or soreness along the sides and far back

✓ Cheek	Look for …	Feel for …
	• White patches or soft velvet-red spots • Ulcers	• Bumps or lumps • Swelling • Painful areas

FIGURE 21-9

Oral cancer self-examination. Alert your family dentist to any changes in the six major areas of your mouth that remain for more than 2 weeks. (Courtesy University of Louisville School of Dentistry, Louisville, Kentucky).

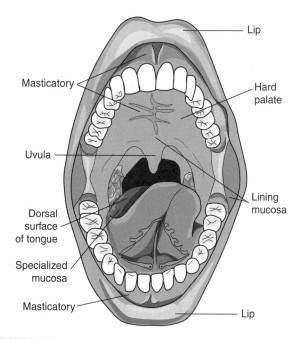

FIGURE 21-10

Anatomical locations of parts of the oral cavity, including the oral mucosa.

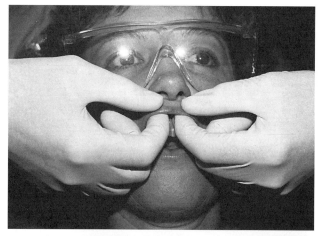

A

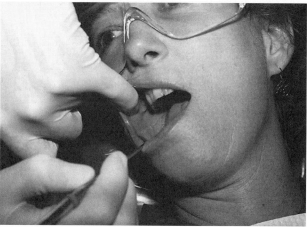

B

FIGURE 21-11

A, The lip is inverted and palpated. **B,** The cheek is retracted to examine the buccal mucosa.

and smooth to the touch. The masticatory mucosa is keratinized. It is immovable and resists compression, which means that it is firm to the touch. The specialized mucosa is made up of papillae and taste buds.

In order to complete an examination of the oral mucosa, the examiner will need a tongue depressor, an angled mouth mirror, sterile 2 x 2 gauze and a direct light source, such as an illuminator head lamp or penlight. Before beginning any intraoral examination, ask the patient to remove any appliances that are not fixed, for example, full dentures or partial dentures.

Lips and Vestibule

The lips are the muscular folds that surround the opening of the mouth. In health the lips will have a smooth texture and appear pink in color. The lips are inspected for size, form, color, edema, lesions, or indurate areas. Indurate areas feel hard to the touch. The corners or commissure of the lips should be examined for flexibility. If the lips appear dry or cracked, apply a thin layer of lubricant to those areas before continuing the examination. Using a direct light source, observe the labial mucosa. When completing an examination of the lips and vestibule, invert (or turn outward) the upper and lower lips. Palpate the lips with light pressure while the patient's teeth are in a closed position (Figure 21.11, *A*). There are minor glands inside the lips that produce fluid to keep these tissues moist.

The buccal and labial mucosa make up the space known as the *vestibule*. Buccal mucosa line the cheeks and labial mucosa line the lips. With the patient's mouth in an open position, inspect the buccal mucosa on each side of the mouth (Figure 21.11, *B*). Swelling in this area could indicate an infection at the apex of a tooth. Using direct vision, use two fingers to palpate and reflect the tissue. The mucobuccal fold begins as the mucosa turns toward the gingiva. This tissue should be loose and movable.

Located at the midline of both upper and lower lips is a fold of tissue known as the *labial frenum.* If the upper frenum extends too close to the alveolar ridge it may cause a **diastema** or open space between the teeth. If corrected early, this condition can be avoided. The lower frenum may contribute to gingival recession if it extends too close to the gingiva. Any abnormal color, texture, or lesion should be described and documented.

Diastema
A space between teeth

Occlusion

To check the occlusion, the examiner will retract the cheeks as the patient bites in a normal position. This is called *centric*

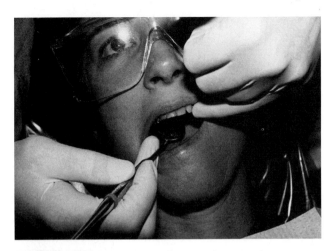

FIGURE 21-12

The hard palate is observed by using a mouth mirror.

occlusion, which means the teeth are in the position of physiologic rest. In a normal bite the anterior maxillary teeth will extend over the mandibular anterior teeth. The buccal cusp of the maxillary posterior teeth should be external to the buccal cusps of mandibular posterior teeth. This position protects the lips and cheeks from being bitten.

Palate and Uvula

The palate is made up of hard and soft tissue that forms the roof of the mouth. The anterior of the palate or hard palate is supported by bone. The posterior portion is made up of the soft palate, which is not supported by bone and is muscular tissue. It is flexible and changes shape when relaxed.

The hard palate may be viewed by direct observation or indirectly with the mouth mirror (Figure 21.12). The patient should be placed in a supine position. The posterior hard palate, soft palate, and uvula may be directly viewed when the tongue is depressed. The shape of the hard palate varies with each individual. It may be contoured with a high vault or it may be flat. It is covered with masticatory mucosa. The area appears pale pink in color, sometimes having a bluish-gray tint. The hard palate should feel firm when touched. Sometimes a raised bony structure, called torus palatinus, may be found in the midline area. This is not normal and can interfere with the adaption and retention of dentures. A narrow white line or streak normally appears at midline, this is the palatine raphe.

The soft palate is covered with lining mucosa, which appears darker than the hard palate. The boundary between these two areas can be easily observed by having the patient say "ah." This will cause the soft palate to rise. During swallowing, the soft palate seals the area of the nasopharynx and pharynx to prevent food from entering the respiratory tract. If a patient wears a full denture or a partial denture, a color

change may occur because of pressure exerted by these devices. The soft palate terminates with a downward, cone-shaped projection known as the *uvula*. The uvula prevents food or liquid from entering the nasal cavities. The uvula may be examined by depressing the tongue. The length of the uvula varies from just visible to almost touching the tongue. Any deviation from midline should be noted. Absence of the uvula could be caused by a congenital condition or surgical procedure.

Tongue, Alveolar Ridges, and Floor of Mouth

The tongue is a muscular organ that connects to the floor of the mouth and extends into the pharynx. The tongue assists in the chewing process, begins the swallowing process, and is necessary for speech. Before examining the tongue, explain the procedure to the patient. The dorsal surface, or back of the tongue, is inspected first. This is where the taste buds are located and the only area of specialized mucosa. The examiner will look for swelling, color variations, coating, or ulcerations. The dental assistant will ask the patient to extend his or her tongue for evaluation of any deviation, tremor, or constriction of movement. The tongue may appear broader if the patient has no teeth (is edentulous) (Box 21.6). The tongue is examined by placing the patient in an upright position and using a sterile 2 x 2 gauze; wrap it around the tip of the patient's tongue and, by using pressure, pull the tongue from side to side to observe all surfaces (Figure 21.13, *A*). The patient is then asked to touch the tip of the tongue to the palate to expose the lower surface of the tongue (ventral). The lower surface of the tongue should appear smooth and shiny. On inspection any swelling or varicosities should be identified and recorded. The lingual frenum can also be observed for any restrictions of the tongue.

After the tongue examination is completed, the alveolar ridges should be checked by retracting the cheek tissue (buccal mucosa) and depressing the tongue to view the lingual side of the alveolar ridge. The ridges should be palpated using the index finger of each hand (bi-digital compressions). Any indurate (hard) areas, swellings, lesions, color abnormalities, or tenderness indicated by the patient should be recorded.

The floor of the mouth is the next area to be observed. Using bi-digital palpations, place one finger inside the mouth on the posterior floor of the mouth under the tongue and place the other finger on the skin under the chin. Press up into the mandible (Figure 21.13, *B*). The fingers are moved from the posterior area forward toward the chin. When both fingers are pressed together, the floor of the mouth can be palpated. This procedure is repeated from the lower midline area outwardly and bilaterally. Any irregularities in color, surface texture, lumps, bumps, ulcers, or anatomical abnormalities should be documented

Box 21.6

Procedure

Procedures for Examination of Tongue, Alveolar Ridges, and Floor of the Mouth

1. Place patient in an upright position.
2. Explain examination procedure to the patient.

Tongue

3. Wrap a sterile 2 x 2 gauze around the tip of the patient's tongue.
4. Inspect the dorsal surface first by retracting the tongue, turning it, exposing each side, and observing all surfaces.
5. Use one hand to stabilize the tongue, while bi-digitally palpating the lateral borders from posterior to anterior.
6. Inspect the ventral surface by asking the patient to touch the tip of the tongue to the roof of the mouth.
7. Observe the lingual frenum.
8. Record any findings.

Alveolar ridges

9. Retract the cheek tissue and depress the tongue, examining the lingual side of the alveolar ridge.
10. Palpate the ridges with bi-digital compressions.
11. Record any findings.

Mouth floor

12. Place one finger inside the mouth on the posterior floor under the tongue and the other finger on the skin under the chin.
13. Use bi-digital palpations and press up into the mandible moving fingers from the posterior area forward toward the chin.
14. Repeat palpations from lower midline area outward and bilateral.
15. Record any findings.
16 Report findings to dentist.

A 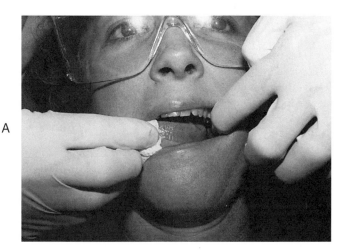 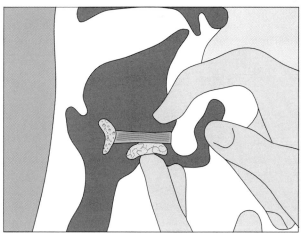 B

FIGURE 21-13

A, A sterile 2 x 2 is wrapped around the tip of the tongue and the tongue is gently pulled forward so that the entire dorsal and lateral surfaces can be examined. **B,** Correct placement of fingers in palpation examination of the floor of the mouth.

and reported to the dentist. The examiner must be careful because the oral tissue in this area of the mouth is thin and easily traumatized. Disorders of the tongue are discussed in Chapter 11.

The clinical examination also includes a visible observation of the surface of the tongue and observation during swallowing and speech. By teaching the patient how to make these observations and how to follow the steps for this

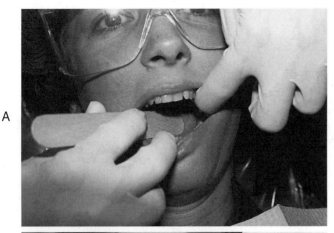

A

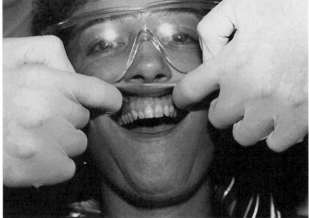

B

FIGURE 21-14

A, The lingual gingiva can be examined by retracting the tongue with a sterile tongue depressor. **B,** The facial gingiva can be examined by retracting the lips and cheeks with the index fingers.

examination, the dental assistant can make an important contribution as a health care provider.

Gingiva

The gingiva is the tissue that immediately surrounds the teeth. Indirect lighting, using an angled mouth mirror, may be necessary for observation of lingual surfaces. The tongue usually has to be retracted with a mirror or tongue depressor in order to observe the mandibular lingual gingiva (Figure 21.14, *A*). The gingiva should appear firm and should contour around each tooth. Free gingiva should appear light pink in color. When the gingiva tissue is healthy the sulcus depth should not exceed 2.5 mm (see Chapter 25). The sulcus depths are examined, measured, and recorded during the charting of periodontal tissue. The attached gingiva varies from light to dark pink. Generally the darker a person's complexion the darker the gingiva tissue (Figure 21.14, *B*).

The gingiva tissue is a masticatory mucosa, because it aids in the breakdown of food and the digestion process.

Pharynx and Tonsils

The pharynx is also referred to as the throat. It is a fibrous tube that extends from the soft palate to the esophagus and serves both the respiratory and digestive systems. The pharynx receives food and the muscles of the pharynx drive the food downward into the esophagus. To observe the pharynx the examiner will place the patient in a horizontal position and have the patient inhale while saying "Ah." The pharynx normally appears pink and moist. The tonsils can be observed at this time for any enlargement or discoloration. The tonsils are located between the oral cavity and the pharynx and act as filters against disease. They should appear pink and equal in size under normal conditions.

Larynx

The larynx, or voice box, is located below the pharynx. It has two functions; one as an airway and another as an instrument of speech. The larynx can be examined by placing the fingertips bilaterally over the structure, applying pressure against it, and having the patient swallow. The larynx should move freely, up or down, as the patient swallows. The inability to move freely suggests an abnormal condition.

Salivary Glands

Salivary glands produce saliva that contributes greatly to the oral health of the patient. Saliva aids in cleaning the mouth and teeth and the salivary glands produce enzymes that help control infection. There are three pairs of major salivary glands: (1) parotid, (2) submandibular, and (3) sublingual (see Figure 8.29). The pairs can be identified by the secretion consistency of the saliva coming from the ducts underneath the tongue or the cheek near the maxillary molars. For instance, the parotid gland produces a thin watery secretion; the submandibular gland produces a thick, sticky secretion; and the sublingual gland also secretes a sticky substance. The operator will be checking the consistency of flow, excessive secretion flow, or decreased secretion flow, and any presence of swelling under the chin or in front of the ears.

Excessive secretion is referred to as *sialorrhea*. Excessive secretion may be associated with an infection. A dry mouth may be caused by medical treatments, a systemic disease, or the natural process of aging. A dry mouth is referred to as *xerostomia*.

Lymph Nodes

Lymph nodes are found along the lymph vessels (see Figure 8.23). The nodes are small bean shaped bodies. The function of the lymph nodes is to filter the lymphatic fluid. They also

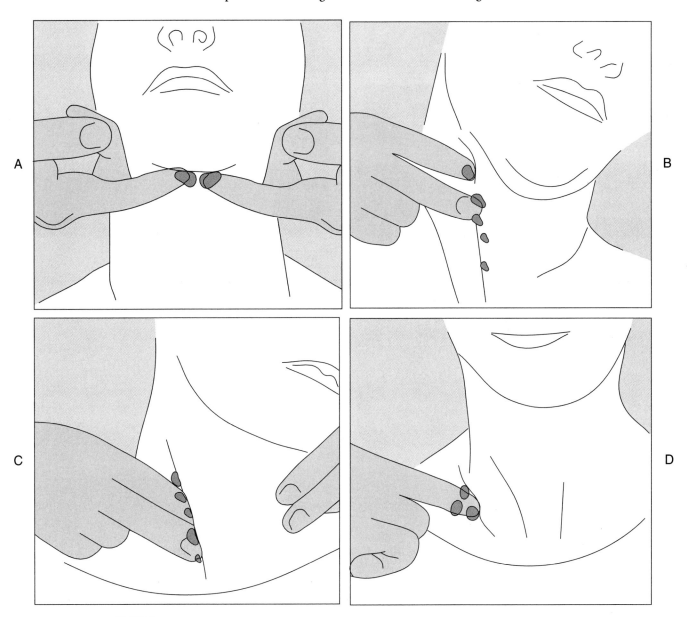

FIGURE 21-15

The examiner will palpate along the chain of lymph vessels (**A**) beneath the chin, (**B**) place fingers along the anterior margins of the sternocleidomastoid muscles of the neck, (**C**) press the fingers below this muscle, (**D**) move fingers down to the clavicle area and press firmly.

produce white blood cells, which the body uses to fight infection. These vessels are generally not palpable or detected if the patient has healthy lymph nodes. The examiner begins by placing the fingers in front of the ear and continuing down the neck to the clavicle (Figure 21.15). This will allow the examiner to palpate along the chain of lymph nodes beneath the chin and sternocleidomastoid muscles of the neck (see Figure 21.15). It is important for the examiner to press the fingers below this muscle, forcing the fingers gently beneath the anterior margins of this muscle of the neck to detect swelling or tenderness. If palpation reveals swelling or

tenderness in this area it usually suggests the presence of infection. This infection may be traced to a dental abscess, tonsillitis, or a condition much more serious, such as tuberculosis or cancer. Next, the fingers are moved down to the clavicle area and pressed firmly. Abnormalities must be recorded and inspected by the dentist (Box 21.7).

Temporomandibular Joint

When the mouth is opened, the mandible moves forward and downward. The disc between the ball and the joint stays

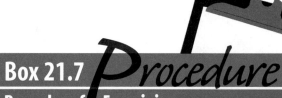

Box 21.7 *Procedure*

Procedure for Examining the Lymph Nodes

1. **Place patient in an upright position.**
2. **Explain examination procedure to the patient.**
3. **Place fingers in front of the ear, palpate and continue down the neck to the clavicle.**
4. **Palpate along the chain of lymph nodes beneath the chin.**
5. **Press fingers below the sternocleidomastoid muscle, forcing the fingers gently beneath the anterior margins of this muscle of the neck to detect swelling or tenderness.**
6. **Move fingers down to the clavicle area and press firmly.**
7. **Record any abnormalities and report them to the dentist.**

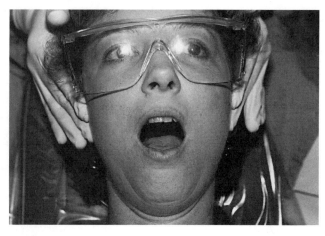

FIGURE 21-16

The examiner will palpate the joint and listen as the patient opens and closes the mouth.

between the bones of the joint (Figure 21.16). The left and right temporomandibular joints (TMJ) will move in unison or synchrony. If the movement of the joints is not together, the disc separating the jaw from the skull can slip out of place and dislocation can result. In these instances there is limitation of opening. The patient may indicate a tenderness of the jaw muscles, aching in front of the ear and possibly a clicking of the joint.

Clinical examination involves palpation of the joint, auscultation (listening during various movements), and observation for any deviations. An abnormal bite or bruxism can cause inflammation of the temporomandibular joint. Occasionally psychologic factors are responsible for the pain. For example, a clenched jaw may be caused by tension or anxiety and can cause discomfort. Based on the examination and input from the patient, the dentist will determine the best treatment.

The examiner may place the little finger of each hand into the patient's auditory canal opening or the index and middle finger in front of the auditory canal to test the range and smoothness of motion as the mouth opens and closes (see Figure 21.16). The mouth should open at least 40 mm to 50 mm. A stethoscope placed in front of each ear may reveal popping, clicking, or grating noises.

Thyroid Gland

The thyroid gland can be palpated with the examiner standing behind the patient and placing the index and middle finger over the thyroid gland (Figure 21.17, *A*). With the index and middle fingers, gently move the tissue to the other side of the neck, using the other hand palpate for enlargements or tenderness (Figure 21.17, *B* and *C*). As the patient swallows, observe the gland for ease of movement.

DIAGNOSTIC AIDS

Diagnostic aids may be necessary to assist the dentist to accurately make an accurate diagnosis and to determine treatment. These aids include (1) radiographs, (2) photographs, (3) diagnostic models, and (4) laboratory tests. Such aids are valuable in explaining the condition or treatment to the patient.

Radiographs

A full-mouth set of radiographs should be taken of each new patient (Chapter 13). The radiographs are viewed as the patient's oral conditions are charted. Clinical observation along with radiographs allow for a more accurate assessment of the patient's oral condition. A panoramic radiograph may be taken if it is of diagnostic value. An edentulous patient, for example, can benefit from the information obtained through a panoramic radiograph and usually a panoramic radiograph is required during treatment for orthodontic and oral surgery patients. See Chapters 26 and 27.

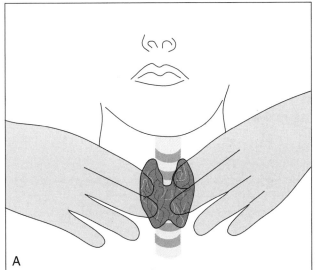

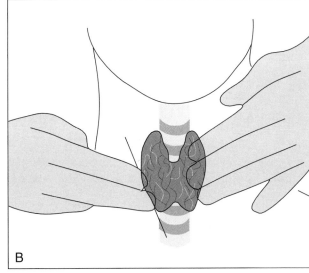

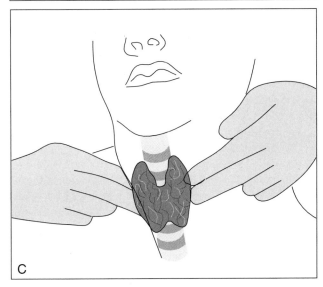

FIGURE 21-17

Anatomical location of the thyroid gland and examination: (**A**) index and middle fingers over the thyroid gland, (**B**) gently move the tissue to one side of the neck and (**C**) to the other side.

Photographs

While radiographs reveal some underlying conditions, photographs can give a vivid account of the patient's dental condition. Intraoral video systems are valuable aids when presenting a treatment plan.

Diagnostic Models

Diagnostic models offer the patient a three-dimensional view of the mouth. Study models help the patient visualize his or her oral condition during a treatment plan presentation. These models also aid in the dentist developing the treatment plan.

Biopsy

A **biopsy** is used to confirm the presence and nature of neoplastic disease. A biopsy is a simple procedure that may be completed by removing or excising the entire area or incising a small section of a suspect area. A biopsy may be excisional (removal of the entire suspect area) or incisional (removal of a small section of the suspect area). The equipment and materials that will be needed for a biopsy procedure are antiseptic, syringe, anesthetic, tissue

Biopsy

The removal of living tissue for microscopic examination

scissors, tissue forceps, hemostats, needle, needle holder, sutures, scalpel handle, scalpel blade, and specimen bottle, with preservatives. It is important to label the specimen bottle with all pertinent information.

Blood Test

A RIA-radioimmunoassay test is often requested by the dentist for a patient who has a positive history of hepatitis. It should be noted that dentists (oral surgeons in particular) have a higher incidence of hepatitis than the general population. Hepatitis vaccine should be taken by all dental personnel.

Cytologic Smear

A surface tissue smear is taken for microscopic evaluation in cases of suspicious nonbacterial organism. This procedure is used to collect a sample of superficial cells. It is a painless and simple procedure. The procedure begins by marking a glass slide with the patient's name and account number. The suspicious area is scraped with a sterile, wet tongue blade or metal spatula. The cells are smeared onto a glass slide and completely covered with a prepared fixative spray and air dried. The slides are then prepared according to laboratory instructions.

Cultures

A **culture** is the growth of living cells under laboratory con-

Culture

The growth of living cells on an artificial media

ditions. The examiner will take a sample of oral fluid and plaque to test for bacteriologic oral infections. The culture is taken with a sterile swab. Each specimen must be labeled with care. If the presence of other systemic problems is found through the oral examination, the dentist may request that the patient's physician help determine jointly what test should be administered.

Other tests that may be used to motivate the patient toward better oral hygiene include the Phase Contrast Microscopy and the Modified Snyder Test. Such visual evidence can help to convince the patient of the need for good dental care. These aids are discussed in more detail in Chapter 17.

CHARTING

As conditions are identified, they must be recorded systematically through the use of a tooth identification system. Several numbering systems are described in Chapter 9. The information in this chapter will be based on the Universal Numbering System. The use of a system allows uniform interpretation of a patient's dental chart information. There are symbols used that indicate certain oral conditions; refer to the charts illustrated in Table 21.2. A uniform system enables staff to recall the patient's dental conditions and status.

When communicating with specialists or other offices it may be necessary to identify a particular condition. A numbering system eliminates the necessity to use a complete verbal or written description. This is important when completing an irreversible procedure, such as an extraction. Anatomical and geometric charts are available (Figure 21.18, A and B). Both charts rely on the dental health personnel having a comprehensive understanding of the tooth surfaces (see Chapter 9).

The word restoration refers to any procedure that returns a defective area to its normal form and function. All restorations are charted in blue. A defect of a tooth indicates the existence of a condition that requires treatment. All defects are charted in red. A defect includes cavities, extractions to be made, restorations that are faulty, and fractured teeth. The chart below illustrates the charting of both restorations and defects.

The dental chart of patient restorations and defects may be used for the following aspects of patient care:
- Treatment planning: The graphic representation of the existing conditions of the patient's mouth is needed to organize dental procedures into a plan of treatment.
- Treatment: The charting is useful as a reference during appointments.
- Evaluation: Comparisons may be made between existing conditions and future examinations and charting in order to evaluate the outcome of the treatment.
- Protection: In the event of legal proceedings the records and chartings are realistic evidence.
- Identification: In case of an emergency, accident or disaster, a patient may be identified by his or her dental chart.

TREATMENT PLAN AND PRESENTATION

Data Gathered

The data gathered during the initial interview and the clinical examination, along with any additional information, such as outside consultations and laboratory test reports, must be evaluated thoroughly before an accurate and complete assessment of the patient's dental needs can be determined. All data must be considered comprehensively. The overall well being of the patient is considered, not just the patient's dental needs.

The information checklist includes the following:

Table 21-2

Charting of Existing Restorations and Defects

Restoration	Description	Illustration
Amalgam	Solid blue shading Class I on tooth #2 Class II on tooth #4 Class V on tooth #3	
Composite	No shading #9, 11 Class III on tooth #10 Class V on tooth #12	
Full gold crown (FGC)	Crown marked with blue diagonal lines FGC on tooth #29 FGC on tooth #30	

Continued

Table 21-2—Cont'd.

Charting of Existing Restorations and Defects

Restoration	Description	Illustration
Porcelain fused to metal (PFM)	Porcelain area dotted, metal area diagonal lines PFM crown on tooth #26	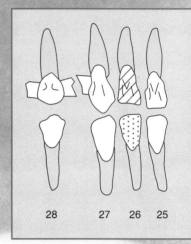
Bridge	Abutment teeth and pontic charted according to material Root of pontic tooth marked with blue X PFM crown on tooth #20 FGC pontic tooth #19 FGC on tooth #18 Bar indicates connection of abutment teeth to pontic	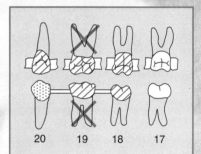
Removable partial denture (RPD)	Bracket is used to indicate teeth replaced by RPD Missing teeth marked with blue X RPD replaces teeth 2 to 5 - 15 and 14	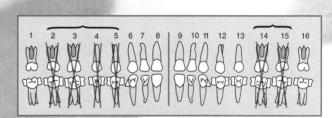
Complete denture (CD)	All teeth in arch marked with one blue X Maxillary CD	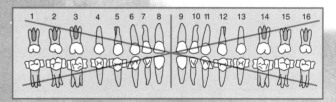
Cavity	Decayed surfaces are shaded in red Class I on tooth #3 Class III on tooth #8 Class V on tooth #6	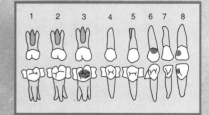

Table 21-2—Cont'd.

Charting of Existing Restorations and Defects

Restoration	Description	Illustration
Extractions	The tooth to be extracted is marked with a red X Tooth #17 to be extracted	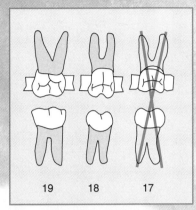
Fracture restoration of tooth	The fracture is outlined in red Incisal edge of tooth #8 Cusp of tooth #2	

Charting symbols

Missing	X
Cavity	Red
Food impaction	↑
Open contact	‖
Furcation open	▲
Periapical area	Ꝗ
Drift-extruded	D → ↑
Mobility	1-2-3
Restorations	Blue
Muco-gingival stress	ᙡ
Margin irregular	⟋ᙡ
Contact irregular	ᙡ

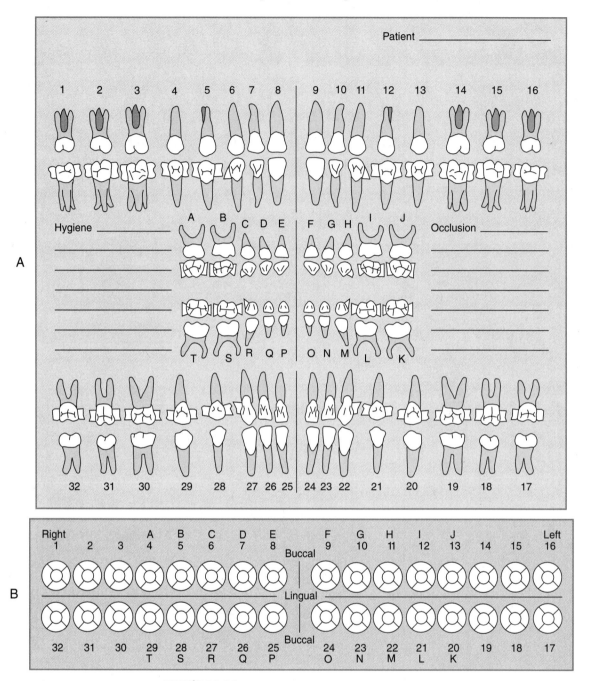

FIGURE 21-18

A, Sample anatomical chart. **B,** Sample geometric chart.

1 Personal history: General information (address, phone, and so on.)
2 Medical history: The patient's physical condition will play an important role in the formulation of the treatment plan.
3 Dental history: The chief complaint must be addressed *first.* Present oral conditions, as well as conditions that existed before the patient's initial visit are a factor.

4 Extraoral examination: Any abnormal conditions must be investigated. Abnormal conditions may influence dental treatment.
5 Intraoral examination: The findings of teeth and tissue must be evaluated.
6 Laboratory test: Conclusions of any blood test, biopsies, or culture smears are needed.

7 Radiographs: Full mouth periapical and bitewings are viewed.

8 Photographs: Preoperative photographs documenting conditions are examined and later used to compare with postoperative photographs.

9 Chartings: Intraoral conditions of teeth and tissues are interpreted.

Treatment Planning

The dentist will compare what is found clinically with radiographs taken. Chartings of restorations and defects will be examined as well as soft tissue evaluations and diagnostic models. Problems and conditions will be identified and the course of treatment will be determined. The dentist will develop a summary of problems found using the information gathered. From this summary the objective of the treatment plan will be determined. The decision will be made as to the priority of each procedure. The dentist will begin with the best available plan of treatment based on the dental conditions only, this would be considered an ideal plan. From this plan the dentist will develop a more realistic plan, one that takes into consideration the individual patient. The following factors will determine the plan of treatment:

- Patient's medical condition
- Patient's age
- Desires of patient
- Time required for treatment
- Patient's financial status

The patient's health and age are factors in the planning of treatment. A patient's medical condition might require modifications of dental treatment, such as placing a limit on the amount of time that a patient can spend in the dental chair for each appointment. It is generally agreed that a patient under the age of 18 years has not completed his or her oral development and any crown and bridge procedures should be postponed. It may also be a challenge to convince an older patient to accept the best treatment planned for them. An older patient will probably have different priorities than a younger patient. The sequence of the treatment should be based on the desires of the patient, taking into consideration completion of essential conditions. However, the patient's desires may be influenced by many factors: past dental experiences, finances, and the value they place on appearances. A patient's work schedule may influence the amount of time they have available for dental appointments. The financial status of the patient will be a major factor in the patient's acceptance of the plan. If the patient cannot afford the best plan of treatment it may be necessary to consider an alternative plan. Alternative plans usually allow the patient some financial options. Different dental materials may be used or perhaps a different procedure; the fee for a removable par-

tial denture might be lower than the fee for a gold bridge. The patient should be offered the best treatment plan and available alternatives. After all procedures have been identified the dental assistant or other office personnel will add fees and procedure numbers to complete the treatment plan.

The law requires that patients be given enough information to make an informed decision concerning their health care; the health care provider has a legal obligation to obtain the patient's informed consent. Informed consent can only be given with the provision of the following information:

- Description of the problem conditions
- Recommended treatment
- Risks involved
- Alternative treatment available
- Estimated fees
- Estimated time

The above listed information must be determined before presenting the plan to the patient.

Treatment Plan Presentation

Just as it is important to have an established sequence for the clinical examination it is equally important to be systematic about the treatment plan presentation. The allied dental personnel presenting the treatment plan must allow the patient to ask questions and be able to answer these questions with knowledge and confidence. The guidelines for establishing informed consent must be followed. The patient should be presented with a summary of the problems or conditions found. Radiographs and study case models can be used to help the patient see what conditions need to be corrected and to understand the effect of not correcting the conditions. An explanation of the cause and the effect of each condition must be given in terms of the patient's understanding. The recommended treatment must be explained along with the advantages or disadvantages of alternative treatment plans. Any significant risk must be explained. The estimated fees and the amount of time needed to complete the treatment must be discussed. Whether the plan is presented by the dentist or the dental assistant it must be given in terms that are clearly understood by the patient. Understanding the treatment plan is essential to the successful outcome of the presentation.

The patient should understand that the treatment plan can change. The treatment plan is just a plan; plans are always subject to change. A dentist cannot positively predict the outcome of any treatment. *If any additional treatments are included or the treatment plan is changed it is necessary to obtain an informed consent for these changes.* The patient's signature or the signature of the patient's guardian must be obtained. It should be documented in the patient's chart that

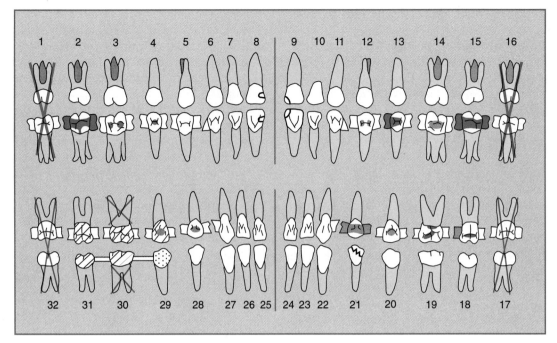

FIGURE 21-19

Completed chart of a patient's dental conditions.

the patient gave informed consent for treatment. A series of appointments should be made at this time.

The patient's acceptance of the treatment plan must be based on the education they have received concerning their oral health. Dental education of the patient begins when the patient enters the dental office. Patient education is most often the responsibility of the dental assistant.

A completed charting of a patient's oral condition is shown in Figure 21.19. Figure 21.20 is a treatment plan based on those conditions.

Proposed completion date ___9/15/94___   Actual completion ___9/15/94___

Patient name ___Dr. Smith___   Doctor name ___J. B. Sloan___

Patient number ___461-89-4780___

Summary of problems _____

_____

_____

_____

Treatment objectives _____

_____

_____

_____

Treatment prescription

ADA code	Area/ tooth	Surface	Treatment prescription	Est. net fee due	Date	Approved changes
4 3 4 1	41		Scaling & RT planning		/	
4 3 4 1	43		Scaling & RT planning		/	
4 3 4 1	44		Scaling & RT planning		/	
4 3 4 1	46		Scaling & RT planning		/	
2 1 4 0	12	0	Amalgam - one surf. AD		/	
2 1 4 0	14	0	Amalgam - one surf. AD		/	
2 1 4 0	20	0	Amalgam - one surf. AD		/	
2 1 4 0	28	0	Amalgam - one surf. AD		/	
3 3 3 0	18		RCT, three or more C		/	
2 9 5 2	18		Cast post & core		/	
2 7 9 0	18		Crown, full cast, HI		/	
3 3 1 0	21		RCT, one canal		/	
2 9 5 2	21		Cast post & core		/	
2 7 9 0	21		Crown, full cast, HI		/	
0 1 5 0			Reevaluation & recall examination		/	
					/	

I have been presented a plan of treatment (chart # _____ . Dated _____).

I understand that the estimated fee for the above is $ _____ . I also understand that the quoted fee is only an estimate and is subject to change.

Date _____ Patient signature _____ Dentist _____

FIGURE 21-20

Treatment plan.

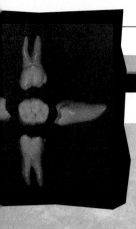

Points for Review

- Initial interview records
- Examination methods
- Procedure for taking vital signs
- Types of common emergency treatment encountered in practice
- Dental assistant's role in detecting medical problems
- Procedure for performing intraoral and extraoral examination and recording findings
- Diagnostic aids available to the dentist and personnel
- Charting and assisting in treatment planning presentation

Self-Study Questions

1. A patient's blood pressure is obtained using which one of the following examination techniques?
   a. Palpation
   b. Auscultation
   c. Percussion
   d. Olfaction

2. The diastolic blood pressure reading is recorded during which phase of listening?
   a. Phase 1
   b. Phase 2
   c. Phase 3
   d. Phase 5

3. Which of the following is not considered to be a patient's vital sign?
   a. Pulse
   b. Weight
   c. Respiration
   d. Temperature

4. If a patient's respiration is classified as hyperventilation how would you describe his or her breathing?
   a. Normal
   b. Slow
   c. Rapid
   d. Difficult

5. What is the normal range for the pulse rate of an adult patient?
   a. 30 to 50 beats per minute
   b. 40 to 60 beats per minute
   c. 60 to 100 beats per minute
   d. 70 to 110 beats per minute

6. What area of the oral cavity would be covered with masticatory mucosa?
   a. Gingiva
   b. Tongue
   c. Oral surface of the cheeks
   d. Soft palate

7. How would an alloy restoration be charted?
   a. Solid blue shading
   b. Solid red shading
   c. Outlined in red
   d. Blue diagonal lines

8. How would a full gold crown be charted?
   a. Blue shading
   b. Red shading
   c. Outlined in red
   d. Blue diagonal lines

9. What would a tooth surface shaded in red indicate?
   a. Extraction
   b. Cavity
   c. Full gold crown
   d. Composite

10. What is the summary of dental problems called?
    a. Consent form
    b. Treatment plan
    c. Contract
    d. Estimate

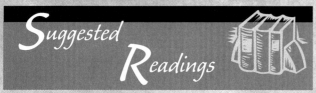

Becker, Steven, Langlais, Robert P, and Miller, Craig S: *Oral diagnosis, oral medicine, and treatment planning,* Philadelphia, 1994, Lea & Febiger.

Kinn, Mary E: *Medical assistant: administrative and clinical,* Philadelphia, 1988, W B Saunders.

Krutchfiff, David J: The clinical diagnostic process, *JADA* 124 (2): 122-124, 1993.

Minden, Nick J, Fast, Thomas B: The patient's health history form: how healthy is it? *JADA* 124:(8) 95-100, 1993.

Woodall, Irene: *Comprehensive dental hygiene care,* St Louis, 1993, Mosby.

Chapter 22

Management of Dental Office Emergencies

Key Points

- Possibility of medical emergencies in dental practice
- Prevention of medical emergencies in dental practice
- Basic life support and cardiopulmonary resuscitation (CPR)
- Causes, signs, symptoms, and treatment of possible medical emergencies
- Occupational hazards in the dental office
- Ethical and legal responsibilities related to medical emergencies in dental practice

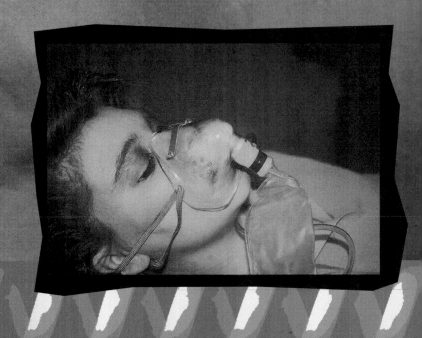

Chapter Outline

Responding to a Medical Emergency
   Office preparation for a medical
     emergency
   Emergency protocol
   Supplies and equipment
   Emergency kit
   Basic life support
   Emergency cricothyrotomy
   Cardiopulmonary resuscitation
Causes and Treatment of Possible Emergen-
   cies in the Dental Office
   Vasodepressor syncope (fainting)
   Hyperventilation
   Swallowing or aspiration of a foreign
     body
   Allergic reactions
   Diabetes mellitus

   Epilepsy and convulsive disorders
   Heart disorders
   Stroke
Occupational Hazards in the Dental Office
   Human immunodeficiency virus and ac-
     quired immunodeficiency syndrome
   Hepatitis B virus
   Herpetic whitlow
   Radiation hygiene
   Mercury hygiene
   Nitrous oxide
   Acrylic monomer and polymer
   Eye protection in the dental office
   Cuts, needlesticks, and soft tissue
     injuries
   Asbestos
   Other emergencies

Learning Objectives

On completion of Chapter 22, the student should be able to do the following:

- Define key terms.
- Describe the responsibilities of the dental team in responding to a medical emergency.
- Describe the preparations that must be made to prevent or reduce the chance of a medical emergency during dental treatment.
- Describe when, how, and why the various BLS and CPR techniques should be performed.

- Describe the medical emergencies most likely to occur in the dental office and ways to respond to them.
- Describe the occupational hazards of the practice of dentistry.
- Describe the legal and ethical responsibilities of each member of the dental team in responding to a medical emergency.

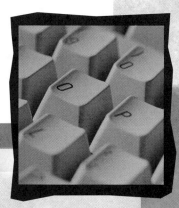

Key Terms

Aspiration

Basic Life Support (BLS)

Cardiopulmonary Resuscitation (CPR)

Dyspnea

Edema

Emergency Protocol

Heimlich Maneuver

Vital Signs

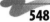

RESPONDING TO A MEDICAL EMERGENCY

To properly respond to a medical crisis in the dental office, the entire dental staff must thoroughly understand the four Ps of dealing with emergencies: prevention, planning, preparation, and practice (Box 22.1).

Office Preparation for a Medical Emergency

Vital signs

Indicators of the state of the body's basic functions: pulse rate, respiratory rate, temperature, and blood pressure

The best way to prevent an unexpected medical problem and the most basic rule of health care is *know your patient.* This usually is accomplished through the health history or medical history, the physical evaluation, and monitoring and recording of the patient's **vital signs** (see Chapter 24).

Emergency Protocol

The dental team uses a thorough medical history, physical evaluation, assessment of vital signs, and consultation with the patient's physician to avoid a medical emergency. However, despite their best efforts, everyone in the office must expect that an emergency will occur. The office must prepare for such an event by developing a protocol for responding to medical crises.

A protocol is a specific plan of action that outlines a series of steps to be taken should a certain event occur. The protocol should be part of the office manual. Every member of the dental staff should be thoroughly knowledgeable about the **emergency protocol** to be used in case of a medical emergency in the office. The roles of the dentist, the dental assistant or hygienist, and the receptionist in a medical emergency are outlined below.

Emergency protocol

Preplanned roles and behaviors to be followed by those responding to a medical emergency

Role of the Dentist

1 Assume primary responsibility for the patient's care.
2 Diagnose the problem and begin appropriate first aid treatment:
   a Supplemental oxygen
   b Basic life support

Box 22.1

Four Ps of Dealing with a Medical Emergency

The dental staff *must:*
Prevent a medical crisis by becoming knowledgeable about the patient.
Plan for the possibility of a medical emergency.
Prepare the necessary supplies and equipment in advance.
Practice and rehearse the duties of office personnel in an emergency.

---

   c Advanced life support
   d Administration of drugs and other medications
3 Call for appropriate assistance:
   a Emergency medical service (EMS)
   b Patient's physician
   c Local hospital
4 Stay with the patient until qualified personnel have assumed responsibility for the person's welfare.
5 Thoroughly document the event in the patient's record.
6 Perform a follow-up analysis of the event to determine how and why it occurred and how such an occurrence could be prevented in the future.

Role of the Dental Assistant or Hygienist

1 Advise the dentist immediately of the emergency.
2 Provide basic life support (BLS) if required until the dentist arrives:
   a Establish or maintain an open airway
   b Provide artificial respiration if the patient is not breathing on his or her own
   c Support the circulation by means of external heart compressions if no pulse can be detected.
3 Retrieve the office emergency kit and make it available to the dentist (the kit should be readily available to all).
4 Retrieve the oxygen tank and mask and make them available to the dentist.
5 Retrieve a hard backboard and assist the dentist in placing the patient either on the backboard or on the floor if CPR is necessary (CPR cannot be performed satisfactorily in the dental chair).
6 Maintain the contents of the emergency kit according to the dentist's instructions.

Role of the Receptionist

1 Post emergency telephone numbers by the telephone (EMS, local hospital, local medical clinic).
2 Call EMS (usually 911) and advise paramedics of the following:

a That there is an emergency and the rescue unit is needed

b The nature of the emergency (such as an unexplained loss of consciousness, cardiac arrest, or diabetic crisis)

c The patient's name, age, and gender

d The exact location of the office, with directions

e The receptionist's name and the office telephone number

3 Calm any patients in the waiting room or other treatment rooms. These patients should be advised only that the dentist must attend to a patient who is having a medical problem. No specifics of the problem should be provided, such as its nature or the patient's name. If the situations warrants, any patients who are waiting should be rescheduled.

4 Provide whatever other assistance the dentist may require.

Supplies and Equipment

Two essential pieces of emergency equipment should be readily available in every dental office: (1) an oxygen tank with a regulator, hose, and mask and (2) an emergency kit that contains a positive-pressure ventilation mask, emergency drugs, and other supplies.

Oxygen

Pure oxygen (100%) is the perfect agent for resuscitating unconscious patients who are still breathing on their own. It can be administered by anyone trained in the use of the equipment. The procedure for operating oxygen equipment is outlined in Box 22.2, and precautions for oxygen therapy are listed in Box 22.3.

Oxygen equipment includes the following components:

1 *Oxygen tank:* Oxygen is supplied in cylinder tanks, which are always green. The office should have two tanks, one primary and one back-up. A designated staff member, such as a dental assistant, should be given the responsibility to make sure that the tanks are full, that they are replaced when necessary, and that they are always in their proper place.

2 *Regulator:* The regulator is a valve that allows oxygen to be released from the tank at a specific rate (Figure 22.1). The regulator may be opened either by a small wheel, which can be turned by hand, or by a special wrench, which often is attached to the regulator by a cable. Turning the wrench *counterclockwise* opens the regulator valve; turning it *clockwise* closes the valve.

3 *Pressure gauge:* Attached to the regulator is a pressure gauge, which indicates the amount of oxygen in the tank, measured in pounds per square inch (psi). This gauge usually has areas marked in green and red. The green zone indicates that oxygen remains in the tank. The red zone indicates that the tank is empty or almost empty.

4 *Flowmeter:* The flowmeter is a gauge attached to the regulator tubing that registers the amount of oxygen, measured in liters per minute, delivered from the tank. This

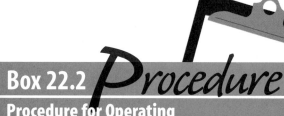

Box 22.2 Procedure

Procedure for Operating Oxygen Equipment

1. If the tank is new, use the attached wrench to crack the seal slightly to release a little oxygen, thereby clearing dirt or debris from the valve.
2. Attach the regulator and flowmeter (special grooves and threads allow these to be attached in only one way).
3. Open the regulator completely (turn it counterclockwise) and then turn it back one turn. This prevents damage to the equipment by a staff member who may think the regulator is closed and try to open it further.
4. Adjust the rate of flow to 4 to 6 liters per minute (see Figure 22.1).
5. Make sure that the hose has no knots or twists.
6. Place the mask over the patient's face, making sure that it fits with a good seal. If the patient is receiving oxygen, a clear mask probably will fog up, confirming that the patient is receiving oxygen.
7. Monitor the patient during the administration of oxygen. When oxygen therapy has been completed, remove the mask, turn off the oxygen, close the regulator valve, and disinfect or dispose of the mask and tubing.

Box 22.3 Take note

Precautions for Oxygen Therapy

Although oxygen therapy usually is very safe, three precautions must always be observed:

1. Although oxygen gas is not explosive, it is flammable and supports combustion. It therefore should not be used near an open flame.
2. Grease or oil can explode in the presence of oxygen and a flame. Staff members must make sure that there is no grease on the tank, on their hands, or in the vicinity.
3. Oxygen therapy should not be given to a patient who is hyperventilating because it will only worsen the problem.

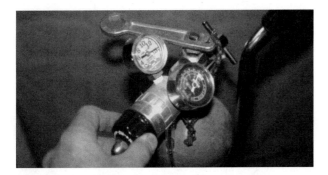

FIGURE 22.1

E-size oxygen tank with regulator valve, volume gauge, and flowmeter. To open the tank, the wrench is twisted counterclockwise (to the left). The person using this tank is adjusting the flowmeter.

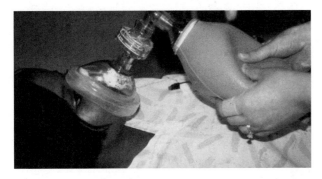

FIGURE 22.2

Use of an Ambu-bag.

gauge usually is a round, aneroid gauge, although some systems may use a pressure-compensated flowmeter, which is a vertical glass tube with a ball float that rises and falls with the volume of oxygen actually passing through the tube.

5 *Face mask:* Oxygen can be delivered to the patient by a face mask or nasal cannula (a loop of tubing that hooks over the ears and has two small prongs that fit directly into the patient's nostrils to deliver the oxygen). If a face mask is used, it should be made of clear plastic so that the patient's mouth and nose can be seen.

Ambu-Bag

If the patient is not breathing on his or her own, a positive-pressure inflation bag may be attached to the oxygen tube. This device, often called an Ambu-bag, consists of a rubber or plastic bag attached to a face mask. The face mask is placed snugly over the person's nose and mouth, and the bag is squeezed to force air into the lungs (Figure 22.2). If the bag is attached to the oxygen hose, oxygen can be forced directly into the patient's lungs.

Components of an Emergency Kit

1. A pocket mask for mouth-to-mouth ventilation. The mask is placed over the victim's mouth and nose, and a one-way valve allows the rescuer to blow air into the mask without coming into direct contact with the patient (Figure 22.3).
2. Ammonia inhalant ampules for syncope (fainting).
3. Nitroglycerine tablets or sublingual spray for angina (chest pains).
4. Ampules of antihistamines and adrenaline for allergic reactions.
5. A bronchodilator for asthma.
6. A preloaded epinephrine syringe for anaphylactic shock.
7. Disposable plastic syringes.
8. A tourniquet for intravenous (IV) injections.
9. Sugar cubes or cake frosting for insulin shock.
10. Drugs to treat conditions such as convulsion, loss of blood pressure, slow pulse, and extreme pain.
11. A cricothyrotomy needle to create an emergency airway.

Emergency Kit

Each dental office should have an emergency kit containing emergency drugs, syringes, a tourniquet, a positive-pressure mask, a cricothyrotomy needle, and so on. Selection of these items is the responsibility of the dentist (Box 22.4).

Although only licensed, trained personnel, such as the dentist, may legally administer the drugs in the emergency kit, the dental assistant often is responsible for checking the kit regularly to make sure that the contents are complete and current.

Emergency Drugs

Dr. Stanley F. Malamed, a nationally recognized expert in medical emergencies in dentistry, recommends that the basic emergency kit contain only six drugs, just two of which are injectable. These drugs are:

1 Oxygen in positive pressure, to support oxygenation of compressed tissues.
2 Epinephrine (1:1000): 0.3 to 0.5 ml, preloaded; administered intramuscularly (IM) for an immediate allergic response such as anaphylaxis.
3 Diphenhydramine HCL (Benadryl): 50 mg/ml for delayed allergic response.
4 Nitroglycerin spray for angina (not exposed to air, this form stays fresh until it is used).
5 Bronchodilator, such as isoproterenol or metaproterenol, for asthma attacks.
6 Orange juice or cake icing for hypoglycemia or insulin shock.

If desired, an ammonia ampule may also be kept on hand to treat syncope.

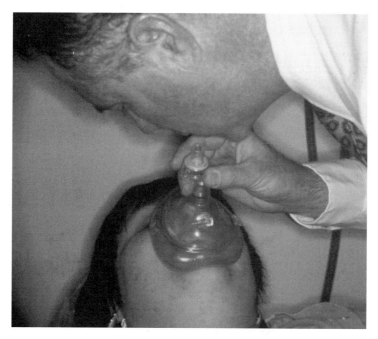

FIGURE 22.3

Use of the pocket mask for mouth-to-mouth ventilation. The mask has a one-way valve that allows the rescuer to blow air into the mask without coming into direct contact with the patient.

If the dental office is within minutes of an EMS base, administration of other drugs is best left to trained paramedics. The six drugs listed previously will maintain a patient until EMS personnel arrive. Although the dentist and dental auxiliaries must be knowledgeable about medical emergencies and the medications used to treat them, their primary responsibilities in dealing with such emergencies are (1) to recognize the problem; (2) to stabilize the patient's condition and prevent the problem from getting worse; and (3) to call for expert help *immediately.* The dentist and staff are not expected to be EMS technicians or emergency medicine physicians.

Basic Life Support

Brain damage begins when the brain has been deprived of oxygen for 4 minutes. Lack of oxygen to the brain occurs if breathing stops or the heart stops beating, or if both occur at the same time. After 6 to 10 minutes, brain death becomes certain. Because brain death can occur so quickly, the most basic and important skill of all health care professionals is **basic life support (BLS).**

Basic life support

Artificial support of vital life processes; includes the ABCs: *airway* opening, *breathing*, and *circulation* of the blood

Airway, Breathing, and Circulation

The three critical elements of basic life support are keeping the airway open, aiding the breathing function, and supporting circulation.

- *Airway:* A closed or blocked airway must be opened. The Heimlich maneuver is one means of accomplishing this.
- *Breathing:* The lungs must be ventilated manually if the patient is not breathing on his or her own. This is known as rescue or artificial breathing.
- *Circulation:* Manual pumping of blood (artificial circulation) is necessary if the patient's heart has stopped beating.

The last two elements usually are combined into the process of cardiopulmonary resuscitation. All members of the dental team should complete a yearly refresher course in BLS taught by an instructor certified by the American Red Cross or the American Heart Association. In many areas this is a requirement for licensure or certification.

Management of a Blocked Airway

If air cannot get to the lungs, the beating of the heart becomes irrelevant. In a conscious patient, obstruction of the airway usually is caused by a foreign body lodged in the throat. In most cases, the treatment for this problem is a version of the **Heimlich maneuver.** In an unconscious patient, obstruction often occurs because of regurgitation or

Box 22.5

Procedure

Procedure for Abdominal Compressions (Heimlich Maneuver)*

Conscious, standing patient:

1. Have a bystander call paramedics.
2. Quickly move behind the person and place your arms around the patient's upper waist.
3. Make a fist with one hand and place the thumb of that hand midway between the person's rib cage and navel.
4. Cover the fist with your other hand (Figure 22.4, *A*).
5. Tell the patient to lean forward slightly over your arm and hand.
6. Make several (6 to 10) sharp, quick *inward and upward* abdominal thrusts with the locked fist and hand, with a slight pause between thrusts.
7. Repeat as necessary until the object is dislodged and the person is breathing freely or emergency medical help arrives.
8. When the technique is successful, the dislodged object often flies forcibly out of the patient's mouth.
9. If the patient is seated, the technique is basically the same: squat or kneel behind the patient so that you can wrap your arms around the person and repeat the procedure described above.

Unconscious patient:

1. Place the patient in the supine position (on his or her back) on a flat, hard surface such as the floor.
2. Open the airway, using the head tilt–chin lift method from CPR to pull the tongue away from the back of the throat.
3. Attempt to ventilate using the CPR technique. If this is unsuccessful, turn the patient's face to one side to make removal of the material easier and, using the index finger like a hook, sweep the mouth from one side to the other, reaching to the back of the tongue and pulling forward to remove the object, if possible.
4. Straddle one or both of the patient's legs, facing the head.
5. Place the heel of one hand on the patient's abdomen between the navel and the lower part of the breastbone (xiphoid process of the sternum).
6. Place the heel of the other hand on top of the first hand and interlock the fingers (Figure 22.4, *B*).
7. Thrust vigorously several times (6 to 10) *inward and upward* toward the patient's diaphragm.
8. Repeat the finger sweep of the oral cavity and attempt to ventilate.
9. Repeat abdominal thrusts, until the object is dislodged or emergency medical help arrives.
10. If the object is dislodged, turn the patient's head to the side and remove the object carefully to prevent it from falling back into the throat.

*These guidelines also apply to children over 8 years of age. For a child 1 to 8 years of age, adult techniques are used but with proportionally less force.

Heimlich maneuver

An emergency maneuver performed to expel a foreign body from the airway; a quick thrust is used to squeeze the upper abdomen and force residual air from the lungs, ejecting the object

aspiration of vomit or because the tongue has collapsed into the back of the mouth. Resolving the airway obstruction is the first goal of CPR.

A patient who is obviously choking or who suddenly cannot speak and begins to turn blue should be asked, "Can you speak?" If the person is getting air, he or she will be able to speak somewhat and probably cough forcibly. If this is the case, the dental staff should *do nothing* until the person coughs up the object or until it becomes obvious that the patient needs further assistance. However, if the patient fails to cough up the object or cannot speak and begins to turn blue, the dental staff must act *immediately* to save the person's life (Box 22.5).

Aspiration

Ingestion of a foreign body into the airway tree; also, negative pressure in a hypodermic syringe

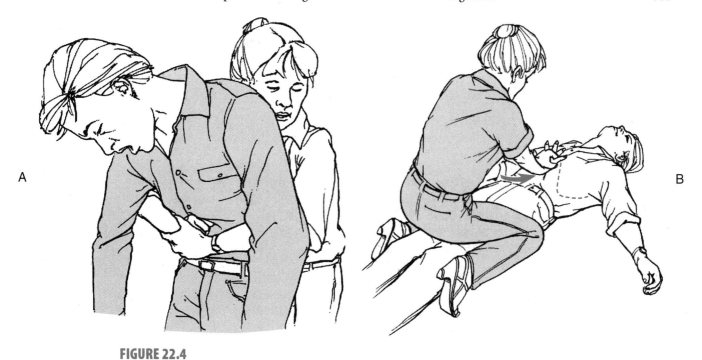

FIGURE 22.4

A, The Heimlich maneuver as performed on a conscious standing or sitting individual suffering from airway obstruction by a foreign body. **B,** The Heimlich maneuver as performed on an unconscious victim. (Courtesy American Heart Association.)

Chest thrusts, rather than abdominal thrusts, should be used to compress the lungs if the patient is (1) severely obese or (2) in the latter stages of pregnancy. With either condition it often is impossible for the rescuer's arms to go around the patient's waist. Also, abdominal thrusts could easily damage a developing fetus. In these cases proper compression of the patient's chest can work as effectively as abdominal compression (Box 22.6).

Finger Sweeps in an Unconscious Patient

Removing a foreign object from the oral cavity of a conscious patient is very difficult. However, in an unconscious patient the mouth and throat muscles relax, making it possible to attempt to remove something from the mouth (see Box 22.6). This must be done carefully to avoid worsening the problem by pushing the object farther down the throat.

Airway Obstruction in Infants and Children

Children over 8 years of age are treated according to adult guidelines. For a child (1 to 8 years of age), adult techniques are used but with proportionally less force. Infant guidelines are applied for those under 1 year old. An infant with a complete airway obstruction makes no sounds. The infant simply turns pale and then blue, loses consciousness, and dies. The treatment of airway obstruction in infants is presented in Box 22.7.

Performing the Heimlich Maneuver on Oneself

A person may start to choke when alone and no help is available. Should that occur, the following steps should be taken:

1 Lean over the back of a chair, a railing, a sink, or other similar object.
2 Press quickly against the upper abdomen to try to dislodge the object.

Emergency Cricothyrotomy

Occasionally the Heimlich maneuver, in all its variations, is unsuccessful. In such cases the choking victim will die in a matter of minutes unless an airway can be established *below* the obstruction. In the past the standard technique was the surgical tracheotomy. However, this is a very risky technique that can be performed successfully only by specially trained personnel, usually in ideal circumstances. In an emergency situation the tracheotomy has a poor success rate. For that reason, the cricothyrotomy has become the *surgical technique of last resort* (see Box 26.19).

Cardiopulmonary Resuscitation

Obviously, if a person is not breathing or the heart is not beating, opening the airway is not enough. In such cases the patient's lungs must be artificially ventilated or the

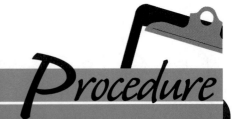

Box 22.6

Procedure for Chest Compressions

Conscious patient (standing or sitting):
1. **Stand behind the patient.**
2. **Place your arms directly under the patient's armpits and around the chest.**
3. **Make a fist with one hand and place the thumb side of the fist over the middle of the sternum (breastbone),** *not* **the edge of the rib cage or xiphoid process at the bottom of the sternum.**
4. **Place the other hand over the fist and administer several quick, backward thrusts until the object is expelled or emergency medical help arrives (Figure 22.5,** *A***).**

Unconscious patient:
1. **Place the patient in the supine position (on his or her back) on the floor or a hard, flat surface.**
2. **Using the head tilt–chin lift technique, open the airway and leave the head tilted back.**
3. **Straddle or kneel beside the patient as in the technique for abdominal thrusts (see Box 22.5).**
4. **Place the heel of one hand over the victim's lower sternum (not the xiphoid process),** **place the other hand over the first, and interlock the fingers. This will be the same position you will use if doing CPR.**
5. **Administer 6 to 10 quick downward chest compressions.**

Finger sweeps in an unconscious patient:
1. **With the patient in the supine position, open the person's mouth using the head tilt–chin lift technique or by inserting the thumb and index finger between the teeth on each side of the mouth.**
2. **Place the index and middle fingers of one hand at the corner of the mouth and move them along the inside of the cheek to the back of the mouth (on the side) near the base of the tongue (Figure 22.5,** *B***).**
3. **Using a hooking motion of the fingers, make a sweep across the back of the mouth to the other side and pull forward. Proceed carefully to avoid forcing a foreign body farther down the airway.**
4. **Repeat twice. If unsuccessful, repeat chest compressions and finger sweeps until recovery or emergency medical assistance arrives.**

Cardiopulmonary resuscitation (CPR)

Artificial ventilation of the lungs and pumping of the heart

heart artificially pumped through **cardiopulmonary resuscitation (CPR).** All health care providers, including dental auxiliaries, have a professional responsibility to know CPR. The sequence of steps in CPR is summarized as the "ABCs"—*a*irway, *b*reathing, and *c*irculation.

nique. If the victim is unconscious but breathing and has a detectable pulse, the rescuer should call for emergency medical help and stay with the victim until that assistance arrives. However, if the victim is not breathing and has no pulse, CPR must begin immediately (Box 22.8).

Calling for Help

Once the rescuer has determined that CPR is necessary, he or she should call for help from bystanders, assuming that other individuals are in the area. This should be done while the rescuer prepares to start CPR.

Determining Consciousness (Shake and Shout)

The rescuer should tap the patient firmly on the shoulder and shout in the person's ear, "Are you all right? Are you all right?"; this is often referred to as the *shake and shout* tech-

Opening the Airway

In an unconscious victim, the airway must be opened if artificial respiration is to succeed. Therefore the rescuer's next task is to move the tongue away from the back of the throat to open the airway.

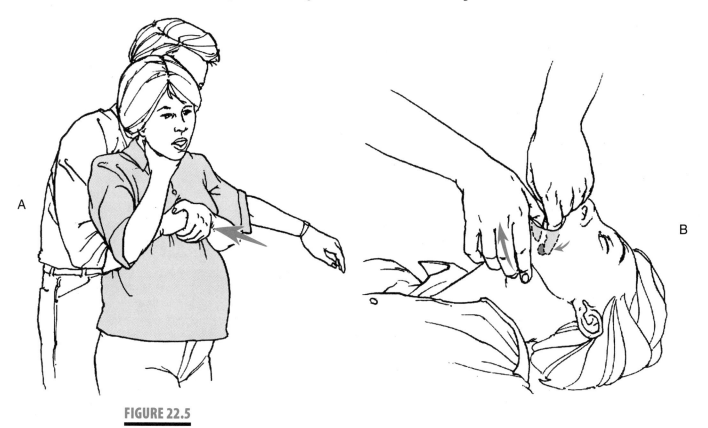

FIGURE 22.5

A, Chest thrusts should be used on a conscious victim of foreign body obstruction who is pregnant or obese. **B,** Finger sweeps. (Courtesy American Heart Association.)

Head Tilt–Chin Lift

The customary and most effective technique for opening the airway is the *head tilt–chin lift* method. The victim is positioned flat on the back on a firm surface. The rescuer approaches the victim from the side and places the palm of one hand on the victim's forehead and the fingertips of the other hand on the *bony* portion of the chin. While applying firm backward pressure on the forehead to tilt the head back, the chin is lifted *forward and up* with the fingertips on the bony portion *only* of the chin. In this process, lift the tongue away from the back of the throat and airway.

Airway Check

At this point the rescuer must check the victim's airway to determine if any air is passing through and if the victim is breathing on his or her own; this is done with the *look, listen, and feel* technique. The rescuer places an ear next to the victim's mouth to hear any sounds of breathing and to feel any air passing against the side of the face. At the same time the rescuer must look down for the rise and fall of the chest. If the airway is open but no breathing can be detected, the rescuer must begin artificial respiration.

Face Mask with One-Way Valve

A face mask with a one-way valve may be used to prevent contact with the victim's body fluids. Many emergency kits contain a small, heart-shaped face mask that forms an air seal over the victim's nose and mouth (see Figure 22.3). This mask has a one-way valve, which the rescuer may blow into without coming into direct contact with the victim. A face mask connected to an Ambu-bag, described previously, also can be used to ventilate the lungs while avoiding direct contact with the victim.

Verification of a Pulse

After the first two ventilations of the victim's lungs, the rescuer must check to see if a pulse is present. The *carotid artery* in the neck is used to verify the pulse because it is close to where the rescuer is working and is accessible without removing any clothing. *For an adult or child, the pulse is detected using the tips of the index and middle finger over the carotid artery for 5 to 10 seconds. For the infant, the brachial artery on the inside of the arm halfway between the shoulder and elbow is used. To feel the brachial pulse, place the thumb on the outside of the infant's arm with the index and middle finger on the inside over the brachial artery. If no pulse can be felt within 10 seconds, the rescuer should assume cardiac arrest*

Box 22.7

Procedure for Dislodging a Foreign Body in an Infant*

Conscious infant:

1. Cradle the infant on your forearm, face down, with the head lower than the trunk.
2. Using the heel of the opposite hand, give four back blows between the shoulder blades (Figure 22.6, *A*).
3. If the object is not dislodged, turn the infant face up, supporting the head and neck with your hand and cradling the body on your forearm.
4. With the index and middle fingers of the opposite hand, give four quick chest thrusts in the area of the midsternum between the nipples.
5. Check for the foreign object by placing a thumb in the mouth over the tongue and lower incisor region and opening the mouth. *Only if you see it,* attempt to remove the foreign object with a finger sweep of the index finger.
6. Repeat until the foreign body is dislodged or the infant loses consciousness. In the latter case, proceed to the next section.

Unconscious infant:

1. Place the infant in the supine position (face up) on your lap, supporting the head and neck with your forearm (the head should be lower than the trunk). As an alternative, place the infant on a hard surface, such as the floor.
2. Open the infant's airway and attempt to ventilate twice.
3. If ventilation is not possible, place the tips of the index and middle fingers midway between the infant's rib cage and navel.
4. Press *inward and upward* into the abdomen with four quick movements (Figure 22.6, *B*).
5. Turn the infant over and cradle the child on your forearm with the head again lower than the trunk. Give four back blows between the shoulder blades in the same manner as described for a conscious infant.
6. Check the infant's mouth as described above; if the foreign object is visible, make two sweeps with your index finger to try to dislodge it.
7. Repeat the process until the infant recovers or emergency medical assistance arrives.

*These guidelines apply to infants under 1 year of age. For a child 1 to 8 years of age, adult techniques are used (see Box 22.5) but with proportionally less force.

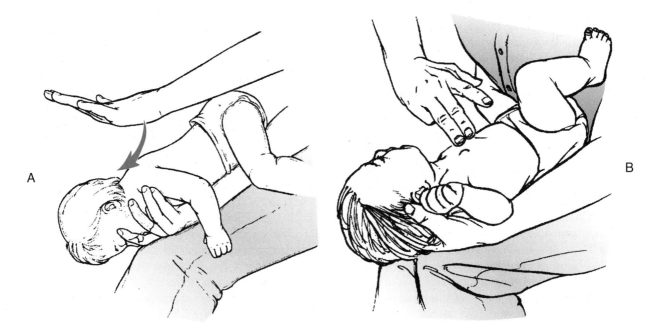

A

B

FIGURE 22.6

A, Back blows are used to dislodge a foreign body in a conscious infant. **B,** The chest thrust should be used on an unconscious infant. (Courtesy American Heart Association.)

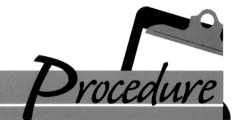

Box 22.8

Procedure for Providing Artificial Respiration

Adult:

1. Kneel alongside the patient.
2. Open the airway using the head tilt–chin lift technique.
3. Maintaining the head tilt with backward pressure on the forehead, use the thumb and forefinger of the same hand to seal the patient's nostrils.
4. Take a deep breath, open your mouth, and place it completely over the patient's mouth, making an airtight seal (Figure 22.7).
5. Blow two or three puffs of air gently but firmly into the patient's mouth.
6. Allow the patient to exhale passively, with gravity deflating the lungs.
7. Repeat the cycle immediately.

Infant or child:

1. Use the same techniques for a child 1 to 8 years of age if a good seal around the mouth can be made. For an infant, less than 1 year of age, it is often possible to cover and seal the mouth and nose at the same time.
2. To inflate the lungs, use greater force because of the smaller air passages in infants and children.
3. In both cases, reduce the volume of air provided to the victim to accommodate the smaller lung capacity.
4. The rescuer must carefully observe the rise of the chest to avoid overinflation, which could cause regurgitation or injury.
5. Determine consciousness of the child by "shake and shout" technique used for

the adult. For infants, shout the baby's name while thumping on the sole of their foot.
6. If the child or infant does not immediately respond, the rescuer should assume they are unconscious and proceed to the next step.
7. If the child or infant is unconscious, position them on a hard, flat surface.
8. Use the head tilt-chin lift technique to open the airway even further. Place two or three fingers beneath the lower jaw at the angle and lift the jaw upward (forward) and outward. If no evidence of neck injury exists, a slight head tilt may be used if the jaw thrust alone does not open the airway.
9. Determine if there is air exchange, using the "look, listen, feel" technique.
10. If there is no detectable breathing, check for blockage and repeat the process. Once the airway is opened, give two rescue breaths at the correct volume (judged by the rise of the chest) and rate (once every 3 seconds for an infant and once every 4 seconds for a child) and verify the pulse.
11. Two person CPR: one rescuer provides ventilation to the lungs while the other performs chest compressions.
12. The ratio of compressions to ventilations in two person CPR is usually five compressions to one ventilation. To combat fatigue, the rescuers can reverse roles at the end of a ventilation cycle by a prearranged signal.

has occurred and immediately begin CPR measures to artificially circulate the blood throughout the body.

Circulation (External Chest Compressions)   If a pulse is not present, despite satisfactorily opening the airway and ventilating the lungs, the rescuer must begin to artificially circulate the blood. This is done by a rhythmic

compression of the sternum that forces blood out of the heart (Boxes 22.9 and 22.10). It is done while simultaneously ventilating the lungs with air. The rescuer can begin external chest compressions by appearing alongside the patient and locating the proper pressure point for administering chest compressions (the lower portion of the sternum).

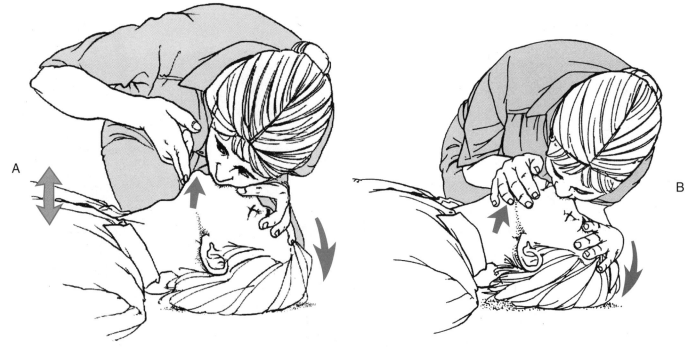

FIGURE 22.7

A, Mouth-to-mouth rescue breathing. The breathing rate for adults is 12 times per minute (every 5 seconds); for children, 15 times per minute (every 4 seconds); and for infants, 20 times per minute (every 3 seconds). **B,** If a seal cannot be maintained with the mouth, mouth-to-nose rescue breathing could save a victim's life. (Illustrations courtesy American Heart Association.)

CAUSES AND TREATMENT OF POSSIBLE EMERGENCIES IN THE DENTAL OFFICE

Vasodepressor Syncope (Fainting)

The common type of fainting is known medically as *vasodepressor syncope,* which is a general term that describes a sudden, temporary loss of consciousness. This loss of consciousness is the result of a loss of adequate blood flow to the brain, and it is one of the most common medical emergencies in the dental office. It is also one of the easiest emergencies both to prevent and to treat (Box 22.11). However, if not properly and promptly treated, the prolonged loss of consciousness associated with fainting could lead to brain damage or even death.

Hyperventilation

Hyperventilation is an abnormal increase in the depth and rate of respiration in a *sedentary* individual. Because it is associated with stressor anxiety, it is a common occurrence in the dental office. Treatment measures are outlined in Box 22.12.

Swallowing or Aspiration of a Foreign Body

Dental treatment creates the perfect environment in which a patient can swallow or aspirate (inhale) a foreign body. Four-handed sit-down dentistry, with the patient in a reclined or supine position, greatly increases the likelihood of such an event. With the patient in this position, a variety of wet, slippery objects (such as crowns or inlays, amalgam particles, clumps of dental cements, teeth or fragments of teeth, impression materials, and cotton rolls) may fall to the back of the patient's throat, where they may be swallowed or aspirated. The proper use of rubber dams and throat packs, where appropriate, are affective methods to prevent the incident from happening. Box 22.13 lists the signs and symptoms of airway obstruction, as well as treatment measures.

Allergic Reactions

Allergic (hypersensitivity) reactions may be immediate or delayed in onset. A reaction is considered immediate if it occurs within seconds to 1 hour of exposure to the antigen; the reaction is considered delayed if it occurs hours to days after

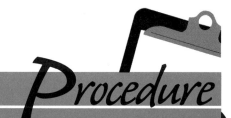

Box 22.9

Procedures for Providing External Chest Compressions

Adult:

1. Place the index and middle finger of the hand closest to the victim's feet along the lower border of the rib cage on the side closest to the rescuer.
2. Trace or follow the margin of the rib cage with the fingertips to the notch in the lower chest where the ribs from the right and left side meet at the midline.
3. Place the middle finger in the notch with the index finger alongside it on the lowest portion of the breastbone. (This is the xiphoid process of the sternum.) *Do not* press here; this part of the sternum is fragile and easily fractured. A fracture could cause severe internal damage, such as a laceration of the liver.
4. Place the heel of the opposite hand (located closest to the patient's head) on the sternum directly alongside the index finger. This will be the area for chest compressions.
5. Remove the first hand and place on top of the hand resting directly on the sternum.
6. Interlock the fingers to keep the fingers off of the chest during compressions. The ribs could easily be damaged by fingers pressing on them during chest compressions.
7. Lock elbows and position the shoulders over the hands to use the body weight instead of arm muscles for force.
8. Compress an adult victim's chest about 1.5 to 2 inches at a rate of 80 to 100 compressions per minute (15 compressions in 9 to 11 seconds).
9. Following compression, release pressure to allow the heart to refill, without removing the hands to not lose correct hand position.
10. Maintain a smooth, even rhythm with equal time allowed for compression and release.
11. One-person CPR: administer 15 compressions, counting aloud during each compression, "1 and 2 and 3 and 4 and . . . . 15."
12. On reaching 15, administer two, slow and full rescue breaths, relocate the correct hand position, and provide another 15 chest compressions.
13. After three or four cycles of chest compressions and rescue breaths the rescuer should check for a carotid pulse. If a pulse is felt but the victim is not breathing spontaneously, rescue breathing should be continued. If no pulse is felt, rescue breathing and chest compressions should be continued.
14. Repeat sequence until the victim begins to recover; others qualified in CPR are able to take over; medical assistance arrives; or the rescuer is physically exhausted and can no longer continue.

Child:

1. The location for administering external chest compressions for a child is the same as for an adult (i.e., on the lower portion of the sternum but above the xiphoid process).
2. The method for determining this location is also the same.
3. Because the bones of a child are smaller and more fragile than those of an adult, the *amount* of force and subsequent chest compressions are proportionally less.
4. For a child, the heel of *one* hand, not both, is used to compress the sternum about 1.0 to 1.5 inches.
5. Because a child has a higher heart rate than an adult, the *rate* of chest compressions must be faster (about 80 to 100 per minute) or five compressions every 3 to 4 seconds, counting "1 and 2 and 3 and 4 and 5" as for the adult.
6. One rescue breath should be administered every five compressions (instead of two breaths per 15 compressions in the adult).

Continued

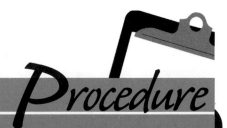

Box 22.9—Cont'd.

Procedures for Providing External Chest Compressions

Infant:

1. The infant's heart is located higher in the chest, beneath the middle of the sternum between the nipples. This is the location for chest compressions.
2. Because an infant's bone structure is fragile, compressions are made with only the tips of the index and middle finger and only to a depth of 0.5 to 1.0 inches.

3. The rate is even higher than that of a child, closer to 100 beats per minute or five compressions every 3 seconds. To maintain this pace, the rescuer should count "1, 2, 3, 4, 5," with a compression for each count.
4. After every five compressions, a ventilation "puff" is made to inflate the lungs.

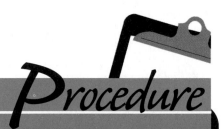

Box 22.10

Procedure for Recognizing and Treating Cardiac Arrest

Cause: Sudden failure of respiratory and circulatory systems; may be caused by anaphylaxis, electric shock, or heart attack.

Signs and symptoms:

1. *Pulse:* None detected in carotids
2. *Blood pressure:* None detected
3. *Respiration:* None
4. *Pupils:* Fixed, centered, dilated
5. *Skin:* Ashen gray or blue (cyanotic)

Treatment:

1. If arrest event is observed, deliver a sharp blow to the sternum.
2. Position the patient level (horizontal) on a firm, flat surface, such as the floor.

3. Open the airway with the head tilt–chin lift technique.
4. Inflate the lungs with four quick breaths (mouth to mouth, Ambu-bag); supplemental oxygen also may be used.
5. Provide external cardiac massage.

Summary of external cardiac massage (adult patient):

1. Place heel of one hand on midsternum.
2. Place heel of other hand on top of first hand.
3. Lean forward, use body weight to apply pressure downward (Figure 22.8). Two rescuers: 5:1 compressions to ventilations; one rescuer: 15:2 compressions to ventilations.

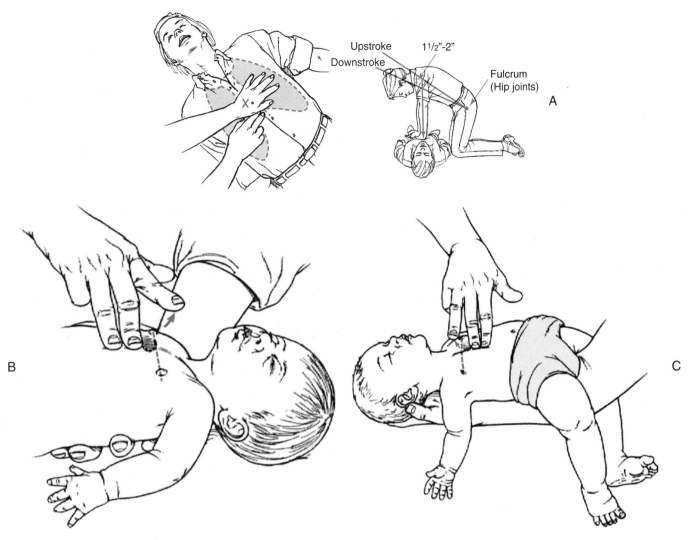

FIGURE 22.8

A, Proper position for rescue effort. The rescuer's shoulders are directly over the victim's sternum, with the elbows locked. **B,** Chest compression for an infant. The infant is placed on his or her back in the palm of the rescuer's hand. **C,** A larger infant or small child should be held on the rescuer's forearm with the head supported in the rescuer's palm. The infant's head and torso must be kept level. (Illustrations courtesy American Heart Association.)

exposure. A reaction that occurs suddenly is likely to be more serious than one that does not appear for several hours or days.

Skin Reactions

Skin reactions to allergens may take several forms and range from mild to severe.

Contact Dermatitis

Contact dermatitis is the result of exposure of the skin or a mucous membrane, such as the mucosal lining of the mouth, to an allergen. The allergen may be a plant (poison ivy), a cosmetic (lipstick), a metal (nickel), an impression material (alginate), or a latex examination glove. As the name suggests, the dermatitis continues as long as exposure to the allergen continues. The signs and symptoms of contact dermatitis usually are pruritus (itching) followed by erythema (redness and rash), **edema** (swelling), and vesicle (blister) formation. The reaction usually is confined to the area where the antigen made contact, but occasionally it may spread.

Edema
Swelling, usually caused by accumulation of fluid in the tissues

Box 22.11

Procedure for Recognizing and Treating Syncope

Procedure

Cause: Lack of blood flow to the brain.

Signs and symptoms:
1. *Pulse:* Initially rapid, then slow and weak
2. *Blood pressure:* Normal to slightly depressed
3. *Respiration:* Shallow and rapid; possibly yawning
4. *Pupils:* Dilated
5. *Skin:* Pale, moist, cool, ashen gray
6. *Other signs:* Lightheadedness, dizziness, nausea
7. Mild convulsions possible

Treatment:
1. Cease treatment.
2. Place the patient in the Trendelenburg position (supine with the feet slightly higher than the head).
3. Ask patient to move legs to help pump blood back to heart.
4. Maintain an open airway.
5. Give the patient a brief sniff of aromatic spirits of ammonia.
6. Loosen ties, collars, or belts if they are tight.
7. Provide supplemental oxygen.
8. Provide gentle restraint if convulsive movements or seizure occurs.
9. Place a cool towel on patient's forehead and cover with blanket if patient is cold.
10. Monitor vital signs and recovery.
11. Minimize noise, lighting, and commotion.
12. Patient should not leave office unescorted. Call a friend, relative, or cab.

Treatment of a delayed contact dermatitis reaction involves the following steps:
1 Removal of the offending allergen
2 Administration of antihistamines to counteract the effect of the histamine response
3 Administration of corticosteroids to suppress the body's inflammatory response
4 Obtaining a medical consultation

If the reaction is immediate and severe, administration of epinephrine also may be necessary to counteract the effects of the histamine. Continuous reexposure to a contact allergen, such as the latex in examination gloves, can result in chronically indurated (hard), dry, scaly lesions, which are difficult to treat unless the allergen is removed completely.

Urticaria

Often called hives, urticaria is a skin response to an allergen that is either ingested or placed on the skin. Unlike contact dermatitis, which tends to be a localized reaction, urticaria often is a generalized skin response. The signs and symptoms usually appear as intense pruritus, the formation of wheals (smooth, slightly elevated patches of skin), erythema, and edema. The primary treatment is removal of the allergen, al-though antihistamines and corticosteroids may be used to assist recovery.

Angioedema

Angioedema is a localized swelling that occurs in response to an allergen; it involves the skin, subcutaneous tissue (tissue beneath the skin), muscle, or mucous membranes. It occurs without inflammation, and pain and itching are uncommon. Angioedema results when an antigen enters or contacts the body, triggering a release of histamine, which causes capillaries to expand and leak, filling tissue spaces with fluid. The most common areas of occurrence are the face, hands, feet, and genitalia.

In dentistry, angioedema is a concern as a serious allergic response because it may occur on the lips, tongue, pharynx, or larynx, and it has the potential to constrict or obstruct the airway. The progressive signs and symptoms of respiratory reactions are a feeling of tightness in the chest, coughing and wheezing as the bronchioles constrict, shortness of breath, cyanosis (blue color of the skin, lips, and nails) as the blood loses oxygen, and laryngeal edema as swelling constricts or closes the airway.

Treatment of angioedema consists of removing the cause and administering antihistamines. Unless the prob-

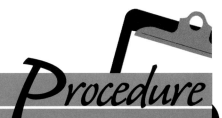

Box 22.12

Procedure for Recognizing and Treating Hyperventilation

Cause: Change in blood chemistry associated with a lack of carbon dioxide.

Signs and symptoms:

1. *Appearance:* Tense, hyperalert
2. *Hands:* Cold, damp, possibly having a slight tremor
3. *Face:* Moist with beads of sweat; may be pale or flushed
4. *Pulse:* Significantly elevated, pounding
5. *Blood pressure:* Significantly elevated
6. *Respiration:* Very rapid (25 to 30 per minute) and deep, almost uncontrollable
7. *Other signs:* Dry mouth, numbness in the extremities, chest pain, sense of suffocation, stomach pain, muscular rigidity or cramps, loss of control, severe anxiety

Note: Because cardiac arrest and hyperventilation are caused by changes in the respiratory and circulatory system or blood chemistry, the signs and symptoms may appear similar. A key difference is an elevated pulse and blood pressure associated with hyperventilation, whereas the pulse and blood pressure may not be detectable with cardiac arrest.

Treatment:

1. Terminate the dental procedure and remove anything from the patient's vision that may trigger the problem (for example, syringe, forceps, or sharp instruments).
2. Remove foreign objects from patient's mouth.
3. Place patient in upright position.
4. Loosen patient's clothing that may restrict breathing.
5. Calm the patient and explain what is happening.
6. Have the person do the following:
   a. Slow down the breathing rate
   b. Hold the breath for a few seconds
   c. Breathe into a paper bag or into cupped hands held over the nose
7. Be prepared to administer diazepam (Valium) if the patient's anxiety cannot be controlled.
8. *Do not* administer oxygen because this can worsen the condition.
9. Determine if treatment is to be continued.
10. Document incident.

---

lem constricts the airway, it usually is not serious in itself and the dentist may choose not to treat it directly. Instead, the dentist may elect to refer the patient to a physician or allergist for follow-up care. The real danger associated with angioedema, as with other allergic skin reactions, is that they may be the beginning of other life-threatening allergic reactions, such as anaphylactic shock. If so, they are warning signs of an impending emergency situation.

Respiratory Reactions

Asthma and anaphylactic disorders are allergic reactions that can affect the respiratory system (Box 22.14). An anaphylactic reaction (anaphylaxis or anaphylactic shock) is an especially severe allergic reaction that occurs in an individual who has been previously sensitized to a particular antigen.

Asthma

Asthma is a disorder of the tracheobronchial tree, which comprises the trachea, bronchi, and bronchioles. The signs and symptoms are sudden, periodic episodes of **dyspnea** (difficulty breathing) and wheezing, caused by bronchospasm (constriction of the walls of the bronchioles), edema of the bronchial wall, and oversecretion

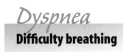

Dyspnea

Difficulty breathing

by the mucous glands (Box 22.15). Although most asthma "attacks" are moderate and controllable with medication, several hundred people die each year in the United States from this problem.

During the attack the bronchioles are constricted because of the contraction of the smooth muscles surrounding them.

Box 22.13

Procedure

Procedure for Recognizing and Treating Airway Blockage

Cause: Aspiration of a foreign object.

Signs and symptoms:
1. Difficulty breathing (patient may signal choking by pressing the hands to the throat)
2. Inability to make any sound (complete laryngospasm or complete obstruction)
3. High-pitched, crowing sounds (partial laryngospasm or partial blockage)
4. *Skin:* Blue, cyanotic
5. Loss of consciousness (unrelieved obstruction)

Treatment:
1. Have a bystander call for help.
2. For a conscious patient:
   a. Do not allow the patient to sit up, as this will allow the object to move further down the throat.
   b. Position chair in a head down, Trendelenburg position to allow the object to be coughed up.
   c. Have patient lie on right side and cough forcefully.
   d. Strike the patient repeatedly between the shoulder blades with the heel of your hand.
   e. Perform the Heimlich maneuver (abdominal thrusts) (see Box 22.5).
   f. If unable to recover the object, accompany the patient to a medical facility for radiographs.
3. For an unconscious patient:
   a. Establish the airway.
   b. Attempt to breathe for the patient and observe for chest movement (CPR, Ambubag, supplemental oxygen).
   c. Check for a foreign body.
   d. Aspirate oropharyngeal secretions.
   e. Roll the patient on the side and strike between the shoulder blades.
   f. Repeat Heimlich maneuver.
   g. Perform cricothyrotomy if above measures are unsuccessful.

Added to this restriction is an overproduction of mucous, which produces the clogging of air passages that makes breathing difficult.

Diabetes Mellitus

Diabetes mellitus is a disease that disrupts the body's ability to properly use (metabolize, or burn) glucose, the simplest of all carbohydrates and the simplest sugar. Glucose is the body's primary fuel, the only fuel that the brain can use, and it is made from the foods we eat. It is carried throughout the body by the bloodstream. However, to metabolize glucose, the cells of the body must have *insulin,* a hormone produced by the pancreas. They must also have special chemical *receptors* that allow them to use this available insulin. Without either insulin or insulin receptors, glucose cannot penetrate the cell membranes of many of the cells of the body, and the result is diabetes.

Diabetes has been classified into two types:
- *Type I diabetes* is also called insulin-dependent diabetes. The more severe form of the disease, it affects about 5% of the diabetic population.
- *Type II diabetes* is called non-insulin-dependent diabetes. The more common and milder form of diabetes, it affects the majority of the diabetic population.

Dental assistants should familiarize themselves with procedures for treating hypoglycemia (insulin shock), which can arise from patient oversight in the control of diabetes (Box 22.16).

Epilepsy and Convulsive Disorders

Epilepsy is a disorder in which the patient suffers from periodic and recurrent seizures (convulsions). Seizures are defined as sudden, usually brief disorders of brain function characterized by an attack involving changes in state of consciousness, motor activity, or sensory phenomena (Box 22.17).

Grand Mal Seizure

A grand mal seizure is a classic tonic-clonic seizure (*tonic* meaning rigid body position and *clonic* meaning uncon-

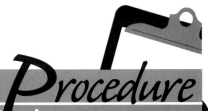

Box 22.14

Procedure for Recognizing and Treating Respiratory Allergic Reactions

Cause: Antigen-antibody reaction; may be induced by medications.

Signs and symptoms

MILD REACTION:

May develop from 1 hour to days after administration of medication

1. Watering of the eyes
2. Nasal obstruction, runny nose, sneezing
3. Skin rash, redness, and itching
4. Swelling of the eyelids, face, hands, and larynx
5. Stable vital signs
6. Anxious, nervous, restless, sweating, weak, and faint

SEVERE REACTION:

Anaphylactic shock; develops immediately or up to 1 hour after administration of medication

1. *Pulse:* Rapid and thready
2. *Blood pressure:* Significantly decreased
3. *Respiration:* Coughing, wheezing, shortness of breath
4. *Skin:* Redness, itching, swelling, hives
5. *Secretions:* Increased salivation, watering of eyes, increased nasal secretions
6. *Gastrointestinal signs:* Cramps, nausea, vomiting, diarrhea, urinary incontinence.

7. Swelling of tissues around the larynx, causing partial or complete obstruction of airway.
8. Pallor, light-headedness, unconsciousness, cardiac arrest, and death.

Treatment

MILD REACTION:

1. Remove allergen.
2. Administer antihistamine, for example, diphenhydramine (Benadryl), 50 mg.
3. Administer epinephrine (1:1000), 0.125 to 0.3 mg intramuscularly or subcutaneously.

SEVERE REACTION (ANAPHYLAXIS):

1. Place patient in Trendelenburg position.
2. Establish the airway.
3. Administer oxygen.
4. Administer epinephrine (1:1000), 0.125 to 0.3 ml intravenously if possible (sublingually if IV administration is not possible) (Figure 22.9).
5. Call for medical assistance.
6. Administer antihistamine diphenhydramine, 50 mg, and hydrocortisone, 100 mg.
7. Monitor vital signs and maintain CPR until medical help arrives.
8. Be prepared to perform CPR or a cricothyrotomy, if necessary.

---

trolled muscle movements). This is the type of seizure most people picture when they think of epilepsy.

Petit Mal Seizure

A petit mal seizure usually occurs in children; these are also called *absence attacks.* For a few moments the patient loses awareness of the surroundings and may appear confused or distracted; this is followed by a blank stare.

Partial Seizure

A partial seizure affects one hemisphere (side) of the brain. The patient experiences an involuntary jerking movement of an arm or leg but remains conscious. If the disorder crosses to the other hemisphere, level of

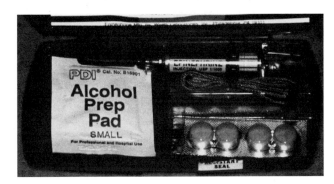

FIGURE 22.9

Emergency treatment kit for anaphylaxis.

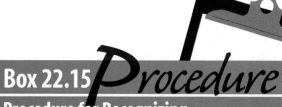

Box 22.15 *Procedure*

Procedure for Recognizing and Treating Asthma

Cause: Bronchial spasm and constriction caused by allergen or anxiety.

Signs and symptoms:
1. *Pulse:* Rapid (tachycardia)
2. *Blood pressure:* Normal to slightly elevated
3. *Respiration:* Rapid, labored breathing (tachypnea, dyspnea) with coughing and wheezing. Very difficult exhalations assisted by chest muscles. Feeling of thickness and congestion in the chest as bronchioles constrict and fill with mucous. Patient needs to be positioned upright.
4. *Skin:* Pale; blue tinge (cyanosis) develops as blood loses oxygen. Cyanosis also is seen in the nails and mucous membranes if the attack worsens.
5. *Mental state:* Anxiety that becomes fear as the attack progresses.

Treatment:
1. Stop treatment and remove all materials from the mouth.
2. Seat patient upright.
3. Use bronchodilator if available (Figure 22.10).
4. Administer oxygen, 4 to 6 liters per minute.
5. Administer epinephrine by inhaler, or 0.125 to 0.3 mg intramuscularly or subcutaneously.
6. Summon medical assistance.

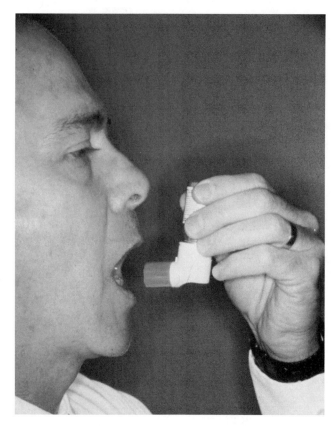

FIGURE 22.10
Use of a bronchodilator in treating asthma.

Heart Disorders

Diseases of the heart are the leading cause of death in the United States. Although dentists cannot treat an underlying heart disease directly, they must have sufficient knowledge about the more common types to reduce the likelihood of an emergency heart problem during dental treatment and to respond correctly should such an emergency occur.

Angina Pectoris

Angina pectoris is a choking or strangling pain of the heart. It is caused by a period of inadequate blood flow through the coronary arteries, which temporarily deprives the heart of oxygen (Box 22.18).

Myocardial Infarction

Myocardial infarction can be defined as a reduction in or loss of the blood supply to a portion of the heart muscle that is so severe it results in death and necrosis of that part of the heart muscle. In lay terms, a myocardial infarction is a heart attack. The consequences of myocardial infarction can be shock, heart failure, cardiac arrest, and death (Box 22.19).

consciousness and ability to respond to external stimuli are impaired.

Status Epilepticus

Status epilepticus is the most dangerous and life-threatening type of seizure. It consists of one continuous seizure or repetitive seizures without recovery between them. These seizures can last hours or days and can be fatal in as many as 20% of cases.

Box 22.16

Procedure

Procedure for Recognizing and Treating Hypoglycemic Shock

Insulin shock (hypoglycemia)

Cause: Excess insulin and lack of glucose in the blood, usually a result of excess activity, stress, or skipping a meal.

Signs and symptoms

1. *Pulse:* Rapid
2. *Blood pressure:* Normal to decreased
3. *Respiration:* Rapid, shallow
4. *Skin:* Pale, cold, wet
5. *Behavior:* Sudden change, with confusion, lethargy, and stupor developing as brain is deprived of glucose
6. Loss of consciousness if condition goes untreated

Treatment

1. *Conscious patient:* Administer glucose orally; for example, orange juice with 2 to 4 tablespoons of sugar added, or a sugary soft drink.
2. *Semiconscious patient:* Administer cake icing or honey in the buccal vestibule.
3. *Unconscious patient:* Administer 50 mg glucagon intramuscularly, followed by an intravenous drip of dextrose solution.

Diabetic coma (hyperglycemia)

Cause: Excess glucose in the blood.

Signs and symptoms

1. Dehydration, thirst, excess urination
2. Loss of appetite, nausea, fatigue
3. Sweet, acetone breath
4. Physical discomfort

Treatment

1. *Conscious patient:* Administer patient's usual dose of insulin.
2. *Unconscious patient:* Transport to hospital, where insulin administration can be carefully monitored.
3. Dental staff should never administer insulin to a patient suspected of being hyperglycemic.

Note: Treat all diabetic crises as hypoglycemia, which is the faster acting and more serious disorder. Glucose given to a hyperglycemic patient will not aggravate the problem significantly in the short term.

Congestive Heart Failure

Congestive heart failure can be classified into two categories, left heart failure and right heart failure. In *left heart failure,* the left side of a diseased or weakened heart lacks the strength to pump blood satisfactorily throughout the body. *Right heart failure* is the inability of the right side of the heart to pump blood through the lungs; it is often associated with pulmonary edema, which is an accumulation of fluid in the lungs. The two disorders often occur together. They usually are caused by a longstanding illness, such as diabetes, obesity, hypertension, coronary artery disease, or bacterial or viral infections of the heart, and they are often seen in the elderly (Box 22.20).

Stroke

Transient Ischemic Attacks

A transient ischemic attack (TIA) is a "ministroke" that is brief and has only a temporary effect. TIAs are similar to attacks of angina pectoris in that they often precede complete strokes. They usually last 2 to 10 minutes and, depending on the area of the brain affected, may cause a weakness, numbness, or partial paralysis of the arms, legs, and fingers, often described as a feeling of "pins and needles."

Cerebral Embolism

A cerebral embolus is a clot that usually begins in the heart or aorta and travels to the brain, where it becomes lodged,

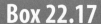

Box 22.17

Procedure

Procedure for Recognizing and Treating Epileptic Seizures

Cause: Unknown.

Signs and symptoms

1. Subtle change in emotion or behavior
2. "Aura'" of sight, sound, or smell
3. Epileptic "cry" or "gasp" with loss of consciousness
4. Tonic (rigid) movements followed by clonic movements (uncontrolled spasms)
5. Loss of bladder and bowel control possible
6. Respiration inadequate and irregular
7. Excess salivation and "frothing at the mouth"

Treatment:

1. Place patient in supine position.
2. Remove foreign (including dental) objects from the patient's mouth.
3. Remove glasses and ties and loosen tight clothing.
4. Place a pillow under the patient's head.
5. Place a soft item in the patient's mouth, if possible, and *gently* restrict movement to prevent injury.
6. Suction oral secretions if necessary and if possible
7. Monitor vital functions and open airway; administer oxygen if cyanosis is present.
8. Allow the seizure to run its course, and reassure and calm the patient.
9. Discharge patient into custody of a responsible adult.
10. Summon medical assistance if necessary.

---

causing a cerebral embolism, or blockage. The symptoms usually are an abrupt, mild headache followed by neurologic symptoms, which develop within the next several hours. The severity of the neurologic symptoms may slowly diminish if the clot begins to break up or dissolve. The person usually is awake and conscious when the cerebral embolism occurs.

Cerebral Thrombosis

A cerebral thrombus is a clot that forms within a cerebral artery itself. It usually results when an atherosclerotic deposit in the artery breaks away and forms a clot. Cerebral thrombosis, or blockage caused by the thrombus, often occurs during sleep, and the individual frequently wakes up with neurologic symptoms, such as stuttering. Those symptoms tend to reach their maximum effect within 1 or 2 days.

Cerebral Infarction

A cerebral infarction is a loss of blood supply to a portion of the brain, leading to death of those brain tissues. Although infarction can be caused by either an embolus or a thrombus, it usually is caused by atherosclerosis, which results in a gradual decrease in the diameter of the artery involved. When the amount of oxygenated blood supplied to the tissues served by that artery falls below the amount needed to keep the tissues alive, death and necrosis of those tissues result.

Cerebral Hemorrhage

A cerebral hemorrhage is the rupture of an artery in the cranium, the portion of the head that contains the brain. The bleeding can cause displacement and destruction of brain tissue. This type of stroke often occurs during a period of physical or psychologic stress (such as a dental procedure) that causes a significant rise in systolic blood pressure. Because the hemorrhage happens suddenly, the initial symptoms also appear immediately and usually include an intense, excruciating headache that starts in one area of the head but becomes generalized (Box 22.21).

OCCUPATIONAL HAZARDS IN THE DENTAL OFFICE

The environment of the dental office presents several possible hazards to the patient and the dental staff. These hazards include the possibility of disease transmission from patient to staff, staff to patient, and patient to patient; physical injury to the patient or staff; and chemical injury to patients or

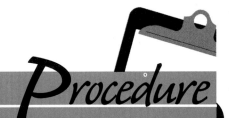

Box 22.18

Procedure for Recognizing and Treating Angina Pectoris

Cause: Inadequate blood supply (i.e., oxygen) to the heart.

Signs and symptoms:

1. Dull, aching pain or pressure beneath the sternum that may spread to the shoulders or arms; usually triggered by physical, emotional, or environmental stress
2. *Pulse:* Rapid, strong
3. *Blood pressure:* Slightly elevated
4. *Respiration:* Shortness of breath, difficulty breathing
5. *Other signs:* Anxiety and a feeling of impending death

Treatment:

1. Calm the patient.
2. Place the patient in the most comfortable position (usually upright).
3. Administer 0.3 mg nitroglycerin (vasodilator) beneath tongue; a second dose may be administered in 2 to 3 minutes if discomfort continues.
4. Administer oxygen, 4 to 6 liters per minute.
5. If no relief is obtained, allow patient to breathe vapors of amyl nitrite (crushed 0.3 mg ampule).
6. Monitor vital signs and call EMS if recovery is not seen.

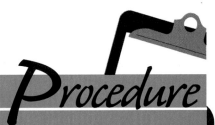

Box 22.19

Procedure for Recognizing and Treating Myocardial Infarction

Cause: Blockage of blood supply to the heart, leading to damage or death of part of the heart muscle.

Signs and symptoms:

1. Pain resembling that of angina but much more severe; often occurs at rest (a small percentage of individuals have little or no pain)
2. Pain unrelieved by nitroglycerin therapy
3. *Pulse:* Weak, thready, rapid (occasionally slow)
4. *Blood pressure:* Varies; sometimes increased but if decreased condition is more serious
5. *Respiration:* Difficulty breathing (dyspnea), shortness of breath; patient will want to sit up.
6. *Skin:* Cold, clammy, moist; pale or ashen gray in color and may turn blue as the level of oxygen in the blood decreases

7. *Other signs:* Severe anxiety, sense of impending doom; restlessness, weakness; nausea and vomiting (common)

Treatment:

1. Calm the patient.
2. Administer oxygen, 4 to 6 liters per minute.
3. *Call for medical assistance.*
4. Administer 0.3 mg nitroglycerin beneath the tongue if systolic blood pressure is above 100.
5. If pain is acute: administer morphine, 10 to 15 mg intramuscularly or subcutaneously; or meperidine, 50 to 100 mg intramuscularly.
6. Monitor vital signs.
7. Transfer to hospital.

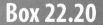

Box 22.20

Procedure for Recognizing and Treating Congestive Heart Failure

Cause: Progressive weakness of the heart muscle.

Signs and symptoms (right heart failure):
1. Swelling of the feet or ankles during the course of the day
2. Swollen areas remain "pitted" if depressed
3. Extreme weakness and fatigue
4. Bluing (cyanosis) of nails and mucous membranes

Signs and symptoms (left heart failure):
1. Weakness; patient cannot do a short, mild activity (such as taking a short walk or climbing a flight of stairs) without shortness of breath, extreme fatigue, and chest pain.
2. Frequent nightly urination
3. Need to sleep in the upright position
4. *Pulse:* Rapid, although may alternate between rapid and weak (pulsus alterans)
5. *Blood pressure:* Elevated, especially diastolic pressure
6. *Respiration:* Rapid
7. *Skin:* Cool, pale, and moist

Treatment:
1. Help the patient into a comfortable position.
2. Administer oxygen, 3 to 4 liters per minute (use nasal cannula to avoid a feeling of suffocation).

---

staff members. If these hazards are recognized and managed properly, the risk should be reduced almost to zero. That reduction comes about through the use of common sense and through strict attention to and discipline in infection control and environmental safety measures.

Human Immunodeficiency Virus and Acquired Immunodeficiency Syndrome

Perhaps no disease strikes greater fear in people today than acquired immunodeficiency syndrome (AIDS), which is caused by the human immunodeficiency virus (HIV). The fear is legitimate, because HIV eventually causes death in virtually 100% of cases. HIV usually is spread through direct contact or exchange of body fluids contaminated with the virus. Thus blood-to-blood contact is a common means of transmitting the virus; such contact may involve a blood transfusion, being stuck with a contaminated instrument or hypodermic needle, or bleeding directly into a nick or wound in the skin. This type of transmission poses a very real risk to members of the dental team because most dental procedures can cause at least some bleeding of the oral tissues. (Unlike blood, saliva has proved to be one of the few body fluids that does not seem to be able to carry enough of the virus particles to cause infection.) For that reason, when following ap-

propriate infection control standards, HIV is not transmitted easily and there are few documented cases of health care workers becoming infected while treating HIV-infected patients.

Hepatitis B Virus

Hepatitis B (HBV) is a highly contagious virus that can permanently damage the liver. It is several hundred to several thousand times more infectious than HIV and can be transmitted by any body fluid or tissue, such as blood, saliva, or mucus. Cross-infection with HBV can be prevented by strict observance of infection control measures.

Herpetic Whitlow

Most adults carry the herpes simplex virus, which causes the common oral "cold sore." When these sores are active, the fluid oozing from them is filled with the herpes simplex virus. Should the fluid from the cold sore get into a nick or cut on the hand of the dentist or auxiliary, a serious infection can result. Besides making the dental provider ill with flulike symptoms, the infection can seriously damage a hand or finger, causing swelling, blistering (vesicle formation), drainage, and intense pain. If the dental provider wipes his or her eyes after touching the fluid from a cold sore, the virus can be transmitted to the eye and cause a serious eye infection.

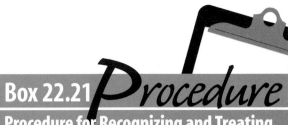

Box 22.21 *Procedure*

Procedure for Recognizing and Treating Strokes (Cerebrovascular Accidents)

Cause: Loss of blood flow to parts of the brain, usually caused by clots, hemorrhage, or hypotension.

Signs and symptoms:

1. Severe headache, weakness, numbness or paralysis on one side, loss of speech, confusion, or disorientation are possible, depending on the severity of the stroke and the area of the brain affected.
2. *Pulse:* Decreased
3. *Blood pressure:* Elevated (with diminished pulse, a very serious sign)
4. *Respiration:* Decreased
5. *Temperature:* Elevated
6. *Other signs:* Nausea, vomiting

Treatment:

1. *Conscious patient:* Seat upright.
2. *Unconscious patient:* Maintain airway.
3. Administer oxygen *only* if the patient is in respiratory distress.
4. Monitor vital signs.
5. *Call for medical assistance immediately.*

Radiation Hygiene

The proper use of radiography (x-rays) is an essential part of modern medical and dental diagnosis. Although the use of radiographs in dentistry has become so commonplace that it is now taken for granted, the dangers associated with radiation should always be respected. Radiographs present a very real risk, especially to the office staff, if the equipment is defective or operated in an unsafe manner or unsafe environment. Long-term exposure to low levels of radiation "leaking" from a defective machine can increase the likelihood of cancer, infertility, genetic defects, birth defects, and stillbirths. Fortunately, such risks can be eliminated simply by using a properly operating machine in the correct manner (see Chapters 12 and 13).

Mercury Hygiene

Dental amalgam is made up of various silver, copper, and tin alloys mixed with free mercury. Once the mercury is "tied up" by the alloys, it is considered reasonably safe. However, in its free or liquid state, mercury is a poison and it poses a serious health and environmental risk if it touches the skin or is exposed to air, allowing it to give off mercury vapor. For these reasons, the methods used for routine preparation and handling of dental amalgam have changed over the past 20 years. Box 22.22 presents guidelines for safe preparation and handling of amalgam.

Nitrous Oxide

Nitrous oxide-oxygen is a commonly used dental gas. However, it poses some risk to pregnant women and to those who might abuse it. It therefore should be used in the following manner:

1. All nitrous oxide/oxygen equipment should be periodically checked by a certified technician to ensure that all components of the system are working properly.
2. The system itself should be used only as designed and as recommended by the current scientific thinking on the subject.
3. All systems should have an active nitrous oxide scavenger to remove exhaled and leaking nitrous oxide from the atmosphere. This scavenger is usually connected to the central suction system.
4. The gas should not be used on pregnant patients, nor should pregnant staff members be in the room when nitrous oxide is administered.
5. *Nitrous oxide should not be used as a recreational drug.* It is not completely benign, as was once thought, and cases of addiction and ruined careers have been documented.

Acrylic Monomer and Polymer

Dental acrylics are used for a wide range of devices, including temporary restorations, denture bases, and occlusal splints. These materials are usually prepared as a mixture of a liquid (acrylic monomer) and a powder (acrylic polymer), which creates a "dough" that is hardened chemically or by means of a light-curing mechanism. Although safe when used properly, these materials present some risks to both the patient and the staff.

The monomer and polymer mixture generates a significant amount of heat as it "sets." This heat can be sufficient to burn the oral soft tissues or damage the pulp of teeth. When these materials are used, care should always be taken to avoid hard or soft tissue injury as the acrylics are adapted within the mouth.

A much more serious threat to the dental provider is the flammability of the monomer liquid and the possibility of damage to the lungs from the polymer powder. Monomer

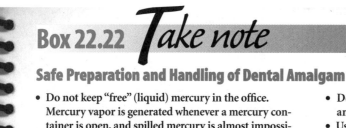

Box 22.22 Take note

Safe Preparation and Handling of Dental Amalgam

- Do not keep "free" (liquid) mercury in the office. Mercury vapor is generated whenever a mercury container is open, and spilled mercury is almost impossible to remove completely, especially from such areas as carpeting and floorboards.
- Do not mix alloy powder and free mercury in the open air because this generates mercury vapor.
- Use only premeasured, enclosed capsules of mercury and alloy prepared and sold by the manufacturer.
- Activate and mix the alloy capsules strictly according to the manufacturer's instructions.
- Use an amalgamator with a cover to control any vapors that might leak from the capsule during the trituration process.
- Manage any vapors that do occur by directing a high volume of fresh air *into* the operatory and then venting it directly *outside* without going through any other part of the office.
- Wear latex or vinyl gloves at all times when handling mixed dental alloy. Never touch mixed dental alloy with bare hands.

- Do not squeeze mercury from freshly mixed amalgam.
- Use a high-volume vacuum, water spray, and rubber dam when removing old amalgam restorations from teeth, because significant mercury vapors are generated during this procedure. Change the face mask after removing the old amalgam.
- Collect scrap amalgam from the trap in the suction lines and unused amalgam from dental procedures and store it under radiographic fixer solution in covered glass or vinyl containers.
- Return scrap amalgam to the manufacturer for refining in sealed plastic bags provided for that purpose. *Do not* dispose of scrap amalgam with the normal refuse and trash. Even in small amounts the mercury in scrap amalgam poses a hazard to the environment.
- Immediately clean up amalgam or mercury spills, using trap bottles, absorbent tape, fresh mixes of amalgam, or commercial clean-up kits to pick up mercury droplets. *Do not* use a household vacuum cleaner.

liquid is highly flammable. Severe accidents have occurred in dental laboratories when a glass container of monomer has broken and spilled its contents on an open flame. The liquid flashes almost explosively, inflicting life-threatening burns on dental personnel. *Liquid monomer should never be handled or stored near or above an open flame.*

The fabrication of acrylic splints usually involves some grinding and adjusting, either in the laboratory or at chairside. This grinding creates an ultrafine dust of acrylic particles that, if inhaled, can seriously and permanently damage the lungs. In fact, there have been reported cases of untimely death among dentists whose practices largely involved occlusal splints and who spent a great deal of time adjusting those splints. For these reasons, acrylic splints or temporaries should always be adjusted *away* from the patient, and the person doing the adjusting should *always* wear an effective particle mask, such as the protective masks worn during most dental procedures (Box 22.23).

Eye Protection in the Dental Office

The dental operatory presents several hazards to the eyes of the patient, the dental auxiliary, and the dentist. The high-speed cutting of teeth, metal, porcelain, or composite can produce flying debris that can cause severe or permanent eye damage. Over the years numerous eye injuries to dentists or members of their staff have been recorded during these procedures.

The mist of water droplets created by the turbine handpiece or ultrasonic cleaner or even backscatter from the three-way syringe can be loaded with microorganisms from the patient's oral cavity. If sprayed on the conjunctiva of the eye, serious eye infections can result.

The passing of sharp instruments or strong chemicals over the patient's face poses many risks. The list of instruments or materials dropped on patients includes explorers, endodontic files and spreaders, scalers and curettes, burrs, enamel chisels and hatchets, copal varnish, enamel etchant, bonding agents, monomer, and virtually anything else used in the practice of dentistry.

Because of these risks, regulations set forth by the federal Occupational Safety and Health Administration (OSHA) require all dental personnel to wear protective eyewear (face shields or eyeglasses *with side shields*) when performing procedures that may produce splash or scatter. The way to prevent eye injuries is simple and obvious: *Everyone—patient, dentist, and dental auxiliary—wears*

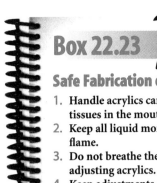

protective eyewear. There is simply no justification or excuse for anyone to suffer an eye injury in the modern dental office.

Cuts, Needlesticks, and Soft Tissue Injuries

Daily use of needles, scalpels, explorers, scalers, files, spreaders, burrs, elevators, and other such instruments presents numerous opportunities for members of the dental team to incur soft tissue injuries. These blood-borne injuries can be very serious. Several documented cases of HIV infection in health care workers have been attributed to an accidental stick with a needle or scalpel that had been used on a patient who was HIV positive. In such tragedies, as with airplane or automobile accidents, prevention is the best medicine.

Soft tissue injuries are prevented by rigorous practice of the strict discipline involved in the use and management of sharp instruments. Most soft tissue injuries occur because of a split second of thoughtlessness; therefore the handling of sharp instruments must be done not only in the right way but also with the proper mind set. This requires strict attention to detail and complete awareness of what is happening at the moment. As with any hazardous activity, the risk of human error can be reduced completely by following the preventive measures that include the following:

1 Completing the HBV vaccination series
2 Keeping tetanus immunity current
3 *Always* using gloves, masks, glasses, and proper barrier protection
4 Ensuring that all items used on the patient have been properly sterilized or disinfected according to infection control directives

If a cut or needlestick occurs despite the preventive measure efforts, the response is almost the same as that for any cut or wound (Box 22.24).

Asbestos

Asbestos should not be a threat to anyone in the workplace today. Its ability to cause fatal lung cancer has been universally recognized, and current commercial building codes, as well as OSHA regulations, forbid its use in building materials, insulation, ceiling tiles, and other materials. However, in a small area of dental practice, asbestos could still be a risk.

A small percentage of dental practices still make their own dental castings. Until about 15 or 20 years ago, an accepted part of this process was the use of an asbestos liner on the inside of the casting ring to allow for setting expansion of the investment material. When the dangers of asbestos became known, nonasbestos liners were developed; these liners are now the industry standard. If the office in which a dental auxiliary works casts its own crowns and inlays, the auxiliary should check to make sure that the liner used is a nonasbestos product and that any old asbestos liners are properly and safely disposed of according to environmental regulations.

Other Emergencies

Many of the products commonly found in the home and workplace are poisonous. All health care professionals must know the steps to take if a poisoning emergency occurs. A form such as the one shown in Figure 22.11 can be used as a quick reference for antidotes to common poisonous products.

LIFESAVING ANTIDOTE GUIDELINES

TYPE OF POISONING	WHAT TO DO
Swallowed poisons	If the person is awake and able to swallow, give milk or water only. Then call the poison center or doctor. *Caution:* Antidote labels on products and antidote charts may be out of date and incorrect. *DO NOT* give salt, vinegar or citrus fruit juices.
Poisons on the skin	Remove any affected clothing. Flood involved parts with water, wash with soap and water, and rinse. Then call the poison center or doctor.
Poisons in the eye	Flood the eye with lukewarm (never hot) water, poured from a pitcher held 3-4 inches from the eye for 15 minutes. Then call the poison center or MD.
Inhaled poisons	Immediately carry or drag the person to fresh air and give mouth-to-mouth resuscitation if necessary. Ventilate the area. Then call poison center or MD.

Always keep on hand syrup of ipecac which induces vomiting, and epsom salts which acts as a laxative. Do not use either one unless instructed to do so by the poison center or your doctor, and *follow their directions for use.*

SOME COMMON SUBSTANCES AND POSSIBLE SYMPTOMS OF OVERDOSE
The following is a list of some of the potentially toxic substances in the environment. Always call for assistance immediately after a poison exposure. NEVER wait until symptoms appear.

MEDICINES
Amphetamines-hyperactivity, agitation, convulsions
Antibiotics-allergic reaction, such as swelling, skin eruptions, breathing difficulty, shock
Anticonvulsants-coma
Antidepressants-coma, convulsions, hallucinations, heart irregularities
Antidiarrheals (prescription)-coma
Antihistamines-hallucinations, agitation, convulsions, coma, fever, depression
Aspirin-fast breathing, ringing in ears, shock, sweating, fever, convulsions
Camphor-convulsions, excitement, coma, feeling of warmth
Cold preparation-hyperactivity, convulsions, coma
Iron, vitamins with iron-bloody vomiting and diarrhea, shock, coma
Oil of wintergreen-fast breathing, ringing in ears, shock, sweating, fever, convulsion
Sleeping pills-coma, convulsions, respiratory depression
Tranquilizers-coma, convulsions, respiratory depression

CLEANING PRODUCTS
Ammonia, bleach, dishwater soap, disinfectants, drain cleaners, toilet bowl cleaners-irritation or chemical burns in mouth and esophagus
Furniture polish, bleach mixed with other cleansers-burning irritation, coughing

Laundry detergents, soaps-vomiting and/or diarrhea

GARAGE AND GARDEN PRODUCTS
Acids, adhesives-chemical burns
Antifreeze-coma, blindness, convulsions, drunkenness
Fertilizers-vomiting and/or diarrhea
Gasoline, kerosene, turpentine, paint thinners, solvents, thinners, degreasers, charcoal lighter fluid-coughing, coma, burning irritation
Insecticides-headache, increased body secretions, vomiting, diarrhea, convulsions
Strychnine-convulsions

PERSONAL PRODUCTS
Nail polish remover-irritation and dryness inside mouth and esophagus
Perfume, after shaves, mouthwashes, rubbing alcohol-incoordination, depression, coma
Shampoo, soap, lotions-vomiting and/or diarrhea

PLANTS
There are thousands of poisonous plants. The poison control center should always be called if any plant is ingested.
Mushrooms-Symptoms vary, and may be delayed. Always call the poison center if it is thought a poisonous mushroom may have been eaten.

Unknown poisons: Call the poison center or doctor immediately.
POISON CONTROL CENTER   PHONE:

POISON CONTROL CENTER PHONE:
FAMILY DOCTOR PHONE:
HOSPITAL EMERGENCY UNIT PHONE:
FIRE DEPT. PHONE:
POLICE DEPT. PHONE:

FIGURE 22.11

Quick reference for lifesaving antidotes.

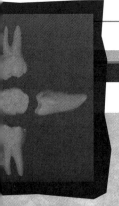

Points for Review

- Factors that contribute to the likelihood of a medical emergency in the dental office
- The legal and ethical responsibilities of the dental team in responding and managing medical emergencies
- The four "Ps" of a proper response to a medical crisis
- The importance of an emergency protocol
- The contents of an emergency kit
- The signs, symptoms, and treatment for described medical emergencies
- The role of the dental auxiliary in preventing medical or legal problems associated with medical emergencies in the dental office

Self-Study Questions

1. What is a protocol?
   a. An instrument used to record temperature
   b. A preplanned response to a certain situation
   c. A tool used to open an oxygen tank
2. The Heimlich maneuver is performed on a person having what kind of difficulty?
   a. Coughing
   b. Choking and unable to breathe at all
   c. Choking but still able to partly breathe
3. What is the rescuer's first step in CPR?
   a. Calling for help
   b. Ventilating the lungs
   c. Head tilt–chin lift
   d. Determining consciousness
   e. Checking the airway
4. Where should the pulse of an unconscious adult patient be checked?
   a. Brachial artery
   b. One of the carotid arteries
   c. Both carotid arteries
   d. Radial artery
   e. Femoral artery

5. What is the ratio of chest compressions to ventilations performed in two-person CPR?
   a. 15:2
   b. 12:2
   c. 10:2
   d. 8:1
   e. 5:1
6. What is the ratio of chest compressions to ventilations performed in one-person CPR?
   a. 15:2
   b. 12:2
   c. 10:2
   d. 8:1
   e. 5:1
7. What is the rate of chest compressions for adults receiving CPR?
   a. 60 to 80 per minute
   b. 80 to 100 per minute
   c. 100 to 120 per minute
   d. 120 to 140 per minute
8. What is the rate of chest compressions for children receiving CPR?
   a. 60 to 80 per minute
   b. 80 to 100 per minute
   c. 100 to 120 per minute
   d. 120 to 140 per minute
9. Syncope can be caused by what factor or factors?
   a. Psychological stress or fear
   b. Sitting upright suddenly
   c. Standing still for a long period
   d. Hunger
   e. All of the above
10. Hyperventilation usually is caused by what factor?
   a. Physical stress
   b. Psychologic stress
   c. Hunger
   d. Drug interaction
11. What should be done for a patient who is hyperventilating?
   a. Have the person breathe into a plastic bag
   b. Have the person breathe into a paper bag
   c. Give the person supplemental oxygen
   d. None of the above
12. What is the most serious consequence of anaphylaxis?
   a. Severe itching
   b. Swelling of the mucous membranes

    c. Watering of the eyes
    d. Shortness of breath
    e. Death
13. What drug is the first choice for treating anaphylactic shock?
    a. Diphenhydramine
    b. Benadryl
    c. Epinephrine
    d. Hydrocortisone
14. A person who goes into a blank stare for 30 to 60 seconds may be experiencing what type of disorder?
    a. Grand mal seizure
    b. Petit mal seizure
    c. Status epilepticus seizure
    d. All of the above
15. What should the dental staff do for a person undergoing an epileptic seizure?
    a. Prevent the person from injuring himself or herself
    b. Administer oxygen
    c. Administer diazepam
    d. Force the person's mouth open
16. What is a common symptom or symptoms of a stroke?
    a. Severe headache
    b. Feeling of numbness or paralysis on one side
    c. Loss of speech
    d. Mental deficits, such as confusion
    e. All of the above

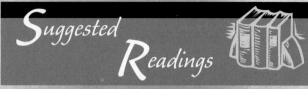

Suggested Readings

American Heart Association: *Healthcare provider's manual for basic life support,* 1988, 1990, The Association.

American Heart Association: *Textbook for basic life support for healthcare providers,* Dallas, 1994, National Center.

Chernega, Bridger J: *Emergency guide for dental auxiliaries,* ed 2, Albany, 1994, Delmar Publishers.

Chilco V, Strong M, Borea G: *Life-threatening emergencies in dentistry,* Padova, Italy, 1988, Ishiyaku Euroamerica.

Malamed SR: *Medical emergencies in the dental office,* ed 5, St Louis, 2000, Mosby.

McCarthy FM: *Emergencies in dental practice prevention and treatment,* ed 2, Philadelphia, 1972, WB Saunders.

Page G, Mills K, Morton R: *A colour atlas of cardiopulmonary resuscitation techniques,* London, 1986, Wolfe Medical Publications.

Unit V

Specialty Principles and Techniques

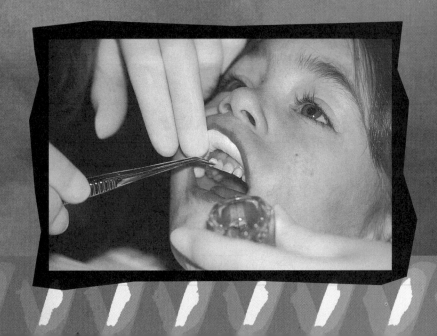

Chapter 23

*E*ndodontics

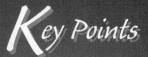
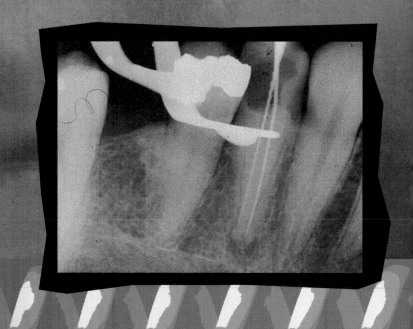

Chapter Outline

Scope of Endodontics
  Role of the dental assistant in endodontics
Pulp
  Pulpalgia and pulpitis
  Conditions that cause dental pain
Root Canal Therapy
  Indications
  Contraindications
  Endodontic examination
  Endodontic instruments
  Basic Endodontic Setup
  Other endodontic armamentaria
Procedure for Root Canal Treatment
  Isolation of the tooth
  Gaining access to the pulp chamber and
    canal
  Measurement of the tooth

Sterilization of the pulp chamber and
  canal
  Filling of the root canal
Other Endodontic Procedures
  Vital pulp capping
  Pulpectomy
  Pulpotomy
  Incision and drainage
  Bleaching of nonvital teeth
Specific Types of Endodontic Surgery
  Apicoectomy
  Retrofilling
  Root resection
  Periapical curettage
  Replantation
Endodontic Surgical Technique

Learning Objectives

On completion of Chapter 23, the student should be able to do the following:

- Define key terms.
- Describe the purpose and scope of endodontics.
- Describe and identify conditions that result in pulpal pain.
- Discuss the indications and contraindications for endodontic treatment.

- Identify instruments and procedures for assisting during endodontic procedures.
- Discuss the role of the dental assistant in endodontics.
- Discuss the role of antibiotic therapy in endodontics.

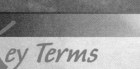

Key Terms

Apicoectomy	Medicaments	Pulpitis
Carcinogenic	Pulp Capping	Pulpotomy
Debridement	Pulpalgia	Retroprep
Endodontics	Pulpectomy	Vitalometer

SCOPE OF ENDODONTICS

Endodontics is the branch of dentistry concerned with treatment of the pulp and the surrounding periapical tissues. Root canal therapy, a primary aspect of endodontics, makes it possible to save a tooth that otherwise would require extraction. A general dentist may provide this treatment or may refer the patient to an endodontist, a dentist who has had advanced training in treating pulpal pain. The goal in root canal therapy is to remove bacteria from the pulp, pulp chamber, and root canals and to fill the canals and pulp chamber with a solid material, such as gutta-percha, to prevent problems and save the tooth.

Endodontics
The branch of dentistry concerned with treatment of the pulp and surrounding periapical tissues

Role of the Dental Assistant in Endodontics

In some states, advanced endodontic procedures can be delegated to expanded-function dental personnel. Some of these advanced procedures include the following:

- Pulp testing
- Placement of a rubber dam
- Irrigation and drying of canals
- Fitting of trial gutta-percha points
- Placement of temporary fillings
- Placement of medicament packing
- Suture removal

A trained dental assistant may take radiographs of the trial sizing of files and trial fitting of gutta-percha points. Dental personnel who assist with endodontic procedures must become familiar with the various instruments used for endodontic treatment.

PULP

The dental pulp consists of a network of tissue fibers that branch from the arteries and veins in both the maxillary and mandibular arches (Figure 23.1). The pulp receives nourishment through the blood supply from the arteries and veins, and the blood supply also provides the source of defense against infection.

Pulpalgia and Pulpitis

Pulpalgia and **pulpitis** are similar in that both terms refer to pulpal pain, yet the two are very different diagnoses of the condition. *Pulpalgia* refers to the clinical description of pulpal pain, and *pulpitis* refers to the histologic "laboratory fea-

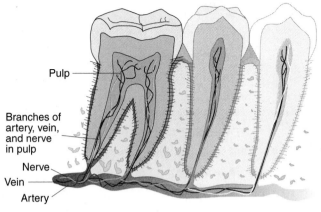

FIGURE 23.1

The pulp of the tooth consists of arteries, veins, and connective tissue, which nourish the tooth and protect it against infection.

tures" that microscopically reveal signs associated with pulpal pain. Dental assistants should be aware that these words are often interchanged because they both refer to pain and the possible need for root canal therapy. Pulpalgia is the term more commonly used in dental offices. Pulpalgia is often classified according to its severity (Box 23.1).

Pulpalgia
The clinical symptoms of pulpal pain

Pulpitis
Infection of the pulp that causes pulpal pain

Conditions That Cause Dental Pain

A number of conditions can cause dental pain. For example, a decayed tooth that has been left untreated can cause severe pain (Figure 23.2). Although bacteria are a common source of dental pain, other conditions also can irritate the pulp, causing pain. Some of the terms related to dental pain are listed in Box 23.1.

ROOT CANAL THERAPY

Most often, a tooth can be restored through treatment of the pulp performed in root canal therapy. If root canal therapy is unsuccessful, however, surgical treatment may be required. Intraoral conditions determine whether root canal therapy should be performed.

Indications

The indications, or reasons for, root canal therapy include the following:

Box 23.1

Classification of Pulpalgia and Terminology Related to Dental Pain

Classification of pulpalgia

Incipient pulpalgia: A condition in which the pulp may be irritated by a stimulus such as cold, sugar, or occlusal problems.

Moderate pulpalgia: Pulp tester elicits an immediate response from the tooth.

Advanced pulpalgia: Pain and heat act as irritants on the inflamed pulp.

Chronic pulpalgia: A history of pain that may have persisted for some time.

Terminology related to dental pain

Hyperreactive pulpalgia: Sudden, sharp pain that lasts for a short period.

Hyperemia: The presence of an increased amount of blood flow in the pulp that occurs when heat is applied, which may cause a transient dull pain.

Hyperplastic pulpitis: Pulpal pain that results from compression of the exposed pulp during eating. Hyperplastic pulpitis may also occur as a result of extreme temperature changes with hot or cold liquid or food.

Necrotic pulp: Pulp that has been destroyed, usually by decay. The pulp is said to be necrotic if a stimulus, such as a pulp tester, elicits no response. If the pulp is only partly necrotic, some response may occur.

Hypersensitivity: Pain experienced as a result of exposure to cold, stimulation of exposed dentin or tooth surface structure, or the contact of two different kinds of metal.

Internal resorption: The destruction of the dentin within the tooth.

Traumatic occlusion: Can be caused by a filling that is too high or a tooth that is not in occlusion with the rest of the dentition.

Incomplete fracture: A split or crack in a tooth that usually causes intermittent pain.

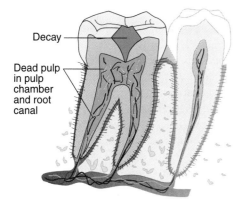

FIGURE 23.2

Decay usually begins in pits and fissures or interproximal areas.

- Necrotic pulp
- Fractured tooth or tooth knocked out of the socket
- Possibility of restoring tooth to natural function
- Periodontal-related condition
- Esthetics

Contraindications

The contraindications, or reasons against, root canal therapy are as follows:

- Tooth unable to be restored to natural function
- Tooth unable to be maintained periodontally
- Patient's medical condition
- Refusal of treatment

Endodontic Examination

Endodontic patients are often emergency patients who come to the dental office because they are in pain. The pulpal pain may be acute or intermittent, or the patient may have only vague symptoms. The diagnosis is based on the symptoms described by the patient and the dentist's clinical observations.

Before any treatment is given, the patient's medical-dental history is taken. Also, a periapical radiograph of the suspected tooth, including all surrounding tissues, is imperative (Figure 23.3). The initial endodontic radiograph is used for diagnosis and for measuring the length of the root canal.

Once a thorough medical-dental history has been obtained and the periapical radiograph is available, the dentist continues with the examination and diagnostic testing.

An endodontic examination focuses on the following elements:

- *Mobility:* The tooth is tested for looseness in the socket, which can be caused by infection or injury that has persisted for some time.
- *Thermal sensitivity:* The tooth's response to hot and cold stimuli is tested.
- *Percussion:* The tooth is tapped to test its sensitivity.
- *Palpation:* The face and neck are lightly pressed with the fingers to detect sensitivity or tissue enlargement.
- *Transillumination:* High intensity light can be illuminated through the anterior teeth to detect fractures or decay.
- *Tooth cavity:* The preparation that results from removal of caries.
- *Pulp vitality test:* A high-frequency electrical instrument is used to test the sensitivity of the pulp.

The subjective symptoms described by the patient, the objective symptoms noted by the dentist, and the results of the examination all assist in determining the required treatment.

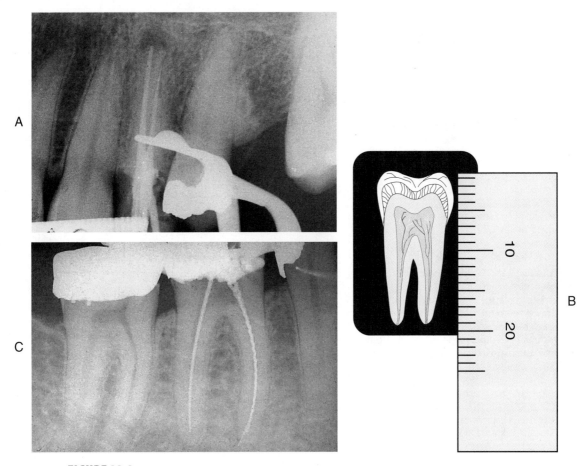

FIGURE 23.3

Dentists use periapical radiographs to (**A**), check the endodontic filling (**B**), measure the length of the root canal and (**C**), check for root canal completion.

Pulp Vitality Testing

A **vitalometer** is a high-frequency electrical device used to test a tooth's level of sensitivity, or vitality. This test enables the dentist to determine if endodontic treatment should be completed. Pulp vitality testing, which are described in Box 23.2 and Table 23.1, may be delegated to dental assistants.

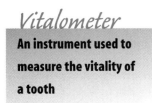

Vitalometer

An instrument used to measure the vitality of a tooth

Endodontic Instruments

Broaches

Endodontic broaches (Figure 23.5) are finger-operated instruments used primarily for extirpation of the pulp and gross fragments. Because they are inflexible in the canal, they are used with a push-pull action. Broaches are avail-

able in six sizes: xxx-fine, xx-fine, x-fine, fine, medium, and coarse.

Files and Reamers

Endodontic files are finger-operated instruments that are used in gradually increasing sizes to enlarge, shape, and smooth the walls of the canal. Files are available in three lengths: 21 mm, 25 mm, and 30 mm. Two basic types are used in most endodontic procedures, the K-type file and the Hedstrom file (Figure 23.6).

Reamers are finger-operated instruments that are inserted into the pulp canal and pulled out with a twisting action to enlarge it (Figure 23.7).

Files and reamers come in 20 different sizes, ranging from #06 (the smallest) to #140 (the largest). Six basic colors are used to code the size of the instruments, and the colors are reused to accommodate all available sizes. The smaller files and reamers (#06, #08, and #10) are delicate and can break easily. The colors used to code these smaller

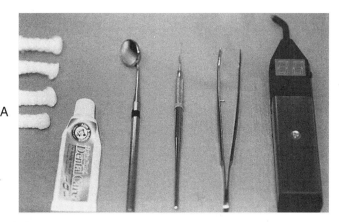

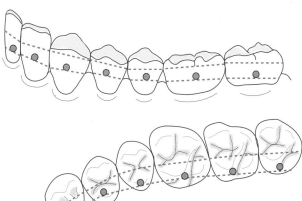

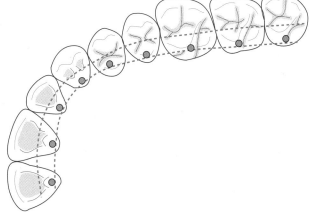

A   B

FIGURE 23.4

A, Pulp testing setup. **B,** The tip of the vitalometer is placed firmly on designated areas of the enamel.

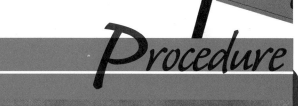

Box 23.2

Procedure for Pulp Vitality Testing

Instruments
Vitalometer (Figure 23.4)
Toothpaste
Cotton roll
Basic endodontic setup

Technique

1. Describe the procedure to the patient. Explain that a feeling of warmth may be experienced, and that the patient should lift a hand when a stimulus is felt on the tooth.
2. Identify the tooth in question and then select the identical tooth on the opposite side to be the control tooth (this tooth is tested for comparison readings).
3. Isolate the involved teeth with cotton rolls and keep them dry with the air syringe.
4. Assemble the tip of the pulp tester, adjust the indicator to zero, and turn on the vitalometer.
5. Apply a small amount of toothpaste to the tip of the pulp tester to act as a conductor for contact with the tooth.
6. Place the tip of the pulp tester firmly against the enamel of the control tooth. (Never place the tip on a metallic restoration, because it will cause the patient discomfort and produce a false reading.)
7. Move the indicator lever from zero upward to increase the stimulus and record these readings.
8. Isolate the tooth in question as was done with the control tooth.
9. Test each tooth twice for accuracy.
10. Testing will be inconclusive if the tooth has had a pulp cap, is necrotic, or, if mulit-rooted, is vital in only one root.

Table 23.1					
Evaluation for Pulp Vitality Testing					
Pulp Vitality Testing	4	3	2	0	X
1. Secure materials.					
2. Describe procedure.					
3. Identify teeth.					
4. Isolate involved teeth.					
5. Assemble pulp tester.					
6. Adjust indicator.					
7. Turn on vitalometer.					
8. Apply conductor.					
9. Place tip against enamel.					
10. Move indicator lever.					
11. Test twice.					
12. Clean equipment.					

The numeric criteria: 4 Excellent; 3 Good but some improvement can be made; 2 Below average, usable, needs to improve skill; 0 Unsatisfactory; X Not able to evaluate.

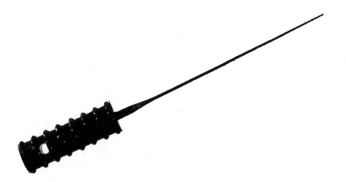

FIGURE 23.5

Broaches are used to remove pulpal tissue.

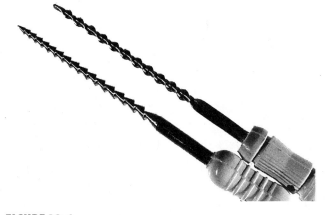

FIGURE 23.6

Files vary in size and are used to enlarge the root canal and to shape and smooth its walls. *Top*, K-type file. *Bottom:* Hedstrom file.

instruments are not included in the basic group of six, which makes them easy to identify. The dental assistant should become familiar with all file and reamer sizes and their color codes (Table 23.2).

File Box

Endodontic files are kept in a sterile file box. A standard file box usually has room to maintain three sets of K-type files (#10 through #140) and one set of Hedstrom files (#15 through #100). The file box also usually has space for other endodontic instruments, such as a #2, a #4, and a #6 round burr; a #557 burr; a #18 safety-tipped diamond burr; Gates Glidden drills (#1 through #6); and peeso drills (#1 through #6).

Spreaders

Spreaders are smooth, pointed, tapered instruments. Depending on the dentist's preference, a spreader can be a finger-operated instrument or a hand-operated instrument. Spreaders are used to pack gutta-percha points into the prepared canal.

Condensers

Condensers are elongated instruments with a pointed tip. Also known as pluggers, they may be finger-operated in-

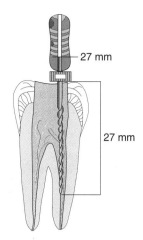

- 27 mm
- 27 mm

FIGURE 23.7

Reamers and files are used in the root canal to remove hard and soft tissue.

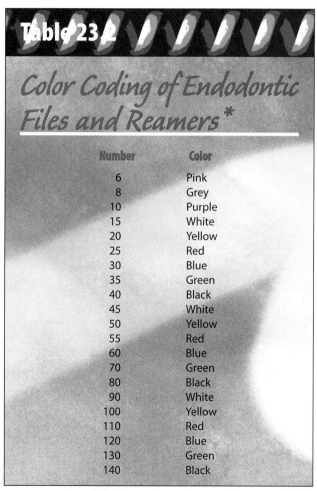

Table 23.2

*Color Coding of Endodontic Files and Reamers** *

Number	Color
6	Pink
8	Grey
10	Purple
15	White
20	Yellow
25	Red
30	Blue
35	Green
40	Black
45	White
50	Yellow
55	Red
60	Blue
70	Green
80	Black
90	White
100	Yellow
110	Red
120	Blue
130	Green
140	Black

*Endodontic files and reamers are color coded according to size. The table is arranged from smallest to largest.

struments or hand-operated instruments. Condensers are used to compress gutta-percha filling material. Hand-operated condensers may have a straight tip or a tip that is offset by an angle at the long axis of the instrument (Figure 23.8).

Gates Glidden Drill

Gates Glidden drills are used with a slow-speed, contraangle handpiece to enlarge the root canal. Endodontic files normally are used for this purpose, but Gates Glidden drills are often used when enlargement with a file is difficult (Figure 23.9).

Basic Endodontic Setup

Endodontic instruments and their accessories are usually prepared in sterile cassettes and trays (Figure 23.10). These cassettes are made of durable plastic capable of withstanding the heat necessary for sterilization, whereas the endodontic file boxes are made of metal. The cassette and file box provide a good method of infection control. Endodontic instruments are flexible and very delicate and must always be examined for signs of wear and weakness. Broken instruments should immediately be removed from cassettes and replaced. Sponges in the file boxes should be checked regularly and changed as needed.

The instruments found in a basic endodontic setup include the following:

- Broaches
- Reamers
- Endodontic file box
- High-speed or contraangle handpiece (or both)
- Paper points
- Sterile cotton gauze, cotton pellets, and cotton-tipped applicator
- Disposable irrigating syringe
- Glass bead sterilizer

Other Endodontic Armamentaria
Glass Bead Sterilizer

The glass bead sterilizer is a small electrical unit used for sterilizing endodontic instruments. The device is used at chairside to sterilize reamers, broaches, and any finger-held instrument that is not contained within the sterile endodontic file box. Nowadays most practitioners use steam to also sterilize these endodontic instruments, but because some practitioners may still use the glass bead sterilizer, a brief description is given.

The sterilizer has a well in the top section that is filled with glass beads, and a thermostat that allows the temperature to be set up to 450°. The instruments are inserted into the well, sharp point down, for 10 seconds before being used

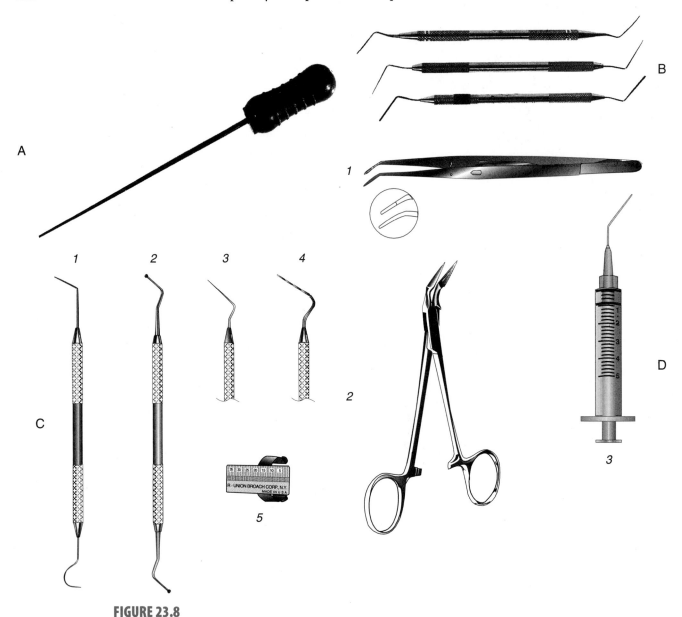

FIGURE 23.8

A, Finger condenser (plugger). **B,** Handheld condensers are used to compress gutta-percha filling material into the canals. **C,** *(1)* Root canal explorer, *(2)* excavator, *(3)* handheld spreader, *(4)* root canal plugger, and *(5)* endodontic ruler. **D,** *(1)* Endodontic pliers, *(2)* root and silver point forceps, and *(3)* irrigating syringe.

in the root canal (see Chapter 18 for more information on infection control).

Microhead Attachment

A microhead is an attachment that connects to the slow-speed handpiece and is used in apical surgery (Figure 23.11). Because of the space constraints involved in apical surgery, the microhead's size allows it access to extremely circumscribed areas.

Ultrasonic Surgery Unit

The ultrasonic unit has miniature microtips that allow even greater access and maneuverability than the microhand piece (Figure 23.12). Ultrasonic microtips are able to (1) complete the preparation faster, (2) reduce the amount of root bevel, (3) make a more accurate **retroprep**,

Retroprep
Preparations located on the apex of the tooth

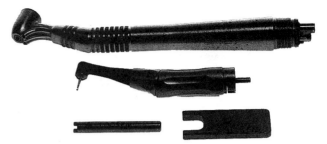

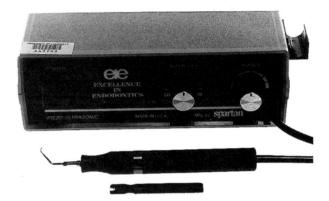

FIGURE 23.11

Because of its small size, the microhead allows access to extremely circumscribed areas. Compare the microhead *(bottom)* to the regular handpiece *(top)*.

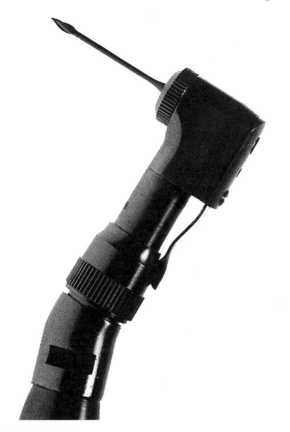

FIGURE 23.9

The Gates Glidden drill, which is available in several sizes, is used with a slow-speed contraangle handpiece to enlarge the root canal.

FIGURE 23.12

The ultrasonic surgery unit provides greater access to the periapical area.

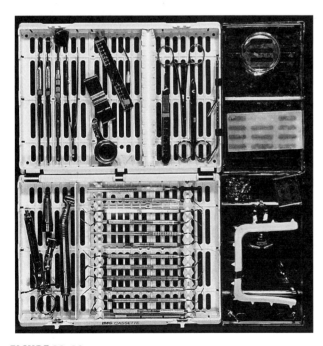

FIGURE 23.10

Basic endodontic setups are prepared in sterile cassettes and trays.

(4) remove points, hard pastes, and obstructions from the canal, and (5) reach the full length of the canal. Some ultrasonic handpieces can be sterilized in the autoclave.

Miniaturized Retromirrors

Miniaturized retromirrors are available for use with surgical microscopes or high-power loupes. These retromirrors allow the operator to visualize root ends, inspect the retroprep, and look behind roots.

Surgical Microscope

The surgical microscope is a new optical system designed to magnify and illuminate the surgical site. It allows the surgeon to refine operative techniques while providing clarity of the periapex, fractures, or accessory canals. Illumination of the surgical field provides more image detail and eliminates shadows, especially in deep cavities (Figure 23.13).

The microscope can be a floor-standing model, wall mounted, or ceiling mounted. Some surgical microscopes are available with fiberoptic or halogen light sources. They are also available with a variety of accessories for the assistant and for documentation purposes. For instance, some

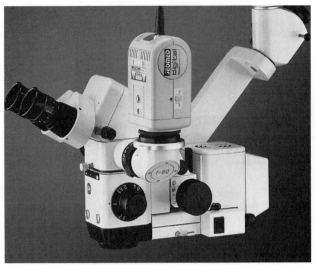
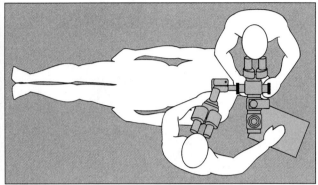

FIGURE 23.13

The surgical microscope allows the assistant as well as the operator to view a magnified surgical site. (Courtesy JEDMED Instrument Co.)

surgical microscopes are available with dual inclinable binoculars, which allow both the operator and the assistant to view the operating site in a comfortable position. They are also available with video and recorder systems that can magnify and record the image.

PROCEDURE FOR ROOT CANAL TREATMENT

Isolation of the Tooth

Use of a rubber dam is essential in endodontic treatment, and the dental assistant may be responsible for preparing the tooth for root canal therapy by placing the rubber dam. The tooth first is isolated by placing a rubber dam clamp on it. (It is important that the dental assistant become familiar with the various sizes and shapes of rubber dam clamps in order to select the proper clamp.) The rubber dam is prepared by punching a hole in it corresponding to the tooth to be isolated. The punched hole is then placed over the tooth that has been clamped (for more detailed instructions on rubber dam placement, see Box 23.3 and Chapter 33).

Gaining Access to the Pulp Chamber and Canal

A tapered fissure or round carbide burr (or both) usually is used to open the pulp chamber and canal. The size of the burr used always depends on the size of the chamber and canals of the tooth.

After gaining access, the operator removes the pulp and pulpal remnants. The barbed broach is the standard instrument for removing the pulp (Figure 23.15). Remaining pulpal tissue is removed through the process of shaping and cleaning the canals. After the pulp and any remaining pulpal tissue have been removed, the root canal is debrided. **Debridement** is the progressive removal of debris within the root canal. During the process of debridement, the canal is enlarged and shaped in preparation for the permanent filling (gutta-percha). Debridement can be accomplished either by mechanical instrumentation or by use of chemicals combined with mechanical instrumentation. Regardless of the method chosen, mechanical instrumentation is essential to complete debridement of the tooth.

Debridement

The removal of pulpal tissue and debris from the pulp canal of a tooth

Mechanical Debridement

Mechanical debridement of a canal is performed with endodontic reamers and files. The operator selects the sizes of reamers and files to be used, and these instruments are sterilized in a glass bead or salt sterilizer before use. A reamer is used to open and enlarge the canal. A file can aid in enlarging the canal and removing debris. Unlike the reamer, the file also smoothes and shapes the canal. Irriga-

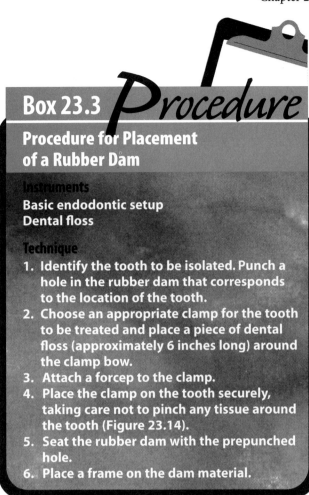

Box 23.3 *Procedure*

Procedure for Placement of a Rubber Dam

Instruments
Basic endodontic setup
Dental floss

Technique
1. Identify the tooth to be isolated. Punch a hole in the rubber dam that corresponds to the location of the tooth.
2. Choose an appropriate clamp for the tooth to be treated and place a piece of dental floss (approximately 6 inches long) around the clamp bow.
3. Attach a forcep to the clamp.
4. Place the clamp on the tooth securely, taking care not to pinch any tissue around the tooth (Figure 23.14).
5. Seat the rubber dam with the prepunched hole.
6. Place a frame on the dam material.

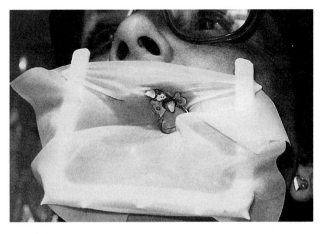

FIGURE 23.14
Set up and placement of rubber dam for endodontic procedures.

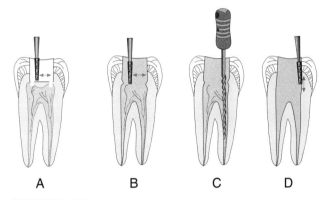

A B C D

FIGURE 23.15
Endodontic instruments help the operator to (**A**), gain access to the pulp chamber (**B**), debride (**C**), enlarge and shape the root canals and (**D**), smooth the canals.

tion is used with the instrumentation to ensure adequate cleansing of the canal.

A periapical radiograph is made with either the file or the reamer in the canal. This radiograph helps provide a starting measurement of the length of the root canal. The root canal is measured on film, and stops are placed at the points representing the distance from the apex to the occlusal surface or incisal edge. Radiographs are exposed incrementally with instrumentation to ensure that a correct working length has been established.

Chemical Debridement

In chemical debridement, also referred to as "chelation," decalcifying chemicals are used to soften the tooth structure in the canal so that the canal can be properly cleaned and widened. Paper points are dipped in the chemical and then placed in the canal. The chemicals used in debridement (commonly metacresol acetate, beechwood creosote, formocresol, or eugenol) must be confined to the canal to avoid irritating periapical tissue. The operator chooses which chemicals to use. Mechanical instrumentation is used with chelation.

Measurement of the Tooth

An accurate measurement of the length of the tooth is essential to endodontic treatment (see Figure 23.3, *B*). Failure to obtain an accurate measurement may result in apical perforation and overfilling. The x-ray films taken during endodontic treatment must be clear and without error because these films can show incomplete instrumentation or underfilling.

An initial x-ray film, called the preoperative radiograph, is used to determine the length of the tooth root (Figure 23.16). The tooth is measured from the radiograph with an endodontic millimeter ruler, a gauge used to measure endodontic files, reamers, and broaches to the appropriate length. A tooth that has more than one root may be radiographed from various angles to determine the alignment and number of roots. The length of the tooth is estimated and then verified by exposing another radiograph with a test file in place. The measurement obtained from the second radiograph provides an estimated working length. Once the length has been determined, the endodontic files are measured and marked by the placement of stops, which are round pieces of rubber that are placed on files to mark the length of the tooth. Stops are used to prevent an instrument from being placed too far into the canal. To ensure accuracy, the stop attachment should be placed at a right angle.

The endodontic assistant can measure the files with the stops in place. After this, the files should be arranged in order of size.

Sterilization of the Pulp Chamber and Canal

The pulp chamber and canals are sterilized using a combination of chemical and mechanical techniques. Sterilization by chemical means involves the use of irrigation and **medicaments,** which aid in the destruction of microorganisms. Sterilization by mechanical means is accomplished through debridement, which aids in

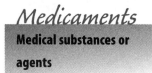

Medicaments
Medical substances or agents

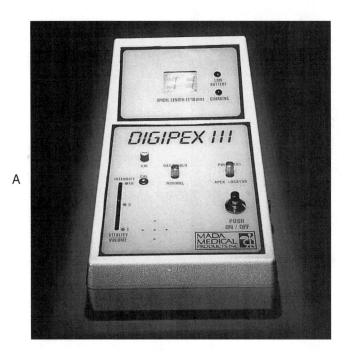

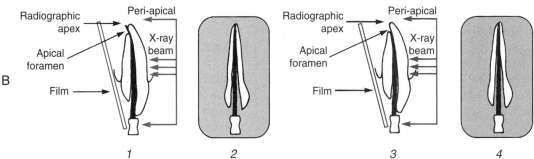

FIGURE 23.16

A, Electronic equipment, such as the DIGIPEX, help the operator determine the distance to the apical foramen. **B,** *(1)* The apical foramen opens on the lingual surface; the instrument protrudes into the periapical tissues 2 to 3 mm beyond the apical foramen. *(2)* The radiograph is misleading, indicating that the tip of the instrument is at the apical foramen. The foramen deviates from the root tip in at least two thirds of all teeth. *(3)* Clinically, the instrument is exactly at the apical foramen. *(4)* Another misleading radiograph, which shows the instrument to be 2 to 3 mm short of the apex. If this radiograph were used, the root canal might be overinstrumented. (Courtesy MADA Medical Equipment.)

the physical removal of the microbial mass with instrumentation.

Irrigation of the Tooth

Root canals must be irrigated and dried during the process of instrumentation and canal enlargement. Irrigation is the process of aspirating solutions such as solvents or disinfectants into the root canal and then drying the canals with air and absorbent points. The purpose of irrigation is to remove all pulpal remnants, disinfect the canals, and lubricate the canal walls.

Solutions used for irrigation include sodium hypochlorite and saline water. Sodium hypochlorite is an excellent disinfectant and solvent for necrotic tissue. It can be used directly from the bottle or diluted with one to two parts water. Saline water is an aqueous solution of sterile water mixed with salt. The preferred irrigating solution is basically a choice of the operator. In the past hydrogen peroxide was used to irrigate the pulp canal, but this solution is no longer recommended because of the incidence of pericementitis associated with it. Pericementitis is the inflammation of the periodontal ligament and the tissues surrounding the apex of the root. Some studies also have shown hydrogen peroxide to be **carcinogenic,** or a cancer-causing substance.

Carcinogenic

A term referring to cancer-causing substances

Irrigation is most often performed with a disposable syringe with a blunt 20- to 23-gauge needle. Often the dentist may bend the needle to an angle to facilitate access to the canal. After the canals have been irrigated, they are dried out with paper points. Advanced-function dental assistants may be delegated the responsibility of irrigating and drying the canals (Box 23.4 and Table 23.3).

Placement of Medicaments

Medicaments may be placed in the pulp chamber between visits to help eradicate infective organisms. Antimicrobial agents

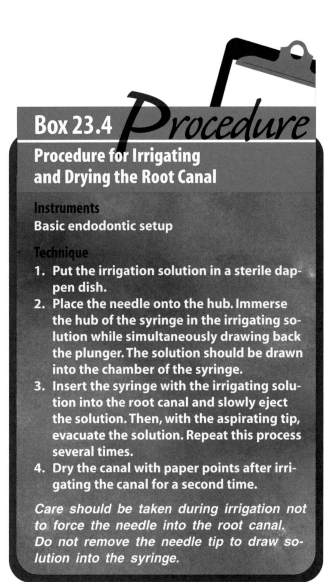

Box 23.4 *Procedure*

Procedure for Irrigating and Drying the Root Canal

Instruments
Basic endodontic setup

Technique
1. Put the irrigation solution in a sterile dappen dish.
2. Place the needle onto the hub. Immerse the hub of the syringe in the irrigating solution while simultaneously drawing back the plunger. The solution should be drawn into the chamber of the syringe.
3. Insert the syringe with the irrigating solution into the root canal and slowly eject the solution. Then, with the aspirating tip, evacuate the solution. Repeat this process several times.
4. Dry the canal with paper points after irrigating the canal for a second time.

Care should be taken during irrigation not to force the needle into the root canal. Do not remove the needle tip to draw solution into the syringe.

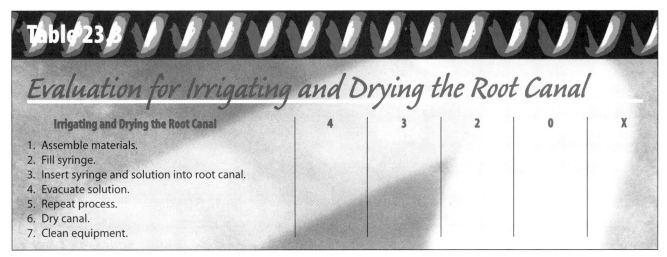

Table 23.3

Evaluation for Irrigating and Drying the Root Canal

Irrigating and Drying the Root Canal	4	3	2	0	X
1. Assemble materials.					
2. Fill syringe.					
3. Insert syringe and solution into root canal.					
4. Evacuate solution.					
5. Repeat process.					
6. Dry canal.					
7. Clean equipment.					

The numeric criteria: 4 Excellent; 3 Good but some improvement can be made; 2 Below average, usable, needs to improve skill; 0 Unsatisfactory; X Not able to evaluate.

Box 23.5

Procedure for Placing Medicaments and Temporary Fillings

Instruments
Basic endodontic setup

Technique

1. After thoroughly drying the root canal with paper points, take a sterile cotton pellet, tear it in half, moisten it with medication, and blot it dry with a sterile gauze.
2. Place the treated pellet on the floor of the pulp chamber over the orifice of the canal. Place the other, untreated half of the cotton pellet on top of the treated piece (Figure 23.17).
3. Mix the temporary filling according to the manufacturer's instructions or, if using Cavit, squeeze out just enough to fill in the opening of the tooth.

4. Use a carver (discoid/cleoid) to adjust any excess material while the filling material is still soft. The temporary filling material must be flush with the natural surface of the tooth.
5. Put a piece of articulating paper in the articulating holder. Ask the patient to gently bite down and to grind the teeth as in natural chewing. Check the tooth to see if any marks are present, indicating that the filling material is too high.
6. If the filling material has not set, adjust the temporary filling using a carver. If the material has hardened, inform the dentist so that the filling can be adjusted with a handpiece.

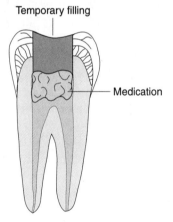

Temporary filling

Medication

FIGURE 23.17

Medicated cotton pellets are placed on the floor of the pulp chamber.

that may be used are calcium hydroxide and 2% iodine potassium iodide. The medicament is placed on the floor of the pulp chamber and a temporary filling material is placed over it. This procedure, which is described in Box 23.5 and Table 23.4, may be performed by an advanced-function dental assistant.

Filling of the Root Canal

After the pulp and other debris have been removed and the chamber and canal have been shaped and sterilized, the

tooth is filled. This procedure may require several more steps, depending on the condition of the canal. These steps include the trial point, the final filling, and permanent restoration of the tooth.

Trial Point

After the root canal has been irrigated and dried, the canal is filled in with gutta-percha. Gutta-percha, which is a solid material, has been used in dentistry for more than 130 years. It has been used as a temporary restoration, as an impression material (bite registration), and as a root canal filler.

Before the tooth is filled, a trial gutta-percha point, called a master cone, is selected and placed in the canal. The tooth is radiographed to check how the master cone fits into the canal. The selected point must not extend beyond the apex of the root. A properly fitted point should be tight in the canal, no farther than 1 to 1.5 mm from the apex of the root tip. The dentist may make a slight mark on the master cone at the point where it is even with the opening of the tooth. This provides a guide for how far the master cone should be seated in the canal.

Final Filling

After the trial points have been placed, the tooth is dried thoroughly and preparations are made for the final fill. The operator has a choice of methods for filling the root canal, including lateral condensation, vertical condensation, therma-fil, and sargenta paste. The method discussed in this chapter is lateral condensation.

Table 23-4

Evaluation for Placing Medicaments and Temporary Fillings

Placing Medicaments and Temporary Fillings	4	3	2	0	X
1. Assemble materials.					
2. Dry canal.					
3. Place medicament.					
4. Mix temporary filling.					
5. Place temporary filling.					
6. Remove excess material.					
7. Articulate bite.					
8. Adjust filling if necessary.					

The numeric criteria: 4 Excellent; 3 Good but some improvement can be made; 2 Below average, usable, needs to improve skill; 0 Unsatisfactory; X Not able to evaluate.

Lateral Condensation

After inserting the master cone, the dentist selects accessory gutta-percha points or cones to place in the root canal beside the master cone. The dental assistant prepares the cement material to be used to seal the gutta-percha. The cement powder and liquid should be mixed according to the manufacturer's directions. The cement should be thick and creamy in consistency but thin enough to evenly coat the gutta-percha cones.

The master cone is placed in the canal. Then an endodontic spreader is used to apply pressure to condense the gutta-percha and make room for the accessory cones. The gutta-percha is packed tightly into the canal until it is full. A condenser, or plugger, is then heated, and the excess gutta-percha is removed.

A successfully treated tooth can then be permanently restored. The restoration most often recommended for an endodontically treated tooth is a full crown, because such teeth are more likely to be brittle and prone to fracture. Molars, for example, are more likely to fracture than lateral or central teeth because of the chewing pressure exerted on molars. The practitioner selects the appropriate permanent restoration. The tooth may be radiographed at intervals of 6 months to 1 year so that the progress of the endodontic treatment can be checked.

OTHER ENDODONTIC PROCEDURES

Vital Pulp Capping

In cases involving deep caries in which the pulp is inflamed and has degenerated, even though the patient feels no pain, the dentist often is faced with the problem of saving the pulp. Research shows that when carious dentin extends down to the pulp, a more or less inflammatory condition will exist within the pulpal tissue. Elimination of carious dentin, which is an inflammatory irritant, permits a condition called regressiveness, in which the tooth remains vital although the pulp is scarred. In such cases, attempts are made to save the pulp through a procedure known as **pulp capping.**

Pulp capping
Treatment of exposed pulp to maintain tooth vitality

Indirect Pulp Capping

Indirect pulp capping is a technique in which the dentist leaves a thin layer of dentin between the pulp and the capping material. This procedure helps to maintain the vitality of the pulp while hardening the remaining soft dentin. The materials most commonly used for indirect pulp capping are calcium hydroxide and zinc oxide and eugenol cements. After completion of the procedure, the tooth can be permanently restored. The dentist may choose to check the tooth periodically to make sure that no problems persist.

Direct Pulp Capping

Direct pulp capping is a treatment in which a dressing is placed in direct contact with the exposed pulpal tissue. This method can maintain pulpal vitality when the pulp is exposed accidentally during the removal of dental decay. The materials used for direct pulp capping are the same as those used for indirect pulp capping.

Pulpectomy

Pulpectomy is the surgical removal of vital pulp tissue.

Pulpectomy
Surgical removal of pulpal tissue from the pulp chamber

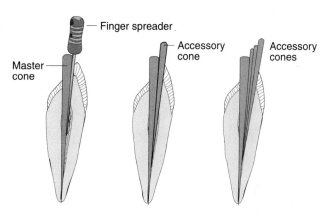

FIGURE 23.18

Gutta-percha points or cones are condensed into the root canal.

The steps involved are the same as those for endodontic treatment of nonvital pulp.

Pulpotomy

Pulpotomy is the removal of pulp from the chamber of the crown; the pulp in the root portion of the tooth is not removed, which allows the pulp in the root canal to remain vital. Pulpotomies usually are performed on young patients with the purpose of stimulating the pulp tissue in the root canal to form dentin over the pulpal tissue.

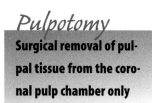

Pulpotomy

Surgical removal of pulpal tissue from the coronal pulp chamber only

Incision and Drainage

Incision and drainage is a procedure performed on a tooth that has an acute apical abscess. The abscess usually is accompanied by severe pain and swelling. This procedure is effective when the infection is localized and is clearly defined on the mucosa. The incision is made at a point that allows drainage of the infection that created the swelling. Instant relief often accompanies the incision. A drain may be placed in the infected area to keep the site open and allow complete drainage, and antibiotics are normally prescribed to eliminate any remaining infection. Once the infection has been eliminated, the tooth can undergo endodontic treatment (Figure 23.18).

Basic Setup for Incision and Drainage

The instruments and accessories used for incision and drainage are shown in Figure 23.19. The dental assistant can prepare for this procedure by first cutting a drain, usually in the shape of an "I." The drain is then connected with the su-

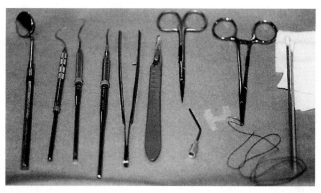

FIGURE 23.19

Basic endodontic surgical setup. Instruments: mouth mirror, explorer, endodontic explorer, periodontic probe, cotton pliers, Bard-Parker holder, suture holder, suture scissors, surgical aspirator tip. Accessories: 2 × 2-inch gauze sponge, cotton-tipped applicator, #15 blade, antiseptic solution, sterile rubber dam, topical anesthetic, suture material.

ture, usually at the tip, and is placed back on the sterile tray. The incision site is swabbed with an antiseptic solution, and to minimize discomfort, a topical anesthetic may be used on the site. The dentist is now ready to make the incision and place the drain if indicated.

Bleaching of Nonvital Teeth

Often a nonvital tooth may become discolored as a result of a traumatic injury that causes pulpal hemorrhage into the dentinal tubules. Teeth can also be discolored or stained by medicaments used in root canal therapy. Bleaching the discolored teeth can produce dramatic improvement. Several bleaching or whitening products are available (see Chapter 24). Often a mixture of hydrogen peroxide and sodium perborate is used on the tooth. The technique most often used to bleach an endodontically treated tooth is a "walking bleach." With this technique, a mixture of sodium perborate and hydrogen peroxide is placed on a cotton pellet and sealed in the pulp chamber for a 3 to 7 days.

SPECIFIC TYPES OF ENDODONTIC SURGERY

Apicoectomy

Apicoectomy is the surgical removal of the apical portion of the tooth root (Figure 23.20). An apicoectomy may be required for a number of reasons: root canal

Apicoectomy

Surgical removal of the apex of the tooth root

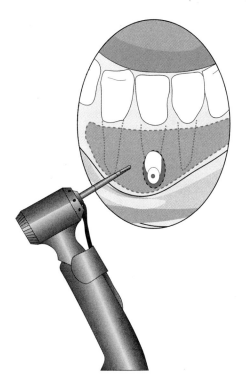

FIGURE 23.20

The apex of the tooth root is surgically removed during an apicoectomy.

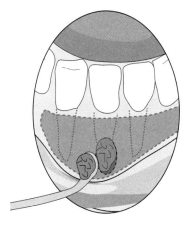

FIGURE 23.21

The removal of periapical tissue by surgical scraping is called curettage.

therapy or other dental treatment that fails to control infection; lodging of a broken instrument in the canal; unfilled or improperly debrided root canals; and discomfort after endodontic treatment. The apicoectomy is accomplished through a surgical opening made in the overlying bone and gingival tissues.

Retrofilling

Retrofilling is a surgical procedure that can be performed at the time of an apicoectomy. It involves filling the root canal from the apex of the tooth. Amalgam is the material most often used for retrofilling.

Root Resection

Root resection involves the amputation of a root when it is not treatable but the rest of the tooth is restorable and able to function adequately. Resection may also be necessary if the root is fractured, a canal is obstructed, or a pathologic conditions exists that is not treatable in one root.

Periapical Curettage

Periapical curettage is the surgical scraping away of periapical soft tissue (Figure 23.21). This is accomplished through a

surgical opening made in the gingiva and alveolar bone. Periapical curettage can be done during an apicoectomy.

Replantation

Replantation allows the dentist to extract a tooth, perform endodontic treatment on it, and replant it in the socket. This procedure can also be performed on a tooth that has been accidentally knocked out. A temporary splint is placed around the tooth to help stabilize it in the dental arch. In both cases it is important to complete the procedure within a short period of time.

ENDODONTIC SURGICAL TECHNIQUE

Figure 23.22 presents the basic instrument setup for endodontic surgery. During an apicoectomy, the dental assistant prepares the scalpel and passes it to the dentist after administration of a local anesthetic. The dentist prepares the site by creating a mucoperiosteal flap parallel to the apex of the treated tooth. The dental assistant retracts the flap, revealing the cortical bone of the alveolus that covers the apex of the tooth to be treated. The dentist then uses the handpiece and surgical burr to remove the cortical plate, allowing access to the root tip. A rongeur forceps is used to remove tissue fragments and smooth the area. The dental assistant irrigates the surgical area with saline solution and aspirates the area. Curettage is performed to remove all infectious tissue. If indicated, retrofill is completed at this time.

If a retrofill was to be performed with the apicoectomy, the operator will have already removed the root tip at an angle in order to prepare the blunted apex for the retrofill. The site is irrigated and aspirated. Sterile cotton pellets can be used to dry the area.

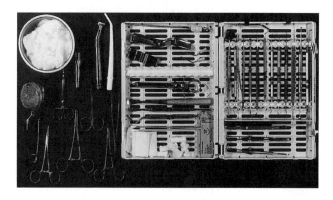

FIGURE 23.22

Basic endodontic surgical setup.

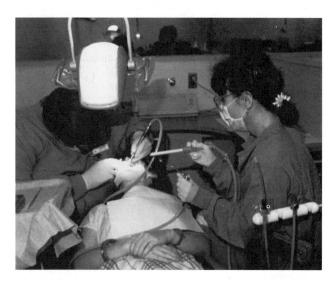

FIGURE 23.23

The chairside assistant aids the operator by keeping the work area dry and free of debris.

The dental assistant's main function during the surgical procedures is to keep the operating site clean so that the dentist can see the work area (Figure 23.23). After the area has been aspirated, a gauze is placed to help catch any scrap amalgam. The alloy is triturated and placed in the amalgam well, from which the dental assistant loads the alloy into the messing gun. The alloy is then placed in the prepared apex concavity and condensed with the reverse-action plugger. The amalgam is condensed and finished flush with the completed apex. The assistant then removes the gauze to avoid dropping the amalgam debris into the incision. A radiograph may be taken before the tissue is sutured to ensure that no amalgam particles have been left in the surgical area. The tissue is then reposi-

Box 23.6

Postoperative Instructions for Endodontic Surgery

1. After the surgery, rest for the balance of the day, and avoid strenuous activity. When you want to lie down, prop your head up with two pillows; do this for the first day and night.
2. Do not lift or pull on the lip to look at the area and the skin. This can pull out the sutures, cause bleeding, and retard healing.
3. Many patients experience swelling in the area, and the skin may look bruised. The swelling can be greatly controlled by holding an ice pack on the area, applying and removing it every 15 minutes for the first 6 to 12 hours.
4. If swelling persists after 12 hours, apply warm, moist heat (not a hot water bottle) to the swollen area, alternating 15 minutes on and 15 minutes off as often as possible. Also, exercise the jaw muscles by slowly moving the jaw from side to side as the warm, moist heat is applied. Swelling usually subsides in 3 to 6 days.
5. For the first 2 days, eat a soft diet and avoid chewing and brushing the gum tissue near the surgical site. It is very important to drink lots of liquids and eat nutritious foods. Do not smoke for 4 hours and do not eat yogurt for 2 days. Starting on the second day, gently rinse the area with warm (not hot) saltwater, especially after meals (mix 1 teaspoon of salt in an 8-ounce glass of warm water). Do not use commercial mouthwashes for several days. You should be able to resume normal brushing without discomfort by the fifth day.
6. Have your prescriptions filled, and take the medicine as directed. Do not drink any alcoholic beverages while taking the medications. Also, do not drive while taking pain medications stronger than aspirin or Tylenol.
7. The following are expected and should not cause concern:
   a. Discomfort or mild to moderate pain
   b. Slight oozing of blood for 36 to 48 hours (saliva may be pink)
   c. Swelling and discoloration of the skin
   d. Mouth odor and an unpleasant taste
8. Please call the dental office anytime you have questions or problems and be sure to keep your next appointment.

tioned and sutured. After the procedure has been completed, the dental assistant gives the patient postoperative instructions for home care (Box 23.6). At a subsequent visit, usually 7 to 10 days later, the sutures are removed (Box 23.7 and Table 23.5).

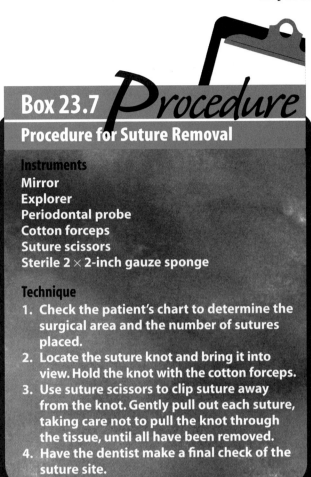

Box 23.7 *Procedure*

Procedure for Suture Removal

Instruments
Mirror
Explorer
Periodontal probe
Cotton forceps
Suture scissors
Sterile 2 × 2-inch gauze sponge

Technique
1. Check the patient's chart to determine the surgical area and the number of sutures placed.
2. Locate the suture knot and bring it into view. Hold the knot with the cotton forceps.
3. Use suture scissors to clip suture away from the knot. Gently pull out each suture, taking care not to pull the knot through the tissue, until all have been removed.
4. Have the dentist make a final check of the suture site.

Table 23.5

Evaluation for Suture Removal

Suture Removal	4	3	2	0	X
1. Assemble equipment.					
2. Check patient's chart.					
3. Locate suture knot.					
4. Hold knot with cotton forceps.					
5. Clip suture.					
6. Pull out sutures.					
7. Obtain final check from dentist.					
8. Clean equipment.					

The numeric criteria: 4 Excellent; 3 Good but some improvement can be made; 2 Below average, usable, needs to improve skill; 0 Unsatisfactory; X Not able to evaluate.

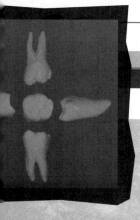

Points for Review

- The dental assistant's role in endodontics
- Pulpal disease and conditions that cause dental pain
- Endodontic examination, instruments, other armamentaria, and types of procedures
- Isolation of the tooth for endodontic treatment
- Endodontic surgical procedure, suture removal, and postoperative instructions

Self-Study Questions

1. A vitalometer is an instrument used to measure the length of a canal.
   a. True
   b. False

2. The dental pulp receives nourishment from what supply?
   a. Heart
   b. Arteries and veins
   c. Iron buildup
   d. Dentin

3. What is the most common cause of dental pain?
   a. Hypersensitivity
   b. Bacteria
   c. Hyperemia
   d. Hyperthermia

4. For what purpose is the initial endodontic radiograph useful?
   a. Diagnosis
   b. Measurement of the length of the root canal
   c. Examination of surrounding tissues
   d. All of the above

5. Endodontic files are used primarily for extirpation (removal) of the pulp and gross fragments.
   a. True
   b. False

6. How is debridement of the root canal accomplished?
   a. Chemical means
   b. Mechanical means
   c. A and b
   d. None of the above

7. What solutions are used to irrigate endodontically treated teeth?
   a. Sodium hypochlorite
   b. Saline water
   c. Alcohol
   d. A and b
   e. All of the above

8. What type of pulpalgia is considered to exist when the patient exhibits acute pain to heat irritation?
   a. Incipient pulpalgia
   b. Moderate pulpalgia
   c. Advanced pulpalgia
   d. Chronic pulpalgia

9. What term is used for the procedure in which the pulp is removed from the chamber of the crown only?
   a. Pulpotomy
   b. Pulpectomy
   c. Pulp capping
   d. Pulpitis

10. What term is used for the procedure in which all of the vital pulp is removed?
    a. Pulpotomy
    b. Pulpectomy
    c. Pulp capping
    d. Pulpitis

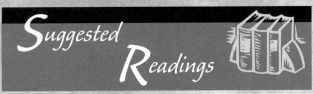

Suggested Readings

Berns JM: *Why root canal therapy?* Chicago, 1986, Quintessence.

Gutman JL, Dumsha TC, Lovdahl PE: *Problem solving in endodontics,* ed 3, St Louis, 1997, Mosby.

Keate KC, Wong M: A comparison of endodontic file tip quality, *J Endodontics* 16(10), 1990.

Sargenti AG: *Endodontics,* Switzerland, 1993, Endodontic Educational Service.

Selbt AG: Understanding informed consent and its relationship to the incidence of adverse treatment events in conventional endodontic therapy, *J Endodontics* 16(8), 1990.

Sjoren U et al: Factors affecting the long-term results of endodontic treatment, *J Endodontics* 16(10), 1990.

Trowbridge HO: Pathogenesis of pulpitis resulting from dental caries, *J Endodontics* 7(2), 1981.

Weine FS: *Endodontic therapy,* ed 5, St Louis, 1996, Mosby.

Chapter *24*

Pediatric Dentistry

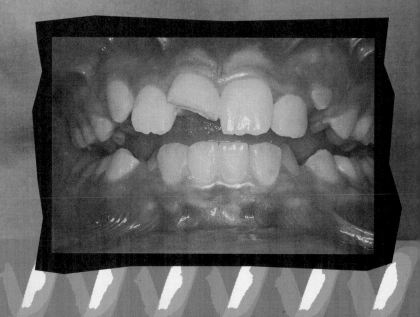

Chapter Outline

Learning Objectives

On completion of Chapter 24, the student should be able to do the following:

- Define key terms.

- Identify the stages of child development and discuss some of the characteristics.

- Identify the types of fear presented by children and list ways that a child can be prepared for dental treatment.

- Explain the role of dental auxiliaries in behavior management of children.

- List the important features of office environment in a pediatric office.

- Identify how offending oral habits can be treated.

- Describe the process of tooth development.

- Identify three appliances fabricated in a pediatric dental office and list the procedures essential to constructing a space maintainer and mouth guard and placing a stainless steel crown.

- List the procedures for bleaching vital teeth.

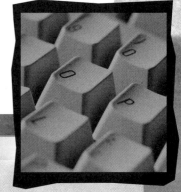

Key Terms

Adverse Conditioning

Bruxism

Empty Habit

Frenectomy

HOME (Hand-Over-Mouth Exercise)

Necrosis

Objective Fears

Pulpectomy

Pulpotomy

Subjective Fears

PEDIATRIC DENTISTRY

Pediatric dentistry refers to dentistry for children. Although pediatric dentistry was initially established to reduce dental decay, pulpal inflammation, and pain associated with children, it has always promoted prevention. Sealants and fluoride treatment have been instrumental in reducing dental decay for children and interception and treatment of malocclusion has helped to manage orthodontic problems. Although there is an increase in the number of children using dental services and a reduction in dental decay, there still remains a large number of unmet dental needs for children in the inner cities and special-population areas. See Table 24.1 for stages of child development.

BEHAVIOR MODIFICATION OF CHILDREN

The dental assistant should understand what techniques are used for child behavior management. Behavior is an observable act that can be described or measured reliably. Behavior modification means changing or shaping behavior in a beneficial way. *Motivation* is providing an incentive to cause an action or to help reach a specific goal. Motivation can include positive reinforcement, negative reinforcement, or **adverse conditioning.**

Adverse conditioning

A negative reinforcement method used to stop an undesirable behavior

Positive Reinforcement

Positive reinforcement is giving something the patient wants for obtaining the goal (that is, a reward).

Negative Reinforcement

Negative reinforcement means taking something away from the child that he or she does not want. Removing the pain from a toothache is a negative reinforcement that encourages the child to visit the dental office in the future.

Adverse Conditioning

Adverse conditioning, in the dental office, means the patient is given something that is not wanted, for instance, punishment to stop undesirable behavior. This may include using the hand-over-mouth exercise (HOME), which is used as a physical restraint to stop the child's undesirable behavior (screaming). The dentist will usually continue this method of conditioning until the bad behavior is dis-

continued, at which time the hand is removed (extinction). Children will usually learn to control their behavior with this technique.

TECHNIQUES USED TO MANAGE CHILDREN

There are a number of techniques that are used in the dental office to help children with their behavior. The American Academy of Pediatric Dentistry has developed a Standard of Care for Behavior Management (Table 24.2).

Desensitization

A method used to accustom a child to the dental practice is desensitization. Desensitization refers to beginning an experience a little at a time and increasing the experience until the child is no longer anxious. This is why it is important to orient the child to the dental office before beginning any treatment. One of the primary roles of the dental assistant in pediatric dentistry is to help the child learn to control his or her fears and any anxiety he or she may be feeling about the visit to the dental office. An observant dental assistant can recognize the child's level of discomfort and help the child relax and feel more comfortable.

The dentist will determine if the parent will be allowed to accompany the child during dental treatment. The dental assistant and dentist must establish this preference before seating the child or allowing the patient into the operatory with the child (Box 24.1).

Communication

The primary technique used to manage behavior is establishing communication and demonstrating a caring attitude with the child. This involves both verbal and nonverbal communications. The classical approach to communications and reconditioning is based on "Tell-Show-Do."

1 *Tell* the child exactly what you are going to do before you do it, while you're doing it, and after you've done it in a soft (yet firm), confident voice.
2 *Show* the child what to expect. For instance, when placing a rubber dam, tell the child what you are going to do and show him how it will feel. Pinch the arm or hand to demonstrate how the pinch of the clamp will feel in the mouth.
3 *Do* what you said you would do using the same voice and describing what you are doing while you are doing it. Don't proceed until you feel the child is clear in understanding.

Association (Mentoring)

Children will often model or imitate another child or adult in the dental practice. If a parent sits in the chair first and

Table 24.1

Stages of Child Development

Age	Behavior	Management
Birth to 2 years	Child has freedom to explore, touch, feel, and see.	Dental assistant should ask parent before the child is nurtured, held, touched, and cuddled. Parent may need to be present, so check dentist's preference.
2 to 3 years	Child usually able to walk, explore, and get into things and asks, "Why?" Afraid of noises and sudden movements. Child timid, shy, and bashful but can communicate fairly well. Limited vocabulary may lead to frustration and tantrums.	Dental assistant plays with child during first visit. Allows child to touch the mirror, rubber cup, water syringe, and smell toothpaste. Time for dental assistant to develop a good relationship.
3 to 5 years	Child begins to seek adult attention and likes to talk, tell stories, is easier to please and asks questions. Four-year-old exaggerates and can be incorrigible and defiant and will listen and respond to non-complicated directions if explained well, usually cooperative and willing helpers.	Dental assistant should praise child and help hold water syringe or a cotton roll.
5 to 7 years	Because of preschool, child will usually be well adjusted and compliant. Will enjoy group activities and play and is responsive to praise, compliments about hair, clothing, or school. At 5 years old will generally have no fear of going into the operatory alone. At 6 years, the child is moving away from family dependency and exhibits some anxiety with new situations. Beginning to lose primary teeth and may be conscientious about loss of "two front teeth" and may have temper tantrums. At 7 years old, anxiety decreases, behavior improves, and is anxious to please again. Little moody and needs reassurance and praise. May not like to be touched; becoming self-conscious of bodies.	Dental assistant must be truthful to maintain child's trust. Dentist may have to take control with firmness and voice control followed with a reward and praise. Dental assistant needs to reassure child and show kindness and appreciation. Praise and compliment child about personal appearance.
8 to 10 years	Child is sensitive and interested in relationships and likes to be treated as an adult. Has fewer fears, is adaptable, and is critical of self and others. Has tendency to dramatize situations and has more verbal aggressive behavior. The 9-year-old is more responsible, independent, cooperative, and competitive but uncertain. Child is self-critical, lacks confidence, may appear depressed, and is upset by mistakes. May also sob. Does not like to be told what to do and is sensitive to correction. The 10-year-old is easier going, well balanced, and more confident. If angry, child may be violent but can quickly resolve problems. Generally shrugs responsibility and wants to have good time. Seeks adult relationships.	Dental assistant should not demean child by saying, "act like a big boy or girl." Dental assistant should compliment the 9-year-old when cooperative or has had a successful event in school. Dental assistant should carry on conversation with 10-year-old about things that are fun and what is going on. Discuss likes and dislikes. Note special events in child's record and bring it up during the next appointment.
11 to 16 years	Child understands the what and why of procedures but worries. Afraid of unknown experiences, especially injections. Proud and competitive but afraid; often resentful and belligerent. A 12-year-old is more adjusted and happy and wants to be treated as an adult. Enthusiastic, overgenerous, outgoing, factual, and down to earth. Preoccupied with food and eating. The 13-year-old is often argumentative but by 14 years old is again outward and well adjusted. A 15-year-old may slam doors, hate authority, and often is defiant. Craves freedom but is locked into dependency. By 16 years old again happy and well adjusted because of driving and gaining some freedom to get around.	Dental assistant should explain what will take place and allow questions. Communicate humorously with 12-year-old. Talk about school and future plans as child nears 16 years old.

(Courtesy University of Louisville School of Dentistry, Department of Orthodontic, Pediatric, and Geriatric Dentistry.)

Table 24.1

Standards of Care for Behavior Management
American Academy of Pediatric Dentistry

Management Type	Description	Objectives	Indications	Contraindications
I. Communicative management **a. Voice control**	Controlled alteration of voice volume, tone, or pace to influence and direct patient's behavior.	a. Gain patient's attention and compliance. b. Avert negative or avoidance behavior. c. Establish authority.	May be used with any patient.	None
b. Nonverbal communications	Reinforcement and guiding behavior through contact, posture, and facial expression.	a. Enhance the effectiveness of other communicative management techniques. b. Gain or maintain the patient's attention and compliance.	May be used with any patient.	None
c. Tell-Show-Do	*Tell:* Verbal explanation of procedures in phrases appropriate to the developmental level of the patient. *Show:* Demonstrations for the patient of the visual, auditory, olfactory, and tactile aspects of the procedure in a carefully defined, nonthreatening setting. *Do:* Without deviating from explanation and demonstration, completion of procedure	a. Teach the patient important aspects of the dental visit and familiarize patient with the dental setting. b. Shape the patient's response to procedure by desensitization and well-described expectation.	May be used with any patient.	None
d. Positive reinforcement	Method to reward desired behaviors and thus strengthen the recurrence of those behaviors. Positive voice modulation, facial expression, verbal praise, and appropriate physical demonstrations of affection from dental team, e.g., tokens and toys.	Reinforce desired behavior.	May be used with any patient	None
e. Distraction	Diverting the patient's attention from what may be perceived as an unpleasant experience.	Decrease the perception of unpleasantness. a. Gain the patient's attention and compliance. b. Avert negative or avoidance behavior.	May be used with any patient.	None
f. Parental presence/absence	Communications between dentist and child paramount. Presence or absence of parent may be beneficial or detrimental. Must optimize the treatment setting recognizing operator's skills, abilities of child, and the desire of the parent.	a. Gain child's attention enabling communications with dentist so appropriate behavior expectations can be explained. b. Eliminate inappropriate avoidance responses to dental treatment and establish appropriate learned responses. c. Enhance the child's self-confidence in coping with the treatment. d. Ensure the child's safety in the delivery of quality dental treatment.		
II. Hand-Over-Mouth Exercise (HOME). Informed consent must be obtained and documented in the patient record.	Hand is placed over the child's mouth and behavioral expectations are calmly explained. The child is told that the hand will be removed as soon as appropriate behavior begins. When the child responds the hand is removed and the child's appropriate behavior is reinforced. Must take into consideration: (1) Alternative methods. (2) Patient dental needs. Quality of dental care. Patient's emotional development. (3) Anxiety-provoking. (4) Stimuli of dental treatment. (5) Patient's physical considerations.		A healthy child, who is able to understand and cooperate but who exhibits defiant, obstreperous, or hysterical avoidance behaviors to dental treatment.	a. In children who, due to age, disability, medication, or emotional immaturity are unable to understand and cooperate. b. When it will prevent the child from breathing.

Table 24.1—Cont'd.
Standards of Care for Behavior Management American Academy of Pediatric Dentistry

Management Type	Description	Objectives	Indications	Contraindications
III. Treatment immobilization. Informed consent and type of immobilization used, indication for immobilization, and duration of application in the patient record.	Partial or complete immobilization of the patient to protect the patient, practitioner, and dental staff from injury while providing dental care. Performed by the dentist, staff, or parent, with or without the aid of an immobilization device. Must take into consideration: (1) Alternative methods. (2) Dental needs. (3) Quality of dental care. (4) Patient's emotional development. (5) Patient's physical considerations.	a. Reduce or eliminate movement. b. Protect patient and dental staff from injury. c. Facilitate delivery of quality dental treatment.	a. A patient who requires diagnosis/or treatment and cannot cooperate due to lack of maturity. b. A patient who requires diagnosis/or treatment and cannot cooperate due to mental or physical handicap. c. A patient who requires diagnosis/or treatment and does not cooperate after other behavior techniques have failed. d. When the safety of the patient and practitioner would be at risk without the protective use of immobilization.	a. A cooperative patient or a patient who cannot be immobilized safely due to underlying medical or systemic conditions.
IV. Nitrous oxide-oxygen inhalation sedation	A conscious sedation technique that is safe and effective. Onset of action is fast, its depth of sedation is easily titrated, and recovery is rapid and complete. Provides a variable degree of analgesia for some patients. Must take into consideration: (1) Alternative methods. (2) Patient dental needs. (3) Quality of dental care. (4) Patient's emotional level of development. (5) Patient's physical considerations.	a. Reduce or eliminate anxiety in dental patients so safe, comfortable, quality dental treatment can be rendered. b. Reduce untoward movement and reaction to dental treatment. c. Enhance communication and patient cooperation. d. Raise the pain reaction threshold. e. Increase tolerance to longer appointments. f. Aid in treatment of the mentally, physically, or medically compromised patient. g. Reduce gagging.	a. Fearful, anxious, or obstreperous mentally, physically, or medically compromised patients. c. A patient whose gag reflex interferes with dental care. d. A patient for whom profound local anesthesia cannot be obtained.	a. May be contraindicated in some chronic obstructive pulmonary diseases. b. May be contraindicated in certain patients with severe emotional disturbances or drug-related dependencies. c. Patients in the first trimester of pregnancy. d. Patients with drug-induced or disease-induced pulmonary fibrosis.
	Used for patients unable to receive dental care for reasons of age or mental, physical, or medical condition. Must take into consideration: (1) Alternative methods. (2) Patient dental needs. (3) Quality of dental care. (4) Patient's emotional development. (5) Patient's physical considerations.	a. Reduce or eliminate anxiety in dental patients so that safe, comfortable, quality dental treatment can be rendered. b. Reduce untoward movement and reaction to dental treatment. c. Enhance communication and patient cooperation. d. Increase tolerance for longer appointments. e. Aid in treatment of the mentally, physically, or medically compromised patient.	a. Patients who are ASA Class I or II. b. Patient requiring dental care who cannot cooperate as a result of a lack of psychological or emotional maturity. c. Patients requiring dental care who cannot cooperate due to a mental, physical, or medical disability. d. Patients requiring dental care for whom the use of sedation may protect the developing psyche.	

Continued

Table 24.1—Cont'd.

Standards of Care for Behavior Management American Academy of Pediatric Dentistry

Management Type	Description	Objectives	Indications	Contraindications
V. Conscious sedation. Parental or guardian informed consent must be obtained and documented prior to use of conscious sedation.		Provide safe, efficient and effective dental care.		
VI. General anesthesia. Parental or guardian informed consent must be obtained and should be documented prior to the use of general anesthesia. Record should include informed consent and indication for use.	General anesthesia can be done in an ambulatory care setting, same day surgery center, an out-patient surgery area of a hospital or an inpatient hospital setting with the use of preoperative or postoperative patient admission to the hospital. A controlled state of unconsciousness accompanied by a loss of protective reflexes, including the ability to maintain an airway independently and respond purposefully to physical stimulation or verbal command. Must take into consideration: (1) Alternative methods. (2) Patient dental needs. (3) Quality of dental care. (4) Patient's emotional development. (5) Patient's physical considerations. (6) Patients requiring dental care for whom the use of general anesthesia may protect the developing psyche.		a. Patients with certain physical, mental, or medically compromising conditions. b. Patients with dental needs for whom local anesthesia is ineffective because of acute infection, anatomic variations, or allergy. c. The extremely uncooperative, fearful, anxious, or uncommunicative child or adolescent with dental needs deemed sufficiently important that dental care cannot be deferred. d. Patients who have sustained extensive orofacial and dental trauma. e. Patients with dental needs who otherwise would not obtain necessary dental care. f. Patients requiring dental care for whom the use of general anesthesia may protect the developing psyche.	a. The cooperative patient with minimal dental needs. b. Medical contraindication to sedation. c. A physical contraindication to general anesthesia.

Courtesy of American Academy of Pediatric Dentistry, 1996.

Box 24.1

When Parents Should Accompany a Child in the Operatory

Reasons for parents to be in the operatory

1. Increases dentist-parent contact for more personal relationship for child.
2. Parent can experience child's behavior.
3. Saves time, dentist can answer parent's questions.
4. Under 3 years, the child may respond more positively and benefit psychologically from parent's presence.

Reasons for parents not to be in the operatory

1. Parent's anxiety may be transmitted to the child.
2. Parent may repeat verbal orders from dentist thus annoying the dentist and child.
3. Parent may interject orders to child causing barrier between dentist and child.
4. Dentist may not be able to use firmness in tone of voice with parent near.
5. The dentist must be in control of the child, which may be difficult with parent present.
6. Parent may use wrong vocabulary.

shows the child how comfortable it is, the child will often model or follow the parent's example.

Relaxation

The use of conscious sedation such as nitrous oxide-oxygen inhalation is a method of relaxation used to reduce or eliminate anxiety and decrease the potential of reactions. Inhalation sedation is used for relief of fear and apprehension and not relief of pain or as a substitute for routine proven methods of child management.

Voice Control

Voice control is using the tone and volume of the dentist's voice to interrupt inappropriate behavior by the child. It requires increasing the volume and conviction (sternness) of the voice, for example, saying loudly, "Stop that. That's not allowed here!"

Hand-over-mouth exercise (HOME)

A physical restraint used by dentists with small children to gain attention and protect the child during a temper tantrum

Hand-Over-Mouth Exercise

There are occasions when the operator can use the **hand-over-mouth exercise**

(**HOME**) to get the child's attention in order to gain communication and ensure the child's safety during treatment. It is important to consult with the parent and gain permission before using this method.

Restraints

Sometimes it is also necessary to use physical restraints to prevent the child from moving the head, hands, feet, and body and to protect them from injury (See Table 24.2). The Pedi-Wrap, a nylon mesh cover wrapped and fastened around the child's body or a sheet will immobilize the arms and legs. A mouth prop is often used to control jaw movement and help the child keep his or her mouth open.

WELCOMING CHILDREN TO THE DENTAL OFFICE

During the initial telephone contact with the dental office, the business assistant will often need to determine if the child should be seen immediately for an emergency visit or for a scheduled routine visit. Before scheduling either appointment, the following information should be obtained and recorded:

1 Patient's name (nickname)
2 Parent's or guardian's name
3 Address
4 Telephone number (both business and home)
5 Patient's age
6 Referring person (if another dentist, ask why the child is being referred in case of a behavior problem)
7 Grade in school and progression (to indicate if dealing with retarded child)

When scheduling, provide the parent with two choices of time that suits the office, one in the morning and one in the afternoon unless the dentist treats children at a certain time of day. In this case give the appropriate suggested times. At this time explain any first visit procedure and fee requirement.

A previsit letter is often sent to parents confirming the appointment and explaining office philosophies. The advantages of the previsit letter is to establish the day and time of the appointment and to educate parents in communities where children's dentistry is not readily known or accepted. The letter will prepare the parent and child for the appointment. This letter can let them know about office policies on parents being permitted in the treatment area or management of behavior problems. These letters often include the following information:

1 Confirmation of date and time of appointment
2 Appreciation for the parent's confidence in selecting your office to schedule an appointment for the child
3 What will be accomplished the first visit and in what manner

4 Any specific information related to the appointment

5 Education material to prepare the child for the dental visit
Letters can also be sent to the child at his or her level of understanding. The business assistant should call the day before to prevent broken appointments and lost operating time.

First Appointment

Children should be taught not to fear a dental office. Orienting the child to the dental office is part of communication and begins by observing appointment times. Scheduling children early to assure they are rested and not missing a nap time is recommended. It is also important not to rush a child and to provide some time for the child to become accustomed to the office. Greeting children at their level in a friendly manner and using play therapy (providing a short play time) will help the child minimize his or her fear.

The business assistant is often the first person to greet the child in the dental office but he or she is usually an unfamiliar face. Wearing a white gown may represent a hospital or medical clinic and may be suggestive of a painful experience in the past. Therefore, the appearance and behavior of staff can affect the child's perception of what is going to occur. Although aseptic techniques require clinical attire for personnel, the clothing worn by dental assistants in pediatric practices can be colorful and appealing to children.

Extreme quietness in the waiting room may be as strange and disturbing as over enthusiasm, which may arouse suspicion and fear. As the child becomes more familiar with the dental office and the operatory, this fear of the unfamiliar should disappear. As with adults, it is important that the child is told what the various infection control barriers are and why they are used in the operatory. Children usually understand the concept of washing their hands and catching a cold. Keep in mind, aseptic techniques are as important when working with children as with adults. Children have the same diseases as adults and there is the same need to control infection transmission (see Chapter 18).

VERBAL COMMUNICATION WITH CHILDREN

The child can be introduced to (not entertained by) the dental chair (up, down, back), handpieces, syringes, light, and so on. The child should be guided and "told" (not "asked") because of the following reasons:

1 Children usually find comfort in knowing specifically what to do.

2 If "asked" the child may say "NO!" Then what do you do?

3 Because this may be a new experience, it is unfair for the child not to know what is expected.

4 Children need constant and repeated instruction.

5 Tell the child where to sit. Don't waste time and encourage children to seat themselves quickly.

6 Avoid sudden movements.

7 When approaching the child with napkins, clips, and so on, explain positively what is happening.

8 Do not show instruments to apprehensive children.

9 If asked about procedures, explain that the dentist will explain everything that is going on.

10 Remain silent when the dentist is present to explain the treatment.

11 Remain with the child if the dentist leaves the area.

12 Do not let the child touch the equipment without the dentist's permission.

Communicate at the child's level of comprehension, in terms that the child understands. For instance, most young children can relate to plastic and metal toys and can understand having "Mr. Decay" taken out and a nice white plastic filling or metal filling placed in their teeth. Putting a "rain coat" over the tooth is better than "placing a rubber dam"; a mosquito itch or a pinch is less sensitive than a "shot."(Box 24.2).

INFORMED CONSENT

It has been more important in recent years to make sure parents understand what treatment is being prescribed and what alternatives they have to the treatment plan. Making sure that informed consent is obtained before providing dental treatment as well as handling any behavior problem for a child is the dentist's responsibility and can be critical if there is a misunderstanding in how a situation was managed (see Chapter 3).

RECOGNIZING CHILD ABUSE

Since 1966, it has been the responsibility of professionals to report any suspicions of child abuse that may be recognized. This includes trauma such as burns, bruises, cuts,

Box 24.3

Pediatric Terminology Substitution

Sustitute terminology for explaining procedures to children

Dental Terminology	Word Substitute
Air	Mr. Wind
Impression material	Mashed potatoes
Anesthetic	Sleepy water
Bur	Brush
Caries	Brown spot, Mr. Tooth Decay
Explorer	Tooth counter
Evacuator	Vacuum cleaner
Matrix	Fence
Prophylaxis paste	Special toothpaste
Rubber dam	Raincoat
Rubber dam clamp	Ring
Rubber dam frame	Raincoat hanger
X-ray equipment	Camera
Radiograph	Picture of tooth

Planning ahead for children

DOs

1. Make sure everything is ready before the child is seated in the operatory.
2. Be relaxed with children.
3. Tell the child your name.
4. Call the child by his or her name or nickname.
5. Pay attention to the child.
6. Let small children hold your hand.
7. Have children go to the bathroom before treatment is started.
8. Have children climb into the chair themselves.
9. Explain the equipment and its use.
10. Discuss the child's favorite game or toy.
11. Start on time.
12. Be truthful with children.
13. Do not get angry or sound angry with children.
14. Speak with the child according to age level.
15. Make the first visit special.
16. Talk with parents about the child's history.
17. Be kind and understanding but firm and positive.
18. Keep instruments out of sight.
19. Always try to educate children and parents.
20. Give the child lots of attention.
21. Show, tell, and do.
22. Communicate with the child.
23. Be consistent.
24. Compliment the child on dress, shoes, and so on.

DON'Ts

1. Don't use a loud voice around children.
2. Don't use baby talk.
3. Don't pick up children or grab them.
4. Don't be overenthusiastic or overbearing.
5. Don't carry the child without the parent's permission.
6. Don't ignore the child.
7. Don't adjust the chair without notice.
8. Don't provide too much sympathy to the child.
9. Don't criticize children.
10. Don't leave the child alone.
11. Don't discuss treatment in front of the child.
12. Don't provide children with the opportunity to be disagreeable.
13. Don't let children view sharp or harmful instruments.
14. Don't get mad.

poor nutrition, or observing lack of medical and dental care. The professional is protected if an innocent parent or guardian seeks legal litigation because of the report. However, the law addresses the legal implications for dentists who knowingly and willfully fail to report suspected child abuse. If the dental assistant suspects child abuse, do not confront the parent. It is important to make the dentist aware of the observation for further action. Dental offices should have an office policy on steps to be taken if child abuse is suspected. The dental assistant does have a responsibility to follow through with the dentist to make sure any suspicions are recorded, discussed, and reported if concerns appear to be substantiated. The local Center on Child Abuse and Neglect can provide information if needed (see Chapter 4).

COMMON TRAUMA PROBLEMS OF CHILDREN

Trauma or interference during the stage of tooth development may result in missing teeth or extra teeth. Figure 24.1 identifies deformities. Box 24.4 will familiarize you with a number of the terms used to describe tooth development, and Figure 24.2 shows the stages of tooth development.

HEAD AND FACE DEVELOPMENT

The growth and development of the head and face is complex. Until the fourth week (the presomite stage of development) the embryo has no significant appearing face. However, raised masses and processes begin to merge and form into five enlargements, the initial facial features. These processes are the frontal-nasal process, (two) maxillary processes, and (two) mandibular arches.

During the next 4 weeks the maxillary processes move toward the midline and attach to the lateral nasal fold of the frontonasal process. At this same time, the mandibular processes fuse at the midline and the mandible begins to develop. As osseous development takes place and the muscles of mastication and trigeminal nerves form, approximately 60 days after gestation, the fetal period is reached.

The cranial portion of the embryo, one half the total body, develops rapidly when compared with the caudal portion of the embryo. By the fifth month the head is reduced to about one third the total body length. During this fetal period, the eyeballs, brain, and nasoseptal structures expand and there is an osseous buildup of the facial bones.

During the embryonic stage the mandible is larger than the maxilla but during the fetal stage the maxilla is more developed than the mandible. During this 7 months of fetal life there is a fast and expansive growth of the cranium. At birth, the mandible appears to be retrognathic to the maxilla. Newborns have small mouths and almost no chins. Although

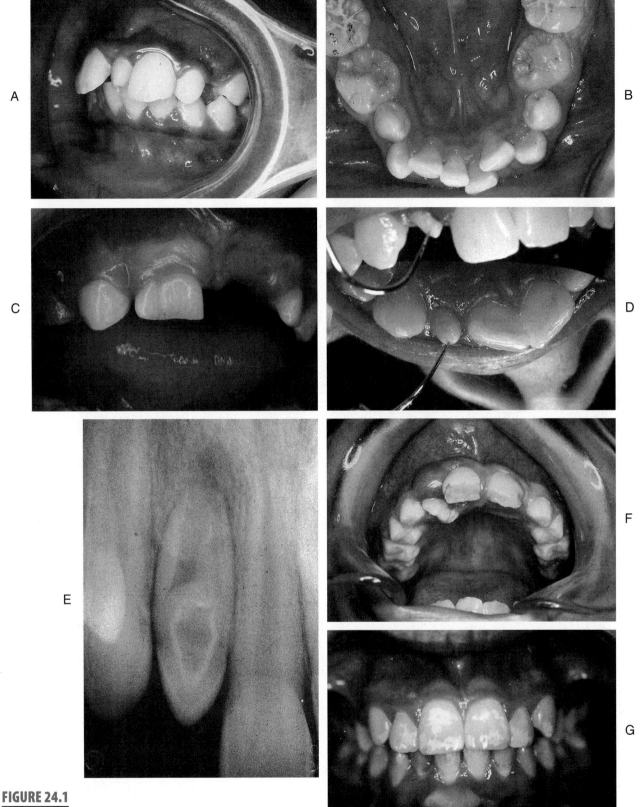

FIGURE 24.1

Interference during the stages of tooth development can cause deformities in the dentition. **A**, Supernumerary teeth can develop, for instance, if the interference takes place during the initiation stage of tooth development. Deformities during proliferation stage could include (**B**) extra cusps on teeth (molars) or (**C**) fusion of the teeth (central and lateral incisors). Disturbances during morphodifferentiation may cause the following deformities: **D**, Peg-shaped teeth (lateral incisor). **E**, Dent-in-dente (lateral incisor). Interference during apposition may cause: **F**, Hypoplasia or **G**, Hypocalcification.

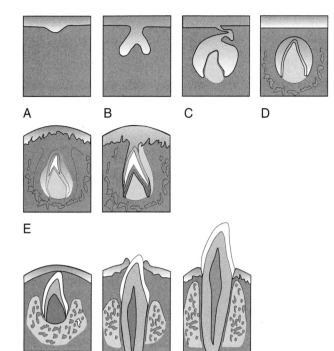

FIGURE 24.2

Stages of tooth development. **A**, Initiation "bud stage." **B**, Proliferation "cap stage." **C**, Histodifferentiation "bell stage." **D**, Morphodifferentiation. **E**, Apposition and calcification. **F**, Eruption.

their faces appear small, their eyes, forehead, and cranium are large in comparison (Figure 24.3).

ORAL HABITS OF CHILDREN

During the first year, infants (neonates) exhibit an oral and clinging behavior because the oral cavity is one of the primary sensory organs. Early reflexes and basic needs center around sucking, grasping, and rooting. This allows the infant to satisfy the nutritional needs. As the infant learns and matures, this biologic need becomes a pleasurable experience and the thumb is often substituted for the nipple if the nipple is not available. When the infant is hungry or frustrated, thumb sucking often becomes an alternative source of security and satisfaction.

Digital Sucking

Digital (or finger and thumb) sucking is one of the most common oral habits of children. It can be a meaningful habit from a psychologic cause or an **empty habit** with no detectable cause, which can be discontinued without psychologic trauma. Children generally stop oral habits around 3 to 4 years of age if they are secure and have emotional support. They usually receive gratification and a feeling of well-being (emotional support) from the various activities they are involved in and from their personal environment. If the dentist diagnoses a meaningful habit, the parent, along with the family physician and psychiatrist, should be consulted.

Empty habit

A habit that has no detectable cause and can be discontinued without psychologic trauma

Effects of Digital Sucking

The ability for self-correction of the effects of digit sucking will depend on the type and severity of the sucking. The long-term clinical effects of thumb sucking are anterior open bite and overjet, labial flare of the maxillary anterior teeth, and lingual inclination of the mandibular anterior teeth (Figure 24.4, *A*).

Correction with Digital Sucking Appliances

The dentist may choose a fixed type appliance or a removable type of correction appliance. The fixed type of appliance, most common for digital sucking, uses orthodontic bands around the maxillary first permanent molars for retention with an upper lingual arch and a palatal U-shaped crib to prevent the child from placing his thumb against the hard palate (Figure 24.4, *B*). The removable type of appliance uses ball clasps, circumferential clasps, or modified arrowhead clasps for retention. Blunt wire loop reminders are embedded in the acrylic to remind the child whenever the thumb is placed in the mouth.

Tongue Thrust and Swallowing Habits

Abnormal tongue position, tongue thrust, and deviation (change) from the normal movement of the tongue during

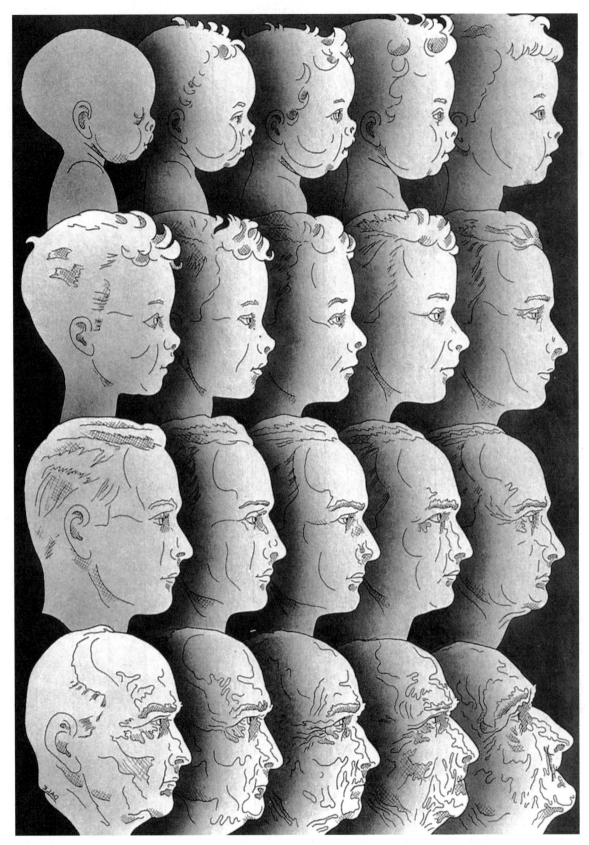

FIGURE 24.3

Growth and development of the human face from birth to old age. Top row, birth to 4 years. Note that a newborn will appear to have a small chin and the baby's mandible is smaller than the maxilla. Second row, 6 to 20 years; third row 25 to 50 years; bottom row, 60 to 80 years. (From Ten Cate, AR: *Oral histology: development, structure, and function*, ed 5, St Louis, 1998, Mosby)

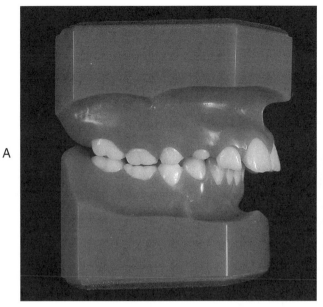
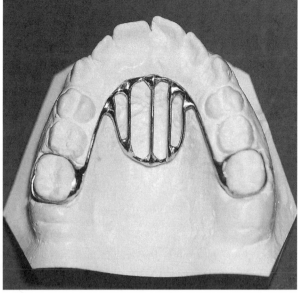

FIGURE 24.4

A, Thumb sucking can cause anterior overbite and overjet. Model indicating malocclusion caused by digital sucking. **B,** A *fixed palatial crib* appliance can be used to discourage digital sucking.

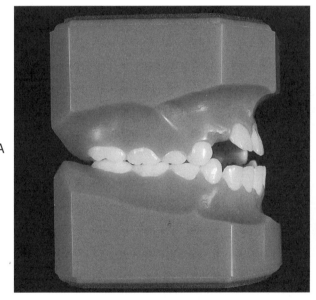
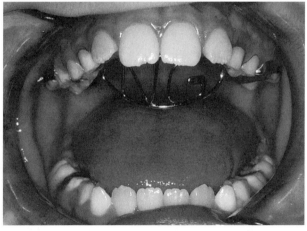

FIGURE 24.5

A, Model indicating malocclusion caused by a tongue thrust habit. **B,** Fixed tongue thrust appliance in oral cavity.

swallowing are associated with anterior open bite, protrusion of the maxillary incisors, and lisping. Normally the tongue is placed to the anterior in the mouth at rest and during swallowing.

Effects of Tongue Thrust

It is believed that most of the time tongue thrusting does not cause malocclusion but skeletal relationships as well as other factors do. Therefore, myofunctional therapy may not only be directed at the tongue and swallowing but extend to altering the resting posture of the tongue. Younger children may only need to be observed while completing swallowing maturation while older children who have not shown spontaneous progress toward adult swallowing may need therapy. This therapy may be carried out by promoting changes in resting tongue position and orthodontic treatment (Figure 24.5, *A*).

Correction and Use of Appliances

It has been observed that open bites originate in the primary dentition and usually close by the age of 10 years in 90 percent of children. Therefore, it may be advised to wait until the child is 10 years of age before actively attempting to correct the anterior open bite. Functional therapy may be attempted by having the patient practice swallowing correctly 20 times before each meal in front of a mirror. The child can sip water with the teeth in occlusion and the tip of the tongue against the incisive papilla while swallowing. This can be followed by relaxation of the muscles and repeated until swallowing progresses smoothly. A mint or lemon drop can be held between the tip of the tongue and roof the mouth until it melts. As saliva flows it will be necessary for the child to swallow correctly.

After the child has trained the tongue and muscles to function properly during swallowing, a mandibular lingual arch with a crib or acrylic palatal retainer with a "fence" can be constructed (Figure 24.5, B). This will be a reminder to position the tongue properly during swallowing.

Fingernail Biting

Fingernail biting is another type of oral digital habit. Nail biting usually begins around 3 years of age and serves as a need for oral gratification and is also considered a response to stress.

Effects of Fingernail Biting

There is little harm done to the occlusion by nail biting. However, there is damage done to the nail beds of the fingers and often there can be some deformity to the incisal surfaces of the central and lateral incisors.

Correction or Treatment

Children are usually self-conscious and embarrassed by this habit. The social pressure of parents, teachers, and friends often causes this habit to be discontinued. Punitive treatment will not usually be effective, but it may lead to resentment. The best approach is to treat the emotional problem rather than the habit itself. Emotional support from the family and helping the child to groom the fingernails and eliminate the ragged edges may be beneficial. Often when teenagers give up this habit they may begin chewing gum and pencils, picking their nose and nails, chewing the inside of the lips, and cheeks, or using tobacco to substitute.

Lip Habit

Two basic types of lip habits are wetting the lips with the tongue and pulling the lips into the mouth between the teeth. Lip sucking is more commonly associated with the lower lip (Figure 24.6). This can cause reddened, irritated, and chapped areas below the vermilion border of the lips.

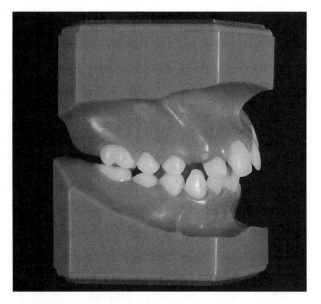

FIGURE 24.6
Model indicating malocclusion caused by lip biting.

Effects of Lip Habits

The wedging of the lip between the upper and lower incisors will cause a muscular imbalance that, if practiced with sufficient intensity and frequency, can cause the maxillary incisors to move labially with interdental spacing and the lower incisors to collapse lingually with crowding. If a Class II Division I malocclusion exists, the overjet may be increased. The habit may also cause an anterior dental open bite.

Correction or Treatment

Self-discipline may help break the habit. However, a lip bumper will make the practice of pulling the lower lip between the anterior teeth more difficult while reminding the child. Lip wetting, although able to cause soreness, will not usually cause malocclusion.

Mouth Breathing

Breathing through the nose is an instinct with the function of removing foreign particles (dust, pollen, bacteria), warming the air, and adding moisture to the air before being received by the lungs. When air is inspired through the mouth, it is not cleaned, warmed, or moistened as it would be through the nose. Mouth breathing is common in children between 5 and 15 years of age (Figure 24.7). This may be due to (1) an obstruction such as enlarged adenoids, hypertrophy of the turbinates, or a deviated septum, (2) an anatomical deformity such as a short upper lip, or (3) a habit causing the child to breathe through the mouth.

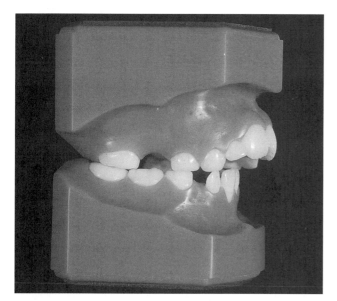

FIGURE 24.7

Model indicating malocclusion caused by mouth breathing.

Effects of Mouth Breathing

If pharyngeal tonsils (adenoids) are large enough, they may cause nasal breathing to be difficult and they may need to be removed. Although the palatine tonsils (pharyngeal lymphoid tissues) enlarge until ages 10 to 12 years of age they will rarely cause nasal airway obstruction. However, engorged and swollen nasal turbinates can obstruct nasal airflow. This swelling is often caused by allergic hypersensitivity of the nasal mucosa to airborne particles and particular climate conditions. Usually an otolaryngologist will manage the treatment. Nasal polyps and a deviated septum may also cause breathing problems, usually, later in adulthood. Some children who have not had a nasal airway obstruction may develop an open-mouth posture or breathing habit as an acquired habit to imitate family or friends.

Mouth breathers may develop an open-mouth posture. This may influence the occlusion because mouth breathers hold their tongue low and forward to keep the oral airway open and the cheeks will exert force against the buccal surfaces of the maxillary posterior teeth as a result of the imbalance of the tongue position. The lip will become flaccid (lack tone) because of not being held in a closed position. This will decrease labial support of the maxillary anterior teeth causing a flaring of the maxillary incisors and the potential of an anterior open bite. Dry mouth from mouth breathing can also cause gingivitis and an increase in dental caries.

Correction or Treatment

Several common treatments include employing an oral screen, taping the lips together at night, or using other reminders to change the mouth breathing habit.

Bruxism

It is quite common for children to grind their teeth while sleeping. **Bruxism** and clenching the teeth can be caused by both physiologic and occlusal origins. Occlusal interference can cause bruxism.

Bruxism

The grinding of teeth while sleeping

Effects of Bruxism

Bruxism causes occlusal wear of the primary teeth. An examination will often show that the enamel on the cusps has been worn away and there is exposed and thin dentin. Rarely will abrasion expose the pulp.

Correction or Treatment

Occlusal interference can be corrected by removing the interference. If bruxism is caused by a psychologic condition, oral exercises, soft occlusal guards, and biofeedback can be used as therapy.

Self-Mutilation

Occasionally children will purposely traumatize their oral structures. Self-inflicted lesions may be incorrectly diagnosed. Dentists and staff should be aware of the incidence of this condition and approach the problem as with other habits. It will be important to determine the cause. Dental factors can be corrected but emotional problems are often involved and the family must be directed to competent consulting services.

Effects of Self-Mutilation

Children may traumatize the free and attached gingival tissues with a fingernail and even destroy the supporting alveolar bone. Biting of the inner surface of the cheek, producing a large necrotic area, has been documented.

Treatment

Treatment begins with recognizing the condition. Psychologic therapy is often necessary because these conditions are often caused by unhappy and poorly adjusted children with tension and conflicts in the home. Self-mutilation is often an escape from reality.

Pacifier Use

The use of pacifiers can cause traumatic gingival recession in infants because the unconventional sucking habit can cause a segment of the plastic shield to be embraced by the infant's lower lip allowing the shield to press against the labial aspect of the incisors and the gingival tissues. The sucking movement will cause the edge of the shield to move with an abrasive action across the gingival causing injury, recession, and loss of alveolar bone. There are a number of nipples and pacifiers on the market today that are designed close to the shape of the human breast and are able to eliminate the objectionable feature of the non-physiologic ones.

PEDIATRIC DENTAL PROCEDURES

It is important that preventive services and good restorative dentistry are provided for children to preserve the teeth and surrounding tissues and prevent future orthodontic problems. Refer to Chapter 26 to review preventive dentistry, oral hygiene instruction, pit and fissure sealants, and topical fluoride use. It is extremely important to maintain good radiographic records of the patient before planning and initiating treatment.

Space Loss and Space Maintenance

The teeth are held in position in the dental arch by the controlling forces of the tongue, opposing teeth, lips, cheeks, alveolar process, and periodontal tissues. It is important that each tooth is maintained in good condition in order to (1) maintain contact and tooth support; (2) prevent loss of arch length; (3) prohibit increased overbite, crowding, or tooth malposition; and (4) avert impactions and arch asymmetries.

If the primary molars are extracted before the eruption of the first permanent molars, there will be a greater chance of drifting. Most space loss occurs in the first 6 months following a tooth extraction. Closure of the space is faster in the maxilla than the mandible. It is important to place a space maintainer immediately after the loss of a tooth to avoid the need for space regaining. By preventing space loss, the dentist can avert many children and adults from needing orthodontic treatment or from being further compromised.

Effects of Space Loss

There are a number of reasons why there could be a loss of space in the primary and permanent dentition. Permanent teeth may be congenitally missing or they may erupt in abnormal positions (ectopic eruption) or in an abnormal eruption sequence. Primary teeth may be ankylosed (tooth is anchored or attached to the bone). Space loss can also occur when contact is lost as a result of fractured teeth, interproximal caries, premature loss of primary or permanent teeth or any combination of these conditions.

If there is premature tooth loss and a lapse of time before the space is filled, teeth may drift, shift, or rotate, causing crowding and other space-related problems. These conditions can also interfere with proper occlusion, the eruption process, muscle and soft-tissue formation, and appropriate craniofacial growth. In other words, if space is lost, permanent teeth will not be able to erupt into normal positions

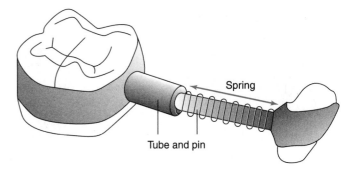

FIGURE 24.8
Sample space regainer.

causing malocclusion, potential future loss of teeth, and possible facial deformities.

The different types of space maintainers used for space control are classified as removable, fixed, or semi-fixed. Appliances may initiate action to move the teeth (active), for instance, or they may be inactive so as to cause no movement (passive) but be placed to hold the teeth in position. They may have bands or no bands and be functional or nonfunctional. There is also a need to regain space if there is not enough space to allow the eruption of the specific tooth. There may have been enough space to allow the proper eruption but the teeth may have begun to drift and close the space. The appliance used to regain this space is called a space regainer (Figure 24.8).

Correction and Treatment

Distal Shoe
The distal shoe appliance may be used on a primary posterior tooth, usually primary first molar, to guide the path of eruption of the permanent first molar when the second primary tooth has been lost prematurely (Figure 24.9, A).

Band and Loop
A band is placed around a primary tooth with a loop to the anterior abutment when a tooth has been lost (Figure 24.9, B).

Crown and Loop
A crown and loop is similar to the band and loop except a crown will be placed on a primary tooth and the loop will be welded to the crown to maintain space for the proximal erupting tooth (Figure 24.9, C).

Lingual Arch
A lingual arch can be used when a mandibular primary tooth has been lost and there has been a shift in the midline toward the direction of the loss (Figure 24.9, D).

Stainless Steel Crown
The dentist may place a stainless steel crown on a tooth that has been prepared because of dental caries in order to main-

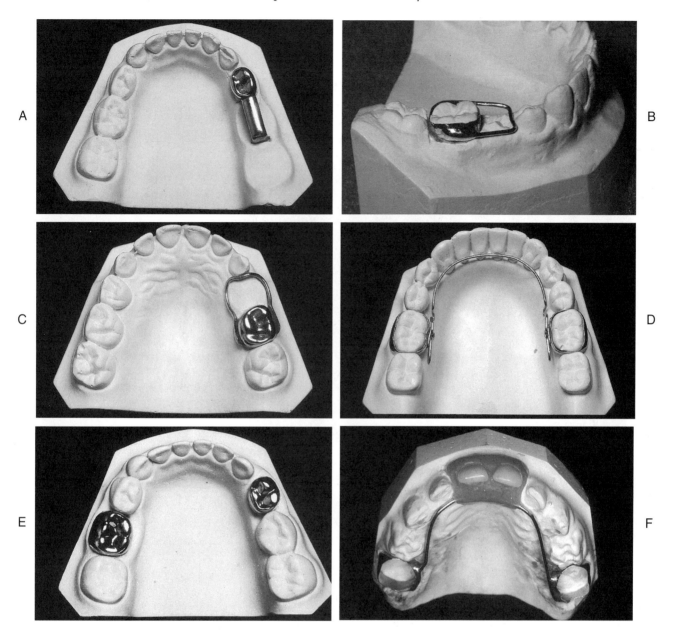

FIGURE 24.9

Space maintainers. **A,** Distal shoe. **B,** Band and loop. **C,** Crown and loop. **D,** Lingual arch.
E, Stainless steel crowns. **F,** Pedo partial.

tain the tooth and the space for the permanent teeth (Figure 24.9, *E*).

Pedo Partials

Pedo partials may be used when teeth are lost to maintain the space (Figure 24.9, *F*).

Fabricating a Band and Loop Fixed Space Maintainer

The dentist may choose to have the dental assistant fabricate space maintainers, such as the band and loop, because

of their ease of construction, service to children, and time savings if completed in the dental office. The teeth will need to be cleaned before cementing any appliance to the teeth. The materials and steps listed in Box 24.5 and Table 24.3 will be necessary to fabricate a band and loop fixed space maintainer.

Traumatic Injuries

When children or adults present in the dental office with traumatic injuries, it is important to take a complete medical

Box 24.5

Procedure

Procedure for Fabricating a Band and Loop Space Maintainer

Materials needed (Figure 24.10, *A*)

Band or crown
Band pusher
Band biter
Impression tray
Compound or alginate impression material
Band-removing pliers
Sticky wax
Stone
Stainless steel orthodontic wire (9.936)
Bird beak pliers or clasp-contouring pliers
White arch-marking pencil
Heavy wire-cutting pliers
Silver solder
Stainless steel flux
Soldering flame
Heatless stone
Burlew disks
Robinson bristle brush
Tripoli and rouge
Cement, mixing pad and spatula

1. Select band. (see Chapter 26)
2. Adapt band to abutment tooth.
3. Prepare an impression.

4. Remove band from tooth and seat into impression.
5. Secure band in impression material (Figure 24.10, *B*).
6. Pour impression in stone.
7. When set, remove model from impression.
8. Form a loop by bending stainless steel wire. (Figure 24.10, *C*)
9. Contour loop wide enough to allow underlying tooth to erupt and to contact surface of proximal tooth (Figure 24.10, *D*).
10. The loop should rest lightly (passively) on the on the gingival tissue.
11. Secure loop to stone cast so it will not move when soldering (Figure 24.10, *E*).
12. Solder loop buccally and lingually to band with flux and solder.
13. Remove appliance from model.
14. Polish with heatless wheel, white stone, rubber point, and felt wheel with polishing compound.
15. Check fit of maintainer in mouth before cementing.

---

history. When there has been an accident, the dental assistant should question the patient thoroughly about their general health as well as possible cardiac or bleeding disorders, seizures, allergies, and medications taken. The dental assistant should also find out about tetanus immunization. If the child has not had a tetanus immunization in the past 5 years, they should be referred to a physician within 24 hours for tetanus toxoid. If there is no history of tetanus immunization and a cut is deep and dirty, the child should be referred for toxoid and antitoxin.

The following questions should be asked if the parent or guardian calls about an injury to his or her child:

1 When did the accident occur?
2 How did the accident happen?
3 Where did the accident occur? (indoors, outdoors)
4 Was there soil contamination?
5 Has the child been disoriented, unconscious, vomited, or had a headache?

6 Are any teeth missing or is there a change in occlusion?

The dental assistant should know the office procedures for handling traumatic injuries; if the assistant is unsure, they should always consult the dentist before taking any action.

Fractured and Displaced Teeth

When a child presents with a fractured tooth or other injury it will be necessary for the dental assistant to aid the dentist in recording any extraoral or intraoral injuries. The lips and face will need to be examined for the presence of foreign fragments and the teeth will need to be checked for fractures, pulp exposure, and discoloration. If the pulp is exposed the dentist will dry the dentin with a cotton roll (because of sensitivity, do not use air) and place a temporary calcium hydroxide dressing to protect the pulp.

The dentist will palpate (lightly tap) the tooth to check if the tooth is sensitive to percussion. Since vitality testing is

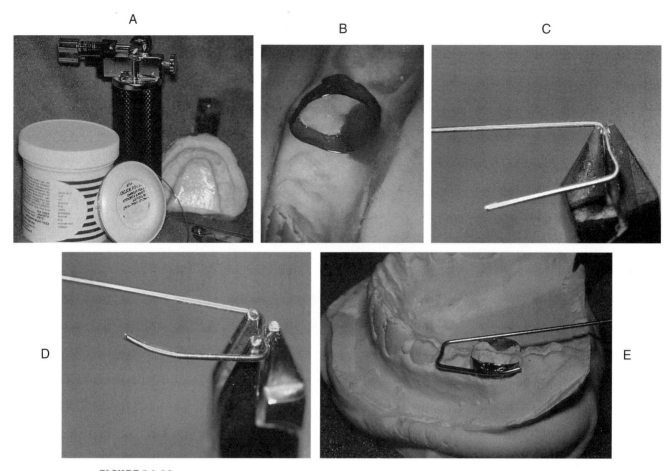

FIGURE 24.10

A, Materials needed to fabricate a band and loop fixed space maintainer. **B,** Secure band in impression material. **C,** Form a loop by bending stainless steel wire. **D,** Contour the loop wide enough to allow the underlying tooth to erupt and to contact surface of proximal tooth. **E,** The loop should rest lightly (passively) on the gingival tissue.

not as reliable in children, the dentist will often use heat and cold to evaluate tooth sensitivity. The dental assistant will record all data, and several radiographs of the area will usually be taken. Depending on the trauma, the dentist will often take extraoral and intraoral photographs.

If the tooth is displaced, the dentist will evaluate and record how far the tooth is displaced (out of place). This may be horizontally or vertically. There will be an increased chance of root resorption, loss of the tooth, or need for root canal therapy the further the tooth is displaced from it's normal position. The dentist will check for bone fractures, TMJ injury, and tooth sensitivity. Initial trauma appointments, depending on severity, will usually be followed-up within 2 to 3 weeks in an attempt to detect any pulp **necrosis** or resorption. This may be followed by a 6-week check-up to detect any further problem.

Necrosis
The morphologic change indicating cell death caused by infection

Children will also present with broken cusps or cavities that are so large that they cannot be filled. It is important to save the tooth if possible to preserve the space. This can be accomplished by performing a **pulpectomy**, if necessary, and excavating (removing) the decay, preparing the tooth, and shaping a chrome steel crown (cap) to the tooth. The chrome steel crown is a preformed crown that is trimmed and fitted over the entire tooth. This procedure will usually take only one appointment and the crown will usually last for the life of the primary tooth. This crown will prevent the teeth from drifting and restore proper function. If the tooth is in the anterior, an acrylic resin crown can also improve esthetics. Remember, although deciduous teeth are temporary, they do have a specific pediatric function that must be maintained and they preserve space for the permanent teeth, which must last for a lifetime.

Pulpectomy
The removal of the complete pulp

Table 24.3

Evaluation of Fabricating a Band and Loop Space Maintainer

Fabrication of Band and Loop Space Maintainer	4	3	2	0	X
Secure materials and equipment.					
Select band.					
Adapt band to abutment tooth.					
Prepare an impression.					
Remove band from tooth and seat into impression.					
Secure band in impression material.					
Pour impression in stone.					
Remove model from impression.					
Form a loop.					
Contour loop.					
Place loop in resting position.					
Secure loop to stone cast.					
Solder loop to band.					
Remove appliance from model.					
Polish appliance.					
Check fit of maintainer.					
Cement maintainer in place.					

The numeric criteria: 4 Excellent; 3 Good but some improvement can be made; 2 Below average, usable, needs to improve skill; 0 Unsatisfactory; X Not able to evaluate.

After the dentist has prepared the tooth, the clinical dental assistant can select, trim, contour and cement the preformed chrome steel crown. The steps taken for this technique are listed in Box 24.6 and Table 24.4.

Common Trauma Reactions to the Teeth

Apioectomy: Removal of the apical portion of the root through an opening in the bone.

Calcific metamorphosis: The buildup of dentin in the pulpal areas causing the pulp chambers to become calcified and to appear yellow.

Diastema: A narrow opening, space, or cleft in the midline area between two adjacent teeth in the same dental arch.

Direct pulp capping: Covering or capping exposed pulp as soon as possible after injury.

Fistula: The abnormal passage leading from a periapical abscess to the intraoral surface of the labial vestibule or lingual area.

Fracture Class I: Refers to only an enamel fracture, which may be repaired by smoothing rough areas or using the acid etch technique.

Fracture Class II: Refers to a fracture involving both the enamel and dentin. However, the dentin can be covered with a composite "band-aid" temporarily.

Fracture Class III: Refers to enamel and dentin fractures with pulp exposure. The exposure should be covered as soon as possible.

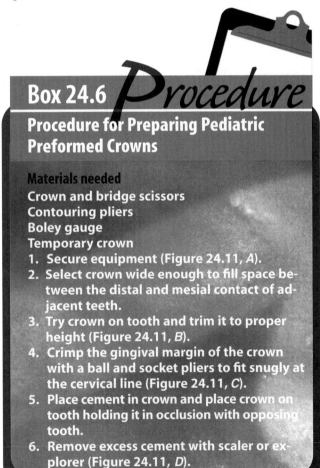

Box 24.6 *Procedure*

Procedure for Preparing Pediatric Preformed Crowns

Materials needed

Crown and bridge scissors
Contouring pliers
Boley gauge
Temporary crown

1. Secure equipment (Figure 24.11, *A*).
2. Select crown wide enough to fill space between the distal and mesial contact of adjacent teeth.
3. Try crown on tooth and trim it to proper height (Figure 24.11, *B*).
4. Crimp the gingival margin of the crown with a ball and socket pliers to fit snugly at the cervical line (Figure 24.11, *C*).
5. Place cement in crown and place crown on tooth holding it in occlusion with opposing tooth.
6. Remove excess cement with scaler or explorer (Figure 24.11, *D*).

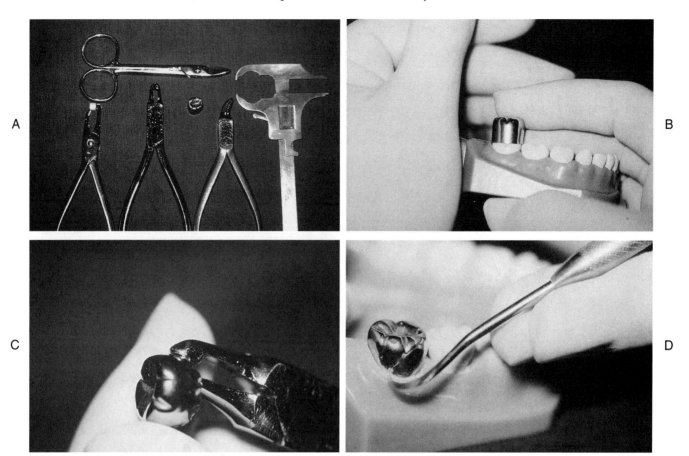

FIGURE 24.11

Procedures for preparing pediatric preformed crowns. **A,** Select crown wide enough to fill space between the distal and mesial contact of adjacent teeth. **B,** Crimp the gingival margin of the crown with a ball and socket pliers to fit snugly at the cervical line. **C,** Place cement in crown and place crown onto tooth holding it in occlusion with opposing tooth. **D,** Remove excess cement with scaler or explorer.

Table 24-A

Evaluation of Preparing Pediatric Preformed Crowns

Preformed Crowns	4	3	2	0	X
Secure materials and equipment.					
Select crown.					
Try crown on tooth.					
Trim preformed crown.					
Crimp gingival margin of crown.					
Place cement in crown.					
Place crown on tooth.					
Remove excess cement.					

The numeric criteria: 4 Excellent; 3 Good but some improvement can be made; 2 Below average, usable, needs to improve skill; 0 Unsatisfactory; X Not able to evaluate.

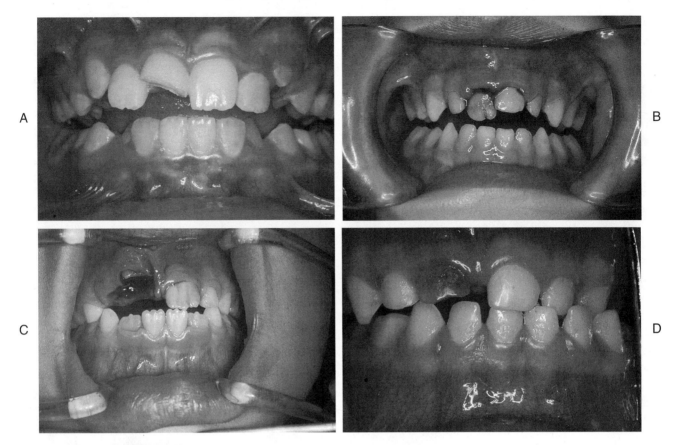

FIGURE 24.12

Traumatic injuries to primary dentition. **A**, Before treatment of a fractured maxillary central incisor. **B**, Extrusion of a central incisor. **C**, Intrusion of a central incisor. **D**, Photograph of a fractured central incisor.

Fracture Class IV: Refers to fracturing the total crown with a large exposure (Figure 24.12, *A*). The crown may be cemented in place as a temporary measure.

Fracture of root: May involve a fracture in the apical, middle, or cervical third.

Internal hemorrhage: The blood vessels rupturing causing blood to enter into the dentinal tubules and discoloring the tooth. The tooth often remains vital.

Pulpal hyperemia: A pink discoloration of the tooth caused by an abnormally large blood supply to the tooth as a result of minor trauma.

Pulpotomy

The removal of the coronal pulp because of exposure of the pulp

Pulpal necrosis: The devitalization (death) of the pulp tissue caused by severe pulpal hyperemia, hemorrhage, or crushing of the apical tissue.

Pulpectomy: The removal of the entire dental pulp.

Pulpotomy: The removal of the coronal portion of the pulp.

Resorption phenomena: Early resorption of inflamed periodontal dental ligament and necrotic pulp, which often results in root canal therapy.

Common Trauma Reactions to Supporting Structures

Avulsion: The total displacement of the tooth from the socket.

Concussion: Caused by trauma to the tooth and supporting structures in which there is no loosening or movement of the tooth but there is response to percussion (tapping).

Extrusion: Caused by partial displacement of a tooth axially out of its socket with little bony destruction (Figure 24.12, *B*).

Extrusion laterally: Caused by partial displacement of a tooth, not axially, out of its socket, which involves bone destruction.

Intrusion: Caused by the tooth being displaced into the alveolar bone and will include fracture of the socket (Figure 24.12, *C*).

Subluxation: Caused by an injury to the tooth-supporting structures causing loosening of the tooth without displacement (Figure 24.12, *D*). However, long-term effects could be tissue irritation and possible bone resorption.

Prevention of Trauma to the Teeth by Using Mouth Guards

Children who play contact sports should wear protective mouth guards. According to the American Dental Association, more than 200,000 oral injuries can be prevented annually by the use of mouth guards. The National Youth Sports Foundation also estimates that there will be more than 5 million teeth knocked out during sport activities. The benefits of mouth guards that cover all maxillary teeth, in conjunction with helmets and face masks, has been well documented. In addition to protecting the dentition, mouth guards will also reduce breathing interference. The American Society for Testing and Materials classifies mouth guards as Type I (Stock), Type II (Mouth-formed), and Type III (Custom-fabricated).

Type I Mouth Guards

The use of Type I mouth guards are discouraged because they are preformed, purchased over the counter, and do not properly fit the dentition. They are often bulky, interfere with breathing and speech, and provide the least amount of protection.

Type II Mouth Guards

Type II, thermally moldable mouth guards are recommended for children who are in the active stage of tooth development because they can be reformed. However, Type II mouth-formed mouth guards, purchased over the counter can cause tissue damage if they are heated and placed in the mouth at too hot a temperature. It is important that parents understand that adolescents wearing fixed orthodontic appliances or who have congenital abnormalities should only be provided with mouth guards while under the supervision of the dentist.

Type III Mouth Guards

Type III custom-fabricated mouth guards are preferred over the other types because they are properly adapted to the individuals mouth, have retention, best protect the dentition because of fit, and allow for proper breathing and speech. The dental assistant may construct mouth guards.

Mouth protectors or guards can be fabricated by the dental assistant and provided to growing teenagers and adults who play contact sports. This service can be a practice builder. A simple method of fabricating a mouth guard is by using a vacuum adapter (Box 24.7 and Table 24.5).

Note on construction of mouth guards:

1 The thinner the material the quicker it softens.
2 Wear safety glasses and mask when cutting any acrylic resin material.

Pediatric Periodontal Problems

As with adults, children are faced with a number of periodontal problems. Some of these problems are directly related to eruption factors while others are related to poor oral hygiene education and techniques. Problems associated with the eruption of primary teeth will usually be eliminated on appearance of the teeth and inflammatory disease can be reduced and eliminated by proper oral hygiene.

Eruption Factors

Eruption hematoma: Caused by an accumulation of fluid in the follicular sac around the erupting tooth, which will be eliminated on eruption.

Eruption periocoronitis: Inflammation caused by a thin layer of tissue (operculum), which often covers the occlusal surface of erupting teeth.

Eruption gingivitis: Caused by inflammation from debris during eruption of a tooth.

Frenum Factors

A **frenectomy** is the surgical removal of the frenum (the median fold of mucous membrane connecting the inside of each lip to the corresponding gingivae tissue) (Figure 24.14).

Frenectomy

The surgical removal of the frenum (median fold of mucous membrane connecting the inside of each lip to the gingivae tissue)

Gingival Factors

Gingivitis: Caused by inflammation of the gingiva and is common in 90% of all children as a result of poor oral hygiene.

Primary herpes: Caused by the herpes simplex virus (small white vesicles appear, rupture, and leave) in which there may be fever, discomfort, and gingival inflammation, which may last 10 to 14 days.

Recurrent aphthous ulcers: May be caused by stress and appear as a sensitive (burning) pit surrounded by inflammation. These ulcers will heal within 2 weeks.

Localized juvenile periodontosis: Infection involving more than one "permanent" tooth in adolescents, may be some localized bone loss and the presence of plaque.

Dilantin gingival hyperplasia: The abnormal increase in gingival cell growth associated with medication to treat seizures (Dilantin therapy), more often in young patients (Figure 24.14, *C*).

Pediatric Oral Surgery

Special care and planning must be undertaken for any minor intraoral surgery for children to avoid possible injury to the underlying permanent dentition (Box 24-8). Removal of

Box 24.7

Procedure

Procedures for Constructing a Mouth Guard

Materials needed
Prophy materials
Alginate impression
Dental stone model
Vacuum
Mouth guard resin
Lubricant
Dental knife

Preliminary procedures
1. Clean the teeth.
2. Secure an alginate impression of the maxillary arch.
3. Wash under cool water and disinfect.
4. Remove excess liquids gently with air.
5. Pour impression immediately with thick mix of dental stone.
6. After setting, separate and trim removing bubbles and filling voids.
7. Relieve specific areas if orthodontic appliances are worn.

Construction of mouth guard
1. Prepare the vacuum adapter (Figure 24.13, *A*).
2. Select resin material for fabricating the mouth guard. Vacuum materials are used to construct mouth guards, base plates, and custom trays.
3. Lubricate the vacuum adapter press (Figure 24.13, *B*)
4. Place acrylic resin material into press and secure.
5. Wet the dental model and place plaster model on adapter table and turn heating element on.
6. Check acrylic resin with instrument or Q-tip to test slumping or softening state of material.
7. When material is softened sufficiently, bring press and material over model and turn adapter off.
8. Cool acrylic resin materials under cold running water.
9. Check to see if adapted correctly and remove excess acrylic resin material and smooth any rough edges (Figure 24.13, *C*).
10. The palatal area may be cut out with utility knife.
11. Trim the peripheral areas short of the mucobuccal fold and relieve the frenum areas carefully.
12. Rough edges can be smoothed with a polishing stone or rubber wheel and flamed lightly with an alcohol torch.
13. After try-in adjust if necessary.

---

primary roots, for instance, may interfere with the developing permanent tooth bud. The removal of primary teeth may depend on the presence of acute infection. If there is acute systemic infection, blood disease, uncontrolled diabetes mellitus, irradiated bone, or acute oral infection, tooth removal may be contraindicated (undesirable, not recommended).

Dental assistants in pediatric practices must know how to take children's blood pressure. A pediatric blood pressure cuff will need to be used if a child is small or less than 10 to 12 years of age. This will be necessary in order to obtain a true reading. Normal pediatric values and vital signs should be maintained with the equipment (Tables 24.6 through 24.8).

Cosmetic Dentistry for Children

Children and adolescents are as cognizant (aware) of their physical appearance as adults are of theirs in today's society. Often, "looking good" is directly related to personal self-image. Physical appearance is idealized by a bright shining smile with attractive well shaped, "white" teeth.

Several techniques are available to improve appearance. Good home oral health care, dietary management, fluoride administration, treatment of diseases of the dentition, and maintaining dental checkups can help to maintain and improve one's appearance. It is important for children to have a preventive assessment completed to determine fluoride us-

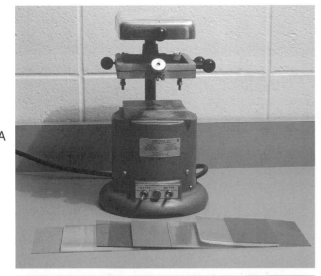

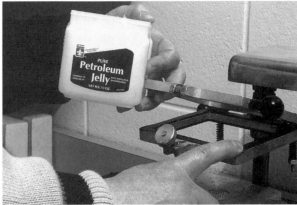

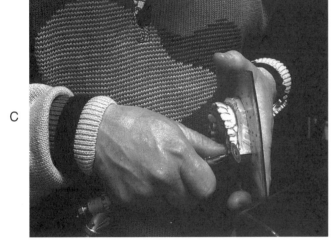

FIGURE 24.13

Procedures for constructing a custom fabricated mouth guard using vacuum adaptation. **A**, Prepare the vacuum adapter. **B**, Lubricate vacuum adapter press. **C**, Check to see if adapted correctly and remove excess acrylic resin materials and smooth any rough edges.

age, proper home tooth cleaning care, diet, condition of the dentition, PHP factors, and recommendation for improvement or correction (Figure 24.15).

There may also be occasions when alternative methods must be used to improve appearance because of discolored anterior teeth. It is important that the dentist and patient discuss the choice of material and technique to be used because of the wide variety. The methods used to improve anterior esthetics include bleaching vital and nonvital teeth, veneering teeth with preformed veneers, using acid etch composites, or enamel microabrasion.

Causes of Discoloration of Vital Teeth

Discoloration of vital teeth can be caused by trauma, enamel dysmineralization, enamel hypoplasia caused by fluorosis, and administration of tetracycline antibiotics during childhood. The teeth are especially vulnerable during tooth formation. This is when staining of the enamel will most likely occur (Table 24.9).

Enamel dysmineralization causes small white or yellow flecks on the enamel, tetracycline staining varies from a light yellow-brown to a dark bluish-gray color within (intrinsic) the enamel, and hypoplasia causes white or yellow-brown spots on the enamel. Discoloration of endodontically treated teeth can occur when teeth are nonvital.

Bleaching Vital and Nonvital Teeth

There are two types of vital bleaching techniques used to increase the whiteness of teeth: power bleaching and night guard vital bleaching. It has been noted that bleaching is more effective with the lighter stains. It is recommended that the dental assistant take a pretreatment photograph to document the treatment and to use for patient education (Box 24.9 and Table 24.10).

Power Bleaching Technique

When using the power bleaching technique, a heavy rubber dam is applied for isolation to avoid potential chemical burn

Table 24-5

Evaluation of Constructing a Mouth Guard

Constructing a Mouth Guard	4	3	2	0	X
Secure materials and equipment.					
Preliminary procedures					
Clean teeth.					
Secure alginate impression.					
Rinse impression.					
Pour impression.					
Separate and trim model.					
Remove bubbles and fill model voids.					
Relieve model.					
Construction of mouth guard					
Prepare vacuum adapter.					
Select resin material.					
Lubricate vacuum adapter press.					
Place resin into press and secure.					
Wet dental model.					
Place model onto adapter table.					
Turn heating element on.					
Test slumping.					
Secure press and material over model.					
Turn adapter off.					
Cool resin materials.					
Remove excess resin and smooth rough edges.					
Trim palatal, peripheral, and frenum areas.					
Smooth rough edges.					
Try in and adjust if necessary.					

The numeric criteria: 4 Excellent; 3 Good but some improvement can be made; 2 Below average, usable, needs to improve skill; 0 Unsatisfactory; X Not able to evaluate.

of the soft tissue while the hydrogen peroxide solution is placed on the darkened teeth. Then heat is applied to the area with an electric light or probe with a cotton pellet attached. The heat helps to oxidize the H_2O_2 and increase the effects of bleaching. This is repeated three or more times with periodic retreatment to maintain the whiteness.

Night Guard Vital Bleaching Technique

The night guard vital bleaching technique uses a custom mouth guard with a milder form of hydrogen peroxide. This is a patient home method that is usually placed over the teeth at night when sleeping. This method causes less sensitivity to thermal change than power bleaching, although there is some concern as to the effects of peroxide solution to the soft intraoral tissue when used for long periods of time. There are numerous commercial brands

available over the counter today. Caution should be taken when using these bleaches because of the lack of long-term studies.

Enamel Microabrasion

Superficial enamel coloration defects can be caused by enamel dysmineralization during tooth development. This discoloration appears as a white chalky decalcification lesion on the surface of the enamel. Decalcification on the anterior teeth may also appear as an orange brown. The dentist, using a low-speed, high-torque rotary handpiece, can remove this discoloration and a compound of hydrochloric acid and a fine grit abrasive. By polishing with the compound a small layer of enamel is abraded away leaving the smooth, glasslike finish. The enamel will remineralize to form a new outer layer of enamel.

Text continued p. 630

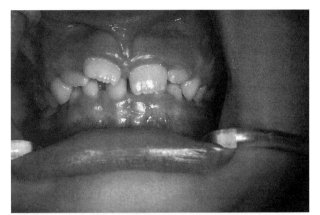

A

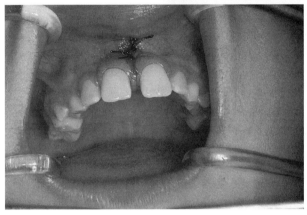

B

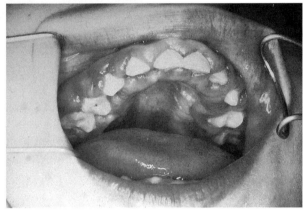

C

FIGURE 24.14

Pediatric periodontal problems. **A**, Before frenectomy. **B**, After frenectomy. **C**, Dilantin gingival hyperplasia.

Box 24.8

Pediatric Surgical Conditions

Ankylosed teeth: Care must be taken to remove a primary tooth that has been ankylosed (joined to the alveolar bone) because of the potential of injury to the developing dentition.

Over-retained primary tooth: Caused by root resorption not taking place in the primary tooth, causing it not to loosen and exfoliate. Because the erupting permanent tooth may become displaced, the retained primary tooth will need to be removed.

Nonrestorable carious primary tooth: Should be removed and space maintenance undertaken

Natal or neonatal primary tooth: The natal tooth (erupted before birth) and the neonatal tooth (erupted after birth) may be supernumerary teeth and are usually extracted if they are mobile, irritating to tissue or tongue, or interfere with breastfeeding.

Impacted tooth: May be a supernumerary tooth, a malformed tooth, or an unerupted ectopically placed tooth in which treatment may be complicated and take the skilled decision of a well-trained dentist or specialist.

Sectioning primary molar teeth: Sectioning and removing a tooth, one half at a time, may be necessary if the primary molar roots are adjacent to the developing tooth bud.

Supernumerary teeth: Which supernumerary (extra) tooth to remove must be carefully considered.

Postoperative considerations

There should be minimum discomfort for well children who have primary teeth removed. Usually a mild analgesic such as aspirin or Tylenol can be used if necessary. A clean gauze pack is usually placed for 10 minutes and a soft diet is recommended the first day so as not to disturb the blood clot. Warm saline mouth rinse can be used four to five times the following day. The child should be watched so he or she does not chew on his or her lip, tongue, or cheek.

Table 24.6

Growth and Development: Normal Values

Height and weight

Standard charts are available for pediatric offices to determine if a pediatric patient is within the norm for height and weight. The following table will help to identify averages.

Weight		Height	
Birth	7 lb. 6 oz.	Birth	20 inches
3 to 12 months	Age (mos) + 11	1 year	30 inches
1 to 16 years	Age (yrs) $\times$ 5 + 17	2 to 14 yrs	Age (yrs) $\times$ 2^1/$_2$ + 30
6 to 12 years	Age (yrs) $\times$ 7 + 5		

8-year-old average weight is 57 lbs ($8 \times 5 = 40 + 17 = 57$ lbs.)
6-year-old average height is 45 in ($6 \times 2^1/_2 = 15 + 30 = 45$ in.)

Table 24.7

Normal Vital Signs for Children

Use a pediatric blood pressure cuff if the child is small or less than 10 to 12 years of age to obtain a true reading. The following tables provide normal vital sign values.

Mean Blood Pressure

Age	Systolic	Diastolic	Heart Rate	Respiratory Rate
2	99-100	54-60	89-151	22-31
4	102-110	63-67	80-120	21-27
6	105-113	69-64	75-115	18-24
8	109-116	72-78	70-110	17-23
10	112-119	75-81	70-110	17-21
12	112-123	78-82	65-105	16-22
14	121-128	79-83	60-100	15-21

Table compiled from data courtesy Jane A. Soxman, DDS, PA.

Table 24.8

Pulse Rates

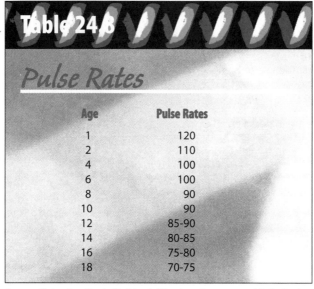

Age	Pulse Rates
1	120
2	110
4	100
6	100
8	90
10	90
12	85-90
14	80-85
16	75-80
18	70-75

Courtesy University of Louisville School of Dentistry, Department of Orthodontic, Pediatric, and Geriatric Dentistry.

Preventive assessment* _____

Fluoride inventory:
    Water fluoridation: ☐ Yes   ☐ No   ☐ Unsure
    Fluoride supplements: ☐ Yes   ☐ No
    Fluoride rinse: ☐ Yes   ☐ No
    Fluoride toothpaste: ☐ Yes   ☐ No

Tooth cleaning:
    Frequency: Times per day _____ When? _____
    Type of toothbrush: _____
    Dental floss: ☐ Yes   ☐ No
    Disclosing tablets: ☐ Yes   ☐ No
    Who is responsible for tooth cleaning? ☐ Parent   ☐ Child   ☐ Both
    Have you received instruction in tooth cleaning? ☐ Yes   ☐ No

*Information provided by _____
_____

    Diet counseling indicated: ☐ Yes   ☐ No
    Sealants indicated: ☐ Yes   ☐ No
    Water analysis indicated: ☐ Yes   ☐ No
    Caries experience: ☐ Minimal   ☐ Moderate   ☐ Severe
    Gingival condition: ☐ WNL   ☐ Red   ☐ Enlarged
                    ☐ Bleeding   ☐ Stain/calculus

Initial PHP results __ __ __ __ | __ __ __ __ | __ __ __ __ = _____

Attitude level: P = Parent; C = Child
    Interest: Low _____   Average _____   High _____
    Understanding: Low _____   Average _____   High _____

Results and recommendations

Subsequent PHP scores

Date							
Score							

Teeth recommended for sealants: _____
Tooth cleaning recommendations:
    Brush type: _____
    Floss: _____
    Frequency of cleaning: _____
    Disclosing: _____
    Supervision/responsibility: _____
Diet counseling recommendations: _____
_____
Fluoride recommendations: _____

FIGURE 24.15

Preventive assessment. (Courtesy University of Louisville School of Dentistry, Orthodontic, Pediatric, and Geriatric Dentistry)

Table 24.9

Treatment of the Discolored Dentition

Treatment	Indications	Conditions
Vital bleaching	Light yellow or gray tetracycline strains, fluorosis superficial stains, hemorrhagic discoloration	Ultraconservative, predictable, least costly; little or no regression; can not be used alone for extremely dark tetracycline stain
Nonvital bleaching	For all discolored nonvital teeth	Ultraconservative, predictable; least costly; Slight regression may occur
Direct composite labial veneers	Labial wear, hypoplasia; fluorosis	Conservative, excellent esthetic veneer; normal labial contours; excellent gingival response; easily repairable; not highly technique-sensitive; moderate cost
Direct composite labial veneers using opaquers and tints	Hypoplasia; fluorosis; dark tetracycline discoloration	Conservative, excellent esthetiacs, normal labial contours; excellent gingival response; easily repairable; cost moderate; requires extensive clinical experience regarding proper use of opaquer-tints; technique-sensitive;
Direct composite labial veneers combined with bleaching	Moderate; tetracycline stain, fluorosis	Ultraconservative, predictable; affordable cost; little or no regression; easily repairable; not highly technique sensitive; not usually applicable to extremely dark tetracycline stain
Indirect porcelain veneers	Dark tetracycline discoloration and otherwise extensive involvement	Conservative; excellent esthetics and gingival response; technique sensitive; most costly method; repair difficult
Indirect composite veneers	Dark tetracycline discoloration and otherwise extensive involvement	Conservative; very good esthetics; not highly technique sensitive; easily repairable; moderate cost; esthetic result not as good as porcelain veneers

If dysmineralization or decalcification is too deep, a tooth-colored bonded restoration can be used over the abraded enamel to cover the discoloration more thoroughly. Another technique is to use carbamide peroxide or hydrogen peroxide bleach in a custom tray at home after the enamel has been abraded to further remove the discoloration. The procedure will take 45 to 60 minutes and the initial step for treatment is similar to the above procedures. No local anesthetic is needed. The tray setup and materials needed are listed below:

Rubber dam setup
Suction tip
Saliva ejector
Mirror
Explorer
Scaler
Prophy paste
Fluoride/dappen dish

Microabrasion instruments
Slow speed handpiece with microabrasion cup

A rubber dam is placed on the teeth to be treated. The patient, dentist, and dental assistant must wear safety glasses because the chemical used may damage tissues; and personnel must wear gloves. The procedures are followed by applying microabrasion compound with the handpiece using firm pressure on the tooth for 60 seconds. Rinse with water, assess results, and reapply as needed.

Dark stains will require increased abrasion time (15 to 30 minutes). If the discoloration is too deep, causing concavity, a composite resin restoration can be placed. After the lesion has been removed, the tooth can be polished with a fine grit abrasive and fluoridated, prophylactic paste can be used. The tooth can be saturated with neutral sodium fluoride gel for 4 to 8 minutes following the polish. Refer to Chapter 17 for further information on coronal polish and topical fluoride treatment.

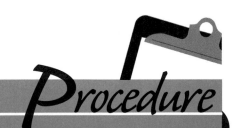

Box 24.9

Procedure for Vital Bleaching

Materials needed

Cotton tip applicator	Chloroform
Vaseline	Bleaching solution
Heavy rubber dam	Gloves
Rubber dam frame	Mask
Safety glasses	Mouth mirror
Rubber dam punch	Explorer
Waxed dental floss	Probe
Plastic instrument	X-ray
Rubber cup	Cotton pliers
and pumice	and pellets
Dappen dish	

First visit

1. Use gloves to protect hands and safety glasses for self and patient. Patient should also be draped.
2. Do not anesthetize the tooth as the patient will need to communicate if the tooth gets uncomfortable.
3. Pumice the teeth.
4. Test vitality and take radiographs of teeth to be treated.
5. Place rubber dam, avoiding any leakage when possible.
6. Ligate teeth with waxed floss.
7. Place Vaseline on gingiva by folding dam forward.
8. Wipe teeth with chloroform, rinse, and dry.
9. Etch each tooth for 1 minute.
10. Wash for 20 seconds.
11. Dry lightly for 20 seconds.
12. Bleach tooth with selected bleaching solution, rinse well and remove the rubber dam (Figure 24.16).
13. Tell the patient the treated teeth may be sensitive to hot and cold for 24 to 48 hours. The discoloration will return in a few days but will disappear as treatment is continued. If there is any chemical burn it will heal and be virtually painless.

Second visit

1. Repeat same procedures.
2. The patient should know some sensitivity may exist as before but the whiteness will remain longer.

Third visit and fourth visit (if necessary)

1. Same as first visit.
2. After final visit, rinse with rubber dam in place and complete the optional steps if desired:
   a. Acid etch the teeth.
   b. Place plastic matrix strips between the teeth.
   c. Paint a thin coat of clear sealant on labial of bleached teeth being careful not to leave raised areas of sealant adjacent to the matrix strips.
   d. Let the patient know the teeth will be sensitive to hot and cold for a few days and the color should be more stable.

Table 24-10

Evaluation of Vital Bleaching

Vital Bleaching	4	3	2	0	X
First visit					
Secure materials and equipment.					
Seat and drape patient.					
Present safety glasses to patient.					
Wear gloves, mask, and eye wear.					
Polish teeth (See Chapter 17).					
Test tooth vitality.					
Take radiographs.					
Place rubber dam.					
Ligate teeth.					
Place Vaseline on gingival.					
Wipe teeth, rinse, and dry.					
Etch appropriate teeth (60 seconds).					
Rinse (20 seconds).					
Dry (20 seconds).					
Bleach appropriate teeth.					
Remove rubber dam.					
Instruct patient.					
Final or optional steps					
Acid etch the teeth.					
Place matrix strips between teeth.					
Paint clear sealant on bleached teeth.					
Instruct patient.					

The numeric criteria: 4 Excellent; 3 Good but some improvement can be made; 2 Below average, usable, needs to improve skill; 0 Unsatisfactory; X Not able to evaluate.

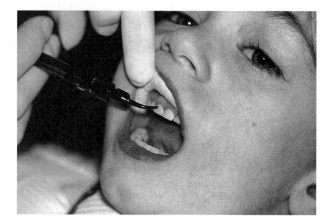

FIGURE 24-16

Bleach tooth and rinse well.

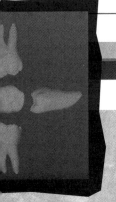

Points for Review

- Stages of child development
- Managing children's fear of the unknown
- Behavior modification of children
- Welcoming children to the dental office
- Verbal communications with children
- Informed consent
- Recognizing child abuse
- Physiologic process of face and tooth development
- Oral habits of children and corrective appliances
- Pediatric dental procedures

Self-Study Questions

1. Children should be first seen in the dental office at what age?
   a. Birth to 2 years of age
   b. 2 to 3 years of age
   c. 3 to 5 years of age
   d. When they are not frightened

2. What type of behavior modification is providing a little experience at a time?
   a. Extinction
   b. Restraint
   c. HOME
   d. Desensitization

3. What is the "cap stage" in which cells increase in number rapidly called?
   a. Initiation
   b. Proliferation
   c. Differentiation
   d. Calcification

4. Hypoplasia can be caused by the ingestion of excess fluoride during which stage of tooth development?
   a. Initiation
   b. Proliferation
   c. Apposition
   d. Eruption

5. What are habits that have a psychologic cause called?
   a. Meaningful habit
   b. Empty habit
   c. Noncompulsive
   d. Infantile habit

6. The ability for a child to "self-correct" a habit will depend on which of the following?
   a. Length of time the habit continues
   b. Emotional support
   c. Type of appliance used
   d. A and b

7. What type of habit can occlusal interference cause?
   a. Tongue thrust
   b. Lip habit
   c. Bruxism
   d. Mouth breathing

8. What is the devitalization or death of the pulp tissue called?
   a. Pulpal necrosis
   b. Pulpal hyperemia
   c. Pulpotomy
   d. Apioectomy

9. What is the removal of the coronal pulp called?
   a. Pulpal necrosis
   b. Pulpal hypermia
   c. Pulpotomy
   d. Pulpectomy

10. What are teeth called that are joined to the bone?
    a. Supernumerary
    b. Ankylosed
    c. Over-retained
    d. Calcified

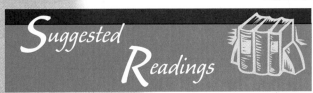

Suggested Readings

Freeman M: *Standard operating procedures for pediatric dentists*, Santa Maria, Calif, 1995, Dental Communication Unlimited.

Furnish GM, O'Toole TJ, Parkins FM: *Pediatric dentistry I*, 1996, Sophomore, University of Louisville School of Dentistry, Orthodontic, Pediatric and Geriatric Dentistry.

McDonald RE, Avery DR: *Dentistry for the child and adolescent*, ed 7, St Louis, 2000, Mosby.

Pinkham JR et al: *Pediatric dentistry: infancy through adolescence*, ed 3, Philadelphia, 1999, WB Saunders.

Proffit WR: *Contemporary orthodontics*, ed 3, St Louis, 2000, Mosby.

Soxman JA: Local anesthesia for pediatric patients, *Dentistry Today* 16 (1): 40, 1997.

Snawder KD: *Handbook of clinical pedodontics*, St Louis, 1980, Mosby.

University of Louisville, School of Dentistry, Department of Orthodontic, Pediatric and Geriatric Dentistry, *Pediatric dentistry II*, 1995.

Chapter *25*

Periodontics

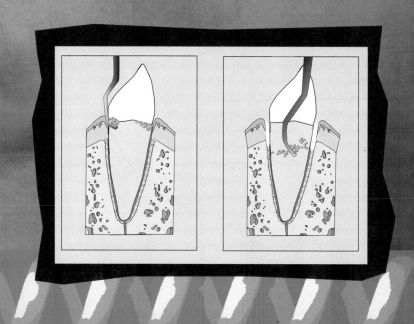

Learning Objectives

On completion of Chapter 25, the student should be able to do the following:

- Define key terms.
- Discuss the anatomy and physiology of the normal periodontium.
- Discuss the clinical characteristics of healthy and inflamed gingival tissues.
- Discuss the etiology of periodontal disease.
- List indications and contraindications for periodontal treatment.
- Define the procedures used to diagnose and treat periodontal problems.
- List the functions of instruments used in periodontal therapy.
- List the sequencing of periodontal treatment procedures.
- Discuss the principles of assisting during periodontal surgery.
- Describe how to mix, place, and remove periodontal dressing material.
- State the postoperative instructions given to a patient after periodontal scaling, Actisite placement, and periodontal surgery.
- Discuss the procedures used in periodontal surgery

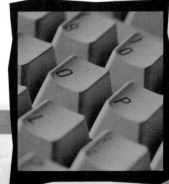

Key Terms

Acute

Attachment
    Apparatus

Etiology

Gingivectomy

Gingivitis

Inflammation

Mobility

Pericoronitis

Periodontal Diagnosis

Periodontal Disease

Periodontal Ligament

Periodontics

Periodontitis

Periodontium

Prognosis

Regeneration

Resorption

Root Planing

Scaling

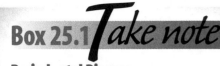

Box 25.1

Take note

Periodontal Disease

The predominant cause of inflammatory periodontal disease is bacterial plaque. Preventive measures, including thorough, regular oral hygiene practiced by the patient and periodic, periodontal scaling of the teeth performed by dental professionals, can prevent most periodontal diseases and the consequent loss of teeth.

PERIODONTICS AND PERIODONTAL DISEASE

Periodontics
The branch of dentistry concerned with the cause, treatment, and prevention of periodontal disease

Etiology
The study of the cause or origin of a disease

Periodontics is the branch of dentistry concerned with the characteristics of the normal periodontium; the **etiology**, treatment, and prevention of periodontal disease; and the establishment and maintenance of periodontal health. **Periodontal disease** can be defined as any pathologic process that affects the tissues of the periodontium (Box 25.1).

CHARACTERISTICS OF THE NORMAL PERIODONTIUM

Periodontal disease
The various diseases that affect the periodontium, especially gingivitis and periodontitis

Periodontium
The tissues that surround and support the tooth and anchor it to the bone

The **periodontium** is an anatomic term that refers to the tissues that surround and support the tooth in the jaws. These tissues are (1) the gingiva, (2) the dentogingival junction, (3) the cementum, (4) the periodontal ligament, and (5) the alveolar bone.

Functionally, these components can be divided into three categories: the *covering gingival tissue* (gingiva), which protects the underlying structures; the *dentogingival junction*, which seals the gingiva to the tooth and

protects the anchoring components of the periodontium; and the **attachment apparatus** (the cementum, the **periodontal ligament,** and the alveolar bone, which anchors the teeth in the jaws. The cementum is included as part of the periodontium because it functions as a support for the fibers of the periodontal ligament.

Gingiva
Anatomic Features

The gingiva is the part of the oral mucosa that surrounds the necks of the teeth and covers the alveolar process of the jaws (Figure 25.1). The anatomic landmarks are as follows:

- The *free,* or *marginal, gingiva* is the small portion of the gingiva adjacent to the tooth that surrounds it like a collar. It is usually about 1 mm wide, not directly attached to the tooth, and forms the soft tissue wall of the gingival sulcus. The coronal edge of the free gingiva is called the free gingival margin.
- The *free* (or *marginal*) *gingival groove* separates the free gingiva from the adjacent attached gingiva. The marginal gingiva is held firmly against the tooth by various gingival collagen fibers, which anchor the marginal gingiva with the cementum and prevent food from entering the sulcus during eating. The gingival fibers are arranged into bundles or groups according to their orientation and insertion into the tissues. As can be seen in the cross section in Figure 25.2, some fibers extend obliquely to the crest of the gingiva, some horizontally into the free gingiva and from tooth to tooth, some obliquely and external to the alveolar bone, and some around the tooth.
- The *attached gingiva* is continuous with the free gingiva and extends apically to the mucogingival junction. It is relatively firm, thick, and tightly bound to the underlying bone.
- The *mucogingival junction* is the line that separates the attached gingiva from the alveolar mucosa. It is relatively loose, thin, and moveable.
- The *interdental groove,* a depression between the roots of the teeth, usually appears in the interdental area of

Attachment apparatus
The portion of the periodontium that connects the tooth to the bone (that is, the cementum, the periodontal ligament, and the alveolar bone)

Periodontal ligament
The connective tissue fibers that surround the root of the tooth and attach it to the alveolar process

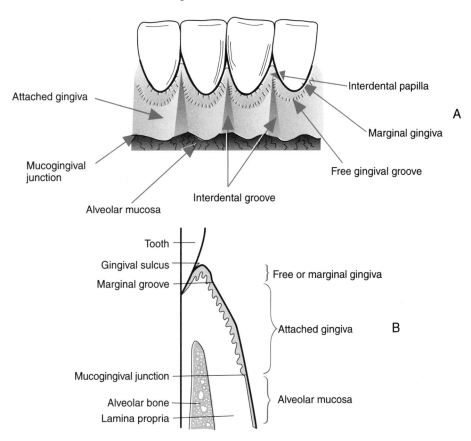

FIGURE 25.1

A, Gingiva (facial surface). **B,** Diagram of the gingival tissues.

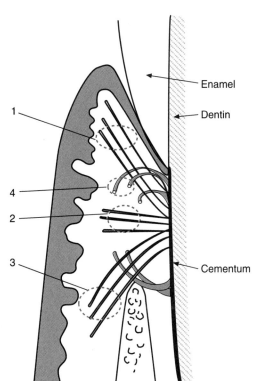

FIGURE 25.2

Diagram of gingival fibers. As seen in cross section, some of the fibers extend obliquely to the crest of the gingiva *(1)*, horizontally into the free gingiva and from tooth to tooth *(2)*, obliquely and external to the alveolar bone *(3)*, and around the tooth *(4)*.

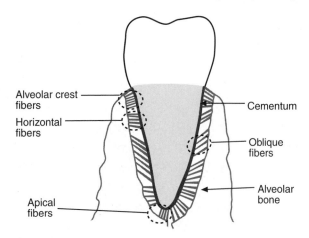

FIGURE 25.3

Periodontal ligament, with the principal fiber groups indicated.

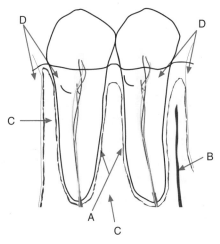

FIGURE 25.4

Parts of the alveolar process. **A,** Alveolar bone proper (cribriform plates). **B,** Blood vessel within a nutrient canal in the interdental area. **C,** Cancellous (spongy) supporting bone. **D,** Roots of the teeth.

the attached gingiva, running parallel to the long axes of adjacent teeth.

- The *interdental papilla* is the part of the gingiva that fills in the interproximal space between adjacent teeth beneath the area of tooth contact. It usually is pyramidal in shape when viewed from the front surface, especially in the anterior region of the mouth.
- The *gingival sulcus* is the open, shallow crevice or space bounded by the surface of the tooth on one side and the free gingiva on the other. It is V shaped, barely permitting the entrance of a probe. The gingival sulcus contains fluid that seeps into it from the underlying gingival connective tissue. This fluid helps keep the sulcus clean and also has antibacterial properties.
- The *alveolar mucosa* is the loose, elastic tissue immediately apical to the attached gingiva. It is continuous with the oral mucous membrane of the lips, cheeks, and floor of the mouth. The palate has no attached gingiva or alveolar mucosa; all palatal tissue is called masticatory mucosa, which is firm, tightly bound tissue similar to the attached gingiva.

Attachment Apparatus

The attachment apparatus, which comprises the tooth-supporting structures of the periodontium, consists of the periodontal ligament, the cementum, and the alveolar bone.

The *periodontal ligament* surrounds the root of the tooth and connects it with the alveolar bone. The ligament consists of a network of principal fibers, which are collagenous bundles arranged in various groups, that attach the tooth to the bone, cushion its resistance to occlusal forces (shock absorption), and protect the vessels and nerves in the ligament from injury by mechanical forces. The fibers have different orientations and functions at various levels on the tooth root (Figure 25.3). For example, the alveolar crest group prevents tooth extrusion, the horizontal group resists lateral move-

ment, and the more numerous oblique fibers act as a sling to resist downward pressure.

Cementum is the calcified outer covering of the anatomic root of the tooth. It is similar to bone tissue in that it has both a cellular and a fibrillar structure, and deposition continues throughout life; however, it lacks blood and lymph vessels and does not undergo physiologic **resorption** and remodeling. Cementum performs several

Resorption
The loss of osseous (bone) tissue that occurs with periodontitis

functions: it attaches the periodontal ligament fibers to the root and permits a continuous rearrangement of these fibers; it contributes to the process of repair after damage to the root surface; it compensates through growth for loss of tooth structure; and it facilitates the mesial drift of teeth.

The *alveolar process* is the portion of the maxilla and the mandible that supports and forms the sockets of the teeth (Figure 25.4). It forms when the tooth erupts to provide the bony attachment to the emerging periodontal ligament and gradually disappears if the teeth are lost. The alveolar process consists of three parts: an outer plate of mostly thick, compact bone; an inner, socket wall of thinner, compact bone, called the alveolar bone proper (also known as the cribriform plate, or lamina dura); and cancellous or spongy bone found between the two compact layers, which acts as supporting alveolar bone.

Blood is supplied to the supporting structures of the teeth by the superior and inferior alveolar artery (a.a.), which runs through the maxilla and the mandible, respectively (Figure 25.5). The dental artery (d.a.) branches from the alveolar artery and splits into the intraseptal artery (i.a.), which runs

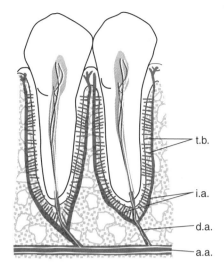

FIGURE 25.5

Blood supply to the teeth and periodontium.

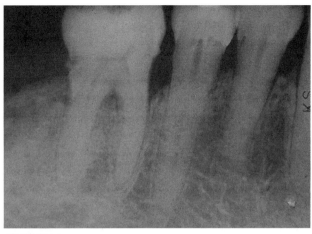

FIGURE 25.6

Periapical radiograph of a molar tooth showing calculus deposits as tiny white spicules projecting into the interproximal area.

through the alveolar process. Terminal branches (t.b.) of the intraseptal artery penetrate the cribriform plate of the alveolar process at all levels of the socket. As the dental artery enters the tooth socket, it also puts out branches that supply the apical portion of the periodontal ligament. Ultimately, the dental artery enters the root canal of the tooth.

PERIODONTAL DISEASE

Plaque

Plaque bacteria cause **inflammation** by producing substances (enzymes and toxins) that destroy the periodontal tissues and minimize host defenses. One objective of periodontal therapy is to limit or control the destructive nature of these bacteria. Plaque is necessary to initiate periodontal disease, but a small amount of plaque in an otherwise healthy individual can be controlled by the body's defense mechanisms. In fact, when periodontal tissues are healthy, little plaque accumulates.

Inflammation

The protective response of the body's tissues to irritation or injury

Calculus

As early as the first day of plaque formation, both supragingival and subgingival plaque may become calcified, or hardened, by deposition of mineral salts (mostly calcium phosphate) from the saliva (Figure 25.6). However, all plaque does not necessarily undergo calcification and become calculus, or tartar in lay terms. Once plaque becomes mineralized, it can no longer be removed by the patient and must eventually be removed by the dentist or hygienist with appropriate scaling instruments. Regular, effective plaque control measures can minimize or eliminate the buildup of calculus.

Other Tooth Deposits

Bacterial plaque and calculus are not the only material that accumulates on tooth surfaces. Other tooth deposits include the following:

- *Acquired pellicle:* A thin protein film that rapidly forms on erupted teeth. It can be removed with an abrasive, such as the prophy paste used for coronal polishing.
- *Materia alba ("white material"):* A yellow to greyish white, loose, soft mixture of bacteria, salivary proteins, epithelial cells and blood cells, and food particles. Unlike plaque, materia alba is visible without the use of disclosing materials and can be flushed away with a water spray. It is common in individuals who have poor oral hygiene.
- *Food debris:* Particles of food that remain in the mouth after eating. Most food debris is liquefied by bacterial enzymes and cleared from the mouth by the action of the oral musculature and saliva within minutes after eating. Any remaining food debris usually is impacted between the teeth or within periodontal pockets. Contrary to common belief, food debris does not simply become dental plaque and is not an important cause of gingivitis. However, if sugars are present, the food debris may contribute to dental caries if it is not removed.

• *Dental stains:* As is pointed out in Chapter 14, dental stains are predominantly a cosmetic problem and are relatively harmless.

GINGIVITIS

Inflammatory periodontal disease begins as **gingivitis**. The

Gingivitis

Inflammation of the gingiva

free gingival margin is usually the first area involved. It takes only 9 to 21 days for a healthy mouth to regress to a clinically observable gingivitis. The gingival color changes from pink to red,
the contour progresses from knife edged to enlarged, and the tissue consistency changes from firm to spongy. Eventually the gingival sulcus may bleed when examined with a periodontal probe. Sometimes the patient may complain of pain or soreness in the gingival area, especially when brushing.

Treatment of gingivitis usually includes instruction in oral hygiene and professional prophylaxis of the teeth (scaling and coronal polishing). The dental assistant can provide the oral hygiene instruction, but the dentist or dental hygienist is usually responsible for the scaling procedure. In some states the dental assistant, with proper training, may perform coronal polishing.

PERIODONTITIS

Periodontitis, an inflammation of the supporting structures

Periodontitis

Inflammation of the periodontium that involves alveolar bone loss and deepening of the gingival sulcus (pocket)

of the teeth, is not as common as gingivitis. It affects about one fourth to one half of the adults in the United States and most other developed countries. In periodontitis, the periodontal sulcus deepens from its normal depth of 2 to 3 mm and becomes a periodontal pocket, and loss
of alveolar bone occurs (Figure 25.7). Other supporting structures of the tooth may also be affected, including the cementum and the periodontal ligament.

Periodontal Examination

A complete periodontal examination consists of taking and recording the patient's vital signs, a medical and dental history, and examination of the soft and hard structures of the oral cavity, including the mucous membranes, the teeth, and the periodontal structures (that is, the gingiva and the gingival sulcus, or pocket).

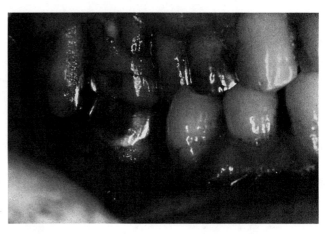

FIGURE 25.7

Signs of periodontal destruction evident in this clinical photograph include gingival recession and root exposure of tooth #3, revealing the furcation area.

A critical element in the periodontal examination is probing and recording the depth of the periodontal pockets with a periodontal probe, a calibrated instrument designed to measure in millimeters the amount of bone loss around a tooth.

Traditional Periodontal Probing and Charting

The operator (in some states this can be the dental assistant) inserts the probe into the periodontal pocket in line with the vertical axis of the tooth until resistance is encountered. The operator then "walks" the probe around each tooth, calling out to the recorder the numerical readings in millimeters that correspond to the "probing depth" in each area. Probing depths of 1 to 3 mm are considered shallow and normal. Shallow probing depths are usually associated with periodontal health.

In the traditional method of probing and charting, six probing depths are examined and recorded on each tooth; these are the distolingual, midlingual, mesiolingual, mesiofacial, midfacial, and distofacial measurements (Figure 25.8, *A*). Bleeding of the gingival tissues on probing is noted and recorded at the same time, such as by underlining the probing depth number in red. The findings of the examination are recorded on a periodontal chart, such as the one shown in Figure 25.8, *B*.

A Nabors probe is used to detect any furcation involvement, which is a space near, at, or through the root furcation. The root furcation is the area between two or more roots of the same tooth at the point where the roots separate. Any furcations found can be marked in red on the charted tooth as a triangle in the area of the furcation involvement, corresponding to the actual location of the problem area. Other charting symbols can be used to indicate other problems, such as missing teeth, caries, open or irregular contact areas,

A   B

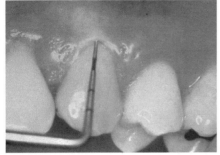
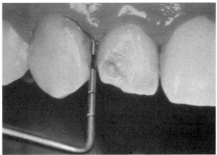

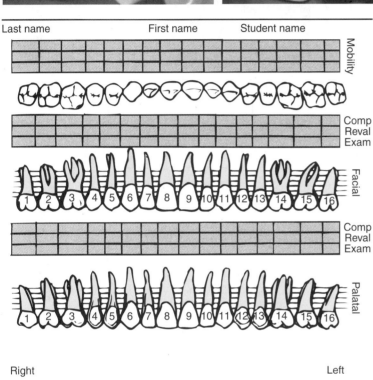

Last name   First name   Student name

Mobility

Comp
Reval
Exam

Facial

Comp
Reval
Exam

Palatal

Right   Left

C

Lingual

Exam
Reval
Comp

Facial

Exam
Reval
Comp

Mobility

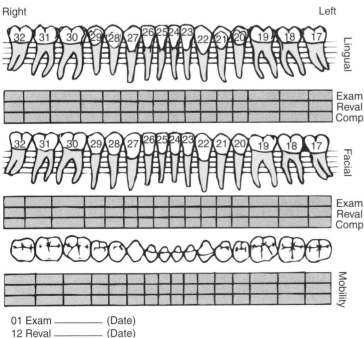

01 Exam ————— (Date)
12 Reval ————— (Date)
35 Completed
     treatment ————— (Date)

FIGURE 25.8

Probe placement; (**A**) midfacial on #11 and (**B**) mesio-facial on #6. **C**, Periodontal chart for recording pockets. The probing depths are written in each box, with three measurements per box. Three rows of boxes are provided for recording three series of measurements: those made at the initial examination ("exam"), those recorded at the reevaluation ("reval") several months later, after all scaling has been completed, and those taken upon completion of treatment ("comp").

Table 25.1	
Tooth Mobility Codes	
Code	**Degree of Mobility**
0	No mobility
1	Slight mobility
2	Moderate mobility
3	Extreme mobility

Mobility

> **The degree of movement of the tooth within the socket, expressed by a number rating (0, 1, 2, 3) designating no mobility to extreme mobility**

periapical pathologic conditions, drifted or extruded teeth, and irregular contacts (see Chapter 21).

Mobility, or the movement of the tooth within the socket, is also recorded on the chart. Often each tooth is given a number rating, from 0 to 3, which corresponds to the degree of tooth mobility, ranging from no mobility (0) to extreme mobility (3) (Table 25.1).

Periodontal Screening and Recording

An alternative to the traditional method of probing and recording the depth of every periodontal pocket in the manner described above is the periodontal screening and recording (PSR) system. It was developed by the American Academy of Periodontology and the American Dental Association. Compared to traditional probing and charting described above, PSR is a cost-effective, quick, and easy way to determine if patients have periodontal disease (Figure 25.9).

This "early detection system" uses a specially designed probe with a 0.5-mm balled tip that is color coded from 3.5 to 5.5 mm (Box 25.2). In summary, shallow periodontal depths and the absence of inflammation (including redness of the marginal gingiva and bleeding on probing) are associated with periodontal health. Initiating full-mouth debridement before a periodontal examination may be necessary (Figure 25.10).

Radiographic Films

Radiographs are valuable as an adjunct to the oral examination but are not a substitute for it. A key factor in radiographic evaluation of periodontal disease is the appearance and relative position of the lamina dura (the "white line" in

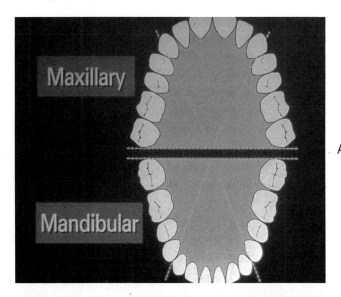

A

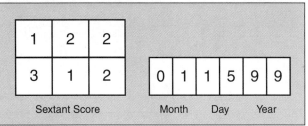

B

FIGURE 25.9

A, For the periodontal screening and recording (PSR) system, the mouth is divided into sextants. **B,** Sticker used to record a patient's PSR score.

the radiograph, which represents the bone surface lining the tooth socket). In a healthy patient the lamina dura appears as a relatively thin, almost continuous white line surrounding the roots of the teeth. The crest of the lamina dura interproximally is relatively close (about 1 to 2 mm) and generally parallel to a line between the cementoenamel junctions of the approximating teeth; this would indicate a "high" crest of interproximal bone. The absence of bone loss is associated with periodontal health and a lower risk of future periodontal disease.

A patient with periodontitis interproximally has a bony crest that is lowered on the roots interproximally, usually indicating alveolar bone loss. However, because radiographs are only two dimensional, this is not diagnostic and must be confirmed with other clinical information to reach a definitive diagnosis. Breakdown in the continuity of the lamina dura also may be seen as a result of the inflammation extending from the gingiva into the bone. In such cases the lamina dura appears more fuzzy and broken.

During the periodontal examination, the dental assistant records all findings described by the clinician in the appropriate places on the periodontal chart.

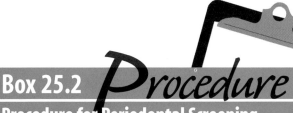

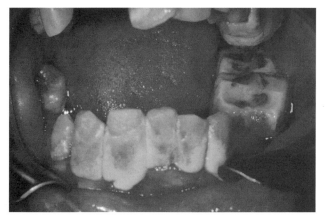

FIGURE 25.10

Extensive calculus deposits may require full-mouth debridement before a comprehensive periodontal examination can be performed.

Procedure for Periodontal Screening and Recording (PSR)

1. The mouth is divided into sextants: maxillary right, anterior, and left; and mandibular left, anterior, and right (see Figure 25.9, *A*). All teeth in each sextant are checked with the special probe.
2. As with traditional probing, six sites on each tooth in a quadrant are examined. However, instead of the charting associated with a comprehensive, full-mouth examination, only the deepest probing depth of each sextant is charted in the patient's record, using a unique PSR code (see Table 25.1).
3. The PSR code is determined by how much of the colored band on the PSR probe is visible when the probe is placed in the gingival crevice. The code varies from 0 to 4, which also represents the level of health or periodontal disease in each sextant of the mouth. Code 0 indicates periodontal health, and code 4 indicates a probing depth greater than 5.5 mm. An asterisk (*) is added to the sextant score whenever the findings indicate clinical abnormalities, such as furcation involvement or recession.
4. The numbers obtained for each sextant and the date are recorded on a special sticker (see Figure 25.9, *B*), which is placed in the patient's chart.

odontal diseases fall into two general categories: those that affect the gingiva (gingival diseases) and those that affect the supporting structures of the teeth.

Gingival Diseases

The following disorders are some of the more common gingival diseases:

- **Chronic** gingivitis (the most common type)
- Gingival recession
- Gingival enlargement
- Acute necrotizing ulcerative gingivitis (ANUG)
- Acute herpetic gingivostomatitis
- **Pericoronitis**
- Desquamative gingivitis

Periodontal Diseases

Diseases of the tooth-supporting structures include the following:

- Adult periodontitis (the most common type)
- Prepubertal periodontitis
- Juvenile periodontitis
- Rapidly progressing periodontitis
- Periodontitis associated with systemic disease
- Necrotizing ulcerative periodontitis

Periodontal Diagnosis

Periodontal diagnosis

The determination of the type of periodontal disease present, including its extent, distribution, and severity

Based on the patient's history and the results of the periodontal examination, the dentist makes a **periodontal diagnosis** and a **prognosis.** This allows an appropriate treatment plan to be established that is geared to the patient's particular needs. Most peri-

Prognosis

A prediction of the duration and course of a disease and the likelihood of its response to treatment

Chronic

A disease or condition that develops gradually and persists for a long period

Pericoronitis

Inflammation and infection of the gingival tissue surrounding the crown of an erupting tooth

- Refractory periodontitis
- Trauma from occlusion

Chapters 11 and 17 further discuss the periodontal diseases that appear in this section.

Periodontal Treatment

The aim of periodontal treatment is to establish and maintain a healthy periodontium throughout the patient's lifetime. The primary goals of periodontal treatment are to eliminate gingival inflammation and to correct the conditions that caused it. The rationale for periodontal therapy is tied to the remarkable healing capacity of the periodontal tissues. Periodontal treatment can (1) eliminate gingival inflammation, infection, pain, bleeding, and pus formation; (2) reduce periodontal pockets, tooth mobility, and tooth loss; (3) arrest soft tissue and bone destruction; and (4) reestablish the gingival contours needed to preserve periodontal health and prevent the recurrence of disease. To achieve these objectives, good rapport with a cooperative patient is necessary.

After the diagnosis and the prognosis have been made, the treatment is planned. The periodontal treatment plan includes all procedures needed to establish and maintain good oral health and functioning, including, in sequential order, oral hygiene instruction, **scaling** and **root planing,** extraction of hopeless teeth, reevaluation, other nonsurgical and surgical procedures, and recall maintenance.

Scaling

The removal of calculus from the tooth with various mechanical and hand instruments

Root planing

A procedure for smoothing roughened root surfaces that is performed after the scaling procedure

Emergency Care

Conditions considered periodontal emergencies include the following:

Acute

A disease or condition that begins abruptly with marked intensity and then subsides after a relatively brief period

- **Acute** necrotizing ulcerative gingivitis
- Acute pericoronitis
- Acute herpetic gingivostomatitis
- Periodontal abscess
- Severely mobile teeth

Conditions such as these often are associated with pain and infection. Immediate treatment is directed at alleviating the acute symptoms and comprehensive follow up to prevent a repeat episode. Some teeth may require extraction at this point. If this creates a significant esthetic liability, an immediate temporary prosthesis may be necessary.

Phase I: Initial Therapy

Phase I of periodontal treatment includes the following elements:

- Plaque control and follow-up reinstruction
- Dietary planning

Calculus removal and root planing and polishing, including:

- Adult prophylaxis (gingivitis)
- Periodontal scaling and root planing (periodontitis)
- Periodontal maintenance
- Treatment of defective restorations and carious lesions (temporary or final)
- Strategic extraction of hopeless teeth (may necessitate a temporary prosthesis)
- Antimicrobial therapy
- Occlusal therapy
- Minor tooth movement
- Splinting of loose teeth

Surgical Therapy

Surgical treatment involves the following:

- Corrective periodontal procedures
- Placement of implants

The primary purpose of periodontal surgery is to eliminate or correct problems in the periodontium that make it difficult or impossible for the patient to remove plaque and for the therapist to remove calculus (see Figure 25.10), such as deep or complex pockets and furcation involvements. Surgery sometimes is necessary for other reasons, such as to provide more surface area for crown attachment (crown lengthening), for esthetics (tissue grafts), or to place implants.

Phase II: Restorative Therapy

Phase II of treatment includes the following:

- Extraction of nonmaintainable teeth
- Final restorations
- Creation of fixed and removable prosthodontics (bridges, partials)
- Active periodontal maintenance

Recall Periodontal Maintenance Therapy

Periodic Recall Visits

To help ensure the benefits of a healthy, well-functioning periodontium and other oral structures, patients who have completed all active and corrective therapy are recalled at intervals appropriate for their individual needs. Commonly, patients with gingivitis are seen approximately every 6 months, whereas patients with periodontitis are recalled every 3 to 4 months. At each recall appointment, the periodontal tissues are reevaluated and an adult prophylaxis or

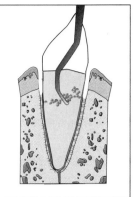

Box 25.3

Responding to the Patient's Questions

1. Begin responses positively.
2. Use terms lay people understand, not dental jargon.
3. Give any bad news gently.
4. Follow bad news with reassurance.
5. Be a good listener.
6. Keep answers brief and to the point
7. Personalize responses for that patient.
8. Obtain feedback.

Never tell an apprehensive patient, "There's nothing to be afraid of." It's much better to tell the patient something like, "This office caters to cowards."

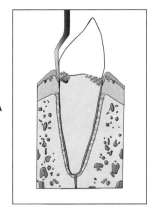

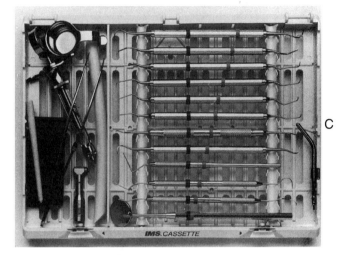

periodontal prophylaxis is performed. Periodontic radiographs are taken when indicated.

Answering Patient Questions on Treatment Plans

During the diagnostic and treatment planning phase of dental care, the dental assistant has the primary role of assisting the dentist during the history and examination, recording the findings in the patient's chart, and perhaps taking the medical and dental history directly, including vital signs. (As mentioned previously, in some states the dental assistant may perform periodontal probing.) At this point the patient may have many questions but may be reluctant to ask the dentist and may decide to ask the assistant instead, such as when the dentist leaves the operatory. The dental assistant's answers could make a difference in the patient's acceptance or rejection of the treatment plan. Box 25.3 presents some suggestions for dealing with a patient's questions about the diagnosis, prognosis, and treatment options.

Plaque Control

Teaching the patient to remove plaque efficiently and thoroughly is a treatment goal of considerable importance in initial therapy. A well-trained dental assistant is ideally suited to perform this task. Training in oral hygiene ordinarily requires several visits for instruction, repetition, and reinforcement. The various aids and procedures are described in Chapter 17.

Dietary Planning and Use of Supplements

Chapter 16 discusses ways to help a patient choose foods that will promote and enhance oral health. It should be emphasized that dietary counseling, if indicated, plays a secondary role in the treatment of periodontal disease. However, some periodontal conditions warrant a stronger nutritional focus. For example, a patient with ANUG may have considerable difficulty eating firm, chewy foods such as raw fruits and vegetables. This painful condition may cause the patient to

FIGURE 25.11

A, Scaling removes supragingival and subgingival plaque and calculus from the teeth. **B,** Root planing smoothes the root to allow the supportive tissues to reattach to the tooth. **C,** Root planing setup: mirror, explorer, probe, sickle scaler, root planing curettes, universal curettes, dressing pliers, sharpening stone, pumice cup, prophy angle, suction tip, aspirating syringe, and air and water syringe tip. (*C,* courtesy Hu-Friedy, Chicago, Ill.)

avoid these and other such foods, leading to a diet inadequate in vitamins B and C, which in turn could exacerbate an already aggravated gingival response. Supplementing the diet with vitamins B and C has been shown to lessen recurrences of this acute condition.

Calculus Removal, Root Planing, and Polishing

Calculus has a rough surface that provides retentive areas in which oral bacteria can accumulate, promoting the buildup and retention of dental plaque. Unfortunately, even the most diligent patient usually cannot remove all plaque, which continually collects on tooth surfaces and on and within calculus deposits (especially subgingivally). For this reason, periodic scaling to remove plaque and calculus is a practical necessity to ensure effective plaque control (Figure 25.11).

Box 25.4

Dental Assistant's Role in Scaling and Root Planing Procedures

For scaling and root planing procedures, the dental assistant has the following responsibilities:

To carry out infection control measures in the operatory, preparing it for the patient

To escort the patient to the operatory and explain the procedure and the reasons for it

To teach, review, and reinforce plaque control before the surgery

To assist the clinician chairside with the procedure

To give the patient appropriate postoperative instructions and then dismiss the person

To prepare the operatory for the next patient and sterilize the instruments used

Box 25.5

Postoperative Instructions for Scaling

The patient should be given the following instructions after a scaling procedure:

1. If bleeding occurs, use a sterile gauze sponge to apply heavy finger pressure to the bleeding area for 10 minutes.
2. For pain after the anesthesia subsides, take one or two tablets of a nonprescription pain medication, such as aspirin, Tylenol, Advil, Nuprin, or Motrin, every 3 or 4 hours or as the dentist has directed. These medications should not be taken on an empty stomach.
3. If the dentist has prescribed a chlorhexidine mouth rinse to control bleeding, it should be used as follows:
   a. Rinse with $1/2$ oz for 30 seconds twice a day after meals, in the morning and evening.
   b. Do not rinse with water immediately after using the mouth rinse.
4. For mild discomfort the day after scaling, rinse the mouth gently with 1 tsp salt in an 8-oz glass of warm water several times a day.
5. Call the office if any problems develop.

Box 25.6

Postoperative Instructions for Patients Treated with Actisite

A patient who has been treated with Actisite fibers should be given the following information and instructions:

1. The Actisite fiber slowly releases an antibiotic under the infected gum.
2. Do not brush or floss the teeth being treated with Actisite, because this may dislodge the fibers. However, be sure to brush and floss the rest of the teeth.
3. Do not touch the treated area with your tongue or fingers, because the fiber may fall out.
4. Avoid eating hard, crunchy, or sticky foods that may loosen or dislodge the fiber. Such foods include hard bread, toast, nuts, raw vegetables, chewing gum, and candy. Also, to avoid getting food stuck under the gumline, do not eat foods with seeds (such as poppy seeds) or foods such as popcorn or oat bran.
5. Return to the office as scheduled to have the fiber removed and the progress of the treatment checked.

for reduction or elimination of gingival inflammation. Large, overhanging margins must be eliminated by replacing the restoration when correcting the contour of the existing restoration is difficult or impossible. Carious lesions are removed and restored (at least temporarily), not only to eliminate the infected area of the tooth but also to allow for proper cleansing in an area that otherwise may be impossible to clean.

Antimicrobial Agents

Antimicrobial agents, which include antibiotics, mouth rinses and topical fluoride, are sometimes used in the treatment of periodontal diseases. These products can be effective when used by the patient as a daily oral rinse, either conventionally or as an irrigant in an oral irrigation device equipped with a marginal irrigation tip. Stannous fluoride has also been shown to have antibacterial effects when used as an oral irrigating solution in the treatment of advanced periodontitis.

Actisite (tetracycline-impregnated plastic fibers) can be placed in the periodontal pockets of teeth that do not respond well to scaling and root planing in an effort to reduce or eliminate pocket depth, or it can be used as an adjunct to those procedures to enhance their results. The fiber is placed in a manner similar to that for gingival retraction cord, and it is secured by superficial application of a cyanoacrylate adhesive (medical glue) and a periodontal dressing. The fiber is left in place for 10 days and then removed. Actisite may be useful for patients who refuse periodontal surgery or when such surgery is contraindicated.

Resorbable devices of a similar nature are under development. Postoperative instructions for patients treated with Actisite can be found in Box 25.6. When used in conjunc-

After scaling has been completed, the roots of the teeth, if exposed, must be planed until smooth; this aids in optimal plaque control and helps minimize the accumulation of plaque. Scaling and root planing usually are completed at the same visit by the dentist or the hygienist (Boxes 25.4 and 25.5).

Treatment of Defective Restorations and Carious Lesions

Restorations that are not well contoured and smooth tend to accumulate plaque and therefore are associated with periodontal inflammation and alveolar bone loss. Because such restorations interfere with efficient plaque control, they must be removed and smoothed during phase I treatment to allow tion with scaling and root planing, these products slightly raise clinical attachment levels and decrease probing depths and bleeding.

Occlusal Therapy

The term *occlusion* refers to the way the upper and lower teeth come together in function. If no pathologic condition results from the biting relationships or functioning of the teeth, the person is considered to have a physiologic (healthy) occlusion. On the other hand, if any disturbance or injury is caused by occlusal functioning, the occlusion is classified as traumatic.

If occlusal trauma can be established to have occurred as a result of a traumatic occlusion, occlusal treatment (perhaps in addition to other forms of periodontal therapy) may be indicated. Some examples of occlusal therapy include occlusal adjustment (coronal reshaping of teeth), splinting (immobilization) of teeth, construction of an occlusal stabilization splint (bite guard appliance), and orthodontic treatment.

SURGICAL TREATMENT

The effectiveness of periodontal therapy depends primarily on the elimination of factors that favor plaque accumulation and on daily removal of plaque by the patient. The purposes of periodontal surgery are to:

1　Create access for proper professional scaling and root planing and daily cleaning by the patient
2　Correct gingival contours so that the patient can remove plaque adequately
3　Reduce probing depths
4　Regenerate periodontal tissues lost to or damaged by destructive disease
5　Improve esthetics
6　Enhance restorative and cosmetic dentistry
7　Place implants

Measures for helping to keep the patient comfortable during periodontal surgery are presented in Box 25.7.

A periodontal dressing (pack) often is used after surgery to cover the areas treated; to lessen the likelihood of postoperative hemorrhage and infection; to reduce postoperative pain; to prevent trauma during healing by protecting the operative site from the oral musculature and from hot and spicy foods; to support slightly mobile teeth; and to help give contour to regenerating gingival tissue. Many states allow dental assistants to place and remove periodontal dressings.

The most commonly used periodontal surgical dressing is Coe-Pak, which comes in two tubes that are mixed together immediately before use (Box 25.8, Table 25.2, and Figure 25.12). The dressing is secured by interlocking the pack into the interdental spaces and by blending the facial and lingual segments when placing the material so that they are locked

Box 25.7

Steps for Enhancing the Patient's Comfort During Periodontal Surgery

1. Put petroleum jelly on the patient's lips before surgery and, using separate gauze squares, periodically alternate applications of water (or mouthwash) and petroleum jelly.
2. Periodically irrigate the patient's mouth with water and suction with a disposable saliva suction tip. Do not use the surgical aspirator for this purpose.
3. Be gentle and careful when retracting and manipulating soft tissue, including the lips, cheek, and tongue. Roughness can cause tissue injury and postoperative discomfort and can delay healing.
4. Watch the patient and occasionally ask if the person is doing all right. The patient may need a drink of water, suction, less lip pressure, or more anesthesia or may need to go to the toilet. The dentist may get preoccupied with surgical details, although a good operator also asks this question.
5. Maintain a positive attitude with the patient and the dentist. Periodically tell the patient—with feeling—that he or she is doing a great job.
6. It may help to make small talk with the dentist as the surgery proceeds. This may take the patient's mind off the procedure, thereby relaxing the patient, and it usually doesn't do the dentist any harm, either.

and stabilized when hardened. Isolated teeth may require additional reinforcement, such as tying a piece of floss around the tooth and pack.

Postoperative Care

Postoperative care should be provided after the periodontal pack has been placed and the patient has been given an ice bag to put on the outside of the face over the surgically treated area. The dentist may give the patient prescriptions for pain medication or antibiotics at this time. Postoperative instructions are given to the patient both orally and in printed form. Box 25.9 presents an example of written instructions.

Dressing and Suture Removal

The patient usually returns to the office approximately 1 week after surgery for removal of the pack and sutures, evaluation, and possible repacking. If the law permits, the dental assistant may remove the pack and sutures and repack (if necessary). The dentist should evaluate the surgical site after the pack has been removed. A postoperative kit for dressing and suture removal is shown in Figure 25.13. Particles that adhere to a tooth may need to be removed with a scaler. If sutures were placed, these may be caught in the pack, therefore care must be taken in removing the dressing. Superficial debris, sloughed cells, and bits of food usually will have

Box 25.8

Procedure

Procedure for Mixing and Applying Periodontal Dressing (Coe-Pak)

1. Place an equal amount of dressing mix and catalyst on a mixing pad (about a 2-inch strip per quadrant) (Figure 25.12, *A*).
2. Put warm water in a plastic cup with 1 drop of soap.
3. Spatulate the dressing material together with a tongue blade into a homogeneous mix and then gather the mix onto one side of the tongue blade. Place the tongue blade with the mix in the cup of warm water briefly to hasten the setting time.
4. After the pack has lost its tackiness (this may take a few minutes), test it to see if it is sticky (Figure 25.12, *B*). The mix is ready when it feels smooth.
5. Put on gloves and lubricate the fingers with petroleum jelly. Take a small amount of pack off the tongue blade and roll it with the fingers into a small cylinder as wide or as large as the operative sight. Dry the teeth with gauze.
6. Place the pack on the facial segment as needed to cover the surgical site, then repeat the process for the lingual area until all surgical sites have been covered with pack.
7. Use a cotton applicator lubricated with petroleum jelly or moistened with water (or use a plastic instrument) to mold the pack interproximally to conform to gingival contours so that the pack stays in place. Blend the facial and lingual segments so that they are locked and stabilized when hardened (Figure 25.12, *C*).
8. Make sure the pack covers the gingiva but not the uninvolved mucosa; covering the mucosa might be irritating to the patient and may interfere with tongue movement. Trim away any portion that interferes with the occlusion.
9. Do not overpack; this only interferes with the patient's comfort, and excess pack tends to break off, dislodging additional pack.

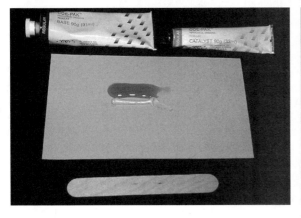

A

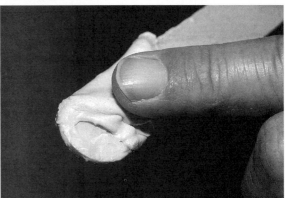

B

C

FIGURE 25.12

A, Equal strips of the dressing mix and catalyst are placed on the mixing pad. **B,** The pack is tested for stickiness. **C,** The facial and lingual segments are blended so that they are locked and stabilized when hardened.

Table 25.2

Evaluation for Mixing and Applying Periodontal Dressing

Periodontal Dressing (COE-PAK)	4	3	2	0	X
1. Assemble materials.					
2. Proportion mix and catalyst.					
3. Spatulate.					
4. Check consistency.					
5. Roll pack.					
6. Dry teeth.					
7. Position pack over site.					
8. Mold dressing.					
9. Secure dressing and trim excess.					
10. Check coverage.					

The numeric criteria: 4 Excellent; 3 Good but some improvement can be made; 2 Below average, usable, needs to improve skill; 0 Unsatisfactory; X Not able to evaluate.

Box 25.9

Postoperative Instructions for Periodontal Surgery

The patient should have an escort home and be given the following instructions after a periodontal surgical procedure:

To prevent swelling:

1. Hold the provided ice pack on the outside of your face over the surgical area for 20 minutes, then remove it for 20 minutes.
2. When you arrive home, begin using the ice pack (20 minutes on, 40 minutes off) until bedtime.
3. For the next 24 hours, use additional pillows to keep your head elevated when lying down or sleeping.

To preserve the surgical dressing:

1. The puttylike material around the teeth is a surgical dressing. Don't worry if small pieces break off, but call the dentist if the dressing comes off in the first 48 hours.
2. Avoid eating anything hot for a few hours. Protect the dressing by not eating hard, sticky, or grainy foods, such as carrots, gum, candy, or toast. Also avoid citrus fruits, fruit juices, and highly spiced foods. For a few days, try to avoid eating on the side where the surgery was performed.
3. If a graft has been placed, the dressing should stay in place until the sutures are removed.

For pain or discomfort:

1. Take pain medication before the anesthetic wears off.
2. Aspirin usually is more effective than Tylenol; Motrin, Advil, or Nuprin is also very good for pain.
3. An adult can take up to two aspirins every 3 hours, or three Motrin, Advil, or Nuprin every 6 hours.

4. Do not take pain medication on an empty stomach.
5. Take the pain medication even if you don't have pain, because it minimizes inflammation.
6. If a narcotic has been prescribed, *do not operate a motor vehicle or machinery under its influence.*

To prevent infection and promote healing:

1. An antibiotic may be prescribed to reduce infection. The patient will take a prescribed amount at specific times according to the dentist's prescription.
2. If a mouthwash has been prescribed, start using it tomorrow. *Do not rinse today.* The mouthwash helps reduce the chance of infection and speeds healing.
3. Extra vitamin C (up to 500 mg) per day may also aid healing.

Diet and oral hygiene:

1. Twenty-four hours after surgery, begin bathing the surgical area with warm salt water ($^1/_2$ tsp in an 8-oz glass of water). Try to bathe the mouth for 5 minutes each waking hour for the first 2 or 3 days and then several times a day until the next visit. *Rinse gently.*
2. *Do not use peroxide.*
3. Brush and floss the teeth in the unoperated areas as usual. Beginning on the second day after surgery, gently brush the dressing.
4. Maintain a nutritious diet with liquids at first (such as Ensure, or milk with a multiple vitamin/mineral supplement) and progress to regular foods as tolerated.
5. *Avoid using alcohol and tobacco, which retard clotting, circulation, and healing.*

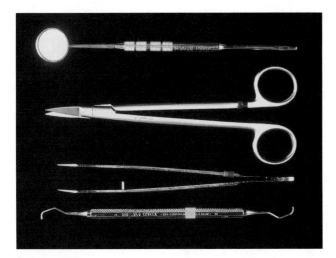

FIGURE 25.13

Periodontal postoperative kit includes *(top to bottom):* mouth mirror, tissue scissors, tissue pliers, and curette.

seeped under the pack, creating a distinct odor. The area should be cleaned gently using warm water from a syringe or moistened Q-tips, which may be saturated in a mix of hydrogen peroxide and water or mouthwash.

When removing the sutures, care should be taken always to cut and pull out the sutures in such a way as to avoid pulling the knot through the tissue. Also, care should be taken not to make so many cuts that suture material would be left in the tissue and could not be pulled out. The tissues should be cleaned before the sutures are removed so that bacterial debris is not pulled into the delicate, healing tissue, possibly causing infection. The sutures are cut next to the knot with scissors and then pulled out with the pliers, knot first. The sutures may need to be gently pulled away from the tissues before they are cut.

Oral Hygiene

If the pack does not need to be replaced, the patient should be given postoperative oral hygiene instructions, which can be provided by the dental assistant. The patient should be instructed to avoid vigorous brushing and to keep the area as clean as possible to promote healing. Brushing can be attempted with a "sensitive" (very soft) toothbrush in a very gentle manner, with the bristles directed away from the tender, healing gingival tissues. If this proves too difficult or causes significant bleeding, the patient should be encouraged to allow the area to heal for a few more days and then to attempt brushing again.

Root Sensitivity

A common problem among patients after periodontal surgery is root sensitivity. This sensitivity usually disappears by itself over time. A number of nonprescription desensitizing toothpastes that have been accepted by the American

Dental Association (ADA) can help with this condition and are available for the patient to use (see the section on dentifrices in Chapter 17). These toothpastes should be used twice a day for at least several weeks. ADA-accepted products for controlling hypersensitivity also are available, such as Gel-Kam, a 0.4% stannous fluoride gel that can be used at home (see the section on fluoride brush-on gels in Chapter 17). Gel-Kam has been accepted by the ADA for both caries and sensitivity control. It is well to remember that it may take several days of use for these anti-hypersensitivity products to exert their effect.

Postoperative Prevention of Root Caries

Another concern after periodontal surgery is the potential for root caries. The roots of the teeth are more susceptible to decay than the crowns because the exposed cementum is softer and less calcified than enamel and probably has considerably less fluoride. Many periodontal surgical procedures leave the roots exposed, making them especially prone to decay immediately after surgery because it is difficult for the patient to keep the newly exposed surfaces clean.

A new prescription product, Gel-Kam Oral Care Rinse, addresses these concerns (see the section on fluorides in periodontal therapy in Chapter 17). The rinse is a 0.63% stannous fluoride concentrate that the patient mixes with water and uses as a mouth rinse or adds to the reservoir of a home irrigating device (Box 25.10).

Instruments Used in Periodontal Surgery

Periodontal surgery and the instruments required for it often involve the common procedures and instruments listed

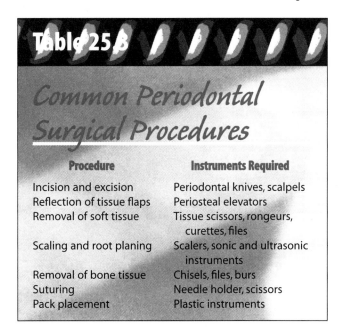

Table 25.3

Common Periodontal Surgical Procedures

Procedure	Instruments Required
Incision and excision	Periodontal knives, scalpels
Reflection of tissue flaps	Periosteal elevators
Removal of soft tissue	Tissue scissors, rongeurs, curettes, files
Scaling and root planing	Scalers, sonic and ultrasonic instruments
Removal of bone tissue	Chisels, files, burs
Suturing	Needle holder, scissors
Pack placement	Plastic instruments

in Table 25.3. The procedures are shown in the order in which they are performed and the instruments in the order in which they are used.

Instrument Storage and Maintenance

The instruments used for the various surgical procedures are stored in ready-to-use packs or trays, such as the Hu-Friedy IMS Cassette system. The instruments must be managed to prevent the interchange of sterile and nonsterile devices. It also is important to maintain the instruments in good working condition. This means that all sharp instruments (scalers, curettes, and knives with fixed blades) must be sharpened regularly and that hinged instruments (scissors, rongeurs, and needle holders) must be properly lubricated.

Instrument Trays

Figure 25.14 shows a tray system frequently used for periodontal surgery. A set of instruments frequently used in oral surgery and some commonly used periodontal surgical instruments are combined into a basic "pack."

Specific Surgical Instruments

The surgical instruments below are discussed in the approximate order in which they are used in many periodontal surgical procedures. Several common periodontal surgical procedures are described more fully at the end of this chapter.

Gingivectomy

A surgical procedure in which a portion of the gingival tissues are excised, or removed

The periodontal pocket marker (Figure 25.15) is used when starting a **gingivectomy** to punch small

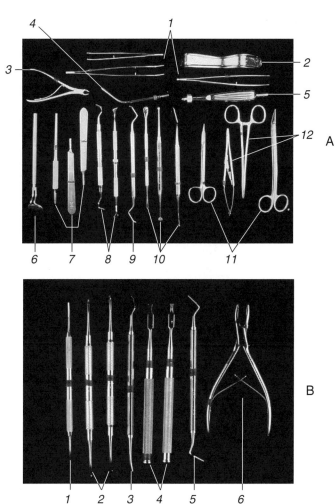

FIGURE 25.14

A, Instruments included in a primary surgery tray, arranged in approximate order of use. *(1)* Tissue and cotton pliers. *(2)* Cheek retractor. *(3)* Nipper. *(4)* Aspirator tip. *(5)* Aspirator and retractor. *(6)* Mouth mirror. *(7)* Scalpel handler. *(8)* Perio knives. *(9)* Surgical currette. *(10)* Molt currette/elevators. *(11)* Tissue and cotton scissors. *(12)* Needle holders. **B,** Supplemental surgery tray. *(1)* Wedelstaedt chisel. *(2)* Fedi chisels. *(3)* Kirkland chisel. *(4)* Ochenbein chisels. *(5)* Sugarman interproximal file. *(6)* Rongeur forcep.

holes into the gingival tissue to mark the shape and depth of the periodontal pockets in the area to be treated. Especially when they start to bleed slightly, these punch marks act as a guide to indicate the bottom of the pockets and the line of the scalpel incision, the next step in the procedure. The pocket marker resembles a tissue pliers with two tips, a rounded tip and a cutting tip. The rounded tip is inserted into the pocket with the cutting tip on the outside of the gingiva. As the rounded tip is moved along the depth of the pocket, the cutting tip is pressed against it intermittently to cut the tissue, leaving a guide for the scalpel incision.

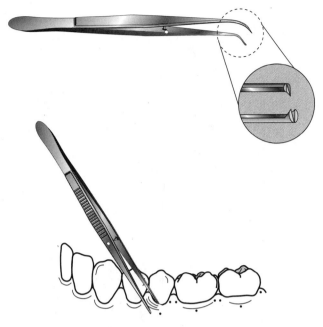

FIGURE 25.15

Periodontal pocket marker is used to make a puncture mark on the gingiva indicating the bottom of a pocket and the line of incision.

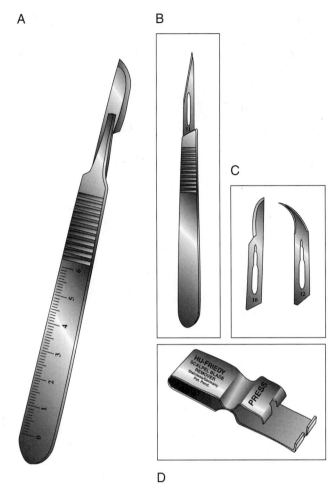

FIGURE 25.16

Scalpel handle and blade styles. *Care must be taken when inserting and removing surgical blades, which are very sharp.* **A,** #15 blade in a scalpel handle. **B,** #11 blade in a different scalpel handle. **C,** #15 blade *(right)* and #12 blade *(left)*. **D,** Blade remover.

As surgery begins, knives (scalpels) are used either to cut into the gingiva to expose the underlying tissue (flap surgery) or to excise gingival tissue (gingivectomy, gingival graft, or biopsy). Scalpels are available with either fixed or removable blades (Figure 25.14 shows fixed-blade scalpels, which are also called gingivectomy knives). After the pocket marker has been used to establish the depths of the periodontal pockets, gingivectomy knives are used to excise and remove the gingival tissue. They are also used to recontour the remaining gingival tissue around the tooth at the end of the surgical procedure (gingivoplasty). The blades are angled and shaped to reach into interdental and posterior areas.

Scalpels with removable, disposable blades are available in different shapes (Figure 25.16). These scalpels usually are used to make releasing incisions in flap operations. The blades are made of surgical carbon steel and come in several sizes and styles. Great care must be taken when inserting the scalpel blade into the handle and when removing it. For safety, a hemostat can be used to hold the scalpel blade when inserting it into the handle, and a scalpel blade remover is helpful for removing it (see Figure 25.16).

Scalpel handles, which hold the removable scalpel blades, are available in a number of designs. They are shaped according to their use. Angled handles are available in addition to the handles shown in Figure 25.16.

Periosteal elevators (Figure 25.17, *A*) are used in flap operations to push the gingival tissue away from the bone after the initial releasing incisions have been made with the scalpel. This procedure exposes the roots of the teeth and the bone, which is usually the purpose of elevating a flap. The operator or dental assistant may also use the instrument to retract soft tissue flaps, allowing good visibility of the operative site. The blades of the periosteal elevator have a blunt cutting edge that is rounded (and suitable for retraction) or pointed at the tip. These devices are primarily double-ended instruments with combination blades, and they are available in a wide variety of sizes and shapes.

Surgical curettes are similar to scaling instruments but are somewhat larger, less flexible, and have heavier cutting blades (Figure 25.17, *B*). Besides being used for scaling and root planing the teeth during periodontal surgery, they also are used for removing soft tissue. For example, in periodontal surgery, after the flap has been elevated, the infected soft tissue lining the periodontal pocket wall (granulation tissue)

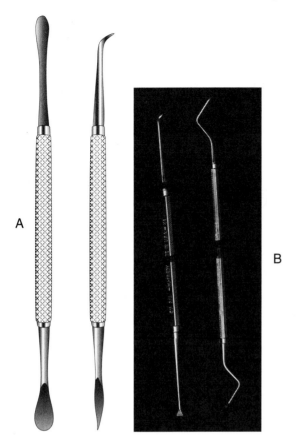

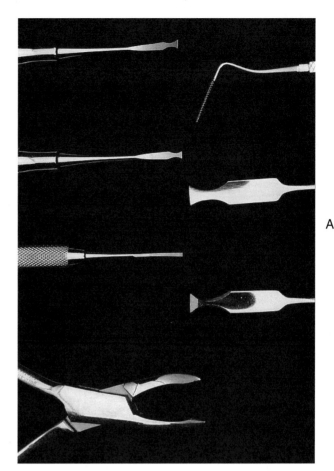

FIGURE 25.17

A, Periosteal elevators with rounded tips *(left)* and pointed tips *(right)*. Only the rounded-tip style should be used for retraction. **B,** Surgical curettes. *(Left)* Molt and *(right)* Prichard.

is removed with surgical curettes. This procedure helps expose the roots of the teeth and the underlying bone, giving the operator a clear view. The roots may have hidden calculus and rough areas, which are now revealed. Periodontal disease may have left the bone with rough, irregular margins or bony pockets in need of recontouring, bone grafting, or regenerative procedures.

Bone Removal Instruments

Many instruments are available for removing and reshaping bone that has various defects as a result of bone resorption (loss). Among these instruments are files, chisels, and rongeurs (see Figure 25.14, *B*). Figure 25.18, *A* presents a closer look at the tips of these instruments.

Periodontal files, also called bone files, are used to smooth rough areas of bone and to remove small areas of osseous tissue, especially in interproximal areas (Figure 25.18, *B*).

Chisels are straight instruments with a flat, beveled cutting blade and a large, broad handle. They usually are used to remove and smooth small areas of bone around the tooth. The chisel is used with a broad, small push stroke with the handle supported by the palm of the hand.

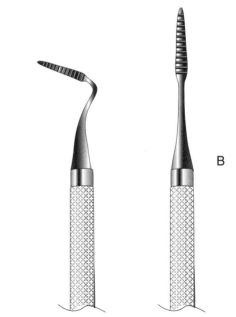

FIGURE 25.18

A, Instruments for removing and reshaping bone. *Top to bottom, right:* Sugarman file, Ochenbein chisels; *left:* #1 and #2 Fedi chisels, Wedelstaedt chisel $^3/_4$, mini-Friedman rongeur. **B,** Interproximal periodontal bone files.

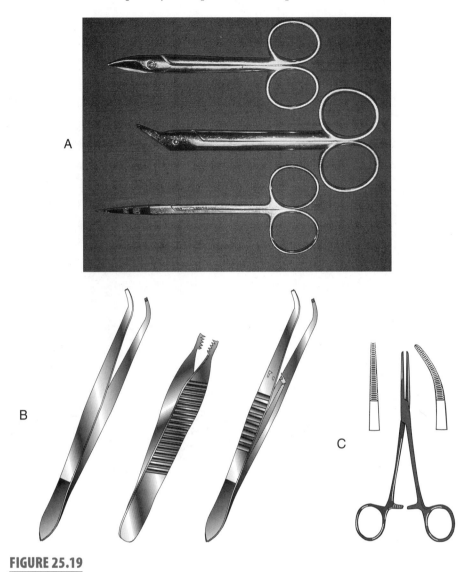

FIGURE 25.19

A, *Top and bottom:* tissue scissors; *middle:* suture scissors. **B,** *Left and center:* nonlocking tissue pliers; *right:* locking tissue pliers. **C,** Hemostats may have either straight or angled serrated beaks.

The rongeurs have a large handle, like an extraction forceps, and two sharp beak tips that are used for removing small pieces of bone. As bone is removed with these instruments, the dental assistant must use sterile water and suction to remove the bone debris from the operative site and maintain a clear field of view for the operator.

Surgical burs are also used for bone removal. As the burs are operated in the slow handpiece, the dental assistant rinses the area with sterile water to ensure adequate cooling and aspiration for removal of tissue remnants. However, if a bur or other bone removal instrument is used to remove osseous tissue that will be used for a bone graft, the dentist must tell the assistant not to rinse or aspirate this material.

Tissue and suture scissors are used to trim tissue and cut sutures (Figure 25.19, *A*). The scissors are small and have fine,

sharp cutting surfaces. Some tissue scissors may have blunt, rounded tips, and they may be straight, angled, or slightly curved to reach difficult areas. Some scissors have one serrated blade to eliminate slippage when cutting, and others have narrow beaks for removing interproximal tissue and sutures.

Instruments for Handling Flaps

If periodontal tissues are to heal properly after surgery, tissue damage must be minimized by manipulating soft tissue flaps very gently. The dentist takes care in using the scalpel, curettes, files, chisels, rongeurs, burs, and scissors, and the dental assistant must do likewise when handling the following instruments for flap management.

Tissue pliers and forceps are used to grasp, retract, and secure the periodontal tissues to provide greater visibility during

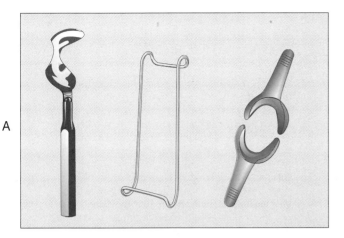

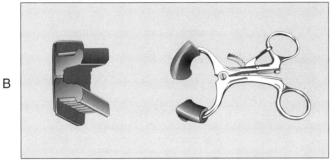

FIGURE 25.20

A, Tongue and cheek retractors. **B,** Mouth props; rubber bite block *(left)*, and molt mouth prop *(right)*.

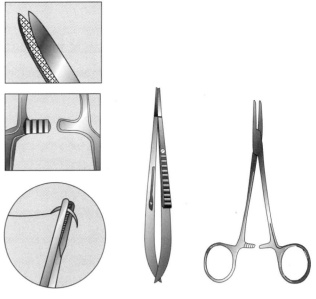

FIGURE 25.21

Needle holders *(right)* and illustration of serrations, lock, and a needle in a holder *(left)*.

surgery (Figure 25.19, *B*). They are also used to grasp bone and tissue fragments. The pliers may be straight or slightly curved with serrated working tips that help to grasp the tissue. The forceps have the appearance of locking scissors or hemostats.

Hemostats, which are similar to needle holders, are used to grasp and hold soft tissue and bone particles for removal (Figure 25.19, *C*). They should not be used on tissues not destined for removal, because this would cause unnecessary tissue damage. Hemostats have straight or angled serrated beaks in various lengths. The handles have a multiposition ratchet to provide controlled grip pressure and release.

Other Instruments

Tongue and Cheek Retractors and Mouth Props As their names imply, tongue and cheek retractors are devices used to pull back the tongue and cheek and hold them out of the way while the operator is working in the mouth (Figure 25.20, *A*). Retractors are made of plastic or metal and are available in various shapes and sizes for children or adults. Some retractors are used for intraoral photography. Rubber mouth props (Figure 25.20, *B*) and mouth gags are used to make sure that the mouth stays open during treatment. These props are also sized to fit a child or an adult. Molt mouth gags are ratchet gags designed to lock the prop in place to prevent slipping.

The needle holder, which resembles a hemostat, is used to solidly grasp and hold the needle in place during suturing (Figure 25.21). The needle holder must prevent any movement of the needle. The holder is available in several lengths and designs and contains a groove for the needle. The holder tips are serrated, and the handles are interlocking.

ROLE OF THE DENTAL ASSISTANT IN PERIODONTAL SURGERY

Box 25.11 outlines the various duties of the dental assistant in periodontal surgery in the approximate order in which they are usually performed.

Surgery usually involves opening or removing the gingival tissues to expose the roots of the teeth and remove infected soft tissues. In some cases the bone is also exposed and may also require corrective surgery. Tissues and synthetic (artificial) bone and membranes (barriers) may be placed in or over the tissues to regenerate periodontal structures that are diseased or have resorbed. The gingiva is then repositioned and sutured so that the periodontal pockets are eliminated and the healed tissues will be easier to keep clean. As a result of the surgery, the gingival margin may be lower on the tooth when it heals, exposing more tooth structure and possibly creating some spaces between the teeth. This does not always occur, but if it does, the appearance of the teeth may be slightly altered and some root sensitivity may be present for a brief period while the tissues heal.

Box 25.11

Duties of the Dental Assistant in Periodontal Surgery

The following are the dental assistant's duties in peri-odontal surgical procedures.

Preparing the operatory:

1. Use a head bonnet, safety glasses, mask, and sterile gloves.
2. Place surgical kits on the surgical tray and open them:
   a. Scaling and root planing kit
   b. Primary and supplemental surgical kits
3. Within each kit, arrange the instruments in the order the dentist will be using them; remove water syringe tips from the kit and place them on the water syringes on the unit; cover them with plastic sleeves.
4. Place disposable scalpel blades on the surgical tray.
5. Place Cavitron tip, sterile gauze, and sutures on the surgical tray; do not open the sutures packet.
6. Assemble the suction apparatus (tubing, plastic or metal tip) and place a plastic sleeve over the suction apparatus.
7. Put sterile water in the sterile water bowl and put it with the operative armamentarium.
8. Put the syringe needles and needle protector on the surgical tray with the anesthetic carpules.
9. Put the topical anesthetic on a cotton applicator and place on the surgical tray.
10. Insert a sterile, high-speed handpiece onto the unit, cover with a plastic sleeve, and place a sterile bur block on the surgical tray.
11. Tape a small biohazard bag to the assistant's cart.
12. Place tongue blades and additional cotton applicators on the surgical tray; put petroleum jelly on one tongue blade, which will be used to periodically moisten the patient's lips. The other cotton applicators are used to place periodontal dressing material.
13. Put some antimicrobial solution in a plastic cup and place it on the assistant's cart. During surgery, periodically moisten a piece of gauze with the solution and clean the patient's lips and tongue.
14. Put a sterile towel over all instruments, plastic sleeves on light handles, and a protective plastic covering over chair buttons.
15. Put periodontal dressing paste and a mixing pad, a disposable patient head bonnet, napkin, alligator chain clip, and sterile safety glasses on the countertop.
16. Remove your gloves.

Assisting in surgery:

1. Bring the patient into the operatory and seat the person.
2. Place the head bonnet, safety glasses, and napkin on the patient.
3. Take the person's temperature, pulse, and blood pressure and record them in the patient's chart.
4. Have the patient rinse the mouth with antimicrobial solution for 30 seconds, then suction the mouth.
5. Put on a surgical mask and sterile gloves. Remove the sterile towel covering the instruments and place it on the patient. Give the dentist the topical anesthetic on a cotton applicator and retract soft tissue as needed with a mirror.
6. After the dentist places the topical anesthetic, take the applicator from the dentist. Place the appropriate needle with a needle protector on a syringe; slightly loosen the needle and then hand the dentist the syringe. Place the needle holder with protector on the surgical tray and take the used carpules from the dentist. Place the used carpules in the biohazard bag and give the dentist fresh carpules as needed.
7. The dentists uses a needle sweep to place the syringe back on the surgical tray, with the needle and holder loosely attached to the syringe.
8. Wait for the anesthetic to take effect
9. Hand the dentist the surgical instruments as required while retracting and suctioning as needed.
10. Periodically irrigate the surgical site and the patient's mouth with sterile water and suction as needed.
11. Periodically moisten the patient's lips and cheeks with gauze moistened with antimicrobial solution and with petroleum jelly on a tongue blade.
12. Periodically put blood-saturated gauze in the biohazard bag.
13. If a handpiece is requested, insert the desired burr and hand the handpiece to the dentist; change the bur if requested. During use of the bur, retract the soft tissue and periodically use a syringe filled with sterile water to moisten the area, control heat, and maintain a clear visual field
14. When surgery is complete, dip sterile gauze in sterile water and place the gauze on the operative site; hold it in place with firm pressure for a few minutes to approximate gingival tissues and to control bleeding.
15. Open the suture materials as required.
16. Retract the soft tissues and suction periodically as suturing proceeds.
17. When requested, cut the sutures a few millimeters from the tied knot; suction cut suture material as necessary.
18. When the suturing is complete, place gauze on the site to control bleeding and to dry the teeth.
19. Mix and place a periodontal dressing if requested.
20. After placing the periodontal dressing, use water to lightly irrigate the patient's mouth, including the pack. Check to make sure that no bleeding is occurring through the pack. Clean the patient's face and lips with gauze moistened with sterile water.
21. Remove your gloves and place them in the biohazard bag. Activate and place an ice pack on the

Box 25.11—Cont'd.

Duties of the Dental Assistant in Periodontal Surgery

patient's face opposite the operative site if the dentist so instructs. Retake and record the patient's temperature, pulse, and blood pressure.

22. Remove the patient's head bonnet and safety glasses

23. Give the patient sterile gauze and provide postoperative instructions orally and in writing. Confirm that the patient has the necessary prescriptions or that they have been called into the patient's pharmacy. Confirm the next appointment, and give the patient an extra ice pack to use later if the dentist requests it.

24. Dismiss the patient and always commend the person for excellent cooperation by saying something such as, "You've been a great patient!"

25. Clean and disinfect the operatory and prepare it for the next patient. Sterilize the used instruments.

The patient also may have some temporary loosening of the teeth and mild to moderate postoperative pain for a short period, but the latter problem can be controlled with medication.

SPECIFIC PERIODONTAL SURGICAL PROCEDURES

Except for the gingival graft, all the procedures described below are aimed at reducing the depth of the periodontal pockets.

Gingivectomy

A gingivectomy is a basic surgical procedure for simply cutting away excessive gingival tissue (Figure 25.22). This can be performed with gingivectomy knives or a dental laser. Removal of the tissue overgrowth eliminates the periodontal pockets that have developed, making it easier for the patient to keep the teeth and gingival tissues clean and healthy. The procedure also eliminates a "gummy" smile but does not increase the clinical attachment level.

Periodontal Flap Surgery

Periodontal flap surgery can be used alone or combined with other techniques, such as osseous surgery, guided tissue

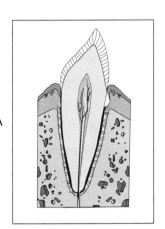
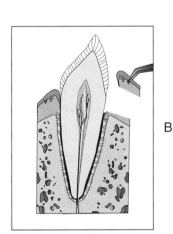
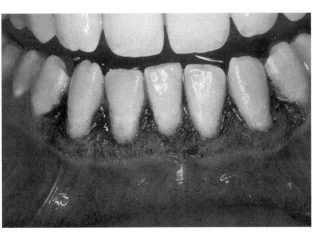
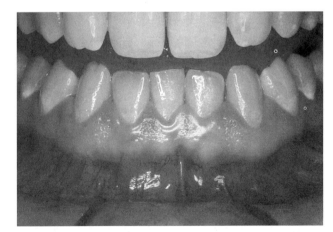

FIGURE 25.22

Gingivectomy performed with a dental laser. **A,** Excess tissue and a gingival pocket are evident on the facial area of the tooth root. **B,** Redundant tissue is removed, eliminating the gingival pocket. **C,** Affected area before surgery. **D,** Area after surgery. (Courtesy Dr. John Dodge.)

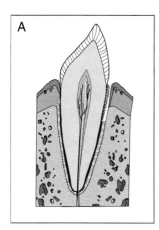

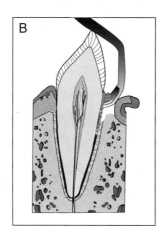

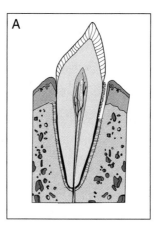

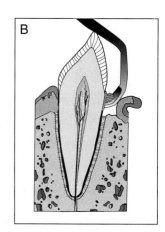

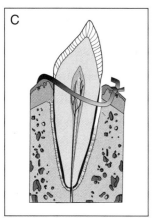

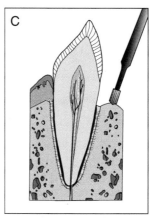

FIGURE 25.23

Periodontal flap surgery. **A,** Calculus can be seen embedded in a deep pocket on the facial surface of the tooth root. **B,** Flap is reflected, allowing access for removal of plaque and calculus. **C,** Flap is apically repositioned on the bone, eliminating the pocket.

FIGURE 25.24

Osseous (bone) surgery. **A,** Periodontal pocket, bone destruction, and a crater can be seen on the facial side of the tooth. **B,** Flap is reflected, and plaque and calculus are removed. **C,** Bone is recontoured, eliminating the crater.

regeneration, and bone grafts. With flap surgery, the gingiva is cut and then separated and lifted from the tooth but not removed. This creates a gingival flap of tissue and provides access to the deep, infected periodontal pockets and bone tissue, allowing the dentist to remove plaque, calculus, and diseased tissue from the roots and pockets around the tooth that were not otherwise accessible (Figure 25.23, *A* and *B*). When it is replaced and sutured back in place, the flap tissue may be positioned apically (a little lower on the tooth), which helps eliminate the periodontal pocket that was there (Figure 25.23, *C*).

Osseous (Bone) Surgery

Osseous surgery is done as part of the periodontal flap surgery described above. It is used when part of the bone has been destroyed by periodontal infection, leaving periodontal pockets, bony craters, and other defects requiring surgical correction (Figure 25.24, *A*). After a flap has been reflected

to obtain access to the periodontal pockets and diseased bone, the plaque and calculus are first removed from the root of the tooth (Figure 25.24, *B*). The bone is then recontoured, which removes the craters and rough, irregular margins (Figure 25.24, *C*). The gingival tissues are positioned and sutured back over the reshaped bone, which allows the tissues to heal in a pattern that gives better access for proper daily home care. The procedure is aimed at reducing the pocket depth and raising the clinical attachment level.

Bone Graft

In bone grafting, the gingival flap is first reflected, and then tiny pieces of bone from human or synthetic (artificial) sources are placed in the areas of resorbed bone (Figure 25.25). In some cases antibiotics are mixed in with the bone material to prevent infection. The bone fragments serve as a platform for growth and attachment of new bone and attachment, which supports and stabilizes the weakened tooth. Medical-grade plaster of paris and other tissues or mem-

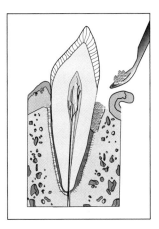

FIGURE 25.25

Bone graft material is placed in a bony pocket.

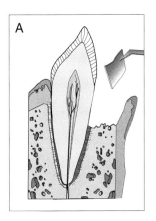
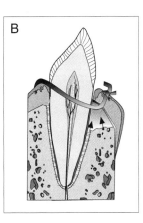

FIGURE 25.26

Guided tissue regeneration. **A,** Flap is reflected, exposing the bony defect and a membrane. Membrane barrier is placed over the bone and tooth. **B,** Arrows show the eventual growth of a new attachment apparatus.

branes (barriers) may be placed over the bone graft to help hold it in place and to prevent the gingival tissues from growing into the area, which would interfere with healing. Finally, the gingival flap is repositioned and sutured in place.

Guided Tissue Regeneration

Guided tissue **regeneration** is a new periodontal procedure

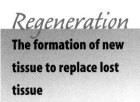

Regeneration

The formation of new tissue to replace lost tissue

in which an artificial barrier membrane is strategically placed in the periodontium to help new attachment tissue grow into the pockets created by disease. First, a gingival flap is raised, exposing the bony defects, and all infected tissue is removed (Figure 25.26, *A*). A special membrane is then placed over the defect (Figure 25.26, *B*). This membrane acts as a physical barrier that prevents the gingival tissue from growing into the area and allows new supporting fibers and bone to grow into the diseased area under the barrier. This process eliminates pockets and establishes a new attachment apparatus to strengthen and support the weakened tooth. Connective tissue from a human donor also can be used as a barrier material for this procedure. Guided tissue regeneration sometimes is used in conjunction with bone grafting to help prevent the gingival tissue from moving into the space where the bone graft was placed.

Gingival Graft

The surgical procedures described previously usually are directed at eliminating periodontal pockets. In most such cases, esthetics is not the primary concern. With a gingival graft procedure, however, improving the appearance may

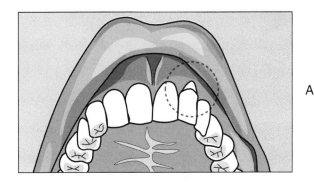

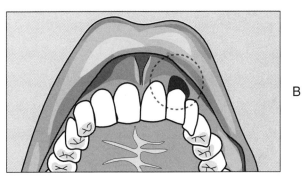

FIGURE 25.27

Gingival graft. **A,** Recession and exposed root are seen on tooth #10. **B,** Gingival graft covers the defect and prevents further recession.

be a major objective. For this reason, this type of surgery often is performed on teeth in the anterior region of the mouth. Because of periodontal disease or toothbrush abrasion, a tooth or a group of teeth may show gingival recession (Figure 25.27). To cover the exposed root of the

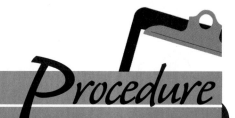

Box 25.12

Procedure for Periodontal Surgery

The procedure described below is for a periodontal flap with a bone, plaster, and dermis graft on tooth #11

Preparation:

1. The primary surgical instrument setup and a supplemental tray is prepared. The supplemental tray should include the water irrigator, a bowl of sterile water, and a cup of mouth rinse for defogging mirror.
2. The scaling and root planing setup tray is prepared; it includes anesthetic carpules, a syringe needle and protector, gauze, an anesthetic syringe, a mirror, a periodontal probe, a Nabors probe, explorers, Gracey curettes, a universal curette, and sickle scalers.
3. The operator, patient, and assistant are positioned properly to begin surgery.

Surgical procedure:

1. After obtaining anesthesia and making the initial incisions with the scalpel, the operator elevates a gingival flap while the assistant suctions blood and debris with the aspirator tip.
2. The assistant periodically flushes the aspirator tip with sterile water to keep it clean and clear.
3. The assistant retracts the cheek with the mirror and aspirates the area.
4. The assistant holds a 2×2-inch sponge while the operator curettes the soft tissue.
5. The operator periodically dries the tissue with sponges while the assistant aspirates the area.

6. In this case, a severe bony defect exists on teeth #11 and #12. The facial and distal portion of the root of tooth #11 is almost completely exposed. Although the tooth has a poor prognosis, the patient has requested treatment in an attempt to save the tooth.
7. The assistant places the contents of an antibiotic capsule in the dish with the synthetic bone graft material.
8. The assistant adds saline to the contents of the dish and mixes the solution.
9. The assistant periodically moistens the patient's lips and mouth with a 2×2 sponge dampened with water.
10. The assistant helps the operator place the bone graft/antibiotic mixture in the defect. *Caution: The assistant must not suction in this area to avoid displacing the graft.*
11. The operator fills the defect with bone graft material.
12. The assistant adds saline to the calcium sulfate material (medical-grade plaster of paris) and mixes it.
13. The operator places the mixture over the graft to stabilize it.
14. Dermis (connective tissue) is removed from the sterile package, measured to the appropriate size with a calibrated probe, cut, and placed over the defect.
15. Several layers of dermis are used to cover the defect.
16. The operator places the sutures while the assistant suctions and retracts with a mirror.
17. The assistant freshens up the patient, explains the postoperative instructions, and then dismisses the patient.

tooth and prevent further recession, a piece of soft tissue is removed from some other place in the mouth (usually the palate) and the "new" tissue is placed and sutured over the recessed area.

PROCEDURES FOR PERIODONTAL SURGERY

Box 25.12 presents the procedures involved in periodontal surgery. Figure 25.28 shows the surgical instrument setup (primary and supplemental trays).

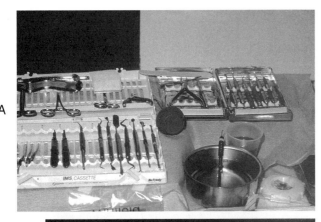

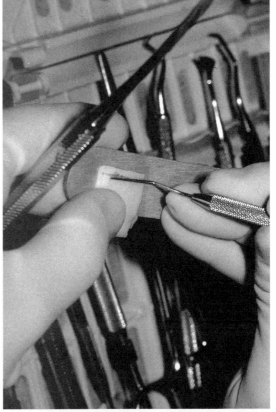

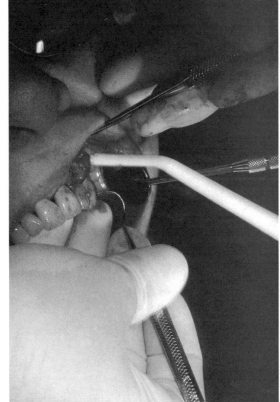

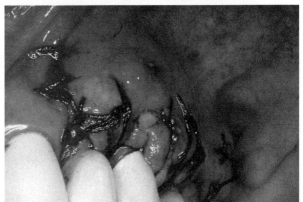

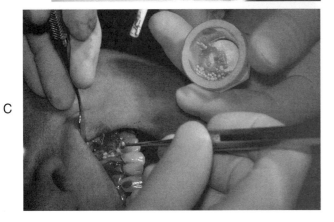

FIGURE 25.28

A, Surgical instrument setup (primary and supplemental trays) with water irrigator, bowl of sterile water, and cup of mouth rinse for use as a mirror defogging agent. **B,** Assistant retracts the cheek with the mirror and aspirates the area. **C,** Operator places the bone graft/antibiotic mixture into the defect. *The assistant should not suction in this area to avoid displacing the graft.* **D,** Tissue is measured to the appropriate size with a calibrated probe. **E,** Sutures are placed.

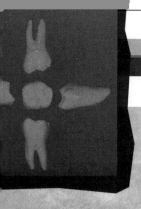

Points for Review

■ The differences between a normal and a diseased periodontium

■ The etiology and prevention of periodontal disease

■ The elements of the periodontal examination

■ The instruments used in periodontal examination and treatment

■ Common periodontal diagnoses

■ Periodontal treatment procedures, including surgery

Self-Study Questions

1. What is the primary cause of inflammatory periodontal disease?
   a. Calculus
   b. Plaque
   c. Smoking
   d. Diet
   e. Stress

2. How can most periodontal diseases be prevented?
   a. Regular professional prophylaxis daily
   b. Use of mouthwash
   c. Regular oral hygiene
   d. Proper diet
   e. A and c

3. What structure is part of the attachment apparatus?
   a. Periodontal ligament
   b. Gingiva
   c. Dentogingival junction
   d. Tooth
   e. Alveolar mucosa

4. What is the small portion of the gingiva that surrounds the tooth called?
   a. Gingival groove
   b. Attached gingiva
   c. Alveolar mucosa
   d. Free gingiva
   e. Mucogingival junction

5. What is the part of the gingiva that fills the interproximal space called?
   a. Interdental groove
   b. Interdental papilla
   c. Gingival sulcus
   d. Mucogingival junction
   e. Dentogingival junction

6. What is the shallow crevice that surrounds the tooth called?
   a. Gingival sulcus
   b. Fissure
   c. Interdental groove
   d. Interdental papilla
   e. Pit

7. What is the gingival connective tissue that contains gingival fibers, blood vessels, and nerves called?
   a. Attached gingiva
   b. Mucosa
   c. Lamina propria
   d. Alveolar mucosa
   e. Collagen

8. What is the radiographic term for the alveolar bone proper?
   a. Outer cribriform plate
   b. Lamina dura
   c. Cancellous bone
   d. Spongy bone
   e. Alveolar process

9. The periodontium has receptors for pain, touch, pressure, and proprioceptors.
   a. True
   b. False

10. Systemic factors responsible for periodontal disease include plaque, calculus, and faulty dentistry.
    a. True
    b. False

11. Adults with the highest levels of periodontal disease tend to be smokers.
    a. True
    b. False

12. Bacterial plaque and calculus are the only materials that accumulate on tooth surfaces.
    a. True
    b. False

13. What common type of disease is associated with supragingival plaque formation?
    a. Periodontitis
    b. Gingivitis
    c. Abscess
    d. Pericoronitis
    e. Acute necrotizing ulcerative gingivitis

14. What is considered the category for prevention of disease?
    a. Cause-related measures
    b. Corrective measures
    c. Maintenance measures
    d. Surgical measures
    e. None of the above

15. What is the primary purpose of periodontal surgery?
    a. To correct problems relating to removal of plaque and calculus
    b. To remove pockets
    c. Esthetics
    d. To improve crown-root ratios
    e. C and d

16. Many states allow dental assistants to place and remove periodontal dressings.
    a. True
    b. False

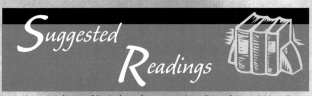

Suggested Readings

American Academy of Periodontology, American Dental Association, Procter & Gamble: Periodontal screening and recording training program, Chicago, 1992, ADA.

American Academy of Periodontology: *Periodontal disease management*, Chicago, 1994.

American Academy of Periodontology: World workshop in periodontics, *Ann Periodontol*, 1996.

Carranza FA, Newman MG: *Clinical periodontology*, ed 8, Philadelphia, 1996, WB Saunders.

Carranza FA, Perry DA: *Clinical periodontology for dental hygienists*, Philadelphia, 1986, WB Saunders.

Hardin JF: *Clark's clinical dentistry*, vol 3, Periodontics/oral and maxillofacial surgery, St Louis, 1997, Mosby.

Genco RJ, Goldman HM, Cohen DW: *Contemporary periodontics*, St Louis, 1990, Mosby.

Harris NO, Christen AG: *Primary preventive dentistry*, ed 5, Norwalk, Conn, 1999, Appleton & Lange.

Lindhe J: *Textbook of clinical periodontology*, ed 2, Copenhagen, 1989, Munksgaard.

Rateitschak KH: *Color atlas of dental medicine*, vol 1, Periodontology, ed 2, New York, 1989, Thieme Medical Publishers.

Wilkins EM: *Clinical practice of the dental hygienist*, ed 8, Philadelphia, 1999, Lea & Febiger.

Chapter 26

The Professional Orthodontic Assistant

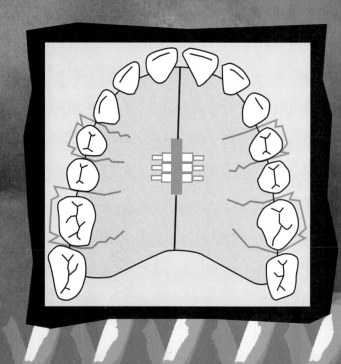

Chapter Outline

Learning Objectives

On completion of Chapter 26, the student should be able to do the following:

- Define key terms.
- Identify the orthodontic instruments and equipment.
- Identify various orthodontic appliances.
- List the infection control procedures for an orthodontic office.

Key Terms

Angulation	Cephalometrics	Orthodontics
Appliance	Malocclusion	Occlude
Articulate	Model	Rotate

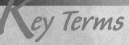

ORTHODONTICS

In the modern **orthodontic** practice the dental assistant may, where state laws provide, perform all the tasks involved in the orthodontic procedure. This allows the dental assistant to work more in a one-on-one interaction with the patient. Less use of four-handed dentistry disciplines would be applied. In addition to being involved in the task of placing **appliances**, the orthodontic assistant has the unique opportunity for the education and motivation of the patients concerning the nature of their diagnosis and treatment. Assurance and understanding at the beginning of treatment will help decrease the patients apprehension and will prepare them for the treatment that lies ahead. The dental assistant is usually responsible for presenting visual aids and demonstrations on proper wear and care of the appliances, as well as proper brushing techniques. The dental assistant may also provide instruction on the use and wear of removable appliances, headgear, facemasks, and elastics.

Orthodontics
The specialty of dentistry that deals with the causes, prevention, and correction of irregularities or malocclusion of the teeth and jaws

Appliance
A mechanical device for changing tooth position

Many general practice dentists provide a broad range of orthodontic treatment for patients. Therefore, dental assistants need to have a good understanding of orthodontic procedures and a certain level of skills in orthodontic treatment. Individual state dental practice laws regulate what the dentist can delegate to dental assistants in the area of taking impressions for working **models** and more advanced orthodontic procedures. It is important for dental assistants to know what orthodontic procedures they can perform in their state. Some more advanced functions include orthodontic banding, bonding, debonding, removing and retying arch wires, and orthodontic laboratory procedures.

Model
A replica of the mouth, usually in plaster or stone

Need for Orthodontic Treatment

Orthodontics has been described by Robert H.W. Strang as "that science which has for its objective the prevention and correction of **malocclusion** of the teeth and associated dentofacial disharmonies." Normal occlusion may be described as the normal relationship of the occlusal planes with the bones of the face and jaw in normally functioning tissues. Malocclusions are any variation from the norm. These variations can be minor or severe.

Most patients feel their greatest need for treatment is to achieve cosmetic improvements in facial appearance. Malocclusion can strongly influence a person's self-esteem and positive feelings about himself or herself.

Another need for orthodontic treatment is oral function, which may be compromised in all aspects if the teeth do not meet (**occlude**). There can be difficulty in chewing when only a few teeth meet or **articulate** together. Swallowing can become difficult when there are jaw discrepancies or TMJ (temporomandibular joint) dysfunction. TMJ pain is often caused by muscle fatigue and spasm, which usually correlates with the patient holding their jaw forward, laterally, clinching or grinding their teeth. All of these can be triggered by minor malocclusion.

Malocclusion
Poor positioning of the teeth so that they do not meet correctly, interfering with efficiency

Occlude
To close or bring the teeth together

Articulate
In orthodontics, to place teeth in their proper "bite" position for esthetic and functional purposes

Perhaps one of the most important needs for orthodontic treatment is good oral health. With malocclusion it is more difficult for the patient to clean his or her teeth, therefore the caries rate and health of the periodontium can be affected by their inability to care properly for the teeth.

Types of Orthodontic Treatment

Three types or phases of orthodontic treatment are preventive, interceptive, and corrective.

Preventive

Preventive orthodontics is the phase of treatment concerned with eliminating irregularities and malposition in the developing dentofacial structure. This includes the control of caries, early detection of genetic and congenital abnormalities and maintaining space for erupting permanent teeth. Also included in this category is the correction of bad oral habits such as thumb-sucking, mouth breathing, tongue-thrusting, and bruxism (Chapter 24).

Interceptive

Interceptive treatment signifies the interruption of a condition before it develops into a problem or correcting problems while they are developing. Some primary conditions and measures used to correct them are listed next.

Missing Tooth

If a tooth is missing, that space needs to be maintained for the erupting permanent tooth. Teeth on either side tend to drift into the opening, closing the space for erupting teeth. A space maintainer can be made that will preserve the space or move drifted teeth apart (see Figure 24.9). If the condition exists where there has been a loss of primary dentition on both sides of the arch, a lingual holding arch may be used to keep the space available for permanent dentition that has not yet erupted. Usually the lingual holding arch is used to hold space in the area of the first and second permanent bicuspids but can be for other areas of the dentition also. The lingual holding arch may be fabricated with loops in the wire just mesial to the solder joint and bands. This would allow the dentist to make adjustments to the arch wire or to activate it.

Crossbite

Single tooth crossbite is when only one tooth in the dentition is erupting or has erupted into the incorrect position, such as maxillary central incisor erupting lingual to the mandibular central and lateral incisor. This condition can be intercepted with a removable finger spring appliance to push the incisor forward (Figure 26.1, *A*). Another example is when the lower anterior teeth are trapped in front of the upper anterior teeth causing the lower jaw to slide forward and in front of the upper jaw. This can be treated at an early age with a bite jump appliance (Figure 26.1, *B*).

A posterior crossbite is when the buccal aspect of the maxillary teeth are positioned inside the mandibular teeth. This is a result of a narrowing of the maxillary arch sometimes as a result of a prolonged sucking habit. Interception of the posterior crossbite may be accomplished with fixed or removable appliances. This condition may be treated as soon as a child has complete primary dentition. Sometimes dental interferences can cause mandibular teeth to shift into crossbite. Posterior crossbites may be treated with bilateral maxillary expansion appliances.

Fixed Appliances In the fixed appliance category there is a W-arch and the quad helix. Both are made of wire soldered to bands that are cemented to molars. The appliances are activated with bends until the crossbite is corrected. This treatment may be followed by retention with a removable appliance (Figure 26.2). When the posterior crossbite is a skeletal as opposed to a dental condition the treatment of choice is to use the RPE (rapid palatial expander) to open the midpalatine suture. This transverse maxillary expansion is best accomplished during or before adolescence. The RPE is a fixed appliance using a heavy jack-screw soldered to two molar bands and two premolar bands. After about 10 days of activation, a large diastema can be seen between the maxillary central incisors. The expansion is usually completed within 2 weeks and the screw is tied off with a brass separating wire to hold the expansion until the palate has had sufficient time to fill in the suture (Figure 26.3).

Removable Appliance A removable appliance, which is used for posterior crossbite, is a split-plate appliance, incorporating retentive clasps, a skeleton type expansion screw and an acrylic base. The removable appliance is sometimes not as successful as the fixed because it depends on patient compliance. (Figure 26.4). Some of these springs include the following:

- Springs: Stainless steel shapes designed to move and **rotate** the teeth, usually to the mesial, distal, or facial. Orthodontic springs are named for their use and shape.

Rotate
The movement of a tooth in a circular direction.

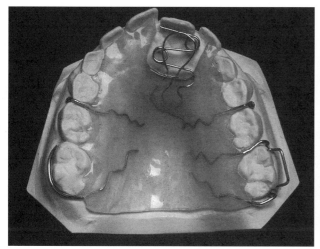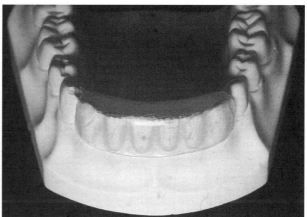

A

B

FIGURE 26.1

A, Removable appliance with a finger spring. **B,** Facial view of an anterior biteblock.

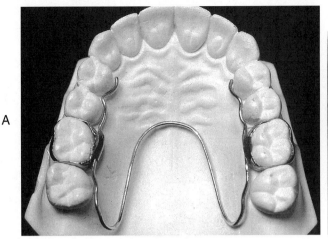

FIGURE 26.2

Fixed expansion appliances. **A**, W arch appliance. **B**, Quad Helix appliance.

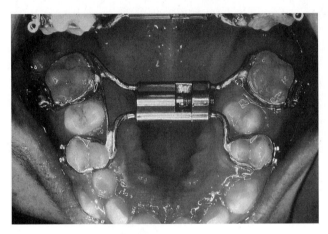

FIGURE 26.3

Rapid palatal expander.

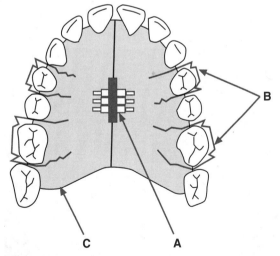

FIGURE 26.4

Removable expansion appliance. **A**, Skeleton type screw expands 5 to 7 mm. **B**, Adams clasps. **C**, Acrylic base with slot cut anterior and posterior to the screw.

- Overlapping springs: To round out and guide the incisors and anterior teeth forward.
- S-springs: To correct tooth rotation and to stabilize tooth movement.
- Finger springs: To keep teeth from drifting and to move teeth mesially or distally.
- Mousetrap springs: To align incisors or to round out the anterior arch.
- Springs with helixes: An S-shaped spring used to move the teeth with light pressure.
- Expansion screws: Used for tooth movement and expansion of the maxillary arch. Expansion screws include the transverse, sagittal, one-tooth, micro screw, fan-type, and three-way.
- Acrylic bite plates: Anterior bite plates and posterior bite plates are used to open the bit and cause the posterior teeth not to occlude.

Openbite

An anterior openbite is when the posterior teeth are in contact and the anterior teeth are bowed open leaving the incisors, cuspids, and sometimes the premolars unable to come together. This condition is usually caused by a habit such as thumb- or lip-sucking; however, tongue thrust swallowing is often an adaptation to make a seal because the openbite is not always the cause of it (see Chapter 24).

Corrective

Corrective orthodontics is appliance therapy by primarily mechanical means. Surgical and psychological methods may also be employed. Corrective treatment is indicated for the following reasons: (1) disharmony between teeth and the skeleton, (2) malocclusion, and (3) bad oral habits.

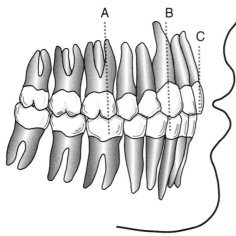

FIGURE 26.5

Characteristics of dentition. **A,** Class I molar relationship.
B, Crown angulation. **C,** Crown inclination.

Classification of Occlusion and Malocclusion

There have been many systems developed to classify occlusion. The root of the word occlusion is *occlusio,* which means to close or bring together. In a normal, healthy mouth the maxillary and mandibular teeth will come together. However, many patients have malocclusion and the teeth do not come together.

In the 1960s, Dr. Lawrence F. Andrews studied hundreds of people with "normal dentition" and from the study of 120 people identified six common characteristics of the dentition that could be considered normal occlusion. These characteristics are considered the Six Keys to Normal Occlusion and are the goals of orthodontic treatment.

1 Class I molar relationship (Figure 26.5, *A*): The mesial-buccal cusp of the maxillary first molar occludes opposite the buccal groove the mandibular first molar.

Angulation

Moving the tooth root backward or forward to correct the tooth angle

2 Crown **angulation** or tip (Figure 26.5, *B*): The gingival portion of the long axis of each crown is distal to the incisal or occlusal portion of the axis.

3 Crown inclination or torque (Figure 26.5, *C*): The incisal portion of the maxillary central and lateral incisor crowns are labial to the gingival portion of the tooth crown. However, for the cuspid and posterior teeth, the incisal and occlusal portion of the tooth crown is lingual to the gingival portion of the tooth crown.

4 No rotation: Teeth are not rotated. Rotated teeth take up more or less space than they should.

5 No spaces: All teeth have tight contact points with no space interproximally.

6 Flat to slight curve of Spee: A flat curve of Spee represents normal occlusion, whereas a deep curve provides less space for the upper teeth.

Normal Occlusion

Normal occlusion is the accepted relationship of the teeth in one arch to those teeth in the opposing arch when the teeth are in centric occlusion. When classifying deviations from normal occlusion, the following characteristics are considered:

- The overjet and overbite of the anterior teeth (Figure 26.6, *A*)
- The relationship of one arch to the other
- The relationship of all the teeth in their normal position
- The axial position of all the teeth of the arch

In the Angle system, the permanent first molars were selected for identifying the normal relationship of the mandibular to the maxillary arch. The reason for this is because they are the first permanent molars to erupt, they have long roots, and they tend to be in a stable position in the arch.

When the teeth are in occlusion and the jaws are at rest, the mandibular arch is in normal occlusion or mesiodistal relationship to the maxillary arch if the following apply:

1 The mesiobuccal cusp of the upper permanent first molar occludes in the buccal groove of the lower first molar and the rest of the teeth are aligned.

2 The mesiolingual cusp of the upper permanent first molar occludes with the occlusal fossa of the lower permanent first molar.

It is important to note that it is the relationship of the permanent first molars that determines classification (Figure 26.6, *B-D*).

Class I Malocclusion

There is a normal Class I molar relationship but the teeth are crowded in the rest of the arch.

Class II Malocclusion

The lower arch and the body of the mandible are in a distal relationship to the upper arch by half the width of the permanent first molar. In other words the mesiobuccal cusp of the upper first molar occludes in the space between the lower second premolar and the mesial cusp of the lower first molar. Often this causes the maxillary anterior teeth to look like they protrude.

Class II, Division 1

The lower lip is tucked behind the upper incisors and the lips are usually flat and parted. The upper lip is drawn up over protruding maxillary anterior teeth and appears short. The upper incisors extend beyond (slanted outward) the normal overlap of the incisal edge of the lower incisors.

Class II, Division 2

The jaw, molar, and cuspid relationships are the same as described for Class II malocclusion. This relationship places the maxillary central incisors close to a normal position or they may be tipped slightly lingually (slanted inward). The maxillary lateral incisors may be tipped labially and mesially and they often overlap the central incisors.

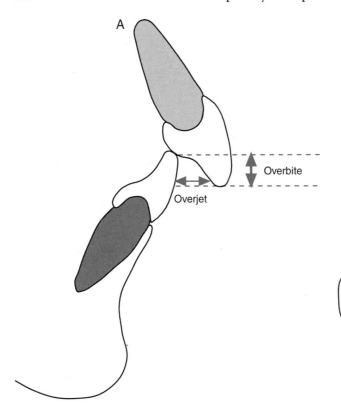

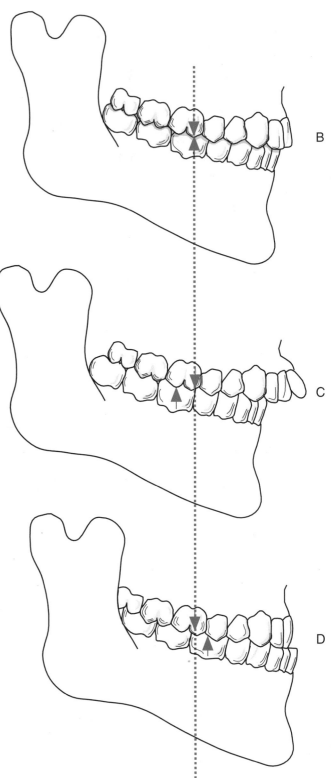

FIGURE 26.6

A, Overjet and overbite. Classification of malocclusions: **B,** Class I. **C,** Class II. **D,** Class III.

Class III Malocclusion

The mandibular arch and the body of the mandible are in mesial relationship to the maxillary teeth. This frequently makes it appear that the mandible protrudes. The mesiobuccal cusp of the upper first molar occludes in the space between the distal cusp of the lower permanent first molar and the mesial cusp of the lower permanent second molar. For malocclusion to be Class III, the body of the mandibular arch must be large or positioned mesially to the maxilla.

Orthodontic Appliances

Orthodontic appliances can greatly improve malocclusion and other types of improper tooth positioning. Patients can enjoy efficient mastication, improved appearance, and greater personal satisfaction and well-being through corrective bands or braces, patient dedication, and staff support. Throughout the orthodontic treatment it is important that the teeth as well as the appliance are clean and that good eating habits are maintained. Many appliances can be fabricated to meet the requirements of each patient. Various types of appliances will be described in this chapter.

Splints

Splints are used for temporomandibular joint dysfunction. This condition is caused when the temporomandibular joint

relationship does not match with the occlusion of the teeth. The teeth may not occlude properly and the muscles may become sore. This malocclusion can cause headaches, clicking jaw movements, sinus pain, neck and shoulder pain, and eventually degenerative joint disease. Splints are also used to prevent bruxism.

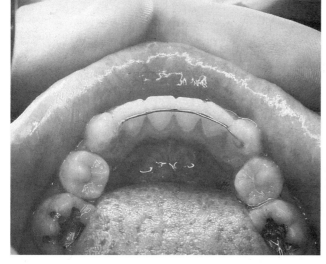
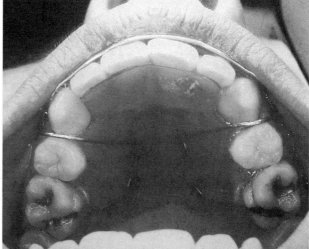
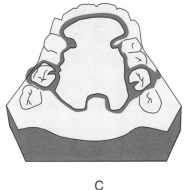
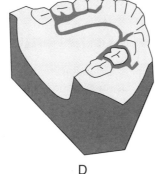

FIGURE 26.7

A, Bonded lingual arch retainer. **B,** Hawley retainer. **C,** Upper crozats. **D,** Lower crozats.

Centric Relation Splint

Centric relation splints are usually fabricated of clear cold-cure acrylic resin material to fit over the arch. Incisal guidance and cuspid protection may be provided by forming a ramp or extra acrylic to the anterior portion of the splint.

Incline Bite Plate Splint

Upper incline bite plates are used to reposition the mandible forward and lower incline bite plates are used to slide the maxillary anteriors forward out of crossbite.

Flat Occlusal Plane Splint

This splint is often referred to as a nightguard to maintain tooth position or as a splint to prevent bruxism. It provides full coverage for either the maxillary or mandibular arch and has a flat occlusal surface that occludes with the opposing teeth.

Space Maintainers and Retainers

These appliances are shaped to the contour of the treated teeth to maintain the position of the teeth as well as to adjust the teeth or to activate movement. Retainers may be removable or they may be bonded to the selected teeth to hold them in place. Space maintainers are used in edentu-

lous areas to prevent drifting of adjacent teeth, prevent molar drift or rotation, or to facilitate expansion of the molars.

Lingual Arch

Lingual arches are fabricated in various lengths according to need. These arches may include loops for adjustment or they may be bonded. The advantage of bonded retainers is that they do not have loops and, therefore, can not be seen (Figure 26.7, *A*).

Band and Loop Retainer

The band and loop retainer is a space maintainer that is used to prevent drifting in an area in which a tooth has been extracted or exfoliated (see Chapter 24).

Hawley Retainer

The Hawley retainer (Figure 26.7, *B*) is used after completion of treatment to hold the teeth in their new position. The retainer can be either fixed or removable.

Crozat Appliance

The Crozat appliance is designed to retain either maxillary or mandibular teeth after treatment or put gentle force on them during treatment (Figure 26.7, *B-D*). The appliance has a wire body with molar cribs, molar clasps, occlusal rests, and lingual arms. Additional springs and hooks may be added if needed.

Nance Holding Appliance

The Nance holding appliance is cemented to the upper molars. It prevents unwanted overeruption of upper molars and serves as an anchor in the movement of cuspids.

Positioner

The orthodontic positioner is constructed of a hard rubber material and is custom made for each patient following treatment. It is designed to retain the teeth and permit the alveolus to rebuild support around the teeth.

Space Regainers

Space regainers are used to push apart adjacent teeth that have drifted into a space developed by the loss of a tooth (see Chapter 24).

Habit Appliances

Habit appliances prevent the patient from thrusting the tongue forward against the anterior teeth or from thumb- and finger-sucking. These appliances may be passive or aggressive in design.

Tongue Appliance

This appliance is cemented to the teeth until the habit is broken. This usually takes 6 months to a year. It may impair the speech temporarily but it will reorient the tongue to its proper position.

Thumb Appliance

The thumb appliance is also a permanent appliance that is cemented to the teeth. It may make the tongue sore for a short time and may interfere with speech but the child can adapt to this appliance quite rapidly. It prevents the sucking action and serves as a tongue training device. This can take a few months or as long as a couple of years.

Expansion Appliances

Expansion appliances correct crossbites by expanding and separating teeth that are crowded or expanding the palatal suture. The appliances may be fixed (bonded to the teeth) or removable.

Palatal Expander

The palatal expansion device is used to widen the maxillary arch. The maxilla, or upper jaw, has a suture down the center, which allows it to be separated and widened. The expansion device is cemented into place and the patient (or parent if the child is young) turns the screw once or twice a day, until the desired expansion is achieved (see Figures 26.3 and 26.4).

Lip Bumpers

This appliance takes advantage of the maxillary or mandibular lip muscle to distalize or move the first permanent molars distally. They also help to disengage or relax and hyperactive mentalis or orbicularis oris muscle.

Orthopedic Correctors

Orthopedic correctors are used to correct malocclusions, reduce overbites, increase arch width and length, close an open bite, and increase mandibular advancement.

Orthodontic Head Gear or Facemask

A lightweight stainless steel head or facial device used to attach an orthodontic appliance and pull the maxillary or mandibular dental arches forward. The device is usually made up of a forehead rest, mouthbow, and chin or cheek rest. A headstrap may be used to provide increased stability.

Orthodontic Impression Trays

Orthodontic impression trays are used to take impressions for study models to be used for diagnosis and treatment planning and for working models to construct orthodontic appliances. The facial and lingual sides of these trays are often deeper than general perforated impression trays to allow for better reproduction of the soft tissue, mucobuccal fold. Some operators prefer aluminum trays that are perforated for retention and others may select nonperforated trays or trays that are Teflon coated for easy cleaning. Plastic disposable trays are also available. Both types of trays are accessible in many assorted sizes. The sides of the trays are extended to allow for deeper impressions needed by the orthodontist for ortho study models.

Orthodontic Instruments

Band Seater

The band seater (Figure 26.8, *A*) is used for seating bands with the aid of the patient's biting force. The handle and tip is one piece or it may have a replaceable nylon tip to cushion the biting force. The tips are available in several shapes and usually serrated to allow a positive grip on the edge of the band.

Mershon Band Pusher

The Mershon band pusher is used to seat and position the band on the tooth. It can also be used to contour the edges of the band around the tooth and to tuck in the metal ligature wires (pigtails). This stainless steel band pusher has a large tapered handle and an angulated, rectangular, serrated tip to prevent slippage during use.

Ligature Wire Cutter

The ligature wire cutter (Figure 26.8, *B*) is used to cut thin ligature wires. The tapered beaks have sharp cutting edges, which are available with carbide inserts that can be replaced or sharpened when worn. Ligature wire cutters are manufactured in different sizes with various tip tapers and cutting angles.

Arch-Forming Pliers

Arch-forming pliers (Figure 26.8, *C*) are used to smoothly form and contour archwires. They can be used on either round or rectangular wire. The pliers have a concave, cylindrical shaped beak that may be grooved or smooth.

Light-Wire Pliers

Light-wire pliers (Figure 26.8, *D*) are used primarily for contouring loops in orthodontic wire. They are also used to place spring separators and add minor bends in the archwires. The beaks of the pliers differ, one has a pyramid shape and the other is conical shaped. The pyramid beak may have grooves at the tip to make loops and a cutting edge at the back of the beak.

Band-Contouring Pliers

Band-contouring pliers (Figure 26.8, *E*) are used to recontour and adapt the O-band around the tooth. The beaks are tapered with a slight bow. One beak tip is concave and one is convex. This allows them to fit together for contouring orthodontic bands. They are constructed of stainless steel and the tips vary with manufacturers.

Bird-Beak Pliers (No. 139)

Bird-beak pliers (Figure 26.8, *F*) are used for seating separating springs and bending wire. The opposing beaks are conical and pyramidal and available in various lengths.

Distal end Cutting Pliers and Holder

The distal end cutting pliers (Figure 26.8, *G*) are used for cutting the distal ends of the archwires and preventing the end of the cut archwire from cutting into the gingival tissue. The right-angled beaks have opposing cutting edges. There is a safety hold located distal to the cutting edges to catch the loose end of the cut archwire. These pliers will cut round wires and rectangular wires.

Tweed Loop-forming Pliers (Omega)

These pliers (Figure 26.8, *H*) are used to form the omega loop and various other loops. They have one round and one concave opposing parallel beaks. There are three sections of

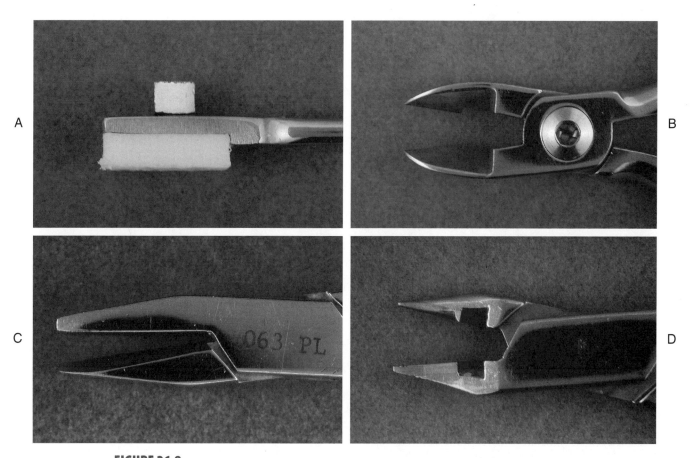

FIGURE 26.8

Orthodontic instruments. **A**, Band seater. **B**, Pin and ligature cutter. **C**, Arch forming pliers. **D**, Light wire pliers.

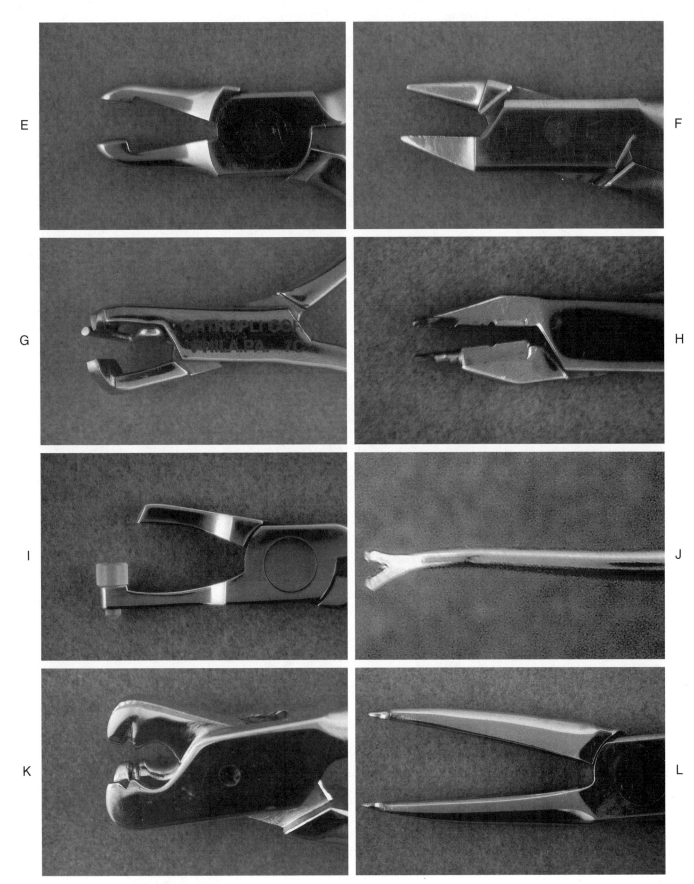

FIGURE 26.8, cont'd

Orthodontic instruments. **E**, Band contour pliers. **F**, Bird beak pliers. **G**, Distal end cutter. **H**, Tweed loop forming pliers. **I**, Posterior band remover. **J**, Ligature director. **K**, Face-bow pliers. **L**, Howe utility pliers.

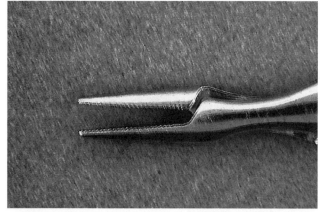

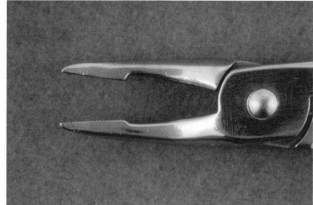

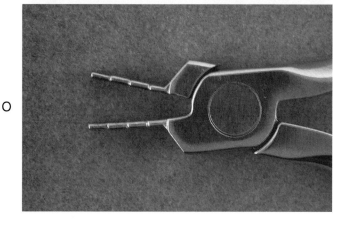

Orthodontic instruments. **M**, Mathieu ligature pliers. **N**, Wiengart utility pliers. **O**, Tweed arch adjusting pliers.

various diameters are on the round beak and the outer third of the concave beak is serrated. They are available with replaceable tips.

Posterior Band-Removing Pliers

Posterior band-removing pliers (Figure 26.8, *I*) are used to remove posterior bands. They have two stainless steel beaks. One beak is cylindrical with a replaceable nylon-tip and the opposing beak is curved with a carbide insert. The cylindrical beak is placed on the occlusal surface and the curved beak is placed on the gingival surface of the band.

Ligature Director

The ligature director (Figure 26.8, *J*) is used to press the ligatures under the archwire and to push the archwires into proper placement. The tips are notched and may be straight or angled to enable the operator to hold the wires. They may be double-ended or in combination with other tips.

Face-Bow Adjusting Pliers

The pliers (Figure 26.8, *K*) are used to contour large-diameter wires of various shapes and to adjust the inner and outer arches of face bows. These adjusting pliers have three parallel beaks; two beaks opposite the beak that is positioned between the two beaks when the pliers are closed. Each beak has a notch on the opposing surface near the tip of the beak.

Howe Utility Pliers

The utility pliers (Figure 26.8, *L*) are used for placing bands, tying ligature wire and holding and adjusting the archwire during placement and removal. Howe pliers have two long, round beaks that are tapered and end with serrated pad tips.

Ligature Pliers (Mathieu Style)

Ligature pliers, (Figure 26.8, *M*) of this style, are used most often for tying metal ligature wires and placing Alactics. They are constructed of stainless steel and are available in small or regular sizes with tips that vary in length and taper. The tips are serrated and the handle has a positive-locking ratchet and spring to aid in opening and closing the pliers quickly.

Weingart Utility Pliers

Weingart utility pliers (Figure 26.8, *N*) are used to hold orthodontic archwire and to place it into the mouth and also to remove it from the mouth. They are also used for holding the archwire while bending it. They are stainless steel and have an adjustable screw joint. The two opposing beaks have serrated tips. The tips are pointed and may be straight or curved. These shapes allow for different types of adjustments to be made in the oral cavity.

Tweed Arch-Adjusting Pliers

The tweed arch-adjusting pliers (Figure 26.8, *O*) are used for holding and adjusting archwires. They have opposing

Table 26.1

Attachments Used To Fabricate Orthodontic Appliances

Attachment	Purpose
Pontics	Artificial teeth selected to match patient's natural teeth and used to replace missing teeth on an appliance.
Arch wires	Orthodontic wire that comes in various shapes (ovoid, tapered, square), composition (stainless steel most common), configuration (single strands, twisted or braided) and diameter (gauge varies by use). Most archwires are preformed by the manufacturer, however the operator can bend and form straight wire to fabricate the orthodontic appliance.
Elastomeric rotation wedges	Added to archwire to help rotate tooth and move into correct position.
Open coil springs	Added to archwire to correct spacing for erupted teeth or open spaces for erupting teeth.
Closed coil springs	Added to archwire to maintain spaces between teeth.
Labial bow	The wire part of a removable retainer that is used for retention and to correct tooth alignment and protrusion.
Bands	The stainless steel rings commonly placed around the first and second molars.
Buttons and cleate	Attached to bands to secure elastics.
Seating lugs	Attached to bands to aid in seating the band on the tooth.
Sheaths	Mechanism attached to band to aid in applying force (e.g., quad helix).
Tubes	Tube shaped devices named for their use (headgear tubes, utility tube, buccal tube, double tube) used to place archwire through.
Brackets or clasps	Attachments bonded to the teeth (sapphire or ceramic) or welded (stainless steel) to bands that are cemented onto the teeth to attach archwires and auxiliaries in order to guide tooth movement. Sapphire and ceramic brackets are chemically treated to adhere to the teeth whereas stainless steel brackets have a mesh pad welded in place to help adhere to tooth enamel. Clasps are named for their shape or use.
Buccal tube	A type of bracket that is placed on the buccal side of a molar band in a horizontal position, containing a slot for the archwire or a tube for holding the ends of a facebow or both.

parallel beaks that have either smooth or scored tips. The carbide insert tips are replaceable.

Orthodontic Attachments

There are various attachments used to fabricate orthodontic appliances. Each attachment has a specific purpose and must be applied to the teeth or appliance itself. Table 26.1 lists the attachments with which you should be familiar.

INITIAL EXAMINATION APPOINTMENT

Medical and Dental History

As with any new patient in the office it is important to gather basic personal information, medical and dental history, and to record the information accurately and thoroughly (Figure 26.9, *A*). It is important to find out the patient's attitude toward orthodontic treatment, who referred the patient, and if they have consulted with another orthodontist. Both the patient and the parent, if the patient is a child, must be in-

volved in the first visit. This visit has a separate fee, which should be quoted to the responsible party making the appointment. Most patients will not have a very good understanding of orthodontics at this time and will be very apprehensive. A warm smile and friendly atmosphere will help to make them feel more comfortable and relaxed.

The patient is also examined to determine how many and which teeth they have, and they are charted on the initial examination form (Figure 26.9, *B*). Also recorded is the permanent first molar and cuspid classifications using Angle's classifications. The arch length is determined as to whether it is normal, deficient, or excessive. The midline frenums, crossbites, and eruption patterns are checked for any deviations from the norm. Measurements are taken to determine an overbite or overjet.

Overbite is estimated as a percentage, for example, the patient has a 20% overbite, meaning the overlap of the maxillary incisors covers 20% of the incisal edge of the mandibular incisors. A 100% overbite would mean that the maxillary incisal edge is at the gingival margin of the mandibular anterior. This could be known as an *excessive deep bite*. Overbite is a vertical relationship of the incisors. The overjet is

Orthodontic acquaintance form

Date _____

Date of birth _____

Patient's name _____ Age _____ Sex _____

Address _____ Zip _____ Phone _____

School _____ Grade _____ Nickname _____

Patient's dentist _____ Physician _____

Referred by _____

Father's name _____ Mother's name _____

Employed by _____ Employed by _____

Business address _____ Business address _____

_____

Business phone _____ Business phone _____

Emergency person and phone number _____

Person financially responsible _____ Soc. Sec. # _____

Address _____ Phone _____

Name of dental insurance co. _____ Medical assoc. no. (if app.) _____

Names and ages of other children in family _____

Medical history

Is patient in good health? _____ ☐ Yes ☐ No

Does patient have any history of major illness? _____ ☐ Yes ☐ No

Has the patient ever been under the care of a physician for illness? _____ ☐ Yes ☐ No

Check any of the following for which the patient has been treated

Diabetes .... ☐	Tuberculosis.............. ☐	Endochine problems .... ☐
Pneumonia.............. ☐	Anemia .... ☐	Prolonged bleeding.............. ☐
Heart trouble .... ☐	Epilepsy.................... ☐	Fainting or dizziness............. ☐
Rheumatic fever......... ☐	Asthma .... ☐	Nervous disorders .... ☐
Bone disorders .... ☐	Sicca .... ☐	Glaucoma.......................... ☐

Does patient have tendency of: colds ☐ sore throats ☐ ear infections ☐ _____ ☐ Yes ☐ No

Have tonsils and adenoids been removed? What age? _____ ☐ Yes ☐ No

List any drugs or medications now being taken; give reasons: _____

Do you wear contact lenses? _____ ☐ Yes ☐ No

List any allergies or drug sensitivity: _____ ☐ Yes ☐ No

Has the patient reached puberty? Girls: Has she started menstruation _____ ☐ Yes ☐ No

Boys: Has his voice changed _____ ☐ Yes ☐ No

Height: _____ Weight: _____

Dental history

Have any injuries to the face, mouth, or teeth occurred? _____ ☐ Yes ☐ No

Has the patient ever sucked a thumb or fingers? Until what age? _____ ☐ Yes ☐ No

Does the patient have any speech problems? _____ ☐ Yes ☐ No

Is the patient a mouth breather? While awake? _____ ☐ Yes ☐ No

While asleep? _____ ☐ Yes ☐ No

Have you ever been informed of any missing or extrapermanent teeth? _____ ☐ Yes ☐ No

Has an orthodontist been consulted previously? _____ ☐ Yes ☐ No

Has either parent had orthodontic treatment? _____ ☐ Yes ☐ No

List any musical instruments played: _____

Reason for consultation: _____

_____

Signature: _____ Date: _____

FIGURE 26.9

Continued

A, Orthodontic acquaintance form.

Name _____ Age _____ Sex _____ Case number _____

1. Angle classification and relation of segments

	Right side		Left side	
	Molar	Cuspid	Molar	Cuspid
Class I				
Class II				
Div II				
Class III				

2. Dentition

R I G H T			E	D	C	B	A		A	B	C	D	E				L E F T
8	7	6	5	4	3	2	1	1	2	3	4	5	6	7	8	
8	7	6	5	4	3	2	1	1	2	3	4	5	6	7	8	
			E	D	C	B	A	A	B	C	D	E				

3. Arch length max _____ mm
   man _____ mm
4. Overbite _____ %
5. Overjet _____ mm
6. Crossbite- max _____ (buccaulingual)
   man _____ (buccaulingual)
7. Median line- _____|_____ amt. _____ mm
   amt. _____ mm
8. Tooth to lip _____ mm
9. Missing teeth _____
10 Eruption pattern _____
11. Abnormal frenum _____
12. Airway _____
13. Tongue _____
14. Condition of gingiva _____
15. Periodontal condition _____
16. Oral hygiene _____
17. Path of closure _____
18. TMJ _____
19. Lip posture _____
20. Lip muscle tone _____
21. Profile _____
22. Facial type _____
23. Musculature _____
24. Habits _____
25. Disposition of case _____
26. Estimate _____
27. Comments _____

C-Caries
X-Extracted
S-Supernumerary
O-Congenitally missing
A-Atypical form
I-Impaction
D-Decalcification
M-Missing

Key factors in TX

Date		Fee	Date		Fee

FIGURE 26.9, cont'd

B, Initial examination form. (Courtesy Dr. Kimberly R. Foushee, Louisville, Kentucky.)

the horizontal relationship of the maxillary and the mandibular incisors and is measured in millimeters. The periodontal probe is an instrument that has millimeter markings on the tip. It is usually for measuring the depth of a periodontal pocket in the gingiva; however, it is every useful for measuring the millimeters of distance between the incisors for overjet.

The patient is examined for supernumerary teeth, unusual eruption patterns such as rotations or eruptions of a tooth labial or lingual to the arch, and abnormal movement of the tongue such as anterior or lateral tongue thrust. The TMJ is palpitated as the mandible is going through its exertions (lateral, protrusive, retrusive) to try and determine the extent of any existing habits such as thumb-sucking, fingernail biting, lip-sucking, pen or pencil chewing, mouth breathing, and clinching or grinding.

Preliminary Diagnosis

Once the initial examination and medical history is complete, the orthodontist will be ready to give a preliminary and brief diagnosis. It may be explained to the patient that some cases needed treatment are skeletal problems that may involve the size and growth of the lower jaw or the upper jaw and how they relate to each other. Some cases are dental only and they involve changing the relationship of the teeth and how they occlude. Then again, the case may involve both a skeletal and a dental discrepancy. The orthodontist can relate to the patient what can be determined simply by looking in the patient's mouth; however, a true diagnosis can only be arrived at when, after the records appointment, the orthodontist has been able to study the radiographs, photos, and models and design an effective treatment plan. The cost and length of treatment will also be determined. The patient is now ready to schedule the records appointment. The medical history and initial examination form become a part of the patient's permanent record and the examination is recorded and dated on the treatment card.

RECORDS APPOINTMENT

It is important that the orthodontic assistant is able to collect and record all information essential for the dentist to analyze the patient's condition and to make treatment decisions. The records appointment involves taking radiographs requested by the orthodontist, intraoral and extraoral photographs, and impressions for diagnostic study models.

Radiographs

The orthodontic assistant will obtain the diagnostic records. The radiographs usually taken in orthodontic treatment are full mouth periapicals and bitewings, occlusal, panagraphic,

and **cephalometric**. Refer to Chapter 12 and 13 for further information on radiographs.

The following are examples of radiographs:

Cephalometrics
The science of measuring the cranial bones in the head

- Full mouth periapical radiographs are used to examine each tooth and surrounding bone.
- Interproximal radiographs help to detect interproximal caries.
- Occlusal radiographs help to identify root fragments, unerupted teeth, and ectopic eruption of teeth.
- Panagraphic radiographs provide a complete radiograph of the patient dentition from right or left. The panagraph helps to identify the relationship between the teeth present and the surrounding bone structure as well as the eruption sequence. The panagraph can help the dentist determine any abnormalities in eruption patterns, existence of the necessary permanent dentition in a mixed dentition patient, and complete formation of the apeses of the roots. If the apesis is not complete in its formation, force should not be applied to the tooth as it may cause damage to the tooth.
- Cephalometric radiographs are used to study the growth and development of the head and face and skeletal-dental landmarks. It is used to determine skeletal relationships and discrepancies by measuring the upper and lower jaw on the cephalometric tracing. The cephalometric radiograph is a lateral view of the patient's face, neck, and dentition (Figure 26.10). The patient must be in occlusion when the cephalograph is exposed. The orthodontist may also ask for the posterior-anterior radiograph of the face and head or a hand-wrist radiograph (used to determine where the patient is on the growth chart).

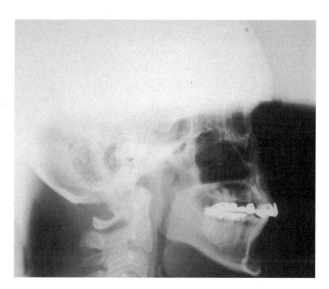

FIGURE 26.10

Cephalometric film.

Photographs

Extraoral Photographs

Extraoral photos are taken involving two frontal shots, one smiling one not smiling; and two profile shots one smiling and one not smiling. In the profile shots the patient must place any long hair behind the ear so that the angle of the mandible is visible. Intraoral photographs are taken using mirrors and cheek retractors to hold the lips and cheeks away from the teeth. Begin with a frontal intraoral with the teeth in their normal occlusion and six anteriors in focus. Next take a shot of the right and left buccal segments in their normal occlusion and the first molars in focus. Occlusal shots of the maxillary and mandibular arches follow, being sure to include the most distal aspect of the last molars whatever they may be in that dentition. There are several common procedures that can be followed.

Box 26.1 *Procedure*

Procedures for Taking Extraoral and Intraoral Photographs

Material needed

Camera
Film

Extraoral photographs

1. All views are taken with the camera held vertically.
2. Check camera for focus and correct exposure.
3. Have patient remove glasses.
4. View should be from top of head to middle of neck.
5. All extraorals should be the same distance.
6. Photograph should be taken at eye level of patient (not above or below).
7. Point flash at top for frontal view.
8. Point flash on facial side for lateral views.
9. Camera should be focused on eyes on frontal view.
10. Camera should be focused on outer canthus of eye on lateral view.
11. Head not tilted (Frankfort plane is parallel to bottom of frame).
12. Take 4 views:
Frontal: Lips together*
Frontal: Smiling
Lateral: Lips together*
Lateral: Smiling
* If there is excessive strain to close the lips, an extra photo should be taken with the lips apart.

Material needed

Camera
Film
Cheek retractors
Intraoral mirror
Mouth mirrors

Intraoral photographs

1. All views are taken with the camera held vertically.
2. Patient is seated in upright position.
3. Remove glasses.
4. Place cheek retractors in patient's mouth and ask patient to hold lips and cheeks out of the way with the retractors (if patient is young have an assistant hold the retractors).
5. Teeth in occlusion on frontal and lateral views.
6. Teeth centered in photograph.
7. Patient pulls lips up or down with retractors in mirror shots.
8. Only show teeth in upper mirror photo - no nose.
9. Five (5) views: Figure 26.11, *A-E*
10. Use mirror on the mandibular occlusal surface to photograph the maxillary occlusal surface and focus on middle of palate.
11. Photograph the mandibular occlusal surface direct without mirror.
12. If patient can keep tongue out of the way, take photo with tongue down.
13. If patient can not control tongue, push tongue back with mirror or tongue blade.
14. On lateral views, have patient pull retractor as hard as possible on the photo side and relax the retractor on the other side.

Intraoral Photographs

Intraoral photographs are pictures of the inside of the mouth and extraoral photographs are pictures of the face. It is important that the orthodontic assistant is able to take these photographs with a 35 mm camera. It is important that the camera is set. This means to check the shutter speed, focus, distance, lens opening, and point or ring flash. The orthodontic assistant will need to practice taking these photographs because cameras will vary in settings. There are several common techniques that can be followed (Box 26.1 and Table 26.2).

Occlusal Bite Registration

The orthodontic assistant will next secure the occlusal bite registration. A wax bite registration is to be taken with the patient in their normal occlusion to be used when trimming the models together. Usually a prescription is written for the diagnostic study models, which included the patient's name, date of records, age or date of birth of the patient, and a due date of completion of the models. It is important to get an accurate recording of how the maxillary and mandibular occlusal surfaces contact one another (see Chapter 15).

Impressions and Orthodontic Models

Usually impressions for orthodontic models are made of alginate. Impressions are taken during the records appointment and they are used for diagnostic study models. Explain this to the patient and have a set of finished models on hand for demonstration purposes so the patient will have a better understanding of how the impressions are used. Show the patient the impression trays, try the empty trays in the mouth for proper size and let the patient get an idea of how it will feel when the tray is inserted. Explain to them how the impression material is mixed and how it will feel in their mouth as pressure is applied to the tray. Ask the patient to breath in and out of their nose when the tray is inserted. It is a good idea to explain and practice this when the tray is tried in for size without the impression material.

Study Models

Diagnostic study model impressions must have full and complete extensions into the sulcus facial and lingual around the entire arch. The impressions must have complete posterior extensions that include the maxillary tuberosities and the mandibular retromolar pads and the junction of the

Table 26.2

Evaluation for Extraoral and Intraoral Photographs

Task	4	3	2	0	X
Extraoral photographs					
Materials secured					
Patient instruction					
Camera settings and exposure					
Distance					
Patient positioning on film					
Lighting					
Frontal views (extraoral)					
Lateral views (extraoral)					
Intraoral photographs					
Cheek retractor use					
Teeth position on film					
Frontal views (intraoral)					
Lateral views (intraoral)					
View					
1 Frontal					
2 Right lateral					
3 Left lateral					
4 Maxillary occlusal					
5 Mandibular occlusal					
Use of mirror					

The numeric criteria: 4 Excellent; 3 Good but some improvement can be made; 2 Below average, usable, needs to improve skill; 0 Unsatisfactory; X Not able to evaluate.

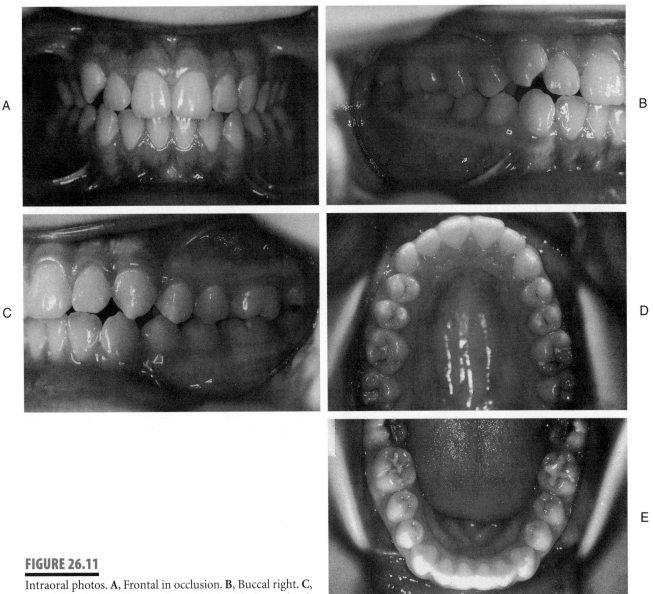

FIGURE 26.11

Intraoral photos. **A**, Frontal in occlusion. **B**, Buccal right. **C**, Buccal left. **D**, Maxillary occlusal. **E**, Mandibular occlusal. (Courtesy Dr. Kimberly F. Foushee.)

hard and soft palate. Ask the patient to raise their tongue before complete insertion of the mandibular tray in order to achieve full extensions of the lingual sulcus. The lips must be lifted and pulled forward over the border of the tray to achieve full extensions of the labial sulcus mandibular and maxillary.

It is important that the impressions of the teeth and surrounding soft tissue is as complete and exact in detail as possible. The following techniques are followed in preparation for case presentation (see Chapter 15). Please review this chapter for (1) selecting impression trays, (2) taking a bite registration, (3) taking alginate impressions, (4) mixing gypsum, and (5) pouring up impression trays.

After the orthodontic models have been secured, all bubbles and obstructions must be removed from the tooth surfaces. As with most study models a good rule of thumb for the desired proportions of a model after trimming is $^1/_3$ tooth portion, $^1/_3$ anatomic portion and $^1/_3$ base portion (see Chapter 15 for an illustration). Because trimming orthodontic models requires greater detail than for trimming general study models, further instructions are given (Box 26.2 and Table 26.3).

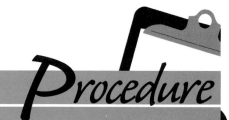

Box 26.2

Procedure

Procedures for Trimming Orthodontic Study Models

Materials needed

Compass
Ruler or protractor
Colored pencil
#600 Fine wet/dry sandpaper
Centric and reclusal record
Orthodontic model trimmer
Orthodontic work table and accessories
Angle guide
Vertisquare

Upper model

1. Trim gross excess around periphery of upper model no closer than $^1/_2$ inch from facial surfaces of the teeth. Place the maxillary cast on a flat tabletop and with the aid of a compass, draw a line $1^1/_2$ inch (38 mm) above the table top, completely around the base of the upper model.
2. Using the Vertisquare, trim away excess base material down to the previously drawn line. There should be no rocking of the model when it is placed flat on its base.
3. Draw a line over the midpalatal raphe to serve as the main reference line for the rest of the model trimming procedure (Figure 26.12, *A*). All future cuts will be in reference to this midline, so it is very important to accurately draw a line over the raphe that is clearly discernible.
4. Trim the upper heel just distal to the depth of the hamular notch. Before making this cut it is important to see if the lower arch has any anatomical landmarks (i.e., third molars) that may necessitate a lesser amount being trimmed from the heel of the upper model.
5. Set the Angle Guide onto the Degree Plate and then set the Degree Plate to 25 degrees as indicated by the white indicator mark on the front of the Orthodontic Tray.
6. With the heel of the upper model against the Angle Guide, trim the left and right anterior segments of the upper model from roughly the mid-point of the cuspids to an imaginary extension of the mid-palatal raphe. The apex of the two anterior cusps should be about $^1/_4$ inch (7 mm) from the teeth.
7. With the Angle Guide in place, rotate the Degree Plate to 65 degrees. Hold the base of the upper model against the Angle Guide and with steady pressure trim the left and right buccal segments until the anterior segments are of equal length (midline of the canines on the symmetric arch). The buccal cuts should be to the deepest portion of the buccal vestibule and should measure approximately $^3/_{16}$ inch (5 mm) from the buccal surface of the teeth. Asymmetric arches require special consideration that can be found in the manufacturer's instruction manual (Figure 26.12, *B*).
8. With the Angle Guide in place, rotate the Degree Plate to 115 degrees. Hold the heel of the upper model against the Angle Guide and trim the left and right posterior corners symmetrically to a width of about $^5/_8$ inch.

Lower model

9. Trim the gross excess around the periphery of the lower model no closer the $^1/_2$ inch (12 to 13 mm) from the buccal surface of the teeth.
10. With the models articulated and the centric record in place, carefully invert them on the tray table, so that the lower model is on top of the maxillary model. Next, carefully trim the heel of the lower model parallel and flush with the upper model. It is important that the upper model heel not be accidentally trimmed during this process.
11. With the models in occlusion, the Vertisquare is used to trim the lower base parallel to the upper base. Slide the Vertisquare into the Degree Plate and with the base of the upper model against the pad of the Vertisquare trim the base of the

Continued

Box 26.2—Cont'd.

Procedure

Procedures for Trimming Orthodontic Study Models

lower model until the pointer on the side of the Vertisquare reaches the 70 mm mark on the Degree Plate. This cut will leave the articulated models at the desired height.

12. Remove the Vertisquare and slide the Angle Guide onto the Degree Plate. Rotate the Degree Plate, trim the mandibular anterior segment in a semi- circle. The anterior segment is trimmed no closer than $\frac{1}{4}$ inches from the facial surface of the anterior teeth. The cut should be sharp and distinct. To insure that the buccal segments are of equal length, the distance from the cut to the heel should be the same on each side (Figure 26.12, *C*).

13. Return the Angle Guide to the Degree Plate and set the degree plate to 115 degrees. With the upper and lower models together, place the heel of the lower model against the Angle Guide. Gently push the model and Angle Guide until each lower posterior trimmed corner is trimmed flush with the opposing upper posterior corner.

14. The upper and lower models should remain in occlusion when resting on the heels of the models (Figure 26.12, *D*).

15. The upper and lower models should remain in occlusion when resting on the left or right posterior corners of the models (Figure 26.12, *E*).

16. All bubbles and voids should be filled with stone and the flat surfaces of the model be smooth. Any overlying base portion should be trimmed away so that the entire facial anatomical view may be viewed. Line angles should be sharp and parallel and trimmed at the angles indicated on the slide (Figure 26.12, *F*).

17. The upper and lower models should be labeled before soaping. The patient's name, age and date the impressions were taken should be printed on the model. Using a sharp pencil, the lettering should be in capitol letters and should not exceed $\frac{1}{8}$ inch in height.

18. To give models the best appearance possible, they should be soaked in a soap solution, such as Whip Mix Model Glow, after they have been allowed to dry. It is important to rinse any excess soap off after soaping and polish with a dry cloth once the models have dried.

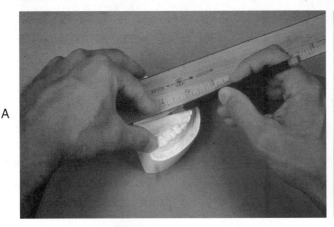
A

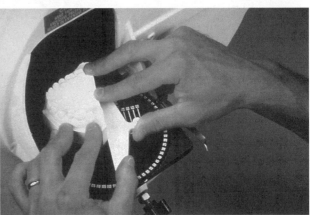
B

FIGURE 26.12

A, This midline mark will serve as the main reference line for the rest of the model trimming procedure. **B,** With steady pressure trim the left and right buccal segments until the anterior segments are of equal length.

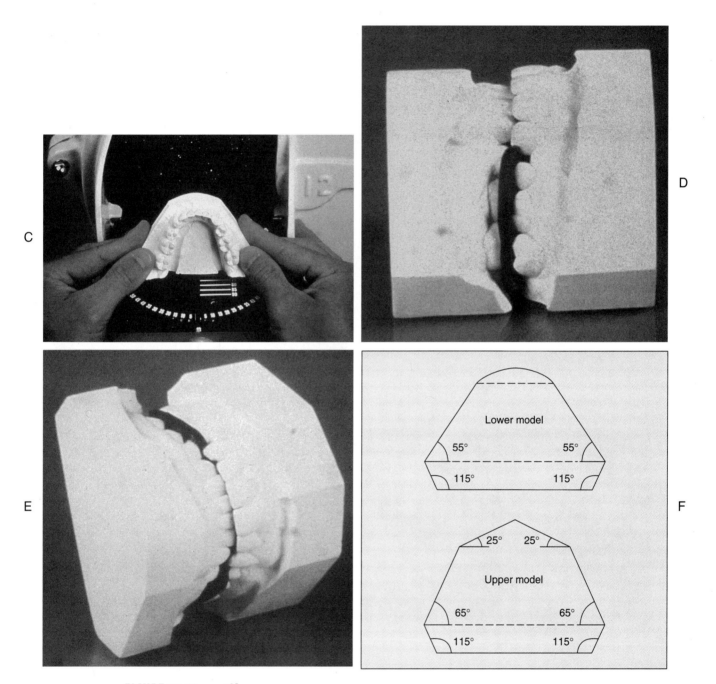

FIGURE 26.12, cont'd

C, The anterior segment is trimmed no closer than $1/4$ inch from the facial surface to the anterior teeth. **D,** The upper and lower models should remain in occlusion when resting on both the heels. **E,** Resting on the left or right posterior corners of the models. **F,** Correct line angles.

Table 26.8

Evaluation for Orthodontic Model Trimming

Task	4	3	2	0	X
Trim excess and draw line 1¹/₂ inches from table top on model-upper.					
Trim base to line making base parallel to occlusal plane.					
Draw line over midpalatal suture; trim upper heel perpendicular to line.					
Trim upper anterior segments at 25 degrees.					
Trim upper posterior segments at 65 degrees.					
Trim upper corners at 115 degrees.					
Trim excess from lower model, articulate, and invert.					
Trim heels of upper and lower flush.					
Trim lower base to parallel with upper base to 70 mm mark.					
Trim lower buccal segments at 551.					
Trim lower anterior segment in semicircle.					
Trim comers together at II 5A upper and lower in occlusion.					
Keep models in occlusion on table top resting on heels and corners.					
Line angles sharp and parallel.					
Models *soaped and labeled*.					

The numeric criteria: 4 Excellent; 3 Good but some improvement can be made; 2 Below average, usable, needs to improve skill; 0 Unsatisfactory; X Not able to evaluate.

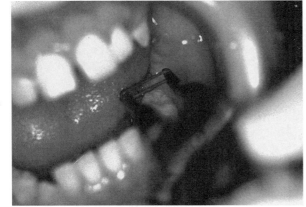

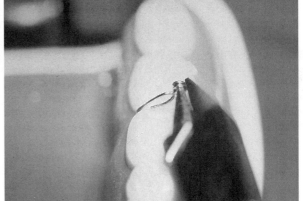

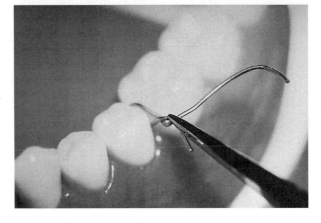

FIGURE 26.13

A, Elastic separator: place the elastic separator on the tip of the pliers and stretch. **B**, Stainless steel separator: hold with pliers, need the helix and insert curved portion below contact or buccal. Then bring the short arm over the marginal ridge to snap in place. **C**, Brass separators: after threading through the embrasure on the lingual, grasp brass wire on facial and pull half way through the contact, then bring the wire over occlusal and twist.

CASE PRESENTATION

After careful study of the patient records and diagnostic aids, the orthodontist will develop a treatment plan and an estimated cost. During the case presentation, the diagnosis and treatment plan is explained to the patient. The approximate length of treatment and a clear explanation of the patient's responsibility helps to ensure successful treatment. Usually thirty minutes is allowed for this appointment, but some individual cases may require more time. Treatment is begun after the patient's case has been worked up and presented to the patient for approval. Several different types of appointments are made.

Separating Appointments

The purpose of the separation appointments are to create space between the teeth to be banded. The patient will need to be informed that there will be some discomfort involved. It is important to consider the patient's concerns at this time and to reassure them that any discomfort will only last a few days. Several types of separators may be used (Figure 26.13): (1) elastic, (2) steel spring, or (3) brass wire. The procedures for placement of the separators follow in Box 26.3 and Tables 26.4, 26.5, and 26.6.

Box 26.3

Procedure

Procedures for Placement of Orthodontic Separators

Placement of elastic posterior separators

Materials needed

Mirror
Explorer
Cotton forceps
Probe
Elastic posterior separators
Separating pliers

1. Select large ring separators for the posterior teeth and place them using the elastic separating pliers or dental floss.
2. Squeeze the separating pliers and stretch the separators through the contact using a seesaw motion as if flossing (Figure 26.13, A).
3. Remove the pliers and make sure the separator surrounds the contact on all sides.
4. Record the exact position of each separator and the number of them placed in the patient's chart.

Placement of steel spring separators

Materials needed

Mirror
Explorer
Cotton forceps
Probe
Long beak pliers
(Long and short) molar steel spring separators

1. Using long beak pliers choose a long separator for molars and a shorter one for premolars.
2. With pliers near the helix coil on the shorter arm, insert the curved portion beneath the contact on the lingual (Figure 26.13, B).

3. After hooking the curved portion in the embrasure on the lingual, bring the short arm over the marginal ridges, the contact area and into the embrasure on the buccal side.
4. Gently push it into place after it has been engaged in the contact. The separator will snap into place because of the tension of the helix.

Placement of brass wire separators

Materials needed

Mirror
Explorer
Cotton forceps
Probe
Brass separator wire
Hemostats

1. Cut a small piece of wire and bend it into the shape of a hook.
2. Grasp the brass wire just above the hood with a pair of hemostats. Thread the wire through the embrasure from the lingual to the facial taking care not to damage the tissue.
3. Grab the brass wire on the facial side, pulling half of it through the contact.
4. Bring the rest of the wire over the occlusal surface and cross the ends of the wire on the buccal side (Figure 26.13, C).
5. Grasp the ends of the brass wire with the hemostat and turn clockwise until it is snug around the contact.
6. Cut the excess wire leaving a small pigtail on the buccal. Tuck the pigtail gingivally.

Table 26.4

Evaluation for Placement of Elastic Separators

Task	4	3	2	0	X
Place elastic separator on pliers and stretch through contact.					
Place two pieces of floss through one separator and stretch through contact; remove floss.					

The numeric criteria: 4 Excellent; 3 Good but some improvement can be made; 2 Below average, usable, needs to improve skill; 0 Unsatisfactory; X Not able to evaluate.

Table 26.5

Evaluation for Placement of SS Spring Separators

Task	4	3	2	0	X
Grasp spring with the tip of pliers near helix coil.					
Place long curved arm through gingival buccal embrasure.					
Bring short arm over marginal embrasure into place to snap under contact.					
SS spring is secure.					

The numeric criteria: 4 Excellent; 3 Good but some improvement can be made; 2 Below average, usable, needs to improve skill; 0 Unsatisfactory; X Not able to evaluate.

Table 26.6

Evaluation for Placement of Brass Wire Separators

Task	4	3	2	0	X
Grasp brass wire with pliers and bring through gingival lingual embrasure; grasp on facial and pull half way through.					
Bring wire over occlusal and cross ends of wire on buccal.					
Twist to tighten, clip, and tuck.					
Brass wire is secure.					

The numeric criteria: 4 Excellent; 3 Good but some improvement can be made; 2 Below average, usable, needs to improve skill; 0 Unsatisfactory; X Not able to evaluate.

APPLIANCE PLACEMENT APPOINTMENT

Fixed orthodontic appliances are attached to the teeth by cementing bands in place or by chemically bonding the brackets and pads directly to the teeth. Generally, molar bands are cemented into place and brackets are selected and bonded to the anterior teeth and bicuspids. Before either of these procedures, however, the teeth must be cleaned for smooth surface adhesion.

Band Placement

Banding is the cementing of bands, usually, on the molars to stabilize the brackets and pads. The archwire is attached to these brackets and force is applied to move the teeth.

Band Selection

Bands range in size and are usually preformed to the shape of the tooth. The occlusal edge of the band is slightly contoured, whereas the gingival edge is straight. The band is adapted to the contours of the teeth and cemented in place. The purpose of the band is to secure auxiliary devices such as lingual attachments (buttons, cleats, seating lugs and sheaths) or buccal attachments (buccal tubes), which are routinely placed on the bands. This provides a secure grasp on the tooth and allows for tooth repositioning. The band must fit the tooth as closely as possible, to prevent washing out of the cement. The band is made of material, usually stainless steel, that is highly resistant to deformation and tarnish.

Bands may be selected by any of three methods. First before the patient arrives, a plaster cast is used to select the approximate band sizes. This method is time consuming and much time will be spent later in selecting the exact band size. The second method is to take the plaster cast and measure the teeth. This is also time-consuming but fairly accurate. The third method is the most efficient. The bands are selected by the assistant and placed on the patient's teeth. This method can be used only in areas where state laws allow dental personnel to aid the orthodontist or dentist in the placement of bands.

Band Fitting

At the banding appointment the separators are removed. The teeth will be moved apart slightly with elastic separators before band placement to make room for the bands to be seated. The teeth that will receive bands are cleaned and rinsed. The bands are fitted to the teeth. Use of cotton pliers will aid in picking the bands from the tray but must not go into the mouth. The proper fitting band will almost fit using finger pressure, but not completely.

Use the flat end of the bite stick and place it completely across the surface buccolingual of the band and have the patient bite. This will seat the band down to the occlusal surface. The band pusher may also be used to push the band between the mesial or distal contacts. Use the small metal attachment of the bite stick to further seat the band placing it on the occlusal edge of the band lingual and buccal asking the patient to bite down each time.

The band fits properly when it is seated evenly mesial, distal, buccal, and lingual with no more than 1 mm of the marginal ridges showing occlusal to the edge of the band. The band should not rock back and forth buccally or lingually and there should be no spaces between the band and the tooth surface. Before cementing the bands please make sure there are correct bands available for that quadrant (right or left and upper or lower).

Make sure there are bands with the correct attachments for the appliances being used in the procedure. If the patient will be wearing a lip bumper the bands must have a tube that will accept the lip bumper. The lip bumper can be placed in and out by the patient. It is worn full-time and its purpose is to hold the muscle of the lip away from the teeth. This stretches the lip muscle and allows some expansion of the arch. The lip bumper can be preformed or made chair side with .045 stainless steel wire. A plastic tube is placed over the wire. Another attachment that maybe used is a removable transpalatal arch (TPA). This wire goes from one first molar to another across the palate and can be fixed or removable. Its purpose can be to rotate the molars or for anchorage. Band for anterior or premolar teeth will have a bracket with wings as an attachment instead of a tube on the buccal.

Band Cementation

Once the correct bands are fitted they are ready to be cemented (Box 26.4 and Table 26.7). Usually a zinc phosphate or glass isomer cement is used. Mix to the proper consistency. A thicker mix will be less likely to wash out. Be sure to dry the inside of the band thoroughly. It is a good idea to wax the tubes and slots of the bands so that cements do not get in them, making it difficult to place wires. After cementation of the bands clean off all excess material with a scaler, being careful not to remove occlusal edge of the band between the band and the tooth.

Bracket Placement

Today, the advantages of bonding has made this procedure more popular. Placing bands on fewer teeth eliminates the discomfort of separating as many teeth and bonding directly to incisors, cuspids, and bicuspids is more esthetic than bands. Bonding is also easier and quicker.

Box 26.4

Procedure

Procedures for Cementing Bands

Materials needed

Mouth mirror	Band removal pliers
Explorer	Bite stick
Cotton forceps	Wax
Probe	Cotton rolls
Scaler	Dental floss
Prophy paste	2 x 2 gauze
Low speed handpiece	Cement
Prophy angle	Cement spatula
Bands	Mixing pad
Band pusher	Model
Band contouring pliers	

1. Check the oral cavity and remove any separators. Clean teeth and apply fluoride.

2. Select and try in bands. After approval of orthodontist, arrange bands on flat surface according to placement in dental arch (Figure 26.14, *A*).
3. Clean and dry bands.
4. Protect brackets and buccal tubes from cement by covering them with orthodontic wax. Isolate and dry the tooth to be banded. Mix cement by following manufacturers directions.
5. Place cement on the inside of the band and hand to orthodontist to be seated (Figure 26.14, *B*).
6. With scaler and floss remove excess cement from the band and between the teeth.

Table 26.7

Evaluation for Cementation of Bands

Task	4	3	2	0	X
Secure proper tray setup.					
Remove separators and prophy teeth.					
Select and fit proper size bands.					
Clean, dry, and wax bands.					
Isolate tooth to be banded.					
Mix cement and load band.					
Clean excess cement from tooth and band.					

The numeric criteria: 4 Excellent; 3 Good but some improvement can be made; 2 Below average, usable, needs to improve skill; 0 Unsatisfactory; X Not able to evaluate.

Stainless steel brackets are backed with a mesh pad that aids in bonding the bracket to the tooth. The sapphire and ceramic brackets have a smooth back that is treated with a chemical that reacts with the bonding material for a stronger bond. It is important to wear gloves when working with these brackets and not to touch the bracket back with bare hands because the contamination of body oils effects the bonding ability.

The first step in the bracketing procedure is to clean all teeth that will receive a bracket. A nonfluoridated prophy paste must be used when light cure bonding materials are

used. Cleaning the teeth helps remove the thin protein layer on the tooth surface. After cleaning the teeth, rinse well and apply the etchant.

An *etchant* (acid etch) is used to help prepare the tooth surface for bonding. Cheek refractors or cotton rolls are used to isolate the area to be worked on. The etchant is placed on each tooth, rinsed thoroughly, and dried. The etchant should only be placed on the surface of the tooth that will receive a bracket (a small square on the facial). After the entire process is finished you should be able to see a chalky surface on the enamel of the tooth that has been

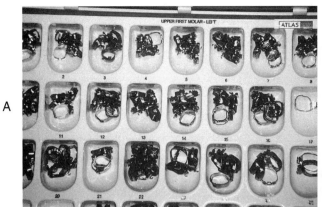
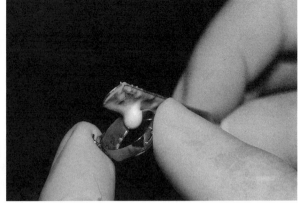

A   B

FIGURE 26.14

A, Select bands. **B**, Place cement on the inside of the band.

etched. The tooth is now ready to receive the bonding resin, which is painted on and then light cured.

The patient is now ready for bracket placement. Each bracket is placed individually on the tooth it was designed for (lateral, cuspid, and so on). When using a light cure material, a small amount is placed on the mesh pad of the bracket. The bracket is lifted by the wings with a pair of bracket tweezers. Then the material can be placed on the pad. Be sure that the bonding material does not slump over the edge of the pad into the wing area. This will cause a problem when trying to tie the wire into the bracket. The bracket is placed in its correct position on the tooth and cured with the light. Shine the light from all aspects of the tooth surface to ensure complete bonding of the material (mesial, distal, gingival, and occlusal).

Once the brackets are placed (Box 26.5 and Tables 26.8 and 26.9), the patient is ready for wired and ties. Usually the first wire placed is the smallest in diameter of all the wires used. This allows more flexibility as the teeth are malaligned. When the teeth become more aligned the wires graduate to a larger size. Once the wire is placed in the band slot and the bracket slots it is ready to be tied in. *Tied into* means that after the wire is placed in the slot of the bracket, a tie is wrapped around the wings on the facial surface of the bracket locking the wire into place.

There are many forms of ties from elastic to stainless steel, but they all serve the same purpose: to hold the wire securely in the slot of the bracket. This is called ligating or using ligature ties. Once the wire is ligated it is necessary to check the length of the end of the wire at the distal aspect of the buccal tube of the band. Any wire extending beyond that point should be cut with a distal end cutter (pliers).

The orthodontist can use many different brackets, which are designed per prescriptions by the manufacturers. Most orthodontists choose to use popular prescriptions already being manufactured; however an orthodontist could write his or her own prescription and the bracket would be manufactured that way.

Wire Placement

There are also many types of wire. Nickel titanium is very flexible and popular for use during treatment of malalignment. Stainless steel wires are more ridged and can be placed as the teeth become more aligned. The wires are alternated and graduated throughout the treatment starting with the smallest and most flexible and ending with the largest and most rigid. Many variations of wire used in orthodontic treatment: twistoflex, reverse curve, and closing loop arch wire, to name a few.

Ligation

Once the archwire has been placed, it is necessary to secure the wire in the slot of the brackets. This is accomplished with ligation or tying into place (Box 26.6 and Tables 26.10, 26.11, and 26.12). There are many choices of materials for ligation: stainless steel ties, elastomeric modules, or elastomeric chain.

Patient Education and Appliance Maintenance

One of the most important responsibilities delegated to the orthodontic assistant is patient education and oral health evaluation. The success of treatment often depends on the assistant's ability to effectively communicate to the patient the importance of good oral hygiene and appliance maintenance (Boxes 26.7 and 26.8 and Table 26.13). The assistant will need to create an environment of cooperation, achievement, and patient satisfaction through caring, praising, and encouragement. *The assistant must be professional at all times through their knowledge of the subject, skills, attitude, and the understanding of the patient's personal and orthodontic treatment needs.*

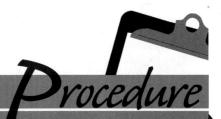

Box 26.5

Procedures for Bonding Brackets and Placement of Archwire

Materials needed

Mouth mirror
Explorer
Cotton forceps
Probe
Scaler
Prophy paste
Low speed handpiece
Prophy angle
Cotton rolls
Bracket placement forceps
Brackets
Bonding material
Plastic spatula

1. Brackets are selected and arranged on a bracket tray for easy identification during cementation
2. The teeth are polished free of plaque with a rubber cup and pumice.
3. The teeth are rinsed thoroughly with plenty of water, dried well and cotton rolls or cheek retractors are used for isolation.
4. Etching is on the enamel surface of the teeth. Do not rub the surface with the etching solution and take care not to get it on the gingival tissue.
5. After 60 seconds, rinse the solution thoroughly with water (Figure 26.15, A), cotton rolls are removed and teeth are dried. They should appear chalky, but if they don't they must be re-etched. Isolate the teeth to be bonded with cotton rolls and cheek retractors and place a saliva ejector in the patient's mouth.
6. Dry the teeth and apply the sealant or bonding agent. Let the sealant dry or light cure.
7. Apply the bonding material to the base of the bracket.
8. Place the bracket on the tooth surface and remove excess material (Figure 26.15, B).
9. Allow at least 5 minutes for the material to completely harden or light cure then place a light force archwire.

Procedures for placement of archwires

Materials needed

Mirror
Explorer
Cotton forceps
Probe
Archwire
Wire cutters
Buccal tube archwire slot in places
Ligature pliers

10. Secure the archwire and use the selected archwire and determine the proper length. Slide one end of the archwire into the molar buccal tube archwire slot with the pliers. Carefully slide the archwire evenly into the bracket slots and seat firmly.
11. Clip the long ends of the wire at the distobuccal aspect of the tube with distal end cutter pliers.
12. Choose ligation material.

Table 26.8

Evaluation for Bonding Brackets

Task	4	3	2	0	X
Select tray setup and bracket setup.					
Clean and dry teeth, isolate.					
Apply etchant to facial surface, rinse, and dry.					
Apply bonding agent and cure.					
Apply bonding material to bracket.					
Apply bracket to tooth and remove excess material.					
Cure bonding material; secure.					

The numeric criteria: 4 Excellent; 3 Good but some improvement can be made; 2 Below average, usable, needs to improve skill; 0 Unsatisfactory; X Not able to evaluate.

Table 26.9

Evaluation for Placement of Archwire

Task	4	3	2	0	X
Select archwire and determine approximate length.					
Slide wire into buccal tubes.					
Seat wire into bracket slots.					
Clip distal end.					

The numeric criteria: 4 Excellent; 3 Good but some improvement can be made; 2 Below average, usable, needs to improve skill; 0 Unsatisfactory; X Not able to evaluate.

A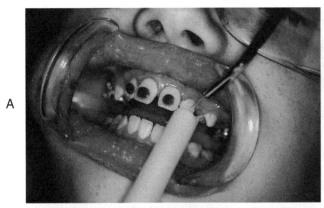

B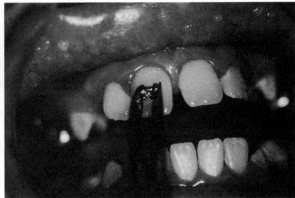

C

FIGURE 26.15

A, 60 seconds after placing etchant on the enamel, rinse the solution thoroughly with water. **B**, Place the bracket on the tooth and remove excess material. **C**, Ligature, elastic modules, elastic chain, stainless steel ties, power thread, open coil, and auxiliary hooks.

Table 26.10

Evaluation for Placement of SS Ligature Ties

Task	4	3	2	0	X
Secure materials.					
Bend end of tie 90A and slide under bracket wings.					
Twist-tie and tighten.					
Clip and tuck tail.					

The numeric criteria: 4 Excellent; 3 Good but some improvement can be made; 2 Below average, usable, needs to improve skill; 0 Unsatisfactory; X Not able to evaluate.

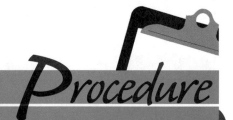

Box 26.6

Procedures For Placement Of Ligature

Placement of stainless steel ligature

Materials needed
Mouth mirror
Explorer
Cotton forceps
Probe
Preformed stainless steel ligature wire
Forceps
Pin and ligature cutter
Ligature director
Distal end cutter
Model with braces and archwire
1. Secure materials.
2. Bend the end of the ligature wire to a 90 degree angle with fingers. Slide the ligature wire under the bracket, tie wings and pull tightly with fingers. With fingers twist the ends of the ligature wire (Figure 26.16, *A*).
3. Grasp the ligature wire with the ligating forceps and lock forceps, twist and tighten. Seat the archwire completely in the bracket slot (Figure 26.16, *B*). Cut the wire with the ligature wire lingually so that it is smooth. Use end cutter to remove any excess archwire.

Ligation of elastomeric modules

Materials needed
Mirror
Explorer
Cotton forceps
Probe
Elastomeric modules
Hemostat
Distal end cutter with lock

Model with braces and archwire
(Figure 26.16, *C*).
1. Secure materials.
2. With the hemostat, grip the elastomeric ligature and lock the hemostat.
3. Place the ligature wire under the gingival bracket tie wing.
4. Connect the tie wing by rotating the hemostat over the archwire and release the hemostat lock.
5. Check for secure ligation and remove any excess archwire (Figure 26.16, *D*).
6. To remove ligature, place scaler tips between the archwire and the bracket under the elastomeric and lift it out.

Ligation of elastomeric chain

Materials needed
Mirror
Explorer
Cotton forceps
Probe
Elastomeric modular
Hemostat
Scaler
1. Secure materials needed. Cut off the needed number of elastomeric links. Grip the end link with hemostat and place the end link over the most distal bracket tie wing (Figure 26.16, *E*).
2. Grip next link and repeat ligation until the entire chain is placed. Check for excess archwire. To remove ligature, place scaler tip between the archwire and the bracket under the elastomeric and lift it out.

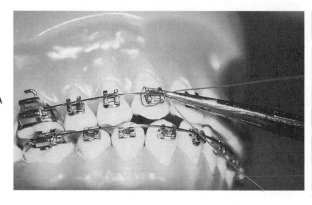

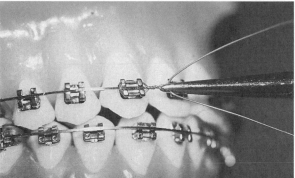

A / B

FIGURE 26.16

A, Place stainless steel ligature: make a 90 degree bend in loop and slide under bracket over wire, pull and twist with fingers. **B**, Grasp with forceps and tighten twist.

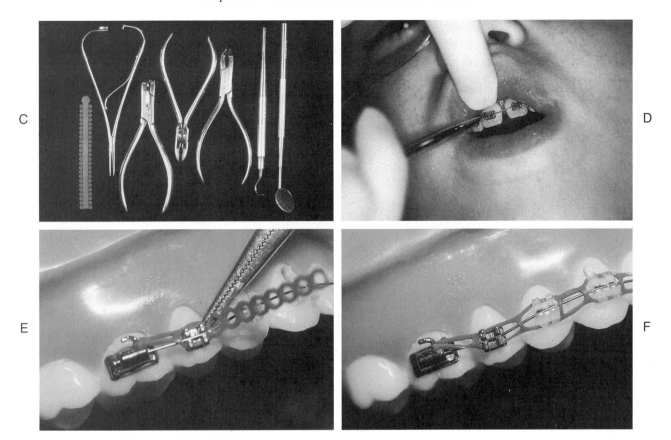

FIGURE 26.16, cont'd

C, Placing elastic modules: tray set up, **D**, check for secure ligation. **E**, Elastic chain: after cutting the length needed and placing it on the most distal attachment. **F**, Grasp the next link and pull over the next bracket, continue until completion of the arch.

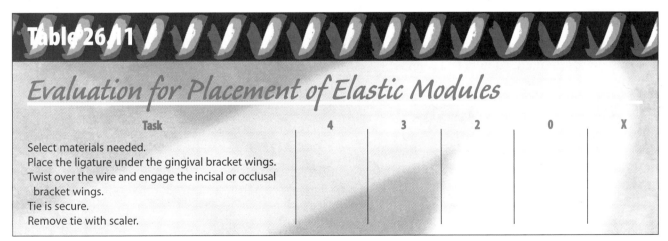

Table 26.11

Evaluation for Placement of Elastic Modules

Task	4	3	2	0	X
Select materials needed.					
Place the ligature under the gingival bracket wings.					
Twist over the wire and engage the incisal or occlusal bracket wings.					
Tie is secure.					
Remove tie with scaler.					

The numeric criteria: 4 Excellent; 3 Good but some improvement can be made; 2 Below average, usable, needs to improve skill; 0 Unsatisfactory; X Not able to evaluate.

Table 26.12

Evaluation for Placement of Elastic Chain

Task	4	3	2	0	X
Secure material needed.					
Cut needed length of chain.					
Place end loop on most distal attachment.					
Place next loop on next bracket.					
Continue until completed arch.					
Chain is engaged under all four wings of all brackets and secure.					

The numeric criteria: 4 Excellent; 3 Good but some improvement can be made; 2 Below average, usable, needs to improve skill; 0 Unsatisfactory; X Not able to evaluate.

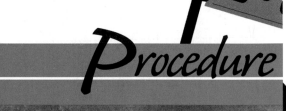

Box 26.7

Procedure

Procedures for Giving Oral Hygiene Instruction

Materials needed
Typodont with orthodontic appliance
Tooth brush
Interproximal brush
Floss
Disclosure tablets
Mouthwash (with fluoride)
Orthodontic wax
Instruction sheet

1. Use typodont with appliances to give instructions.
2. Show patient how to angle the bristles of the tooth brush to remove food and plaque around the gingival margin from all appliances and reaching all the way to the back of the mouth.
3. Show the patient how to brush the lingual of the teeth and all appliances and to angle the tooth brush up to get food and plaque away from the occlusal aspect of the appliances.
4. Show the patient how to brush the lingual of the teeth and all appliances and to use the tooth brush straight up and down to reach the lingual of the anterior.
5. Show the patient how to use the interproximal brush to reach the tooth surface below the arch wire and between the teeth.
6. Show the patient how to thread the floss under the arch wire so that they may floss interproximal between brackets.
7. Show the patient how to use disclosure tablets to find plaque that may have been missed the first time around.
8. Instruct the patient to use a mouthwash with fluoride daily
9. Show the patient how to do a self-examination before and after disclosure tablets and with daily brushing.
10. Show the patient how to check the appliances for cleanliness and maintenance and instruct them to come in immediately if they find anything broken, loose, or out of place.
11. Show them how to use patient wax and medications for any soreness that may develop.
12. Instruct them on proper eating and chewing habits.

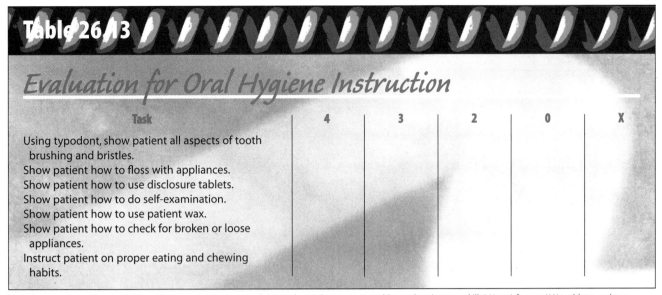

Table 26.13

Evaluation for Oral Hygiene Instruction

Task	4	3	2	0	X
Using typodont, show patient all aspects of tooth brushing and bristles.					
Show patient how to floss with appliances.					
Show patient how to use disclosure tablets.					
Show patient how to do self-examination.					
Show patient how to use patient wax.					
Show patient how to check for broken or loose appliances.					
Instruct patient on proper eating and chewing habits.					

The numeric criteria: 4 Excellent; 3 Good but some improvement can be made; 2 Below average, usable, needs to improve skill; 0 Unsatisfactory; X Not able to evaluate.

Box 26.8

Food to Avoid During Orthodontic Treatment

Sticky food

Caramels
Chewing and bubble gum
Sticky candy

Sugary food

Sweet desserts
Soft drinks
Jam or jelly

Hard food

Apples
Raw carrots, celery, and so on
Ice cubes
Popcorn

ROUTINE ADJUSTMENT APPOINTMENT

The assistant will need to follow through during the entire treatment period to evaluate the patient's oral health condition. The assistant will check the patient's oral health, such as presence of plaque or irregularities in hard and soft tissue, and decide if they are brushing correctly, using interproximal aids, and eating properly (Box 26.9 and Table 26.14).

If the patient comes to an appointment with poor oral hygiene it may be necessary to have the patient use a disclosure tablet (see Chapter 17). This will allow both the assistant and the patient to see what areas need attention. Have the patient work the bristles of the toothbrush into trouble spots and tell them to pay attention to these areas when they are brushing at home.

Ligature and Archwire Removal

As treatment progresses, the patient will get a change of wire (Box 26.10 and Table 26.15). Each time the wire is changed the ties will be changed. The procedure will be to remove the ties, remove the wire, place a new wire in the slots, and place new ties around the wing tips of the brackets. To remove the elastic ties from the bracket a scaler can be used. Place the tip of the scaler under the elastic and lift and pull the elastic off each wing tip until the elastic is free from the bracket.

Headgear

During treatment the patient may need to wear headgear or facemask devices to provide extraoral force to achieve the desired treatment results. The headgear consists of a facebow and a large outer bow soldered to a smaller inner bow.

Box 26.9

Procedure

Procedures For Checking Oral Hygiene

Materials needed
Mirror
Explorer
Cotton forceps
Probe
Large face mirror
Toothbrush
Floss
Disclosure tablets

1. Pull the lips and cheeks away from the patient's teeth for direct vision.
2. Look at the gums for redness or swelling.
3. Check the teeth, tissue and bone for plaque.

4. Check for decay or problem areas.
5. Disclosure tablets to identify plaque.
6. Check all orthodontic appliances:
    Archwires
    Brackets
    Bands
    Ligatures
    Headgear
    Removable
7. Discuss oral cavity conditions, appliance conditions, and review and reinforce any unsuccessful or incomplete instructions.
8. Record results in the patient's record.

Table 26.14

Evaluation for Oral Hygiene Check

Task	4	3	2	0	X
Check all teeth and tissue for plaque, irritation, decay, or inflammation.					
Provide disclosure tablets.					
Recheck for plaque after disclosure.					
Check all appliances for cleanliness.					
Discuss conditions, review, and reinforce.					
Record results.					

The numeric criteria: 4 Excellent; 3 Good but some improvement can be made; 2 Below average, usable, needs to improve skill; 0 Unsatisfactory; X Not able to evaluate.

The inner bow fits into the buccal tubes of the bands on the first molars. There are several traction devices used that attach to the outer bow. They are high-pull traction, cervical traction, and chin cap.

High-pull traction is like a cap worn over the top of the head that is hooked up perpendicular to the occlusal plane. This may be used to control growth of the maxilla. Cervical traction is a strap worn at the base of the skull around the neck and it hooks up parallel to the occlusal plane. This may be used to stabilize or distalize the first molars. High-pull and cervical traction can be used in combination and this will provide an external force upward and backward. The chin cap is a combination of a chin cup and high-pull cap. It may be used to control growth of the mandible. A facemask can be worn for extraoral force. Its components are a vertical bow that is attached to a chin pad and a forehead pad. The vertical bow has a small horizontal bow that allows elastics to be attached to the buccal hooks on the first molar bands to the facemask. This device can be used to encourage growth of the maxilla.

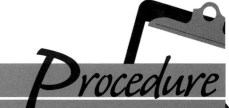

Box 26.10

Procedure

Procedures for Removing Stainless Steel Ligatures

Materials needed
Mirror
Explorer
Cotton forceps
Probe
Ligature cutter
Wiring cut pliers

1. Secure the ligature cutter and gently grip the ligature wire opposite the pigtail and cut it (Figure 26.17).
2. Grip the opposite pigtail cut end and carefully lift the wire off the bracket and archwire.

Procedures for removing the archwire

1. Secure the Weingart pliers to remove the archwire.
2. The distal ends of the archwire must be straightened before trying to remove it.
3. Once the ends of the archwire is checked and straightened, if necessary, grip the archwire mesial to the cuspid with the Weingart pliers.
4. Carefully ease and remove the wire from the anterior bracket.
5. If the archwire does not slide easily check the distal ends and the last band again while gently easing the wire from the brackets.

Table 26.15

Evaluation for Removing Stainless Steel Ligature Ties

Task	4	3	2	0	X
Tips of pin and ligature pliers placed on tie opposite the pigtail.					
Tie clipped and removed.					

The numeric criteria: 4 Excellent; 3 Good but some improvement can be made; 2 Below average, usable, needs to improve skill; 0 Unsatisfactory; X Not able to evaluate.

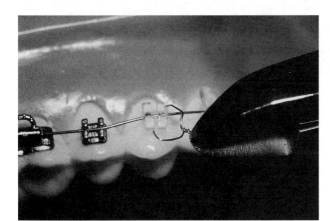

FIGURE 26.17

Removal of stainless steel ties: place tips of ligature cutter opposite pigtail and clip, then lift the wire off the bracket.

Elastics

Intraoral force can be applied with the use of intraoral elastics (Box 26.11 and Table 26.16). They come in variety of sizes or forces. They are classified as Class I, Class II, Class III, and Class IV. To use the intraoral elastics, there needs to be hook attachments on the brackets and bands. There are hooks made on some brackets but if there is not a hook where one is needed, you can add one. One way of doing this is to add a *Kobayashi tie,* which is a small loop on the end of a stainless steel tie. This can be tied around the bracket just like a ligature tie and you've added a hook.

The roots of the teeth may also need to be torqued (tipped) into a more ideal position; this can be done by placing bends in the wire or repositioning the brackets. The teeth may look great just looking in the mouth but it is necessary to take a Panorex radiograph to see if the roots are in the correct inclination.

Box 26.11　　　　　　　　　　　　　　　　*Procedure*

Procedures For Placing Intraoral Elastics

Materials needed

Mirror
Explorer
Cotton forceps
Probe
Intraoral elastics (Class I, II, III, and IV)
Hemostat
Scaler

1. Class I elastics are attached from the anterior to the posterior of each same arch. They may be used for the purpose of retracting canines to close space from the extraction of a first premolar (Figure 26.18, *A*).
2. Class II elastics are worn from the anterior canine maxillary arch to the posterior first molar mandibular arch. They are used to correct the occlusion of the opposing arches (Figure 26.18, *B*).
3. Class III elastics are worn from the posterior first molar of the maxillary arch to the anterior canine of the mandibular arch. They are also used to correct the occlusion of opposing arches (Figure 26.18, *C*).
4. Class IV elastics-are used to correct a crossbite and they are attached from the lingual cleat of one tooth to the buccal hook of the band of the opposing arch (Figure 26.18, *D*).
5. Intraoral elastics may also be used in the shapes of triangles or boxed or zigzag. The shapes would be used in opposing arched and for specific corrections required for completion of treatment.

Table 26.16

Evaluation for Placement of Intraoral Elastics

Task	4	3	2	0	X
Place Class I elastics.					
Place Class II elastics.					
Place Class III elastics.					
Place Class IV elastics.					
Place triangle elastics.					
Place boxed elastics.					
Place zigzag elastics.					

The numeric criteria: 4 Excellent; 3 Good but some improvement can be made; 2 Below average, usable, needs to improve skill; 0 Unsatisfactory; X Not able to evaluate.

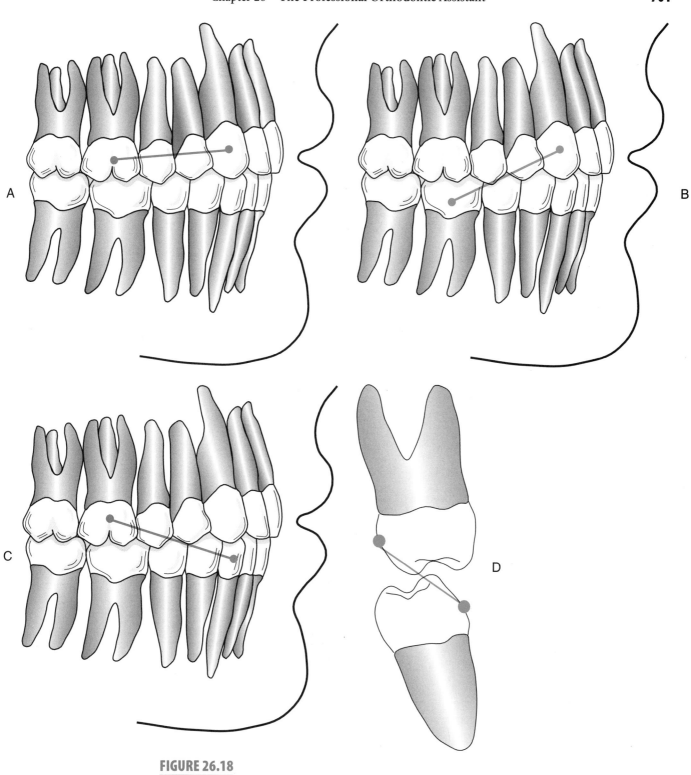

FIGURE 26.18

A, Class I elastics. **B**, Class II elastics. **C**, Class III elastics. **D**, Class IV elastics.

Orthodontic Wire Bending

There are two basic types of wire used in orthodontic treatment: the round wire and the rectangular wire. The most popular wires are made of stainless steel or nickel-titanium. Orthodontic treatment usually involves taking the patient through progressive phases using round, square, or rectangular wire of varying sizes and force.

Treatment Phases

Phase One

The first phase is the alignment of the teeth in the dental arch using a series of round wires and working up to rectangular wire.

Phase Two

Phase two is the leveling of the teeth into their proper vertical alignment and the curve of Spee.

Phase Three

Phase three is the closing of spaces usually using rectangular wire and elastic forces.

Phase Four

Phase four is the finishing phase or final phase of treatment. This is the phase in which finishing bends are placed in the archwire. The 0.018 x 0.025 inch stainless steel wire is a good finishing wire. Special bends can be placed in the finishing wire to place the crowns or the roots of the teeth in their most ideal position.

Wire Bending Technique

Special pliers are used for wire bending. The wire is held with the pliers but is actually bent with the fingers or thumb. Orthodontic pliers usually have round tips, square tips, or a combination of both. The most important aspect of wire bending is the proper orientation of the wire and the pliers. The pliers should be held in the palm of the hand in a position that makes it perpendicular to the floor. The wire should then be held by the pliers tip in a position that is parallel to the floor. The archwire should lie flat on the table as it is in its correct arch form. After each bend is placed in the wire it should again lie flat on the table.

Compensating Bends

First Order Bends

First order bends are placed in the wire in and "in-out" position or on the "horizontal plane." These are called "offset" bends. An offset bend will move the tooth in a buccal direction. An "inset" bend will move the tooth in a lingual direction (Figure 26.19, *A* and *B*).

Second Order Bends

Second order bends are in the "up-down" position or in the "vertical plane." These bends may be used to bring one or more teeth down or up occlusally (Figure 26.19, *C*).

Third Order Bends

Third order bends are used to move the roots of the teeth buccally or lingually. To do this a twist is placed in the archwire. This is also called "torque." Usually a special set

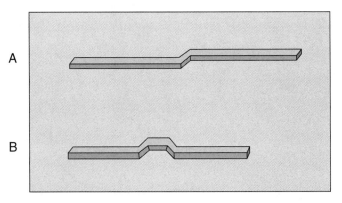

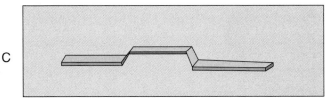

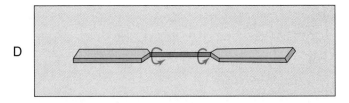

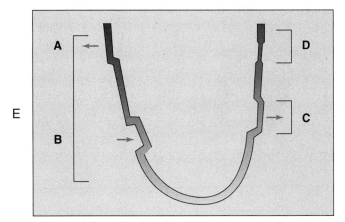

FIGURE 26.19

Compensating bends. First order bends: **A**, Bend toward facial. **B**, Bend toward lingual. Second order bends: **C**, Bend toward occlusal. Third order bends: **D**, Twist. **E**, Wire arch indicating the four bands.

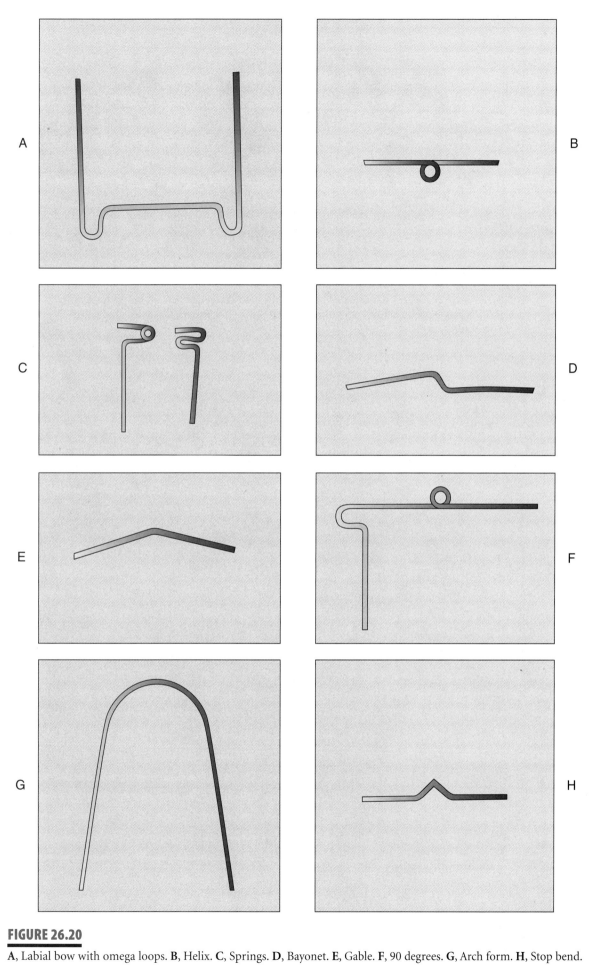

FIGURE 26.20

A, Labial bow with omega loops. B, Helix. C, Springs. D, Bayonet. E, Gable. F, 90 degrees. G, Arch form. H, Stop bend.

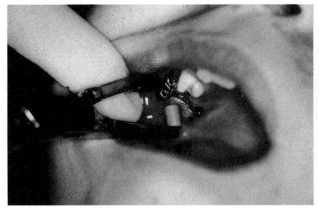
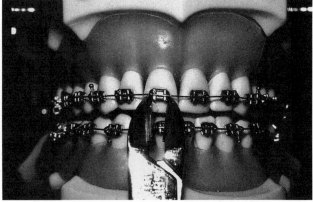

FIGURE 26.21

A, Band removal: place beak of pliers on band with the plastic base of pliers on the occlusal surface of tooth and squeeze. **B,** Bracket removal: after archwire is removed, place tips of pliers under bracket and squeeze.

Procedure

Box 26.12

Procedure for Removing Bands and Brackets

Removing bands	Removing brackets
Materials needed	**Materials needed**

Removing bands

Materials needed

Mouth mirror
Explorer
Cotton forceps
Probe
Scaler
Band removing pliers
Ligature cutter
Model with bands, brackets, and archwire

1. Secure materials.
2. Remove the archwire.
3. Place the plastic beak of the band removing pliers on the occlusal surface and the metal beak on the facial surface under the gingival margin part of the band. Squeeze the handles of the pliers together and the cement bond will usually separate. If not, the band may need to be cut from the tooth.
4. Lift the band from the tooth.
5. The old cement is scaled from the teeth and then the teeth are cleaned.
6. Check the gingiva carefully to make sure all cement has been removed and rinse the patient's mouth thoroughly

Removing brackets

Materials needed

Mirror
Explorer
Cotton forceps
Probe
Howe pliers
Band removing pliers
Scaler
Handpiece
Bur
Sandpaper disk
Model with brackets

1. Secure materials.
2. Remove the archwire.
3. Using the Howe pliers, press the bracket tie wings together and lift the bracket from mouth or use band removing pliers by placing tips under bracket and press together. Debonding "guns" are also available for debonding.
4. Carefully remove remaining composite from the subgingival surface with a scaler and from the enamel with the scaler or the low speed handpiece, fluted bur, and extra-fine sandpaper disk.
5. Prophy the enamel surface with a rubber cup and pumice.

of pliers is used to place the torque in the archwire (Figure 26.19, *D*).

It is important to mark the midline of the archwire when making any bends and to see that the midline of the archwire is matched up to the midline of the dentition.

Remember that detailing bends are usually used in the last phase of treatment. Up to that point it is necessary to let the wire slide easily through the bracket slots to accomplish space closure and to more effectively use the mechanics that are fashioned into the bracket slot prescription.

Wire Bending for Appliances

Wire bending is also used for the fabrication of orthodontic appliances. Orthodontic appliances are worn during and after treatment. The same rules apply as in bending archwire. The pliers are held perpendicular to the floor and the wire is held parallel to the floor. Some of the components of an orthodontic appliance are clasps, springs, and labial bows. A labial bow uses an arch form with two omega loops at the middle of the cuspids. It is most commonly used to passively hold the anterior teeth in the ideal shape of the arch. The clasps are designed to give retention to the appliance and hold it in place. Springs may be used to move teeth by applying force to designated areas.

Some of the more popular exercises in wire bending involve omega loops, helix or continuous loops, bayonet gable, 90- and .45-degree bends, and of course the smooth curve or arch form (Figure 26.20).

APPLIANCE REMOVAL APPOINTMENT

After the treatment has been completed and malocclusion has been corrected, the bands and brackets are removed (Box 26.12, Tables 26.17, 26.18, and 26.19 and Figure 26.21). It is important to take care in removing the cemented bands and bonded brackets from the teeth. Once all of the appliances have been removed from the teeth as well as all of the bonding material, the teeth are cleaned and fluoride is applied. Before the fluoride treatment however, impressions must be taken for retainers. Using a perforated metal impression tray and alginate impression material, take an upper and lower impression. The retainers will be made from these impressions and will be delivered in 1 to 5 days.

RETAINER APPOINTMENT

The purpose of the retainer is to hold the teeth in their correct alignment for a certain length of time so that there will be no relapse of rotations or malalignments. They are usually worn full-time for 6 to 12 months. If the habit that has caused the malocclusion has not been eliminated, retention may fail. Retainers may be removable or fixed. Removable retainers are made of acrylic and wire and the patient may take them out for eating or brushing. Fixed retainers are bonded to the lingual aspect of the upper or lower anteriors (Figure 26.22).

Table 26.17

Evaluation for Removing Bands

Task	4	3	2	0	X
Secure tray setup.					
Remove archwire.					
Place plastic beak of band removing pliers on occlusal surface of tooth with metal beak of pliers under the gingival margin of the band.					
Squeeze the handles of the pliers and separate the cement bond.					
Remove band from tooth.					
Clean off remaining cement.					

The numeric criteria: 4 Excellent; 3 Good but some improvement can be made; 2 Below average, usable, needs to improve skill; 0 Unsatisfactory; X Not able to evaluate.

Table 26.18

Evaluation for Removing Archwire

Task	4	3	2	0	X
Grasp archwire mesial to the buccal tube and pull.					
Straighten or clip distal end of archwire if necessary.					
Grasp archwire at the mesial of opposite band and pull.					
Ease archwire out of bracket slots in the anterior.					
Remove archwire.					

The numeric criteria: 4 Excellent; 3 Good but some improvement can be made; 2 Below average, usable, needs to improve skill; 0 Unsatisfactory; X Not able to evaluate.

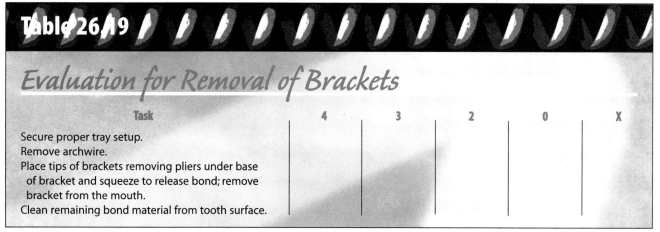

Table 26.19

Evaluation for Removal of Brackets

Task	4	3	2	0	X
Secure proper tray setup.					
Remove archwire.					
Place tips of brackets removing pliers under base of bracket and squeeze to release bond; remove bracket from the mouth.					
Clean remaining bond material from tooth surface.					

The numeric criteria: 4 Excellent; 3 Good but some improvement can be made; 2 Below average, usable, needs to improve skill; 0 Unsatisfactory; X Not able to evaluate.

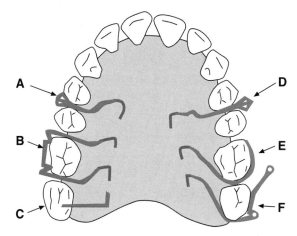

FIGURE 26.22

Retention appliance: **A,** ball clasp: placed in the interproximal embrasure. **B,** Arrowhead clasp: placed in the interproximal embrasure. **C,** Adams clasp: placed in the interproximal embrasure. **D,** "C" clasp: placed below the height of contour. **E,** Occlusal rest: placed in lingual groove carried over to occlusal. **F,** Band clasp fits in buccal slot between tubes.

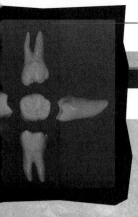

Points for Review

- General qualifications of an orthodontic assistant
- Need for orthodontic treatment
- Etiology of malocclusion
- Types of orthodontic treatment
- Mechanism of realigning teeth
- Classification of occlusion and malocclusion
- Orthodontic appliances and orthodontic armamentarium
- Types of appointments

Self-Study Questions

1. Orthodontics is the branch of dentistry concerned with which of the following?
   a. Disease of the tissues surrounding the teeth
   b. The causes, prevention, and treatment of malocclusion of the teeth and jaw
   c. Developing prosthetic devices for people who have lost their natural dentition
   d. Root canal therapy

2. What must an individual do to become an orthodontist?
   a. Straighten the teeth of at least 50 people
   b. Have worked in at least two states as a general dentist
   c. Complete 2 years of formal education in an accredited university after receiving their dental degree
   d. Have a good reputation for straightening teeth

3. The majority of orthodontic practices include patients who are of what ages?
   a. Young children
   b. Adults
   c. Teenagers
   d. All ages

4. What reason(s) support the need for orthodontic treatment?
   a. Proper oral function

   b. More pleasing esthetics
   c. Good oral health
   d. All of the above

5. In the Angle's system of classification, which permanent teeth were selected for identifying the normal relationship of the mandibular to the maxillary arch?
   a. First molars
   b. Second premolars
   c. Second molars
   d. All of the above

6. What is a removable appliance that can correct crossbites by separating teeth?
   a. Lip bumper
   b. Hawley retainer
   c. Expansion appliance with skeleton screws
   d. Lingual holding arch

7. Orthodontic impression trays are used to do which of the following?
   a. Measure the length of the tongue
   b. Expand the palate
   c. Make negative duplicates of the patient's dentition
   d. Correct malocclusion

8. The initial examination may try to determine the existence and extent of which of the following bad habits?
   a. Thumb-sucking
   b. Fingernail biting
   c. Mouth breathing
   d. All of the above

9. The panagraphic radiograph is a complete radiograph of the patients dentition in which of the following cases?
   a. On the upper arch only
   b. From right to left
   c. When the patient is lying down
   d. For the deciduous teeth only

10. Why are the permanent first molars selected for identifying the normal relationship of the mandibular and the maxillary arch?
    a. Because they are the largest teeth in the arch
    b. Because they are the first permanent molars to erupt, they have long roots, and tend to be in a stable position
    c. Because they have the most permanent cusp tips
    d. Because they can be moved with the least amount of resistance

11. How can a Class III malocclusion be recognized?

   a. Forward or protrusive inclination of the mandible

   b. Backward or retrusive inclination of the mandible

   c. Ability of the mandible to open beyond 13 mm

   d. The shortness of the chin

12. Which bone is effected by the use of a rapid palatal expander fixed appliance?

   a. The frontal bone

   b The maxilla

   c. The tibia

   d. The zygomatic process

13. Which pliers would be used for cutting the archwire that is too long after being placed in the mouth?

   a. Weingart utility pliers

   b. Ligature pliers

   c. Tweed arch-adjusting pliers

   d. Distal end cutting pliers with holder

14. What things might be done to a patient on their first visit to the orthodontic office?

   a. Removal of band and brackets from the teeth

   b. Ligation of the arch wire into the brackets

   c. A medical and dental history

   d. Oral hygiene instruction for how to take care of their appliances

15. What form of intraoral force can be applied to help correct the occlusion?

   a. Pushing on the anterior teeth with the ball of the thumb at least 10 times a day

   b. Pressing the tongue against the lingual aspect of the teeth as often as possible

   c. Using intraoral elastics that are attached to hooks on the bracket and bands

   d. Occlusal registration wax bites

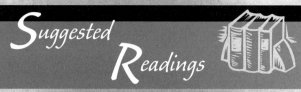

Suggested Readings

American Heart Association: *Heathcare provider's manual for basic life support,* 1988, 1990.

Bennet JD, Dembo JB: *The dental clinics of North America: medical emergencies in the dental office,* Philadelphia, 1995, WB Saunders.

Chandra NC, Hazinski M: *Textbook of basic life support for heathcare providers,* Dallas, Tex, 1994, American Heart Association.

Chernega JB: *Emergency guide for dental auxiliaries,* ed 2, Albany, New York, 1994, Delmar Publishers.

Chilo V, Strong M, Borea G: *Life threatening emergencies in dentistry,* Padova, Italy, 1988, Lshiyaku Euroamerica.

Garcia B, editor: *Mosby's emergency dictionary: EMS, rescue, and special operations,* ed 2, St Louis, 1998, Mosby.

Graber, TM: *Orthodontics current principles and techniques,* ed 3, St Louis, 2000, Mosby.

Little JW, Falace D: *Dental management of the medically compromised patient,* ed 5, St Louis, 1997, Mosby.

Malamed SR: *Medical emergencies in the dental office,* ed 5, St Louis, 2000, Mosby.

Malamed SR: Physical evaluation and the prevention of medical emergencies: vital signs, *Anesth Pain Cont Dent* 2 (2):107-113, 1993.

McCarthy FM: *Essentials of safe dentistry for the medically compromised patient,* Philadelphia, 1989, WB Saunders.

Nanda R, Burstone CJ: *Retention and stability in orthodontics,* Philadelphia, 1993, WB Saunders.

Protzman S, Clark J: *The dental assistant's management of medical emergencies,* Chicago, 1995, American Dental Assistants Association.

Salyer SW: *The physician assistant emergency medicine handbook,* Philadelphia, 1997, WB Saunders.

Terezhalmy G, Batizy LF: *Urgent care in the dental office: an essential handbook,* 1997, Quintessence.

Chapter 27

Oral and Maxillofacial Surgery and Introduction to Hospital Dentistry

Key Points

- Preoperative and postoperative surgical considerations
- Pain and anxiety control
- Oral surgery armamentarium
- General and hospital oral surgery procedures
- Role of the dental assistant in oral surgery

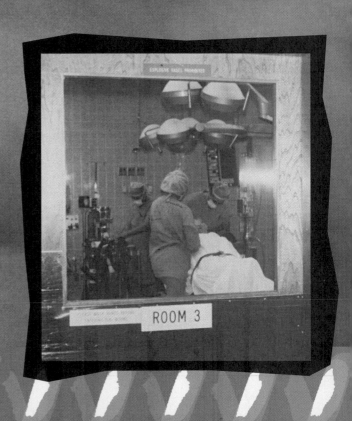

ROOM 3

Chapter Outline

Overview of Oral Surgery
Indications and Contraindications in Oral Surgery
Examination and Consultation
  Medical history
  Radiographs
  Oral examination
  Financial arrangements
  Informed consent
Pain Control
  Electronic anesthesia
  Nitrous oxide
  Local anesthesia
  General anesthesia
Instruments Used in Oral Surgery
  Basic oral surgery setup
  Scalpel handle and disposable blade
  Elevators
  Bone file
  Surgical curette
  Forceps
  Hemostats
  Tissue and suture scissors
  Needle holder
  Tongue and cheek retractors, molt mouth prop, and intraoral mouth props
  Surgical bur
  Mallet and chisel
  Sutures and surgical needles
  Throat pack
  Sterilization of surgical instruments
  Crash cart

Role of the Dental Assistant in Oral Surgery
  Preparing the operatory
  Preparing the patient
  Surgical scrub techniques
  Passing surgical instruments
  Suture placement
  Removal of sutures
  Preoperative instructions
  Postoperative instructions
  Postoperative medications
Selected Oral Surgery Procedures
  Incision and drainage
  Alveolitis
  Alveoloplasty
  Exostoses (tori)
  Biopsy
  Frenectomy
  Fractures
  Implants
  Gingival grafts
  Third molar extractions
Oral Surgery Procedures Involving Extractions
  Role of the dental assistant in extraction procedures
  Role of the dental assistant in administration of a general anesthetic
Hospital Dentistry
  Hospital outpatients
  Admissions
  Discharge
  Role of the dental assistant in hospital dentistry

Learning Objectives

On completion of Chapter 27, the student should be able to do the following:

- Define key terms.
- Identify the instruments and equipment used in oral surgery.
- Explain the role of the dental assistant in oral surgery and in hospital dentistry.
- Give preoperative and postoperative instructions and explain why it is important that the patient follow them
- Identify different forceps and explain their functions.
- Explain why a biopsy is performed.
- List the types of drugs used for preoperative and postoperative medication of surgical patients.
- List the indications and contraindications for oral surgery.

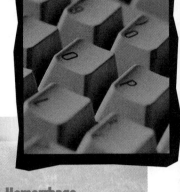

Key Terms

Alveoloplasty   Biopsy   Hemorrhage

OVERVIEW OF ORAL SURGERY

Oral surgery is the area of dentistry that involves the removal of teeth, as well as other surgical procedures of the jaws, oral tissues, and adjacent tissues. The procedures performed by oral surgery are (1) extraction of teeth, (2) bony and soft tissue surgery, (3) treatment of jaw fractures, and (4) surgical correction or treatment of other abnormalities of the jaws and immediate associated structures.

An oral surgeon is a dental specialist who has had at least three years of advanced dental training and often additional medical school training. (A general dentist can legally perform several of the oral surgery procedures but has limited training in many of those areas.) Oral surgeons treat patients with various facial deformities, and they often work with other medical specialists to correct physical conditions such as cleft palate, cleft lip, or children's facial syndromes.

Oral surgeons also treat patients who have been injured in accidents. Such treatment includes suturing of lips or repair of facial fractures. Because they are receiving medical degrees, more oral surgeons are involved in these types of surgical procedures.

INDICATIONS AND CONTRAINDICATIONS IN ORAL SURGERY

A dentist must consider many factors, pro and con, before performing surgical procedures. These factors are called indications and contraindications. The indications, or reasons for, oral surgery include the following:
- Carious teeth that cannot be restored
- Teeth that have little or no bone support

- Removal of root tips
- Removal of teeth for orthodontic treatment
- Removal of teeth that cannot be orthodontically aligned
- Removal of infected teeth that do not respond to treatment
- Removal of unrestorable teeth because of fractures or root resorption or because teeth are in line with a jaw fracture
- Removal of teeth before radiation treatment
- Removal of tumors, cysts, and other abnormalities
- Removal of bone overgrowth

The contraindications, or reasons against, oral surgery include the following:
- Teeth that are restorable
- Pregnancy (surgery should be delayed during pregnancy especially until after the first trimester and until after delivery if possible)
- Medical history (surgery should not be initiated until the medical history has been received and, if the patient has a tendency to bleed or **hemorrhage**, until preparations have been made for this contingency)
- Patient's health (surgery should be delayed if the patient's health condition, such as heart or kidney disease, diabetes, or high blood pressure, indicate the need to contact the person's physician).

Hemorrhage
Flow of blood caused by trauma

EXAMINATION AND CONSULTATION

A patient's first dental visit is very important (see Chapter 21). During this appointment the patient's health history is collected, and this information is kept in the patient's chart and used for future visits. It is essential to review the patient's health history at each visit to see if any changes have occurred.

Medical History

Upon arriving at the office, the patient should first fill out a medical history form (Figure 27.1). This form contains various questions about the patient's health condition. After reviewing the medical history form, the dentist may contact the patient's physician or send a consultation form to the physician. Consulting with the physician may delay the patient's treatment, but this contact may eliminate unnecessary risks.

Radiographs

The dentist usually has the dental assistant take radiographs (x-ray films) during the first visit. The radiographs most commonly taken for extractions are the periapical or panoramic films. However, the dentist may request an occlusal, cephalometric, or temporomandibular radiograph for specific procedures.

Oral Examination

On the first visit the dentist also performs a thorough oral examination of the patient's mouth, which includes checking other areas of the head and neck for related problems or abnormalities.

Financial Arrangements

Once the course of treatment has been determined, the treatment plan and a cost estimate are presented to the patient so that financial arrangements can be made. If the visit is an emergency appointment and the patient is in pain, the dentist will relieve the pain and then provide whatever appointments and care are needed to improve the patient's oral health in the future. In such cases emergency treatment is rendered first to relieve pain, and financial arrangements are made before the next appointment for further treatment.

Informed Consent

The oral surgery procedure should always be explained to the patient before treatment begins. This explanation should describe the procedure and any possible risks or complications. The following types of information should be discussed with the patient:

- Bleeding is normal after oral surgery. The patient should leave the gauze pack on for approximately 30 minutes. However, if slight bleeding continues after the pack has been removed, the patient can add another pack in the surgical area. If the bleeding becomes excessive, the patient should return to the office for further treatment.

- Swelling may also occur and usually reaches its peak 48 to 72 hours after surgery. Any considerable swelling that develops should be checked by the oral surgeon.
- Numbness may occur if the surgery is performed close to the inferior alveolar nerve. If this nerve is bruised or cut, the patient may have temporary numbness of the lip or tongue. This numbness is rarely permanent.
- Infection is a possibility with any type of surgery. If infection is present at the time of surgery, the procedure may be postponed and an antibiotic prescribed to clear up the condition. If infection develops after surgery, antibiotics may be prescribed or further surgical treatment may be needed.
- Damage to adjacent teeth or jaw fracture may occur because of the pressure exerted in removing a tooth. If this should occur, the oral surgeon will provide further treatment.

Once these points have been discussed with the patient, the person is asked to sign a consent form (Figure 27.2). This form should identify the tooth that is to be removed or the procedure that is to be performed. The signed consent form indicates that the patient has agreed to have the listed procedure completed and understands the possibility of complications. The dental assistant often signs the form as a witness that the procedures and any potential complications have been explained to the patient before the start of treatment and that the patient has willingly signed the consent form.

PAIN CONTROL

Professional control of dental pain is discussed in Chapter 14. However, it is important to note that oral surgeons are trained in advanced pain control techniques, and the dental assistant should be knowledgeable of these procedures.

Electronic Anesthesia

Electronic anesthesia currently is used effectively to control pain and discomfort during restorative treatment; however, it is not effective at this time for surgical procedures.

Nitrous Oxide

Many patients are very anxious about having a tooth extracted. Therefore a dentist may choose to use an oral type of sedation to help the patient relax. The pain control method most commonly used to help a patient relax is nitrous oxide/oxygen. This gas is easy to use, relaxes the patient quickly, and is easily removed from the body after treatment (also see Chapter 14).

Local Anesthesia

Local anesthesia is a primary component in providing pain relief during oral surgery (see Chapter 14).

UNIVERSITY HOSPITAL DENTAL SERVICE

Comprehensive ☐   Limited ☐
CARE STATUS: _____
CHIEF COMPLAINT: _____   REFERRED BY: _____

1. What is your present health status? _____   Yes No   Remarks
2. Have you recently been under medical treatment? ....   ☐   ☐
3. Has a physician ever informed you that you had:

	Yes	No		Yes	No		Yes	No
A heart ailment	☐	☐	Hepatitis	☐	☐	Kidney disease	☐	☐
Rheumatic fever	☐	☐	Blood disease	☐	☐	Thyroid disease	☐	☐
High blood pressure	☐	☐	Diabetes	☐	☐	TB	☐	☐
Lung disease	☐	☐	EENT	☐	☐	Arthritis	☐	☐
Asthma or bronchitis	☐	☐	Glaucoma	☐	☐	Tumors or growths	☐	☐
Liver disease	☐	☐	Stomach or intestinal disease	☐	☐	Nervous disorders	☐	☐

4. Have you had any major operations? ....   ☐   ☐
5. Have you had any bleeding or healing problems? ....   ☐   ☐
6. Are you presently taking any medication? ....   ☐   ☐
   List _____
7. Are you allergic to any foods or drugs? ....   ☐   ☐
                                    Penicillin? ....   ☐   ☐
8. Have you had any difficulties with general anesthesia? ....   ☐   ☐
                                    Local anesthesia? ....   ☐   ☐
9. Have you ever had x-ray therapy? ....   ☐   ☐
10. Do you wear contact lenses? ....   ☐   ☐
11. Are you pregnant? ....   ☐   ☐   At risk _____
12. Last intake of food or liquid? _____

Family physician _____   Family dentist _____

	N	AB			N	AB	
			1. Facial bones				6. Buccal mucosa
			2. Skin				7. Palate
			3. Neck				8. Tongue
			4. Salivary glands				9. Floor of mouth
			5. Lips				10. Gingiva
							11. Oral hygiene

Significant laboratory and radiographic findings:

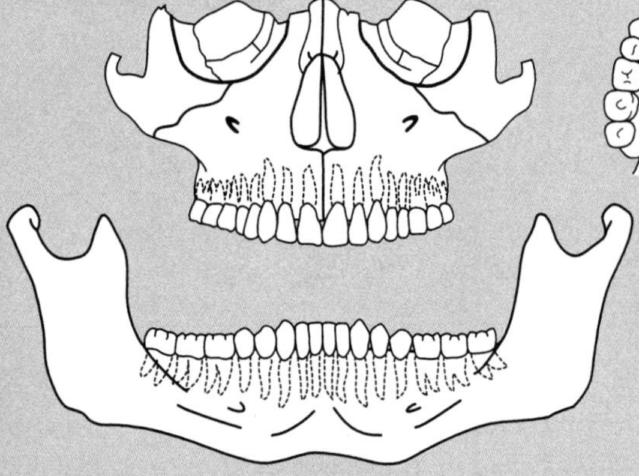

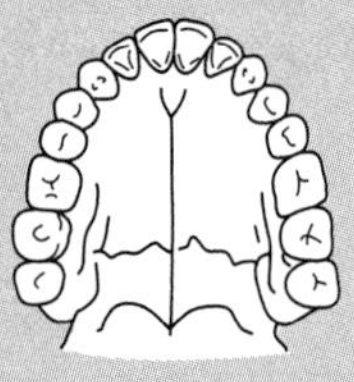

Comments:

_____ BP
_____ Pulse
_____ Temp.

Diagnosis: _____
_____
_____
_____
_____
_____
_____

Signature   Date

FIGURE 27.1

The medical history form used for oral surgery is a complete record of the patient's health history. (Courtesy University of Louisville School of Dentistry, Department of Oral and Maxillofacial Surgery.)

UNIVERSITY OF LOUISVILLE
DEPARTMENT OF SURGICAL AND HOSPITAL DENTISTRY

INFORMED CONSENT

You have the right to be informed about your condition and the recommended treatment plan to be used so that you may make an informed decision as to whether to undergo the procedure after knowing the risks and hazards involved. This disclosure is not meant to alarm you but is rather an effort to properly inform you so that you may give or withhold your consent.

This is my consent for Dr. _____ and any dentist or physician who is working with him or her to perform the following treatment, procedure, or surgery: _____
_____
_____

Dr. _____ has explained to me that certain inherent and potential risks exist in any treatment plan or procedure and, in this specific instance, such operative risks include but are not limited to the following:

A. Postoperative discomfort and swelling that may necessitate several days of at-home recuperation.
B. Heavy bleeding that may be prolonged.
C. Injury to adjacent teeth and fillings.
D. Postoperative infection requiring additional treatment.
E. Stretching of the corners of the mouth with resultant cracking and bruising.
F. Restricted mouth opening for several days or weeks.
G. Decision to leave a small piece of root in the jaw when its removal would require extensive surgery.
H. Fracture of the jaw.
I. Injury to the nerve under the teeth resulting in numbness or tingling of the chin, lip, cheek, gums, and tongue on the operated side, which may persist for several weeks, months, or in rare instances, permanently.
J. Opening into the sinus (a normal cavity situated above the upper teeth) requiring additional treatment.
K. Other _____

I understand that certain anesthetic risks that could involve serious bodily injury are inherent in any procedure that requires a general or intravenous anesthetic. I consent to the administration of _____ anesthesia.

I have been made aware that certain medications, drugs, anesthetics, and prescriptions that I may be given can cause drowsiness, incoordination, and lack of awareness that, also may be increased by the use of alcohol and other drugs. I have been advised not to operate any vehicle or hazardous machinery and not to work while taking such medication or until fully recovered from the effects of the same. I understand this recovery may take up to 24 hours or more after I have taken the last dose of medication. If I am given sedative medication during my surgery, I agree not to drive myself home and will have a responsible adult drive me home and accompany me until I am fully recovered from the effects of the sedation.

If I am a female using oral contraceptives, I understand that antibiotics and other medications may interfere with the effectiveness of oral contraceptives. Therefore I understand that I will need to use some additional form of birth control for one complete cycle of birth control pills after the course of antibiotics or other medication is completed.

IV sedation and general anesthesia are commonly used in oral and maxillofacial surgery for patient comfort and pain control. Anesthetics given in an ambulatory setting are considered safe, but you should know that certain risks are associated with the procedure. Below are some of the known risks of anesthesia:

Allergic reactions (previously unknown) to any of the medications used in the procedure.

Discomfort, swelling, or bruising at the site where the intravenous drugs are placed into a vein.

Vein irritation, called *phlebitis,* where the needle is placed into a vein. Sometimes this may progress to a level where arm or hand motion may be restricted temporarily and medications may be required.

Nausea and vomiting, although not common, are unfortunate side effects of general anesthesia. Bed rest, and sometimes medications, may be required for relief.

General anesthesia is a serious medical procedure in a hospital or office setting, and risks of brain damage, heart attack, or death exist.

Because of the potential for nausea and vomiting under anesthesia, I understand that I am not to eat or drink *anything* (or have had anything) by mouth for at least 6 to 8 hours before my surgery. *To do otherwise may be life-threatening.*

Continued

FIGURE 27.2

An informed consent form is provided for the patient to sign before surgery. (Courtesy University of Louisville School of Dentistry, Department of Oral and Maxillofacial Surgery.)

If any unforeseen condition should arise in the course of the operation, calling for the doctor's judgment or for procedures in addition to or different from those now contemplated, I request and authorize the doctor to do whatever deemed advisable.

No guarantee or assurance has been given to me that the proposed treatment will be curative and successful to my complete satisfaction. Because of individual patient differences, a risk of failure, relapse, selective retreatment, or worsening of my present condition exists despite the care provided. However, it is the doctor's opinion that therapy would be helpful and that a worsening of my condition would occur sooner without the recommended treatment.

I have had an opportunity to discuss with Dr. _____ my medical and health history including any serious problems and injuries.

I agree to cooperate completely with the recommendations of Dr. _____ while I am under care, realizing that not complying could result in poor results.

PLEASE ASK YOUR DOCTOR IF YOU HAVE QUESTIONS CONCERNING THIS CONSENT FORM.

Patient's (or legal guardian's) signature   Date

Witness' signature   Date

Doctor's signature   Date

FIGURE 27.2—Cont'd

For legend see p. 715.

General Anesthesia

General anesthesia may be indicated because a patient is very apprehensive or the procedure is very complex. Children often require a pain-relieving agent, such as the gas halothane, to induce general anesthesia. Halothane produces sleep through inhalation and is often used for short procedures, such as simple extractions. This provides pain relief without the need for intravenous (IV) administration of an anesthetic.

INSTRUMENTS USED IN ORAL SURGERY

Like other dental instruments, oral surgery instruments are made of steel. These instruments must be strong because of the pressure exerted during surgical procedures and because they must be cleaned and sterilized properly after each use (see Chapter 18).

Many general dentists have relatively simple surgical setups because they primarily perform minor surgical procedures, such as simple extractions and root planing. They also have specific instruments that meet their particular surgical needs. However, some general dentists do perform complicated oral surgery procedures. Dental assistants must have a general knowledge of the various surgical instruments and their purposes, but they also must be familiar with the specific instruments used by the dentist for whom they work.

Because of the large number of instruments available, the following list and Figure 27.3 are not intended to present all surgical instruments, but rather the most commonly used types and styles:

1 Mirror
2 Suction handle
3 Suction tips elevator (#73)
4 Periosteal elevator
5 Seldon elevator
6 Currette
7 Bone file
8 Hemostat
9 Rongeur forceps
10 301 forceps
11 11A forceps
12 Crane elevator
13 Potts root tip elevator (#73)
14 Potts root tip elevator (#74)
15 Maxillary universal forceps (#150)
16 Mandibular universal forceps (#151)
17 Syringe
18 Scalpel handle and blade
19 4 x 4-inch gauze sponge
20 Tissue pickup
21 Needle holder
22 Dean scissors

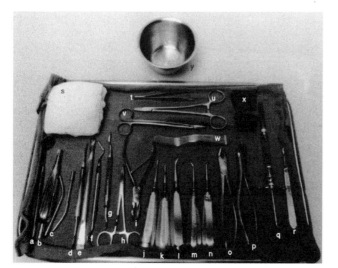

FIGURE 27.3

Surgical tray setup. (Courtesy University of Louisville School of Dentistry, Department of Oral and Maxillofacial Surgery.)

23 Minnesota retractor
24 Bite block
25 Irrigating bowl

Basic Oral Surgery Setup

The mouth mirror and suction handles and tips are part of most instrument setups, including the basic oral surgery setup. The mouth mirror, for instance, is used in oral surgery in the same way it is used in other procedures, that is, to retract the cheek or tongue, for light reflection, and for indirect vision. The suction handle and tips also serve a purpose similar to that in general dentistry, which is to remove blood, saliva, and debris from the oral cavity. Removal of those substances is the dental assistant's primary role during surgical procedures.

Scalpel Handle and Disposable Blade

The scalpel, or "knife," consists of a handle and a blade (see Figure 25.16). The scalpel handle may be made of steel or plastic. A steel handle can be sterilized and used many times, but a plastic handle usually is discarded after surgery. Scalpel blades are extremely sharp so as to allow the dentist to make incisions in the soft gingival tissue. The blades are available in a variety of shapes and sizes, and the selection is determined by the type of procedure and the operator's choice. Surgical blades are discarded after the surgical procedure. A scalpel blade should be removed with dental forceps or a scalpel blade remover; as with any sharp, disposable instrument, it should be disposed of in an approved container (Box 27.1).

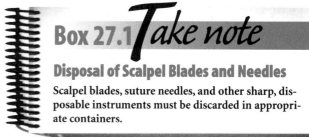

Box 27.1 Take note

Disposal of Scalpel Blades and Needles

Scalpel blades, suture needles, and other sharp, disposable instruments must be discarded in appropriate containers.

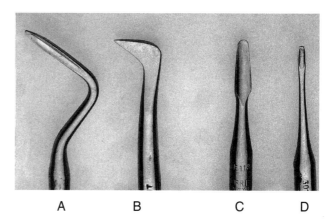

A	B	C	D

FIGURE 27.4

Elevators. *Left to right:* **A,** 303 Apical elevator. **B,** East-west elevator (R). **C,** E11A straight elevator. **D,** 301 elevator. *(R),* Indicates that the instrument is used on the right side of the oral cavity.

Elevators

Elevators can be described as levers because they allow the operator to apply a large amount of force to the tooth or root (Figure 27.4). Because of the force or pressure that is applied to the tooth with the elevator, the operator must have good control of the instrument. A firm fulcrum or finger rest may prevent trauma to the adjacent teeth, gingiva, or alveolar bone.

301 Elevator

The 301 elevator is a small, straight instrument that is used to loosen the tooth and create space. The space allows the tooth to be luxated, or moved back and forth, so that it can be removed from the socket without damage to the adjacent teeth. The 301 elevator is also used to remove large tooth fragments and at times to check the degree of anesthesia. The handle is either bulbous or T shaped to fit the operator's hand for easy control.

11A Elevator

The 11A elevator is also known as the large straight elevator. It is often used after the 301 elevator to create more space to help remove the tooth. The 301 and 11A elevators have the same functions.

Crane Elevator

The Crane elevator, sometimes called a pick because of the shape of the tip, is a specialty instrument that resembles a large ice pick. It is used to aid in the removal of a tooth. The operator places the tip of the elevator into a prepared hole on the surface of the tooth, and the tooth is then lifted from the socket.

Potts (Millers) Elevator

The Potts, or Millers, elevator is used to remove the maxillary or mandibular root tips. The elevator is available in pairs, which are often used when a multirooted tooth is retained.

East-West Elevator

The sharp point and inclined plane of the east-west elevator are positioned to remove the interseptal bone and lift out the root tip. This instrument must be used with great care, or the bone and adjacent teeth can be damaged.

Root Tip Elevator

The root tip elevator looks like a fragile, delicate instrument because of the shape of the working end of the instrument. It may be single or double ended, and the shank may be straight or contraangled. This instrument is very important because root tips often break away from the main body of the tooth during removal. This elevator is used to remove the fractured root tips from the socket.

Periosteal Elevator

The periosteal elevator is a long, circular, double-ended instrument that is sharp on one end and rounded on the other. This elevator often serves two purposes, which are to push and reflect the gingival tissue from the bone, and also to retract the gingival tissue, allowing better visual and working access to the surgical area.

Seldon and Henahan Elevators

The Seldon and Henahan elevators are similar in appearance except that the Seldon is double ended and the Henahan is single ended. Both have flat, broad, rounded ends that allow the operator to retract the elevated soft tissue with minimal trauma. This makes the surgical area more accessible.

Bone File

The bone file is a double-ended hand instrument with serrations or grooves that allow the operator to file or smooth the bone. It is used with push-pull action. The bone file is used after an extraction or during an **alveoloplasty** to smooth rough or sharp areas of bone. It is also used to contour and reshape the bone. During these procedures the dental assistant removes the bone chips from the grooves of the file. After each pull or stroke, the dentist holds the file end of the instrument toward the assistant, who wipes away the bone fragments with a piece of gauze.

Alveoloplasty

Surgical preparation, shaping, and smoothing of socket margins and alveolar ridges after extraction of teeth; it is done to ensure optimal healing for the placement of dentures.

Surgical Curette

The curette is a double-ended instrument (see Figure 25.17, B) that may have a straight or a contraangled shank with spoon-shaped ends. The spoon-shaped ends are available in a variety of small and large sizes. The curette is used primarily to remove, or scoop out, granulation tissue or other abnormal tissue. It is also used to loosen cervical gingival tissue from around a tooth.

Forceps

Oral surgery forceps are used to extract or remove teeth (Figure 27.5). The shape of the handles allows the operator to hold the instrument with a palm grasp, giving greater leverage when removing a tooth. Some forceps have a contoured handle with a hook or curved end to provide a rest for the small finger and better stabilization and leverage. The beaks of forceps are designed to fit into the curve of the tooth or in the gingival one-third area or cervical area. Some forceps are the universal type, which means that they can be used on the right or left side of the mouth and on the upper or lower arch (Figure 27.6).

Maxillary Incisor Forceps

Three main types of forceps are used to remove maxillary incisors. They are the 99A, the 99C, and the 150 Universal Cryer forceps. Some maxillary forceps, such as the 99A model, have a contoured handle that gives the operator better stabilization and leverage. The 150 Universal Cryer forcep may be used on the left or right side of the maxillary arch. The shape of the 99C forcep allows for a firm grip while removing a tooth.

Maxillary Cuspid and Premolar Forcep

The 286, or bayonet, forcep is considered a universal forcep. It is used to remove the maxillary cuspids or premolars.

Maxillary Molar Forceps

The most commonly used maxillary molar forceps are the 24, 88R/88L, 23R/23L, 18R/18L, and 53R/53L models. The letter "R" after the number (for example, 88R) means that the forceps is used on the right side of the oral cavity; the letter "L" means that it is used on the left side.

Mandibular Incisor Forcep

The 151 Cryer forcep is the universal forcep used for the mandibular central and lateral incisors. The beak is con-

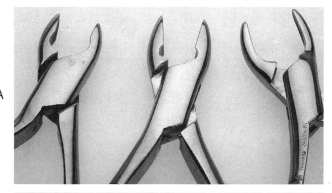

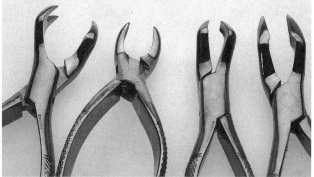

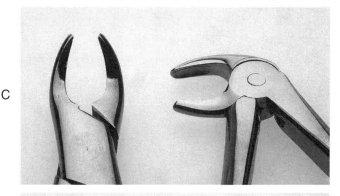

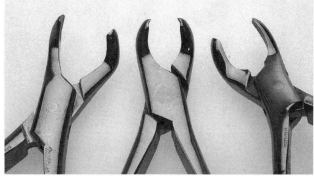

FIGURE 27.5

A, Maxillary incisor, cuspid, and premolar forceps. *Left to right:* 99A forcep, 99C forcep, 150 Universal Cryer forcep. **B,** Maxillary molar forceps. *Left to right:* 88L Nevius forcep, 18L forcep, 210 forcep, bayonet forcep. **C,** Mandibular incisor, cuspid, premolar, and root tip forceps. *Left to right:* 151 Universal forcep, MD3 forcep. **D,** Mandibular molar forcep. *Left to right:* 222 forcep, 17 forcep, 24 forcep.

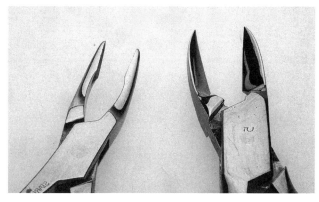

FIGURE 27.6

Rongeur forceps. *Left to right*: Mead rongeur forceps; side cutting rongeur forceps.

toured so that when the handle is held with a palm-down grasp, the beak angles slightly downward.

Mandibular Cuspid and Premolar Forcep

The 103 forcep has a thinner beak to fit the curvature of the cuspid and premolar teeth. The curved handle allows the operator to exert more leverage.

Mandibular Molar Forceps

The MD4 forcep has an offset beak to allow for a more secure hold. The beak of the #23, or Cowhorn, forcep, fits into the bifurcation of a two-rooted molar.

Mandibular Third Molar Forcep

The #222 forcep is another universal model that is used to extract erupted third molars. The beak extends farther than those of other forceps, allowing for a firm grasp on the tooth.

Rongeur Forceps

Rongeur forceps resemble pliers but have a spring mechanism between the handles. The beak is sharp, which allows the operator to remove or cut the sharp edges of bone left after an extraction. The beak of the rongeur forceps may have a sharp tip, or the side of the beak may be sharp. Rongeur forceps must be cleaned and sterilized after each use and kept sharpened. The Mead rongeur forceps tip is used to cut small pieces of bone; the side cutting rongeur forceps is used to cut larger sections of bone.

Hemostats

Hemostats, which are similar to needle holders (see Figure 25.19, *C*), are used to grasp and hold soft tissue and bone particles. Hemostats are available in several shapes and sizes and with straight or angled serrated beaks in various lengths. The handles have a multiposition ratchet to provide controlled grip pressure and release. They are used to hold or clamp objects and to remove debris from the tooth socket. They may also be used to stop hemorrhage by clamping off a blood vessel or tissue.

Tissue and Suture Scissors

Tissue and suture scissors (see Figure 25.19, *A*) are used to trim tissue and cut sutures. The scissors are small and have fine, sharp cutting surfaces. Some tissue scissors may have blunt, rounded tips. They may be straight, angled, or slightly curved so as to reach difficult areas. Some scissors may have one serrated blade to prevent slipping when cutting, and others may have a narrow beak for interproximal tissue and suture removal. These scissors are often used for **biopsy** procedures.

Biopsy

Gross and microscopic examination of tissues or cells removed from a living patient for diagnostic purposes.

Needle Holder

The needle holder (see Figure 25.21) resembles a hemostat but is larger and has a longer shank. The needle holder is used to solidly grasp and hold the needle during the placement of sutures. Needle holders have interlocking handles, and the beak may have a groove for the needle, as well as small serrations to help hold the needle and prevent needle movement. Needle holders are available in several lengths and designs.

Tongue and Cheek Retractors, Molt Mouth Prop, and Intraoral Mouth Props

Tongue and cheek retractors are used to hold the tongue and cheek out of the way while the operator is working in the mouth. Retractors may be made of plastic or metal and are available in various shapes and sizes for children and adults. Cheek retractors are used to pull back the lips and cheeks during intraoral photography (Figure 27.7, *A*). Intraoral mouth props are used to hold the mouth open during treatment to allow the operator more space in which to work (Figure 27.7, *B*). These mouth props are sized to fit a child, an adult, or an edentulous patient. Molt mouth props are designed with a ratchet so that the prop can be locked in place to prevent slipping (Figure 27.7, *C*).

Surgical Bur

A #8 round surgical bur or a #103 fissure bur is often used with the Hall handpiece to remove bone surrounding a tooth or to cut the tooth in half for easier removal.

Mallet and Chisel

Bone chisels and the surgical mallet are used to chisel at or remove the bone surrounding the tooth to be removed and to cut the tooth in half for easier removal. They are also used to remove maxillary and mandibular tori. The dental assistant must make sure to keep surgical chisels sharp (see Figure 19.19).

Sutures and Surgical Needles

Sutures are surgical stitches, which are placed to hold tissue together (unite two surfaces) after an incision has been made and the surgical procedure is complete. Suture material looks like sewing thread and is made of silk, nylon, or gut materials. Silk and nylon sutures are nonabsorbable and must be removed by the dentist or dental assistant. Gut suture material is absorbable and need not be removed.

Surgical needles may be curved or straight and are available in different sizes. The operator must select the appropriate needle for the specific procedure. The needle must be small enough not to tear the thin soft tissue or damage the flap.

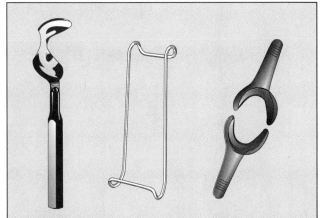
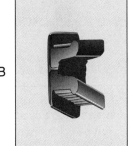
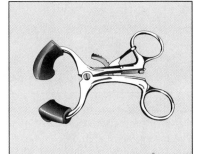

A

B

C

FIGURE 27.7

A, Cheek retractors. **B,** Intraoral mouth prop. **C,** Molt mouth prop.

Throat Pack

Throat packs (Figure 27.8) are not always used during surgical procedures. However, use of throat packs is a good practice to follow, because it may prevent a patient who has been given a general anesthetic from swallowing a tooth or other materials during the surgical procedure. The operator places a piece of surgical gauze in the oral cavity in the throat area, and the dental assistant should continually check the pack to make sure that it stays in place during the procedure.

Sterilization of Surgical Instruments

Sterilization of surgical instruments is very important. First, all blood and debris must be cleaned from the instruments. This can be accomplished by soaking the instruments in a Sterall solution for at least 10 minutes and then scrubbing away all debris. The instruments should then be placed in an ultrasonic machine for at least an additional 10 minutes. They must then be rinsed and dried. After this process has been completed, the instruments may be placed on a tray or packaged individually.

Crash Cart

Every employee must be familiar with the crash cart and the contents of each of its drawers (Figure 27.9). A small index card listing the materials in each drawer may be attached to the cart or kept in one of the drawers. The crash cart is an important piece of oral surgery equipment because emergencies can occur at any time in the dental office. Emergencies range from a simple episode of syncope (fainting) to more life-threatening situations that require more intensive treatment. A crash cart stores the medicines and equipment that may help during an emergency.

The dental assistant is usually responsible for keeping the crash cart stocked with current medications and equipment, and the assistant also is expected to be properly trained in providing immediate emergency treatment if necessary. The event of an emergency is not the time to realize that the crash cart is not up-to-date. The cart must be kept current and should be checked monthly to ensure that necessary medications are available and have not expired.

The crash cart can be organized according to the operator's preference. Usually each drawer is categorized to avoid confusion when using the emergency materials. For instance, the first drawer may contain items such as suture materials, blades, and bandages. The second drawer may have equipment for securing the airway, such as mouth props and the laryngoscope. The third drawer may contain the drugs considered essential for emergency procedures, and the fourth drawer might contain intravenous fluids, an Ambu bag, and other oxygen equipment.

ROLE OF THE DENTAL ASSISTANT IN ORAL SURGERY

The general duties of the dental assistant in an oral surgery procedure are outlined below.

1 Provide the preoperative instructions.
2 Prepare the operatory.
3 Prepare the patient.
4 Take the patient's vital signs.
5 Attach monitoring devices.
6 Place the nitrous oxide mask.

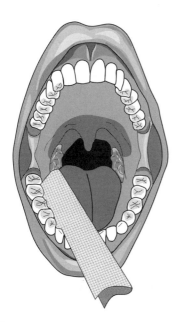

FIGURE 27.8

Throat packs are placed in the patient's mouth as a protective guard.

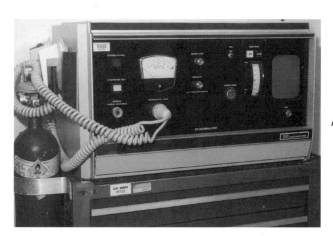

A

FIGURE 27.9

A, The crash cart is equipped with a portable oxygen tank and a defibrillator. (Courtesy University of Louisville School of Dentistry, Department of Oral and Maxillofacial Surgery.)

(Continued.)

PRIMARY CARE CENTER

CRASH CART CHECKLIST	
Item	✓
Top of cart	
Defibrillation monitor	
EKG electrodes	
Defibrillation pads	
Contamination container	
Personal Protective equipment (gloves, gowns, mask, eyeglasses)	
ACLS algorithms and drug lists	
Drawer #1: Airway	
Crash cart papers	
Defibrillator EKG paper (one roll)	
Cetacaine spray	
Bite block	
Phenylephrine nasal spray 1/2%	
Lidocaine jelly 2%, 30 g	
10 cc syringe	
Trach tape	
Two D-cell batteries	
Two C-cell batteries	
Two bulbs for blades #04800 and #4104882	
Laryngoscope handle	
#2 and #3 straight Miller blades	
#3 and #4 curved Macintosh blades	
McGill forceps	
Large and medium airways	
Endotracheal tubes (two each), sizes 6, 7, 8, and 9	
Shiley endotracheal tubes numbers 6, 8, and 10	
Two ABG kits	
Yanker suction	
Oxygen flow meter	
Oxygen tubing, mask, and nasal canula	
Flashlight	
Electrodes	
Two defibrillation pads	
Two suction caths	
One set lead wires	
ET tube styletts	
Drawer #2: IV	
One wound tray #5006310	
One sharp blunt scissors #5306925	
Three packages of 2 to 0 silk suture	
Two #11 knife blades	
Betadine solution	
Two #16 ga intracaths	
Two #19 ga intracaths	

Continued

FIGURE 27.9—Cont'd.

B, The crash cart list is used to review the contents of the cart and to ensure that all materials are readily available. (Courtesy University of Louisville School of Dentistry, Department of Oral and Maxillofacial Surgery.)

CRASH CART CHECKLIST		
Item		✓
Angiocaths	Spinal needles	
1 to 14 ga	2 to 18 ga 3½	
2 to 16 ga	2 to 20 ga 3½	
2 to 18 ga	2 to 22 ga 3½	
2 to 20 ga		
Alcohol preps		
Four 18 ga needles		
Four 21 ga needles		
Two 5X7 OPSITE dressings		
One roll 1 inch silk tape		
One roll 2 inch silk tape		
Two to three way stopcocks		
Three microdrip piggyback #6602915		
Two primary clamp piggyback #6604045		
Two Abbott sets #6607505		
Two IV filters		
Two extension sets		
One dial-a-flow		
Drawer #3: First line meds		
Three 30 cc vials of NS		
Four 21 ga needles		
Four 18 ga needles		
Three Sodium Bicarb 50 MEQ Abboject		
Two D50 W Abboject		
Four Atropine 1 mg Abboject		
Two Calcium Chloride 1½ inch Abboject		
Twelve Epinephrine 1 mg 1½ inch Abboject		
One Epinephrine 3½ inch Abboject		
Five Lidocaine 100 mg Abboject		
One Lidocaine 2 g in D5W 500 ml		
Two Dopamine 400 mg in 250 ml		
Drawer #4: Second line meds and labs		
Two 4x4 sterile dressings		
Three tourniquets		
One black marker		
One large red top tube		
Two small red top tubes		
Two blue top tubes		
Two green top tubes		
One purple top tube		
Four 10 cc syringes		
Four 3 cc syringes		
Needles 5 to 18 ga, 5 to 21 ga		
Five Adenosine 6 mg vials		

Continued

FIGURE 27.9—Cont'd.

For legend see opposite page.

CRASH CART CHECKLIST	
Item	**✓**
Four Bretylium 500 mg syringe	
Two Digoxin 0.5 mg amp	
Two Dobutamine 500 mg vials	
Two Dopamine 200 mg vials	
Five Epinephrine 1 mg amp	
One Furosemide 100 mg vial	
One Heparin 1000 u/10 ml vial	
Four Isoproterenol 1 mg amp	
Four Magnesium Sulfate 1 g vial	
Three Naloxone 0.4 mg amp	
One Nitroglycerine 50 mg vial	
One Nitroprusside 50 mg vial	
Four Norepinephrine 4 mg amp	
Three Phenylephrine 10 mg vial	
One Potassium Chloride 40 meq vial	
One Procanimide 1 g vial	
Four Propranolol 1 mg amp	
Ten 5 mg vials Verapamil	
Drawer #5: IV fluids	
One 1000 cc D5W	
Two 1000 cc lactated ringers	
One 1000 cc normal saline	
One 1000 cc D5 ½	
One 500 cc D5W	
One 250 cc D5W	
One 250 cc normal saline	
One pressure cuff	
One 250 cc NS bottle with NTG tubing	
Two 50 cc NS partial ?	
Bottom shelf	
One connecting tube	
One 18 fr. salem sump	
One 60 cc cath tip syringe	
Two packages barrier shields	
Gloves (two each) 6½, 7, 7½, and 8	
One 1000 cc NS irrigation	
One suction liner	
One suction cannister, tubing, and holder	
One 250 cc bottle of sterile water	
Four 16 fr. catheters	
One 12x12 isolation bag	
One triple lumen tray	
Two PAC trays (percutaneous sheath introducer)	
One central venous tray	
Ambu bag with mask	

FIGURE 27.9—Cont'd.

For legend see page 722.

7 Use surgical scrub techniques and infection control barriers.

8 Help the operator prepare the general anesthetic and administer drugs.

9 Pass surgical instruments and maintain good suction and irrigation.

10 Cut the suture material after the operator has finished suturing.

11 Reassure the patient.

12 Take preoperative and postoperative radiographs, if needed.

13 Give the patient instructions for any postoperative medications prescribed, as well as any care instructions, and then dismiss the patient.

Preparing the Operatory

Before seating the patient, the dental assistant must prepare the operatory. The room should be completely wiped down with disinfectant, and plastic infection control covers should be placed on the chair, light, and essential equipment. The instruments are placed on the operator's tray and covered with a sterile wrap.

Preparing the Patient

It is important that the patient be comfortable and relaxed; this is a special responsibility of the dental assistant, who greets and seats the patient. Once the patient has been seated, the dental assistant drapes the patient, takes the vital signs (blood pressure and pulse), and makes any final arrangements before the operator arrives.

Surgical Scrub Techniques

At times general practitioners and oral surgeons may perform surgical procedures that require hand washing or a surgical scrub technique like that required before surgical procedures in a hospital. Box 27.2 and Table 27.1 present a description of the preliminary wash and surgical scrub technique.

Passing Surgical Instruments

Oral surgery instruments are handled in a manner similar to that used in the four-handed dentistry method. This allows the tray to stay organized and the procedure to be completed more quickly and smoothly. Proper passing of instruments helps reduce the risk of injury to the surgeon or the assistant. For this reason, the assistant must be familiar with the instruments and their position on the tray.

Suture Placement

When suturing is required, the assistant places the needle properly in the needle holder and passes it to the operator.

The assistant should maintain a clear operating field by retracting the cheek and tongue, if necessary, and by suctioning any blood or debris during the suturing procedure.

The operator will close the flap so that there will not be a great amount of tension on the soft gingival tissue. The needle and suture are placed from the free gingiva into the attached gingiva with equal amounts of material on each side of the incision (Figure 27.10). After the operator completes the procedure, the suture is tied to the side of the sutured area, not on top of the suture. The assistant then cuts the suture, leaving a short length to make it easier to grasp and remove nonabsorbable sutures after healing is complete. If chromic or catgut sutures or other absorbable suture material is used, the patient will not have to return to the office for suture removal. When nonabsorbable sutures are used, the operator decides when the sutures are to be removed, usually 3 to 7 days after the surgical procedure. Operators may differ in this decision, and suture removal also depends on the individual patient's rate of healing.

Removal of Sutures

A postoperative visit is scheduled so that the surgical area can be checked. If healing is adequate, the sutures are removed. This procedure, which is described in Box 27.3 and Table 27.2, may be performed by the operator or the dental assistant. A mirror, cotton forceps or hemostat, and suture scissors are needed. After the sutures have been removed, the oral cavity is irrigated to remove any debris and to allow reevaluation of the healing process.

Preoperative Instructions

It is usually the dental assistant's role to explain the preoperative instructions (Box 27.4). Some of these instructions must be given at least 1 or 2 days before the appointment; others are given in the office before the patient is sedated or receives general anesthesia. Preoperative instructions are important, and they must be explained simply and clearly. If the patient fails to follow the instructions, the surgery may have to be rescheduled. General instructions usually include the following:

- Have nothing to eat or drink, including water, for at least 6 to 8 hours before surgery.
- Wear clothing with short sleeves and a loose-fitting neckline.
- Wear flat, comfortable shoes.
- Do not wear nail polish, earrings, necklaces, or bracelets for the appointment, because they may be removed for surgery.
- Remove dental appliances, chewing gum, tobacco, and other such items from the mouth.
- Make arrangements for an escort who is responsible for getting you home.

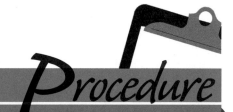

Box 27.2

Procedure for the Preliminary Wash and Surgical Scrub

Materials needed
Scrub attire
Scrub brush attire
Cleaning solution
Sterile tissue

Preliminary wash:
1. Dress in proper scrub attire.
2. Open the scrub brush package and remove the brush or sponge.
3. Rinse the hands and forearms, making sure to keep the hands elevated above the elbows.
4. Lather the hands and arms with the brush or sponge and cleaning solution to remove gross contamination. Do not rinse.
5. Clean thoroughly under and around the nails with the cleaner while supporting the scrub brush in the palm of the hand being cleaned.
6. Rinse off the cleaning solution, working from the fingertips toward the elbows.

Surgical scrub:
The surgical scrub requires *5 minutes* to complete.
1. Nails
   Scrub the nails of each hand with the brush bristles parallel to the nail tips for 20 strokes for each hand.
2. Fingers
   Scrub each finger (four planes) of one hand, following a side to back to front to side pattern to avoid touching a scrubbed plane to an unscrubbed plane; 10 strokes to each plane.
3. Back of the hand and wrist
   Scrub one hand from the finger base through the wrist (three planes) with the fingers flexed; 10 strokes to each plane.
4. Palm and wrist
   Scrub one hand from the finger base through the wrist (three planes) with the fingers hyperextended; 10 strokes to each plane.
5. Change hands and repeat steps 2 through 4; approximately 3 minutes total for both hands.
6. Arms
   Scrub the arms with small, overlapping circles from the wrist (three sections and four planes each), stopping at one brush width above the elbow; 6 circles to each plane.
7. Switch the brush back to the first hand and repeat step 6 under Preliminary Wash; approximately 2 minutes total for both hands.
8. Rinse from the fingertips toward the elbows, making sure to keep the hands and arms elevated and away from the body.
9. Proceed to the operating room and dry the hands on a sterile towel.
10. *Don gown and gloves as appropriate. Note: If at any time during the scrub any part of the brush, hands, or arms becomes contaminated, the entire scrub process must be repeated.*

- Do not drive a car or operate machinery for 24 hours after surgery.

Postoperative Instructions

The dental assistant usually reviews the postoperative instructions with the patient (Box 27.5). These instructions, which should also be given to the patient in writing, may include the following information:

1 Bite on gauze for 30 minutes.
2 Do not spit, smoke, or suck through a straw for 24 hours.
3 Beginning the day after surgery, rinse the mouth with warm saltwater.

All prescriptions must be written by the dentist and should be reviewed with the patient. At this time the patient should be asked again if he or she has any allergies related to prescription drugs.

Table 27.1

Evaluation of Preliminary Wash and Surgical Scrub

Wash and Scrub	4	3	2	0	X
Preliminary wash					
Wear proper attire.					
Assemble materials.					
Secure brush and cleaning solution.					
Wash.					
Rinse.					
Surgical scrub					
Complete in 5 minutes.					
Scrub nails.					
Scrub fingers.					
Scrub palm and wrist.					
Repeat.					
Scrub arms.					
Repeat.					
Rinse.					
Dry.					
Wear proper attire.					

The numeric criteria: 4 Excellent; 3 Good but some improvement can be made; 2 Below average, usable, needs to improve skill; 0 Unsatisfactory; X Not able to evaluate.

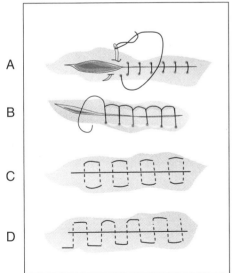

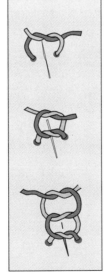

FIGURE 27.10

Suturing techniques. **A,** Interrupted (single) sutures. **B,** Continuous locking sutures. **C,** Continuous sutures. **D,** Interrupted mattress sutures. **E,** Surgical square knots.

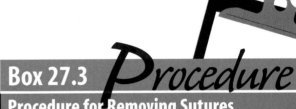

Box 27.3 *Procedure*

Procedure for Removing Sutures

Materials needed
Suture removal setup (Figure 27.11, *A*)
Mirror
Explorer
Cotton forceps
Suture scissors
Hemostat

1. Grasp the end of the suture material with the cotton pliers or hemostat and raise it slightly.
2. Place one blade of the suture scissors under the surface suture material and cut the material (Figure 27.11, *B*).
3. Carefully remove the suture with the cotton pliers or hemostat so as not to pull the suture knot through the soft tissue (Figure 27.11, *C*), which could cause discomfort for the patient and trauma to the tissue.

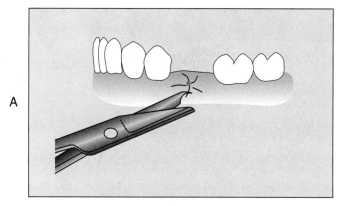

A

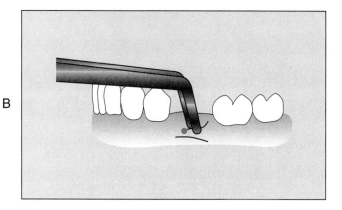

B

FIGURE 27.11

A, One blade of the scissors is placed under the surface suture material, which is cut. **B,** The suture is removed with cotton pliers.

Box 27.4

Preoperative Instructions for Outpatients Who Will Be Receiving a General Anesthetic or Intravenous Sedation

1. Have *nothing* to eat or drink (that is, nothing by mouth, including water) after 12 midnight before your appointment unless otherwise instructed.
2. Dress comfortably in clothing with short sleeves and a loose-fitting neckline. Wear flat shoes.
3. Remove nail polish, earrings, contact lenses, bracelets, and necklaces before your appointment. Do not wear makeup. Remove dental appliances, chewing gum, tobacco, and snuff from the mouth.
4. You must be accompanied to the clinic by a responsible adult who will stay in the immediate area of the clinic during the procedure and who can provide transportation afterward. Preferably, this escort would drive you home.
5. You must plan to have a responsible adult stay with you for 24 hours after surgery.
6. You must not drive an automobile or operate machinery for 24 hours after surgery.
7. Please do not bring more than two escorts, and *no* children, please.
8. Bring your payment of $_____ or a completed and signed insurance form, along with proof of insurance, the morning of your appointment.

Modified from a form provided by the University of Louisville School of Dentistry, Department of Oral and Maxillofacial Surgery.

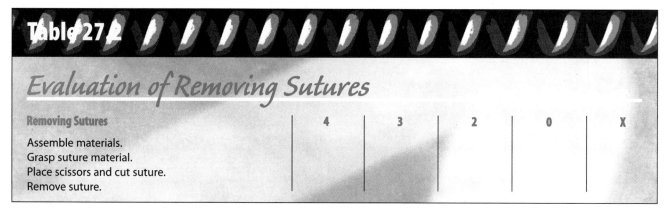

Table 27.2

Evaluation of Removing Sutures

Removing Sutures	4	3	2	0	X
Assemble materials.					
Grasp suture material.					
Place scissors and cut suture.					
Remove suture.					

The numeric criteria: 4 Excellent; 3 Good but some improvement can be made; 2 Below average, usable, needs to improve skill; 0 Unsatisfactory; X Not able to evaluate.

Before the person is dismissed, the patient should be given the dentist's emergency number in case of excessive discomfort or other difficulties. The dentist may schedule a follow-up appointment 5 to 7 days after surgery.

Postoperative Medications

Medication is usually given to patients to help minimize discomfort after oral surgery. Although the medication

Box 27.5

Postoperative Care Following Oral Surgery

1. IMMEDIATELY AFTER SURGERY, keep GAUZE PADS OVER AREA with BITING PRESSURE for 1 hour.
2. SOME OOZING OF BLOOD may occur on the FIRST AND SECOND DAYS FOLLOWING THE PROCEDURE. This type of bleeding may be controlled by first wiping off any old clots and then placing sterile pads over the area and biting firmly for $1/2$ hour at a time.
3. TWENTY FOUR HOURS AFTER SURGERY, RINSE MOUTH WITH $1/2$ TEASPOON OF SALT to a full glass of WARM WATER. Rinse after each meal and before retiring at night. DO NOT RINSE IF THERE IS BLEEDING FROM THE SURGICAL AREA.
4. SWELLING AROUND THE MOUTH, CHEEKS, EYES, and NECK MAY FOLLOW SOME SURGICAL PROCEDURES. This is the body's normal reaction and the swelling usually subsides in several days. TO REDUCE ORDINARY POST-OPERATIVE SWELLING, APPLY AN ICE BAG (15 MINUTES ON AND 15 MINUTES OFF) ONLY FOR THE FIRST 8 HOURS FOLLOWING THE PROCEDURE.
5. To minimize stiffness and to stimulate circulation, exercise jaw periodically by opening and closing.
6. IN SOME CASES DISCOLORATION OF THE SKIN FOLLOWS SWELLING. The purplish color may spread from the skin around the mouth and cheeks to the skin of the neck. The purplish color fades into greenish yellow, then yellow and back to normal. This discoloration is the result of blood elements spreading beneath the tissue layers. This is a perfectly normal post-operative event, especially in individuals who bruise easily.
7. After a general anesthetic, the patient SHOULD FIRST HAVE A SWEET BEVERAGE (SODA or JUICE). Patients may then have a light soft diet.
8. Some individuals experience nausea and vomiting following general anesthesia. If so, sip ginger ale or cola. The nausea usually subsides after several hours.
9. Numbness of the lip occasionally follows oral surgery. This is usually transient and no cause for alarm.
10. FOR MILD DISCOMFORT TAKE usual dosage of aspirin, anacin, bufferin, etc., every four hours. If this is not sufficient, TAKE PRESCRIBED MEDICATION.
11. Nourishment is essential for healing. Drink plenty of liquids (soups or juices) and take more solid foods as you are able, avoiding chewing in the area of operation.
12. BONY EDGES: After teeth are extracted, the patient may feel hard projections in the mouth and think they are roots. This is usually the hard, bony partition which surrounds the roots of the teeth. These generally work themselves out. If not, return to this office for their simple removal.
13. INFREQUENTLY, JAW PAIN, EARACHE, AND BAD TASTE IN MOUTH may develop anywhere from two days to twelve days following extraction. This is the result of the blood clot decomposing or being lost, therefore, leaving the raw bony walls of the socket exposed. Return to this office for simple treatment (insertion of medicated dressing).
14. A BLACK AND BLUE MARK and soreness occasionally develops on the area of THE ARM at the site of intravenous injection. This is to be expected and will disappear.
15. ORAL HYGIENE: Remove all white film from the gums by means of cotton swab or piece of gauze. Brush your teeth with a dentifrice avoiding the operative site.
16. SUTURES (STITCHES) may have been placed in the area of surgery in order to MINIMIZE POSTOPERATIVE BLEEDING AND TO FACILITATE HEALING. They will be removed at a subsequent visit when healing is satisfactory. Removal of stitches usually requires no anesthesia, takes only a minute or so, and has no discomfort associated with the procedure.
17. Please feel free to notify this office of any unusual occurrences or questions. Area Code 502, Telephone 588-5401.
18. Your postoperative visit will be _____ _____ .

From the University of Louisville School of Dentistry, Department of Oral and Maxillofacial Surgery.

can help alleviate some discomfort, it may not relieve all the pain. For instance, during extraction procedures, some teeth are more difficult to remove than others. The degree of this difficulty determines the type of medication or analgesic prescribed. Other factors to consider in prescribing postoperative medication include the patient's health and any history of allergies or drug abuse. It is important to limit the length of time a patient takes prescription pain medication. Antibiotics are not routinely given after oral surgery or extractions. However, they may be required in some cases. For example, antibiotics are given at the time of extraction if infection is present or if the potential for infection exists.

The antibiotics most commonly prescribed are penicillin and erythromycin. Both antibiotics are excellent against infections caused by gram-positive bacteria. Penicillin is routinely preferred unless the patient is allergic to it. (It should be noted that a true allergy exists only if the patient develops a rash or hives or has an anaphylactic reaction.) If the patient is allergic to penicillin, erythromycin (500 mg every 8 hours) may be given as a substitute. The patient should be informed of the possible side affects of erythromycin such as diarrhea and nausea.

SELECTED ORAL SURGERY PROCEDURES

Incision and Drainage

At times a patient may develop an infection that produces a lesion, which is a sore or wound, such as an abscess, that requires immediate attention. In such cases the practitioner may surgically open (incise) the lesion to permit drainage, or the release of pus or other fluids. This procedure is called an I&D (incision and drainage). I&D requires a sterile environment, and the procedure is basically the same whether performed using a local anesthetic or general anesthesia.

Alveolitis

Alveolitis is often referred to as "dry socket." It usually is seen in mandibular extraction sites, although it can occur in maxillary sites. Alveolitis is one of the more common complications of extraction. It can occur after an extraction if the blood clot that has been formed in the socket is lost, and this loss can occur within hours or even several days after the extraction. In such cases the patient may complain of severe pain, which is caused by exposure of the alveolar bone to air. If this happens, the patient must be seen and treated immediately. Pain medication may not provide immediate relief. Although the cause of alveolitis is not clearly understood, some possible contributing factors are trauma during the extraction, infection, lack of vascular blood supply, and use of oral contraceptives. No cure has been found for alveolitis, but treatment can ease the patient's discomfort until the area has healed.

Treatment of Alveolitis

If dry socket occurs, the operator removes any sutures that have been placed and irrigates the extraction site with a solution of sterile saline and hydrogen peroxide or some other similar mixture. Mouthwash may be added to the solution to freshen the patient's mouth and breath. A medicated dressing is placed in the socket after the area has been irrigated; this usually gives the patient some degree of immediate relief. The patient will need to be seen regularly for dressing changes before healing is complete.

Alveoloplasty

Alveoloplasty, or alveolectomy, is the surgical removal of any sharp or protruding alveolar bone that may cause discomfort or prevent dentures from fitting properly. This procedure is routinely performed during the extraction of teeth. Alveoloplasty helps smooth the alveolar ridges, allowing prostheses to be fitted. The ideal ridge is U shaped. The surgeon may achieve this shape simply by using the thumb and finger to compress the alveolar ridges, or a more complex surgical technique may be required. How extensive the alveoloplasty is often depends on the surgeon's judgment. Some surgeons believe that after extractions, nature should be allowed to do its job and the ridges should be left to contour themselves. However, this approach may be very uncomfortable for the patient, because the sharp edges of the ridges can cause pain. Some surgeons therefore smooth over the edges somewhat before allowing nature to take its course.

Simple Alveoloplasty

After the extraction of several teeth, the surgeon may perform a simple alveoloplasty, which is the removal of sharp edges of the buccal alveolar plates and the interseptal bone (Figure 27.12). The surgeon makes an incision along the interseptal crest and uses a periosteal elevator to gently reflect a flap, taking care not to tear the soft gingival tissue. The surgeon then uses a rongeur forceps to trim the alveolar plate of the empty socket to an even height. The rongeur forceps also can be used at a 45-degree angle to remove the interseptal bone. This procedure is repeated on each socket. The bone file then is pulled lightly across the bone in one direction to smooth the bone and remove any chips. After filing, the area is irrigated, and after the debris has been removed, the flap is replaced using interrupted or continuous sutures made of catgut or chromic materials. The sutures may be removed in 7 to 10 days.

Exostoses (Tori)

Exostoses, or tori, are overgrowths of bone, which may occur in either maxillary or mandibular areas of the mouth. Mandibular tori often are described as large bumps or knots found on the lingual surface of the mandibular arch, usually between the right and left bicuspids. Tori are common and rarely have any pathologic significance, but they usually are removed because they can impair the fit of dentures or partials.

The surgical procedures are similar for removing maxillary or mandibular tori (Figure 27.13). Once local anesthesia has been obtained, an incision is made. A periosteal elevator is used to carefully reflect the gingival flap, which is retracted with a Seldon or periosteal elevator. A surgical bur is then used to cut into the tori, after which the area is completely irrigated. Osteotomes or unbeveled or bibeveled chisels and a mallet are used to remove any remaining segments of bone. A bone file is then used to produce a smooth finish. The area is irrigated copiously to remove any bone chips, especially under the gingival flap, and the flap is then trimmed and loosely sutured.

Biopsy

A biopsy is performed to diagnose disease or to confirm normalcy. It also is the most effective method available for determining if a lesion is benign or malignant. Biopsy is the removal of all or some of the suspicious tissue or bone. The

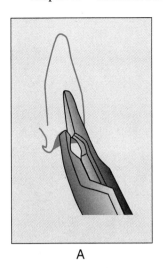
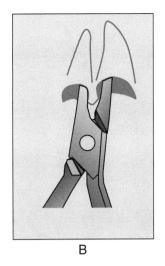
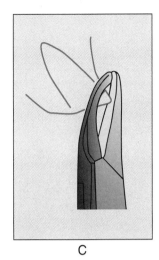

A   B   C

FIGURE 27.12

Alveoloplasty. **A,** A rongeur forceps is used to remove the labial plate. **B,** The interseptal tip is removed. **C,** Side view of the removal of the interseptal tip.

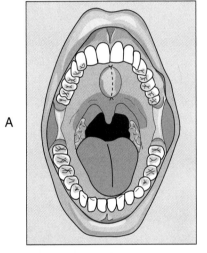

A

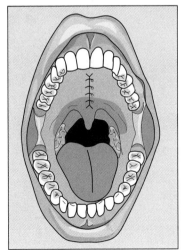

C

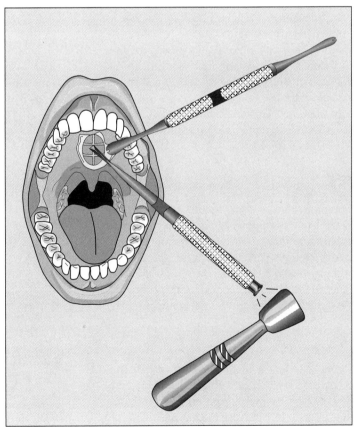

B

FIGURE 27.13

Removal of a palatal torus. **A,** Location of the torus. **B,** A mallet and chisel are used to remove the torus. **C,** Sutures are placed after the torus has been removed.

sample is sent to a pathologist for examination and determination of benignity or malignancy. A biopsy procedure involves the following steps:

1 The history of the lesion or condition is obtained.
2 The patient's past medical history is taken.
3 A physical examination is performed.
4 Pertinent related tests and examinations are done, such as radiographs and blood tests.
5 One of two basic biopsy techniques is performed:

The *excisional* technique involves the removal of the entire lesion, with an adequate margin of normal tissue around and below the lesion.

The *incisional* technique involves the removal of a portion of a larger lesion.

6 The tissue is placed in a specimen bottle in a solution of 10% formalin. The bottle is labeled with the patient's name, an identification number, and the type and origin of the specimen.

Frenectomy

A frenectomy may be performed on a child or an adult. Frenectomy is the surgical repositioning of the frenum, which attaches the lip to the cheek or the tongue to the gingiva. A frenectomy may be done because a patient has speech problems or ill-fitting dentures, and it may be performed in the labial or the lingual area. The procedures for the two locations are similar (Figure 27.14).

To begin either the labial or the lingual procedure, local anesthesia is obtained. The assistant attaches a straight hemostat to the frenum, and the operator makes a V-shaped cut above and below the hemostat with surgical scissors. The labial tissue is smoothed with the periosteal elevator and repositioned so that interrupted chromic sutures can be loosely placed in the gingival tissue.

Fractures

A patient may come to the oral surgery office with a broken jaw or a fracture. Fractures may occur in the maxilla or the mandible. As with any broken bone, the practitioner reduces the fracture. This requires stabilization of the fracture with maxillomandibular fixation, or wiring the mouth shut (Figure 27.15). The patient usually is sedated for this procedure, but it may be performed using only a local anesthetic.

Implants

Dental implants represent a major advance in dentistry. Implants are used to replace teeth that were extracted or lost through accidents or that are physiologically absent (Figure 27.16). Implants are also used to replace full or partial dentures.

Dental implants are considered appropriate for people who want restorations that are as close to natural teeth as

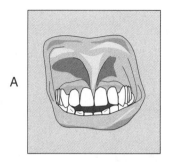
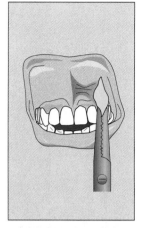
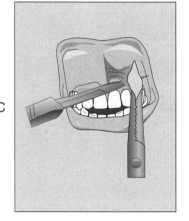
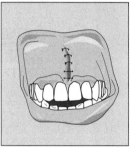

FIGURE 27.14

Frenectomy. **A,** Frenum attachment. **B,** A hemostat is used to retract the frenum to be incised from the midline attachment. **C,** The frenum is incised with a scalpel. **D,** Sutures are placed.

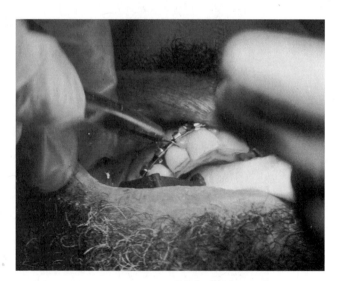

FIGURE 27.15

Placement of maxillomandibular fixation to stabilize a fracture.

possible. Implants can be used to replace a few teeth or all of the teeth. They are placed in the alveolar ridge or jawbone to anchor the prosthetic teeth and to give a more natural appearance. However, dental implants are not for everyone.

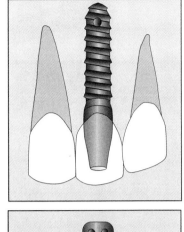

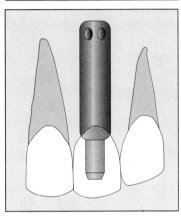

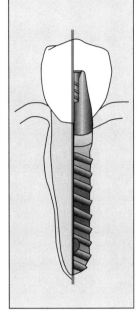

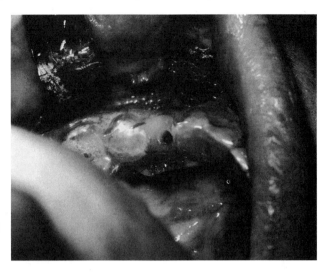

A

B

C

FIGURE 27.16

Implants. **A,** Placement of a threaded implant. **B,** Placement of a cylindric implant. **C,** Relationship of the implant to the tooth.

FIGURE 27.17

A hole in the bone for insertion of the implant is made with a surgical bur.

Each case must be considered individually because of several factors:

• The implant procedure is a 3- to 9-month process.
• Implants require a great deal of care by the patient.
• Regular dental checkups are a must with implants.

The process involved in placing and maintaining dental implants requires a team approach. Oral surgeons, some general dentists, and periodontists place implants. A laboratory technician or a prosthodontist provides the prosthesis that is placed over the implant. A periodontist or a dental hygienist works with the team to help maintain good tissue conditions around the implant. Good dental hygiene is essential to continued good oral health.

When a patient requests an implant, the practitioner performs an oral evaluation. The type of implant and prosthesis to be used are determined, and the risks and possible complications of the procedure are discussed with the patient. Some of those risks and complications are bleeding, infection, and numbness or injury to muscles or nerves in the area of placement. Also, placement of maxillary implants could cause sinus damage, and implants sometimes fail. Af-

ter this discussion the patient signs a consent form, and financial arrangements are made.

Placement of the implant is a rather easy procedure for the patient to endure. Some type of sedation may be needed, or only a local anesthetic may be used. The procedure includes the following steps:

1 An incision is made on the crest of the alveolar ridge.
2 A periosteal elevator is used to reflect the gingival tissue and expose the alveolar bone.
3 A surgical bur is used to make a hole in the bone for insertion of the implant (Figure 27.17).
4 The implant is placed, and the tissues are repositioned with sutures.

Gingival Grafts

Gingival grafting is an oral surgical procedure in which intraoral mucosa is surgically removed from the hard palate or gingivae and sutured into another area of the gingiva. The gingival tissue excised from a donor site can be used to replace granulated tissue or to cover exposed root surfaces. The area where the donor tissue is placed is called the receptor site.

Surgical procedures for gingival grafts involve identifying the donor site, determining the size of tissues to excise, and preparing the patient (Box 27.6). Before surgery is begun, a throat pack must be placed to protect the patient from debris created during surgery. After the gingival tissue has been removed from the donor site, it must be reserved on a piece of sterile gauze moistened with saline solution. The donor tissue is measured, and the callegen tape is trimmed to fit into the prepared receptor site. Callegen tape is placed over the donor site, and the donor tissue is

Box 27.6

Procedure

Procedure for Gingival Grafts

In outline form, the gingival graft technique proceeds as follows:

1. The patient is prepared for the procedure.
2. The throat pack is put in place.
3. The donor site is identified.
4. The amount of tissue to be excised is determined.
5. The gingival tissue is removed from the donor site.
6. The donor tissue is placed on a sterile gauze sponge (Figure 27.18, *A*).
7. The gauze sponge is moistened with sterile saline solution.
8. The donor tissue is measured.
9. The callegen tape is trimmed to fit the donor site.
10. The callegen tape is placed over the donor site.
11. The donor tissue is positioned in the receptor site (Figure 27.18, *B*).
12. The donor tissue is sutured in place.
13. The patient is given postoperative instructions and any prescriptions for medication.
14. An appointment is made for a follow up visit.

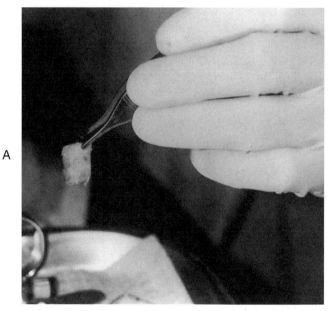

A

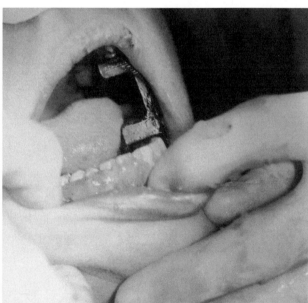

B

FIGURE 27.18

A, The donor tissue is placed on a sterile gauze sponge, which is then moistened with a sterile saline solution. **B,** The donor tissue is positioned in the receptor site and sutured in place.

positioned with the connective tissue side of the graft on the receptor site, where it is sutured into place. An appointment is made for the patient to return to the office in approximately 2 weeks so that the surgical area can be checked and treatment completed.

Third Molar Extractions

For extractions, teeth are classified according to what needs to be done to remove them. Third molars are often classified into four categories:

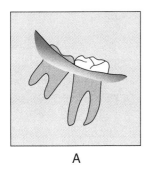
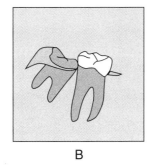
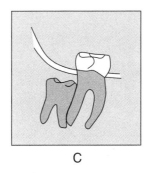
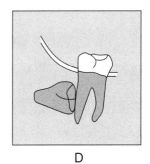

A   B   C   D

FIGURE 27.19

Third molar classification. **A,** I. **B**, II. **C**, III. **D**, IV.

- Class I: An incision is made in the overlying mucosa before the tooth is removed (Figure 27.19, *A*).
- Class II: An incision is made in the overlying mucosa and the flap is reflected before tooth removal (Figure 27.19, *B*).
- Class III: An incision is made in the overlying mucosa, the flap is reflected, and overlying or surrounding bone and the tooth are sectioned before removal (Figure 27.19, *C*).
- Class IV: All the above procedures are performed, as well as specific techniques required for an unusually difficult extraction, such as for a tooth lying sidewise (Figure 27.19, *D*).

ORAL SURGERY PROCEDURES INVOLVING EXTRACTIONS

Before beginning an extraction procedure, the operator reviews the patient's medical history consent form, and reaffirms which tooth needs to be extracted. The operator discusses the potential risks and complications with the patient and then has the patient sign a consent form. Once this has been done, the operator completes the following steps:

1 The patient is anesthetized.
2 An instrument, such as a periosteal elevator, is used to check that adequate anesthesia has been obtained.
3 The patient is told that lots of pressure or slight pain may be felt and to raise a hand if "time out" is needed.
4 The patient is informed that it is important not to make any quick movements because this may cause injury to the patient, the operator, or the assistant.
5 The periosteal elevator is used to loosen the periosteum from the surface of the bone.
6 The 301 elevator or a substitute may be used to create a space around the tooth in order to allow the tooth to be luxated.
7 The 11A elevator is used to create greater space and to help remove the tooth.

8 A selected forceps is used to remove the tooth.
9 If the tooth is fractured or requires additional bone removal, a handpiece and oral surgery bur may be required.

Role of the Dental Assistant in Extraction Procedures

The dental assistant has an extremely important role in oral surgery procedures. The assistant must keep the visual field free of moisture and debris so that the operator can perform the surgical procedure. The assistant must also pass all surgical instruments and deliver necessary materials to the operator. Because of the nature of surgery, the dental assistant can play a significant role in comforting the patient during extractions and other procedures. Many patients become very nervous when they have oral surgery, and the dental assistant can reassure them during the procedure that they are doing very well. The assistant can observe any unusual behavior in the patient and listen to what the person may say. It often is important for the dental assistant to reemphasize what the operator has said, and in some instances, the patient may be more comfortable talking to the dental assistant than to the operator.

Because many patients confuse pain with pressure, it is important to let them know that they may feel a lot of pressure but should not feel any sharp pain. The patient also should be told that if anything sharp is felt, the person should raise a hand and the operator will stop and reevaluate the situation. The assistant should always let patients know that they are doing a great job of helping out.

Role of the Dental Assistant in Administration of a General Anesthetic

The dental assistant is especially important in procedures that require general anesthesia. In addition to assisting the

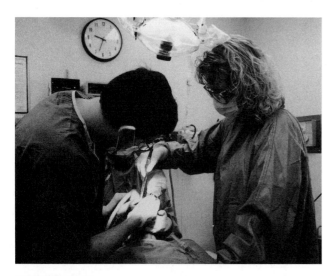

FIGURE 27.20

When general anesthesia is used, one dental assistant is responsible for maintaining the airway while another assistant helps the surgeon during the surgical procedure.

operator, the assistant is responsible for keeping the patient's mouth and airway dry (Figure 27.20). If blood or water is allowed to enter the airway, complications may arise, such as choking or inability to breathe. The dental assistant may need to perform a tonsil suction to remove any water or other fluids.

A dental assistant often is required to monitor the patient's condition and maintain the airway during surgical procedures while another assistant helps the surgeon. Modern monitoring devices have somewhat simplified this requirement during procedures involving general anesthesia. Blood pressure cuffs, electrocardiographic (ECG) monitors, and pulse monitors provide a high degree of patient security and safety and are often also used to measure vital signs before surgery.

In private practice the oral surgeon performs both the roles of surgeon and anesthesiologist. Therefore the surgeon has a great deal of responsibility. During oral surgery, the operator may require one dental assistant to assist with instrumentation while a second assistant assists the patient by holding the head securely, checking the monitors, and maintaining the airway (Figure 27.20).

Dental assisting in an oral surgery office can be very interesting because of the scope of the procedures, ranging from simple extractions to fracture cases, and the high level of responsibility the dental assistant can be assigned. The dental assistant is definitely considered the surgeon's "left hand."

Oral surgery dental assistants should be certified in cardiopulmonary resuscitation (CPR), and practice drills should be held to the staff alert to and current on emergency techniques (see Chapter 22). An emergency can arise at any time during surgical procedures, including cardiac arrest, seizure, uncontrollable bleeding, hypertensive episode, or airway blockage that requires a tracheotomy.

HOSPITAL DENTISTRY

In the 1990s hospital dentistry emerged as a growing trend. Today, the general practitioner may prefer to practice with an oral surgeon in the operating room to meet the patient's oral surgery needs. This is especially true for patients who are severely disabled or mentally impaired. These patient often receive no dental care because it is difficult to accomplish the necessary procedures in a general practitioner's office. Dental assistants are often trained to work with the oral surgeon in the operating room (Figure 27.21).

Hospital Outpatients

Some dental procedures are performed in hospitals as "outpatient" treatment. This treatment may involve general dentistry procedures performed on medically compromised patients or surgical procedures, such as reduction of a fracture, performed on a healthy patient. Some patients have a medical history that requires the more sterile environment of a hospital operating room. The preoperative instructions for office patients also apply to hospital outpatients (see Box 27.4).

Admissions

A patient may be admitted to the hospital the day before or a few hours before the procedure. Necessary laboratory work or tests are done before admission.

Discharge

A patient may be discharged, or released, from the hospital after the practitioner determines that the patient's condition is stable and adequate care can be provided at home.

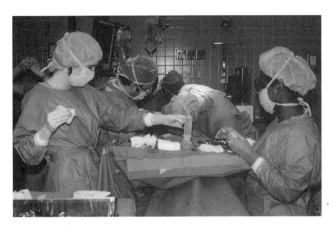

FIGURE 27.21

Oral surgery assistants during surgical procedures.

Role of the Dental Assistant in Hospital Dentistry

The role of the dental assistant on the hospital team is similar to the assisting role in private practice. It involves the following basic steps:

1 Don surgical attire.
2 Perform a surgical scrub.
3 Set up and arrange sterile instruments and equipment.
4 Prepare the patient with complete sterile draping.
5 Assist during procedures (standing for a length of time may be necessary during surgical procedures).
6 Clean up the patient and move the person to the recovery room.
7 Clean up and prepare instruments for sterilization.
8 Complete record keeping.

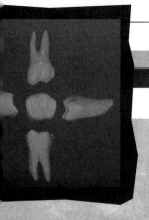

Points for Review

- Examination and consultation procedures
- Methods of pain control for oral surgery
- Oral surgery instruments
- Role of the dental assistant in oral surgery
- Surgical scrub method
- Types of oral surgery procedures

Self-Study Questions

1. Which term below pertains to the jaws and face, particularly with reference to oral surgery?
   a. Periodontics
   b. Maxillofacial
   c. Osteotomy
   d. Prosthodontics

2. What is the microscopic diagnostic procedure in which tissue is removed from the oral cavity?
   a. Hemorrhage
   b. Osteotomy
   c. Biopsy
   d. Alveoloplasty

3. With regard to surgery, how is the first trimester of pregnancy categorized?
   a. Indication
   b. Contraindication
   c. Medical emergency
   d. Abnormality (contraindication)

4. In addition to an explanation of treatment and identification of any risk factors, which of the following should always be included in treatment planning for oral surgery?
   a. Informed consent
   b. Postoperative instructions
   c. Prescriptions
   d. Medications

5. The 150 universal Cryer forceps, the 99A forceps, and the 99C forceps generally are used to remove which teeth?
   a. Maxillary molars
   b. Maxillary incisors
   c. Mandibular molars
   d. Mandibular third molars

6. The 88R/88L and 23R/23L forceps are used to remove which teeth?
   a. Maxillary molars
   b. Maxillary cuspids and premolars
   c. Mandibular incisors
   d. Mandibular molars

7. Rongeur forceps are used for which procedure?
   a. Removing soft tissue around the tooth
   b. Removing pieces of bone
   c. Removing mandibular central incisors
   d. Removing periosteal tissue

8. Which instrument is used to hold soft tissue and bone particles?
   a. Retractor
   b. Rongeur forceps
   c. Elevator
   d. Hemostat

9. If contamination occurs at any time during a surgical scrub, what must be done?
   a. Preliminary wash must be repeated.
   b. Scrubbing of contaminated area must be repeated.
   c. Entire scrub must be repeated.
   d. Surgical scrubs must be changed.

10. Preoperative instructions usually include which of the following rules?
    a. Do not spit, smoke, or suck through a straw for 24 hours.
    b. Do not eat or drink anything for 6 to 8 hours before surgery.
    c. Only water is permitted before surgery.
    d. Driving is permissible if an escort is available.

Archer W, Harry BS: *Oral and maxillofacial surgery*, Philadelphia, WB Saunders.

Blair V, Henry RI: *Essentials of oral surgery*, St Louis, Mosby.

Clark MS, Brunick AL: *Handbook of nitrous oxide and oxygen sedation*, St Louis, 2000, Mosby.

Donoff RB: *Massachusetts General Hospital manual of oral and maxillofacial surgery*, ed 3, St Louis, 1997, Mosby.

Dungman RO, Natvig P: *Surgery of facial fractures*, Philadelphia, WB Saunders.

Kruger GO: *Textbook of oral surgery*, ed 6, St Louis, 1984, Mosby.

Malamed SF: *Medical emergencies in the dental office*, ed 5, St Louis, 2000, Mosby.

Malamed SF: *Sedation: a guide to patient management*, ed 3, St Louis, 1995, Mosby.

Peterson LJ et al: *Contemporary oral and maxillofacial surgery*, ed 3, St Louis, 1998, Mosby.

Smith RG et al: *Dental surgery assistant's handbook*, ed 2, London, 1994, London, Mosby–Year Book Europe.

*F*ixed Prosthetics and Temporary Crown and Bridge

*K*ey Points

- Effect of lost teeth
- Types of fixed prostheses
- Role of the dental assistant in prosthodontics
- Clinical procedures in fixed prosthodontics
- Laboratory procedures

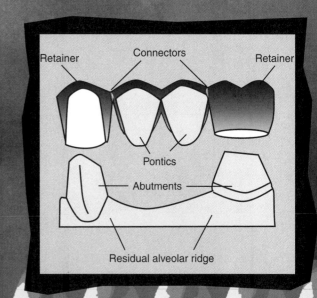

Retainer   Connectors   Retainer

Pontics

Abutments

Residual alveolar ridge

Chapter Outline

Prosthodontics
    Loss of teeth
Types of Fixed Prostheses
    Crowns
    Fixed partial denture (fixed bridge)
    Crown and bridge support
Role of the Dental Assistant in Fixed
    Prosthodontics
Clinical Procedures for Fixed
    Prosthodontics
    First appointment (examination)
    Second appointment (tooth preparation)
    Provisional (temporary) crowns and
      bridges

Third appointment (seating)
Laboratory Fabrication of a Fixed
    Prosthesis
    Pouring the final impression
    Carving the wax pattern
    Spruing the pattern
    Investing the pattern
    Burning out the pattern
    Casting the pattern
    Finishing and polishing the restoration
    Quenching the casting ring
    Porcelain application

Learning Objectives

On completion of Chapter 28, the student should be able to do the following:

◼ Define key terms.

◼ List the consequences of tooth loss.

◼ Identify the types of fixed prostheses.

◼ Define the role of the dental assistant during fixed prosthodontic treatment.

◼ List the procedures performed during the examination, tooth preparation, and seating appointments.

◼ Identify the steps taken for fabricating the fixed prosthesis in the dental laboratory.

◼ List the types of casting alloys and porcelain materials used for fabricating fixed prostheses.

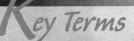

Key Terms

Abutment Teeth	Inlay	Retainer
Casting	Onlay	Retraction
Die	Pontic	Veneer
Fabrication	Provisional	

PROSTHODONTICS

Prosthodontics is a special branch of dentistry, and the dentist who receives additional training in this area is called a prosthodontist. The prosthodontist maintains oral function, comfort, appearance, and health by restoring natural teeth and replacing missing teeth and oral and maxillofacial tissues with artificial substitutes.

Prosthodontics can be divided into four subspecialties: (1) removable prosthodontics, (2) fixed prosthodontics, (3) implant prosthodontics, and (4) maxillofacial prosthodontics.

- *Removable prosthodontics* is concerned with the replacement of teeth and surrounding structures in edentulous or partly edentulous patients with artificial substitutes that can be removed from the mouth.
- *Fixed prosthodontics* is concerned with the replacement of teeth with artificial substitutes that cannot be readily removed from the mouth. A fixed partial denture is luted, or securely retained, to natural teeth, tooth roots, or dental implant abutments.
- *Implant prosthodontics* is concerned with the replacement of missing teeth with implants. An implant is a prosthetic device that is implanted into the oral tissues beneath the mucosa or the periosteal layer in bone (or both). It provides retention and support for a fixed or removable prosthesis.
- *Maxillofacial prosthodontics* is concerned with replacement of missing facial structures with a prosthesis that may or may not be removable, such as a prosthetic eye.

Loss of Teeth

In a functional mouth, a child has 20 teeth and an adult 28 teeth that support each other and provide proper form and function. Each tooth is complemented by opposing and adjacent teeth that help stabilize and strengthen the complete dentition. When part or all of the tooth structure is missing, a process begins that can cause additional tooth damage, pain, and expense for individuals who do not protect their dental health. Box 28.1 lists some of the effects of tooth loss.

TYPES OF FIXED PROSTHESES

If the patient's existing teeth and supporting structures can be preserved, the dentist will design a treatment plan that may involve several types of crowns or fixed partial dentures (bridges). Cast gold usually is the restoration of choice because of its biologic and mechanical properties (see Chapter 18 for further information on the properties of dental materials). However, if esthetics is an essential consideration, tooth-colored materials, such as porcelain or resin, are used to improve the appearance of the ante-

---

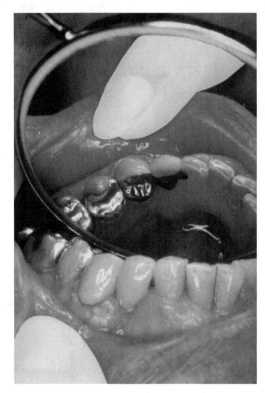

FIGURE 28.1

Patient with multiple fixed prostheses.

---

rior teeth. These artificial replacements are cemented to the natural dentition and will last for many years if they are made appropriately and the mouth is cared for properly by the patient (Figure 28.1).

Crowns

The basic types of artificial crowns are made of gold or other metal alloy, porcelain, resin, a combination of metal with an attached **veneer,** or fused coverage of porcelain or resin. The metals used for crowns and bridges may be a base alloy or a noble white or gold alloy. A fixed crown prosthesis may be an inlay, an onlay, a three-quarter crown, a full gold crown, or a full porcelain crown (porcelain jacket).

Veneer

An overlay or thin layer of acrylic resin or ceramic used to cover the labial surface of a tooth

Inlay

An **inlay** may be made of porcelain, resin, or cast metal. The metal usually considered for this purpose is high noble gold (see Chapter 37 for information on indirect composite acrylic resin inlays). Inlays are designed to restore up to three surfaces of a tooth and are used to restore decayed teeth. Inlays are usually thought of as intracoronal (within the crown) restorations (Figure 28.2, *A*).

Inlay

Intracoronal restoration (within the crown) designed to restore up to three surfaces of the tooth

Onlay

Onlay

A cast restoration that fits largely within the tooth and extends over the cusps; it replaces all or part of the occlusal surface

An **onlay** may be considered if the cusps are to be included in the restoration. An onlay is a cast restoration that fits largely within the tooth but also extends over the cusps and replaces all or part of the occlusal surface of the tooth. An onlay may cover up to five surfaces of the tooth (the mesial, distal, and occlusal surfaces and portions of the facial and lingual surfaces). The tooth is prepared by removing the decay and adjusting the intercoronal surface to receive the onlay (Figure 28.2, *B*).

Three-Quarter (Partial) Crown

A three-quarter crown is usually considered to be a metal crown with natural tooth exposed on the labial or buccal surface (Figure 28.3). The crown covers three axial surfaces. When tooth structure is sufficient, a three-quarter crown allows for natural tooth esthetics with minimum exposure of metal in areas of the mouth readily seen during facial or lip movement.

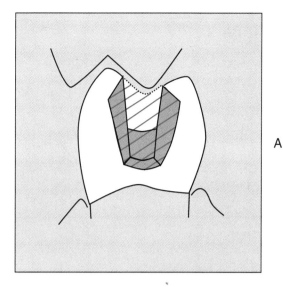

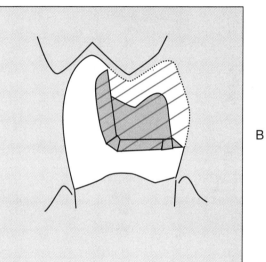

FIGURE 28.2

A, Inlay crown preparation. **B,** Onlay crown preparation.

Grooves that are prepared in the tooth are essential to retention of a partial crown. The grooves are made parallel to each other to help in the seating of the crown. Use of a partial crown is considered more conservative treatment than use of a full crown because the partial crown leaves portions of the tooth's surface intact.

Complete (Full) Crown

A full crown (Figure 28.4) can be constructed to restore the complete crown of a tooth that has broken down or is badly decayed, or it can be used as a retainer for the **abutment teeth** of a

Abutment teeth

The natural teeth that are prepared to support the partial denture

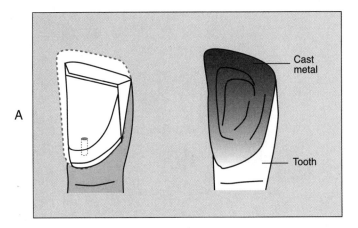

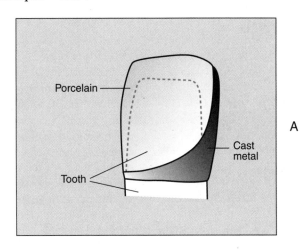

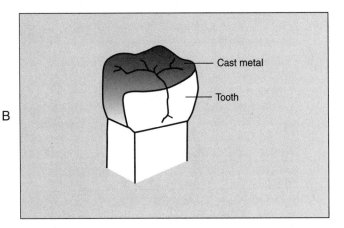

FIGURE 28.3

Three-quarter crowns. **A,** Anterior three-quarter crown. **B,** Posterior three-quarter crown.

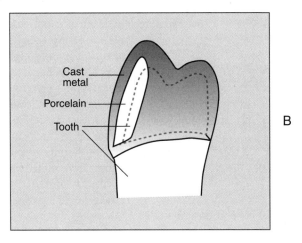

FIGURE 28.5

Full crown with porcelain veneer facing. **A,** Anterior porcelain fused to metal crown. **B,** Posterior porcelain fused to metal crown.

Full Crown with Porcelain or Resin Veneer Facing

A full crown with a porcelain or acrylic resin veneer facing may also be selected to restore anterior and posterior teeth (Figure 28.5). The veneer facing is bonded to the metal substructure and provides both natural looking esthetics and long-term durability. The porcelain may be color matched to the adjacent natural teeth to provide a natural look, particularly in the anterior region of the mouth.

Metal Anterior Crown with Fused Porcelain or Resin

The tooth is prepared using techniques similar to those for a full gold crown. However, only an understructure (coping) or covering of gold or other metallic alloy is formed over the prepared tooth. Varying layers of porcelain or acrylic resin are applied to this coping to reproduce the natural form and esthetics of the crown (Figure 28.6).

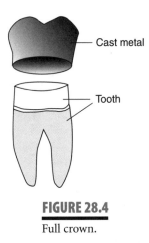

FIGURE 28.4

Full crown.

fixed partial denture. A full crown is a cast restoration that covers the entire coronal surface of a tooth: occlusal/incisal, facial, lingual, mesial, and distal surfaces. The crown can be constructed of a base metal or a high noble alloy.

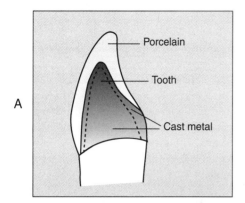

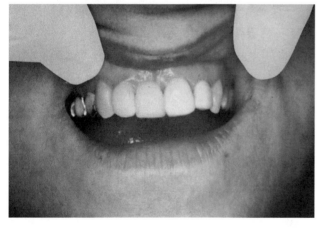

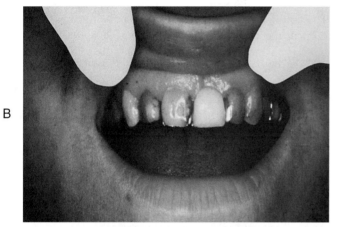

FIGURE 28.6

A, Anterior crown with complete fused porcelain jacket. **B,** Before restoration of anterior teeth. **C,** After restoration.

Complete Porcelain Crown or Jacket

A complete porcelain crown does not have a metal understructure. This type of crown usually is used as a single crown and is often the treatment of choice because of its esthetic qualities. Those qualities are possible because without a metal understructure, the translucency and light-reflecting properties of porcelain are greater. These properties resemble those of the natural dentition.

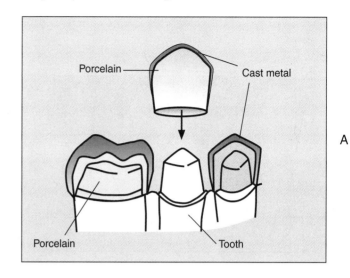

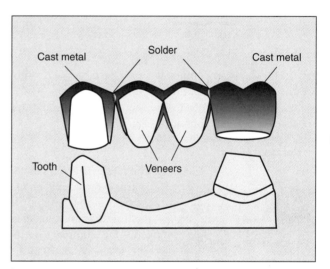

FIGURE 28.7

Two types of fixed bridges. **A,** Solid metal castings with veneers of porcelain or acrylic resin. **B,** Pontics (artificial teeth) soldered to crown retainers to replace missing teeth.

Fixed Partial Denture (Fixed Bridge)

A fixed partial denture or bridge is attached to the dentition by crowns that are cemented to prepared teeth. A bridge may replace an anterior or a posterior tooth, both anterior and posterior teeth, or most of a dental arch. The bridge may be constructed of metal castings or metal castings with porcelain or resin veneers (Figure 28.7). All bridges have fixed attachment support from the natural teeth or from implants (see Chapter 31 for information on dental implants).

Parts of a Fixed Partial Denture

A fixed partial denture may replace one or more missing teeth and is retained by natural teeth or implants adjacent to

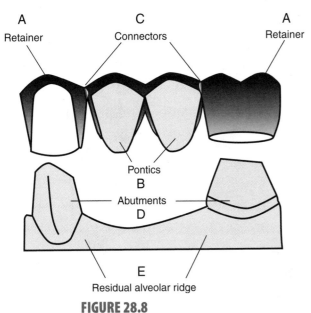

FIGURE 28.8

Parts of a fixed partial denture.

Connectors

The part of the bridge that joins the retainer and the pontic is called the connector (see Figure 28.8, *C*). A fixed partial denture may be cast as a single unit or as separate components that are soldered together into a single unit. A connector that forms a solid unit is called a rigid connector. In some cases, because of alignment problems, for instance, nonrigid connectors may be necessary. These are often called precision attachments or lug and dovetail connectors. They allow some movement when the bridge covers a large portion of the dental arch.

Abutment Teeth

The abutment teeth are the natural teeth that are prepared to support the partial denture (see Figure 28.8, *D*). Two or more teeth may be required to support the bridge if it is placed in a high-stress area. However, in some circumstances one tooth may be sufficient, for example, if the pontic is in a low-stress area.

Residual Alveolar Ridge

The residual alveolar ridge is the edentulous ridge over which the pontic is positioned (see Figure 28.8, *E*). However, the pontic does not sit directly on the gingival tissue; 2 mm of space, or a minimum contact, is left between the tissue and the pontic. This reduces pressure on the tissue and enables the patient to clean both the pontic and the retainers.

Crown and Bridge Support

Additional support and strength may be needed for a full crown or bridge abutment. This can be obtained through the techniques of pin retention, crown core buildup, and post and core construction.

Pin Retention

Retention of a crown may be enhanced by placing pin holes in the tooth preparation. Pin holes and retention grooves must be parallel to the path of insertion of the finished **casting.** The type of crown and the location of the pulp dictate the precise location of the pins and pinholes. Anterior teeth require one hole for each third of the tooth crown. Posterior teeth have one hole for each cusp. Pins are smaller in diameter for anterior teeth and larger for posterior teeth.

Casting

In dentistry, to form into a given shape; the result is a cast restoration, such as a gold crown or bridge

Crown Core Buildup

When the amount of tooth destruction caused by caries or trauma is significant, placing a pin for retention may be impossible. In such cases the coronal crown may need to be built up with amalgam, glass ionomer cement, or composite resin.

the space. The basic components of a fixed partial denture are the retainers, the pontics, and the connectors (solder joints). The abutment teeth and the residual alveolar ridge are also important components (Figure 28.8).

Retainers

Retainer

A device used to preserve space in the dentition or to stabilize a bridge in the dental arch

The **retainers** are the three-quarter crown or full crown portions of the fixed partial denture that are cemented onto the abutment teeth. The retainers attach to the pontics and stabilize the bridge in the dental arch (see Figure 28.8, *A*).

Pontics

A **pontic** is the artificial replacement for a missing tooth. Pontics help to maintain space, stabilize the arch, and ensure proper occlusion. The two types of pontics are the hygienic pontic and the tissue-contacting pontic (see Figure 28.8, *B*). The hygienic pontic is designed to provide space (usually 2 mm) between the pontic and the oral tissue to allow easier access for cleaning around the pontic. It is used most often in the posterior area of the oral cavity. The tissue-contacting pontic may be used in the posterior or anterior region and is the pontic of choice for an anterior bridge because of its esthetic and phonetic qualities.

Pontic

The artificial replacement for a missing tooth; pontics maintain space, stabilize the arch, and aid in proper occlusion

Post and Core Construction

After endodontic treatment, the root of a nonvital tooth may become the support for a full crown or bridge abutment by using a post and core construction. This involves enlarging the root canal and cementing a post, either preformed or custom fabricated, into the canal. The post usually imitates the height of the original natural crown. Self-curing resin is molded over the post to form the core, which is refined and shaped with an acrylic stone and disk. A master impression is then taken. A temporary crown or bridge is worn until the permanent cast post and core is returned by the dental laboratory. The cast restoration is placed over the post and core.

ROLE OF THE DENTAL ASSISTANT IN FIXED PROSTHODONTICS

The dental assistant has a major responsibility in preparing the patient for prosthodontic treatment and assisting the dentist during the procedures. The extent of that role depends on the state dental practice regulations.

CLINICAL PROCEDURES FOR FIXED PROSTHODONTICS

Fixed prosthodontic treatment involves several fundamental clinical procedures, many of which have been covered in previous chapters. The primary procedures are performing a complete examination, preparing the teeth, making impressions, placing temporary restorations, and adjusting and seating the permanent restoration.

First Appointment (Examination)

At the first appointment, the patient's medical-dental history is taken, the patient is examined, radiographs are taken, existing teeth and restorations are charted, periodontal charting is completed, preliminary impressions are made for diagnostic models, and a treatment plan is developed. A subsequent consultation appointment allows the dentist and patient to discuss and decide on the best treatment plan and to make financial arrangements.

The dental assistant sets up the operatory, prepares the patient for the initial appointment, and carries out most of the procedures listed above, if allowed by law. The dental assistant also performs other treatment procedures, such as mixing and using various cements and impression materials used in fixed prosthodontic treatment. (These basic procedures can be reviewed in previous chapters before proceeding with fixed prosthodontic preparation and treatment.)

As part of the examination, the dentist evaluates the condition of the existing teeth and restorations. The best treatment is determined for replacing missing teeth and restoring the oral structures to proper form and function. Sometimes a fixed restoration cannot be used because of certain conditions in the oral cavity. The dentist assesses any possible contraindications, such as the following:

- Insufficient supporting alveolar structures
- Presence of periodontal disease
- Nonvital abutment teeth (unless they have received endodontic therapy)
- Mobility of abutment teeth
- Poor occlusion of the dentition in the opposing arch
- Poor oral hygiene
- Prohibitive cost of treatment

Second Appointment (Tooth Preparation)

After the examination and consultation have been completed and the patient and the dentist have agreed on the treatment plan, the business assistant makes scheduling arrangements with the patient to begin treatment. The patient usually is scheduled for a complete prophylaxis followed by a series of restorative procedures. If the patient is in any dental discomfort, emergency care is provided first. The length of time needed to complete the restorative procedures depends on the comprehensiveness of treatment (Box 28.2).

Initial Preparations

The dental assistant prepares the basic tray setup for tooth preparation, as well as the setups for the local anesthetic, rubber dam, alginate impression, elastomeric-type impression material, bite registration, and temporary coverage material. The operatory is disinfected and prepared for the patient. After the patient has been seated and made comfortable, the dentist administers the local anesthetic. If the restorations require selection of tooth shades, this usually is done before the rubber dam is placed or tooth preparation is begun. Nitrous oxide may be used to relax the patient, and the dental assistant may isolate the working area with a rubber dam, depending on state regulations and the dentist's preferences.

When the patient is ready, the dentist begins tooth preparation, obtains appropriate impressions, and fabricate temporaries. The basic tray setup for crown and bridge tooth preparation is as follows (Figure 28.9):

- High-speed handpiece
- Low-speed handpiece
- Mirror
- Explorer
- Probe
- Dressing pliers
- Cord placement instrument
- Spatula
- Carver
- Plastic filling instrument
- Scaler
- Cavity preparation instruments

Box 28.2

Procedure

Procedure for Tooth Preparation Appointment

Materials needed

Basic setup (mirror, explorer, tissue forceps)
Local anesthetic
Stone and bur assortment
Articulation paper
Cement
Cement placement instruments
Cement spatula and mixing pad
Burnishers
Orangewood stick or tongue blade
Working model and permanent crown
Scalers
Handpieces
Floss

Technique:
1. **Administer the local anesthetic.**
2. **If an anterior restoration is to be done, make a shade selection.**
3. **Obtain a preliminary alginate impression of each arch.**
4. **Place a rubber dam.**
5. **Prepare the tooth.**
6. **Place the retraction cord.**
7. **Obtain the final impression and bite registration.**
8. **Prepare the provisional prosthesis and check the occlusion.**
9. **Cement the provisional prosthesis and remove excess cement.**
10. **Clean up the patient.**
11. **Prepare the impressions and bite registration for delivery to the laboratory.**
12. **Give the patient postoperative instructions and dismiss the person.**

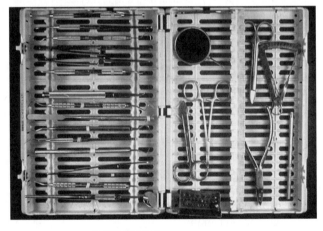

FIGURE 28.9

Crown and bridge tray setup.

- Crown and bridge scissors
- Contouring pliers
- Retraction cord
- Iwanson spring caliper or Boley gauge
- Bur stand (carborundum disks, diamond burs, mandrels, fissure burs [#170 or #169L])
- Articulating paper
- Articulating paper forceps
- Aspirating syringe
- 2 x 2-inch gauze sponges
- Cotton rolls
- Air and water (A/W) syringe tips
- High-velocity evacuation (HVE) suction tip

Preparing the Tooth

The procedures for preparing a tooth for either a crown or a bridge are similar. Therefore the basic procedures for a full crown are outlined in general terms, with additional illustrations and descriptions used to highlight important differences and to emphasize preparations for bridge restorations.

The primary role of the dental assistant during these procedures includes the following:
- Obtaining preliminary impressions before tooth preparation*
- Evacuating debris during tooth preparation

*Delegation of this duty is governed by state regulation

- Retracting the cheek, lips, or tongue as needed
- Cleaning the mouth mirror and rinsing the work area as needed
- Placing and removing packing cord*
- Preparing and seating the temporary crown or bridge*
- Removing cement
- Cleaning up the patient
- Preparing the impression for the laboratory

Making the Preliminary Impression

If a study model was not prepared as part of treatment planning, the dental assistant makes full-arch alginate impressions of both arches before the tooth is prepared. These impressions are put in a humidor or wrapped in a damp towel (see Chapter 15 for further information on alginate impressions). The alginate impressions are used to fabricate the temporary crown or bridge.

Selecting the Tooth Shade

Shade guides provide samples of the various shades of natural teeth. Manufacturers provide guides for their composite resins or porcelain. It is important to select the shade before the rubber dam is placed in the mouth or the tooth is prepared. The shade usually is selected while the dentist waits for the anesthetic to take effect. Because the teeth are usually moist, the shade guide should also be moistened. Natural light offers a more accurate shade. The dentist often turns the operating light off while selecting the shade. After the shade has been selected, the number on the shade guide should be noted in the patient's chart for future reference. The dentist may select several shades to blend and characterize the restoration.

Initial Tooth Preparation for a Full Crown

The dental assistant places the proper diamond bur in the high-speed handpiece. The dentist prepares the teeth while the assistant maintains a clear visual field. The dentist removes enough tooth structure to eliminate any caries or previous restoration or to smooth broken tooth structure while allowing adequate space for a strong restoration. The primary steps involved in preparing the tooth are (1) occlusal-incisal tooth reduction; (2) mesial and distal proximal reduction; (3) facial and lingual reduction; (4) preparation of the shoulder or ledge at the free gingival margin (use of gold or porcelain restorative material determines the width of the margin); (5) smoothing of axial walls and rounding of line and point angles; and (6) cutting of grooves or pin holes.

The dentist prepares the finish line or margin at the cervical area of the tooth. The margin of the preparation is designed to withstand the force of occlusion on the

*Delegation of this duty is governed by state regulation

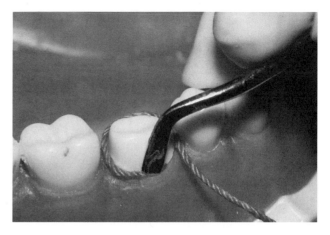

FIGURE 28.10

Use of a retraction cord.

restoration and provide a smooth junction of the margins of the casting with the tooth. The margin of the preparation often extends below the free gingival margin. The dentist is careful not to injure the soft tissue with the bur in this sulcus area.

Gingival Retraction

Retraction usually is necessary to withdraw the gingival tissue from around the tooth and to hold it out of the way. This may be done before tooth preparation because of the depth of the restoration or it may be necessary only to obtain an accurate impression. Retraction is accomplished by electrosurgery, laser surgery, rotary curettage, or use of a surgical knife or retraction cord. The surgical procedures are used to remove hypertrophied or excess tissue that would interfere with placement of the restoration and affect the success of the restoration.

> *Retraction*
>
> **The technique of withdrawing gingival tissue from around the tooth and holding it out of the way**

The removal of gingival tissue with rotary curettage or a surgical knife causes bleeding, which must be controlled by applying an astringent or hemostatic material. The advantage of electrosurgery and laser surgery is that they remove the gingival tissue and also control bleeding.

Use of a retraction cord is a simple method for retracting gingival tissue that helps prevent injury to the free gingival margin. The retraction cord is available plain or with an astringent. The cotton forceps and a plastic instrument can be used to place the cord around the tooth in the gingival sulcus (Figure 28.10). This helps reduce the risk of hemorrhage, with blood flowing into the preparation and distorting the impression. It also helps to extend the free gingiva away from the tooth and the preparation, allowing the impression material to flow unobstructed into the gingival sulcus and the preparation.

After the cord has been placed around the tooth, the ends should overlap and be tucked securely into the sulcus. This reduces the chance of the cord being caught in the bur or cutting instrument. After the cord has been packed securely, the dentist can finalize the cavosurface margins with a chamfered finish line, which provides a detailed impression of the margins and allows for a marginally accurate crown.

Making the Final Impression

The final impression must be accurate in every detail to produce a working cast from which a well-fitting, acceptable anatomic restoration can be fabricated. The impression materials most often used today are the reversible hydrocolloid and elastomeric materials (see Chapter 15 for further information on manipulating these impression materials).

Before the final impression is made, the oral cavity is rinsed and cleansed of debris. The retraction cord that was used to protect the free gingival tissue during tooth preparation may be removed. The tooth is dried, and if the retraction cord was removed, a clean retraction cord is inserted into the gingival sulcus. The dental assistant prepares the impression material and places it in the syringe or impression tray. Just before the dentist places the impression material into the mouth, the dental assistant carefully and quickly removes the retraction cord and makes sure that the area is dry. The assistant also helps the dentist retract the cheeks and lips and place the saliva ejector.

Preparing the Impression for the Laboratory

After the impression has been removed from the mouth, the opposing impression and bite registration are taken. These impressions are rinsed, disinfected, and placed in an appropriate container, with a prescription, and sent to the dental laboratory.

Preparing the Laboratory Prescription

The dentist prepares a work authorization, known as a laboratory prescription, for the laboratory technician (Figure 28.11). Prescription forms vary and are usually supplied by the dental laboratory providing the service. The prescription provides the following information:

- The date the case is presented.
- The dentist's name and address.
- The patient's name, age, and gender.
- The date the case is requested back in the dental office.
- The type of porcelain occlusion, facial margins, metal, and shade variances.
- The type of full cast restoration and metal.
- The pontic design.
- The case design.

- Any special instructions.
- The dentist's signature and license number.

FIGURE 28.11
Sample prescription.

Provisional (Temporary) Crowns and Bridges

The **provisional** crown and bridge is the temporary restoration that is prepared and placed in position until the final restoration has been completed.

Provisional

A temporary restoration

Table 28.1

Provisional Crowns

Types	Primary teeth	Permanent teeth	Posterior	Anterior	Anatomic	Nonanatomic
Permanent						
Gold alloy		X	X	X	X	
Semipermanent						
Chromium	X	X	X		X	
Stainless steel	X	X	X	X	X	
Temporary						
Aluminum	X	X	X	X	X	X
Gold-anodized		X	X		X	X
Silver-tin	X	X	X	X	X	
Polycarbonate	X	X		X	X	
Celluloid	X	X		X	X	
Custom	X	X	X	X	X	X

Although the temporary restoration may not be as strong and precise as the permanent restoration, it should have the critical anatomic characteristics. These include proximal contact, alignment, interproximal spaces, embrasures, occlusion, facial and lingual contours, and curvature of the cervical lines (see Chapter 9 for further information on tooth form and function). The temporary restoration should (1) provide complete coverage of the prepared teeth, (2) maintain the occlusal relationship, (3) render proximal contact and tooth contour, (4) furnish proper esthetics, (5) provide posterior stability, and (6) be smooth and nonirritating to the soft intraoral tissues.

Complete coverage is important so that the temporary can protect the tooth from external fluids, bacterial penetration, and temperature changes. Because temporaries often must last for several weeks and teeth begin shifting quickly, temporaries should be able to provide proper occlusal form and function to eliminate extrusion. Proper contour and proximal contact of the temporary also prevent drifting of the natural teeth and maintain interproximal space integrity until the permanent restoration is seated. It is essential that anterior temporaries be natural and pleasant appearing.

Although posterior temporary restorations are placed in the mouth only for a short period, they must be strong enough to withstand the forces of mastication. Preformed metal crowns are usually used in the posterior areas because of their ease of manipulation and placement. However, resin materials are used for custom-fabricated bridges.

Provisional restorations may be manufactured and preformed or custom fabricated (Table 28.1). A number of manufacturers offer provisionals for posterior anatomic crowns, polycarbonate anterior crowns, and anterior crown forms. Because of the new materials, techniques, and equipment available, the use of acrylic resin for temporaries is increasing. Both anterior and posterior temporaries must be smooth so that they do not irritate the tongue and other soft tissues in the oral cavity.

Types of Temporary Crowns and Bridges

Temporary crowns are made from a variety of materials and are available in various shapes. Stainless steel crowns, which are often considered semipermanent because of their strength, are used for pediatric space maintenance and preservation of remaining tooth structure. They can be used for longer periods but are not strong enough to be considered a permanent restoration. Stainless steel and nickel-chromium provisional crowns are available for both primary and permanent teeth. Temporary crowns include preformed shapes or shells or custom-fabricated crowns and bridges.

Preformed Crowns

Preformed crowns are temporary crowns that are anatomic or shaped like natural anatomic tooth crowns. They are available for both primary and permanent dentition.

Preformed temporary crowns can be made from nickel-chromium alloy, aluminum, gold-anodized aluminum, silver-

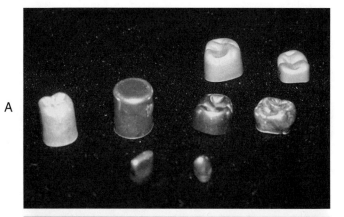

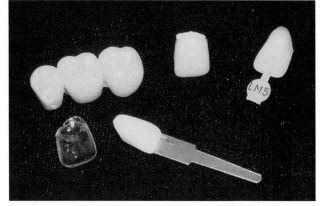

FIGURE 28.12

Custom and preformed provisionals. **A,** Preformed temporary crowns. **B,** Custom bridge and crown, polycarbonate crown, crown form, and shade guide.

tin alloy, or resin. Although stainless steel crowns for anterior teeth are available, metal temporary crowns usually are used for posterior temporary restorations and resin (polycarbonate) temporary crowns are more commonly used for anterior prostheses.

Preformed metal anatomic temporary crowns may be festooned or precrimped, which means that they are manufactured with the contoured shape of that particular tooth and that the cervical curvature duplicates the general outline of the tooth form. These temporary crowns may have either thin or thick walls. They may also have a standard or nonfestooned shape, meaning that the occlusal surface is anatomically correct but the axial surfaces are not contoured. The operator must festoon and contour such crowns by hand.

In addition, both anatomic and nonanatomic metal temporary crowns may be pretrimmed or extended at the cervix. The pretrimmed form eliminates excess trimming around the cervical line, but the extended temporary crown allows more flexibility for the operator to trim the crown to the desired shape. In both cases the cervical margin must be trimmed, smoothed, and festooned to fit the tooth correctly (Figure 28.12).

Resin or polycarbonate temporary crowns are used primarily for anterior teeth and have the esthetic quality of natural teeth (Box 28.3 and Table 28.2). These crowns also have many of the physical characteristics of the metal crowns in that they can be trimmed, crimped, reshaped, contoured, and cemented into place. After the proper size temporary has been selected, the cervix is trimmed and a self-curing or light-cured resin is placed in the crown. The crown is then placed over the lubricated, prepared tooth. After the initial set, the crown is removed and excess material is trimmed away. The provisional is seated again, so that the trimming can be checked, and then removed to cure. When the resin has cured completely, any final finishing is done and the crown is cemented in place. Temporary bridges can also be fabricated with these individual crowns by using a bur to make two holes in the interproximal surfaces and extruding the resin mixture through the holes to fuse the crowns together.

Shell Crowns

Shell crowns, sometimes called "tin cans," are nonanatomic (Box 28.4 and Table 28.3). Shell crowns do not have any occlusal form, and they may have straight axial surfaces or may be precontoured (precontouring means that the axial surfaces are contoured). They are available in different diameters to provide adequate proximal support and contact. Shell crowns may be made from aluminum or silver-tin alloy.

Custom Crown and Bridge Provisionals

Temporary custom crowns and bridges may be fabricated from plastic crown forms or from a matrix or impression obtained from the teeth before tooth preparation.

Preformed Crown Forms

Crown forms are clear plastic forms used for fabricating anterior temporary crowns (Box 28.5 and Table 28.4). They are packaged in a variety of sizes. The selected crown is trimmed and sized to fit the open space. After sizing it is filled with a resin material, placed on the prepared tooth, and held tightly in place until the material has polymerized. Self-curing or light-cured resin may be used. After the initial setting has taken place, the excess material is removed and the crown form is removed. The crown may need to be polished, but minimal contouring will be necessary. These crown forms are also excellent for restoring an incisal angle on an anterior tooth.

Custom Matrix Forms/Light-Cured Resin System

Custom light-cured provisional systems have been introduced for the fabrication of crown and bridge temporaries (Box 28.6 and Table 28.5 on pp. 757-758). Some of the "automix" cartridge temporary systems were introduced only within the past few years.

One of the first steps is to select the shade for the temporary crown. Then vacuum form equipment is used to form a sheet

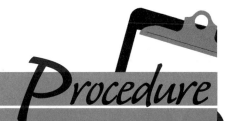

Box 28.3   *Procedure*

Procedure for Preparing a Provisional Crown

Equipment for finishing and polishing crowns and bridges:
Finishing burs
Stone wheels
Stone points
Acrylic polystone points
Rubber wheels
Rubber points
Rubber polishing cups
Mandrel
Sandpaper disks
Polishing brushes
Rag wheel
Pumice
Tin oxide
Tripoli
Rouge

Equipment for preparing an acrylic resin provisional crown:
Plastic temporary crown
Mirror
Explorer
Tissue forceps

Plastic instrument
Scaler
Scissors
Finishing and polishing materials
Resin
Temporary cement
Light-curing equipment

Technique for preparing a resin provisional crown:

1. Select the proper size crown.
2. Trim the cervical contour with scissors, a bur, stone, or diamond bur.
3. Place the resin mix in the crown and seat the crown over the lubricated, prepared tooth (Figure 28.13, *A*).
4. After the initial set, remove the crown and trim away the excess material.
5. Check the crown in position on the tooth for any distortion.
6. Remove the crown and light cure it or allow it to self-cure.
7. Seat the crown with temporary cement.
8. Remove any excess cement and check the sulcus (Figure 28.13, *B*).

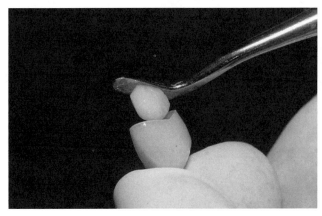
A

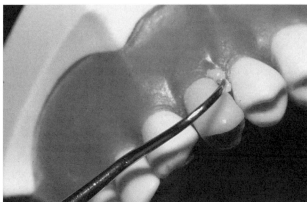
B

FIGURE 28.13

A, After the cervical contour has been trimmed with scissors, bur, stone, or diamond bur, acrylic mix is put in the crown, which is seated over the lubricated, prepared tooth. **B,** The crown is seated with temporary cement, excess cement is removed, and the sulcus is checked.

Table 28.2

Evaluation of Resin Provisional Crown

Resin Provisional Crown	4	3	2	0	X
Secure materials.					
Size crown.					
Trim cervical contour.					
Place in crown.					
Seat crown.					
Remove crown and trim excess.					
Check crown.					
Remove crown and cure.					
Seat crown.					
Remove excess cement.					

The numeric criteria: 4 Excellent; 3 Good but some improvement can be made; 2 Below average, usable, needs to improve skill; 0 Unsatisfactory; X Not able to evaluate.

Box 28.4

Procedure for Preparing a Metal Shell Provisional Crown

Procedure

Materials needed
Aluminum crown
Mirror
Explorer
Tissue forceps
Plastic instrument
Scaler
Scissors
Contouring pliers
Finishing and polishing materials
Temporary cement

Technique:
1. Select the proper size crown (Figure 28.14, *A*).
2. Establish the crown length by scribing a line around the cervical line of the crown with an explorer.
3. Trim the crown 1 mm below the scribed line.
4. Smooth the margins with a heatless stone (Figure 28.14, *B*).
5. Contour the margins with a pliers and crimp.
6. Check the occlusion and contacts (Figure 28.14, *C*).
7. Polish the margins.
8. Isolate the tooth and cement the crown.
9. Remove any excess cement and check the sulcus.

of clear polypropylene coping material on the preliminary model. Once the anatomic shape has been formed into the matrix, the prepared teeth are lubricated, some resin material is injected into the preparation, and the resin-filled matrix is placed over the prepared teeth. After the matrix has been in-serted and the material has cured for approximately 2 minutes, the matrix with the resin can be removed from the teeth and trimmed with scissors to contour the cervical margin. The matrix and resin must be reinserted and light cured for 60 seconds to produce a dense, hard provisional crown or bridge.

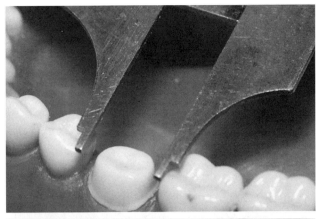

A

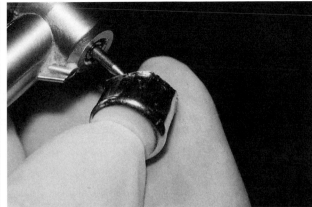

B

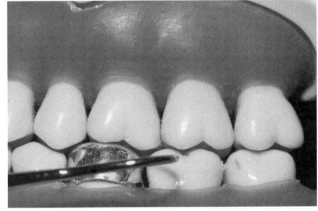

C

FIGURE 28.14

A, The proper size crown is selected by measuring with a Boley gauge or another measuring device. **B,** The crown is trimmed 1 mm below the scribe line, and the margins are smoothed with a heatless stone. **C,** The occlusion and contacts are checked before the excess cement is removed.

Table 28.8

Evaluation of Metal Shell Provisional Crown

Metal Shell Provisional Crown	4	3	2	0	X
Secure materials.					
Select crown.					
Scribe cervical line.					
Trim crown.					
Smooth margins.					
Contour margins and crimp.					
Check occlusional and contacts.					
Polish margins.					
Isolate tooth and cement crown.					
Remove excess cement.					

The numeric criteria: 4 Excellent; 3 Good but some improvement can be made; 2 Below average, usable, needs to improve skill; 0 Unsatisfactory; X Not able to evaluate.

An advantage of this system is the ability to characterize the facial surface of the provisional crown by providing a blended overlay. This is accomplished by removing approximately 0.5 mm of the facial surface of the provisional crown with a carborundum stone or diamond bur, selecting an appropriate shade, and bonding the resin to the prepared surface. The provisional crown must be cured for 60 seconds, finished, contoured, and polished. It is then

Box 28.5

Procedure

Procedure for Preparing Plastic Crown Forms

Materials needed
Crown form
Acrylic resin
Light-curing equipment
Mirror
Explorer
Tissue forceps
Plastic instrument
Scaler
Scissors
Temporary cement
Finishing and polishing materials

Preparing anterior plastic crown forms:
1. Select the proper size crown.
2. Trim and contour the gingival margins, adjust the size if necessary, and check the fit on the prepared tooth.

3. Use an explorer to create air vents by punching a hole in each incisal corner and in the lingual surface (Figure 28.15, *A*).
4. Insert the resin material in one large mass into the crown form to avoid trapping air between layers.
5. Apply force to seat the filled crown on the prepared tooth (Figure 28.15, *B*).
6. Light cure the crown or wait 15 minutes for it to self-cure.
7. Remove the excess material and check the occlusion and contacts (Figure 28.15, *C*).
8. Finish and polish the gingival margins and apply a surface coating.

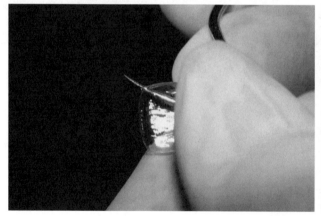

A

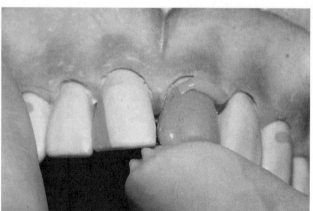

B

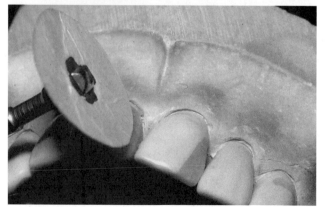

C

FIGURE 28.15

A, Air vents are created by using the explorer tip to punch a hole in each incisal corner. **B,** Force is applied to seat the filled crown on the prepared tooth. **C,** After curing is complete, excess material is removed and the occlusal contacts are checked. The gingival margins are then polished, and a surface coating is applied.

Table 28.4

Evaluation of Anterior Plastic Crown Form

Anterior Plastic Crown Form	4	3	2	0	X
Secure materials.					
Select crown.					
Trim and contour gingival margin.					
Adjust size.					
Check fit.					
Prepare air vents.					
Insert resin material.					
Seat filled crown.					
Cure.					
Remove excess material.					
Check occlusion and contacts.					
Finish and polish gingival margin.					
Apply coating.					

The numeric criteria: 4 Excellent; 3 Good but some improvement can be made; 2 Below average, usable, needs to improve skill; 0 Unsatisfactory; X Not able to evaluate.

Box 28.6

Procedure

Procedure for Preparing a Custom Matrix/Light-Cured Provisional Prosthesis

Materials needed

Mirror
Explorer
Tissue forceps
Plastic instrument
Scaler
Shade guide
Coping material
Vacuum form equipment
Light-curing equipment
Lubricant
Acrylic resin
Scissors
Carborundum stone or diamond bur
Temporary cement
Placement instrument
Finishing and polishing materials

Technique:

1. Select the shade for the temporary crown.
2. Use vacuum form equipment to form a sheet of clear polypropylene coping material on the preliminary model.
3. Lubricate the prepared teeth.
4. Inject some of the resin material onto the teeth (Figure 28.16, A).
5. Fill the matrix and place it over the prepared teeth.
6. Cure for approximately 2 minutes.
7. Remove the matrix with the resin from the teeth and trim the matrix with scissors to contour the cervical margins (Figure 28.16, B).
8. Reinsert the matrix and light cure it for 60 seconds to produce a dense, hard provisional crown or bridge.
9. To characterize the facial surface of the provisional prosthesis, remove approximately 0.5 mm of the facial surface of the prosthesis with a carborundum stone or diamond bur (Figure 28.16, C).
10. Select an appropriate shade and bond the resin to the prepared surface.
11. Cure the provisional prosthesis for 60 seconds.
12. Finish, contour, and polish the provisional prosthesis.
13. Cement the temporary crown and light cure it for 20 seconds.
14. Remove any excess material and cure the provisional prosthesis for 40 seconds.
15. Evaluate the restoration and check the occlusion.

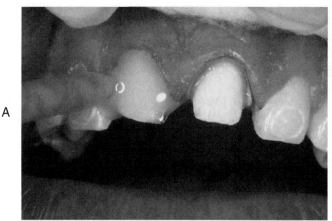

A

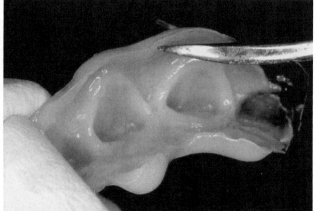

B

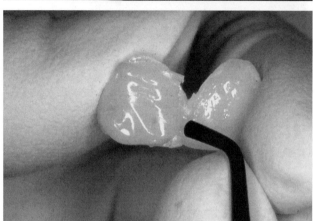

C

FIGURE 28.16

A, Some of the provisional resin is injected into the prepared teeth. **B,** To contour the cervical margins, the matrix is removed with the resin during the elastic phase and trimmed with scissors and a sandpaper disk. **C,** Approximately 0.5 mm of the labial surface must be removed to characterize the facial surface of the provisional prosthesis. (Courtesy JM Braun.)

Table 28.5					
Evaluation of Custom Matrix/Light Cured Provisional					
Custom Matrix/Light Cured Provisional	4	3	2	0	X
Secure materials.					
Select shade.					
Place coping material on model.					
Lubricate prepared teeth.					
Inject resin into teeth.					
Fill matrix and place over teeth.					
Cure (2 minutes).					
Remove cured matrix from teeth.					
Trim and contour cervical margin.					
Reinsert matrix in vacuum former and cure (60 seconds).					
Characterize facial surface.					
Select shade and bond resin to prepared surface.					
Cure (60 seconds).					
Finish, contour, and polish provisional.					
Cement provisional and light cure (20 seconds).					
Remove excess and cure (40 seconds).					
Evaluate and check occlusion.					

The numeric criteria: 4 Excellent; 3 Good but some improvement can be made; 2 Below average, usable, needs to improve skill; 0 Unsatisfactory; X Not able to evaluate.

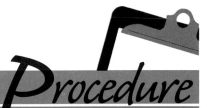

Box 28.7

Procedure for Preparing an Alginate Impression/Self-Cured Provisional

Materials needed

Mirror
Explorer
Tissue forceps
Plastic instrument
Scaler
Alginate
Water
Measuring device
Impression tray
Rubber bowl
Spatula
Acrylic resin
Lubricant
Articulation paper
Finishing and polishing materials

Technique:

1. Obtain an alginate impression before the tooth is prepared. Set the impression aside in a moist container.
2. Prepare the teeth, remove debris, and dry the teeth.
3. Mix acrylic resin and place it in the impression.
4. Lubricate the prepared teeth.
5. Seat the impression with acrylic resin directly over the teeth and cure (Figure 28.17, *A*).
6. Remove the impression from the mouth and retrieve the crown or bridge.
7. Finish, contour, and polish the provisional crown or bridge (Figure 28.17, *B*).
8. Check the occlusion and contacts and cement.
9. Remove excess cement.

A 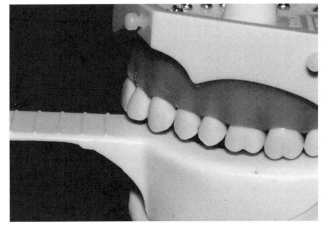 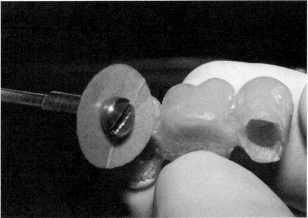 B

FIGURE 28.17

A, The impression is seated with acrylic resin directly over the teeth and cured. **B,** After the impression has been removed from the mouth, the provisional prosthesis is retrieved and finished, contoured, and polished.

cemented in place with a temporary cement and light-cured for 20 seconds. The excess material is removed, and the provisional crown is cured for an additional 40 seconds.

Alginate Impression Form/Self-Cured Resin System

The custom self-cured resin system that uses an alginate impression has been used for many years (Box 28.7 and Table 28.6). It is a simple procedure that requires that an alginate

Table 28.6

Evaluation of Alginate Impression/Self-Cured Provisional

Alginate Impression/Self-Cured Provisional	4	3	2	0	X
Secure materials.					
Secure alginate impression before tooth preparation.					
Assist dentist in preparation of teeth.					
Mix acrylic resin and place into compression.					
Lubricate prepared teeth.					
Seat impression with resin over teeth.					
Remove impression and secure provisional.					
Finish, contour, and polish provisional.					
Check occlusion and contacts.					
Cement provisional.					
Remove excess cement.					

The numeric criteria: 4 Excellent; 3 Good but some improvement can be made; 2 Below average, usable, needs to improve skill; 0 Unsatisfactory; X Not able to evaluate.

impression be obtained before tooth preparation is begun. The alginate impression is used as the form to fabricate the provisional crown or bridge. It is important to remove alginate that has no purpose in the form or that would prevent the impression from seating over the teeth.

After the tooth has been prepared, the acrylic resin material is mixed and placed in the appropriate area of the impression. The teeth are then lubricated. The impression with the resin can be placed directly over the patient's prepared teeth, or it can be placed over a model of the prepared teeth. Because the acrylic resin becomes hot when it polymerizes and some patients are sensitive to resin, the operator may choose to use a working model to fabricate a provisional bridge, especially if several teeth are involved.

Cementing Provisional Prostheses

In some states the dentist can delegate cementing of provisional crowns and bridges to dental assistants. Zinc oxide–eugenol or noneugenol is usually the temporary cement of choice (see Chapter 15 for steps for mixing these cements). After the cement has been mixed according to the manufacturer's directions, a plastic filling instrument is used to carefully line the entire interior surface of the provisional prosthesis (Box 28.8). It is important to use enough cement but also to eliminate any excess, which would have to be removed later from the tooth and gingival sulcus. The provisional prosthesis is completely seated on the prepared tooth, and the occlusion is checked. It is important to remove all excess cement with an explorer, an excavator, or a scaler.

Postoperative Instructions

It is important that the dental assistant remind the patient to chew carefully on the provisional prosthesis and to call the office immediately if the temporary becomes loose. Sticky foods should be avoided. When flossing interproximally, the floss should be brought down gently between the contacts and removed by pulling it out through the lingual or buccal surface and not toward the incisal or occlusal surface.

Third Appointment (Seating)

The third appointment is made to try-in the permanent appliance. The dentist decides if an anesthetic will be used. At this time the provisional prosthesis is removed, and the dentist uses an assortment of stones and burs to make any adjustments to the permanent appliance. The occlusion is checked with articulation paper to identify any interference between the crown or bridge and the opposing teeth.

The dentist may choose to seat the permanent restoration with a temporary cement initially in order to reevaluate the occlusion and the response of the gingival tissue and pulp to the new appliance. However, this is not usually necessary. Before the permanent restoration is seated, the teeth must be isolated and dried, unless a glass ionomer cement will be used. Zinc phosphate cement, zinc polycarboxylate cement, reinforced zinc oxide–eugenol, or glass ionomer cement may be used for permanent cementation.

Proper mixing and application of the cement are vital to the success of the fixed prosthesis. The restoration is seated on the prepared tooth with firm finger pressure initially, followed by heavy pressure. This is accomplished by having the patient bite down on a tongue blade or orangewood stick so that the operator can check the occlusion; this also aids in seating the appliance. It is important to check the margins with an explorer to made sure that the prosthesis has seated completely on the prepared tooth. A

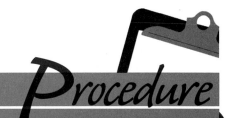

Box 28.8

Procedure

Procedure for Seating a Fixed Restoration

Materials needed
Basic setup (mirror, explorer, tissue forceps)
Anesthetic
Stone and bur assortment
Articulation paper
Cement
Cement placement instruments
Cement spatula and mixing pad
Burnishers
Orangewood stick or tongue blade
Working model and permanent crown
Scalers
Handpieces
Floss

Technique:
1. Confirm delivery of the restoration.
2. Inspect the crown for fit and finish (Figure 28.18, *A*).
3. Administer a local anesthetic if necessary.
4. Remove the provisional prosthesis from the prepared tooth.
5. Clean cement and debris from the tooth.
6. Rinse the tooth.
7. Seat the restoration and inspect it for proper fit.
8. Place a wooden tongue blade on the tooth and instruct the patient to bite down while the marginal fit is checked.
9. Adjust and repolish the restoration if necessary.
10. Dry the tooth (a desensitizing agent may be used on dentin).
11. Mix the cement and place it in the crown.
12. Seat the crown on the tooth while the patient bites down on the tongue blade or crown seater to completely seat the crown.
13. Remove excess cement after it dries, making sure to check the gingival sulcus.
14. Remove debris; rinse the patient's mouth and evaluate the restoration (Figure 28.18, *A*).
15. Clean up the patient and go over the oral hygiene instructions.
16. Dismiss the patient.

A
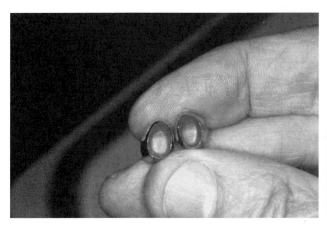

B
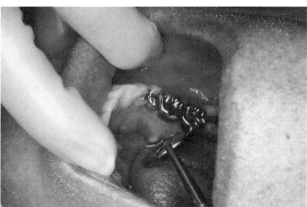

FIGURE 28.18

Procedure for seating a permanent crown. **A,** The crown is inspected for fit and finish. The cement is cleaned from the prepared tooth, the restoration is seated, and the crown is inspected for proper fit (a cotton roll or tongue blade can be placed on the crown, allowing the patient to bite down while the marginal fit is checked). **B,** If the crown fits properly, it is removed from the tooth, the cement is put in the crown, and the crown is seated. After the cement has dried, it is important to check the gingival sulcus and remove any debris.

burnisher can be used to refine the margins. After the restoration has been seated and the cement has become brittle, all excess cement can be removed with an explorer, an excavator, or a scaler. Any excess cement must be removed from the gingival sulcus because it can cause irritation and inflammation.

The dental assistant usually provides the patient with postoperative instructions for oral hygiene and for cleaning and caring for the fixed appliance. The patient usually is scheduled for an appointment in 3 to 6 months so that the fixed appliance can be examined and the condition of the periodontal tissue and occlusion assessed.

LABORATORY FABRICATION OF A FIXED PROSTHESIS

At the dental office, the dental assistant prepares the impressions and the bite registration for transferal to the dental laboratory. All impressions that enter the laboratory must be disinfected by dipping or by spraying with a disinfectant approved by the Occupational Safety and Health Administration (OSHA). Each case that enters the laboratory must be given an assigned number and correlating work plan. The dentist must prepare a prescription to accompany each case with specific details of the work to be completed (see Figure 28.11). After the case has been disinfected and the case number assigned, **fabrication** of the prosthesis begins (Box 28.9).

Fabrication

Construction or molding of a prosthesis

Pouring the Final Impression

The impression is poured with a gypsum die stone, which is very strong and produces good surface detail (Figure 28.19). This process may be performed by the dental laboratory assistant.

Because an accurate working model is essential to the final restoration, immense care must be taken to pour the model cautiously. When the stone is set, it is separated from the impression and the arch is trimmed to a horseshoe shape.

After the arch has been trimmed, one or more holes are drilled in the back of the stone model and the model is boxed with boxing wax. Dowel pins are then placed in the prepared holes, and sheaths are placed over the part of the pin projecting from the back of the model. The back of this model is coated with a separation solution; this prevents the die stone from adhering to the Class II yellow stone that is poured over the back of the working model.

After the Class II stone has set, the working model is cut or sectioned with a small hand saw. This allows the tooth (die) with the crown preparation to be removed from the Class II

stone base. The stone duplicate of the prepared tooth is called the **die** (Figure 28.20).

The die is trimmed around the shoulder or cervical margin; this is called ditching, and its purpose is to provide a clear cavosurface margin from which to fabricate the fine cervical edge of the restoration (Figure 28.21). The die is placed back into the base and is ready for preparation of the wax pattern of the crown. Both the die preparation and base and the opposing model are mounted with the bite registration on an articulator. The articulator represents the maxillary and mandibular arch relationships and guides the models into centric occlusion. This provides a simulation of jaw movement and allows the laboratory technician to restore the artificial teeth to natural form and function.

Die

A form used to fabricated a crown or bridge restoration

Carving the Wax Pattern

Before inlay wax is placed on the die, the fine edge of the margin is carefully marked with a red pencil. This highlights the margin for easier vision. The die is then coated with die lubricant, a sealer that prevents the inlay wax from adhering to the stone die. Some dental laboratories fabricate the die from an epoxy resin or electroplate the die with a coating of copper or silver to protect it from abrasion during carving of the wax pattern. A die spacer may be painted on the die to allow room for the dental cement inside the finished crown. This die spacer cannot be placed on the margins of the die because it would distort the margins. Inlay wax, which vaporizes when heated, is used to carve or build up the crown.

Spruing the Pattern

After the wax pattern has been completed and is anatomically correct, a sprue (pin) is attached to the wax crown. The sprue, which may be made of wax, plastic, or metal, forms the channel through which the molten metal flows after the sprue has been eliminated. The sprue and wax pattern are attached to a crucible former, and all three are placed in a casting ring. The casting ring is made of metal and is lined with a ceramic or paper liner for expansion control. If the ringless technique is used, the mold is removed from the ring and base after 20 to 30 minutes and bench set for 25 minutes. The mold is kept moist until ready for burnout.

Investing the Pattern

The construction of a cast metal crown is a complicated process involving procedures that must be carried out very carefully. A wax replica or pattern of the crown is prepared. This pattern will be surrounded by a material that will form

Box 28.9

Laboratory Preparations at a Glance

1. Pour impression.
2. Prepare die.
3. Build up wax pattern.
4. Sprue the pattern.
5. Invest the pattern.

6. Burn out the pattern.
7. Cast the pattern.
8. Pickle, finish, and polish the casting.
9. Apply porcelain.

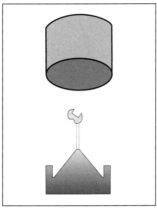

A

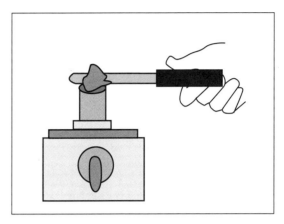

B

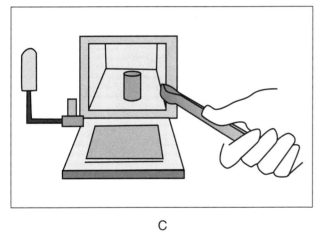

C

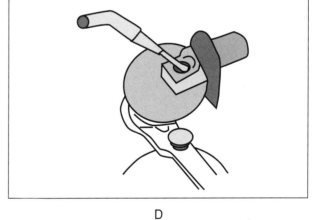

D

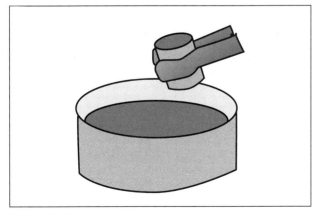

E

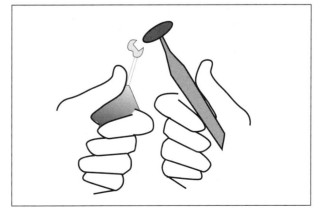

F

A, Spruing of the wax pattern. **B,** Investing of the pattern. **C,** Burning out of the pattern. **D,** Casting of the pattern. **E,** Pickling of the cast crown. **F,** Finishing and polishing of the cast crown.

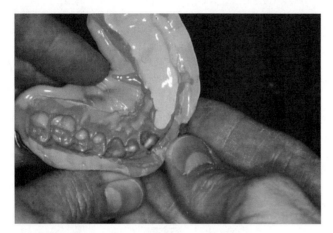

FIGURE 28.19

A variety of die stones are available. However, no matter which is used, care must be taken in pouring. (Courtesy Todd A. Fridrich and Whip Mix Corp.)

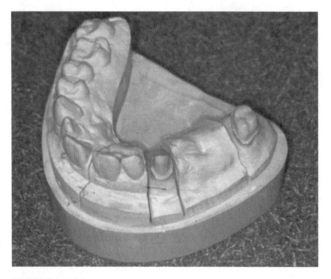

FIGURE 28.20

The die is placed back in the base and is ready for preparation of the wax pattern of the crown. (Courtesy Todd A. Fridrich and Whip Mix Corp.)

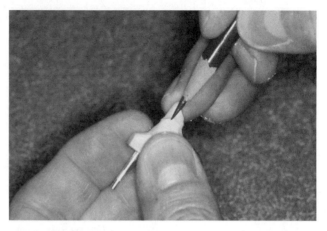

FIGURE 28.21

The fine edge of the margin is carefully marked with a red pencil. (Courtesy Todd A. Fridrich and Whip Mix Corp.)

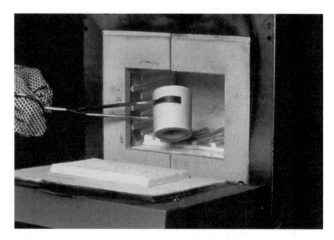

FIGURE 28.22

The casting ring is placed in the burnout oven, which has been preheated to 1300° to 1600° F. The casting ring is left in the over for 40 to 60 minutes. (Courtesy Todd A. Fridrich and Whip Mix Corp.)

an accurate mold of the pattern. This material is called an investment, and many types of investment material are available. They are all designed with specific properties, such as expansion ability, high temperature strength, and porosity. Before the investing process, the wax pattern is coated with a wetting agent, which reduces surface tension, prevents bubbles on the pattern, and helps the investment flow more evenly over the wax pattern.

It is important to use the correct water to powder ratio for the investment, which is mixed with a vac-u-spat to eliminate air bubbles. The investment is vibrated into the investment ring, covering the wax pattern completely. After the investment has been poured, it must bench set for 45 minutes.

Burning Out the Pattern

After the investment has hardened, the sprue is eliminated, producing a hollow mold. The casting ring is placed in the burnout oven at approximately 1300° to 1600° F for 40 to 60 minutes. This eliminates the wax from the investment pattern (Figure 28.22).

Casting the Pattern

After the wax pattern has been sprued and invested, the casting machine is prepared with a clean crucible. Some casting machines have a thermotrol control and centrifuge to melt the metal and must be turned on. Others require the use of a gas-air torch to melt the gold. In either case the casting machine must be wound because it uses centrifugal energy to force the molten metal into the casting ring. The casting arm is wound like a spring and locked. The gold is placed in a crucible and melted. The casting ring is removed from the oven and placed in the casting machine behind the crucible. Flux is added with the metal to reduce oxidation. The torch is used to melt the alloy, and while the metal is molten, the arm of the casting machine is released and the molten alloy is forced into the investment pattern by centrifugal force.

Quenching the Casting Ring

When the casting arm stops, the casting ring is removed from the casting machine with tongs, and the alloy is allowed to bench cool until the metal button looses its red color. The hot casting ring is then quenched or submerged in cool water. This causes the investment material to fall away from the metal casting. Investment remains are removed from the casting. The casting is evaluated and checked for casting defects. It can then be removed from the sprues, trimmed, finished, and polished (Figure 28.23).

Finishing and Polishing the Restoration

The fit of the casting is checked on the working model. The metal crown can be placed on the die, and the button and excess metal can be removed with a separating disk and heatless stones and finished with carbides (see Figure 28.23). The casting may be placed in a pickling acid or cleaned with aluminum oxide to remove surface oxides. A sandblaster may be used to remove investment from the crown. Finishing burs, stones, sandpaper disks, rubber wheels and points, rubber cups and prophy brushes,

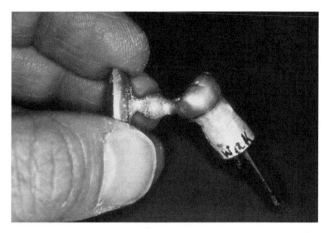

FIGURE 28.23
After the casting has been rinsed, it is inspected for irregularities. (Courtesy Todd A. Fridrich and Whip Mix Corp.)

pumice, and gold rouge can be used to polish the restoration. The restoration must be washed with soap and water to make sure that all oils and debris are removed. It is important always to cover the sink drain when washing the restoration to avoid losing it down the drain. After the crown has been finished and polished, it is ready for delivery to the dental office.

Porcelain Application

If the casting is to contain porcelain, an opaque porcelain is applied to the casting and fired. A multilayer, segmented porcelain buildup can be used to add depth of color. Bisque bake try-in ready for extrinsic staining. The completed restoration is glazed, polished, and cemented.

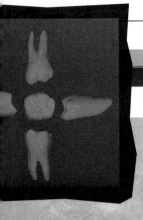

Points for Review

- Dental problems caused by tooth loss.
- Types of fixed prostheses available.
- Clinical procedures performed by the dental assistant during various fixed prosthodontic procedures.
- Steps involved in fabricating provisional restorations.
- Laboratory procedures for fabricating a crown or bridge.

Self-Study Questions

1. What is the purpose of a fixed bridge?
   a. To help move teeth
   b. To prevent movement of the teeth
   c. To make cleaning easier
   d. All of the above
2. What diagnostic aids are used in fixed prosthodontics?
   a. Radiographs
   b. Study models
   c. Clinical examination
   d. All of the above
3. What holds the individual units of a fixed bridge together?
   a. Zinc phosphate
   b. Solder
   c. Zinc oxide–eugenol
   d. Aluminum
4. Why are temporary bridges used?
   a. Esthetics
   b. Space maintenance
   c. Mastication
   d. All of the above
5. For what is electrosurgery used?
   a. To cut tooth structure
   b. To cut bone
   c. To electroplate dies
   d. To remove gingival tissue

6. Why is astringent-impregnated cord used?
   a. To stimulate a patient who has fainted
   b. To dry the prepared tooth
   c. To stop gingival bleeding and retract gingival tissue
   d. To anesthetize
7. What is the advantage of using the elastic impression technique?
   a. No tissue retraction is necessary.
   b. A composite model is obtained.
   c. The material is less expensive.
   d. The material provides a detailed impression.
8. Why is an alginate impression taken during crown and bridge procedures?
   a. To check the fit of the casting
   b. To make temporary crowns
   c. To make a working cast
   d. None of the above
9. What is the purpose of temporary cementation of a fixed bridge?
   a. To check the reaction of the supporting tissue to the prosthesis
   b. To allow the patient to evaluate the prosthesis
   c. To allow the bridge to settle on the abutments
   d. All of the above
10. What type of light is used to select the appropriate tooth shade?
    a. Natural light
    b. Dental light
    c. Fluorescent light
    d. Black light
11. What device smoothes roughness in metals?
    a. Rag wheel
    b. Heatless stone
    c. Rubber wheel
    d. Mandrel
12. What is the purpose of gingival retraction?
    a. To clean the gingival sulcus
    b. To desensitize the gingival sulcus
    c. To widen the gingival sulcus
    d. To prepare the tooth for cementation of a bridge
13. What impression material would least likely be used to obtain a final impression for a fixed restoration?
    a. Compound
    b. Alginate
    c. Rubber base
    d. Hydrocolloid

14. An inlay builds up the occlusal surface, whereas an onlay does not.
    a. True
    b. False
15. Zinc phosphate cement is an acceptable material for permanent cementation of a crown.
    a. True
    b. False
16. Gingival retraction cord is placed after the master or final impression has been obtained.
    a. True
    b. False
17. What are the teeth called that support a fixed bridge?
    a. Abutments
    b. Pontics
    c. Connectors
    d. Partials
18. A pontic is part of a fixed bridge.
    a. True
    b. False

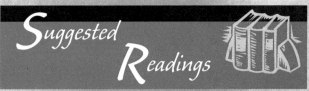

Suggested Readings

Braun JM: Enhanced aesthetics using provisionalization, Signature, Winter 1996 Edition.

Craig RG, O'Brien WJ, Powers JM: *Dental materials: properties and manipulation*, ed 7, St Louis, 2000, Mosby.

Fridrich TA: Perfect partners: ResinRock and PowerCast: a two-part technique article and case presentation. Part 1, Precision working models with ResinRock, Whip Mix Corp, Louisville, Kentucky.

Fridrich TA: Perfect partners: ResinRock and PowerCast: a two-part technique article and case presentation. Part 2, Precision casting with PowerCast, Whip Mix Corp, Louisville, Kentucky.

Glidewell Laboratories: Porcelain and polymer glass to metal: restorative selection guide, 1996.

Naylor WP: *Introduction to metal ceramic technology*, Chicago, 1992, Quintessence Publishing.

Rosenstiel SF, Land MF, Fujimoto J: *Contemporary fixed prosthodontics*, ed 3, St Louis, Mosby (in press).

Chapter 29

*R*emovable Prosthetics

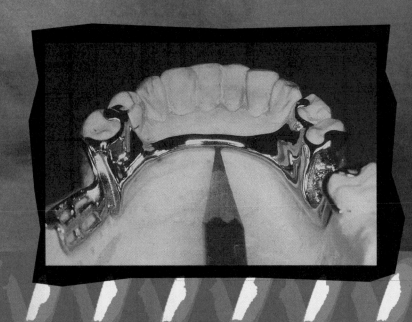

Chapter Outline

Removable Prosthodontics
   The dental assistant's function in removable prosthodontics
   The first appointment with the patient
   The second appointment with the patient
Fixed or Removable Partial Dentures
Planning the Removable Partial Denture (RPD)
Component Parts of the Removable Partial Denture
   Major connector
   Minor connector
   Rests
Appointments Required for Construction of a Removable Partial Denture
   Periodontal therapy
   Endodontics
   Oral surgery

   Restorative dentistry
   Tissue conditioning
Beginning the Partial Denture Phase of the Treatment Plan
   Appointment one
   Appointment two
   Appointment three
   Appointment four
   Appointment five
Permanent Reline of the Removable Partial Denture
   Chairside reline
   Repairing a broken facing
   Adding a tooth to an existing RPD
   Fabrication of record bases and occlusion rims
   Mouth protectors
   Temporary partial denture

Learning Objectives

On completion of Chapter 29, the student should be able to do the following:

- Define key terms.
- Describe the procedures involved in construction of removable partial dentures from patient introduction to delivery and adjustment of the final prosthesis.

- Assist the dentist during removable prosthodontic treatment.

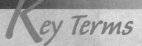

Key Terms

Complete Denture

Facing

Fixed Partial Denture

Implant

Prosthodontics

Removable Partial Denture

REMOVABLE PROSTHODONTICS

Prosthodontics

A special branch of dentistry that maintains oral function, comfort, appearance, and health by restoring natural teeth or replacing missing teeth and oral and maxillofacial tissue with artificial substitutes

Complete denture

A removable dental prosthesis that replaces the entire dentition and associated structures of the maxillae or mandible

Removable partial denture

A prosthesis that replaces one or more teeth in a partially dentate arch and is removable from the mouth

Implant

A prosthetic device implanted into the oral tissues beneath mucosa and periosteal layer and within bone to provide retention and support for a fixed or removable prosthesis

Removable **prosthodontics** are often represented by two types of prostheses: (1) the **complete denture** and (2) the **removable partial denture (RPD)**. A *complete denture* is a removable dental prosthesis that replaces the entire dentition and associated structures of the maxilla or mandible. A *full denture* is supported entirely by the alveolar ridges, hard palate when the maxillary denture is the prosthesis, and oral mucosa.

A *removable partial denture (RPD)* is a prosthesis that replaces one or more teeth in a partially dentate arch and is removable from the mouth (Figure 29.1). It receives its support from the remaining teeth and from the underlying tissues. An *abutment* is a tooth, a portion of a tooth, or that portion of a dental **implant** that serves to support and retain a prosthesis. Removable partial dentures can be divided into two types. The first is the partial denture, which is completely *tooth supported.* It has teeth (abutments) in front of (anterior), and behind (posterior) each edentulous space. This partial denture is supported by the natural teeth at each end of the edentulous space. The second type of removable partial denture is the *distal extension removable denture,* which is supported and retained by natural teeth only at one end of the denture base segment and by the residual ridge beneath the base that holds the prosthetic teeth.

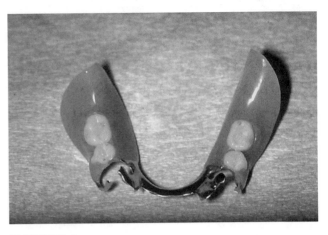

FIGURE 29.1

The removable partial denture is a prosthesis that replaces one or more teeth in a partially edentulous arch with artificial substitutes and is removable from the mouth.

The Dental Assistant's Function in Removable Prosthodontics

The dental assistant is invaluable in all aspects of the treatment of the patient. An assistant may be called on to perform a variety of functions that are outlined in the dental practice legislation of the state in which the dental assistant is employed. Taking x-rays, chairside assisting, tissue conditioning of the prosthesis, patient hygiene education, selection of proper trays to fit the arch, mixing materials, making and pouring diagnostic impressions, fabrication of custom trays, preparation of cases to send to the laboratory, making record bases, trimming casts, taking a facebow record, assisting in the selection of teeth, repairing prosthesis are but a few of the functions that the assistant might be called on to perform in the removable prosthodontic area.

The First Appointment with the Patient

Data Gathering

The first appointment of the patient is usually spent gathering the appropriate data needed for a complete diagnosis, leading to a thorough treatment plan.

Medical and Dental History

A complete medical history of the patient will be taken. Usually a form is provided by the receptionist when the patient registers at the front desk. The assistant is often responsible for seeing that the form is filled out properly by the patient and answering questions that the patient may have while trying to complete the often confusing forms, filled with technical terminology. Many times there is a separate section related to dental history, and, again, the assistant can be helpful in finding out some of the information that is critical to the dentist when determining a treatment plan for the patient. Complete and accurate documentation by the assistant is a necessity.

Radiographs

The dental assistant will take necessary radiographs, which may include a Panorex, periapical, and bitewing x-rays as requested by the dentist. This provides information to the practitioner about impacted teeth, broken root tips, cysts, or other abnormal structures that might interfere with or affect the treatment plan. The x-rays will also provide information about bone support around the remaining teeth.

Charting of Existing Teeth and Restorations

The dentist will need chairside assistance to record the data related to the condition of the remaining natural teeth and oral structures. A charting of decay is often done at the diagnostic data gathering appointment. A patient may also be experiencing sore facial muscles or aching jaws related to temporomandibular dysfunction. All of this information must be accurately recorded. Refer to Chapter 21 in this text regarding the system of recording data in the patient chart.

Periodontal Charting

A complete examination and evaluation of the patient's periodontal condition in general, and of the abutment teeth specifically, must be done in order to make reasonable choices of treatment options.

Impression for Diagnostic Casts

Diagnostic impressions are often made by the dental assistant. The impressions for diagnostic casts for removable partial denture patients are usually recorded with alginate impression material in a prefabricated tray. Information about the hydrocolloid materials, the selection of the proper tray in which to make an impression, details on mixing the alginate and making the impression are discussed in Chapter 15.

Some type of gypsum product is used to fill the impression and create the diagnostic or master model. Refer to Chapter 15 for information about various gypsum products, handling the materials, pouring the impression in gypsum, and trimming the finished cast.

Study casts must reflect an accurate representation of the teeth that remain in the arch as well as a complete duplication of the soft tissues and musculature that will be involved in the final prosthesis. The casts must be free of voids and blebs to allow the dentist to make a thorough and accurate diagnosis. An accurate cast prepared by the assistant may provide the dentist with information that can be attained no other way. The diagnostic casts provide information about the contours of the teeth (which may be used to receive clasps to retain the removable partial denture), may show undercuts in the alveolar ridge (which will need surgery be-

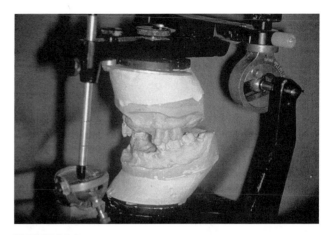

FIGURE 29.2

Diagnostic casts are mounted on the articulator, which is a mechanical instrument that represents the temporomandibular joints and jaws and is used to simulate some of the movements of the mandible.

fore the construction of the prosthesis), and provide visualization to an oral surgeon of the problems and corrections necessary.

Nice-looking study casts provide a wonderful means to educate the patient when presenting the treatment plan, and they are a constant record of the patient's condition when he came for treatment. Sometimes it is advantageous to mount the diagnostic casts on an articulator, (Figure 29.2) a mechanical instrument that represents the temporomandibular joints and jaws and is used to simulate some of the movements of the mandible. It shows the relationship between the maxilla and mandible and provides information about occlusal problems. The maxillary cast is often mounted using a facebow record. The facebow is a simple instrument used to record the relationship of the maxillary arch to some other anatomic reference point on the skull and then to transfer that relationship to the articulator (Figure 29.3).

Base Plates and Occlusion Rims for Removable Partial Dentures

Sometimes when you want to mount a maxillary and mandibular cast on an articulator, it can not be done because there are not enough teeth to support the upper cast against the lower cast while mounting. When this is the case, a record rim, on occlusion rim made with wax, is placed on a record base. A record rim is an interim denture base. A jaw registration record is made to help mount the case (Figure 29.4). The dental assistant or the laboratory technician will be called on to construct the record base(s) with occlusion rim(s). They can be made of a variety of materials, and the method for construction of the record bases will vary somewhat depending on the materials used. See the section under laboratory procedures on Fabrication of Record Bases and Occlusion Rims.

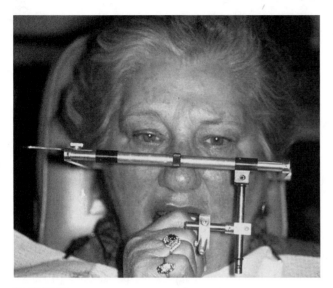

FIGURE 29.3

This facebow is a simple instrument used to record the relationship of the maxillary arch to other anatomic reference points on the skull and then to transfer that relationship to the articulator.

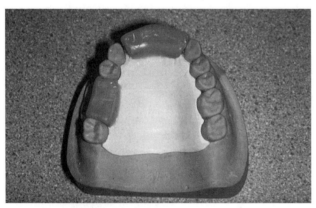

FIGURE 29.4

A maxillary record base with the record rim.

The Second Appointment with the Patient

A Patient's Treatment Plan

When all the information has been collected, the dentist will study the information and construct a set of options for the patient, and the treatment plan options will be presented. Several factors along with medical and dental history will influence the treatment planning choices given to the patient.

Age

The age of the patient and his general physical and mental condition have to be considered before making a treatment plan. An elderly patient confined to a nursing home with poor manual dexterity resulting from arthritis is not a good indication for crown and bridge work that requires difficult oral hygiene procedures.

Caries Activity and Oral Hygiene

The history of caries activity and the oral hygiene of the patient will affect the choice of a treatment plan. A patient with active caries and poor oral hygiene should not have extensive crown and bridge restorations or partial dentures until oral conditions have improved.

Surgical Needs

If a tooth cannot be restored to optimal health, is in the way of a successful treatment for the patient, or is terribly unesthetic, then removal may be necessary to restore the esthetics and function. Teeth are not the only problems when considering a prosthetic appliance. Grossly displaceable soft tissues, inflamed tissue, palatal or lingual tori, other bony undercuts, and sharp areas must be removed before a denture can be constructed.

Other Factors

Orthodontics may be necessary to restore a tooth with either a **fixed partial denture** or a removable prosthesis. It is not uncommon to restore the contours of the teeth or reshape them for use in an abutment for a removable partial denture. If prospective abutment teeth are severely broken down and need *endodontic therapy*, posts and cores, and crowns before using them, this may be a contraindication for use of the tooth as an abutment.

Fixed partial denture

This type of denture is luted or securely retained to natural teeth, tooth roots, or dental implant abutments and is also called a *bridge*

The *financial condition* of a patient should not be something you judge from looking at the patient. Good dental care is quite often a case of priorities rather than ability to afford the treatment. Never assume that a patient will want a specific treatment because of what you think of his financial state. The patient may state to the dentist that he has limitations on the amount he is willing to invest in his reconstruction. This may influence the treatment plan somewhat, but all options should be presented to the patient. Communication between the dentist and the patient should produce the optimum treatment plan that meets the needs of the patient.

Dental assistants are extremely valuable to the dentist at the treatment planning appointment. Assistants can help by explaining treatment such as partial dentures, bridges, or implants to the patient, by showing examples of such prostheses, and, in general, by easing the patient's mind and alleviating apprehension.

A cheerful assistant helps greatly in the management of patients. Through encouragement and positive comments, the assistant can help instill confidence in the patient who is concerned about a treatment plan. By anticipating the questions and concerns of the patient, the dental assistant can often prevent misconceptions about the form of treatment being proposed. In fact, the patient may be more inclined to listen to the dental assistant's comments than to those of the dentist.

FIXED OR REMOVABLE PARTIAL DENTURES

Restoration of total oral health is the goal in treating the partially edentulous patient, because all of the teeth in the opposing arch must be adequately supported so as not to supererupt. The replacement of missing teeth by means of a fixed partial denture (FPD) can be eliminated by such treatment.

PLANNING THE REMOVABLE PARTIAL DENTURE

A dental cast surveyor is a paralleling instrument used in construction of a prosthesis to locate and delineate the contours and relative positions of abutment teeth and associated structures. Beneath the height of the contour, the tooth has an undercut. Clasps must be placed into undercuts to help retain the partial denture.

COMPONENT PARTS OF THE REMOVABLE PARTIAL DENTURE

The framework is the metal skeleton to which the remaining portions of the prosthesis are attached. There are several component parts of a removable partial denture (RPD) (Figure 29.5).

1 Major connector
2 Minor connector(s)
3 Rests
4 Direct retainer(s)
5 Reciprocal component(s) or stabilizing arm
6 Indirect retainer(s) (for distal extension base RPD) It has one or more bases, each supporting one to several teeth.
7 Denture base

Major Connector

A *major connector* is that component part of the RPD that joins the components on one side of the arch to those on the

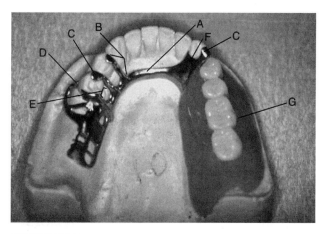

FIGURE 29.5

The component parts of the removable partial denture are shown. **A,** A major connector component part joins the components on one side of the arch to those on the opposite side. **B,** The minor connector unites the major connector with the other component parts of the removable partial denture. **C,** The rest is that unit of the partial denture that provides vertical support for the prosthesis. **D,** The direct retainer is that component of a removable partial denture that is used on an abutment tooth to prevent dislodgement of the partial in an occlusal direction. **E,** The reciprocal arm or stabilizing arm is designed to provide a stabilizing action during removal and insertion of the removable partial denture. **F,** The indirect retainer is the part of the removable partial denture that helps resist rotation of the distal extension partial in an occlusal direction. **G,** The base with artificial teeth is displayed.

opposite side. All of the other parts of the partial denture are either directly or indirectly connected to the major connector.

Minor Connector

The *minor connector* unites the major connector with the other component parts of the RPD such as the rests or indirect retainers. Each rest joins the major connector by means of a minor connector (see Figure 29.5, *B*).

Rests

The unit of the partial denture that rests on a tooth surface to provide vertical support is called a *rest* (see Figure 29.5, *C*). Rests on the partial denture are located on tooth surfaces that have been prepared to receive them. It helps to keep the framework in its planned position and provides resistance to lateral movement of the removable partial.

A rest also helps to prevent the framework from placing unnecessary forces on the soft tissues by preventing movement in a cervical direction. By directing and distributing occlusal loads to the long axis of abutment teeth, it maintains occlusal relationships that are established. As part of the clasp assembly of the partial denture, it prevents the opening of the clasp arm. A rest can keep a tooth from extruding from its socket. Rests are also usually given a descriptive name that gives you immediate visualization of its placement.

Occlusal Rest

The occlusal rest is the rigid extension of a RPD that contacts the occlusal surface of a tooth or restoration. The occlusal surface has been prepared to receive the rest. The shape of the occlusal rest is usually a rounded triangular shape with the apex toward the center of the occlusal surface.

Lingual Rests on Canines and Incisors

The lingual rest is a metallic extension of a RPD framework that fits into a prepared depression within the abutment tooth's lingual surface. It is usually found on maxillary canines on the cingulum. Mandibular canines do not provide good tooth anatomy for lingual rests resulting from the lack of sufficient enamel on the lingual of the tooth in which to prepare the rest. The shape of the lingual rest of a canine is a rounded V-shape with the apex of the "V" directed to the incisal.

Incisal Rest

The incisal rest is a rigid extension of the RPD that contacts a tooth at the incisal edge. These are frequently used on the distoincisal line angle of the mandibular canine. Incisors are not the first choice of placement of incisal rests because of root form, root length, inclination of the tooth and the ratio of the length of the clinical crown to the alveolar support, but when they are used, the rest seat is prepared in the form of a rounded notch at an incisal angle or on the incisal edge.

Interproximal Occlusal Rests

When a clasp assembly must pass between two teeth, then it requires interproximal occlusal rests be used. Individual rests are prepared on each of the teeth. The adjacent rests are used to prevent wedging of the framework between the two teeth.

Direct Retainers and Reciprocal Component

It is impossible to discuss the direct retainer without discussion of the reciprocal component or stabilizing arm at the same time. The *clasp assembly* (Figure 29.6) is the name given to the part of the RPD that is made up of the rest, the direct retainer, and the reciprocal component or stabilizing arm.

The clasp assembly must encompass more than 180 degrees of the greatest circumference of the tooth. When the partial denture is inserted, the direct retainer must flex over the height of contour into the undercut of the tooth for retention of the partial denture. The reciprocal component or stabilizing arm supports the tooth and keeps it from moving when the partial denture is inserted. The rest gives the partial denture positive support on the tooth.

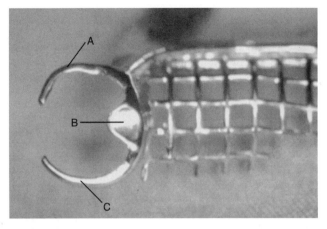

FIGURE 29.6

This clasp assembly is composed of (**A**) the direct retainer, (**B**) the rest, and (**C**) the reciprocal component or stabilizing arm. The direct retainer is the wrought wire at the top, which would engage the buccal surface in the .02-inch undercut.

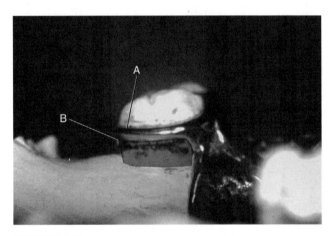

FIGURE 29.7

An example of a partial denture framework. **A,** The reciprocal or stabilizing arm of the clasp assembly. **B,** The area below the reciprocal (shaded black) is below the height of contour.

The direct retainer is that component of a RPD that is used on an abutment tooth to prevent dislodgement of the partial in an occlusal direction (see Figure 29.5, *D*). The direct retainer is used to provide mechanical retention for the partial denture, and the terminal third of the direct retainer is placed below the height of contour to provide mechanical retention.

The reciprocal arm or stabilizing arm is designed to provide a stabilizing action during removal and insertion of the RPD (see Figure 29.5, *E*). It is placed at the height of contour on the tooth and does not provide mechanical retention because it does not go into an undercut on the tooth (Figure 29.7). It braces the tooth when the partial denture is inserted and helps prevent horizontal movement of the denture during function. It does not go beneath the survey line, therefore, it does not provide retention. An example of one type of direct retainer is the intracoronal attachment, which is within the confines of the cusps and normal proximal contours of the abutment tooth, usually in a crown, and consists of a machined key and keyway. The intracoronal attachment is usually regarded as a precision attachment.

Some of the various clasps used as part of the direct retainer include the following.

Circumferential Clasp

The circumferential clasp is a cast clasp that encircles the tooth. It is half round with the flat surface touching the tooth, and it tapers in its shape.

Ring Clasp

The ring clasp is a cast clasp that encircles nearly all of the tooth from its point of origin. It is usually seen with a mesial and distal rest.

Embrasure Clasp

This clasp is a cast clasp that passes through the area where two adjacent teeth touch. It usually has an embrasure rest to prevent wedging of prosthesis between the teeth.

Reverse-Action Clasp

It is designed to permit engaging a proximal undercut from an occlusal approach. Its origin is usually above the retentive area of the clasp arm.

Wrought Wire Clasp

Usually a round 18-gauge wire is tapered and bent to fit the contour of the tooth. It is soldered to or cast to the RPD framework or embedded in the acrylic resin of the RPD base.

Bar Clasp

The bar clasp, sometimes referred to as the *Roach clasp*, arises from the dental framework and approaches the retentive undercut from a cervical direction. Bar clasps may take the form of a Y, T, or modified T.

Indirect Retainer

The indirect retainer is that part of the RPD that helps resist rotation of the distal extension RPD in a cervical direction. It may be in the form of a rest, but it acts to resist rotation and is called an indirect retainer.

Denture Base and Artificial Tooth

Denture Base

The denture base is the part of the partial denture that rests on the foundation tissues and to which teeth are attached (see Figure 29.5, G). Another name given this is the *saddle*. Acrylic resin bases are usually attached to the partial denture framework by a metal minor connector, which looks like meshwork, and it is designed to have a space between it and

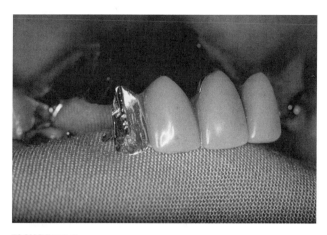

FIGURE 29.8

The central incisor is a facing, which is a denture tooth veneer bonded to the metal framework. Tooth #7 shows the metal backing with some mechanical retention onto which the veneer is cemented.

the underlying tissues of the residual ridge so that it allows for mechanical retention of the acrylic resin. Denture base material made of acrylic resin comes in a variety of colors to match the patient's gingiva.

The denture base may be all metal with metal studs or nail heads used to help hold the artificial teeth. In this case, the metal would be in contact with the alveolar tissues. The area of the acrylic resin or metal that extends from the cervical of the teeth to the denture border is known as the *flange of the denture.*

Denture Teeth

Denture teeth are artificial replacements for the missing oral structures. They are replaced using various materials: metal, acrylic resin, and porcelain artificial teeth. The acrylic and porcelain teeth vary in form and color. A tooth may be an anatomic tooth or a nonanatomic tooth. An anatomic tooth duplicates the anatomic form of natural teeth. Anatomic posterior teeth usually have prominent cusps with cuspal inclinations greater than 0 degrees. Nonanatomic teeth have occlusal surfaces that are not anatomically formed. As applied to posterior teeth, they are formed with mechanical principles in mind. They are represented by teeth that have 0-degree cuspal inclinations.

Artificial teeth must be (1) attached to the denture base by acrylic resin or cement, (2) processed directly to the metal (Figure 29.8), (3) chemically bonded to the framework, or (4) if metal, waxed and cast onto the framework. Denture base material made of acrylic resin comes in a variety of colors.

A denture **facing** is a veneer of any restorative

Facing

A veneer of any restorative material used on a prosthesis to simulate a natural tooth

material used on a prosthesis to simulate a natural tooth. It is bonded to the framework, which provides a metal backing. A tube tooth is an artificial tooth with an internal opening from the center of the base upward in the center of the tooth into which a nailhead will be placed. The nailhead is part of the partial denture framework and is used with some type of luting agent to retain the tooth to the partial denture framework. The metal tooth is waxed into occlusion when the framework is waxed and is part of the framework.

APPOINTMENTS REQUIRED FOR CONSTRUCTION OF A REMOVABLE PARTIAL DENTURE

After the patient has been given a treatment plan, various appointments are necessary to prepare the oral cavity for the final prosthesis.

Periodontal Therapy

It is important that the remaining teeth are sound and that the patient has good oral hygiene. Periodontal surgery may be necessary in areas with deep pockets and where there is chronic inflammation and bleeding. The patient may need to be instructed in oral hygiene procedures; this is often done by the dental assistant.

Endodontics

If the patient has any tooth with a periapical lesion, that tooth should have a root canal done on it to prevent the possibility of an abscess. Some teeth may need to have endodontic therapy so that a post core and crown should be constructed on it.

Oral Surgery

Badly broken down teeth that are not restorable, teeth with severe bone loss that are not treatable with periodontics, and teeth that may be unusable because of their position in the arch will be extracted so that there is time to heal before the construction of the removable appliance. Other soft tissue and bony interferences will also be taken care of.

Restorative Dentistry

Any fillings needing to be done will be completed before the impression for the removable partial is done. Crowns or bridges are constructed at this time and the prescription to the laboratory describes the restorations to be fabricated to meet the plans of the RPD that is to be constructed. A new set of diagnostic casts may be necessary because of the changes that have occurred in the mouth.

Tissue Conditioning

If irritation and inflammation are found in the denture bearing areas, tissue conditioning must be done before taking final impressions for the partial denture. The tissue conditioning materials are elastopolymers that remain soft and allow the inflamed and distorted tissues to return to their normal contour and health.

The dental assistant may be called on to place the tissue conditioner in the denture. The steps are as follows in Box 29.1.

The conditioning procedure should be repeated until the tissues have a healthy appearance. The material should be changed every 4 days. The material will become hard and an irritant if left much longer without a change. The patient may be asked to remove his denture as much as possible. The more the patient can leave the denture out of the mouth, the faster the condition will be resolved. When the tissue-conditioned denture is not in the mouth, it should be kept in a denture case with the lid closed and some moisture in the container. Oral hygiene must be good while this is being done. Warm saltwater rinses three times a day using 1 teaspoon of salt to 1 cup of water may also help the inflamed area. When the tissues are healthy, the final impression may be considered.

It may take three or four changes of tissue conditioner for the tissue to become healthy. Some mouths are even more difficult to manage and may require other treatment, such as a prescription for an antifungal agent.

BEGINNING THE PARTIAL DENTURE PHASE OF THE TREATMENT PLAN

Appointment One

Mouth Preparation of the Abutment Teeth

Diagnostic casts are made and analyzed to verify that the original plan will work. It is time to prepare the abutment, and for teeth to receive the partial denture components.

Guide Planes

The interproximal surfaces of the teeth are prepared first to provide guide planes that are parallel with the path of insertion of the removable partial denture.

Interferences

Interferences will be removed. Any place where the design calls for a component part and the survey line is not ideal on the tooth; the tooth may be altered to provide contours that are in harmony with the design.

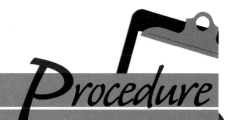

Box 29.1

Procedure for Tissue Conditioning

1. Any area of the denture base that is causing a lesion must be adjusted before tissue conditioning (Figure 29.9).
2. Relieve the tissue side of the denture base by about 2 mm. This allows enough space for an even thickness of tissue conditioning material.
3. Read the instructions completely in the box of materials you are using. You will find correct liquid to powder ratio, time suggestions, and other helpful information.
4. Apply any lubricating agent (provided in most kits) to the areas where you do not want the tissue conditioner to adhere. Apply it to the teeth and flange portions of the denture base to within about 2 or 3 mm of the periphery of the vestibule.
5. Mix the materials, measured to the exact quantities of liquid and powder recommended in the instructions, for the recommended time and to the consistency desired. When placed in the patient's mouth, it should not be runny (Figure 29.10).
6. Apply the material with sufficient thickness to allow for a cushioning effect and to prevent voids in the denture base area (Figure 29.11). When placed in the patient's mouth, it should be runny.
7. Place the denture in the patient's mouth and catch any excess material that is running out the back. The patient should not swallow this material as it will become firm when it sets and could cause an obstruction in the intestinal tract. Ask the dentist if he wants the patient to have the tissue conditioning done with the open mouth technique or with the teeth coming together. Different techniques are used for different types of problems. If the closed mouth technique is used, the patient closes his teeth together while the material sets for the time recommended in the instructions. If the open mouth technique is performed, the framework is held with the rests and major connector in the terminal position against the teeth. The best results are obtained if the patient makes normal movements of the lips, cheeks, and musculature while the material is setting. Border molding is the shaping of the border areas of an impression tray or denture base by functional or manual manipulation of the tissue adjacent to the border.
8. Allow the material to set for the time suggested. Setting time is affected by the liquid to powder ratio and temperature. The more liquid used, the longer it will take to set. With a sharp Bard Parker blade in the laboratory knife handle, trim off the excess material from the denture, trying not to distort the peripheries as the denture is held and trimmed.

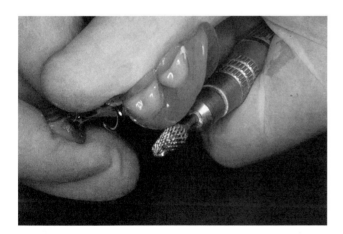

FIGURE 29.9

The denture is adjusted if any lesions are present and to allow for an even thickness of tissue conditioner.

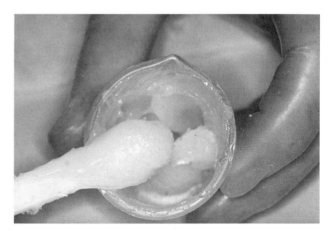

FIGURE 29.10

Mix the material to the desired consistency using the recommended liquid powder ratios.

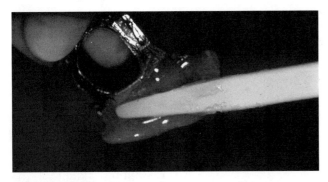

FIGURE 29.11

Apply the mixed material evenly to the tissue side of the denture.

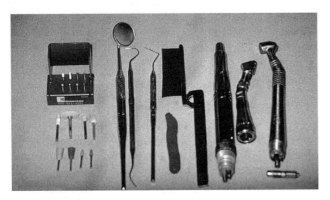

FIGURE 29.12

The tray setup for rest preparations may include: *(left to right)* burs, stones, rubber wheels, mouth mirror, explorer, Perioprobe, articulating paper and holder, low-speed handpiece, and high-speed handpiece.

Rests

Rests may now be prepared. The metal occlusal rest of the RPD must sit in a prepared area on the tooth. If the tooth were not prepared, the occlusal rest would be sitting on top of the teeth. When the patient brings his teeth together, there will be an interference with the rest, which will not allow the teeth to come together naturally.

Enough tooth structure must be removed so that the metal part of the partial denture has a sufficient bulk of metal for strength and rigidity so that it will not break. Burs are used to prepare rest seats and to polish the teeth before a master impression. Figure 29.12 shows the tray setup for rest preps. The setup typically includes the following:

1 Burs and polishing points
2 Mirror
3 Explorer
4 Perioprobe
5 Articulating paper and holders
6 Low-speed handpiece
7 High-speed handpiece

An optional item might be a piece of rope wax. The dentist will ask the patient to bite into a piece of wax after preparing the rest. This enables the dentist to check for sufficient clearance.

Final Impression for the Removable Partial Denture

When all the abutment teeth have been prepared for guide planes on the interproximal surfaces, interferences removed, and rest preparations cut, it is time to take a final master impression for the RPD. Refer to the following topics in Chapter 15: hydrocolloid impression materials, selection of impression tray, procedure for mixing alginate impression material, and procedures for taking alginate impression.

After the master impression is taken, it must be poured using a gypsum product to produce an acceptable master cast on which the final design will be drawn and sent to the laboratory for construction of the denture framework. This is usually poured with a dental model stone. Please refer to Chapter 15 for information on how to handle gypsum products, pour an impression, and procedures for trimming models. This also applies to master casts.

Preparing a Work Authorization

The master cast is surveyed, a design is drawn on the master cast, and a work authorization (order) is written. A *work authorization* is a written set of instructions telling the dental laboratory what procedures are to be performed on the case you are sending to them (Figure 29.13).

It gives the name of the dentist, his license number, the patient name, the date, the service is requested, tooth color, mold, and metal requested, and other special instructions. A work authorization must accompany the master cast with the framework design. A copy of the work authorization should be kept by the assistant in the dental laboratory so that the assistant can keep track of which cases are out, what has already arrived and to help the bookkeeper with billing information.

Appointment Two
Framework Try In

When the framework returns from the laboratory on the master cast, it is tried in the mouth to see that it fits properly. If the case has been sent to the laboratory unmounted, the dentist may or may not have requested that occlusion rims be placed on the framework before try in. If the framework does not fit properly, then adjustment must be completed at that time to see if it can be made to fit properly. The success of the fit is highly dependent on the quality of the impression, the pouring of the master cast, and the quality of the laboratory work.

The occlusion must also be adjusted with the new framework in the mouth. The patient must exhibit the same oc-

Fuhrmann
Dental Laboratory, Inc.

3101 Clays Mill Road, Suite 203
Lexington, Kentucky 40503
(606) 224-4100

Dr. *James Wilson*
432 Forrester Ave.
Louisville, KY 40231
License No.: ___3296___

K.L.R. NO. ___L0591___
Date
sent to lab ___11/6/96___

Due ___11/20/96___   ☒ a.m.
                      ☐ p.m.

Patient: ___John A. Jones___   Sex ___M___   Age ___40___
         (please print)

Shade: _____   Mould: post. _____   plastic porcelain, I.P.N.
Vitallium Metal   ant. _____   plastic porcelain, I.P.N.

C/C IMMEDIATE   **C/C**   **P**   (please circle)

____ Tray (s)   RPD framework try in   ☒ yes ☐ no
____ Baseplate(s)/occlusion Rim (s)   W.W. retainers   ☐ yes ☒ no
____ Arrangement/wax up for try in   Modified cast tray   ☒ yes ☐ no
____ Arrangement/finish
____ Process/finish
____ Remount index and casts
____ Repair
____ Reline
____ Rebase
____ Intermediate denture
____ Modified cast-pour
____ Staple denture
____ OSSEO-integration denture

UPPER

RIGHT   LEFT

LOWER

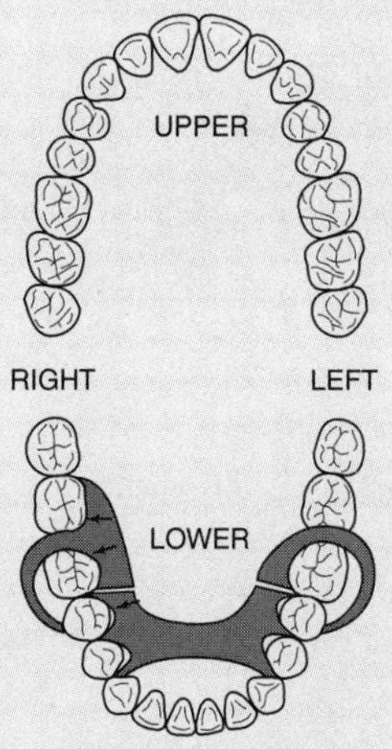

ADDITIONAL INSTRUCTIONS:

Construct RPD framework
#20 | MO rest, distal guide plate
29 | I-Bar w/mid facial 101 Ret.

21
28 | MO rest

Lingual bar mjr. connector, base attachment as indicated
Return for try in

Please send Rx forms ☐
Please send mailing labels ☒

James Wilson, DMD
Signature

FIGURE 29.13

A general work authorization provided by a specific laboratory may be used to write a prescription.

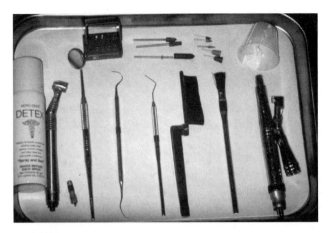

FIGURE 29.14

The tray setup for framework try in may include: mirror, explorer, Perioprobe, articulating paper and holder, high-speed and low-speed handpieces, a spraying medium, such as Detex or Occlude, to detect pressure spots, bur block with burs, stones, rubber wheels, brush, and pliers.

clusion with or without the framework in the mouth. The instrument tray for a framework try in must have the following items (Figure 29.14):

1 Mirror
2 Explorer
3 Perioprobe
4 Articulating paper and holder
5 High-speed and low-speed handpieces
6 Occlude or Detex spray or a similar agent to disclose pressure spots
7 The dentist's bur block used to remove metal that is interfering and polishing points to bring the metal back to a high shine
8 An orthodontic pliers used to adjust clasps, if necessary

When the framework fits and the occlusion has been adjusted, some dentists do a secondary impression of the distal extension area of the RPD. After this is done, it is time to mount the case so that teeth can be set and tried in.

Establishing and Recording the Occlusal Relationship

When there are sufficient remaining teeth to where you can put two casts together and they occlude and the casts are able to stand on each other without any question of where one tooth comes together with the other, then you may mount these without the use of occlusion rims or an interocclusal record. When you can not hand articulate the casts, then occlusion rims are necessary.

Use of Occlusion Rims to Record the Occlusal Relationship

In order for teeth to be set, the case must be mounted on an articulator, so that the proper occlusion can be developed. This is accomplished by the use of occlusion rims

added to the framework(s) in the areas where the patient is edentulous. Sometimes, the dentist mounts the case before having the frameworks made and asks for teeth to be set at the time the framework is made. There is more than one way to get to the completion of a partial denture and the dentist may elect to follow any one of a number of sequences of appointments.

The occlusion rims can be made directly on the cast using the framework for attachment of the wax. Most often, the occlusion rims are constructed by the laboratory. If this is not done, the steps for the assistant would be those listed in Box 29.2 and Table 29.1.

Recording the Occlusal Relationship

The framework(s) with the occlusion rims are placed in the mouth and adjusted to where the patient can get his remaining natural teeth together. If the patient does not have any teeth on one arch, as in the case of the complete denture opposing the RPD, then the rims are adjusted to provide the proper support of the oral musculature and to provide for proper phonetics, function, and esthetics. A facebow record is made to mount the maxillary cast on the articulator. Notches are placed on the occlusion rim to serve as indexes and a soft material, such as compound, is placed on one of the rims, usually the lower, and the patient closes his teeth together and holds until the wax hardens. The use of these records will allow the mounting of the case on the articulator with the mandibular cast in exactly the same relationship to the maxilla in the mouth.

Selection of Teeth

The dental assistant may help the dentist select a tooth that complements the patient. Different manufacturers of teeth have different systems for identifying mold numbers and color. Teeth come in various materials: porcelain, plastic, and composite materials. I will be discussing the teeth supplied by Dentsply International as one example of how to use a company's system. An assistant who becomes familiar with the mold boards, color selection aids, and charts and understands the principles behind selection of teeth can be very helpful to the dentist while adding variety to the assistant's job. Removable partial denture patients usually have remaining natural teeth, and the dentist will try to match the existing natural teeth for an esthetic result.

As a patient ages, his natural teeth will usually turn darker, but with today's bleaching techniques, it is possible for patient's to have a tooth color that is lighter than what their natural teeth were. Teeth should be chosen after any cosmetic bleaching is complete. It will be necessary for the patient to use the bleaching agent periodically if he is to maintain a color acquired through the bleaching technique.

Anterior teeth include central incisors, lateral incisors, and canines. The anterior set is sometimes referred to as a (1 x 6) upper or lower. The mold numbers on the board are shown under different headings. The heading "Square

Box 29.2

Procedure for Fabrication of Occlusion Rims on the Framework

Procedure

1. Apply two coats of tin foil substitute to the cast to prevent the wax from sticking to the cast.
2. Apply one layer of baseplate wax over edentulous area taking care to cover only the edentulous area.
3. Heat up the edentulous area of the framework taking extreme caution not to burn your fingers. Seat the framework into the wax and make certain that the rests and major connector seat completely to their original position. Clean off excess way.
4. Heat up a piece of baseplate wax and fold it on itself until a wax rim is formed that is approximately 8 to 10 mm wide. Heat the

folded wax and press it onto the framework in the area of retention for the base and contour it to the desired shape.
5. Shape the wax using a wax spatula so that it is approximately the same height of the occlusal plane of the remaining natural teeth. It should approximate the width of the natural teeth, if they were present, and be centered over the ridge. The premolar area width of the wax rim is approximately 8 mm wide.
6. Make all the wax neat and clean. Remove any excess wax from the cast. The framework with wax should look acceptable enough that you would allow someone to place it in your mouth.

Table 29.1

Evaluation of Occlusion Rims on the Framework

Occlusion Rims on the Framework	4	3	2	0	X
Secure materials.					
Secure cast.					
Apply tin foil to cast (two coats).					
Apply baseplate wax.					
Heat edentulous area of framework.					
Seat framework into the wax.					
Clean off excess wax.					
Form wax rim (8-10 mm wide).					
Press wax rim into framework.					
Contour and shape wax.					
Remove excess wax from cast.					

The numeric criteria: 4 Excellent; 3 Good but some improvement can be made; 2 Below average, usable, needs to improve skill; 0 Unsatisfactory; X Not able to evaluate.

Tapering" refers to the shape of the face (Figure 29.15). The teeth under that heading would be appropriate on a patient with a square tapering face. The booklet that accompanies the mold board gives information about the width, length, and size of the six anterior teeth. All the anterior molds ending in the same letter, for example "C," have approximately the same length of the six anterior teeth. Measurement of the central incisors will allow you to use the manual to select teeth that are the same size as the original teeth. The cast may be used to select teeth of the same shape and size. The

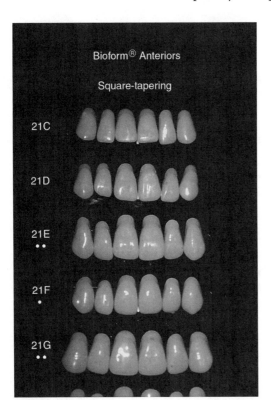

FIGURE 29.15

The mold board shows the l x 6 anterior maxillary molds. They are shown under headings that correspond with shape of face, for example, square tapering.

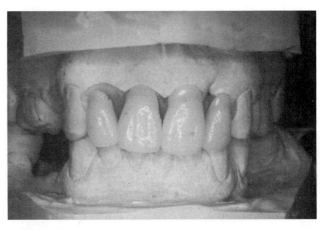

FIGURE 29.16

The anterior teeth may be placed into the edentulous area of the cast to see which mold fits the space and looks best.

Appointment Three
Removable Partial Denture Try In

The dentist may wish to try in the final prosthesis when it is in the wax setup stage. The framework has been sent to the laboratory with the jaw registration. The laboratory mounts the case on the articulator, sets the teeth, and returns the case for the try in. This allows the dentist a chance to check on several things.

1 Verification that the occlusal relationship is the same as it was when it was sent to the laboratory. The occlusion can be verified to see that the patient's teeth come together just like it does on the articulator.
2 The arrangement of teeth can be verified for esthetics and function. The color can be checked to see if it is in harmony with the other natural teeth. The size of the selected teeth can be checked. The dentist may choose to change something at this time. It is easy to move teeth slightly to characterize the denture to the patient.
3 The patient has a chance to voice his opinion. If he does not like something, it can be easily changed because the case is in wax. A verbal or written approval of the case can be obtained from the patient.

The base material shade must be specified at the time the prescription is written. It is important that the shades of the base materials match that of the patient. Feedback from the patient on this selection is important because the patient has a definite feeling about the gingival colors, and their preferred color may differ from the color of their other gingiva. The dentist may need the following instrument setup for this appointment.

1 Mirror
2 Bunsen burner, torch, or some type of flame mechanism and wax spatulas #17 and #3
3 Articulating paper
4 Jaw registration material if the jaw registration has been recorded improperly

mandibular anterior teeth have mold numbers that are different than the maxillary anterior mold numbers.

The posterior teeth include the first and second premolars and the first and second molar. They come in different cusp height: 0, 12, 20, 30 and 33 degrees. The set of posterior teeth is designated as a (1 x 8) upper or lower (maxillary or mandibular). The mold numbers for the upper set and the lower set are the same; therefore, the assistant must specify maxillary or mandibular when ordering the sets of posterior teeth. The first number of the three number posterior mold (in the hundreds position) identifies teeth with a certain degree of cusp. For example the teeth beginning with "4" in the hundreds row are the 0 degree Monoline teeth, the ones beginning with "3" in the hundreds row are the 12 degree Anatoline teeth. The second two numbers, for example, "29," "31," or "33," tell us the length of the posterior teeth from the mesial of the first premolar to the distal of the second molar. If a letter appears, the letter S = short, M = medium, and L = long. In selecting a posterior tooth, select a tooth that is approximately the same size as the ones that remain in the arch. The degree of cusp chosen is slightly steeper than that of the remaining natural teeth. The master cast is beneficial in selecting a tooth that fits into the space (Figure 29.16).

Box 29.3

Procedure for the Try-In

Procedure

1. The prosthesis should be examined for blebs (sharp areas), which must be removed before the prosthesis is placed in the mouth.
2. Pressure indicator paste is placed on the tissue side of the partial and gently inserted, but not forced. Any area that shows pressure on the partial or prevents complete seating of the prosthesis is removed until the prosthesis seats completely and the pressure is evenly distributed on the ridges.
3. The partials are examined in the mouth to see if there is any area of interference between the upper and lower denture. If found, the interference is removed.
4. Any overextended borders are shortened so that the movements of the oral structures do not interfere by lifting of the partial.
5. The occlusion is adjusted and any premature contacts are removed. The goal is to achieve even contact between the maxillary and mandibular posterior teeth, including both the artificial denture teeth and the natural teeth.
6. Finally, the partials are taken to the office laboratory and polished to remove any roughened areas. Pumice and acryluster are used to return the high polish to the denture. The teeth should not be pumiced since it will alter the occlusion and ruin the natural look of the artificial teeth. Any clasp that may not fit properly can be adjusted.
7. The partials are delivered to the patient.

5 The mounted case as it was returned from the laboratory

The accepted case is then sent off to the laboratory to flask, pack, and produce the final prostheses. The dentures are flasked, the wax bailed out, the acrylic resin packed, and the case is processed. The dentures are then broken out of the flasks, finished, and polished to produce a final prosthesis.

The patient is now ready to be reappointed for delivery of the denture. Each laboratory has its own time requirement to finish the partial denture. Check with your laboratory as to how long it will require to process the dentures and return them to you and reappoint the patient.

Appointment Four

Delivery

The delivery appointment is scheduled for the patient and should last about 30 minutes. It is better to schedule it earlier in the day so that the patient who experiences questions or problems may have the chance to get back with the office before it closes for the day. The tray setup for this appointment includes the following (Box 29.3):

1 Mirror
2 Articulating paper and holder
3 Pressure indicator paste used to detect the problem pressure areas of the recently processed dentures and indelible markers for detecting problems

4 The new disinfected and rinsed prosthesis
5 Denture cup for storage of the prosthesis; denture brush and sample soaking and cleaning agents often provided by the manufacturers
6 Handpiece and acrylic burs
7 Pliers for adjustment of clasps

Partial Denture Care Instructions

The dental assistant can take the responsibility for training the patient on care of the new prosthesis. The patient must be made to understand that there will be difficulties and discomfort associated with the new dentures. The patient needs to be informed that there will be soreness, and the 24- or 48-hour appointment is used to take care of some of these problems. The patient must realize that it may take several adjustments to alleviate all the problems. The patient must know how to insert and remove the prosthesis from the mouth before leaving the office. If the office has a set of written instructions for the new prosthesis wearer, it should be given and explained to the patient.

Oral Hygiene

Oral hygiene is of utmost importance in the care of the prosthesis. The partial denture and the natural teeth must be cleaned after each meal and at bedtime. The clasps prevent any natural cleansing by the lips, cheeks and tongue of the natural teeth. The prosthesis may be cleaned in a number of ways; the toothbrush, special denture tooth pastes, soaking agents, ultrasonic cleaners, and water sprays are but a few. Over time, toothpaste high in abrasives and a toothbrush will abrade the artificial resin teeth. A toothpaste made especially for dentures or a mild detergent solution is a good agent to use to brush the debris from the denture. Care must be taken to remove excess detergent from the denture so as to prevent chemical burn to the oral tissues. A number of soaking agents are available to clean the denture. The patient should be instructed not to place the denture in a solution of Clorox and water. The Clorox will tarnish the cast chromium alloy used in the RPD framework.

Sleeping

Sleeping in the denture should be discouraged for the health of the tissues. The patient should leave the prosthesis out of the mouth at night. When it is not in the mouth, it should be kept in a closed container with a wet towelette or gauze in the container to provide a humid environment. Pets may get to a denture left on the nightstand and destroy the acrylic material and the denture. Some patients will not sleep without their prosthesis. If this is the case, then the patient should be encouraged to leave the prosthesis out of the mouth a few hours during the day to allow the tissues to rebound.

Eating

Eating with the new dentures will not come easily. The teeth on the new prosthesis are not in the exact location that they were on a previous prosthesis; therefore, a patient should take it slowly trying to learn how to eat with the new dentures. A steak dinner on the night of insertion is no way to break in a new denture. Soft, fiber-free foods should be eaten the first few days after delivery of the new dentures, while slowly incorporating the tougher foods.

Checkups

The patient should be informed that the denture and the patient will need periodic maintenance. The 24- to 48-hour appointment should be set at this time.

Appointment Five

It is important that the patient be seen 24 to 48 hours after insertion of the prosthesis. The patient will usually experience some difficulty, slight as it may be. This appointment enables the dentist to take care of any problems before they become major problems. A mirror, explorer, articulating paper and holder, pressure indicator paste, indelible ink markers, a slow speed handpiece, acrylic burs, and possibly a set of pliers will be needed at this appointment.

The patient should be questioned about any complaints and sore spots caused by the dentures. The assistant should note the problems for the dentist. A patient usually feels the most severe lesion or sore spot caused by the denture. One should look in the mouth and note all the areas of redness and irritation regardless of what the patient states. A patient often points to an area that is not exactly the offending area. Look, observe, think, and listen to your patient, and make good notes for your dentist.

The dentist will take care of the problems that the patient experiences. When the prosthesis is functioning properly, the patient will be dismissed with an appointment for approximately 1 week. When no more problems or lesions exist, a recall appointment for several months will be established.

PERMANENT RELINE OF THE REMOVABLE PARTIAL DENTURE

The patient may complain of the lower partial not fitting properly, or they may be experiencing lesions caused by changes in the supporting tissues under the base of the denture. A reline is the procedure used to resurface the tissue side of a denture with new base material, thus producing an accurate adaptation to the denture foundation area. It is possible when (1) the occlusion can be corrected with relatively simple adjustment after the reline, (2) the framework is in good condition, (3) the denture base is in good condition and the peripheries are reasonable, and (4) the teeth are not too worn or broken. Before any permanent reline procedure is accomplished, the oral tissues should be in a healthy condition. Tissue conditioning of the denture may be necessary before the reline. A rebase procedure may be requested from the laboratory rather than a reline. A rebase consists of the laboratory process replacing the entire denture base material or the existing prosthesis.

There are two types of reline procedures. One is performed at the chairside and the other is a laboratory procedure and the patient is without his denture for a period of time.

Chairside Reline

This is a one-step procedure using acrylic resins that either harden while in the mouth or are placed into a curing device to achieve final set (Box 29.4).

The operator must be cautious while doing a chairside reline for two reasons. The acrylic resin material will give off considerable heat as it sets. The patient's soft tissue may be damaged by keeping the denture in the mouth too long. Another possible problem is that the denture can get caught in the mouth if excess material flows into an undercut and then goes completely to set while in the mouth. It may have to be cut out.

One of the disadvantages to the chairside reline is that the color stability of these materials is not as dependable as the heat processed acrylic resin completed at the laboratory (Box 29.5).

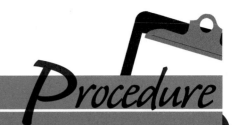

Box 29.4

Procedure for Chairside Relining

1. The denture flanges are adjusted slightly and tissue side of the base is relieved enough to provide space for an adequate thickness of new material. Only about 1 to 2 mm of relief is necessary. The outer layer of acrylic resin is removed to provide a new surface on which to bond new material.
2. A lubricant is applied to the surfaces to which you do not want new material to chemically bond, for example the teeth and acrylic resin of the palatal area.
3. Have the patient rinse his or her mouth with cold water.
4. The liquid and powder are mixed in the desired proportions recommended by the manufacturer; while you are waiting for the desired consistency of the material to be reached, apply some monomer to the tissue side of the base.
5. When the material is sufficiently thick, apply it to the tissue side of the partial denture. Determine whether the open mouth or closed mouth technique will be used for the reline procedure. Place the denture in the mouth and manipulate the oral tissues to border mold the reline material.
6. Remove the denture with the reline material after a short time, well before it is set, and trim the excess material with a scissors or Bard Parker blade.
7. Remove any material that is an undercut so that the partial will not get backed in the mouth.
8. Place the denture back in the mouth and continue to border mold until the material is firm enough to maintain its shape, and reface it.
9. Remove the denture from the mouth and place a pressure pot with warm water or place into a bowl of warm water until it is set.
10. The denture is then tried in the mouth, pressure spots removed, and occlusion adjusted. The denture is then trimmed and polished for delivery.

The patient will have to be without his or her denture for a period specified by the laboratory. Reappoint the patient for delivery and a 24- to 48-hour adjustment will be required, since this is like delivering a new prosthesis to the patient.

Many of the repairs to the RPD are sent out to the local laboratory. They may often pick up the case and deliver it in the same day if necessary. Some of the repairs are quite simple and offer a means of revenue for the office. The dental assistant can be trained to make these simple repairs.

Repairing a Broken Facing

Sometimes a facing comes loose from the metal backing of the framework. A new acrylic or porcelain facing is replaced by fitting a new one of the same mold and shade to the backing using the prosthesis in place in the mouth. Another approach would be to place the framework in the mouth and take an impression. The impression is poured and the new tooth is fit to the stone cast in the laboratory. This will conserve on chair time. There must be sufficient retention in the framework backing and enough surface area of support for the facing for the replacement to be successful. The new facing may be attached with a thin mix of acrylic resin.

Adding a Tooth to an Existing RPD

When a tooth is to be extracted, often the patient would like to have a his partial denture repaired with the new tooth and have it given to him at the time of extraction (Box 29.6). The assistant will need to take an impression with the denture in place (Box 29.7 and Table 29.2). All areas of undercut in the prosthesis must be blocked out except in the area where the tooth is to be extracted. A cast is poured. The tooth to be extracted is cut off of the cast, retention placed in both the existing partial denture and the tooth, and acrylic resin added to retain the new denture tooth. If the tooth is an abutment tooth, then a new wrought wire clasp must be added to the new abutment tooth, before adding the repair acrylic. A 36-gauge, round

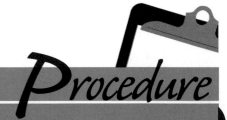

Box 29.5

Procedure for a Laboratory Reline

Procedure

1. The denture flanges are adjusted so that they are 2 to 3 mm short of the tissue and the tissue side of the base is relieved enough to provide space for an adequate thickness of new material and to provide a new surface on which to bond. All undercuts are removed from the base areas.

2. The peripheries are border molded with some type of border molding material, such as compound or polyether impression material, by placing it on the peripheries of the denture and manipulating the cheeks to mold the flange on the cheek side and by asking the patient to make various movements of the tongue to mold the lingual surface of the flange. This is border molding.

3. The border molding material that flows onto the inner surface of the denture is then removed to create a space for the impression material and to take away any material that may place pressure on the tissues.

4. An adhesive material is added to the inside of the denture to help retain the impression material.

5. An impression material is then placed in the denture and the impression is made using either the open mouth technique or the closed mouth technique. An impression material, such as polysulfide, polyvinyl siloxane, or polyether may be used to register an impression of the ridge.

6 A prescription is then written and the denture is sent to the laboratory for it to be relined. The patient will have to be without his or her denture for a period specified by the laboratory.

7. When the newly reline denture is returned, it is fitted to the mouth and the occlusion is adjusted (Figure 29.17).

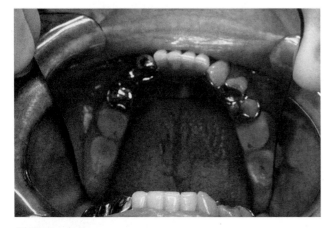

FIGURE 29.17

The newly relined denture is fitted to the mouth and the occlusion is adjusted.

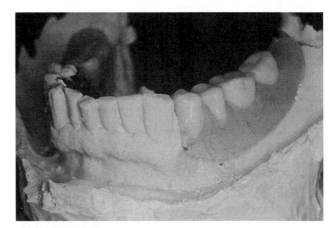

FIGURE 29.18

Stone is carefully vibrated into the impression and allowed to set and a working cast is fabricated.

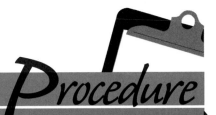

Box 29.6

Procedure for Adding a Clasp to a Removable Partial Denture

1. The partial is placed in the mouth.
2. An impression is made, pulling the partial denture in the impression.
3. Any undercuts are blocked out, the denture is coated with a lubricant to keep stone from getting into the pores of the acrylic resin.
4. Stone is carefully vibrated into the impression and allowed to set, creating a cast (Figure 29.18).
5. Acrylic resin is carefully removed from the flat next to the tooth to which the clasp is being added. Sometimes it is necessary to remove from the tooth next to the abutment tooth.
6. A wrought wire is contoured to fit into the prepared space of the tooth. It is bent with a retentive loop to give it retention when embedded into the acrylic resin.
7. The wire is placed into the area and rested on the tooth. Sticky wax is applied to the wire to hold it into position
8. Acrylic resin repair material is then placed into the preparation and allowed to set in either a pressure pot or a bowl of warm water.
9. When the material is sufficiently hard, it is trimmed and polished.
10. The denture is then cleaned up and delivered to the patient. The wire may need some adjustment in the mouth

Box 29.7

Construction of a Custom Tray for Partial Dentures Using an Alginate Impressions

1. Outline the desired tray on the cast. Usually, a tissue stop is prepared somewhere on the palate of the maxillary custom tray, and on the incisal edges of teeth that are not abutment teeth. A tissue stop is placed on the buccal shelf of the mandibular tray.
2. Place one layer of baseplate wax over all the abutment teeth to act as a spacer for impression material.
3. Place one additional layer of baseplate wax over the teeth and tissues up to the borders of the outline of the tray. Cut any excess wax.
4. Cut tissue stops into the wax relief on the palate of the maxillary cast and on the incisal edges of any teeth that are not abutment teeth. On the mandibular tray, the tissue stops will be cut out on the buccal shelf and the incisal edges of any teeth that are not abutment teeth.
5. Any area of the cast that is exposed should be treated with a tinfoil substitute to avoid damage to the cast. Place tinfoil on the wax surfaces to prevent the wax from getting into the tray material.
6. Mix the acrylic resin tray material to the desired specifications, roll it out on the roller board, using the thick side, and carefully adapt it on the cast to the border of the outline. Trim any excess with a buffalo or Bard Parker blade.
7. Form a handle with excess acrylic resin. The handle should be about 10 to 12 mm wide, 6 mm thick, and a couple of inches long. It should emerge from the tray so as to follow the angulation of the maxillary or mandibular teeth. You will probably have to add additional monomer and powder to get an adequate chemical bond to the tray.
8. When the resin has cured, remove the tray and the wax spacer from the cast. Trim the edges of the tray so that there are no rough edges to irritate the tissues.
9. Use a No. 8 round bur and place holes in the tray every 8 mm. These holes will be used for mechanical retention of the impression material.
10. The finished custom tray must be disinfected before placement in the patient's mouth (Figure 29.19).

orthodontic wire may be bent and added to act as the new clasp. This is a more involved procedure to be done in the dental office and it may be sent to the dental laboratory rather than doing it in the office. This may only work as a temporary measure, but it will allow the patient to have a prosthesis while you are constructing a new one. Occlusion must be adjusted in the mouth before the patient is dismissed.

Fabrication of Record Bases and Occlusion Rims

The following items will be necessary to construct record bases (Baseplates) and occlusion rims. Casts, Vaseline or a lubricating agent for the cast, baseplate wax, sticky wax, acrylic resin or light curing material, pencil, a hot plate, wax spatulas (13 and 17), a Hanau torch, a Bunsen burner and a buffalo knife or laboratory handle with Bard Parker blade (Box 29.8 and Table 29.3).

The record rim is now ready to be tried in the mouth. The maxillary is placed in the mouth and adjusted so that the lower and upper natural teeth come together. The mandibular rim is tried in the mouth and adjusted until the natural teeth are able to come together. A slight space is created between the rims so that the compound or some reaching medium may be placed on the wax rim to record the jaw registration.

Mouth Protectors

Mouth protectors or guards can be fabricated by the dental assistant.

Temporary Partial Denture

A temporary partial denture can be constructed for a patient when something is needed while the remainder of his treat-

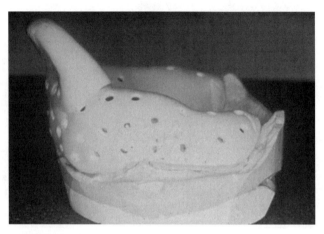

FIGURE 29.19

The finished custom tray should be disinfected before using it.

Evaluation of Partial Denture Custom Tray					
Partial Denture Custom Tray	4	3	2	0	X
Secure materials.					
Secure cast.					
Outline tray on cast.					
Prepare baseplate spacer.					
Place wax over outline.					
Cut tissue steps.					
Place tin foil substitute on exposed areas of cast.					
Place tin foil substitute on wax surfaces.					
Mix acrylic resin material.					
Roll material out.					
Adapt resin material on cast.					
Trim off excess.					
Form a handle.					
Remove tray and wax spacer.					
Trim and smooth edges.					
Place holes in tray and disinfect.					

Table 29.2

The numeric criteria: 4 Excellent; 3 Good but some improvement can be made; 2 Below average, usable, needs to improve skill; 0 Unsatisfactory; X Not able to evaluate.

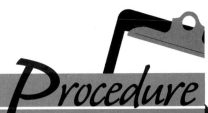

Box 29.8

Procedure for Fabrication of a Record Base and Occlusion Rim

1. Diagnostic casts are obtained and the outline form of the tray is placed in the cast.
2. Block out all the undercut areas on the cast with base plate wax or clay to (1) keep the baseplate from damaging the cast and (2) keep the baseplate from being damaged when removed from the cast.
3. Paint the cast and blockout with tin-foil substitute or Vaseline. If the tin-foil substitute is used, apply a second coat.
4. There are three ways to make the record bases.
   a. Build up the acrylic resin rim by applying a light coating of powder to the desired area and then by dropping the monomer on the powder using a dropper. The rim should be built up to a thickness of approximately 3 mm. Allow the material to set under some type of cover to prevent evaporation of surface monomer. Allow the bases to sit overnight to avoid warping on removal.
   b. Mix the acrylic resin liquid and powder in a waxed paper cup or a glass container. Allow the material to set for a short time. Using a well-lubricated board and roller, roll the material out into the shape of either a horseshoe (for a lower base) or a oval (for an upper). Place the material on the cast and cut the outline that you desire for the record base. Adapt the material to the cast well. Allow the material to set (Figure 29.20).
   c. Using the light cured material, place the material on the cast in the shape of the original desired outline of the record base. Apply the required coating to the material. Place it in the curing oven for the prescribed time.

5. Remove the rim from the cast and take it to the lathe to finish all of the edges so that they are to the desired outlined form and round the sharp edges. Acrylic resin burs work well for this. It may be polished, if desired with pumice and acryluster or a similar polishing material. It is not necessary to polish the record base if the work has been neat.
6. Soften a sheet of baseplate wax and fold the sheet onto itself. Reheat the wax sheet and continue to fold it onto itself until you have a wax roll about $1/_2$ inch in diameter. Preformed wax occlusal rims may be used.
7. Take sticky wax and apply it to the edentulous area of the occlusion rim. This will secure the occlusion rim in place.
8. Apply the softened, molten surface of the wax roll to the edentulous area where you are forming a rim, and press it firmly to the record base.
9. Use the heated wax spatula to seal the wax to the rim where the sticky wax has been applied. The wax should not extend out over onto the cast.
10. Use the hot plate to smooth the occlusal surfaces of the occlusion rim.
11. Smooth the sides of the rim with the #3 spatula.
12. Height of maxilla rim in anterior is 12 mm, the posterior height is 6mm. If teeth are present, use them as a guide for the height of the rim. The width of the rim is about the same as the width of the teeth in that area, 8 mm. (Figure 29.21).
13. Mandibular rim height is 8 mm in the anterior and 4 mm in the posterior. If teeth are present, use them as a guide for the height of the rim. The width of the rim is about 8 mm.

ment plan is progressing (Box 29.9). They are needed for several reasons. The patient may be esthetically conscious and not want to have missing teeth while healing after extractions. They may be used to maintain spaces and prevent teeth from moving. Sometimes the patient needs tissue conditioning and the prosthesis may be used in this process.

Removable partial dentures are and will continue to be an important service provided by the dental office. People

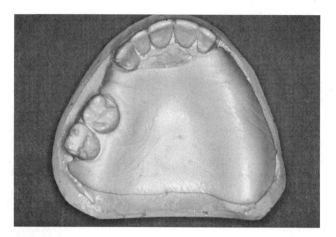

FIGURE 29.20

The material is added to the maxillary cast and trimmed to the desired outline form.

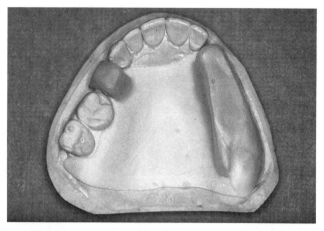

FIGURE 29.21

A maxillary record base with occlusion rim is shown on the diagnostic cast.

Table 29.8					
Evaluation of Record Base and Occlusion Rims					
Record Base and Occlusion Rims	4	3	2	0	X
Secure materials.					
Secure cast.					
Outline form of tray on cast.					
Block out undercut areas on cast.					
Paint cast and black out with tin foil substitute or petroleum jelly.					
Select method and make record base rim on cast.					
Soften base plate wax and form into a roll.					
Apply stick wax.					
Apply wax roll to edentulous area of rim.					
Seal wax to rim.					
Smooth occlusal surfaces of occlusion rim.					
Smooth sides of rim.					
Check height of rim.					

The numeric criteria: 4 Excellent; 3 Good but some improvement can be made; 2 Below average, usable, needs to improve skill; 0 Unsatisfactory; X Not able to evaluate.

Box 29.9

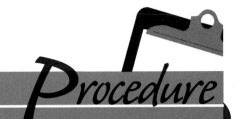

Procedure for Construction of Temporary Partial Denture

Step 1
Get a set of casts on which to construct the partial denture. Do not destroy the diagnostic casts record of treatment. It is not always necessary to mount the case, but if occlusion is a factor, then mounting the case will eliminate some complications that can arise by guessing at the placement of teeth. A color must also be chosen that is in harmony with the remaining dentition, and a tooth may be selected using the patient's teeth as a guide. The existing occlusion, the midline, the length of the vertical and horizontal overlap on the opposing cast must be noted, or a duplicate cast can be made for reference.

Step 2
The teeth are removed from the cast and additional gypsum material is removed, taking into consideration the amount of bone loss that has occurred or will occur when the teeth are extracted. Radiographs will be helpful in estimating this. The cast is prepared so that the ridge is rounded nicely after the removal of the teeth and stone. Some dentists like to select teeth at this time. Any deep undercuts are blocked out by use of baseplate wax.

Step 3
The teeth are then adjusted and set using sticky wax in the edentulous space so that they look natural. The curvature of the facial surface must flow naturally with the remaining teeth. The ridge lap area of the tooth must often be adjusted to give this natural appearance.

Step 4
If mechanical retention is desired, clasps may be added at this time. Ball clasps may be adjusted to add in retention in areas where occlusion is not a problem. Orthodontic wire may also be bent in the shape of a clasp and incorporated into the base material. I use 32- or 36-gauge ortho wire for this purpose. The bent clasp is sticky waxed into place on the facial of the tooth.

Step 5
The cast must be lubricated in the area where a plaster index is to be made. A plaster buccal index is then prepared to record the exact position of the denture teeth. The index must extend over the occlusal surfaces of at least one tooth on each side of the edentulous area to provide support (Figure 29.22).

Step 6
The index is removed, the teeth are removed and all of the wax is cleaned off of the cast and teeth. The cast is then lubricated so that the acrylic resin material does not get cast material in it when processed. Even though the acrylic resin material or light cured material assisted by a bonding agent should bond to the teeth, a retentive lock can be placed in each of the teeth with a tapered fissured bur. The teeth are then placed back into the index and sticky waxed at the incisal area. The index is placed back on the cast.

Step 7
The base material is then added. Acrylic resin may be added or a light cured material may be added to the cast. The acrylic resin material is then placed in a pressure pot containing warm water for 15 minutes and 30 pounds of pressure is added to the pot. If a light curing machine is used, then the steps outlined in the instruction booklet should be followed.

Step 8
The appliance is then carefully removed from the cast and finished using the acrylic resin burs. The teeth adjacent to the edentulous space can be removed before trying to remove the temporary RPD. This lessens the chance of breakage to the new prosthesis when removing it from the cast. After it has been finished, pumice and acryluster are used to polish the prosthesis. The temporary partial denture is delivered to the patient. A 24 to 48 hour appointment is necessary to remove any spots of irritation. Additional adjustments may be necessary.

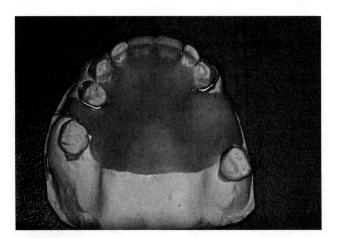

FIGURE 29.22

The cast should be well lubricated before acrylic resin or bonding agent and a light cured material is then added for the base.

are losing their teeth less as a result of dental caries (because of the advent of fluoridated water), but they continue to lose their teeth as a result of periodontal problems. Dental assistants are invaluable to the dental office for provision of care for RPD services. The types of services they provide to the dentist are only limited to the skills and interest of the dental assistant. Knowledge of removable prosthodontics can only enhance your job by allowing you to do interesting and challenging work.

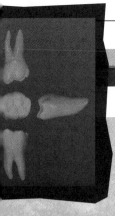

Points for Review

- The role of the dental assistant in removable partial prosthodontics
- Components of a removable partial partial denture
- Repair of partial dentures

Self-Study Questions

1. What is the branch of dentistry called that is concerned with the replacement of teeth and surrounding structures for edentulous or partially edentulous patients with artificial substitutes that can be removed from the mouth?
   a. Implant prosthodontics
   b. Removable prosthodontics
   c. Fixed prosthodontics
   d. Maxillofacial prosthodontics
2. What is the device called that is used to support the upper and lower cast while mounting?
   a. Facebow
   b. Articulator
   c. Base plates and occlusion rims
   d. Diagnostic cast
3. What is a prosthesis called that replaces one or more teeth in a partially dentate arch and is removable from the mouth?
   a. Removable complete denture
   b. Implant
   c. Removable partial denture
   d. Fixed partial denture
4. What is a paralleling instrument called that is used to locate and delineate the contours and relative positions of abutment teeth and related structures when constructing a prosthesis?
   a. Cast surveyor
   b. Facebow
   c. Articulator
   d. Base plates and occlusion rims

5. What is the device called that must be placed into undercuts to help retain the partial denture?
   a. Clasp
   b. Rest
   c. Retainer
   d. Connector
6. What is the unit of the partial denture called that sits on a tooth surface to provide vertical support?
   a. Clasp
   b. Rest
   c. Retainer
   d. Connector
7. What is the name of that clasp that arises from the dental framework and approaches the retentive undercut from a cervical direction?
   a. Ring clasp
   b. Embrasure clasp
   c. Circumferential clasp
   d. Bar clasp
8. What type of artificial tooth duplicates the anatomic form of natural teeth?
   a. Anatomic tooth
   b. Nonanatomic tooth
   c. Tube tooth
   d. Metal tooth
9. What contains the framework design and must accompany a master cast?
   a. Billing information
   b. Work authorization
   c. Dentist's name
   d. Interocclusal record
10. What does the laboratory mount the case on?
    a. Articulator
    b. Cast surveyor
    c. Facebow
    d. Base plates and occlusion rims

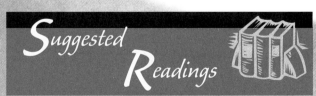

Suggested Readings

Barclay CW, Walmsley AD: *Fixed and removable prosthodontics,* Philadelphia, 1998, WB Saunders.

Bird WF, Hatrick C: *Dental materials: clinical applications for dental assistants and dental hygienists,* Philadelphia, 2000, WB Saunders.

Craig RG, Powers JM, Wataha JC: *Dental materials properties and manipulation,* ed 7, St Louis, 1999, Mosby.

Craig RG: *Restorative dental materials,* St Louis, 1996, Mosby.

Zwemer TJ: *Mosby's dental dictionary,* St Louis, 1998, Mosby.

Chapter 30

Complete Denture Prosthetics

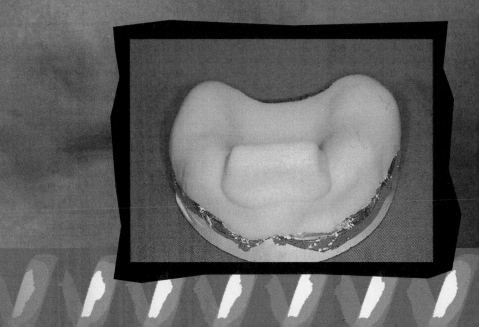

Chapter Outline

Complete Denture Prosthodontics
Indications and Contraindications
Initial Examination
Fabrication of a Custom Impression Tray
   Custom tray try-in
   Final (master) impressions
Vertical Measurements
   Vertical dimension
   Baseplate for maxillary arch
   Maxillary occlusion rim
   Mandibular occlusion rim
   Selection of artificial teeth
Try-in of Trial Dentures
   Role of the dental assistant
   Wax try-in

Delivery of Dentures
   Home care instructions
Immediate Dentures
   Surgical template
   Delivery of immediate dentures
Overdentures
Relining and Rebasing Dentures
   Role of the dental assistant
Denture Tooth and Base Repair
   Technique for denture base repair
   Technique for denture tooth repair

Learning Objectives

On completion of Chapter 30, the student should be able to do the following:

- Define key terms.
- Describe the dental assistant's role in complete denture therapy.
- Explain the procedures involved in the fabrication of complete dentures.
- Describe the maintenance and repair of complete dentures.
- Describe an immediate denture and an overdenture.

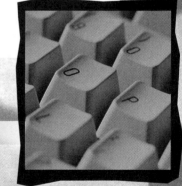

Key Terms

Baseplate (Record Base)

Centric Relation

Complete Denture

Free-Way Space (Interarch Distance)

Immediate Denture

Land Area

Occlusion Rim (Record Rim)

Plane of Occlusion

Posterior Palatal Seal

Vertical Dimension at Rest

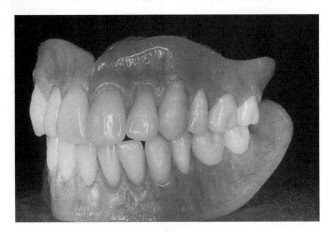

FIGURE 30.1

Complete denture.

COMPLETE DENTURE PROSTHODONTICS

Complete

denture

A removable dental prosthesis that replaces the entire dentition and associated structures of the maxilla or mandible

A **complete denture** replaces the entire dentition in a dental arch. It is a removable prosthesis that derives its support and retention from the underlying tissues of the alveolar ridges, oral mucosa, and hard palate. Complete dentures are artificial replacements for the natural dentition that restore the form and function of the dental arch. The components of a denture are the base of pigmented acrylic resin and the artificial teeth, which are made of either resin or porcelain (Figure 30.1). The base extends from the border of the denture that fills the vestibule of the edentulous arch to the neck or cervical margin of the teeth. The artificial teeth simulate the natural tooth crown.

The artificial teeth are retained mechanically or chemically (or both) with the denture base resin. Anterior and posterior teeth are selected and placed where they will closely mimic the original position of the natural dentition. The posterior teeth, with or without cusps, are selected according to the oral conditions of the edentulous arch and the clinician's preference. Artificial teeth are available through the dental laboratory that provides technical support for the dentist.

INDICATIONS AND CONTRAINDICATIONS

Patients who have lost a considerable amount of bone or who have some difficulty with muscular control may be good candidates for nonanatomic or rational posterior teeth. Indications for complete dentures include the following:

- The patient has no teeth as a result of extraction, trauma, or developmental anomaly.
- The patient has some teeth remaining, but the teeth are severely broken down because of rampant decay, and their prognosis is considered hopeless.
- The patient's teeth are periodontally compromised and would be inadequate as an abutment for either a fixed or removable partial prosthesis; the teeth usually are extremely mobile because of the lack of bone.
- The patient's remaining teeth would be poor abutments for a removable partial denture because of malalignment, root morphology, or their arrangement in the arch.

Contraindications for a complete denture include patients with a debilitating chronic or terminal illness; mentally handicapped patients who are unable to retain the prosthesis; and patients who are sensitive to denture resins.

INITIAL EXAMINATION

The patient is questioned at length to obtain the medical-dental history. Any medications currently taken are documented. Some medications may affect the patient's ability to function and retain complete dentures. If the patient is currently taking these types of medications, the possible effect on denture retention and comfort is discussed during this initial appointment.

The patient's mouth is carefully examined, and notes are made regarding, among other things, the ridge shape, the position of frenum attachments, the activity of the floor of the mouth, the position of the tongue, the consistency of the saliva, the presence of sharp bony areas, the presence of bony undercuts, and the jaw relationship. The instruments needed for the initial examination of an edentulous patient are a mouth mirror, gauze, tongue blade, periodontal probe, cotton forceps, air and water syringe tip, edentulous impression trays, mixing bowl, spatula, irreversible hydrocolloid, and rope wax.

A panoramic radiograph of the edentulous patient usually is taken as an adjunct for diagnosis and treatment planning. With this image the clinician can estimate bone thickness, identify specific anatomic landmarks, and check for pathologic conditions.

After the oral examination and the radiograph have been made, a diagnosis and treatment plan can be developed. In

Box 30.1

Procedure

Procedure for Fabricating a Custom Impression Tray

1. On a diagnostic cast, determine the areas that should be blocked out with wax to allow easy placement and removal of the custom impression tray (areas that commonly require relief are the labial vestibule and the retromylohyoid area).
2. After ensuring sufficient relief of these areas to eliminate any undercut, soften one layer of baseplate wax and adapt it to the cast. It should extend into the depth of the vestibule. Use a hot instrument to sear the wax to the cast and smooth the periphery.
3. Place a layer of tinfoil over the wax. Then apply a thin coat of petroleum jelly to the tinfoil and cast to prevent the acrylic from adhering to the cast.
4. If using *autopolymerizing tray resin*, mix the resin according to the manufacturer's directions and apply it to the cast. The resin must be 2 to 3 mm thick to create a rigid tray. Form a handle from the excess resin, using monomer liquid to moisten the surfaces to be joined. (A cotton swab works

well for moistening the doughy resin when applying the handle before curing is complete.)
   Visible light–cured (VLC) resin can be used instead of autopolymerizing tray resin. VLC resin is packaged in light-proof sheets to simplify handling (Figure 30.2). Remove the VLC resin from the package and adapt it over the cast. As with autopolymerizing resin, the VLC resin must be thick enough to create a sturdy impression tray. Remove any excess resin and repackage it for later use. Adapt a handle to the tray in a manner similar to that for autopolymerizing resin. Use the curing times provided by the manufacturer for the VLC resin (Figure 30.2).
5. After the resin has cured completely, trim the excess with appropriate acrylic burs until the material is smooth. A wet rag wheel and pumice can be used to achieve additional smoothness.
6. Insert the tray into the patient's mouth and check for accuracy of fit. The tray should be stable and comfortable.

some cases surgery is indicated before fabrication of the dentures to ensure a more comfortable fit of the prosthesis. Reduction of tuberosities, removal of mandibular tori, and recontouring of sharp areas are all surgical procedures that should be performed before fabrication of the dentures. Other factors that affect the diagnosis and treatment plan are the patient's age, mental health, physical condition, and expectations.

Construction of a preliminary set of study (or diagnostic) casts is mandatory, especially if any surgery is indicated before the dentures are made. These casts are used to fabricate custom impression trays for the patient. The assistant can easily be trained to make these casts in the laboratory of the dentist's office (Box 30.1 and Table 30.1).

Certain standards must be met to ensure a proper fit for a custom tray. A maxillary custom tray, for example, should

(1) be relieved in the frenum areas; (2) extend to a point 2 mm short of the depth of the vestibule; (3) cover the hamular notches and the posterior palatal seal area; and (4) extend beyond the tuberosities (Figure 30.3).

A mandibular custom tray should (1) be relieved in the frenum areas and over the mylohyoid ridges; (2) extend to a point 2 mm short of the depth of the vestibule; and (3) extend over the retromolar pads.

The instruments needed for master impressions include a mouth mirror, periodontal probe, explorer, cotton forceps, custom trays, impression material, stick compound (depending on the technique), gauze, high- and low-volume suction tips, air and water syringe tip, #7 wax spatula, mixing spatula, low-speed handpiece, scalpel blade, water bath, and any other instruments required by the dentist.

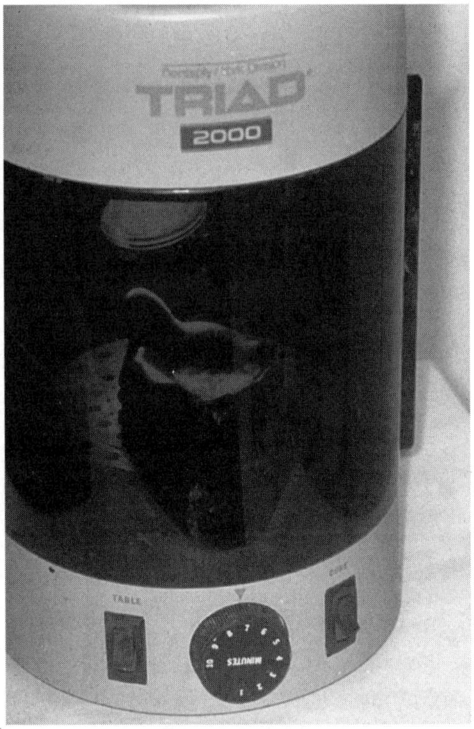

FIGURE 30.2

Tray curing in a visible light–curing (VLC) unit.

Table 30.1

Evaluation of Custom Tray for Complete Denture

Custom Tray for Complete Denture	4	3	2	0	X
Secure materials. Secure diagnostic cast. Block out undercuts. Place tin foil over wax. Place petroleum jelly over tin foil.					
Autopolymer Mix a autopolymer tray resin. Roll to desired thickness (2-3 mm). Form handle.					
Visible light-cured resin Select light proof sheet. Adapt over cast. Remove excess material. Cure.					
Trim excess material and smooth. Try in tray.					

The numeric criteria: 4 Excellent; 3 Good but some improvement can be made; 2 Below average, usable, needs to improve skill; 0 Unsatisfactory; X Not able to evaluate.

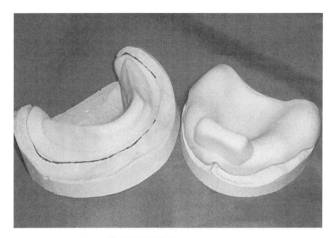

FIGURE 30.3

Tray on a maxillary cast.

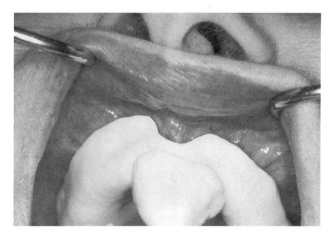

FIGURE 30.4

Properly adjusted impression tray seen in the mouth.

FABRICATION OF A CUSTOM IMPRESSION TRAY

The steps involved in the fabrication of a custom impression tray are presented in Box 30.1.

Custom Tray Try-In

A custom tray is inserted into the patient's mouth, or "tried in," and examined for border extension and stability. If the tray is unstable, the border extensions should be checked, because the borders may need to be trimmed back. After the borders have been adjusted, the tray is tried in again. If instability is still noted and the border extensions are well short of the full extension of the vestibule, the tray may have been distorted during fabrication. A new tray should be constructed.

If the tray is stable after adjustment of the flange, or periphery, (Figure 30.4), the next step is *border molding,* which duplicates the vestibular anatomy in height and thickness. The lips, cheeks, and tongue are moved to "mold" the muscles around the tray. A material such as thermoplasticized wax (stick compound) or a heavy bodied impression material is placed on the shortened flange to capture this detail before the impression procedure. If an impression material is used, an adhesive must be painted on the periphery of the tray so that the impression material will not peel off when the tray is removed from the mouth. After border molding has been completed, the tray is inspected and excess material is removed with a sharp instrument. The internal aspect of the tray is painted with adhesive before the final impression is made.

Final (Master) Impressions

The final, or master, impressions must be accurate because the finished product is fabricated using the master casts cre-

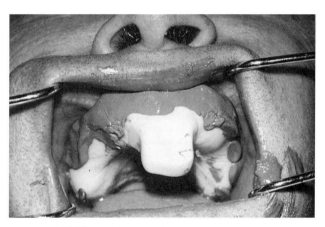

FIGURE 30.5

Impression for edentulous maxillary arch.

ated from these impressions. The impression material should be one that produces fine detail, such as polysulfide, polyvinylsiloxane, or polyether. Once the impressions have been made, they are boxed and poured in a vacuum-mixed dental stone to make the master cast.

The ideal final impression for complete dentures should have an even thickness and should extend slightly beyond the tray margins. It must be well mixed, free of bubbles, and have no streaks (a sign of impression material that was not mixed thoroughly). In a maxillary impression, all details of the arch, such as the frenum attachments, tuberosities, hamular notches, and palate, should be included (Figure 30.5). In a mandibular impression, the retromolar pad area, oblique ridge, mylohyoid ridge, frenum attachments, and genial tubercles should be visible.

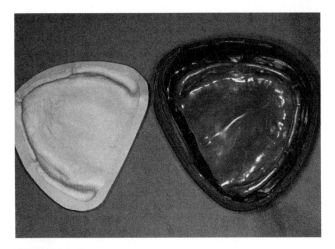

FIGURE 30.6

Final maxillary impression boxed and master cast properly trimmed.

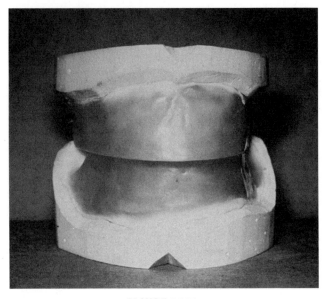

FIGURE 30.7

Occlusion rim.

Land area

The portion of a dental cast that extends beyond the impression's replica surface laterally; it defines the area between the end of the replica's surface and the cast

Impressions are boxed with boxing wax to create a peripheral border, or **land area,** about 5 mm thick (Figure 30.6). The depth of the boxing should be sufficient to create a minimal cast thickness of about 15 to 20 mm. Improved dental stone is mixed according to the manufacturer's directions and then vacuum mixed. The stone mixture is vibrated into the boxed impression and allowed to set for about 1 hour.

After the stone mixture has cooled, the impression can be separated and the model trimmed using a model trimmer.

VERTICAL MEASUREMENTS

Baseplate (record base)

A temporary denture base used to support the record rim material when determining the maxillomandibular relationships

A **baseplate,** or **record base,** is used for establishing and taking vertical measurements, articulation of the casts, and for artificial tooth arrangement so that it can be evaluated once placed into the patient's mouth. Visible fight-cured resin or autopolymerizing tray resin can be used to fabricate the baseplate. The baseplate will cover the area that the finished denture will occupy.

The **occlusion rim,** or **record rim,** is made of baseplate wax and is secured to the baseplate. The occlusion rim helps to establish a **plane of occlusion,** determine the vertical dimension of the patient, and register the occlusal relationship of the arches (Figure 30.7). The occlusion rim may be preformed into a horseshoe shape, or this shape can be made from flat sheets rolled together. In either case, the wax rim is softened and luted to the baseplate with sticky wax.

The height and thickness of the wax should be sufficient to replace the missing dentition and bone. The normal thickness is about 10 to 12 mm in the posterior region, tapering to about 6 to 8 mm in the anterior region. The height of each occlusal rim is about 22 mm for the maxillary rim and about 18 mm for the mandibular rim. The palatal aspect of the maxillary rim and the lingual surface of the mandibular rim are beveled from the occlusal surface to the flange to allow sufficient room for the tongue and the musculature of the floor of the mouth.

Occlusion rim (record rim)

The occlusal surfaces fabricated on a baseplate (record base) to record the maxillomandibular relationship or to arrange teeth

Plane of occlusion

The surface of a wax occlusion rim, which is contoured to guide the arrangement of denture teeth

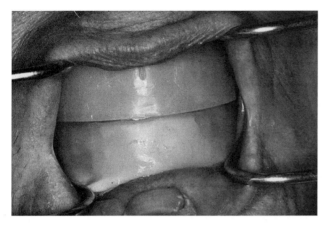

FIGURE 30.8

Occlusion rims in place at the vertical dimension of occlusion.

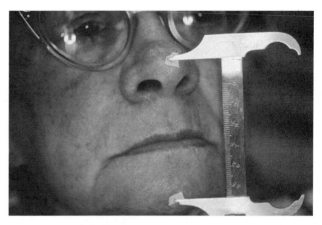

FIGURE 30.9

Measuring the vertical dimension at rest.

Once the master models are ready, with the baseplates and occlusion rims, the next clinical appointment with the patient is used to establish and measure the vertical dimension. The instruments needed to determine the vertical dimension include a mouth mirror, explorer, cotton forceps, periodontal probe, air and water syringe, #7 wax spatula, ball burnisher, cleoid/discoid carver, tongue blade, gauze, wax, compound or other material suitable for bite registration, scalpel blade, shade guide, mold board or mold sheet (for denture tooth selection), and water bath.

Vertical Dimension

Vertical dimension at rest

The postural position between the maxilla and the mandible in which the musculature is in a state of rest

The **vertical dimension at rest** is measured first. This dimension is a postural position between the maxilla and the mandible in which the muscles that open and close the mandible are in a state of equilibrium. At this point there is minimal muscle tonicity sufficient to maintain posture. Some methods commonly used to establish this position include licking the lips and swallowing, repeating certain phrases or sounds, or, if possible, evaluating the patient's current and previous dentures. This position is determined and reevaluated a few times before it is measured (Figures 30.8 and 30.9).

Baseplate for Maxillary Arch

The baseplate for the maxillary arch is tried in and adjusted for comfort and stability. The plane of occlusion is then determined by using external landmarks, such as the distance between the eyes (interpupillary line) and the distance between the ala of the nose and the tragus of the ear (ala-tragus line). The plane of occlusion is used to establish an alignment of the teeth for the maxillary denture. Minor changes can be made according to the patient's preference and smile line.

The **posterior palatal seal** is then determined in the patient's mouth to help create the proper fit for the maxillary denture. The dentist can visualize the vibrating line by asking the patient to say "ahh." The vibrating line is an area of the palate that moves along a line near the junction of the hard and soft palates. The line is marked with an indelible pencil from the hamular notch on one side to the hamular notch on the other side. The baseplate is adjusted until the posterior edge lies over this line. The line is then transferred to the cast and marked to designate the posterior border of the denture.

Posterior palatal seal

The seal at the posterior border of a maxillary prosthesis

Maxillary Occlusion Rim

The maxillary occlusion rim is also used to establish the proper lip contour for the denture. The wax is shaped until appropriate lip support is achieved. Having the patient repeat the sounds of the letters "f" or "v" or words that begin with these letters can help the dentist determine the proper position of the wax and eventually of the denture teeth. The amount of tooth that will be seen is initially determined by using the wax rim as a preliminary guide. On average, 1 to 2 mm of the maxillary incisor tooth is seen below the lip when it is at rest. The patient's input is important when the dentist is adjusting the wax to establish the contour needed.

Mandibular Occlusion Rim

The mandibular occlusion rim is tried in, and flange adjustments are made as needed. The plane of occlusion is adjusted to correspond to the plane previously established with the maxillary rim. With the occlusion rims in place, the dentist reevaluates the previously recorded vertical dimension at rest. The patient is asked to repeat sounds (f, v, s, or th) and to lick the lips and swallow.

Free-way space (interarch distance)

The distance between the occluding surfaces of the maxillary and mandibular teeth when the mandible is in a specified position

The recorded position must be verified again, because the occlusal vertical dimension will have been based on the initial measurement. Normally, an edentulous patient averages 2 to 4 mm of difference between the rest position and the occluded (biting) position; this measurement is the **free-way space,** or **interarch distance.** These measurements are verified again at the next appointment, when the trial denture with the teeth set up in the wax rim are reevaluated in the patient's mouth.

Centric relation

The maxillomandibular relationship in which the condyles articulate with the disks when the articular complex is in its most anterosuperior position against the articular eminence

In order for the laboratory technician to construct the dentures with correct articulation and occlusion, an accurate recording of the centric jaw position, or **centric relation,** must be made. This recording can be obtained in a variety of ways. In the method most often used, wax or compound is interposed between the wax rims, and the patient is asked to close slowly into a retruded position and to hold that position until the wax or compound cools.

A face-bow is used to accurately transfer the relationship of the edentulous arches to the articulator. This puts the maxillary arch in a position on the instrument that closely mimics the jaw opening movement (Figure 30.10).

Another method of recording the centric relation uses the patient's tactile sense with an intraoral tracing device to establish the most retruded position based on markings from the stylus (attached to the maxillary rim) on a blackened surface (attached to the mandibular rim). Once a repeatable point has been established, this position is recorded with wax, compound, or quick-setting plaster. This device can also register other movements of the mandible (Figure 30.11).

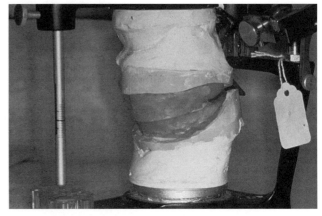

FIGURE 30.10
Centric relation record in place on the articulator.

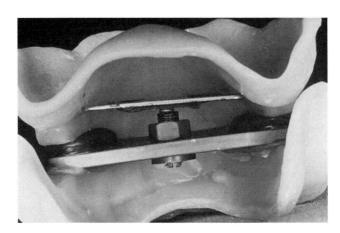

FIGURE 30.11
Use of an intraoral tracing device.

Centric position is the most retruded position of the mandible to the maxilla from which lateral excursions can be made at a given vertical dimension. Protrusion is the most anterior position of the mandible to the maxilla from centric position. Laterotrusion is a sliding position of the mandible from side to side from centric position as it relates to the maxilla. These motions simulate the movements of the mandible as it functions in mastication and speaking.

Selection of Artificial Teeth

In choosing the shade (color) and mold (shape) of an artificial tooth, the dentist must consider the patient's age, skin color, hair color, and lip position and length, as well as the width and length of the space to be occupied by the denture tooth. If the patient desires no change from the previous denture, the dentist can use the existing prosthesis to measure the length and width of the tooth, make a preliminary tracing of the arrangement, and match the shade of the teeth. If the patient wants a change or if the existing pros-

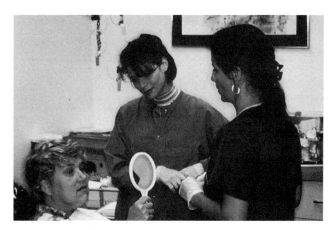

FIGURE 30.12

The dentist, patient, and dental assistant work together to select teeth for the dentures.

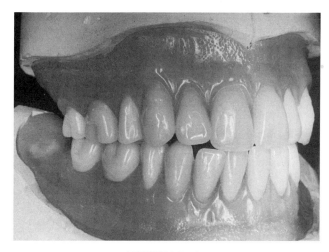

FIGURE 30.13

Wax try-in.

thesis is worn and discolored, the factors mentioned previously can be used as a guide for selecting and arranging the denture teeth. Shades are best selected using the existing overhead lighting in the operatory or natural indirect sunlight (Figure 30.12). Using the operator's light is not recommended, because it is too intense for this purpose.

After the shade and mold have been selected, this information is written in the patient's chart for future reference. Posterior teeth are selected also during this time. Posterior teeth can be flat, fully anatomic, or semianatomic. The type of denture tooth is chosen by conferring with the patient, evaluating the condition of the patient's mucosa, and determining the interarch distance. This information, along with the master casts, occlusion rims, and interocclusal record, is submitted to the laboratory technician for arrangement of the denture teeth for purposes of a try-in.

TRY-IN OF TRIAL DENTURES

The patient is given an appointment for a try-in of the waxed trial dentures (Figure 30.13). The trial dentures consist of the artificial denture teeth, the baseplates, and the wax contoured to simulate the gingival tissue of the finished denture. The teeth are arranged and articulated according to the records submitted to the laboratory technician and the instructions written on the laboratory prescription.

Role of the Dental Assistant

One of the dental assistant's duties is to make sure that the laboratory work is ready to be tried in before the patient arrives for the appointment. Circumstances can arise that may require postponement of the try-in visit. Proper communication between the office and the laboratory can prevent strained relationships between the dentist and the technician.

When laboratory cases are sent out, a return date that is at least 24 hours before the patient's appointment should be specified. This allows sufficient time for rescheduling the appointment if necessary.

Wax Try-In

During the wax try-in visit, several aspects of the setup are evaluated. The tooth mold, tooth shade, and tooth arrangement are checked to determine if they are harmonious with the patient's lips and face. The patient is asked to repeat certain phonetic sounds to evaluate the tooth position with the lips, and the fullness of the cheeks and lips are checked. The vertical dimension is measured again to see if the setup is within the parameters previously established. Muscle attachments are evaluated to make sure that the flanges are not impinging on them, and retention is checked as the patient talks and swallows. Occlusion is verified again and retaken if an inaccuracy is discovered.

Finally, the patient's opinion is requested, to determine if the dentures are acceptable or if any changes are desired, such as in the shade or arrangement. If all aspects of the arrangement are acceptable to the patient and the dentist, the patient is given an appointment for delivery of the dentures.

The dentist prepares a written prescription for the laboratory technician to process, or finish the construction of, the complete dentures. The dentist specifies the type of denture acrylic and acrylic shade to be used. Any final instructions for modifying the setup are also included, and a return date for the case is established based on the appointment time. Most laboratories have a designated time frame for completion of complete dentures. The laboratories in the area can provide the dental office with information about pickup of the case, mailing instructions, and the time allotment for laboratory construction.

DELIVERY OF DENTURES

At the appointment for delivery of the new complete dentures, the patient is seated and the old prosthesis (if one exists) is removed and placed in a container for the patient. Each maxillary and mandibular denture is evaluated by the dentist for any processing errors, such as sharp spicules within the denture or tooth movement. The dentures are placed in the patient's mouth, and the patient is asked to perform a variety of facial movements to make sure the dentures are not creating any impingement or soreness.

The occlusion is checked with articulating paper or ribbon to evaluate the accuracy of the bite. Any gross adjustments are made with a slow-speed handpiece and acrylic burs. Once the occlusion appears even and is comfortable to the patient, any adjustments that were made to the denture base or teeth are polished with flour of pumice and polishing compound to restore the luster to the denture resin (Figure 30.14). Another appointment is made for a checkup on the dentures.

Home Care Instructions

The chairside dental assistant explains the home care procedures to the patient. The patient is instructed to remove and clean the dentures after every meal, when possible. If removal is not possible, the patient should rinse and expectorate to remove food particles from the dentures' surfaces. Dentures should be brushed each day to dislodge food and accumulated plaque.

When cleaning the dentures, the patient should hold them over a sink half-filled with water to minimize damage to the dentures if they are accidentally dropped. Rinsing the mouth at this point with an antiseptic mouthwash is also recommended. When the dentures are not worn, they must be stored in water to avoid warping of the acrylic. Use of effervescent cleansing tablets or other toothpastes is recommended to minimize the accumulation of bacteria and to maintain a fresh feeling for the patient.

IMMEDIATE DENTURES

The term **immediate denture** refers to a denture or dentures that are planned for a patient and that are delivered the same day the remaining anterior teeth are removed (Figure 30.15). This procedure allows the patient to avoid being completely edentulous for an extended period.

In planning for such a procedure, the dental staff must make sure that the patient understands that during the healing process after the loss of the teeth, the bone will change because of resorption, causing the denture to become loose. This change will require a relining procedure or even possibly reconstruction of the entire denture.

Impressions for an immediate denture may require the use of irreversible hydrocolloid as a final impression medium, depending on the mobility of the existing teeth. Some of the more highly accurate materials set up more rigidly than extract the teeth as the impression is removed.

Another impression technique uses a split tray, with the first tray resembling a custom impression tray for a conventional denture impression. This portion of the impression captures the edentulous portion of the dental arch. The second portion of the impression captures the natural teeth and their relationship with the edentulous arch. The try-in of the wax setup before removal of the teeth allows the clinician to

> *Immediate denture*
>
> **A complete denture or a removable partial denture fabricated for placement immediately after removal of the natural teeth**

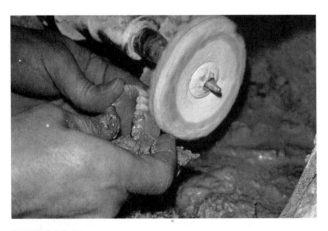

FIGURE 30.14
Polishing teeth and flanges that had been adjusted previously.

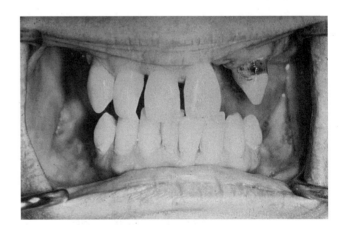

FIGURE 30.15
Immediate denture patient before treatment.

evaluate the occlusal relationship of the posterior teeth and permits the patient to evaluate the shade selection. After these factors have been checked, the remainder of the anterior setup is done in the laboratory without the benefit of a try-in to check the arrangement of the anterior teeth. This is one of the disadvantages of this procedure. If the patient does not like the esthetics of the denture, another prosthesis must be fabricated. The patient must understand that this is a possible outcome of the procedure (Figure 30.16).

To aid in placement of the immediate denture, some bony protuberances may need to be surgically reduced after the remaining teeth have been removed. A surgical template can be constructed when the laboratory constructs the definitive denture.

Surgical Template

A surgical template resembles an impression tray but is made of clear plastic acrylic. Once the teeth have been extracted, this template is placed in the patient's mouth to determine which areas need bone trimming. These areas will blanch, because the template was fabricated after the patient's model was trimmed. The template is meant to act as a guide for the surgeon to facilitate placement of the immediate denture. During healing the denture protects the surgical site and promotes healing, acting as a bandage over the area.

Delivery of Immediate Dentures

The instruments needed for delivery of immediate dentures are the same as those required for the delivery of dentures described earlier. At the time of delivery, the patient is anesthetized, and the remaining teeth are removed. If a surgical template is used, it is tried in at this time to determine the amount of bone to remove before the denture is inserted. Any bony contouring is done, and the mucosa is sutured into

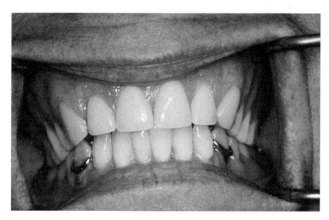

FIGURE 30.16

Immediate denture patient after extractions and placement of denture.

place. The sterilized dentures are rinsed with sterile saline and placed in position. The dentures are then checked for occlusion, and any gross discrepancies are adjusted.

The patient is given a follow-up appointment for the next day, and analgesics are prescribed to ease the pain of the procedure. The patient is advised to wear the denture continuously, except for cleansing, until the next appointment. The patient is usually seen at 24 and 48 hours after extraction of the teeth. Pressure spots are adjusted, and the occlusion is refined as needed. The patient is advised to eat a soft diet until the swelling subsides and the sutures have been removed The person is seen as needed for adjustments.

If the adaptation becomes loose after healing, a tissue conditioner or temporary liner can be placed to help stabilize the denture. After about 3 months, when tissue and bone healing has stabilized, the dentures are reevaluated for a relining or rebasing procedure.

OVERDENTURES

An overdenture is a complete denture that lies over the remaining natural teeth or implants, the residual ridges, and the oral mucosa. The residual tissues, ridges, and tooth roots or implants together provide support for the prosthesis. The denture fits snugly over the teeth or implants and provides a natural relationship for the mandible and maxilla.

Patients who have congenital or acquired intraoral defects, badly worn teeth or only a few teeth remaining, or one or two implants can benefit from overdenture therapy. Maintaining a few teeth can be of psychologic benefit for the overdenture patient. Research has shown that bone levels are maintained and proprioception is enhanced by keeping strategic teeth with an overdenture. A patient whose remaining teeth would be poor partial denture abutments can become an excellent overdenture candidate.

Patients with teeth that will be used for an overdenture require root canal therapy to devitalize the tooth. This prevents any sensitivity when the clinical crown is removed before the denture is delivered. This technique can sometimes be treated as an immediate denture. The teeth that require removal are extracted; the teeth with root canals to be saved are left in the mouth, but the clinical crown is reduced to or near the level of the gingiva.

A primary disadvantage of overdenture therapy is the additional cost of root canal therapy for the tooth or teeth to be saved. If gold copings (thin, smooth gold castings that cover the exposed root face) or other attachments are used, the cost of treatment rises even more. If the patient goes to the added expense to maintain specific teeth, the person must be motivated to practice proper hygiene. Figure 30.17 shows a maxillary overdenture using attachments that allow removal of the denture plate.

Certain key principles must be satisfied to achieve a predictable result with overdenture therapy. First, healthy

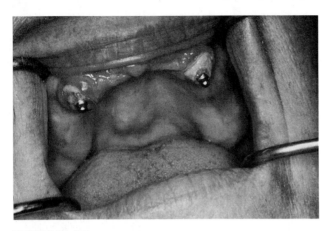

FIGURE 30.17

Attachments used with maxillary canines for overdenture retention.

periodontal tissues are necessary around the prospective abutment tooth. A tooth that is already healthy will be easier for the patient to maintain. Second, minimizing the crown to root ratio of the tooth by reducing the clinical crown helps the prognosis of the tooth and aids in placement of the artificial teeth on the denture. Third, with or without a coping to cover the root face of the tooth, the patient must practice proper oral hygiene continually to minimize decay. Keeping recall appointments with the dentist helps ensure the longevity of the overdenture abutments. If teeth are lost, a relining procedure can be done without much difficulty.

RELINING AND REBASING DENTURES

Changes occur in the supporting tissues underlying complete denture prostheses. Ridge absorption, for example, may cause a patient to complain of loss of retention or a change in the occlusion with the dentures. For this reason, denture patients are counseled to make and keep regular recall appointments so that the dentist can evaluate the dentures and determine if relining or rebasing is indicated.

Relining of complete dentures involves adding a small amount of material to enhance the fit of the prosthesis. This is the treatment required if only a minimal amount of change in the tissues has occurred. The procedure minimally affects the occlusion and esthetics of the complete dentures.

Rebasing of complete dentures is indicated if extensive changes have occurred in the supporting structures. The dentist must replace additional missing tissue and maintain the proper finished product. A closed mouth technique may be used, in which the patient's mouth is closed in the proper centric position while the rebasing material sets. This technique minimizes the amount of time needed to correct the occlusion.

A different technique involves the use of a tissue conditioner as the impression material. The denture is relieved as previously mentioned but is lined with a tissue conditioner. The patient is allowed to wear this for about 1 week. The material molds itself and adapts to the tissues and musculature as the patient goes about the normal routine. This technique is particularly useful if the patient shows signs of tissue irritation. The material helps heal the oral structures in addition to establishing a better fit for the prosthesis.

Both of the above techniques require the denture to be relined or rebased in a laboratory. The patient must understand that he or she will be without the denture for 24 to 48 hours while the denture is processed with the new denture acrylic. A minimum of two visits is required for these procedures.

If being without the denture presents a problem for the patient, a third technique is available in which an autopolymerizing resin or visible light–cured (VLC) resin is used at chairside. This technique allows the patient to wear the finished denture after one appointment. The denture is relieved, and the resin is placed in the denture and seated. The more viscous the resin, the longer it takes to adjust the denture intraorally in its proper position. If this technique is used, care must be taken to ensure proper placement of the denture. The drawbacks of this technique include the following:

- A porous liner retains odor and bacteria.
- Some materials can cause thermal burns because of the heat generated by curing.
- Positioning can be a problem if the material is too viscous or starts setting prematurely.
- Some materials are not color stable.

A minimum of one visit is required to obtain the finished result.

Role of the Dental Assistant

The dental assistant's role in a relining or rebasing procedure is to provide the proper tray setup and materials as requested by the clinician. The assistant may be directed to provide relief in the denture. Care must be taken not to perforate the denture when providing relief in the tissue surface. The assistant also may evacuate saliva as the impression is setting.

If an autopolymerizing or VLC material is used, acrylic burs are needed to trim and finish the borders, in addition to other clinical instruments requested by the dentist. Once the denture has been finished, proper finishing to a smooth surface is necessary using a wet chamois on a lathe with pumice and polishing compound. The assistant must make sure that the surface of the denture is wet while the pumice slurry is used to smooth out any nicks created by the acrylic burs. Light pressure while finishing prevents the pumice from becoming impregnated into the denture base. After polishing, proper disinfection procedures must be followed before the denture is returned to the patient.

At this point the dental assistant should reinforce the oral hygiene instructions. Demonstrations with visual aids to show proper maintenance of the dentures and of the intra-oral structures can help the patient understand the importance of proper oral home care. Providing the patient with brushes, dentifrice, and cleaning solutions helps reinforce the practice of oral hygiene.

DENTURE TOOTH AND BASE REPAIR

Repairs of denture prostheses usually occur on an emergency basis. This type of emergency usually can be handled in the office using autopolymerizing acrylic resin (Figure 30.18). Major fractures, however, may be best handled by a commercial laboratory. In either case, the dental assistant plays a key role in returning the repaired denture to its owner as quickly as possible.

Fractures of teeth or denture base resin may be caused by dropping the denture, or numerous other mishaps, or by changes in the patient's occlusion. When evaluating a fracture, the key is to determine if the pieces return to only one position (Figure 30.19). If concern arises about the positioning of the fractured pieces, it also may be necessary to reline the denture and readjust the occlusion to ensure a proper fit. The patient must be informed of such a development to eliminate any misunderstanding about the treatment.

Technique for Denture Base Repair

If the broken pieces of the denture base can be returned to the original position, they can be held together with an old handpiece bur or tongue blades luted with sticky wax (Figure 30.20). A cast is then formed by vibrating quick-setting plaster into the tissue side of the denture. A very light coating of petroleum jelly is applied to the tissue side to aid in cleaning of the denture after the repair procedure. Once the plaster has set, a groove is cut along the line of fracture down to the plaster and the edges are beveled.

Removal of the denture halves may be required to facilitate the initial preparation. If this is done, care must be taken not to break the cast upon removal and insertion. Care must also be exercised to return the denture to the original position on the cast. Applying a light coating of tinfoil substitute or petroleum jelly to the cast allows easy separation from the cast once the resin has cured. Painting monomer over the fractured ends allows the autopolymerizing resin to bond to the old resin. The new resin is slightly overfilled, and the cast assembly, with the denture, is placed in hot water until the resin has cured. If a pressure pot is available, a denser cured resin can be obtained by putting the assembly into the pressure pot at 20 pounds per square inch (psi) for 15 minutes.

After the resin has set, it is trimmed with acrylic burs and polished first with wet pumice on a rag wheel and then with acrylic compound to achieve a high shine. Box 30.2 and Table 30.2 show procedures and evaluations for denture base repair.

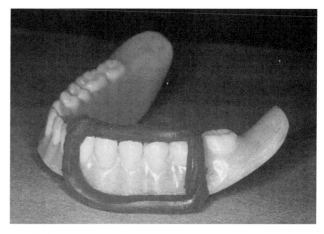

FIGURE 30.18

The tooth is repositioned on the denture and secured with wax; the rope wax is adapted as a matrix for a stone index; the area is coated with petroleum jelly before the stone is added.

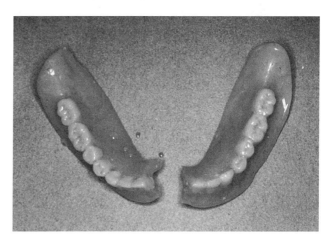

FIGURE 30.19

Denture base repair. Mandibular complete denture broken into two pieces.

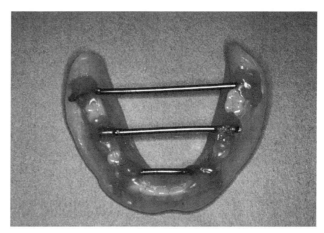

FIGURE 30.20

Denture base repair. Sections of the denture are readapted and secured with sticky wax using wooden or metal dowels.

Box 30.2

Procedure

Procedure for Denture Base Repair

Materials needed
Cast
Sticky wax
Paint brush
Toothpicks
Tinfoil substitute
Denture acrylic resin
Pumice
Acrylic resin compound
Quick setting plaster

1. Cast of mouth or reposition broken pieces.
2. Place brace to secure pieces together.
3. Apply petroleum jelly to the tissue side up.
4. Vibrate plaster into denture.
5. Cut groove along fracture and bevel edges.
6. Paint resin to slightly overfilling in groove.
7. Place cast with resin in hot water to cure (or use pressure pot).
8. After set, trim and polish with pumice on rag wheel.
9. Polish and smooth with acrylic compound.

Table 30.2

Evaluation of Denture Base Repair

Denture Base Repair	4	3	2	0	X
Secure materials.					
Brace pieces together.					
Prepare cast.					
Apply petroleum jelly.					
Cut groove and bevel edges.					
Paint resin into groove.					
Place in hot water.					
Trim and polish.					

The numeric criteria: 4 Excellent; 3 Good but some improvement can be made; 2 Below average, usable, needs to improve skill; 0 Unsatisfactory; X Not able to evaluate.

Technique for Denture Tooth Repair

If a denture tooth fractures from a denture and is not lost or swallowed, it can be replaced simply by adding powder and monomer. The denture is placed in hot water or in a pressure pot, similar to the denture baseplate repair described previously. Once cured, any excess material is trimmed away and the surface is smoothed with wet pumice on a rag wheel and then with acrylic compound.

If several teeth have been fractured from the denture, they can be replaced on the denture in the original position and secured with sticky wax. An occlusal index is made with plaster to gain some record of the tooth position before the fracture.

Once the index has set, it is removed, along with the teeth (see Figure 30.18).

The surface of the denture and the tissue surface of the denture teeth are roughened. The teeth are placed back into the index, and polymer and monomer are poured onto the denture. While the material is doughy, the index containing the teeth is placed back onto the denture. The assembly then is placed in hot water or a pressure pot until it has cured. Acrylic burs are used to remove excess material, and any necessary anatomic contouring of the denture base is done. Surface finishing is accomplished using wet pumice on a rag wheel and acrylic compound as described previously.

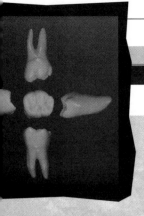

Points for Review

- Steps in the initial examination for complete dentures
- Fabrication of a complete denture custom impression tray
- Construction of a set of baseplates and occlusion rims
- Procedure for the denture try-in
- Techniques for relining and rebasing a denture
- Repair of a denture tooth and a denture base

Self-Study Questions

1. A complete denture gains support and retention from the underlying tissues of what structure?
   a. Alveolar ridges
   b. Oral mucosa
   c. Hard palate
   d. All of the above
   e. None of the above

2. What type of denture is placed immediately after extraction of the natural teeth?
   a. Overdenture
   b. Immediate denture
   c. Transitional denture
   d. Removable partial denture
   e. None of the above

3. Which of the following is *not* an indication for complete dentures?
   a. Patient has no teeth because of extraction, trauma, or developmental anomaly.
   b. Patient has some teeth, but they are severely broken down because of decay, and their prognosis is considered hopeless.
   c. Patient has severe periodontal disease, which has left the teeth extremely mobile.
   d. Patient is healthy and has most of the teeth, which are in reasonably good condition.
   e. Patient's remaining teeth would be poor abutments for a removable partial denture.

4. When a custom tray is made, the baseplate wax is adapted 1 mm short of the depth of the vestibule.
   a. True
   b. False

5. What procedure is used in conjunction with the custom impression tray to accurately duplicate the anatomic configuration of the vestibule?
   a. Border molding
   b. Flange molding
   c. Vestibuloplasty
   d. Frenectomy

6. What postural position is measured when the muscles that open and close the mandible are in a state of equilibrium?
   a. Vertical dimension of rest
   b. Vertical dimension of occlusion
   c. Centric relation
   d. Maximum intercuspation

7. What is the best light source to use when selecting the shade or color of an artificial tooth?
   a. Operatory light shining directly on the patient's face
   b. Indirect natural sunlight
   c. Overhead incandescent light
   d. B and c only
   e. All of the above

8. Home care instructions provided by the dental assistant do *not* include which of the following?
   a. When cleaning the dentures, hold them over a basin or sink that is at least half full of water.
   b. Store the dentures in a dry container when they are not being worn.
   c. Store the dentures in water when they are not being worn.
   d. Use denture toothpastes to help reduce plaque.
   e. Use effervescent cleaning tablets to clean the dentures.

9. Extensive changes in the supporting structure may require what adjustment?
   a. Rebasing, if the dentures are in good condition
   b. Relining, if the dentures are in good condition
   c. Rebasing, if the dentures are severely worn and the teeth are broken
   d. Relining, if the dentures are in poor condition and have cracked or broken teeth

10. Which of the following is *not* an advantage of over-denture therapy?
    a. Cost
    b. Preservation of bone levels
    c. Preservation of some teeth, giving the patient a psychologic boost
    d. Use of roots for better retention of the denture
    e. Improved proprioception

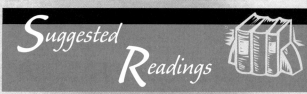

Suggested Readings

Babbush C: *Dental implants: the art and science*, Philadelphia, 2000, WB Saunders.

Barclay CW, Walmsley AD: *Fixed and removable prosthodontics*, Philadelphia, 1998, WB Saunders.

Bird WF, Hatrick C: *Dental materials: clinical applications for dental assistants and dental hygienists*, Philadelphia, 2000, WB Saunders.

Branemark PI: *Tissue-integrated prostheses: osseointegration in clinical dentistry*, Chicago, 1987, Quintessence.

Craig RG, Powers JM, Wataha JC: *Dental materials properties and manipulation*, ed 7, St Louis, 1999, Mosby.

Craig RG: *Restorative dental materials*, St Louis, 1996, Mosby.

Cranin AN, Klein M, Simons AM: *Atlas of oral implantology*, ed 2, St Louis, 1999, Mosby.

Engelman M: *Clinical decision making and treatment planning in osseointegration*, Chicago, 1996, Quintessence.

Hayakawa I: *Principles & practices of complete dentures*, Chicago, 1999, Quintessence.

Lamb DJ: *Problems & solutions in complete denture fabrication*, Chicago, 1992, Quintessence.

McKinney RV: *Endosteal dental implants*, St Louis, 1991, Mosby.

Misch CE: *Contemporary implant dentistry*, St Louis, 1998, Mosby.

Worthington P, Lang BR, LaVelle WE: *Osseointegration in dentistry: an introduction*, Chicago, 1994, Quintessence.

Zarb GA, Bolender CL, Carlsson GE: *Boucher's prosthodontic treatment for edentulous patients*, ed 11, St Louis, 1997, Mosby.

Zwemer TJ: *Mosby's dental dictionary*, St Louis, 1998, Mosby.

Chapter 31

Dental Implantology

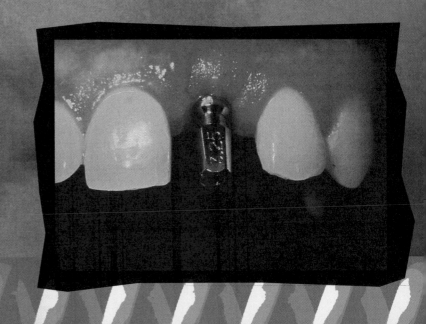

Chapter Outline

Learning Objectives

On completion of Chapter 31, the student should be able to do the following:

- Define key terms.
- Describe the role of the dental assistant in dental implantology.
- Discuss patient selection and treatment planning.
- Describe the surgical role and prosthetic treatment of dental implantology.
- Discuss the importance of maintenance procedures.

Key Terms

Dental Implant

Endosteal Dental Implant

Implant Abutment

Implant Surgery

Impression Coping

Osseointegration

Subperiosteal Dental Implant

Surgical Template

Transosteal Implant

INTRODUCTION TO DENTAL IMPLANTS

A **dental implant** is an artificial device used in the replacement of missing teeth or to enhance the retention of a removable prosthesis. Dental patients may require replacement of teeth that have been lost as a result of caries, periodontal disease, or trauma. Because of recent scientific research, dental implants are now considered a viable treatment alternative. Teeth that once were replaced with fixed, removable partial, or complete denture prosthodontics can now be replaced with bone-anchored implants in either the maxilla or the mandible. Implants can be used for single tooth replacement, fixed bridgework, or to stabilize a removable prosthesis.

Dental implant

> A prosthetic device of alloplastic material implanted into the oral tissues beneath the mucosa and periosteal layer and within the bone to provide retention and support for a fixed or removable prosthesis

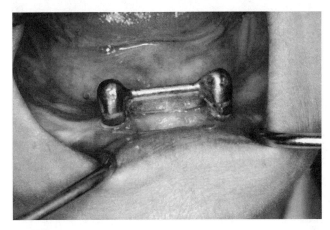

FIGURE 31.1

Clinical view of a transosteal implant. The gold bar pictured is cemented into the implant.

TYPES OF DENTAL IMPLANTS

Dental implants can be classified into three types.

Transosteal

A **transosteal implant** is a type of implant that is placed in the mandible for purposes of securing a complete denture (Figures 31.1 and 31.2). The term *transosteal* means "through the bone." This surgical procedure requires hospitalization and is performed under general anesthesia by an oral surgeon. The device contains a row of screws supported by a plate that butts against the inferior border of the mandible. It is placed after a series of holes are drilled into or through the inferior border of the mandible and the implant is tapped into position. Two extra long screws attached to this device penetrate into the oral cavity. It is this portion of the implant that will be used for attachment of

Transosteal implant

> A dental implant that penetrates both cortical plates and passes through the full thickness of the aveolar bone of the mandible. The term *transosteal* means "through the bone"

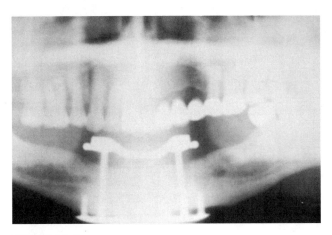

FIGURE 31.2

Panoramic radiograph of another transosteal implant. Notice how part of the implant passes "through the bone."

the complete denture. This procedure is not performed as frequently any more as a result of the evolution of the endosteal or root form implant.

Transosteal implant A dental implant that penetrates both cortical plates and passes through the full thickness of the alveolar bone of the mandible.

Subperiosteal

A **subperiosteal dental implant** is another type of implant that rests on top of

Subperiosteal dental implant

> An eposteal (on top of the bone) dental implant that is placed beneath the periosteum and overlying the bony cortex

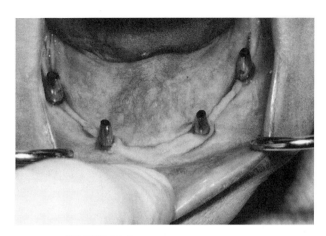

FIGURE 31.3
Clinical view of a subperiosteal implant.

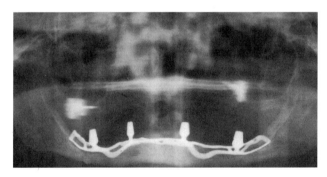

FIGURE 31.4
Panoramic radiograph of a subperiosteal implant. Notice how the implant sets on top of the mandible.

the bone, but beneath the oral tissues (Figures 31.3 and 31.4). This procedure is also usually done in a hospital setting under general anesthesia. The surgical procedure for placement usually calls for two steps.

The first step requires opening the tissue to expose the bone for the purpose of obtaining a direct impression of the bone. From this impression, the framework of the implant is fabricated. The second step involves reopening the gingival flap and placing the implant on top of the bone. The gingiva is then sewn together, thus burying the implant beneath the oral tissues. Recent advances in computer tomography (CT) have been used to obtain a computer-generated model of the mandible for implant framework fabrication, thus eliminating the first surgical appointment. These frameworks have posts that protrude into the oral cavity for purposes of securing the bridgework or denture.

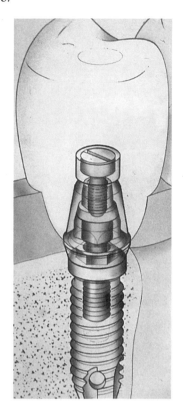

FIGURE 31.5
Diagram of an endosteal screw-shaped implant. (Diagram printed with permission of Nobel Biocare, Inc.)

Endosteal

A third type of implant is an **endosteal dental implant**. Endosteal means "into the bone"; these types can have a variety of shapes (Figure 31.5). Some are blade-shaped, but most that are in use today look like artificial tooth roots. These can be either smooth cylinders, screws, or a combination of both. This type of implant is placed directly into the bone, usually under local anesthesia in the dental office. After making an incision in the tissue to expose the bone, a series of water-cooled drills are used to prepare a hole in the bone where the implant is to be placed. The implant is either pressed into place or screwed into the site. Afterwards, the gingiva is sewn together to allow healing of the surgical site without stress. This area is left undisturbed for up to 6 months, depending

Endosteal
dental implant

Implant placed directly into the alveolar and basal bone of the maxilla or mandible, transacting only one cortical plate. Endosteal means "into the bone"

Osseointegration

The process and resultant direct connection of the surface of an exogenous material and the host bone tissues, without intervening fibrous connective tissue present

on the site. If the healing is successful, a direct bone-to-implant interface will be established, a term called **osseointegration**. After healing and periodic radiographic and clinical examination during this initial phase of treatment, a second minor surgical procedure, called Stage II surgery, is done under local anesthesia to uncover the top of the implant. At this stage, gingival healing caps or abutments are placed to provide some means for securing the final prosthesis to the implants. These components provide a patent opening through the gingiva. The tissue surrounding the implant requires about 2 to 3 weeks of healing.

Patients who inquire about dental implants must be examined carefully, both clinically and radiographically. Time should be taken to explain the procedures associated with the surgery and restorative phases of the treatment. If the patient has unobtainable restorative expectations, psychiatric problems, or is debilitated by disease causing them to be a surgical risk, treatment using dental implants is contraindicated. Only patients who understand the risks in-

Implant surgery

The phase of implant dentistry concerning the selection, planning, and placement of the implant body and abutment.

Most implant systems in use today use a two-stage implant where the implant body is first surgically placed (Stage I) and covered by the oral tissues until healing is complete. Then it is uncovered with a second surgery (Stage II) to attach the abutment.

volved with the procedures and who are motivated to maintain proper oral hygiene around the implant and prosthodontic reconstruction should be considered for such treatment.

ROLE OF THE DENTAL ASSISTANT IN DENTAL IMPLANTOLOGY

The dental assistant plays an important role in the team concept of providing **implant surgery** and implant prostheses for patients. When patients initially inquire about implants for themselves, they will usually ask office personnel, such as the dental assistant. Patient information pamphlets, instructional videos, or pho-

tographs of clinical cases can be helpful adjuncts in answering basic questions concerning the benefits associated with implants. Auxiliaries can obtain necessary information, such as patient medical and dental histories, radiographs, and making impressions. These data aid the dentist in the clinical examination and determination of the plan of treatment for these patients. The clinical examination involves examination of hard and soft tissues (existing teeth and periodontium), vestibular depth, and position of muscle attachments, among other aspects to be evaluated. Special examination forms are sometimes used as diagnostic data is charted for the prospective implant patient.

Diagnostic Evaluation

Radiographs or diagnostic imaging are an important diagnostic tool when evaluating a patient for implant placement and reconstruction. Use of periapical, panoramic, occlusal, and lateral cephalometric radiographs provide important information for the practitioner. They help identify structures, such as the floor of the maxillary sinus, floor of nasal cavity, mental foramen, and the mandibular canal. This aids in measurements to determine the length of implant that can be used in certain areas of the mouth. The dentist can also evaluate trabeculation patterns of the bone by using a quality radiographic image. This can be used to determine if additional implants are necessary or if they can fit in a particular area based on identification of certain structures. If additional diagnostic imaging is necessary, computer tomography is used to provide cross-sectional views of the mandible or maxilla. These images are normally provided by equipment found in hospitals or regional diagnostic imaging centers. A radiographic imaging template is sometimes used to aid the dentist in diagnosis and treatment planning. This is easily fabricated in the office and is commonly delegated to auxiliary personnel (Box 31.1 and Table 31.1).

Certain minimum requirements in bone thickness and height must be followed to obtain a predictable and successful surgical outcome. Opinions vary on the amount of bone needed for placement of implants. Generally, bone that is 6 mm in width buccolingually, 8 mm in width between natural teeth, and 10 mm in height, either above the mandibular nerve or below the maxillary sinus, is necessary to achieve a predictable result. The restorative dentist provides information that will help guide the most ideal placement and position of the implant to the implant surgeon. Commonly, a preliminary diagnostic model using either denture teeth or teeth carved from wax is used to facilitate fabrication of a **surgical template**

Surgical template

Guide used to assist in proper surgical placement and angulation of dental implants

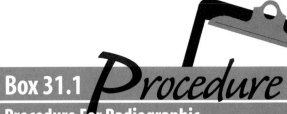

Box 31.1 *Procedure*

Procedure For Radiographic Template Fabrication

1. An accurate impression of the arch in question is made with irreversible hydrocolloid.
2. A model is poured in the dentist's choice of stone.
3. A clear plastic template using a thermoplastic material is formed over the cast under vacuum pressure. Visible light-cured material or autopolymerizing resins can also be used for this procedure.
4. Stainless steel ball bearings of known diameter are secured to the template with cyanoacrylate cement (Figure 31.6, *A*). These should be secured on the template adjacent to where the implants are proposed to be surgically placed. These areas are sited on the cast by the restorative dentist and the oral surgeon.
5. A panoramic radiograph is then taken with the device in place in the patient's mouth (Figure 31.6, *B*). If needed, a lateral cephalometric or an occlusal film can also be taken in those situations where anterior mandibular implants are planned.

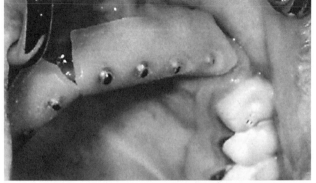

A

B

FIGURE 31.6

A, Radiographic stent in place for maxillary arch. Stainless steel ball bearings have been secured to the stent. **B,** Panoramic radiograph of patient with stent in place. (Photograph reprinted with permission of Nobel Biocare, Inc.)

(guide) before implant surgery. In this way, the implants can be placed in the most esthetic and functional position to ensure a predictable result with the final restoration (Box 31.2).

Table 31.1

Evaluation of Radiographic Template Fabrication

Radiographic Template Fabrication	4	3	2	0	X
Secure materials.					
Secure impression.					
Pour model.					
Form clear plastic template over cast (vacuum pressure or visible light-cured).					
Secure stainless steel ball bearings to template (as sited by operator).					
Take panoramic radiograph.					

The numeric criteria: 4 Excellent; 3 Good but some improvement can be made; 2 Below average, usable. needs to improve skill; 0 Unsatisfactory; X Not able to evaluate.

Box 31.2

Procedure

Procedure for Construction of Diagnostic Templates for Surgery and Treatment Planning

A. For Patients with Fully Edentulous Arches:

1. Impressions of the patient's arches are made in irreversible hydrocolloid or in vinyl polysiloxane impression material.

2. Pour the impressions in dental stone and allow to set completely.

3. After separation and trimming the cast on the model trimmer, baseplates are fabricated either using self-curing poly-methylmethacrylate (PMMA) tray resin or visible light-cured tray material (Figure 31.7).

4. Baseplate fabrication

   a. **PMMA:** Examine the cast with the dentist. Block out with wax any undercuts or thin areas on the cast that are subject to fracture or may interfere with removal of the baseplate. Mix the powder and monomer as per manufacturer's directions allowing the material to reach a doughy consistency. Roll the material on a flat surface to obtain a thickness of about 1 to 2 mm. Apply tinfoil, tinfoil substitute, or petroleum jelly on the model.

   Adapt the material using greased fingers onto the cast, allowing for some excess to extend beyond the borders of the cast. Using a sharp scalpel, trim some of the extra material while it is still doughy.

   After trimming, allow the material to set completely. The tray will feel warm to the touch at the final stage of curing. Remove gently from the cast and trim the borders of the baseplate with acrylic burs using a slow-speed handpiece, laboratory engine, or lathe. Polish the baseplate with wet pumice on a rag wheel to smooth the adjusted flanges.

   b. **VLC trays:** Examine the cast with the dentist. Block out with wax any undercuts or thin areas on the cast that are subject to fracture or may interfere

with removal of the baseplate. Remove a sheet of uncured material from the package. Trim a horseshoe or oval shaped piece of material and begin adapting to a lightly greased stone model. Once the material is adapted to the cast, place the cast into the light curing unit and cure as per manufacturer's directions, usually for 6 to 10 minutes, depending on thickness and type of material used.

   After curing, gently remove from the cast and trim the excess from the baseplate with acrylic burs using a slow speed handpiece, laboratory engine, or lathe. Polish the baseplate with wet pumice on a rag wheel to smooth the adjusted flanges.

   c. Occlusion rims are now adapted to the baseplate by first placing sticky wax on areas of the baseplate that lie over the crest of the ridge. This will allow better adaptation of the baseplate wax and prevent it from coming away from the baseplate. Either using a pre-formed arch of baseplate wax or using a sheet of wax that is warmed and rolled up, adapt the wax to the base-plate to create a rim of wax about 3 to 4 mm in thickness in the anterior and about 6 to 8 mm in thickness in the posterior. The maxillary rim should be about 22 mm in height and the mandibular rim should be about 18 mm in height

4. The dentist will then take measurements from the patient to determine the *vertical dimension of occlusion* that is most comfortable for that patient. After obtaining an interocclusal record and transferring this maxillomandibular relationship to the articulator by means of a *facebow*, dentist and patient will confer on tooth selection. A shade and *mold* is selected that is based on evalua-

Box 31.2—Cont'd.

Procedure

Procedure for Construction of Diagnostic Templates for Surgery and Treatment Planning

tion of the arch size, patient's facial outline, hair color, skin color, and any previous records that will facilitate the selection process.

5. A wax denture try-in appointment is necessary to evaluate phonetics and reevaluate the esthetics and vertical dimension established for the patient at the previous appointment. If acceptable to both patient and dentist, a surgical stent is made based on the tooth position in the trial wax denture.

6. The waxed denture may be modified by the following methods:
   a. In the mandibular waxed denture, remove the molar denture teeth and the underlying baseplate. This provides stability for the stent while in position during the surgical phase of implant treatment.
   b. In the maxillary waxed denture, remove the palate of the baseplate. This will allow direct contact of the stent with the ridge or hard palate of the patient to facilitate stabilization during surgery.

7. Using irreversible hydrocolloid, make an impression of the newly-modified trial waxed denture. These impressions are used to pour clear orthodontic resin, readapted to the cast, and allowed to completely set. The impression is removed from the cast. The clear acrylic denture is removed, trimmed, and polished before disinfection/sterilization.

8. An acrylic template can be fabricated with either vacuum-assisted clear thermoplastic material (.080") or with clear VLC sheet material. A stone model of the

trial denture in wax is needed for this technique. These are easily adjusted as needed with scissors, scalpel, or acrylic burs. It is important that these surgical stents be properly disinfected or sterilized to prevent cross-contamination during implant surgery.

B. For Patients with Partially Dentulous Arches:
   1. After mounting the casts via facebow transfer and interocclusal records on the articulator of choice, wax prosthetic teeth into the edentulous area(s). Spare denture teeth work very nicely for this procedure. They can be easily adjusted with acrylic burs to fit most any arch configuration. The denture teeth are placed using the adjacent teeth and opposing occlusion as a guide to ensure esthetics and function.
   2. Using irreversible hydrocolloid, make an impression of the diagnostic model in a stock tray. The diagnostic model may require soaking in water for 5 to 10 minutes before making the impression so the alginate will not stick to the model. After completely set, separate the impression from the cast and pour the impression in dental stone. This is allowed to set completely. The new cast is removed from the impression and trimmed on a model trimmer.
   3. An acrylic template can be fabricated with either vacuum, assisted clear thermoplastic material or with clear VLC sheet material. These are easily adjusted with scissors, scalpel, or acrylic burs. It is important that these surgical templates be properly disinfected or sterilized to prevent cross contamination during implant surgery.

IMPLANT SURGERY

The surgical aspect of implantology to obtain a predictable result of uneventful healing and successful restoration of the implants depends on the initial phase of implant therapy.

Use of a sterile and standardized implant surgical technique with proper handling of instruments and implant fixtures and, most important, a well-trained surgical dental assistant are necessary to ensure the ease of placement of the implants during surgery.

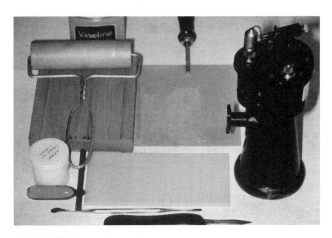

FIGURE 31.7

To fabricate baseplates, materials needed include self-curing tray resin or VLC tray material, baseplate wax, waxing instruments, laboratory knife, petroleum jelly, board, and roller.

Procedures for Implant Surgery

Before seating the patient, the operatory must be properly disinfected and outfitted with the instrumentation necessary for the surgical procedure involved to place the implants. Instruments and materials are unwrapped. Drill motors are appropriately covered and run to dispose of excess oils and to determine that the equipment is operating properly. Syringe, anesthetic, and gauze are made ready. If the patient requires intravenous sedation, the armamentaria for this procedure is available. Any instruments for bone preparation have been placed on a separate tray that is covered until ready for use. This tray includes a mirror, scalpel, periosteal elevator, tweezers, scissors, bone file, Rongeurs, and any other item that the surgeon may require.

A second tray contains all burs and other necessary items to prepare the bone site and place the dental implant. It remains covered or is ready until after the surgeon has prepared the surgical site and is ready to begin the procedure for implant site drilling.

The patient has already been thoroughly evaluated and has been cleared as an acceptable patient for the procedure. The patient may require premedication before the appointment. After the patient is seated and vital signs are taken, he or she is draped and reassured by the dental assistant. Any last minute questions are discussed with the surgeon. An informed consent form is read by the patient, witnessed by the assistant, and signed by both. Box 31.3 explains the procedure for implant surgery.

Follow up Procedures

The patient should be seen routinely during the healing of the implants. The surgical site is examined for signs of swelling, purulence, and redness. Radiographs may be taken once or twice during the healing to ensure no underlying problems are occurring. If the patient is wearing a prosthesis, soft liners can be changed to maintain their softness and minimize stress on the mucosa. The patient should maintain a well-balanced diet to aid overall health and should also refrain from smoking. Patients who smoke show a higher incidence of implant failure.

The surgical site must remain undisturbed for about 4 to 6 months, depending on the operative site. Any pain or swelling noticed during this time must be addressed to minimize risk to the implant or adjacent implants.

Abutment Connection (Stage II)

If proper healing has occurred and the patient has been asymptomatic during the 4 to 6 month healing phase, the patient is now ready to proceed with the next phase of treatment, which involves exposing the implant for abutment connection.

Abutments are screwed, cemented, or tapped into the implant, depending on the system used, to facilitate attachment of the final prosthesis.

The surgical tray consists of instrumentation commonly used, with some additions, in other oral surgery procedures that require removal or manipulation of soft tissue. Anesthetic syringe, mirror, scalpel, cotton forceps, scissors, suture material, elevators, and bone file are among the armamentaria necessary for this procedure. Other rotary instruments are made available in case of need in this procedure. For example, if the doctor finds bone has grown over the top of the implant, preventing easy removal of the cover screw, the bone will have to be removed either by rotary instrumentation or with hand debridement. Copious irrigation is necessary if rotary drills are used. This will prevent the bone and implant from overheating. Care must be exercised to prevent damage to the top of the implant. If damaged, it could prevent proper abutment connection to the implant.

The patient is seated in the dental chair and is draped. Any prostheses that the patient is wearing are removed and set aside. If required, the patient has been premedicated. The surgical site is anesthetized by the doctor, either with local infiltration or using a nerve block.

After palpating the surgical site, the doctor uncovers the implant face by using tissue punch or a scalpel to open a tissue flap to expose the orifice of each implant (see Figure 31.13). As previously mentioned, any bone that covers the cover screw is removed using hand or rotary debridement.

Once uncovered, the cover screw is removed and replaced, usually with a sterile gingival healing cap (see Figure 31.14). Depending on the implant system that is being used, this is screwed into place, temporarily cemented, or press fit to obturate the opening and prevent down

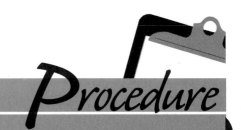

Box 31.3

Procedure for Implant Surgery

1. The patient is anesthetized and given other sedatives, as needed, to ease the anxiety of the surgical procedure. After determining that the patient is comfortable and vital signs are stable, the surgeon is ready to begin.
2. An incision is made in the gingival tissues and a flap is reflected to expose the bone. During this procedure, proper visualization of the site is important. High-speed evacuation is used to retract and to keep the surgical site as clean as possible.
3. If a surgical stent has been prepared, it is placed at this time to determine the site location and angulation of the implant. A pilot or guide drill is then used first to create a pilot hole. This enables the surgeon to use other drills with increasing diameters to establish the proper size and depth for implant placement. It is important to keep copious irrigation on the drill during site preparation. Overheating the bone may lead to implant failure. Research has shown that if bone is heated beyond 47 degrees Celsius, cell necrosis will occur and a fibrous connective tissue may be produced between the implant and the bone. This will lead to a loss of direct contact of the bone to the implant.
4. Once the size has been determined, the site is checked with a *depth gauge* for accuracy. If additional drilling is necessary, it is done at this time, again pious irrigation during drilling. The size is again checked for accuracy of fit (Figure 31.8).
5. If the implant-type, the implant site has to be readied to accept the thread of the screw (Figure 31.9). This procedure uses a slowly rotating bone tap drill in the handpiece. Once the bottom is reached, it is reversed so as to not strip the threads that this instrument is creating. The implant is then removed from its sterile package and threaded into the site. A healing screw is placed in the top of the implant to prevent bone and tissue from growing into the internal threads of the implant (Figure 31.10).
6. If the implant is a press-fit type, the implant is removed from its sterile package and gently placed into the receptor site in the bone (Figure 31.11). Sometimes a gentle tap is necessary using a blunt instrument to ensure that it is completely seated. A healing screw is placed in the top of the implant to prevent bone and tissue from growing into the internal threads of the implant.
7. The surgical site is rinsed. The surgeon then replaces the gingival tissue flap and sutures are placed to ensure primary closure.
8. The patient is given home care instructions and prescriptions to ease postoperative discomfort.
9. The patient is asked not to wear any prosthesis over the surgical site for 1 week. Later, if the patient is wearing a full denture, the denture is adjusted to accept a temporary soft lining material to cushion and protect the surgical site during healing. Sutures are usually removed within 10 to14 days (Figure 31.12).

growth of gingival tissues. If screw-retained, the screw is placed using the instrumentation compatible with the system. A hexagonal wrench or small flat screwdriver are the most common types of instruments used for this purpose.

Healing caps are available in a variety of lengths to allow for differences in thickness of the gingival tissue. Once the healing cap is in place, the tissues are closed with suture material, as needed. The surgical site is reevaluated 1 to 2 weeks later. If the patient is wearing a prosthesis over the implant site(s), the prosthesis is relieved additionally and a temporary liner is placed in the denture to provide patient comfort as tissue healing occurs.

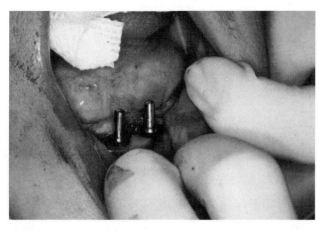

FIGURE 31.8

The implant sites are checked for orientation within the bone and alignment with each other.

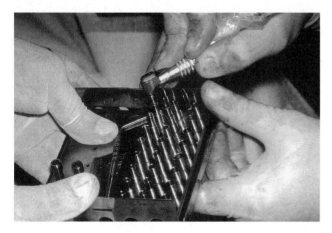

FIGURE 31.9

The assistant helps the surgeon with drill placement into the handpiece.

Prosthodontic Treatment

Healing abutments are usually the primary abutment of choice at Stage II. Following tissue healing, definitive abutment selection and placement can be performed after careful measurement of the tissue surrounding the healing cap. Once the abutment is placed, a provisional restoration can be placed for a single tooth or a multiple implant bridge while awaiting the final prosthesis.

Single Implant/Multiple Implant Restoration for a Partially Dentate Patient

This type of implant restoration is indicated when one or more teeth are missing as a result of trauma, extraction, or

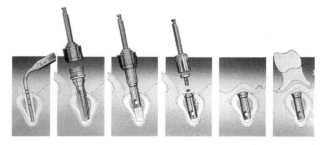

FIGURE 31.10

Diagram of surgical sequence starting with checking the depth of the site preparation; the bone is tapped and the implant is placed using a special tool; the surgical site is closed using sutures; the denture is lined with soft liner and worn until healing is complete, usually 3 to 6 months, depending on the location. (Photograph reprinted with permission of Nobel Biocare, Inc.)

congenital abnormality. With proper planning, implants can be a successful treatment modality for these types of situations.

Assuming a treatment plan of implant surgery was successful and second stage surgery was equally uneventful, the dentist is now prepared to finalize treatment. At this point, the patient is usually anxious to complete treatment. The patient should be reassured that treatment is progressing as planned and their patience is appreciated as the dentist works toward completion.

The tray setup needed for this procedure consists of the following:

- Mirror
- High-speed handpiece
- Large crown and bridge mirror
- Low-speed handpiece
- #23 explorer
- Diamond burs
- #17 explorer
- Abrasive stones
- Cotton forceps
- Sandpaper discs
- Air/water syringe tips
- Implant wrench/driver
- Articulating ribbon forceps
- Impression material
- Cord packing instrument
- Retraction cord
- Curette
- Implant components
- Spoon excavator

Impressions for implant restoration can be performed before or after the dentist selects the type of abutment best suited for the patient. If the dentist decides to select the abutment before the impression, careful measurement of the tissue is necessary after healing has taken place following second stage surgery (see Figure 31.15). This is needed so the

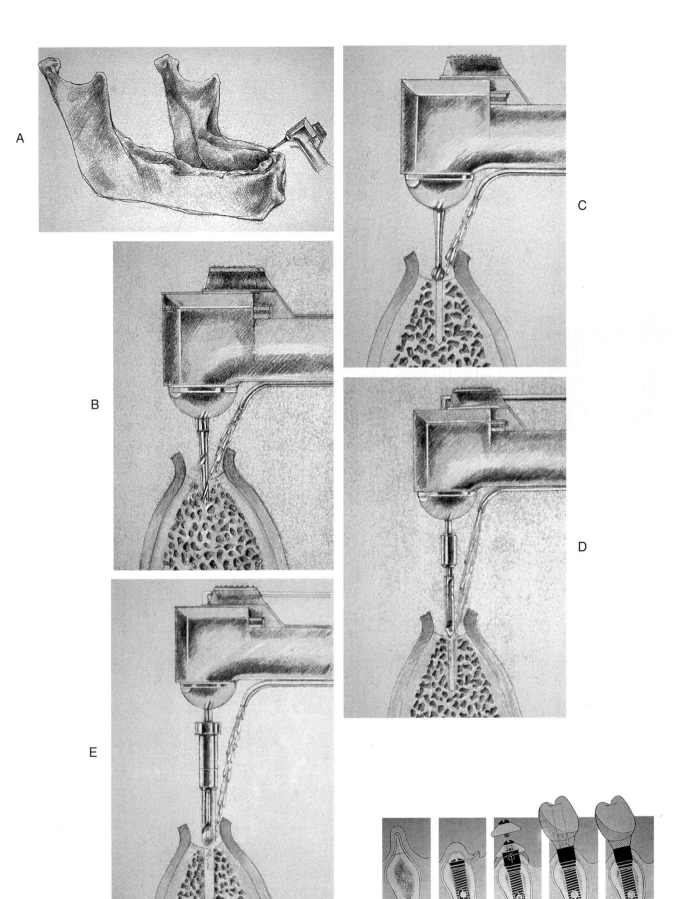

A

B

C

D

E

FIGURE 31.11

Diagram of implant surgery for a press-fit cylindrical implant. (Courtesy Sulzer Calcitek, Inc.)

FIGURE 31.12

Diagrammatic illustration showing sequence before and after implant surgery. (Courtesy Nobel Biocare, Inc.)

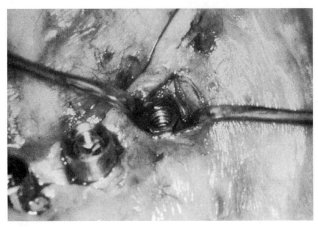

FIGURE 31.13

Dentist uncovers implant to expose the top of the implant.

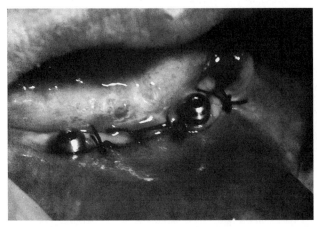

FIGURE 31.14

Healing cuff in place and sutures placed after uncovering implants in mandible.

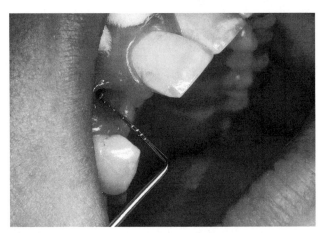

FIGURE 31.15

Measurement of tissue depth using a metal periodontal probe.

proper abutment size, based on tissue thickness, can be placed. The abutment in secured onto the implant either with an abutment seating tool using finger pressure or with a torque wrench set at a predetermined amount of force as described by the manufacturer. These components are highly machined by the manufacturer and provide a precision fit when seated.

If a fixed abutment is used for a cementable prosthesis, the abutment is placed and prepared with a high-speed diamond under water irrigation intraorally to establish the margin thickness and desired design. Some dentists may prefer to remove the abutment after gross reduction has been performed to further refine the margin design. This is one of the advantages of using detachable components with implant systems. The impression is then treated like any conventional crown and bridge impression, including use of retraction cord (Chapter 28).

If the prosthesis is to be screw-retained, the same protocol is followed as for the cementable prosthesis. Before obtaining the impression, an abutment transfer coping is screwed onto the abutment. This arrangement can now be transferred to a model or cast by means of the impression to provide the dentist with the proper relationship of the implant to the remaining teeth in the arch (Box 31.4).

Securing an Impression

The impression is made using either a custom impression tray or a plastic disposable tray with a highly accurate impression material, such as polyvinyl siloxane or polyether. The clinical instrumentation needed for impression procedure is similar to the instruments used for crown and bridge procedures. Usually, no tissue retraction is necessary for implant impressions. A light-bodied material is syringed around the **impression (transfer) coping(s).** The tray is filled with putty or with a heavy-bodied material. The tray is inserted over the implant transfer coping(s) and the material is allowed to set for the allotted time according to the manufacturer's recommendation.

Impression coping

The component of a dental implant system that is used to provide a spatial relationship of an endosteal dental implant to the alveolar ridge and adjacent dentition or other structures. Impression copings can be retained in the impression or may require a transfer from intraoral usage to the impression after attaching the analog or replicas.

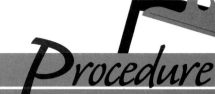

Box 31.4

Procedure for Custom Impression Tray Fabrication

1. On a diagnostic cast, adapt two layers of baseplate wax. These are warmed over a flame or in a hot water bath until soft. Extend the wax over the teeth and about 2 to 3 mm beyond the free gingival margin. Trim away the excess wax with a sharp, warmed knife. Using a hot instrument, sear the wax to the cast and smooth the periphery.

2. On the occlusal surface of the wax, cut squares about 3 mm x 3 mm in four locations, usually one over each canine area and one over each first or second molar. This will help stabilize the tray when it is completely seated in the mouth for the impression.

3. A layer of tin foil is placed over the wax or a thin coat of petroleum jelly is placed over the wax to prevent the acrylic from sticking.

4. Mix autopolymerizing tray resin according to manufacturer's specifications and apply to cast. Small increments of material are first plugged into the holes created on the occlusal surface. Then apply the remainder of the material. A thickness of about 2 to 3 mm of resin is needed for strength. Using excess tray resin, form a handle using some monomer to moisten both surfaces to be joined. A cotton swab works to moisten the doughy resin when applying the handle before complete curing.

   Visible light-cured resin can be used for this, also, in place of the autopolymerizing tray resin. This material comes packaged in light-proof sheets to simplify handling. An adequate thickness of material is also necessary to maintain a sturdy impression tray. This material is removed from the package and adapted around the cast. Any excess material can be removed and repackaged for future use. A handle can be applied to the remainder of the tray before placing in the light chamber for completion. Follow manufacturer's suggested curing times for the material used.

5. After curing, trim the excess material with appropriate acrylic burs until smooth. Additional smoothness can be achieved using a wet rag wheel and pumice.

6. The tray is tried into the mouth to check for accuracy of fit. It should be stable and without noticeable movement when resting on the teeth. If it is determined that the impression coping is too tall and prevents the impression tray from seating, a hole is cut in the tray to allow for additional room for this component (Figure 31.16).

The majority of impression materials available are easily dispensed using the cartridge gun assembly, which controls the flow of material and reduces waste. After the impression is set, it is removed, inspected for accuracy, disinfected before leaving the clinical area, and placed in a container.

Master Cast

The impression or mold is used to fabricate a master cast from which the final restoration is made. The impression is boxed for shipment to a laboratory. A laboratory prescription is enclosed to instruct the dental technician what the dentist wants for the final prosthesis. This is a written directive by the dentist to be followed by the technician for the fabrication of the prosthesis. Included in the text of the pre-

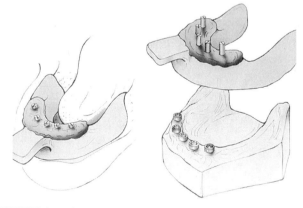

FIGURE 31.16

Screws must be unscrewed to allow removal of impression. This technique achieves a highly accurate impression. (Courtesy Nobel Biocare, Inc.)

scription are such things as porcelain shade, implant type, type of metal to be used, type of abutment that is used or should be included, and other specifications that are deemed pertinent to fabrication of the crown or bridge.

When the restoration is returned from the laboratory, it is checked for accuracy of fit to the cast. The prescription is rechecked to ensure that directions were followed as prescribed by the dentist. If any question arises concerning the prosthesis or prescription, a phone call to the laboratory is necessary. If a multiple unit implant prosthesis is to have porcelain or acrylic veneer, the metal framework must be tried in to insure a proper fit. This will require an additional appointment before treatment is finalized.

Insertion of the Prosthesis

The patient is seated and draped. The tray setup should include any instruments used in crown and bridge procedures, similar to the tray setup that was previously mentioned. If the patient has been wearing a provisional prosthesis, it is removed and any temporary cement is cleaned from the abutments. The prosthesis is placed to determine accuracy and passivity of fit with the **implant abutment.**

Implant abutment

The portion of a dental implant that serves to support and retain any prosthesis

If the prosthesis is to be cemented, it is seated to determine the need for adjustments in occlusion and proximal contacts. Any alterations are made with appropriate stones or diamonds, and the surface is repolished to the previous luster. After the patient has approved the final product, including shape, color, and relationship to adjacent teeth, it is cemented into place onto the implant abutment using either temporary or permanent crown and bridge cement.

If the prosthesis is to be screw-retained, it is seated in a similar fashion, but by using screws to secure the prosthesis into place. Occlusion and proximal contacts are evaluated and adjusted, as needed. The final prosthesis is polished and secured into place with a screw. Waiting 5 to 10 minutes before final tightening is recommended before covering the access hole. A small increment of gutta percha stopping compound or low viscosity impression material works well in obturating the access hole with a final covering of autopolymerizing methylmethacrylate resin or visible light-cured resin.

Occlusion is rechecked if the access hole covering will be involved in the patient's occlusion. Adjustments are performed as necessary and the surface is polished.

Implant Restoration for the Edentulous Maxilla and Mandible

When a patient is totally edentulous (without teeth) and is wearing complete dentures, they may have some degree of

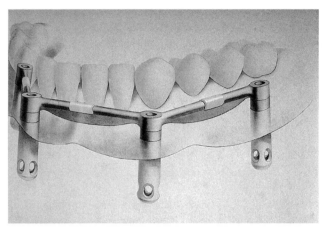

FIGURE 31.17

Diagram of an overdenture. (Courtesy Sulzer Calcitek, Inc.)

difficulty with function, retention, and comfort. A patient with severely resorbed ridges, thin ridges, high muscle attachments, or other anatomical deficiencies may have to resort to adhesives to stabilize the dentures. This sometimes creates other problems in maintenance of the dentures (Chapter 30).

The use of dental implants can aid in securing a complete denture for those patients who otherwise cannot wear and function with a conventional denture. As few as two implants are sufficient to hold an overdenture securely. An overdenture is any complete denture that covers and rests or is partially supported by natural teeth, tooth roots, and dental implants (Figure 31.17). An overdenture can be used with two implants that are freestanding, or can be used if two or more implants are connected by a gold bar. If sufficient bone exists, it is possible to place a number of implants (6 to 8) in an arch to allow a completely fixed prosthesis.

Careful planning through examination of the patient evaluation of diagnostic imaging, consideration of past dental history, and discussion of treatment options with the patient are necessary before surgical and prosthetic treatment using dental implants.

As previously discussed, the diagnostic full denture wax try-in is a critical step in planning. This aids the dentist in the determination of implant site location and the number of implants to be used.

Information obtained will also have an influence on the type of implant prosthesis. For example, if only two or three implants can be placed, the treatment used will be an overdenture with the implants used with an attachment to enhance retention. Where possible, it is best to unite the implants with a bar to distribute the forces associated with mastication more evenly between the implants. Rubber, metal, or plastic attachments are available in a variety of shapes and sizes to facilitate securing the overdenture to the implant bar.

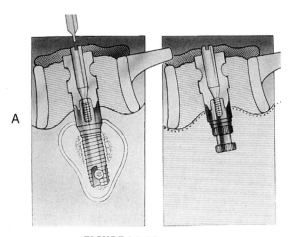

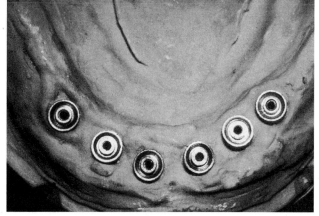

FIGURE 31.18

A, Diagram showing cross-section of impression posts and analogs. **B,** Impression showing position of impression posts and analogs. (Courtesy Nobel Biocare, Inc.)

Impressions

After Stage II surgery, the patient has gingival healing cuffs in place. These can be removed and replaced with implant abutments. If a bar interconnecting the implants is planned, an abutment that is specific for this type of restoration is placed. Usually, a screw-in type that has a finished edge is preferred. The abutments are placed and abutment impression copings are secured to each abutment. A custom tray is then used with the doctor's impression material of choice. This can be polysulfide, polyvinyl Siloxane, or polyether. After determining the impression to be acceptable, the impression copings are removed and temporary housings are placed over the abutments while the bar is being fabricated. If the patient is wearing a prosthesis over the implant site, it must be adapted to allow room for the added height of the abutments. By using autopolymerizing temporary soft lining materials, this not only aids in patient comfort, but can add some retention to the interim prosthesis with the aid of the implant abutments.

Trying in the Gold Bar

The bar is made using conventional crown and bridge techniques and is tried in after receiving it from the laboratory. The fit must be passive. The best way to determine this is to try it in using only one screw at a time. By visualizing the coping on the unsecured side, one can make a determination on the accuracy of fit. It must be flush with the finished edge of the machined abutment. This is similar to checking the fit of a fixed partial denture using natural teeth abutments. When seated completely, it must be stable and have no visible movement when either abutment is depressed. An explorer tip is used to check accuracy as well. No gap should be evident between the gold bar and the abutment.

If an inaccuracy is detected, the bar is sectioned, keyed back to its proper position with a luting agent, and returned to the laboratory for soldering by the technician.

Once a passive fit is obtained, the next step is to finalize vertical relationships for that patient, obtain proper centric relation jaw records, select denture mold and shade (if this has not been done previously), and try-in the trial denture for patient acceptance. Once esthetics and phonetics are determined to be acceptable to both patient and doctor, the dentures are returned to the laboratory for processing in the desired denture base shade.

The attachment mechanism to be employed can be placed by the laboratory during processing of the denture resin. On delivery by the dentist, if the attachments do not align themselves with the bar or abutments that prevents seating of the prosthesis, attachments can be removed and reattached to the denture with autopolymerizing PMMA or with a light-cured resin.

Fixed Detachable Restoration

The impression technique is the same employed for multiple implants using a bar restoration (Figure 31.18). When dealing with multiple implants, care must be taken to accurately reproduce and transfer the implant position onto the master cast. A heavier viscosity impression material may be used to help stabilize the impression transfer copings.

Once the master cast has been poured with the abutment analogs in place, the next step is to measure and establish the vertical relationship for the patient using complete denture prosthodontic principles. Teeth are selected and a centric jaw record is made. The mandibular occlusal rim is usually attached with one screw to the abutment during this recording to prevent movement. A wax try-in is the next appointment to determine if esthetics, phonetics, and the jaw records are acceptable.

The key is to ensure passivity of the superstructure on the implants. Any inaccuracy not corrected can be detrimental to the longevity of one or more implants. Based on the preliminary wax up employed at the diagnostic planning stage of treatment, the superstructure is waxed and cast in a gold alloy. Mechanical retention for PMMA is required to permit the denture teeth and denture base resin to be processed to the superstructure.

The superstructure will usually have distal cantilevers (pontic retained and supported on one end only) to permit placement of posterior teeth. The length of the cantilever will be dependent on the length, diameter, and position of the dental implants, as well as the number of implants in the arch. The shape of the cantilever resembles an I-beam used in building construction. This configuration gives maximum strength to the unsupported portion of the bar.

Similar to planning the position of the bar for implant overdentures, the pattern design for the framework superstructure is dictated by the tooth arrangement previously evaluated during the wax try-in. A silicone-putty index of the denture teeth can provide the technician with the information for positioning the framework in its relationship to the denture teeth. Sufficient space must be present to allow processing of denture resin to attach the teeth. The tissue surface of the superstructure must be of a convex shape to allow easier cleaning by the patient.

Once it is determined that the framework fits passively on the implant abutments, the denture teeth can be waxed into place for one final try-in to reevaluate the tooth position and their functional relationship with the opposing arch. If this is acceptable, the waxed framework is returned to the laboratory for processing and finishing.

Insertion is usually uneventful if care has been taken to ensure an accurate fit of the prosthesis to the implants. Occlusion may require refinement and the teeth can be polished in the office. Access holes in the lingual portion of the prosthesis can be filled with composite. These are finished and polished with appropriate abrasives to a smooth surface. Oral hygiene instructions are given and appropriate follow up visits are scheduled.

MAINTENANCE OF DENTAL IMPLANTS

After completion of the restoration using dental implants, the patient must demonstrate meticulous oral hygiene to minimize plaque accumulation around the implant(s) or prosthesis. Dental implants are no different than natural teeth in regards to hygiene. Both require daily cleaning to remove food debris and plaque. To facilitate plaque removal, a variety of brushes, flossing materials, and irrigation devices are available for the patient. Individual dexterity and ability must be evaluated before recommending a precise regimen of daily home care.

Emphasis on oral hygiene instructions must begin early in the treatment. Patients are instructed on proper wound care following Stage I and Stage II surgeries. As the healing cuffs and abutments are placed, the patient is given instruction with brush and floss to maintain proper plaque control

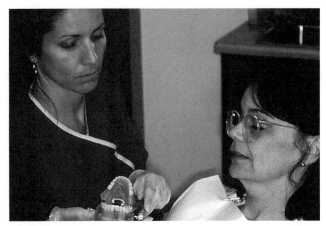

FIGURE 31.19

Assistant demonstrating proper oral hygiene technique to patient.

and gingival health around the implants and the prosthesis (Figure 31.19).

An antimicrobial agent, chlorhexidine, may be recommended and prescribed by the dentist for the patient who has dental implants—it is used to reduce the adherence of plaque to the implant abutment. During the healing phase after Stage II surgery, it can be prescribed as a rinse. Approximately $1/2$ ounce of solution used twice daily has been shown to be effective in minimizing plaque accumulation. However, rinsing with this agent can stain the natural teeth as well as the prosthesis. To avoid this problem following Stage II surgery, the chlorhexidine can be applied with a brush or floss directly onto the abutment.

Role of the Dental assistant in Maintenance

The dental assistant can help the patient in proper oral hygiene techniques. A combination of techniques can be shown to the patient, either directly, with the aid of patient brochures, or other visual aids. Instruct the patient to use a mirror with good lighting to help them visualize what and where they need to clean. Show them how to manipulate floss or ribbon between, under, and around the prosthesis and implant abutments. Demonstration by the dental assistant in the use of an interproximal brush can be another method of cleansing the implant abutments. Whatever the method, careful explanation and demonstration of techniques by the dental assistant is an integral part in the maintenance phase of implant restoration (Figure 31.20). By reassuring the patient as they demonstrate their ability to clean, patients will gain confidence in their ability to adequately clean around the implants without becoming frustrated.

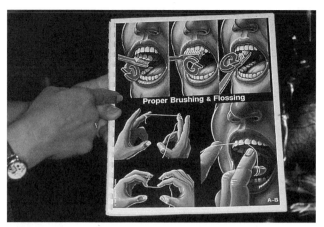

FIGURE 31.20

Dental assistant giving written instructions and home care instructions to the patient.

Another integral part in the maintenance of implants is periodic radiographs of the implant site. This is done to make sure no pathologic condition exists and that the bone level is not deteriorating. It is not unusual to lose a small amount of crestal bone during the first year following implant placement, usually ranging between 1 and 1.5 mm. The radiographic technique is important in recall visits so that the same angulation can be used to adequately determine if bone levels are changing. The paralleling technique is recommended to be used by the dental assistant when these images are taken. No evidence of radiolucency or changes in the pattern of bone trabeculation should be evident in these radiographs. After implant placement, radiographs are recommended every 4 to 6 months during the first year. After 1 year, they can be taken annually.

During recall visits, common findings that require intervention are gingivitis, hyperplastic tissue, surface of the implant exposed, loss of occlusal contact, and a variety of fractures of implant components. One of the most common findings is loose screws. These are easily tightened with the proper tool. However, if screw loosening continues to be a problem in subsequent recall visits, attention should be focussed on the passivity and accuracy of the fit of the prosthesis. In those instances where the prosthesis is screw-retained and better access is needed to clean the abutments, it is recommended that removal of the prosthesis be part of every recall visit. If a patient demonstrates good oral hygiene, this procedure may be performed annually.

Once the prosthesis is removed, especially in the fixed hybrid type of restoration, it can be easily cleaned with an ultrasonic cleaner. Heavier accumulations of calculus can be removed with special scalers that will not scratch the surface of the prosthesis or implant abutments. During this procedure with the prosthesis removed, the abutments should be examined for tightness. Once the prosthesis is cleaned, it is reevaluated for precision of fit. There must be no gap at the interface of the abutment and the prosthesis. Occlusion is again scrutinized to check for unusual wear. If sufficient wear is discovered, corrections are made to equilibrate the occlusion.

Instrumentation that is necessary for recall appointments will vary with each practitioner. The usual instruments required for an examination (miffor, explorers, cotton forceps, plastic periodontal prove) are sufficient with the addition of appropriate hex or slotted wrenches, scalers, or curettes (plastic) that can be used to remove calculus. A slow-speed handpiece with prophy cup may be used to lightly buff the implant abutments using prophy paste. Use caution, though, so as to not damage the interface between the prosthesis and the abutments.

The use of dental implants has revolutionized the practice of dentistry during the past decade. They are no longer considered experimental, and they allow practitioners a treatment alternative to offer their patients. Their success is based on several factors, including proper patient selection, using materials that are biocompatible with the oral tissues, following a precise surgical and prosthodontic regimen, and proper maintenance procedures.

The dental assistant plays an important role is providing this type of care for the dental patient. Educating the patient about dental implants is a job shared by all members of the dental office. It is one of many tasks that are performed by a highly skilled dental assistant. Chairside assistance and laboratory support are other important functions that a dental assistant provides. From initial consultation visit to recall maintenance visit, the dental assistant provides vital assistance in the team effort associated with dental implantology.

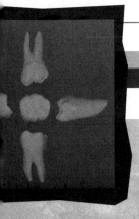

Points for Review

- Differences between the three types of dental implants
- Terminology associated with dental implant surgery
- Terminology associated with dental implant prosthodontics
- Technique associated with template and custom impression tray fabrication
- Maintenance procedures and oral hygiene reinforcement

Self-Study Questions

1. Implants can be used in which of the following indications?
   a. To replace a single missing tooth
   b. To stabilize a removable prosthesis
   c. To replace multiple missing teeth
   d. A and c only
   e. A, b, and c

2. Dental implants can be classified into what three types?
   a. Transosteal, subperiosteal, and endosteal
   b. Transosteal, staple, and endosteal
   c. Epidermal, mesodermal, and endodermal
   d. Eposteal, mesosteal, and endosteal
   e. None of the above

3. What are the possible shapes for an endosteal implant?
   a. Smooth cylindrical
   b. Blade
   c. Screw
   d. A and c only
   e. All of the above

4. Osseointegration is a term that describes which of the following?
   a. The type of healing that occurs when implants are successfully healed and created a direct bone-to-implant interface

   b. The type of healing that occurs when implants are successfully healed and create an interface between the bone and implant that has a periodontal ligament
   c. A way of combining implants and natural teeth with a specific type of bridge
   d. An implant that did not heal properly and was removed
   e. All of the above

5. When evaluating a patient for dental implants, which of the following diagnostic data aid in developing a treatment plan?
   a. Hard and soft tissue examination
   b. Radiographs or diagnostic imaging
   c. Models of the patient's dental arches
   d. Medical and dental history
   e. All of the above are important

6. When evaluating radiographs or diagnostic imaging for determination of implant placement, important structures that require identification do not include which of the following?
   a. Maxillary sinus
   b. Mental foramen
   c. Floor of the nasal cavity
   d. Mandibular canal
   e. Glenoid fossa

7. For implant patients who are completely edentulous, why is a diagnostic wax-up made first?
   a. To determine if the patient can wear dentures
   b. To help determine the proper site to place the implants
   c. To determine if the bite of the patient can be changed
   d. To determine if the patient's wrinkles can be removed
   e. None of the above

8. The surgical phase of implant treatment is extremely critical to ensure predictable healing. The surgical technique includes the all of following except which?
   a. A series of graduated drill sizes that are used with a slow-speed handpiece
   b. A series of graduated drill sizes that are used with a high-speed handpiece
   c. Copious irrigation to prevent the bone from overheating
   d. Maintaining sterile technique
   e. High-speed evacuation to help visualize the field during surgery

9. If the healing after implant surgery is uneventful, the implants are uncovered during Stage II surgery. This usually involves placement of which of the following?
   a. Gingival healing cuff or cap
   b. Abutment
   c. Final prosthesis
   d. Impression post
   e. None of the above

10. Which of the following statements regarding custom tray fabrication is false?
    a. A thickness of 2 to 3 mm of resin is needed for strength of the tray.
    b. One thickness of baseplate wax is required as a spacer over the diagnostic cast.
    c. Two thicknesses of baseplate wax are required as a spacer over the diagnostic cast.
    d. Small squares of wax are removed over three or four teeth in certain areas of the arch to aid in stabilization of the tray on insertion.
    e. Additional resin can be used to form a tray handle to facilitate removal after the impression material within the tray has set.

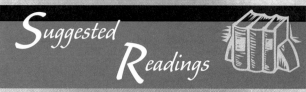

Cranin AN: *Atlas of oral implantology*, ed 2, St Louis, 1999, Mosby.
McKinney RV: *Endosteal dental implants*, St Louis, 1991, Mosby.
Misch CE: *Contemporary implant dentistry*, ed 2, St Louis, 1998, Mosby.
Spiekermann H: *Implantology*, New York, 1995, Thieme Medical Publishers.
Taylor TD, Laney WR: *Dental implants: are they for me?* Chicago, 1993, Quintessence.
Worthington, Philip, Lang, Brien R, and LaVelle WE: *Osseointegration in dentistry: an introduction*, Chicago, 1994, Quintessence.

Chapter 32

Dental Oncology and Maxillofacial Prosthetic Treatment

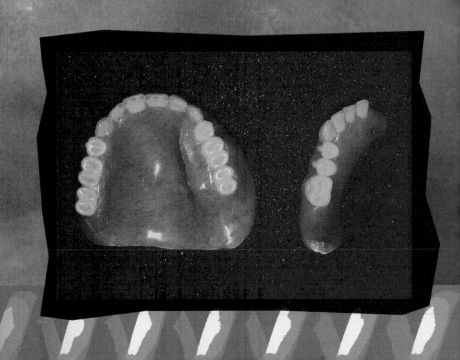

Chapter Outline

Dental Oncology and Maxillofacial Prosthetics
   Treatment of the oral cavity and dentition for patients receiving head and neck radiotherapy and chemotherapy
   Dentist's role in the treatment of head and neck cancer
   Side effects of radiation therapy
   Side effects of chemotherapy
Dental and Oral Health Care Recommendations
   Dental and oral management before radiation therapy

Dental and oral management during and after radiation therapy
Dental and oral management before chemotherapy
Dental and oral management during and after chemotherapy
Use of Maxillofacial Prostheses
   Surgery as a means of cancer therapy
   Intraoral prostheses
   Extraoral prostheses

Learning Objectives

On completion of Chapter 32, the student should be able to do the following:

■ Define key terms.

■ Identify and explain the various intraoral and extraoral maxillofacial prostheses.

■ Discuss the oral and dental care of a patient with head or neck cancer during and after surgery, radiation therapy, and chemotherapy.

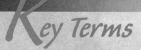

Key Terms

Chemotherapy

Dysgeusia

Immunosuppression

Maxillofacial Prosthetics

Mucositis

Obturator

Osteoradionecrosis (ORN)

Palatal Augmentation (Drop) Prosthesis

Palatal Lift Prosthesis

Radiation Caries

Radiation Therapy (Radiotherapy)

Resection Prosthesis

Speech Aid (Bulb) Prosthesis

Trismus

Xerostomia

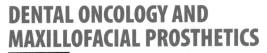

DENTAL ONCOLOGY AND MAXILLOFACIAL PROSTHETICS

Treatment of the Oral Cavity and Dentition for Patients Receiving Head and Neck Radiotherapy and Chemotherapy

Patients who are undergoing treatment for cancer, especially of the head and neck, have special dental needs. The dental assistant should be aware of the following important facts:

- Cancers of the head and neck account for about 4% of all malignant tumors diagnosed in the United States.
- Ninety percent of all cancerous head and neck tumors are squamous cell carcinomas. The remaining 10% comprises adenocarcinomas of a salivary origin, melanomas, or tumors of somatic soft tissues.
- The incidence of head and neck cancer is roughly 1 in 6000 individuals.
- The male to female ratio of head and neck cancer is greater than 3 to 1.
- Use of alcohol and tobacco together is associated with 95% of squamous cell carcinomas of the head and neck.

Dentist's Role in the Treatment of Head and Neck Cancer

Radiation therapy (radiotherapy)
The treatment of disease with ionizing radiation

Chemotherapy
The treatment of disease with chemical agents

Obturator
A device used to restore the continuity of the hard or soft palate or both

The three main methods of treatment for cancer are surgery, **radiation therapy,** and **chemotherapy.** Surgical patients normally require a prosthesis, such as an **obturator,** but radiotherapy and chemotherapy present a number of oral side effects with which the dentist and dental assistant should be familiar. Although some effects are long term, most occur during or immediately after therapy.

Radiation treatment for head and neck cancer can cause many oral complications. Approximately 40% of all patients undergoing chemotherapy also have oral complications. The dentist's role in cancer therapy is to improve and maintain oral hygiene to reduce the risk of these complications.

The dentist can prevent or diminish several of the side effects of cancer therapy, such as **radiation caries, mucositis, trismus,** hemorrhage, **xerostomia,** and **osteoradionecrosis (ORN).** It may be possible to eliminate oral infection before radiation therapy or chemotherapy is begun and to control pain in the oral cavity. Some important dental considerations are (1) maintaining and improving the oral status, (2) preventing deterioration of the natural teeth, and (3) preventing or reducing the incidence of bone and soft tissue necrosis after radiotherapy to the jaws. By providing reconstruction and rehabilitation after surgical procedures, the dental oncologist can improve the overall quality of life for the oncology patient.

Side Effects of Radiation Therapy

Dentists and dental assistants should be alert for side effects of radiotherapy. Short-term effects include mucositis (an oral inflammation), infection (secondary infections, candidiasis, and bacterial, mycotic, and viral infections), trismus (difficulty opening the mouth), **dysgeusia** (change in the sense of taste), xerostomia (dry mouth), and nutritional deficiency.

Long-terms effects include xerostomia (dry mouth), radiation caries (decay caused by tooth demineralization), ORN (infection of the bone) and soft tissue necrosis, trismus (difficulty opening the mouth), tooth sensitivity (rare), and nutritional deficiency caused by xerostomia, mucositis, and dysgeusia. In children, maxillofacial development may be altered.

Side Effects of Chemotherapy

The side effects of chemotherapy are generally short term and similar to those of radiotherapy, but certain long-term

Radiation caries
Decay, mostly at the cervical margins, caused by the loss of minerals that results from radiation therapy

Mucositis
An oral inflammation

Trismus
Difficulty opening the mouth

Xerostomia
Dry mouth

Osteoradionecrosis (ORN)
An infection, or necrosis, of the bones

Dysgeusia
Change in the sense of taste

effects may cause difficulty. Short-term effects are mucositis, xerostomia, infections, and hemorrhage.

Among the long-term effects of chemotherapy is neurotoxicity. Certain chemotherapeutic drugs can cause severe, deep pain that mimics bilateral maxillary and mandibular toothache but that has no dental or oral source. Chemotherapy can also affect maxillofacial development in children.

DENTAL AND ORAL HEALTH CARE RECOMMENDATIONS

Dental and Oral Management Before Radiation Therapy

Informing patients about the possible side effects of radiation therapy is an essential responsibility of the dental staff. This information must stress the need for oral health care and maintenance.

A complete oral and dental evaluation before radiotherapy begins includes taking radiographs, hard and soft tissue examinations, and periodontal and caries examinations and charting. Formulation of a treatment plan is necessary, because all hopeless or questionable teeth (including root fragments) in the field of irradiation must be removed. If preprosthetic surgery is required, it should also be performed before radiation therapy is begun, to allow adequate healing before irradiation. The patient also is given oral prophylaxis and home care instructions.

Upper and lower alginate impressions are made for vacuum-formed vinyl fluoride carriers (0.15-inch thick soft mouthguard material). Current prostheses, if any, are evaluated, and possible sources of irritation are removed. Fabrication of the new prosthesis must be delayed until at least 3 to 6 months after radiation therapy concludes, depending on the mucosal status and the degree of xerostomia present. Nutritional counseling also is necessary.

The radiation oncologist may ask the dentist to fabricate radiation stents and carriers.

Dental and Oral Management During and After Radiation Therapy

Any restorative treatment that was not completed before radiation therapy began may be performed. Other conditions also may need to be treated.

Mucositis

If mucositis develops, the symptoms may be relieved by having the patient use Xylocaine Viscous rinses or a rinse made up of Maalox suspension with equal parts Benadryl Elixir and Xylocaine Viscous. Oratect Gele or Orabase B can be used as a topical oral anesthetic.

Infection Control

For infection control, cultures are done for suspected infectious organisms and treatment is prescribed in cooperation with the radiation oncologist. Peridex (chlorhexidine 0.12%) may be used when necessary as a preventive measure. Treatment also may include: Mycostatin (nystatin), 100,000 U/ml, 5 ml three or four times a day; Mycelex (clotrimazole), 1 troche five times a day for 14 days; Nizoral (ketoconazole), 1 tablet daily for 14 days; Diflucan (fluconazole), 100 mg, tablets for 7 days; or Zovirax (acyclovir), 200 mg, 2 capsules three times a day for 10 days.

Trismus

If trismus occurs, the patient should be instructed to exercise the muscles a few times daily by opening and closing the mouth against pressure as far as possible without pain. Therabite, a mechanical device, may also be used.

Xerostomia

If radiation involves the salivary glands, xerostomia may occur. Relief of symptoms may include use of artificial saliva substitutes (Xerolube, Salivart, Moi-ster). Frequent sips of water are helpful, and sugarless gum and candy may stimulate salivation. Pilocarpine hydrochloride (Salagen), 5 mg three times a day, may also produce saliva.

Radiation Caries

Radiation caries is a rampant form of decay that often occurs at the cervical margins but may be found anywhere in the mouth. The condition is believed to be the result of xerostomia and the accompanying acidogenic shift of the oral environment. Prevention is necessary, because this form of decay is difficult to arrest in a dry mouth.

Silver amalgam restorations perform better under dry conditions, because desiccated composites tend to break down at the margins. Fluoride (Gel-Kam, Prevident, TheraFlur) must be used daily at home with a custom fluoride carrier.

Use and Care of Dental Prostheses

The patient should not wear a removable prosthesis if irritation, mucositis, or ulceration develops. Dentures should be cleaned daily and soaked in an antimicrobial denture-soaking solution, if necessary.

Osteoradionecrosis

Osteoradionecrosis (ORN) develops because of lack of bone healing, which is the result of diminished blood supply to the bone caused by radiotherapy. ORN usually occurs in the mandible after tooth extraction or bone surgery but may be associated with denture sores or may even occur spontaneously.

Teeth in the irradiated field should *not* be extracted for at least 1 year after irradiation. Some researchers believe that the risk of ORN never abates. If tooth extraction is unavoidable, conservative surgery, antibiotic coverage, and hyperbaric oxygen treatment may be necessary.

Dietary counseling is essential, along with excellent home care instructions, including daily use of fluoride; frequent oral prophylaxis; and dental recall.

Dental and Oral Management Before Chemotherapy

As with radiation therapy, it is important to teach the patient about the possible side effects of chemotherapy and the need for oral health care and maintenance before chemotherapeutic treatment begins. A complete oral and dental evaluation should be performed, including radiographs; hard and soft tissue, periodontal, and caries examinations; and charting. A treatment plan also is formulated.

Unrestorable or periodontally compromised teeth, including root fragments, must be extracted to eliminate the risk of infection. This must be done in consultation with a medical oncologist because the patient may be immunosuppressed.

The patient's periodontal status is maintained or improved through scaling and root planing. Indicated restora-

tions may be completed, and removal of orthodontic bands may be considered if chemotherapy is expected to cause problems in the mouth.

If salivary dysfunction is expected, upper and lower alginate impressions are taken for vacuum-formed vinyl fluoride carriers (0.15-inch thick soft mouthguard material). Fluoride prescribed for home use includes Gel-Kam and Prevident.

Oral hygiene instructions include using a soft toothbrush, such as the Biotene Supersoft toothbrush, and dental floss. Frequent recall is necessary, along with dietary counseling.

Dental and Oral Management During and After Chemotherapy

The patient should perform routine dental care as the person's hematologic status permits during chemotherapy (Box 32.1 and Table 32.1). All suspicious lesions should be cultured for bacterial fungus or viral infections. Treatment is

Box 32.1

Daily Oral Hygiene Instructions for Cancer Patients

1. If you have partial or complete dentures:
   a. Remove the dentures and use a denture brush and water to clean them.
   b. Soak the dentures in an antimicrobial denture-soaking solution if necessary.
   c. Do not wear removable partial dentures or complete dentures while sleeping.
2. For natural teeth, use a soft-bristled toothbrush and toothpaste or baking soda to brush your teeth. If your mouth is too sore for a toothbrush, use a Toothette or a cloth.

3. Floss natural teeth by gently placing dental floss between the teeth and sliding the floss up each side of each tooth.
4. Apply a fluoride product, such as Gel-Kam or Prevident, to natural teeth for 5 minutes each evening, using a fluoride carrier or toothbrush. Do not rinse your mouth, eat, or drink for 30 minutes afterward.
5. Do not use over-the-counter mouthwashes or a full-strength peroxide solution because they can dry out and irritate oral tissues. Peridex (chlorhexidine) may be used if prescribed by your dentist.

Table 32.1

Evaluation of Oral Hygiene Instructions for Cancer Patients

Oral Hygiene Instructions for Cancer Patients	4	3	2	0	X
Remove dentures or partials from mouth.					
Clean denture.					
Soak dentures.					
Brush teeth or use Toothette.					
Floss teeth.					
Use fluoride.					
Do not rinse.					
Discuss mouthwashes.					

The numeric criteria: 4 Excellent; 3 Good but some improvement can be made; 2 Below average, usable, needs to improve skill; 0 Unsatisfactory; X Not able to evaluate.

prescribed in cooperation with the medical oncologist (see the section on Infection Control on p. 835 for medications that apply).

After chemotherapy has been concluded, diligent dental home care is required. Follow-up with the dentist is critical to prevent or reduce complications between cycles of chemotherapy.

Immunosuppression

The destruction or impairment of the immune response caused by chemotherapy or radiation therapy

Upon completion of all planned courses of chemotherapy, the patient is closely monitored until all side effects of therapy have resolved, including **immunosuppression.** The patient may then be placed on a normal dental recall schedule. Because these patients may need to undergo additional immunosuppressive therapy if a cancer relapse occurs in the future, it is very important to maintain optimal oral health. Consultation and coordination with the medical oncologist are mandatory because of the patient's hematologic status and the need for antibiotic prophylaxis with indwelling central venous catheters.

Children should receive close lifetime follow-up, with specific attention given to growth and development patterns.

USE OF MAXILLOFACIAL PROSTHESES

Maxillofacial prosthetics

The use of artificial materials to replace parts of the body, such as the eyes, ears, and nose, lost to surgical defects, trauma, or congenital defects

Maxillofacial prosthetics is the science and art of anatomic or cosmetic reconstruction using artificial substitutes for intraoral, paraoral, and extraoral structures that are missing or defective because of surgery, trauma, or developmental malformations.

Surgery as a Means of Cancer Therapy

When surgery is the preferred mode of cancer therapy, portions of the oral cavity and the head and neck region are removed to cure or control a tumor. Surgical defects may not be viable for closure or correction by reconstructive surgery because of the size of the defect, lack of available tissue from the patient, or the possibility of local recurrence of the cancer (leading to inability to monitor a closed defect). These surgical defects require a prosthesis for function and esthet-

ics. The prostheses are classified as intraoral and extraoral prostheses.

Patients with acquired maxillary defects can be restored to normal function and appearance by use of intraoral prostheses. Postsurgical maxillary defects predispose patients to hypernasal speech, food leakage through the nasal cavity, and impaired chewing ability. These can be minimized or eliminated by use of an obturator, with excellent results.

Surgical procedures for cancer can range from a simple soft palatectomy to a maxillectomy encompassing the maxillary hard or soft palate (or both). Normally, the tumor and 2 to 5 mm of margin around it are removed, depending on the histopathology indicated by the biopsy; this can result in defects of different sizes.

The size and location of the defect and whether the patient is dentate or edentulous influence the method of restoration. Small defects of the hard and soft palates can be restored surgically with local flaps, free vascularized grafts and muscle flaps. Larger hard palate defects are better corrected with prosthetic obturation, which allows for easier follow-up checks for local recurrence.

Intraoral Prostheses

Prostheses that are fabricated for the oral cavity include (1) obturators, including surgical obturators, interim obturators, and definitive obturators; (2) mandibular **resection prosthesis;** (3) **palatal augmentation (drop) prosthesis;** (4) **palatal lift prosthesis;** and (5) **speech aid (bulb) prosthesis.**

An obturator is used to close a congenital or acquired hard or soft tissue opening, primarily of the hard palate and contiguous alveolar structures. Prosthetic restoration of the defect includes a surgical interim, and definitive obturator, which are used as follows:

Resection prosthesis

A prosthesis that replaces the missing part of the mandible and associated teeth

Palatal augmentation (drop) prosthesis

A prosthesis that allows the hard or soft palate, or both, to be reshaped

Palatal lift prosthesis

A prosthesis that helps in velopharyngeal closure by elevating an incompetent soft palate

Speech aid (bulb) prosthesis

A prosthesis that restores a congenital defect of the soft palate

- A *surgical obturator* is used to restore the continuity of the hard or soft palate (or both) immediately after surgery or traumatic loss of a portion or all of the hard or soft palate and contiguous alveolar structures.
- An *interim obturator* is made after surgical resection of a portion or all of the maxilla. It often may include replacement of anterior teeth in the defect area for esthetic purposes, with no posterior occlusion. This prosthesis replaces the surgical obturator.
- A *definitive obturator* is a prosthesis that artificially replaces part or all of the maxilla and associated teeth lost to surgery or trauma after healing is complete. The objective is to restore the oral cavity so that the patient can eat and swallow normally.

Fabrication of an Intraoral Prosthesis

A prosthodontist examines the patient before surgery and makes diagnostic impressions and casts. In consultation with the head and neck surgeon, an outline of the presumed defect is drawn and a surgical obturator is fabricated. Retention is achieved using the patient's existing dentition and clasps or bone screws. If the patient is edentulous, the prosthesis is inserted immediately after surgery, thus supporting the surgical packing. The patient is seen several days later and, at that time, the process of creating a bulb with a softer material, such as Coe-Soft or Lynal, is initiated. The patient's comfort is monitored weekly for 4 to 6 weeks, with continual compensation for tissue changes (Figures 32.1 and 32.2).

This prosthesis provides a matrix upon which the surgical packing can be placed. It also prevents contamination of the infected area and ensures close adaptation of the skin graft to the raw surface of the cheek flap. It enables the patient to speak normally by reproducing normal palatal contours and by covering the defect at the surgical site. The prosthesis also allows deglutition so that a nasogastric tube may be removed sooner.

Most important, the prosthesis lessens the psychologic impact of surgery by allowing the patient to speak and swallow. In some situations an existing removable complete or partial denture prosthesis may be modified after surgery to be used as a surgical obturator.

Once the patient has worn a surgical obturator for a few weeks and initial healing has taken place, the prosthesis is converted into a transitional obturator. If a patient is missing anterior teeth, they are added at this time. The soft tissue conditioning bulb portion is replaced with hard acrylic because the change in tissues will be less because of scar contraction. The reason to convert the bulb into acrylic is that this material can be polished to a high shine to prevent irritation of tissues and to prohibit accumulation of food debris and bacteria, which are promoted by soft tissue conditioning material. The transitional obturator (Figures 32.3 and 32.4) normally is worn for 4 to 9 months to accommodate changes in the defective area, especially if the area was lined with a split-thickness skin graft, which might shrink up to 40%. Also, most local recurrences occur within the first 9 months.

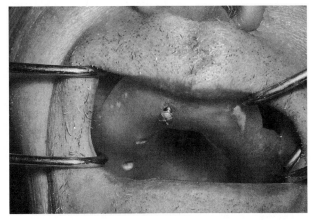

FIGURE 32.2

Surgical obturator held by bone screws.

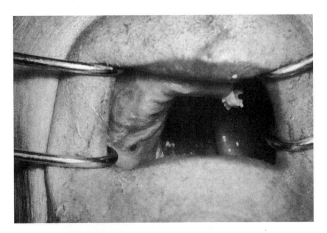

FIGURE 32.1

Intraoral defect of the hard and soft palates.

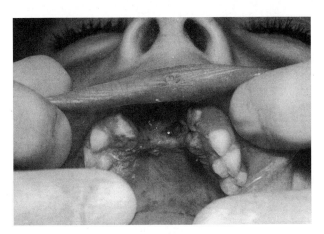

FIGURE 32.3

Intraoral defect of the premaxilla.

After healing is complete, local recurrences have been ruled out, and tissue changes brought about by postsurgical radiation therapy have subsided, a definitive obturator is made in consultation with the head and neck surgeon. Diagnostic casts are made, and fabrication proceeds in the manner of impressions, tracing the bulb, jaw records, face-bow, and a complete wax try-in, followed by processing, finishing, and delivery of the prosthesis. The advantages of a definitive obturator include a better appearance and better function, since the obturator conforms closely to the defect. It also has posterior teeth, which help stabilize the prosthesis and aid in function.

After delivery of the definitive obturator, the patient is followed routinely until all adjustments have been completed. A 1-year recall is established if the patient is edentulous; if the patient is dentate, a 4- to 6-month recall is the norm to provide oral prophylaxis. Designs used for the complete denture obturator prosthesis are modified to accommodate the instability caused by the defect in the palate (Figures 32.5 and 32.6).

Sometimes the defect is limited to the alveolar ridge, with no opening at all into the sinus cavity. In this case a prosthesis is fabricated to replace the teeth and the hard and soft tissues lost to surgery (Figures 32.7 and 32.8).

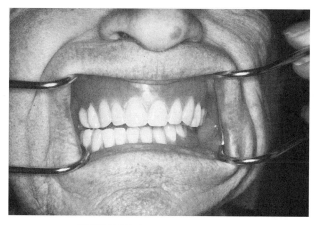

FIGURE 32.6
Prosthesis in the patient's mouth.

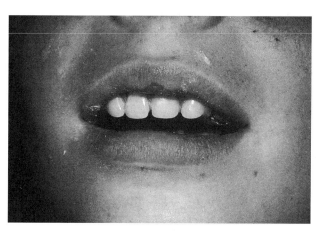

FIGURE 32.4
Prosthesis with satisfying esthetics.

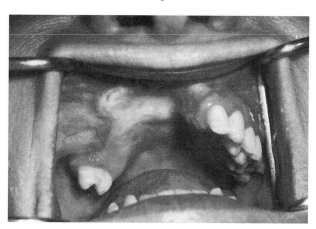

FIGURE 32.7
Maxillary arch after cancer surgery, with no opening into the sinus cavity.

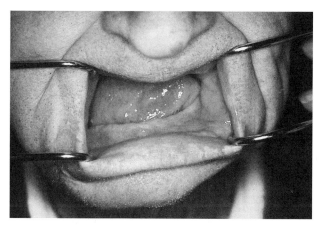

FIGURE 32.5
Intraoral defect of the hard palate.

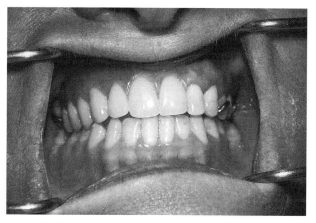

FIGURE 32.8
Completed prosthesis covers a defect intraorally.

Surgical, interim, and definitive obturators for one patient demonstrate different size bulbs, and anterior and posterior teeth being added to the obturator.

Resection Prosthesis

A resection prosthesis (Figure 32.9) is a mandibular prosthesis that replaces the missing part of the mandible and associated teeth. It is delivered after a mandibulectomy to allow the remaining deviated mandibular segment to contact with maxillary dentition. This may require use of a flange guide or a maxillary occlusal platform incorporated into the prosthesis to guide the mandibular segment into optimal occlusal contact.

This prosthesis is made 4 to 6 weeks after cancer surgery for a mandibular defect after initial healing is complete and the patient is able to open and close the mouth adequately.

Palatal Augmentation (Drop) Prosthesis

A palatal augmentation (drop) prosthesis allows reshaping of the hard or soft palate (or both) to improve tongue and palate contact during speech and swallowing. This prosthesis could be a removable partial denture or a complete denture. It is made for patients who have had surgery for cancer involving the floor of the mouth or tongue or for those who have had mandibular cancers. Because of the surgery, the tongue is unable to rise to the maximum potential and movement is restricted. The tongue cannot make contact with the hard and soft palates during speech and swallowing. This may also be the result of trauma or neurologic deficiencies.

Speech Aid (Bulb) Prosthesis

A speech aid (or bulb) prosthesis restores a congenital defect of the soft palate or a defect left by incomplete surgical repair of a cleft palate. A portion extends into the pharynx to separate the oropharynx and nasopharynx during speech and swallowing. This complements the palatal pharyngeal sphincter to improve speech and swallowing. A bulb is created to obturate the nasal escape of air during speech, eliminating nasality.

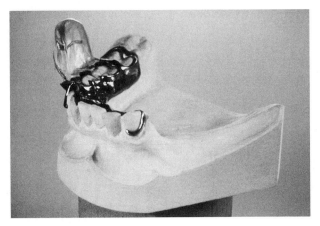

FIGURE 32.9

Mandibular resection prosthesis.

Palatal Lift Prosthesis

A palatal lift prosthesis aids in velopharyngeal closure by elevating an incompetent soft palate. A dysfunction of this sort could be caused by clefting, surgery, trauma, or unknown paralysis. This prosthesis could be a complete denture or a removable partial denture. It enables the patient to swallow and speak. This prosthesis is used mostly for trauma patients. When a patient is involved in an accident such as a closed head injury, a deficit may develop in velopharyngeal competency in which the soft palate does not function normally. In such a case a prosthesis is made to elevate the soft palate posteriorly toward the posterior pharyngeal wall. This helps both with speech and with the effort required to speak. A speech pathologist trains the patient to use the prosthesis to advantage. A palatal lift prosthesis cannot function by itself; rather, it complements a speech therapist's training.

Extraoral Prostheses

Facial defects caused by trauma, cancer surgery, or developmental malformations are usually corrected by surgical reconstruction using the patient's own tissues. Sometimes, however, the defect may be so large that the resulting significant facial deformity prevents reconstruction. Lack of available tissue, a compromised local blood supply (possibly caused by irradiation), or the need to periodically check for local recurrence of a tumor are some of the reasons a patient is referred to a maxillofacial prosthodontist for restoration of the facial deficiency with a prosthesis.

Extraoral prostheses are dependent on adjacent tissue and the size of the defect. Whether a patient is rehabilitated surgically or with a prosthesis, it is of utmost importance to fully inform the patient about future problems and the expected quality of the final result. Patients who are well informed have realistic expectations.

Prosthetic restoration of facial defects caused by surgery can help in the rehabilitation of the disfigured patients by improving their self-esteem and returning them to society. Ideally, a defect in any part of the body should be restored surgically using the patient's own tissues, but in many cases in which the defect is created by cancer surgery, it might be impossible or undesirable. In these situations, prosthetic restorations are achievable for facial defects, including nasal, auricular, orbital, and ocular defects. The materials most commonly used for these prostheses are medical-grade silicones, methylmethacrylate resins, and polyurethanes. These materials are used individually or in combination. A patient's skin tones are matched by the use of pigments in the silicone and acrylic to make a lifelike prosthesis that is barely distinguishable from adjacent tissues.

Medical-grade silicone materials are most commonly used for fabricating facial prostheses because of the excellent physical properties, stability of the material, ease of using coloring agents and pigments, ease of processing, superior esthetic properties, and availability of a wide range of preparations. An example of the use of a nasal prosthesis is shown in Figures 32.10 to 32.12. Drawbacks of silicone prostheses include poor tear strength, inability to be polished, and poor wetting ability. These disadvantages can be overcome by using a polyurethane backing to make a composite prosthesis, which helps in tear strength at the margins and the transition between the skin and the prosthesis, since the urethane by itself is thinner and clear, allowing the adjacent skin color to show through the lining (Figures 32.13 to 32.15).

Retention of the Prosthesis

The retention of a prosthesis is accomplished by using medical-grade adhesives, magnets, tapes, or implants. These are used individually or in combination.

A combination facial prosthesis in which an obturator is attached to an orbital prosthesis with magnets is shown in Figures 32.16 and 32.17. The patient had a maxillary defect that was restored by an obturator prosthesis and an orbital defect that was restored with a silicone and urethane

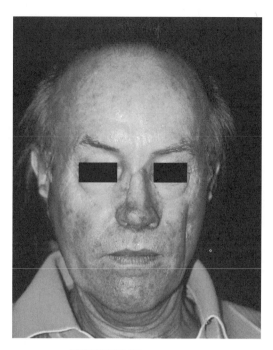

FIGURE 32.12
Prosthesis held by adhesive.

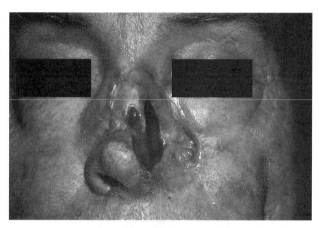

FIGURE 32.10
Small defect of the nose.

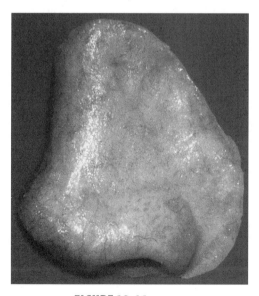

FIGURE 32.11
All-silicone prosthesis.

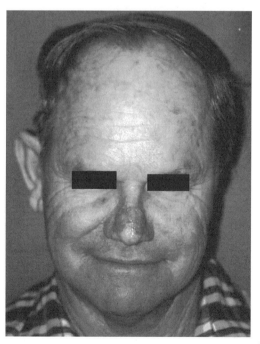

FIGURE 32.13
Patient missing left ear as a result of trauma.

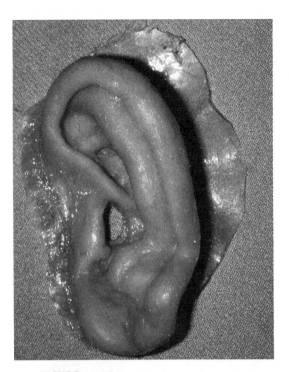

FIGURE 32.14

Silicone-polyurethane auricular prosthesis.

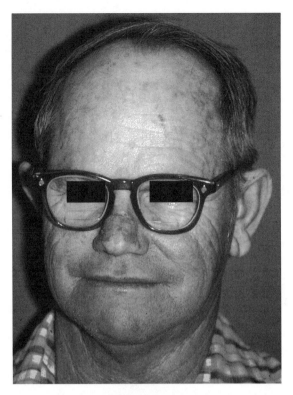

FIGURE 32.15

Prosthesis in position.

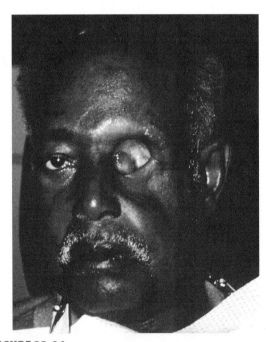

FIGURE 32.16

Patient who has had maxillectomy and orbital exenteration.

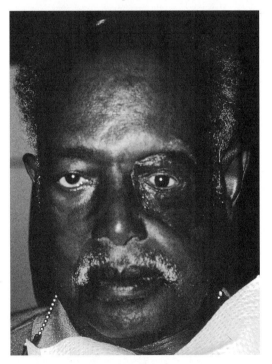

FIGURE 32.17

Orbital prosthesis.

prosthesis using a framework with magnets. The combination prostheses help in ease of manipulation; the patient first inserts the obturator and then, through the defect in the orbit, attaches the framework at one end. The silicone orbital prosthesis is attached to the other end with magnets. Insertion and removal of this prosthesis is easy, and no adhesives are required. This is especially critical in elderly patients and for those who have had radiation therapy, because the skin may be sensitive to adhesives.

Craniofacial osseointegrated implants with special lengths and diameters to be used in skull bones have recently become popular because of the inherent advantages for retaining facial prostheses. Advantages include convenience, consistent positioning, better retention, no adhesive irritation, and better support for combination prostheses in intraoral and extraoral cases. Some orbital prostheses use implants for retention (Figures 32.18, 32.19, and 32.20).

As a final note, patients require other prostheses for defects not located in the head or neck. Fingers can be replaced by a silicone prosthesis held by adhesives. These are made by the maxillofacial prosthodontist in collaboration with plastic or ear, nose, and throat surgeons.

The goal of the specialty of dental oncology is to ensure proper care for dentition and the oral cavity before, during, and after chemotherapy or radiotherapy for head and neck malignancies. Such care prevents or minimizes infections, systemic problems, and the loss of dentition, thereby improving the quality of life for the oncology patient.

The goal of maxillofacial prosthodontics is to replace missing intraoral structures by the use of artificial prostheses to allow patients to speak and swallow normally; for patients in need of extraoral prostheses, rehabilitation and resumption of a normal lifestyle are the goals.

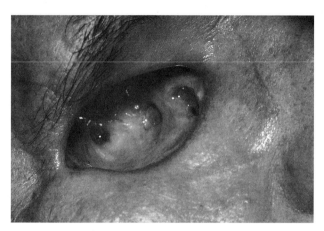

FIGURE 32.18
Orbital defect caused by cancer surgery.

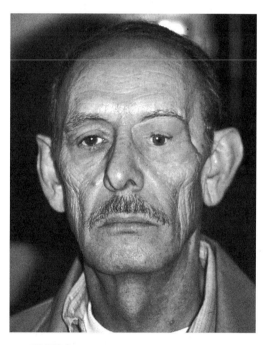

FIGURE 32.20
Esthetic results achieved with prosthesis.

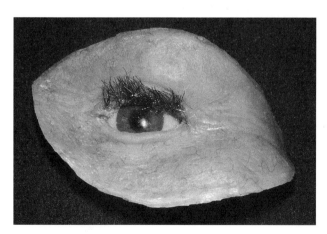

FIGURE 32.19
Orbital silicone prosthesis with gold clip retention.

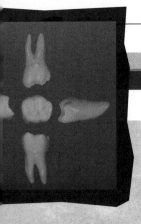

Points for Review

- The dentist's role in the treatment of head and neck malignancies with radiation therapy and chemotherapy
- Dental and oral management before, during, and after radiation therapy and chemotherapy
- Daily oral hygiene instructions for cancer patients and those with dental prostheses
- The use of maxillofacial prostheses to correct cancer, trauma, or birth defects

Self-Study Questions

1. Patients scheduled to receive head and neck radiation should see a dentist before treatment commences.
   a. True
   b. False
2. Which is not a side effect of radiation therapy?
   a. Mucositis
   b. Trismus
   c. Hemorrhage
   d. All of the above
3. What is the term to use for dry mouth?
   a. Mucositis
   b. Xerostomia
   c. Osteroradionecrosis
   d. Trismus
4. What does a home care program for radiation patients include?
   a. Fluoride with carriers
   b. Frequent oral prophylaxis
   c. Frequent recall
   d. All of the above
5. What should patients undergoing chemotherapy do if suspicious oral lesions are present?
   a. Have them removed immediately
   b. Have them cultured
   c. Stop chemotherapy
   d. All of the above
6. A complete denture obturator prosthesis is held in place by adhesives.
   a. True
   b. False
7. A speech aid prosthesis is a bulb which stops the nasal escape of air during speech.
   a. True
   b. False
8. Methods of retention for extraoral prostheses include medical grade adhesives, magnets, tapes, or implants.
   a. True
   b. False

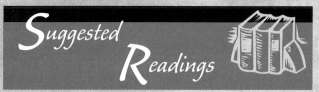

Beumer III J, Curtis TA, Firtell DN: *Maxillofacial rehabilitation, prosthodontics and surgical considerations*, St Louis, 1979, Mosby.

Branemark PI: *Tissue-integrated prostheses-osseointegration in clinical dentistry*, Chicago, 1987, Quintessence.

Chalian VA, Drane JB, Standish SM: *Maxillofacial prosthetics: multidisciplinary practice*, Baltimore, 1972, Williams & Wilkins.

Engelman Michael: *Clinical decision making and treatment planning in osseointegration*, Chicago, 1996, Quintessence.

Laney WR: *Maxillofacial prosthetics*, Littleton, Mass, 1979, PSG.

Laney WR, Tolman DE: *Tissue integration in oral, orthopedic and maxillofacial reconstruction. Proceedings*, Rochester, Minn, 1981, Mayo Medical Center.

Worthington P, Branemark PI: *Advanced osseointegration surgery: application in the maxillofacial region*, Chicago, 1992, Quintessence.

Worthington P, Lang BR, LaVelle WE: *Osseointegration in dentistry: an introduction*, Chicago, 1994, Quintessence.

Unit VI

Advanced Operative Principles and Techniques

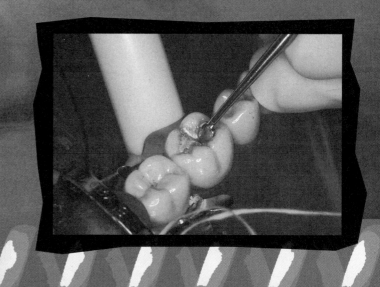

33

Clinical Operative Procedures and Rubber Dam Isolation

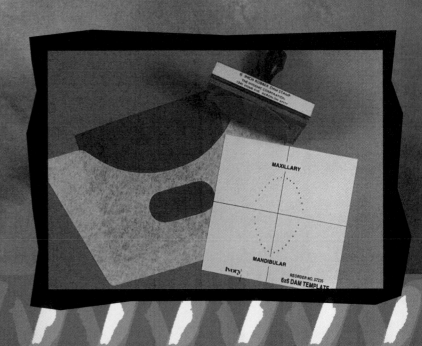

Learning Objectives

On completion of Chapter 33, the student should be able to do the following:

- Define key terms.
- Identify the clinical procedures involved in operative dentistry.
- List the preoperative procedures.
- List the procedures for four-handed rubber dam application.
- Identify the rubber dam armamentarium.
- List the advantages of use of rubber dam.
- Place rubber dam using four-handed application techniques.

- Identify the types of rubber dam clamps and the ways they are used.
- Discuss caries removal and cavity preparation procedures.
- Define cavity classification and nomenclature.
- Complete a self-evaluation of rubber dam placement.
- Identify the indications and contra-indications for clinical application of bases and liners.

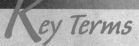

Key Terms

Cavosurface Margin	Invert	Operator
Clamp	Ligate	Point Angles
Interseptal Rubber Dam	Line Angles	Rubber Dam
	Obstruction	Template

OPERATIVE DENTISTRY

Operator

The individual who performs dental procedures directly on the patient. Depending on the procedure, this may be the dentist, expanded-function dental assistant, dental assistant, or dental hygienist

Dentists spend approximately 50% of their operating time replacing or restoring teeth broken down or destroyed by caries or accidents. The chairside dental assistant must have a general understanding of all phases of operative dentistry and restorative procedures to assist the dentist appropriately. Restorative procedures vary in difficulty, and in some states dentists are allowed to delegate many of these procedures to dental assistants and hygienists trained in expanded duties or advanced functions. In order to accept the responsibility of performing operative procedures, the dental assistant must possess both knowledge and clinical skills. For clarity and consistency, the dentist and the expanded-function dental assistant who performs restorative procedures are referred to as the **operator** unless otherwise designated.

Role of the Expanded-Function Dental Assistant

The expanded-function dental assistant who is responsible for restoring the teeth to proper form and function must have basic dental assisting knowledge, technical skills, and preclinical experience in the areas listed in Box 33.1.

Box 33.1

Skills Required for Expanded-Function Dental Assistants in Operative Dentistry

Infection control (see Chapters 10 and 18)
Patient management (see Chapters 4, 14, 20-22)
Principles of instrument design, proper instrument grasp, and equipment use (see Chapter 19)
Operator positioning, so as to gain visibility and access to all areas of the mouth while maintaining the principles of motion economy, mirror use, and finger rest (see Chapter 20)
General characteristics of the teeth and occlusion, cavity nomenclature, and common terminology used in the classification of caries and cavities (see Chapter 9)
Use, manipulation, placement, and finishing of cements and restorative materials, including an understanding of cavity design and the relationship of the cavity design to the restorative material used (see Chapter 15)

Preoperative Preparation

The chairside dental assistant must complete a number of preliminary activities before seating the patient and beginning the operative procedures (Box 33.2 and Table 33.1). The operatory must be prepared using infection control techniques (see Chapter 20 for detailed information on preparatory procedures and Chapter 18 for infection control procedures). To make efficient use of the patient's appointment time, the dentist and dental personnel should review the patient's medical history and records to confirm the treatment plan and procedures to be completed and to identify any special health precautions. The chairside dental assistant makes the diagnostic radiographs available by placing them in the viewbox or bringing them up on the computer monitor for the operator to review.

Restorative instruments are used to restore the teeth to their normal form and function. Restorative cassettes may include several types of setups, such as amalgam, universal amalgam/composite, composite, endodontic, crown and bridge, and porcelain veneer placement systems. Individual tray setups can be designed according to the operator's needs. Restorative cassettes usually contain the basic examination setup instruments, various types of hand cutting instruments, and placement and finishing instruments.

Rubber dam instruments and materials are usually included in the restorative setup. The rubber dam isolation materials and equipment, anesthetic and syringe, and amalgam or composite restorative materials and instrument tray also must be set up (Figure 33.1).

After these procedures have been completed, the chairside assistant attaches the evacuator tip; assembles the anesthetic syringe, matrix band, and retainer, if needed; and inserts the burs into the handpieces. The instrument tray should be covered with a napkin. The patient may then be greeted, escorted to the operatory, and made comfortable as the person is seated, draped, and positioned for treatment. The light must be adjusted and the operator's cart, foot control, and stool positioned (see Chapter 20). After completing these steps, the chairside assistant (1) washes the hands, (2) puts on a mask, glasses, and gloves, (3) positions the assistant's cart, and (4) gets seated in the three o'clock position. If the chairside assistant is trained in advanced functions, the topical anesthetic may be applied while the dentist is en route (see Chapter 14). The dentist is informed when the patient is ready. The assistant should remember to introduce the dentist to the patient if the patient has not yet met the dentist.

After the preliminary procedures have been completed and the dentist is in position, the chairside assistant delivers the mouth mirror and explorer to the dentist for the examination of the operative site. The chairside assistant then retrieves the mirror and explorer from the dentist and returns them to the cassette. The chairside assistant passes the anesthetic syringe and a 2 × 2-inch gauze pad to the dentist or advanced-function assistant (if an expanded

Box 33.2

Outline of Preparation and Procedures for Operative Dentistry

Preparation

1. Prepare the operatory using infection control procedures.
2. Open the patient's record to the treatment plan.
3. Retrieve the diagnostic radiographs.
4. Set out the rubber dam, anesthesia tray, and operative tray.
5. Wash the hands and put on a mask, glasses, and gloves.
6. Attach the evacuator tip.
7. Assemble the anesthetic syringe.
8. Assemble and contour the matrix band if necessary.
9. Insert burs into handpieces.
10. Cover the tray with a napkin.
11. Adjust the light.
12. Position the operator's cart.
13. Position the foot control.
14. Position the operator's stool.
15. Wash the hands and put on a mask, glasses, and gloves.
16. Position oneself and adjust the cart.
17. The operator (dentist or expanded-function dental assistant) applies a topical anesthetic.
18. Inform the dentist that preparation has been completed.

Four-handed operative procedures

The dentist should always examine the patient before beginning restorative procedures.

1. Chairside assistant passes the mouth mirror and explorer.
2. Operator examines the oral cavity and injection site.
3. Chairside assistant retrieves the mirror and explorer from the dentist.
4. Chairside assistant removes the cap from the needle and passes the syringe.
5. Operator administers anesthetic while the assistant supervises the patient's movements.
6. Chairside assistant caps the needle and returns the syringe to the tray.
7. Chairside assistant holds the air and water (A/W) syringe in the left hand and the high-velocity evacuator (HVE) in the right hand to rinse and suction the injection site.
8. Chairside assistant returns the A/W syringe and HVE to the cart.

9. Operator places the rubber dam with the aid of the chairside assistant.
10. Chairside assistant delivers the mouth mirror to operator to use with the handpiece, if needed.
11. Chairside assistant picks up the A/W syringe and HVE and positions suction in the oral cavity.
12. Dentist outlines the cavity preparation with a handpiece and burs and uses cutting instruments to remove caries and form angles.
13. Chairside assistant maintains a clear field and mirror and rinses and dries the cavity preparation.
14. Dentist completes cavity preparation and retention.
15. Chairside assistant flushes debris from the mouth with the A/W syringe and HVE.
16. Operator places and secures retainer and wedges.
17. Chairside assistant prepares pulp protection.
18. Operator dries cavity preparation and applies pulp protection.
19. Chairside assistant prepares restorative material.
20. Chairside assistant passes the amalgam carrier and alloy or acrylic resin filling material and condenser until the cavity preparation has been filled.
21. Operator places the restorative material and uses appropriate carving and finishing techniques and instruments, removing the retainer for final finishing.
22. Chairside assistant passes materials and instruments and uses the A/W syringe and HVE.
23. Chairside assistant clears away debris.
24. Operator and assistant remove the rubber dam.
25. Chairside assistant flushes and dries the area.
26. Chairside assistant disposes of materials appropriately.
27. Operator checks and, if necessary, adjusts the occlusion.
28. Chairside assistant passes and retrieves instruments as needed.
29. Chairside assistant gives the patient postoperative instructions and dismisses the individual.
30. Chairside assistant completes the patient's records and disassembles and disinfects the operatory.
31. Dentist completes a postoperative examination.

The dentist should evaluate the result of the procedure before dismissing the patient.

Rubber dam

A material used in the patient's mouth for protection, to ensure access and visibility in the operating field, and for efficient use of operating time

function). After the injection the syringe and gauze are returned to the tray, and the chairside assistant rinses and suctions the injection site.

The **rubber dam** can then be placed for isolation by the advanced-function assistant. The rubber dam should include enough teeth to provide access and to prevent moisture contamination of the field of operation. Although rubber dam is preferred for isolation and infection control, cotton rolls, a saliva ejector, or a high-velocity evacuator (HVE) or suction tip may be used instead of rubber dam to contain saliva in the operative area.

Note: The operator could be either the dentist or expanded-function dental assistant.

Table 33.1

Evaluation of Operative Dental Procedures

Operative Dental Procedures	4	3	2	0	X
Provision of infection control barriers.					
Position of assistant's chair.					
Position of assistant's cart.					
Anesthetic setup					
Delivery					
Retrieval					
Arrangement of instruments on tray.					
Oral evacuation.					
Use of A/W syringe.					
Mixing of materials.					
Pulp protection.					
Restorative material.					

The numeric criteria: 4 Excellent; 3 Good but some improvement can be made; 2 Below average, usable, needs to improve skill; 0 Unsatisfactory; X Not able to evaluate.

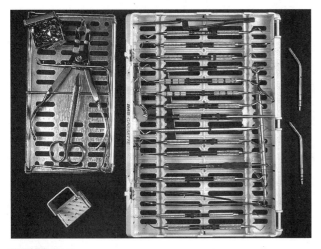

FIGURE 33.1

Amalgam setup: cassette, mirror, explorer, excavator, cavity preparation instruments, placement instrument, amalgam carrier, amalgam plugger, cleoid/discoid, carver, ball burnisher, dressing pliers, accessory box, bur stand, rubber dam clamps, articulating paper forceps, amalgam well, rubber dam forceps, suction tip, aspirating syringe, air and water (A/W) syringe tip, cassette clip, Tofflemire retainer, matrix bands, and color-coded rings.

RUBBER DAM ISOLATION

Various devices and materials are used to control moisture in the operating field and to aid good restorative dentistry. Use of rubber dam should be considered whenever possible for operative procedures because of the many advantages of this technique.

Advantages of Rubber Dam Use

Patient Management and Protection

Rubber dam can help prevent injury to the lips, tongue, cheek, and gingiva by covering the oral cavity and protecting the soft tissues from hand and rotary instruments. Rubber dam also prevents swallowing or aspiration of foreign objects. In endodontic procedures, it can help prevent injury to the soft tissues from medications. It also prevents caustic agents or other chemicals from coming in contact with the soft tissues of the oral cavity. Use of rubber dam is an effective way to maintain sterility during root canal procedures, and it prevents operator and patient exposure to infectious diseases transmitted through the saliva.

Access and Visibility in the Operating Field

Rubber dam is particularly valuable to the operator in terms of access and visibility in the operating field. It protects the lips, tongue, and cheeks, retracts the gingival tissue, and prevents saliva from entering the field. A clean, dry operating field affords improved visibility and allows the restorative materials to reach their optimum physical properties by eliminating saliva contamination. Unobstructed vision, better access, and enhanced patient comfort improve the quality of restorative care while enabling the operator to use the materials to their optimum capabilities.

Optimal Use of Operating Time

Use of rubber dam can reduce operating time because the operator does not have to contend with oral fluids, retraction, and patient interruption. The patient does not need to

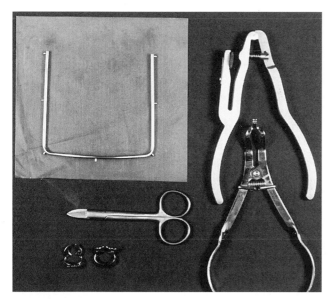

FIGURE 33.2

Rubber dam armamentarium: rubber dam material, frame scissors, clamps, punch, and forceps.

rinse, spit, or talk under rubber dam, which reduces overall operating time. Use of rubber dam also eliminates needless conversation from a nervous patient. A skilled operator should be able to place rubber dam in less than 2 minutes.

The only disadvantage of using rubber dam, as some operators have pointed out, is the time spent in placement. However, the time saved by a clean, visible field more than compensates for the extra effort. The only contraindications for rubber dam could be severe orthodontic problems or partly erupted teeth and third molars. Patients do not usually object to the use of rubber dam if they are informed of the advantages.

Rubber Dam Armamentarium

Rubber dam instruments and materials are included in the restorative setup (Figure 33.2). The rubber dam system includes the following:

- Mouth mirror
- Explorer
- Cotton pliers
- T-ball burnisher or plastic filling instrument
- Rubber dam material
- Rubber dam punch
- Rubber dam forceps
- Rubber dam clamps
- Rubber dam napkin
- Rubber dam frame
- Dental floss
- Rubber dam lubricant (topical anesthetic)
- Crown and bridge scissors
- Hand mirror
- Lubricant for patient's lips

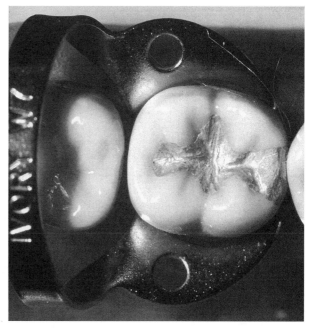

FIGURE 33.3

The clamp must be tried on the tooth to make sure it fits securely around the cervix of the tooth.

Rubber Dam Clamp

A rubber dam **clamp** is made of chrome or nickel-plated steel and is used to secure and stabilize the rubber dam material during an operative procedure (Figure

Clamp

A device used to secure the rubber dam material

33.3). The size and shape of the clamp is chosen depending on where it will be used in the mouth and the shape of the tooth. Molar clamps, bicuspid clamps, labial clamps, and cervical clamps are available. Molar and bicuspid clamps are similar in appearance except that molar clamps have a larger jaw in order to fit around the molar, which is larger than the bicuspid. These clamps are available for the right or left side of the arch. The labial and cervical clamps are similar in that they have two bows that join in the center. They are used primarily for anterior teeth but can also be used for bicuspids in certain circumstances, such as endodontics.

The rubber dam clamp is designed with a bow, or horseshoe shape, that rounds up over the tooth and extends into the flange and jaws of the clamp (Figure 33.4). The bow may be a "high bow," which gives extra clearance over the crown of the tooth. Bows vary in flexibility to achieve a firmer hold on certain teeth.

The flange has points, or jaws, which are flat or festooned. The flat-jawed clamp prevents gum impingement and is often called the "general purpose" clamp. The festooned jaw is contoured, in varying degrees, to fit the size and shape of the cervix, or neck, of the tooth. Some clamp jaws are serrated.

The right and left points, often called beaks, on the jaw of the clamp may have contact points, or they may be spaced. The jaws may also curve subgingivally to fit below the gingival tissue, or they may have a slight reverse jaw bevel to avoid gum impingement. The purpose of these shapes is to allow the clamp to fit around the neck of the tooth, to prevent gum impingement, to conform to gumline curvature, and to provide stable contact by resisting rotation. Irregularly shaped teeth or partly erupted teeth need different clamp shapes.

The selection of a rubber dam clamp also depends on the technique the operator intends to use. Some clamps have dam-engaging projections, and these are called winged clamps. The purpose of the wings is to hold the rubber dam material in place on the clamp while the operator places the material in the patient's mouth. A wingless clamp does not have this capability and is therefore applied after the rubber dam material has been placed around the teeth. The flange has small holes into which the rubber dam clamp forceps fits (Figure 33.5).

Rubber Dam Forceps

Rubber dam forceps are available in various shapes. They are used to place and remove the rubber dam clamp. The forceps work with spring action and have two small projections, or beaks, which fit into the holes of the clamp. The beaks are angled for general application. The forceps also has a sliding ring between the beak and the handle that allows the forceps to lock in a fixed position while the clamp is placed on the tooth or to release when the clamp is removed.

Rubber Dam Punch

The rubber dam punch, which is available in several styles, is used to make holes of varying sizes in the rubber dam material. The working end of the punch has a cutting tip, called a stylus, which is pressed against the punch plate hole. The size of the punch plate hole used depends on the size of the tooth over which the rubber dam must fit. The plate turns so that the proper-size hole can be punched.

Rubber Dam Frame

Most rubber dam frames are U-shaped holders that have attachments to hold the rubber dam material secure. The U-shaped frames are available in metal (Young's frame) or plastic (Whaledent frame). The Nygaard-Otsby plastic frame is circular in shape. Some frames have straps that fit around the patient's head to help hold the frame in place; these can be used for procedures that may take more time or when better security of the dam is desired.

Rubber Dam Material

The rubber dam material is a sheet of flexible rubber. It ranges from thin to a special heavy thickness and comes in a variety of colors. The thickness used is determined by the space between individual teeth to be isolated. The material is punched and used with clamps to isolate the teeth during various dental procedures.

Rubber Dam Face Shield

Some operators like to use cotton face gauze between the rubber dam material and the patient's face so that the material is not lying directly on the patient's face.

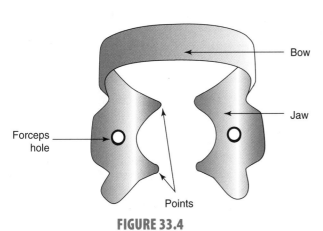

FIGURE 33.4

Parts of the clamp.

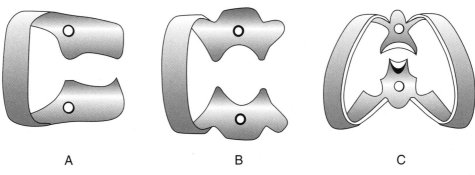

FIGURE 33.5

Types of clamps. **A**, Wingless. **B**, Winged. **C**, Anterior.

Rubber Dam Template and Stamp

Template

The plastic form used to mark the maxillary and mandibular dental arches on the rubber dam material

The **template** is a square plastic measurement guide that is placed over the rubber dam material (Figure 33.6). Both the primary and permanent maxillary and mandibular arches are inscribed on the surface of the template, with varying size holes indicating the position of the teeth. The template is placed over the rubber dam material, and the appropriate holes are marked with a pen.

The rubber stamp is inscribed with the dental arch design in the same way as the template. The stamp is used to print the arch pattern on the rubber dam material.

Considerations in Rubber Dam Use

Several factors should be discussed with the patient before rubber dam is applied. The patient must always be informed that rubber dam is to be used. If rubber dam has not been used for the patient previously, its use and advantages should be explained. Patients usually do not object if they understand the benefits. If the patient has a breathing problem, a hole can be cut in the palatal area of the material, which then can be rolled under the nose, away from the nasal area.

When placing rubber dam over a tooth, these special considerations should be taken into account:

- The material should be stretched to a fine edge so that it can be carried through and beneath the contact area.
- To prevent the dam from lifting, the tooth surfaces can be dried as the material is inverted around the tooth and an immediate coating of copal resin varnish can be applied to the area.

- If any leaks are noted, the dam should be checked to see if it is snagged on part of the clamp or if the holes are too large or unevenly spaced.
- The clamp must be placed on the anchor tooth below the height of contour.
- Floss or a wedge can be used to help carry the rubber dam through the contact areas. If floss is used, it is not lifted back through the contact; rather, it is slid out through the facial surface of the teeth or doubled over itself and slipped out without disturbing the material.
- Difficult contacts are bypassed until the operator is ready to **ligate** the material, a technique that helps secure the rubber dam.
- In general, 3.5 mm of rubber dam should be left between holes, not between centers (Figure 33.7).

Ligate

To secure the rubber dam material with a small piece of the material itself, a double strand of dental floss, a wedge, or an anchor ring

- When convenient, one or two teeth distal and mesial to the tooth to be treated are included in the rubber dam.
- For Class V restorations, the hole for the tooth to be treated is punched 1 mm to the buccal or labial, at the same time allowing 1 mm of extra rubber between adjacent teeth.
- The spacing and position of the teeth, as well as the shape of the arch, will vary.
- Punching the curve of the arch too flat results in folds and stretching of the rubber dam on the lingual side; punching the arch too curved results in folds and stretching on the labial side. This increases the difficulty of inverting the edges of the rubber dam.
- To prevent nicking of the cutting edge of the holes in the punch table, the centering of the hole under the pin is tested slowly and carefully before the dam is engaged in the punch. Also, the dam is pulled up on the shank after each punch.

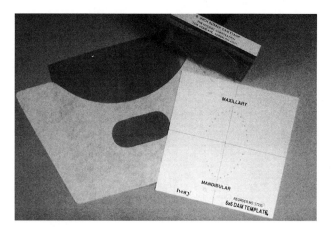

FIGURE 33.6

Rubber dam material, mask, template, and rubber stamp.

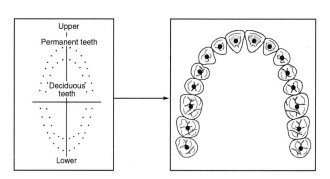

FIGURE 33.7

Template arch form.

Placement of Rubber Dam

The dental assistant makes sure that the rubber dam armamentarium is ready for application. The operator may choose to apply the rubber dam material alone (Box 33.3 and Table 33.2) or with the dental assistant's help. If the operator is aided by an assistant, the equipment and materials are placed on the assistant's cart, with the assistant anticipating the operator's needs and helping throughout the procedure (Figure 33.9). The assistant may have selected the clamp before the procedure and may have punched the rubber dam material for appropriate placement. The following procedures are the steps involved in rubber dam placement whether the rubber dam is applied by the dentist or the dental assistant.

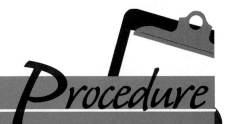

Box 33.3 — Procedure

Procedure for Solo Application of Rubber Dam

Preparation
1. Examine the oral cavity.
2. Remove all calculus and materia alba (hard and soft deposits).
3. Pass dental floss through each involved contact area to remove debris and to evaluate the difficulty of rubber dam placement in these areas.
4. Rinse the affected area.
5. Confirm the area of isolation by checking the contacts, removing irregularities, and flossing the contacts.
6. Select a clamp and tie floss to the bow of the clamp (see Figure 33.9).
7. Try the clamp on the tooth.
8. Place the rubber dam material on top of the template and mark it (see Figure 33.10).
9. Punch the rubber dam material (Figure 33.8).
10. Lubricate the rubber dam material.

Basic wingless clamp technique:
1. Place the clamp on the tooth, lingual first and below the height of contour (see Figure 33.8).
2. Check that the clamp is secure below the height of contour.
3. Place the rubber dam material over the bow of the clamp.
4. Place the rubber dam napkin.
5. Isolate the remaining teeth, remove the corner of the rubber dam material and ligate most anterior tooth to secure rubber dam.
6. Place the rubber dam frame, easing out wrinkles.
7. Floss the rubber dam through difficult contacts.
8. Invert the rubber dam material (see Figure 33.11).

9. Flex and insert the saliva ejector.

Winged clamp technique:
1. Insert the clamp forceps into the clamp.
2. Place the clamp into the rubber dam so that the hole is held open by the wings of the clamp.
3. Attach the frame to the rubber dam material and clamp.
4. Place the rubber dam napkin before applying the clamp and dam.
5. Apply the clamp to the tooth with the rubber dam, clamp, and frame in place.
6. Check that the clamp is secure, and slip the rubber dam off the wings around the cervix of the tooth.
7. Isolate the remaining teeth and ligate the last tooth.
8. Floss the rubber dam material through difficult contacts.
9. Invert the rubber dam material.
10. Insert the saliva ejector.

Alternate winged clamp technique:
1. Place the winged clamp in the rubber dam material.
2. Insert the clamp forceps into the clamp.
3. Place the clamp over the tooth with the rubber dam pulled back; this allows the operator to hold the rubber dam material out of the way for a clear field of vision while placing the clamp over the tooth.
4. Isolate the remaining teeth.
5. Ligate the rubber dam material as described above.
6. Place the rubber dam frame as described above.

Examination of the Oral Cavity

Once the patient is ready and all equipment and personnel are in place, the operator examines the oral cavity. The teeth must be clean and free of debris between the teeth, which can prevent the rubber dam material from sliding through and below the contact areas. Dental floss should be passed through each involved contact area to remove any **obstruction** or irregularity, such as dental calculus and materia alba (hard and soft deposits). The operating area should be rinsed.

Obstruction

An object that blocks, impedes, or interferes with passage

Selection of a Clamp

Many types of rubber dam clamps can fulfill the same purpose. The operator and the dental assistant must be familiar with the various types of clamps and must know how to se-lect them for a procedure and how to order them. The three general types of clamps are discussed in Chapter 22. The operator chooses a winged or wingless clamp according to the technique to be used to place the rubber dam material (see Figure 33.5). Both techniques are described below. The following list of clamps is recommended because most rubber dam applications can be accomplished with this array:

- *Anterior teeth:* #212 and #00 clamps
- *Premolars:* #206, #209, #W8A, and #00 clamps
- *Primary molars:* #W8A, #14, #00, #3A, #4A, and #24 clamps
- *Molars:* #W7, #W8, #W3, #201, #14A, #14, and #24 clamps

Once the clamp has been selected, it must be tried on the tooth to make sure it fits securely (see Figure 33.3). Before the clamp is tried on the tooth, floss must be tied to the bow of the clamp to prevent the patient from aspirating or swallowing it (Figure 33.10).

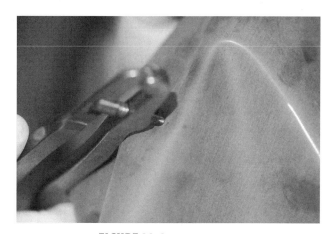

FIGURE 33.8

The rubber dam is punched.

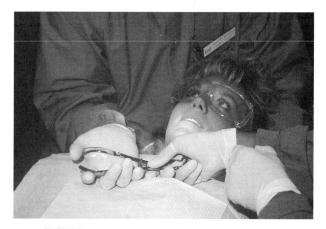

FIGURE 33.9

Dental assistant passing clamp and forceps.

Table 33.2

Evaluation for Rubber Dam Placement

Rubber Dam Placement	4	3	2	0	X
Clamp selection.					
Attachment of floss.					
Absence of tissue trauma.					
Proper distance between holes.					
Hole corresponds to shape of arch.					
Uniform border and unwrinkled material.					
Material below contacts.					
Rubber dam inverted.					
Ligature.					

The numeric criteria: 4 Excellent; 3 Good but some improvement can be made; 2 Below average, usable, needs to improve skill; 0 Unsatisfactory; X Not able to evaluate.

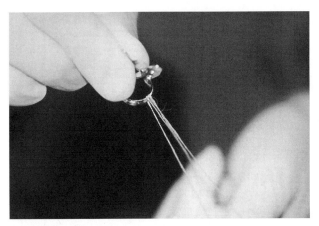

FIGURE 33.10

A clamp is selected, and floss is tied to the bow of the clamp.

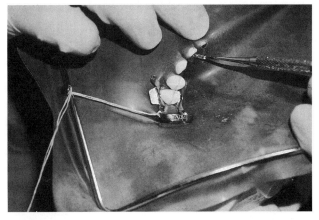

FIGURE 33.12

A plastic instrument is used to help place the rubber dam interproximally.

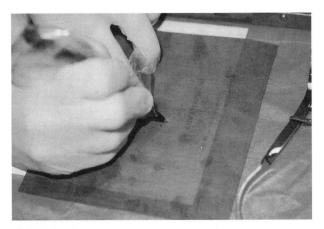

FIGURE 33.11

The rubber dam material is placed on top of the template and marked.

Marking and Punching of the Rubber Dam Material

The rubber dam material may be premarked by the manufacturer. Otherwise, the assistant may mark it using a stamp or template (Figure 33.11). It is important that the holes in the rubber dam material be stamped or marked correctly. The template represents the maxillary and mandibular dental arches and, as mentioned previously, often shows two arch sizes. Using the correct size and spacing helps prevent leakage and unwanted folds and makes the borders more uniform around the patient's face. Usually 3.5 mm of rubber is left between holes (Figure 33.12). The rubber dam material is pulled up over the stylus, or shank, when the holes are punched to ensure that the hole is cut completely through the material. The guide for finding the correct hole size is listed next (Figure 33.13):

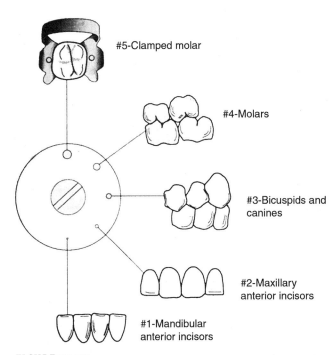

FIGURE 33.13

The rotating punch table guides the selection of the correct hole size.

- #6: (Found only on some punches)
- #5: Largest hole (for clamped molar)
- #4: Molars and large premolars
- #3: Premolars and cuspids
- #2: Maxillary incisors
- #1: Smallest hole (for mandibular incisors)

Some conservative operators prefer to mark and isolate only one or two teeth distal and mesial to the tooth to be restored. However, in the following examples, the quadrant is isolated. Steps for marking and punching the rubber dam material are listed next:

1 Maxillary right posterior isolation to restore the first molar:

Place the rubber dam material on the template.

Mark from the maxillary right second molar to the maxillary right central incisor.

Clamp the maxillary right second molar and isolate to the maxillary right central incisor and ligate.

(When punching the rubber dam material, the largest hole in the punch table [hole #5 on most punch tables] usually is used for the tooth to be clamped, progressing to the smaller holes, or hole #2 for the central incisor.)

2 Mandibular left posterior isolation to restore the second premolar:

Place the rubber dam on the template.

Mark from the mandibular left first molar to the mandibular right central incisor.

Mark the rubber dam.

Clamp the mandibular left first molar and isolate to the mandibular right central incisor and ligate.

(Use hole #5 for the tooth to be clamped and hole #2 for the most anterior tooth, the central incisor.)

3 Maxillary and mandibular anterior isolation to restore the incisors:

Place the rubber dam on the template.

Mark from the right cuspid through the left cuspid.

Clamp the right cuspid and isolate to the left cuspid and ligate.

(Use hole #3 for both cuspids and hole #2 for maxillary incisors or hole #1 for mandibular incisors. One or both cuspids may clamped.)

4 Isolation of a single anterior tooth:

Place the rubber dam on the template.

Mark two teeth mesial and two teeth distal to the tooth being restored.

Isolate the designated area and place an anterior double-bowed clamp over the tooth to be treated (Figure 33.14).

5 Isolation with malaligned or missing teeth:

The holes must be altered according to the malalignment of the teeth or skipped if teeth are missing.

Isolation of the Teeth

The tissue side of the rubber dam material is lubricated before it is slid over the teeth. Lubricating the rubber dam material is an optional procedure for which water-soluble substances such as shaving cream, soap, toothpaste, or petroleum jelly can be used. The lubricant is placed over the holes to help the dam material pass through the contacts.

Basic Wingless Clamp Technique

When the basic wingless clamp technique is used, the clamp is secured in the clamp forceps and then placed on the tooth, lingual first, with the jaws or points of the clamp completely below the height of contour. The bow of the clamp is placed to the distal with all four jaws in contact with the tooth. The

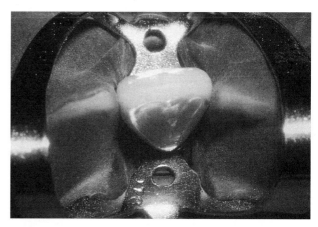

FIGURE 33.14

Anterior isolation with an anterior double-bowed clamp over the tooth to be treated.

clamp must be checked to make sure it is secure on the most posterior tooth to be isolated and that the clamp does not impinge on or cut into the gingival tissue. Next, using the index fingers, the operator or assistant stretches the rubber dam material to a fine edge so as to carry it over the bow of the clamp and through and below the contact area without tearing. The material should not be bunched, and no attempt should be made to try to force it through the embrasures because it may tear. Difficult contact areas should be bypassed until the frame has been placed and the dam ligated.

Winged Clamp Technique

For the winged clamp technique, the clamp is placed into the rubber dam so that the hole is held open by the wings of the clamp. The clamp forceps is placed into the clamp, and the clamp and rubber dam material are conjointly placed over the tooth. After the clamp has been securely placed, the index finger or a plastic instrument is used to slip the rubber dam material off the clamp wings and around the cervix of the tooth.

Alternate Winged Clamp Technique

For an alternate winged clamp technique, the winged clamp is placed into the rubber dam, the hole is held open, the rubber dam is attached to the frame, and the rubber dam forceps is used to place the clamp, rubber dam, and frame over the tooth conjointly.

After the clamp has been placed, the remaining teeth are isolated and the last tooth ligated to secure the anterior portion of the rubber dam material. Waxed dental floss or a wedge can be used to help carry the rubber dam through the contact areas. For the floss technique, about 18 inches of dental floss is cut and wrapped firmly around the two index fingers and held taut. The floss is passed from the labial or lingual surface. The floss should not be snapped through the contacts into the interproximal space because this would cause pain and hemorrhage of the papilla. The floss is looped over the lingual surface and carried through the embrasure again to be doubled through to the buccal surface. Difficult contacts are bypassed until the material has been ligated. Ligation helps hold the rubber dam in place while the more difficult areas are worked on.

Ligation (Anchoring) of the Rubber Dam Material

The rubber dam material must be anchored or secured so that it does not loosen or come off during the restorative procedure. This can be done by stretching a small piece of rubber dam through the contact or by placing a double strand of floss in the contact area mesial to the last tooth isolated. For more difficult areas a wooden wedge can be placed in the contact area, or an O-ring anchor ring can be placed for special applications. Some operators use stick impression compound to secure the material or clamp during lengthy procedures.

Inversion of the Rubber Dam Material

Invert

To turn under the rubber dam material around the neck of the tooth to prevent moisture leakage.

The operator must **invert** the rubber dam material to prevent the leakage of moisture. A plastic instrument can be used to invert the material between the gingiva and tooth (see Figure 33.11). The air syringe is used to dry the tooth surfaces during inversion to prevent the dam from lifting. Copal resin varnish can be applied to the area to help secure the material. The operator should check for leakage from tears, from holes that are too large or unevenly spaced, or from places where the rubber dam material may be caught on the clamp. As mentioned previously, if the patient has a breathing problem with the rubber dam in place, a hole can be cut in the palatal area of the material, which then can be rolled under the nose, away from the nasal area.

Use of the Rubber Dam Napkin, Frame, and Saliva Ejector

The rubber dam napkin is placed under the rubber dam material before the frame is placed. The napkin absorbs saliva at the corners of the mouth and adds to the patient's comfort, particularly when the rubber dam is used for long appointments. It also acts as a cushion at the corners of the mouth and to the lips. It prevents contact between the rubber and soft tissues and reduces the possibility of allergic reactions in sensitive patients. The napkin also provides a convenient means of drying the patient's lips and face when the dam is removed.

When the wingless clamp technique is used, the rubber dam frame is placed after the clamp is secure and the teeth have been isolated and ligated. This is accomplished by holding the frame with the curved portion toward the operator and down or next to the patient's chin with the open portion of the frame at the top, or in the shape of a U. With the frame held securely in one hand, the operator pulls the top corners of the rubber dam material over the projections (points) on the frame. This can be easily accomplished single handed by using one hand to hold the frame, with the index finger securing the material over the top projections on one side of the frame, and pulling the material tightly with the other hand over the top projections on the opposite side. Once this has been done, the bottom projections are secured in the same way and then the center projections. Some operators leave the center projections free to allow for flexibility in the dam. The operator must check to make sure the rubber dam has been flossed through the difficult contacts and that the material has been inverted. The saliva ejector is inserted under the rubber dam.

If necessary, a hole can be cut in the palatal area of the rubber dam material to allow the patient more ease of breathing. The top of the material can be rolled down so that it does not rest too close to the patient's nose. The dam should then be checked for any leaks.

Removal of the Rubber Dam

When the restorative procedure has been completed, the rubber dam is removed (Box 33.4). Any remaining debris must be removed from the operating area with the suction tip. The saliva ejector is then removed. The Young's frame can be removed separately from the rubber dam or, if the winged clamp was used, the frame, clamp, and rubber dam material all can be removed at the same time; this is done by placing the forceps in the clamp and picking up the frame, material, and mask with the other hand, carefully lifting the entire assembly. If the material is to be removed entirely the dam ligature and interseptal dam must be removed first. To remove the rubber dam material from the interproximal area, the interseptal dam is stretched in the buccal or labial direction, the soft tissue is protected with the index fingers, and the interseptal dam is then cut with crown and bridge scissors (Figure 33.15).

If the wingless clamp technique was used, the clamp is removed with the forceps after the frame has been removed. The interseptal dam is removed, and the rubber dam is carefully gathered into the rubber dam napkin; the napkin is used to wipe the patient's lips. The patient's mouth is then rinsed with the water syringe and cleared with suction. The patient may want to swallow some of the water after the mouth has been rinsed. It is important to realign the holes of the rubber dam to check for lost pieces of rubber (Figure 33.16); all interproximal areas must also be checked for small pieces of rubber dam or debris. It is a nice gesture to massage the gingival tissue where the clamp had been placed.

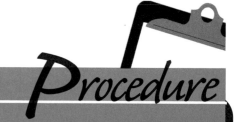

Box 33.4

Procedure for Removal of Rubber Dam

1. Remove all debris from the operating area.
2. Remove the saliva ejector.

Basic wingless clamp technique:
1. Remove Young's frame.
2. Remove the clamp with forceps.
3. Remove the interseptal dam ligature.
4. Stretch the interseptal dam in the buccal or labial direction, protect the soft tissue with the forefingers, and cut the interseptal dam with a crown and bridge scissors.
   a. The assistant helps remove the rubber dam material.
   b. The operator cuts the interseptal material.
5. Gather the rubber dam into the rubber dam napkin and wipe the patient's lips with the napkin.

6. Rinse the patient's mouth.
7. Realign the holes of the rubber dam to check for lost pieces of rubber.
8. Check all interproximal areas for small pieces of rubber dam or debris.

Winged clamp technique:
1. Remove the interseptal dam ligature.
2. Cut the interseptal dam.
3. Attach forceps to the rubber dam clamp and remove the clamp, dam, napkin, and frame in one continuous motion.
4. Rinse the patient's mouth.
5. Realign the holes of the rubber dam to check for lost pieces of rubber.
6. Check all interproximal areas for small pieces of rubber dam or debris.

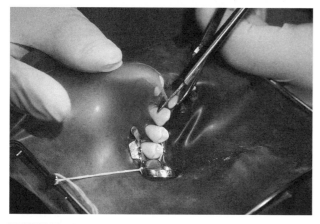

FIGURE 33.15

The assistant helps remove the rubber dam while the operator cuts the interseptal material.

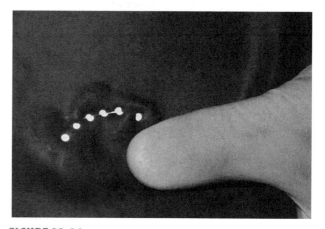

FIGURE 33.16

The holes of the rubber dam are realigned to check for lost pieces of rubber.

Four-Handed Procedures for Rubber Dam Application

The procedures for four-handed application and removal of rubber dam are described next (also see Table 33.1). Once the operator and dental assistant both understand the steps involved, they can gain greater efficiency and effectiveness by working as a team in placing rubber dam.

After the operator and assistant have moved into the proper working positions, the operator establishes a finger rest position and prepares to receive the mirror and explorer to examine the oral cavity. Anticipating readiness, the assistant picks up both instruments and places them at the same time in the operator's hands. The operator checks for any debris, obstruction, or tooth malalignment that could prevent the rubber dam from sliding smoothly over the tooth. After the examination, the operator signals for the assistant to retrieve the instruments (see Figure 33.8). The assistant then passes the dental floss to the operator so that the contacts can be checked or any obstruction removed. A scaler may be needed if the obstruction cannot be removed with floss. The assistant anticipates this need, receives the floss, and passes the scaler. If the contacts are free of obstruction, the assistant passes the rubber dam forceps with the clamp mounted and the mouth mirror, if needed. The forceps should be passed for application to the appropriate arch, and the clamp should be placed in the forceps according to the correct direction of the bow (see Figure 33.8). After trying in the clamp to make sure it fits, the operator signals for the assistant to take the clamp and forceps. Preferably, the rubber dam material is prepunched. If not, the material must be marked and punched according to the conditions or variations of the oral cavity.

The operator may choose to use either of the winged clamp rubber dam placement techniques or the basic wingless clamp technique. As the operator applies the rubber dam, the assistant helps (1) floss the dam below the contacts, (2) invert the dam using the air syringe and a plastic instrument, (3) ligate the dam with floss or a small corner of the rubber dam material, and (4) make any necessary adjustments in the rubber dam material. After the clamp and rubber dam are in place and have been secured, the operator passes the clamp forceps to the assistant. If the frame was not attached to the rubber dam material, it is attached now. If the winged clamp has been used, the operator removes the rubber dam material from the clamp wings and checks the placement of the rubber dam (Table 33.3).

When the procedure is finished, the rubber dam is removed. The assistant passes the scissors to the operator, who removes the ligature and floss and cuts the **interseptal rubber dam.** The assistant can guide the soft tissue and the lip and cheek area away from the interseptal areas and the sharp scissors. After the interseptal rubber dam has been cut, the assistant passes the forceps to the operator for removal of the clamp. The forceps and clamp (and perhaps the entire frame and rubber dam material) are passed to the assistant. The operator inspects the oral cavity for debris and the rubber dam material to check for any missing pieces. The assistant provides a stream of water from the syringe so that the patient can rinse the mouth.

The time saved during the dental procedure far outweighs the several minutes required to place the rubber dam.

> *Interseptal rubber dam*
>
> **The part of the rubber dam material that is positioned between the teeth**

Table 33.3

Four-Handed Rubber Dam Application

Operator	Assistant
Examine tooth and oral cavity.	Anticipate and pass mirror, explorer, and floss.
Floss contacts; identify missing teeth or malaligned teeth and inform assistant if any exist.	Punch dam if it is not prepunched.
Identify appropriate clamp.	Place clamp on forceps and pass to operator.
Try clamp on tooth and pass back to assistant.	Assemble rubber dam, frame, and clamp and pass.
Place clamp on tooth and pass forceps to assistant.	Assist and receive forceps.
Remove rubber dam from wings of clamp.	Prepare to pass plastic instrument and floss; use air syringe.
Floss rubber dam through contacts.	Assist in stretching dam to expose teeth.
Ligate with floss or rubber dam material.	Hold floss with plastic instrument.
Cut ligature if lengthy.	Assist operator.
Invert dam into sulcus area.	Dry with air syringe.
Prepare tooth for restoration.	Assist operator.
Removal of rubber dam	
Cut and remove ligature.	Anticipate and pass scissors and retrieve ligature and scissors.
Cut interseptal rubber dam.	Stretch rubber dam while protecting soft tissues.
Remove clamp.	Pass rubber dam forceps and retrieve forceps and clamp.
Remove rubber dam and frame and inspect for missing parts.	Retrieve rubber dam material and frame.
Rinse patient's mouth.	Spray water and air, then suction.
Evaluate treatment.	Provide any postoperative instructions and dismiss patient.

CARIES REMOVAL AND CAVITY PREPARATION

The dentist determines the proper outline form for the cavity preparation and reduces the tooth surface to achieve adequate access. The air-water coolant is used during caries removal. Large, slow-speed round burs or the spoon excavator can be used to remove the caries and to cut in the deep portions of the preparation. The caries is removed without reducing an unnecessary amount of tooth or damaging adjacent teeth and soft tissue. The dentist extends the cavosurface margins sufficiently to provide cleansible areas. The occlusal grooves, which are susceptible to caries, are prepared as part of the cavity preparation. In order for sufficient bulk of restorative material to be placed in the cavity preparation, the dentin must be reduced. Retention is also placed to help hold the restorative material. When necessary, retention pins or posts may be placed and cut to proper length.

While restoring the missing tooth structure, the operator must have a mental picture of the tooth before its structure and shape were destroyed by disease or accident and altered by cavity preparation. The reader should review the general characteristics of the teeth, presented in Chapter 9, to refresh his or her understanding of caries classification and cavity preparation.

Caries Classification

Classification systems have been developed to help clarify information about the teeth, carious lesions, and the cavity preparation. In the late nineteenth century, Dr. G.V. Black devised a caries and cavity classification system that is still used. Dental plaque causes carious lesions and cavities on various surfaces of the crown. These lesions and the cavity preparations made in treating them are classified according to their location. Some tooth surfaces are smooth and are not as prone to decay as irregular surfaces, such as fossae and grooves, where food often collects in small pits and fissures. However, decay can also be found on smooth surfaces, particularly on the interproximal surface and the gingival one third of the tooth. Lesions are designated "pit and fissure cavities" or "smooth surface cavities" and are identified according to their type and the surface where they are found. Carious lesions are categorized as Class I, II, III, IV, V, or VI.

Class I

Class I cavities are located in the pits and fissures of the occlusal two thirds of posterior teeth and on the lingual surfaces of anterior teeth. These cavities vary in size and can be detected with an explorer (Figure 33.17).

Class II

Class II cavities are located on the proximal surfaces of all posterior teeth (molars and premolars). These smooth sur-

face lesions are detected with dental radiographs (Figure 33.18).

Class III

Class III cavities are located on the proximal surfaces of all anterior teeth (central incisors, lateral incisors, and cuspids). They are smooth surface lesions and can be detected with a dental radiograph or often with a high-intensity light (Figure 33.19).

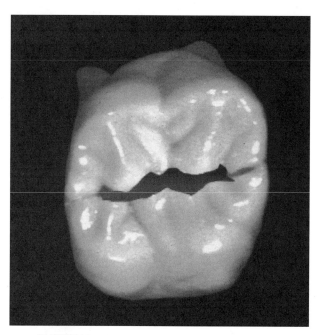

FIGURE 33.17

Class I cavity on the occlusal surface of tooth #31.

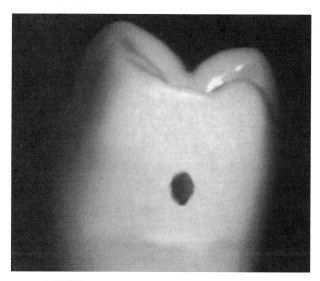

FIGURE 33.18

Class II cavity on the distal surface of tooth #20.

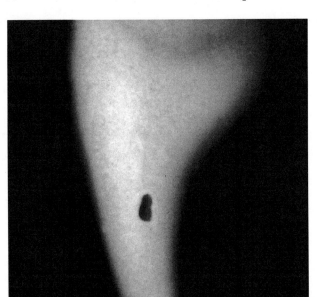

FIGURE 33.19

Class III cavity on the mesial surface of tooth #7.

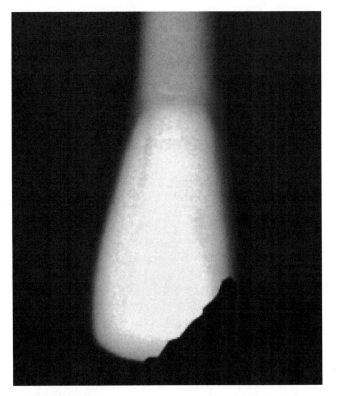

FIGURE 33.20

Class IV cavity involving the mesioincisal angle of tooth #7.

Class IV

Class IV cavities are located on the proximal surfaces of all anterior teeth and include the incisal angle (Figure 33.20).

Class V

Class V cavities are smooth surface lesions located on the gingival one third of the facial and lingual surfaces of all teeth. They vary in size, are found just above the crest of the gingiva, and may involve the gingival one third of the root (Figure 33.21).

Class VI

Class VI cavities are uncommon but occur on the incisal edge or cusp tip.

Cavity Classification and Nomenclature

Line angles

The junctions where two surfaces meet

Point angles

The junctions where three surfaces meet

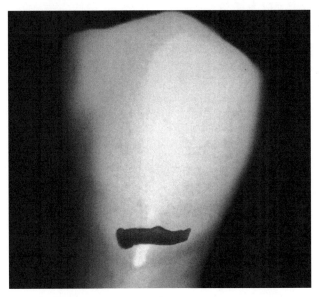

FIGURE 33.21

Class V cavity on the buccal surface of tooth #20.

The operator must have a working understanding of the nomenclature of a cavity preparation in order to properly condense the restorative material into the angles and retentive areas. For example, if the material is not condensed into a point angle, a void will be left that weakens the restoration, causing it to fracture or break down. The operator also places retentive grooves or points in the cavity angles of the dentin to provide mechanical retention. The **line angles** and **point angles** are named after the areas of the tooth where they are located. The walls of the cavity preparation are also named after the surface on which they are located. For instance, the incisal wall is next to the incisal surface. The gingival

Table 33.4

Nomenclature for Dental Features

Term	Location	Definition
Long axis	Axial wall	The line or surface inside the cavity preparation measuring from the crown of the tooth to the root.
Perpendicular wall	Gingival wall	The surface within the cavity preparation that is perpendicular to the long axis of the tooth and coronal to the pulp chamber.
Axial wall	Lingual wall Facial wall Mesial wall Distal wall	A surface within the cavity preparation that is parallel to the long axis of the tooth; it is named for the aspect where it is located.
Cavosurface margin	Mesiocavosurface Distocavosurface Faciocavosurface Linguocavosurface	An angle or junction where the wall of the preparation joins the tooth surface
Point angle	Mesiolinguopulpal Mesiolabiopulpal Distolinguopulpal Linguoaxiogingival Buccoaxiogingival Distoincisoaxial Mesioincisoaxial Distogingivoaxial Mesiogingivoaxial	The junction of three surfaces or the point where three walls meet inside the cavity preparation.
Line angle	Mesiopulpal Distopulpal Faciopulpal Linguopulpal Facioaxial Linguoaxial Gingivoaxial	The junction of two surfaces or the area or line where two walls meet inside the cavity preparation.
Cavosurface angles	Mesiolingual Mesiobuccal Distolingual Distobuccal Mesiogingival Distogingival Mesioocclusal Distoocclusal Buccoocclusal Linguoocclusal Labioocclusal	The junction of two surfaces that meet at the cavosurface margin of the cavity preparation.

Cavosurface margin

The angle or junction where the walls of the preparation join the tooth surface

wall refers to the prepared surface next to the gingiva. The **cavosurface margin** is the finished edge of the cavity preparation or the junction formed where the wall of the cavity preparation joins the external tooth surface.

Two rules govern the terminology used to identify the areas of a cavity preparation:

1. Rule 1: Drop the *-al* ending and replace it with *o* for all connected words except the last word; for example, mesioocclusal.

2. Rule 2: The term *cavosurface* comes last when connecting words that describe the surface of the tooth; for example, buccoocclusocavosurface. The prepared surface above the pulp may be called the pulpal wall or the pulpal floor (Table 33.4).

Class I

Class I cavity preparation is the removal of pit and fissure caries in the occlusal two thirds of the molars and premolars and the lingual surfaces of anterior teeth. The five cavity walls of the occlusal preparation are the buccal, mesial, distal, lingual, and pulpal surfaces (Box 33.5). The eight line angles involved in the occlusal preparation are the mesiobuccal (mb), distobuccal (db), distolingual (dl), mesiolingual (ml), mesiopulpal (mp), distopulpal (dp), buccopulpal (bp), and linguopulpal (lp) line angles. The four point angles are the mesiobuccopulpal (mbp), distobuccopulpal (dbp), distolinguopulpal (dlp), and mesiolinguopulpal (mlp) point angles. The four cavosurface angles are the mesioocclusal, distoocclusal, buccoocclusal, and the linguoocclusal cavosurface angles.

Class II

Class II cavity preparation is the removal of caries on the proximal surfaces of molars and premolars. To remove caries from the proximal surfaces, an occlusal approach must be used. For this reason, caries on the mesial or distal proximal surface (or both) requires removal of a portion of the occlusal surface. The preparation therefore would be described as a mesioocclusal (MO), distoocclusal (DO), or mesioocclusodistal (MOD) preparation.

A two-surface preparation would have four cavity walls, depending on which surface was removed, the distal or the mesial. This description considers the removal of the mesioocclusal surfaces (Figure 33.22), therefore the four remaining cavity walls are the distal, lingual, buccal, and pulpal walls (Box 33.6). The nine line angles are the distobuccal (db), distolingual (dl), distopulpal (dp), buccopulpal (bp), linguopulpal (lp), gingivoaxial (ga), buccoaxial (ba) (retentive area), linguoaxial (la) (retentive area), and pulpoaxial

(pa) line angles. The four point angles are the distobuccopulpal (dbp), distolinguopulpal (dlp), buccoaxiogingival (bag), and linguoaxiogingival (lag) point angles. Because the two-surface preparation extends into the proximal area, the preparation has six cavosurface angles: the distoocclusal, buccoocclusal, linguoocclusal, linguoproximal, buccoproximal, and gingivoproximal cavosurface angles.

Class III

Class III cavity preparation is the removal of caries on the proximal surfaces of the central incisors, lateral incisors, and

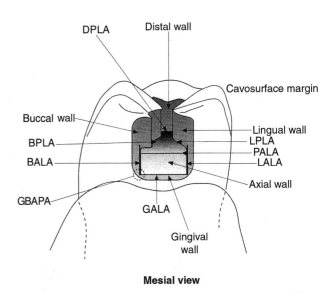

Mesial view

FIGURE 33.22

A Class II cavity preparation involving four walls, line angles, and point angles.

Box 33.5

Nomenclature for a Class I Occlusal Cavity Preparation

Walls or floors	Point angles
Mesial	Mesiobuccopulpal
Distal	Distobuccopulpal
Buccal	Distolinguopulpal
Lingual	Mesiolinguopulpal
Pulpal	
	Cavosurface angles
Line angles	Mesioocclusal
Mesiobuccal	Distoocclusal
Distobuccal	Buccoocclusal
Distolingual	Linguoocclusal
Mesiolingual	
Mesiopulpal	
Distopulpal	
Buccopulpal	
Linguopulpal	

Box 33.6

Nomenclature for a Class II Mesioocclusal (MO) Cavity Preparation

Walls or floors	Point angles
Distal	Distobuccopulpal
Lingual	Distolinguopulpal
Buccal	Buccoaxiogingival
Pulpal	Linguoaxiogingival
Line angles	**Cavosurface Angles**
Distobuccal	Distoocclusal
Distolingual	Buccoocclusal
Distopulpal	Linguoocclusal
Buccopulpal	Linguoproximal
Linguopulpal	Buccoproximal
Gingivoaxial	Gingivoproximal
Buccoaxial	
Linguoaxial	
Pulpoaxial	

cuspids. Depending on the angle of the tooth, the operator may remove the caries directly from the proximal surface or, if this is impossible, from the adjacent surface, the lingual if possible. Removing the caries from the lingual surface preserves the facial tooth structure as much as possible for esthetic purposes. If the area of decay is large, the preparation must be extended onto the labial or facial surface. A Class III cavity preparation generally includes both the proximal and lingual surfaces. This description of a Class III preparation includes the distal and lingual surfaces (Box 33.7).

The walls of a Class III preparation involving the distolingual surfaces are the labial, incisal, gingival, and axial walls (Figure 33.23). The five line angles are the labioaxial,

incisoaxial, gingivoaxial, labiogingival, and labioincisal line angles. The two point angles are the labioaxiogingival and labioaxioincisal point angles. The cavosurface angles are the linguogingival, linguoincisal, mesiolingual, gingivoproximal, incisoproximal, and labioproximal cavosurface angles.

Class IV

Class IV cavity preparation is the removal of caries on the proximal surfaces of the central incisors, lateral incisors, and cuspids; it also involves the incisal angle. The caries removal creates a preparation similar to the Class III type except that the incisal surface is involved (Box 33.8). In Class IV distoincisal preparations, the walls are the gingival, lingual, axial, and labial walls. The line angles are the labiogingival, linguogingival, gingivoaxial, labioaxial, linguoaxial, and incisoaxial line angles. The point angles are the labioaxiogingival and the linguoaxiogingival point angles. The cavosurface angles are the gingivoproximal, labioproximal, and lingual cavosurface angles.

Class V

Class V cavity preparation is the removal of caries on the facial or labial and buccal or lingual surface of anterior and posterior teeth (Figure 33.24). The Class V preparation has five walls: the gingival, mesial, distal, incisal or occlusal, and axial walls (Box 33.9). The line angles are the mesioaxial, distoaxial, incisoaxial or occlusoaxial, gingivoaxial, mesiogingival, mesioincisal or mesioocclusal, distogingival, and distoincisal or distoocclusal line angles. The four point angles are the mesioaxiogingival, mesioaxioincisal or mesioaxioocclusal, distoaxiogingival, and distoaxioincisal or distoaxioocclusal point angles. The four cavosurface angles are the gingivofacial, incisofacial or occlusofacial, mesiofacial, and distofacial cavosurface angles.

Box 33.7

Nomenclature for a Class III Mesioocclusal (MO) Cavity Preparation

Walls
Labial
Incisal
Gingival
Axial

Line angles
Labioaxial
Incisoaxial
Gingivoaxial
Labiogingival
Labioincisal

Point angles
Labioaxiogingival
Linguoaxioincisal

Cavosurface angles
Linguogingival
Linguoincisal
Mesiolingual
Gingivoproximal
Incisoproximal
Labioproximal

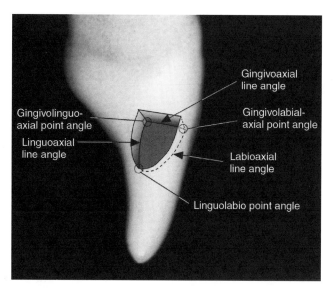

FIGURE 33.23

A Class III cavity preparation involving four walls: labial, incisal, gingival, and axial.

Box 33.8

Nomenclature for a Class IV Distoincisal (DI) Cavity Preparation

Walls
Gingival
Lingual
Axial
Labial

Line angles
Labiogingival
Linguogingival
Gingivoaxial
Labioaxial

Linguoaxial
Incisoaxial

Point angles
Labioaxiogingival
Linguoaxiogingival

Cavosurface angles
Gingivoproximal
Labioproximal

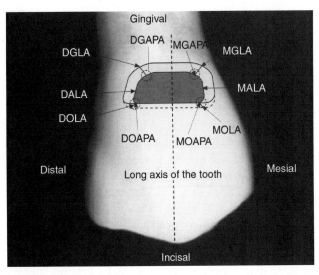

FIGURE 33.24

Class V cavity preparation is the removal of caries on the facial or labial/buccal or lingual surface of anterior and posterior teeth.

Pulp Protection

The operator must make sure the tooth recovers from the damage caused by the dental caries and by preparation of the tooth for restoration. To aid this recovery, a number of dental materials can be used to protect the pulp by acting as a sealant or liner and serving as an obtundant, or stimulant. Glass ionomer liners and bases that release fluoride to provide protection from microleakage are becoming the cement of choice. Bases or insulators, such as zinc oxide–eugenol, zinc phosphate, and the new glass ionomer material, also protect the pulp from thermal irritation and can be used as a strong base from which to compress or condense amalgam alloy. Guidelines for the application of liners are presented in Box 33.10.

Bonding agents, which involve nearly all aspects of restorative dentistry, also are available. These agents are adhesive and can bond to virtually any substance. They are called "universal" bonding agents because they can be used with either alloy or composite acrylic resin materials. Other bonding agents are used only to bond specific

---

Box 33.9

Nomenclature for a Class V Cavity Preparation

Walls

Gingival
Mesial
Distal
Incisal or occlusal
Axial

Line angles

Mesioaxial
Distoaxial
Incisoaxial or occlusoaxial
Gingivoaxial
Mesiogingival
Mesioincisal or mesioocclusal

Distogingival
Distoincisal or distoocclusal

Point angles

Mesioaxiogingival
Mesioaxioincisal or mesioaxioocclusal
Distoaxiogingival
Distoaxioincisal or distoaxioocclusal

Cavosurface angles

Gingivofacial
Incisofacial or occlusofacial
Mesiofacial
Distofacial

Box 33.10

Guidelines for Application of Liners

- Varnish can be used as a liner under moderately shallow amalgam restorations.
- Varnish cannot be used as a liner with composite acrylic resin.
- Varnish is usually applied in two coats and extended over the entire cavity preparation.
- Glass ionomers can chemically bond to the tooth structure, have compressive and adhesive strength, and can be used as either a liner or a base under composites, amalgams, and porcelains.

- Varnish and calcium hydroxide (CaOH) can be used under an amalgam restoration with subpulpal and subaxial extensions.
  a. The calcium hydroxide is placed only on the dentin.
  b. Varnish is placed over the calcium hydroxide and on the enamel walls of the cavity preparation.
- Calcium hydroxide can be used as a liner with composite acrylic resin materials.
- In a near exposure, calcium hydroxide can be used to stimulate the formation of secondary dentin, with varnish applied over the calcium hydroxide and zinc phosphate.

restorative materials, such as composites, directly to the tooth structure. These materials maximize esthetics and are efficient to use. Bonding agents may be used with or without etching the dentin, and they may be self-curing or light-cured. When these bases, liners, bonding agents, temporary filling materials, and pulp-capping agents are used correctly, they can enhance the success of the restoration.

The procedures for applying these materials are presented in Box 33.11.

Because of the increasing variety of materials available, it is extremely important that the dental assistant read the manufacturer's directions and continue to learn about dental materials (these materials and their working conditions are described in Chapter 15).

Box 33.11   *Procedure*

Procedures for Application of Liners, Etchants, and Bonding Agents

Cavity preparation:
1. Remove debris and slightly dry the cavity preparation with light flow of warm air.

Cavity sealants or liners and insulators or bases

VARNISH

Varnish is used to seal the tubules of the exposed dentin and to prevent leakage around the cavosurface margins.
1. With a small wisp or cotton ball held in the cotton pliers, dip into the varnish and apply two light coats *over all walls and cavosurface margins.*
2. Place varnish *over* a zinc oxide–eugenol base but *under* a zinc phosphate base.
3. Do not allow the liner to thicken or pool in the retentive grooves.
4. Replace the cap on the varnish immediately to prevent vaporization.
5. Dry the area with a light stream of air.

CALCIUM HYDROXIDE OR ZINC OXIDE–EUGENOL

Calcium hydroxide or zinc oxide–eugenol is used to help promote the formation of secondary dentin, to soothe the pulp, and to make the tooth less sensitive after the completed restoration.
1. Spatulate the base and catalyst to a uniform mixture.
2. Wipe the spatula, then lightly touch the placement instrument into the mix and flow the material into the deepest area of the preparation; apply in a thin, even coat. Do not flow the material onto the enamel walls or cavosurface margins or into the retentive grooves.

3. If more than one application is needed, be sure to wipe the tip of the applicator between increments.
4. Be sure the pulp is adequately covered, but keep the area dry and do not let the liner become excessively thick.
5. The pulpal floor is coated only in a posterior occlusal preparation; the axial walls are coated only in a Class III preparation.
6. After final set, remove any excess material from the enamel with an excavator or explorer.
7. Allow the liner to dry before placing the restorative material.

GLASS IONOMER

Glass ionomer liners, which release fluoride, are used where microleakage or recurrent caries is probable. These liners may be self-curing or light cured.
1. Apply the glass ionomer evenly to the dentin to a thickness of about 0.5 to l mm.
2. Allow to self-cure, or light-cure for 30 seconds.

ZINC OXIDE–EUGENOL OR ZINC PHOSPHATE BASE
1. Mix the material to a thick, puttylike consistency to provide adequate condensing mass.
2. Place the material into the deepest portion of the preparation only on dentinal surfaces. Do not extend the material to the enamel walls or cavosurface margins or into the retentive grooves.
3. Use light tapping strokes to condense the material.
4. Add sufficient material to make a smooth, even pulpal wall over the floor of the cavity preparation.

Continued

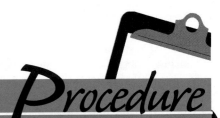

Box 33.11—cont'd

Procedures for Application of Liners, Etchants, and Bonding Agents—cont'd

5. Varnish may be used over a zinc oxide–eugenol base to allow the material to act as an obtundant. However, varnish must be used *under* a zinc phosphate base to protect the pulp from irritation caused by the acidic zinc phosphate material.

Etchants:
Always read the manufacturer's directions.
1. Etch the enamel for 15 seconds, rinse, and then dry.
2. Apply primer to the dentin and enamel (some etchants must not be disturbed, whereas others must be agitated).
3. Air dry (some etchants must not be rinsed off; others must be rinsed off and the tooth dried).
4. Cure for 20 seconds.

Bonding agents:
Always read the manufacturer's directions.
1. Use a brush to apply the bonding adhesives to all surfaces in a thin, uniform layer. Do not thin the adhesive excessively.
2. Do not dry excessively.
3. Cure for at least 20 to 60 seconds.

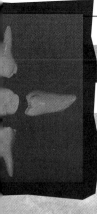

Points for Review

- Rubber dam application
- Four-handed procedures for rubber dam application
- Caries removal and cavity preparation
- Pulp protection

Self-Study Questions

1. Rubber dam isolation offers what advantage or advantages?
   a. Keeps patients quiet
   b. Protects the patient
   c. Controls moisture
   d. All of the above
   e. All of the above except a
2. What technique or techniques can the operator use to help move the rubber dam beneath the contact area?
   a. Use dental floss
   b. Stretch the material to a fine edge
   c. Use a small amount of lubricant
   d. All of the above
3. On which tooth is the anterior clamp usually placed?
   a. The tooth to be treated
   b. Both cuspids
   c. Most posterior tooth
   d. Any tooth except the tooth to be treated
4. What technique helps prevent leakage of the rubber dam?
   a. Clamping the tooth
   b. Inverting the rubber dam
   c. Placing the clamp below the height of contour
   d. Punching the holes in an uneven pattern
5. What is one of the functions of a cavity liner?
   a. Moisture control
   b. Filling the pulpal canal
   c. Soothing the pulp
   d. Strengthening the restoration
6. Which of the following base materials should not be used under a composite resin?
   a. Calcium hydroxide
   b. Glass ionomer

   c. Zinc oxide–eugenol
   d. None of the above
7. Which of the following statements is true?
   a. The bow of the clamp is positioned toward the mesial.
   b. The clamp jaws should contact the tooth at two points.
   c. The lingual clamp jaw should be placed first.
   d. The clamp jaws are above the height of contour.
8. In general, on which tooth should the rubber dam clamp be placed for isolation?
   a. The most distal tooth in the arch
   b. The tooth being treated
   c. The tooth mesial to the tooth being treated
   d. The tooth next to the tooth being treated
9. Which cavity classification includes cavities on the proximal surfaces of all posterior teeth?
   a. Class I
   b. Class II
   c. Class III
   d. Class IV
   e. Class V
10. Which cavity classification includes cavities on the proximal surfaces of all anterior teeth and the incisal angle?
    a. Class I
    b. Class II
    c. Class III
    d. Class IV
    e. Class V

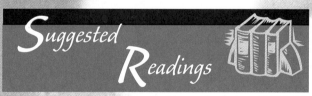

Suggested Readings

Ash MM: *Wheeler's dental anatomy, physiology, and occlusion,* ed 7, Philadelphia, 1993, WB Saunders.

Chasteen JE: *Essentials of clinical dental assisting,* ed 5, St Louis, 1989, Mosby.

Crimm G: *Operative dentistry,* Louisville, Ky, 1995, University of Louisville School of Dentistry.

Council on Dental Materials, Instruments, and Equipment: Choosing intracoronal restorative materials, *J Am Dent Assoc* 1994.

Finkbeiner BL, Johnson CS: *Mosby's comprehensive dental assisting,* ed 1, St Louis, 1995, Mosby.

Jordan RE, Abrams L, Kraus B: *Kraus' dental anatomy and occlusion,* St Louis, 1992, Mosby.

Spohn EE, Halowski WA, Berry TG: *Operative dentistry procedures for dental auxiliaries,* St Louis, 1981, Mosby.

US Department of Health, Education and Welfare: Restoration of cavity preparations with amalgam and tooth-colored materials: Project ACORDE, Castro Valley, Calif, 1979, Quercus Corp.

Zwemer TJ: *Mosby's dental dictionary,* St Louis, 1998, Mosby.

Chapter 34

Matrix Band and Retainer Assembly and Wedge Placement

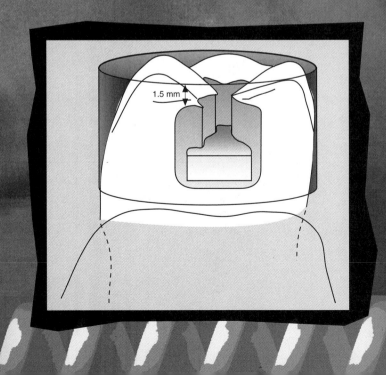

Chapter Outline

Learning Objectives

On completion of Chapter 34, the student should be able to do the following:

- Define key terms.
- Assemble the matrix band and retainer.
- Place the matrix band and retainer.
- Wedge the matrix band.
- Evaluate the placement of the matrix band.
- Identify alternative matrix band techniques.

Key Terms

Matrix Band   Matrix Retainer   Wedge

MATRIX BAND AND RETAINER

A matrix band and matrix retainer are used to form the missing surface of a tooth in a Class II, Class III, or Class IV cavity restoration (review Cavity Classifications, Chapter 33). Although several matrix bands and retainers are identified in this chapter, the Tofflemier matrix band and retainer are discussed in detail.

Matrix Band

Matrix band

A band placed around the tooth to restore the form of the missing tooth structure or wall

A **matrix band** could be considered a temporary wall that encircles the tooth and aids in the restoration of the proximal contours, tooth surfaces, and contacts. The band may be made of metal or plastic. In general, a metal matrix band is used for placing amalgam alloy restorations, and a plastic matrix band is used for composite acrylic resin restorations. The metal matrix band is a thin strip of stainless steel that is available on a roll or precut. The precut bands may be straight or contoured. The universal and the mesioocclusodistal (MOD) matrix bands are used most often, although a variety of other bands and retainers are available (Figures 34.1 to 34.4). The universal band covers most preparations of medium depth. The MOD band can be extended gingivally to cover the gingival interproximal extension of the cavity preparation, and it is wide enough to cover the occlusal height.

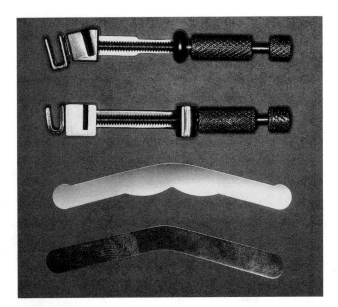

FIGURE 34.1
Tofflemier mesioocclusodistal (MOD) and universal matrix bands and retainers.

Matrix Retainer

A **matrix retainer** holds the metal matrix band in place around the tooth, allowing the operator to mold the amalgam alloy into the cavity preparation. The two mostly commonly used types of Tofflemire matrix retainers are the straight retainer and the contraangle retainer. The straight retainer is placed from the buccal or facial surface of the tooth, and the contraangle retainer is placed from the lingual surface. The contraangle retainer is used if the cavity preparation extends into the buccal surface of the tooth, and the straight retainer is used if the preparation extends lingually.

The matrix retainer can be adjusted. It has two moving parts, an outer nut, which works with the spindle and vise to secure the matrix band, and an inner nut, which works with

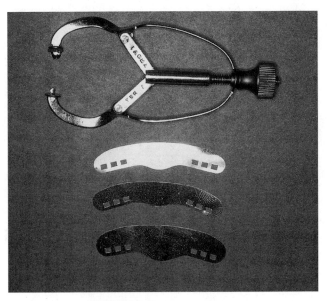

FIGURE 34.2
Ivory matrix band and retainer.

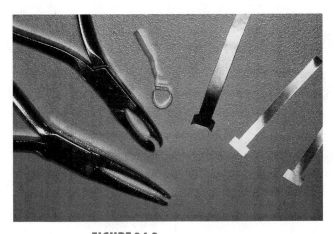

FIGURE 34.3
T-band and contouring forceps.

Matrix retainer

A device that holds the matrix band in place around the tooth

the guide channels to tighten the band around the tooth. The vise diagonal slot holds the band in place when the spindle is tightened. The guide channels direct the matrix band in the appropriate direction. The parts of the Tofflemire matrix retainer are described below (Figure 34.5):

- *Outer nut:* Tightens the spindle and holds the matrix band in position in the diagonal vise slot.
- *Inner nut:* Adjusts the size of the matrix band loop.
- *Diagonal vise:* Holds the ends of the matrix band in the retainer.
- *Diagonal vise slot:* The slanted opening into which the matrix band is placed and secured.
- *Spindle:* A straight screw bit that enters the diagonal vise to tighten and secure the matrix band in the retainer.

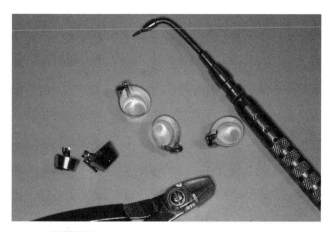

FIGURE 34.4

Auto matrix bands with wrench and side cutter.

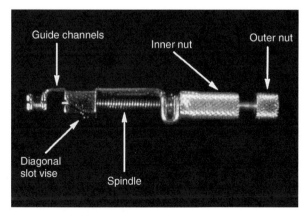

FIGURE 34.5

Parts of the Tofflemier matrix retainer.

- *Guide channels:* Direct the matrix band straight, left, or right depending on the working quadrant.

Once the band has been placed around the tooth, it is adjusted or contoured to achieve a proper interproximal contact, marginal ridge, and cervical adaptation. Contouring can be done with a burnisher while the band is in place, but it is better to contour the band before placement.

Wedge

Although the matrix band is rigid and can support condensing pressure, a **wedge** usually is used with the band to support and adapt the cervical portion of the band to the tooth structure and to separate the teeth slightly. A properly placed wedge ensures that the amalgam alloy can be condensed into the mesial or distal extension of the cavity without flowing into the interproximal space, causing an overhang. It also allows the operator to separate the teeth sufficiently to ensure an adequate contact.

Wedge

A wedge-shaped piece of wood or plastic that helps adapt the matrix band to the cervical position of the tooth structure; it also helps separate the teeth slightly, allowing for a tight margin

Assembling the Matrix Band and Retainer

The amalgam tray setup includes the matrix band and retainer armamentarium for these restorative procedures. The instruments and supplies include the following:

- Locking cotton forceps
- Matrix bands (universal and MOD)
- Retainers (straight and contraangle)
- Mouth mirror
- Explorer (shepherd's hook)
- Ball burnisher
- Wedges (assorted sizes)
- Crown and bridge scissors

Box 34.1 presents the procedure for assembling the matrix band and retainer.

Preparation for Placement of the Matrix Band

Before the matrix band and retainer are placed, a rubber dam is placed in the mouth, the tooth is prepared, a base or liner may be placed in the cavity preparation, any debris or calculus is removed (to allow easy access for placing the matrix band), and the matrix band and retainer armamentarium is set up. Box 34.2 and Table 34.1 detail the procedure for placement of the matrix band and wedge.

Box 34.1

Procedure for Assembling the Matrix Band and Retainer

1. Check the band to make sure that is smooth and has no wrinkles or rough edges.
2. Trim the band for width if necessary.
3. Loop the two ends of the band together evenly.
4. Place the ends of the band into the slit of the sliding vise.
5. Guide the band completely into the left or right slit of the retainer head (Figure 34.6).
6. Turn the outer screw knob clockwise to tighten the vise and hold the band securely (Figure 34.7).

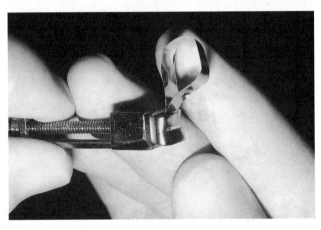

FIGURE 34.6

The band is guided completely into the left or right slit of the retainer head.

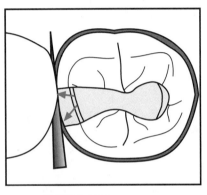

FIGURE 34.8

Placement of the wedge.

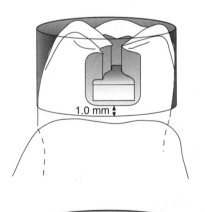

A

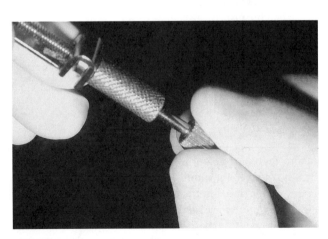

FIGURE 34.7

The outer screw is turned clockwise to hold the band securely in the vise.

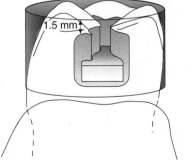

B

FIGURE 34.9

(**A**) The matrix band extends 1 mm to 2 mm gingivally and (**B**) 1 mm occlusally.

Box 34.2

Procedure

Procedure for Placing the Matrix Band and Wedge

1. With the band held securely in the retainer, adjust the size of the loop to fit over the tooth.
2. Carefully press the band around the tooth and below the gingival margin (Figure 34.8).
3. Turn the inner knob clockwise to tighten the band around the tooth.
4. Check the band to ensure that it is 1 to 2 mm above the marginal ridge and approximately 1 mm below the gingival margin of the preparation and that the contact is adapted (Figure 34.9).
5. Position the retainer parallel to the facial or lingual surface of the adjacent teeth.
6. Adapt the band to the gingival cavosurface margin, making sure that no rubber dam material or oral tissue is trapped between the tooth and the band. The band is adapted to the facial and lingual cavosurface margins (Figure 34.10).
7. Check that the band restores the original proximal contour of the tooth and that it is in contact with the adjacent tooth.
8. Burnish the contact surface if necessary.
9. Place the wedge lingually with lock cotton forceps.
10. Make sure the occlusal edge of the wedge is level with the gingival wall of the cavity preparation (Figure 34.11).
11. Evaluate the placement of the band.

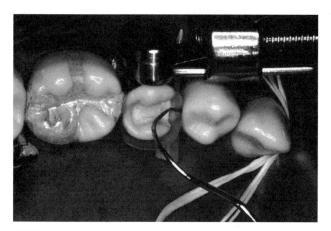

FIGURE 34.10

The band is adapted to the gingival cavosurface margin, with care being taken that no rubber dam material or oral tissue is trapped between the tooth and the band.

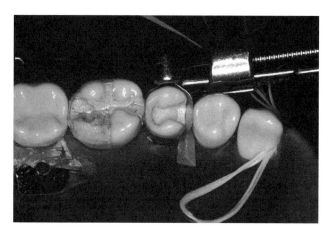

FIGURE 34.11

The retainer should be parallel to the buccal surface of the teeth and the wedge must be placed to hold the band tightly against the gingivocavo surface of the cavity preparation.

Table 34.1

Evaluation for Matrix and Wedge Placement

Matrix and Wedge Placement	4	3	2	0	X
Band smooth and wrinkle free.					
Band secure in retainer.					
Retainer parallel to buccal and lingual surfaces.					
Gingival band edge 1 mm below gingival wall.					
Band adapted to gingival cavosurface margin.					
Rubber dam free					
Band adapted buccally and lingually below the cavosurface margin.					
Proximal contour and contact adapted.					
Occlusal band edge 1.5 mm above marginal ridge.					
Wedge secure.					
Occlusal edge of wedge level with gingival wall of preparation.					
Evaluation of adaptation with explorer.					

The numeric criteria: 4 Excellent; 3 Good but some improvement can be made; 2 Below average, usable, needs to improve skill; 0 Unsatisfactory; X Not able to evaluate.

Placing the Band into the Retainer

Before matrix the band is placed in the retainer, the dental assistant must check the band to make sure that it is smooth and has no wrinkles or rough edges. This can be done by looping the band around an instrument handle and pulling the band carefully, to avoid cutting the fingers on the side of the band. The two ends of the band are then looped together so that they meet evenly. When the band is held between the thumb and index finger in this manner, one side of the loop is smaller than the other. The shorter side of the loop faces away from the retainer, or toward the gingival tissue, when the band has been properly placed around the tooth. Holding the band with the narrow side away from the retainer, the assistant places the ends of the looped band into the diagonal slit of the sliding vise and the head at the end of the retainer. The band must be guided completely into the left or the right slit of the retainer head, depending on the placement of the matrix retainer and band in the mouth (Box 34.3).

The open side of the vise correlates with the narrow opening of the matrix band; therefore the open side of the vise and the small side of the band are placed toward the gingival tissue. The outer screw knob is turned clockwise to tighten the vise and hold the band securely.

Adjusting the Matrix Band around the Tooth

To place the matrix band for restoration of lower right or upper left posterior teeth, the band must be adjusted through the right side of the retainer head while the retainer is held with the open end down or away from the assistant. Conversely, to

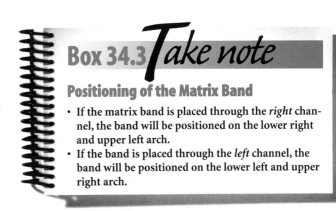

Box 34.3 *Take note*

Positioning of the Matrix Band

- If the matrix band is placed through the *right* channel, the band will be positioned on the lower right and upper left arch.
- If the band is placed through the *left* channel, the band will be positioned on the lower left and upper right arch.

place the band for restoration of lower left or upper right posterior teeth, the band must be placed through the left side of the retainer head while holding the retainer with the open end down. Holding the matrix band and retainer with the small side of the band toward the tissue, the assistant slides the band over the tooth to be restored, carefully pressing, or seating, the band over and around the tooth and below the gingival margin with the index finger or thumb. The inner knob is then turned clockwise to tighten the band. The retainer is parallel to the buccal or lingual surface while the band is tightened.

Some important points to remember when placing a matrix band are:

- Care must be taken not to overtighten the matrix band, because this results in undercontouring of the restoration and eliminates the interproximal contact.
- The rubber dam must be checked to make sure that it has not been caught between the tooth and the matrix band.

- Care must be taken not to bend the edge of the band during placement.
- The matrix band must be checked to make sure that it is wide enough from the occlusal edge to the gingival surface. The band should extend 1 to 2 mm above the marginal ridge and approximately 1 mm below the gingival margin of the preparation (see Figure 34.9).
- The contact area of the band may need to be contoured in the interproximal contact area with a burnisher.
- The band may need to be trimmed on the gingival side for proper width.

Placement of the Wedge

Once the matrix band is in place, the band can be secured with a wedge. A wedge larger than the embrasure is used. More than one wedge can be placed in the embrasure, or the wedge can be cut to fit a smaller embrasure if necessary. The wedge is usually placed from the lingual side in the larger interproximal embrasure with locking tissue forceps and pressed tightly to secure the band around the cervix of the tooth (see Figure 34.11). The band may also be wedged from the buccal side if necessary. If the buccally placed retainer interferes with wedge placement, the retainer must be adjusted. The subgingival and occlusal aspects of the band must be checked from inside the cavity preparation to make sure that the height and depth of the band are satisfactory and that there is no opening that would allow the restorative material to flow under the band. An explorer can be used inside the cavity preparation to check the gingival wall to make sure the band has been wedged or adapted securely. With the band in place, the operator can begin the restoration.

MATRIX BAND TECHNIQUE FOR LARGE AMALGAM CORES

One of the most difficult steps in restoring a badly broken down tooth is the proper adaptation of a matrix band to the remaining prepared tooth. In some cases enough of the tooth remains (one or more cusps) to support a conventional type of retainer and allow adequate enclosure with a stainless steel matrix band. For preparations involving subgingival cavosurface margins in interproximal areas, it is often possible to adapt a stainless steel molar band or copper band to the tooth. In other cases, however, so little tooth structure is left that neither of these two matrices can be used. One possible solution to this problems is to use an anatomically preformed crown as a matrix band.

The clinician should consider using a preformed crown as a matrix band on any posterior tooth that requires a large amalgam core and that cannot be adequately enclosed by a conventional matrix or copper band. Specifically, this includes severely broken down premolars and molars that, when excavated, cannot be banded because of the subgingival position of the cavosurface margins. This technique may

also be considered for cases that would require a preliminary amalgam buildup for an endodontically involved posterior tooth that cannot be adequately isolated because of subgingival margins. In all of these instances the tooth ultimately will receive a full gold crown, and the preformed crown procedure ensures an amalgam core that provides a foundation for this final treatment. The technique described here illustrates how a preformed anatomic crown can be used as a matrix.

Method of Treatment

The badly broken down tooth should be isolated under the rubber dam or with cotton rolls if use of a rubber dam is not possible. The tooth is then prepared: (1) all unsupported enamel should be removed; (2) all jagged cavosurface margins should be planed; and (3) proper retentive features are incorporated in the form of pins, posts, pots, slots, or retentive grooves. If the finished preparation has subgingival areas that are not amenable to matrix banding, a simple electrosurgical procedure should be performed to expose all margins. After all preparation is complete, the tooth is ready to receive a matrix band.

Use of traditional matrix retainers and universal and custom-trimmed bands should be attempted before the preformed anatomic crown technique. If none of these methods yields a stable retainer and adequate occlusogingival band height, the preformed anatomic crown may be considered. A preformed crown that measures slightly larger circumferentially than the prepared tooth is used (Figures 34.12 and 34.13). The occlusal surface of the crown is eliminated with a #556 FG bur (Figure 34.14), and all sharp edges are smoothed with a sandpaper disk to prevent injury to the operator when seating the crown.

The resulting "matrix band" is seated on the prepared tooth so that the operator can determine where changes in band height must be made (Figure 34.15). A curved crown and bridge scissors and sandpaper disks are used to shorten (festoon) the band in areas of excessive length.

The band is the proper height when all cavosurface margins are completely covered, with no tissue pressure (blanching), and the occlusal height is equal to or slightly higher than the adjacent teeth. The band is adapted to the prepared tooth by crimping the cervical portion with #114 contouring pliers until all margins are encompassed. All rough cervical portions of the band are tapered and smoothed with sandpaper disks. The final fit is checked visually and with an explorer. If the band is properly adapted, there should be resistance to occlusal displacement by digital force.

No wooden wedges are used interproximally because they could deform the embrasure areas of the band and possibly dislodge it. The amalgam is triturated, transferred to the preparation, and condensed. Large increments may be used initially. These increments may be placed with the gloved fingers (digitally) or with cotton pliers (Figure 34.16).

Use of a traditional amalgam carrier may not be possible because of difficulty reaching the innermost confines of the

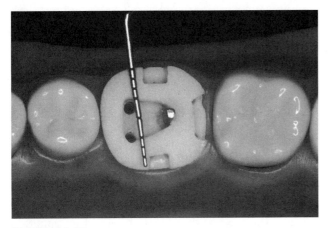

FIGURE 34.12

The prepared tooth is measured from the buccal edge to the lingual edge.

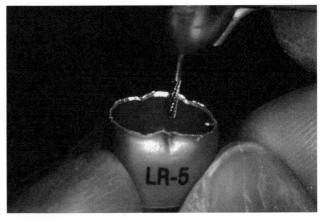

FIGURE 34.14

The center is enlarged by removing the occlusal portion of the shell crown.

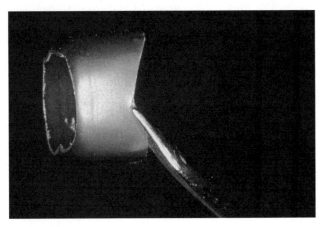

FIGURE 34.13

The proximal cervical margin of a shell crown is contoured to ensure a proper fit over the margin of the tooth.

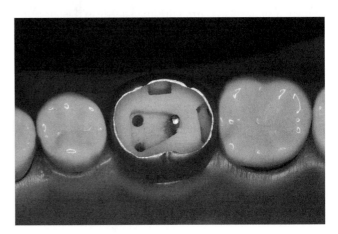

FIGURE 34.15

A properly fitted band should snap into place.

prepared tooth. Initial condensation should be done with hand condensers (Figure 34.17), but as the band is filled, a mechanical condenser serves well to ensure a dense pack free of air voids.

Regardless of the condensation method chosen, care should be taken to direct all packing strokes along the long axis of the tooth. Condensing at any other angle could displace the band, regardless of the tightness of its initial fit.

When the preparation has been adequately overfilled and initial set is complete (Figure 34.18), the band is thinned on both the facial and lingual aspects with a #556 FG bur, and the two resulting band segments are carefully removed with cotton pliers or hemostats (Figure 34.19). Final carving of the amalgam is then completed (Figure 34.20).

In some badly broken-down teeth, the preformed anatomic band can be left intact after occlusal carving of the amalgam. Removal of the band and marginal finishing are done at a later appointment, when the tooth is prepared to receive a crown.

This banding technique is amenable for use with core materials other than dental amalgam. Incremental placement of light-cured composites or light-cured glass ionomer is possible, although the placement and finishing of these materials are more time-consuming and technique sensitive.

The use of a preformed, anatomic crown as a matrix has several advantages. Foremost is the ease of adaptation; unlike copper bands, for example, which are bulky and difficult to crimp, the crown is thin and relatively flexible. Also, little contouring is needed when carving the amalgam core because of the anatomic form of the crown. Most important, overhangs are generally in a horizontal plane and therefore easy to eliminate. The greatest disadvantage of using a preformed crown as a matrix is the difficulty obtaining interproximal contacts. However, if the amalgam core is to receive full-cast coverage, this is not a critical problem.

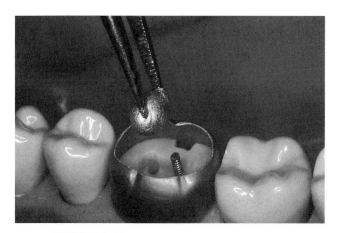

FIGURE 34.16

Initial placement of amalgam with cotton pliers.

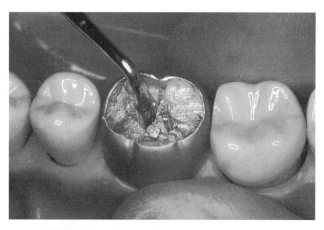

FIGURE 34.17

Incremental fill is done with hand condensers.

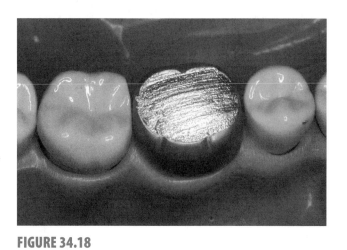

FIGURE 34.18

The occlusal surface is smoothed with a cotton roll before initial set.

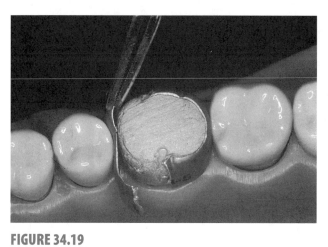

FIGURE 34.19

The band is carefully pulled away from the amalgam alloy, and the mesial portion of the band is removed with cotton pliers or a hemostat.

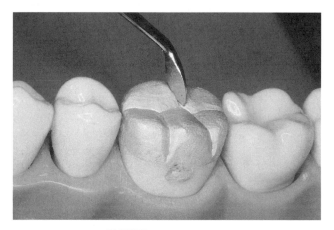

FIGURE 34.20

The grooves are refined.

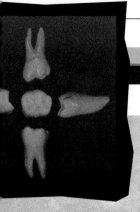

Points for Review

- Assembly of the matrix band and retainer
- Placement of the matrix band and wedge
- Matrix band technique for large amalgam cores

Self-Study Questions

1. What is the term used for an object that blocks, impedes, or interferes with passage?
   a. Guide
   b. Retainer
   c. Obstruction
   d. Wedge

2. Which of the following is used to separate the teeth slightly?
   a. Retainer
   b. Wedge
   c. Obstruction
   d. Matrix band

3. What surface is the contact area on the mesial of the maxillary permanent central incisor?
   a. Mesial third
   b. Gingival third
   c. Middle third
   d. Incisal third

4. What surface is the contact area on the distal of the mandibular first permanent molar?
   a. Occlusal third
   b. Middle third
   c. Gingival third
   d. Distal third

5. What type of matrix band is used most often?
   a. T-band
   b. Universal
   c. Auto matrix band
   d. Tofflemier

6. Which matrix retainer is placed from the lingual surface?
   a. Ivory
   b. Tofflemire straight retainer
   c. Tofflemire contraangle retainer
   d. All of the above

7. Which of the following is used to support and adapt the cervical portion of the band to the tooth structure?
   a. Matrix band
   b. Retainer
   c. Wrench
   d. Wedge

8. What device holds the ends of the matrix band in the retainer?
   a. Guide channels
   b. Diagonal vise slot
   c. Inner nut
   d. Both a and c

9. Which of the following must be done before the matrix band can be placed?
   a. The smaller side of the loop is kept toward the gingival tissue.
   b. The larger side of the loop is kept toward the gingival tissue.
   c. All bands are smoothed before placement.
   d. Both a and c

10. On which arch can the matrix band and retainer be placed if the band is adjusted through the right side of the retainer head while the retainer is held with the open end down or away from the assistant?
    a. Lower right
    b. Lower left
    c. Upper right
    d. B and c

Suggested Readings

Ash MM: *Wheeler's dental anatomy, physiology, and occlusion,* ed 7, Philadelphia, 1993, WB Saunders.

Cohen S, Burns RC: *Pathways of the pulp,* ed 7, St Louis, 1998, Mosby.

Crimm G: *Operative dentistry,* Louisville, Ky, 1995, University of Louisville School of Dentistry.

Gainsford ID: *Silver amalgam in clinical practice,* ed 2, Bristol, England, 1976, John Wright & Sons.

Gordon M, Imber S, Ben-Amar A: *A modified copper band matrix technique for large amalgam restorations,* Chicago, 1985, Quintessence.

Jordan RE, Abrams L, Kraus B: *Kraus' dental anatomy and occlusion,* St Louis, 1992, Mosby.

Knight JS: A matrix solution for severely broken down teeth, *Academy of General Dentistry* 1996.

Lovdahl PE, Gutmann JL: Periodontal and restorative considerations prior to endodontic therapy, *Journal of the Academy of General Dentistry* 28-38, 1980.

Lovdahl PE, Wade CK: Problems in tooth isolation and prosthodontic restorations, *Journal of the Academy of General Dentistry.*

Lovdahl PE, Gutmann JL, Dumsha TC: *Problem solving in endodontics: prevention, identification, and management,* St Louis, 1988, Mosby.

Markley MR: Pin-retained and reinforced restorations and foundations, *Dent Clin North Am* 229-244, 1967.

St Arnault FD, Evins PR: Fabrication of a copper band matrix, *Journal of the Oklahoma Dental Association* 72:18-19, 1982.

Spohn EE, Halowski WA, Berry TG: *Operative dentistry procedures for dental auxiliaries,* St Louis, 1981, Mosby.

Sturdevant CM et al: *The art and science of operative dentistry,* ed 3, St Louis, 1995, Mosby.

US Department of Health, Education and Welfare: Restoration of cavity preparations with amalgam and tooth-colored materials: Project ACORDE, Castro Valley, Calif, 1979, Quercus Corp.

Zwemer TJ: *Mosby's dental dictionary,* St Louis, 1998, Mosby.

Finishing and Polishing Dental Restorations

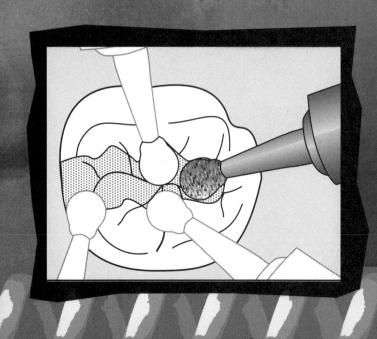

Chapter Outline

Finishing and Polishing
- Finishing and polishing armamentarium
- Rotary trimming and finishing instruments
- Hand instruments and polishing devises
- Abrasive agents
- Restorative problems and corrections
- Recontouring and finishing occlusal surfaces
- Recontouring and finishing proximal surfaces
- Recontouring and finishing facial and lingual surfaces
- Procedures for Finishing and Polishing Restorations

Learning Objectives

On completion of Chapter 35, the student should be able to do the following:

- Define key terms.
- Define the procedures involved in recontouring, finishing, and polishing dental restorations.
- Place, finish, and polish dental amalgam and composite resin restorations.
- Identify the rotary finishing and polishing instruments.
- Identify the hand instruments and polishing devices.
- Identify amalgam restoration problems and corrections.

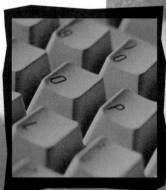

Key Terms

Aesthetics	Intermittent	Recontouring
Flash	Overhang	Submarginal

FINISHING AND POLISHING

The goal of finishing and polishing the dental amalgam is to redefine and recontour, if necessary, the restoration to original anatomical contour of the tooth and to provide a smooth surface. To accomplish this the occlusal and incisal surfaces, proximal embrasures, and facial and lingual contours may need reshaping. The margins of the restoration must be flush with the tooth surface and anatomical landmarks and contours must resemble the natural tooth.

The operator may be able to place, contour, and burnish the dental amalgam perfectly in all respects. However, because of the characteristics of amalgam, it is important that the restoration is finished and polished to a smooth, subtle luster. A well-condensed, smooth, burnished, and polished restoration is stronger because of the reduction of voids within amalgam. Polishing adapts the amalgam and cavosurface margins tighter and makes the restoration easier to keep clean. A smooth surface will resist tarnish and corrosion over a long period of time.

Overhang

Marginal overextension, additional material left at the gingival cavosurface margin caused from the matrix band not being wedged properly and from undercarving

Submarginal

A ditch caused from overcarving or incomplete condensing at the cavosurface margin, which must be corrected

Finishing and polishing the restoration will help to smooth and redefine the grooves, ridges, fossa, cusps, embrasures, and contours of the restoration. These procedures, if completed properly, will assure that the amalgam is flush with the cavosurface margins and there are no voids or **overhangs**. If a very small **submarginal** area is observed with an explorer (0.2 mm or less in depth), it can be removed by smoothing down the enamel lightly. If centric markings made with the articulating paper indicate a difference in density, the operator can adjust or recontour the restoration during the finishing procedure so that it will not feel high to the patient. The teeth should occlude as they did before treatment.

Finishing and Polishing Armamentarium

The finishing and polishing procedures for a dental amalgam restoration cannot begin until 24 hours after the restoration has been placed. Finishing and polishing is accomplished by the use of power-driven rotary cutting instruments and hand instruments. These instruments include finishing burs, stones, finishing discs, rubber points, cups, and brushes. Polishing or abrasive agents such as pumice and tin oxide are also used. However, because of the wide variety of instruments and materials available, operators will have their own finishing and polishing technique and equipment preference. The following armamentarium is generally used for **recontouring**, finishing, and polishing amalgam restorations.

Examination instruments:
- Explorer
- Mouth mirror
- Cotton forceps

Hand instruments and devices:
- Articulating paper and holder
- Finishing knife
- Finishing file
- Abrasive finishing strips

Rotary instruments:
- Low-speed contra-angle and handpiece
- Finishing burs
- Tapered and round green stones
- Tapered and round white stones
- Sandpaper and rubber finishing discs (medium/fine grit)
- Rubber points and cups
- Rubber cup and brush

Abrasive agents:
- Flour of pumice
- Tin oxide

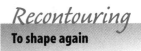

Recontouring

To shape again

Rotary Trimming and Finishing Instruments

It is important to remember that the use of rotary-driven power instruments and abrasives, if not used properly, can cause overheating, pulp trauma, and will weaken the restoration. It is important to use a low speed, **intermittent** strokes, and light pressure on the restoration and tooth during trimming and finishing procedures.

Intermittent

Stopping and starting at intervals

The 12 blade and 40 blade trimming and finishing burs are available in a variety of sizes and shapes. They are different from the cutting burs because they are designed to trim, shape, and finish restorative materials rather than cut hard tooth structure. Finishing burs have fine flutes or blades on the cutting head, which will not remove very much material with each revolution. However, they must be used with care because they can cut the soft gingiva tissue and hard tooth structure if not used properly.

A 12 blade round, flame-shaped, or pear-shaped finishing bur is usually the first rotary instrument used to remove excessive amalgam along the cavosurface margins of the restoration and also to shape the tooth contours and occlusal surface (Figures 35.1 and 35.2). Finishing is usually accomplished using these burs on a low-speed contra-angle handpiece. A low speed will provide the operator greater control reshaping and removing excessive restorative material. The finishing bur is followed by the use of abrasive rotary instruments such as stones and rubber points, cups, and wheels of varying grits. The purpose of finishing and polishing is to use progressively finer abrasives. Refer to Chapter 36 for further detail on the use of each type of finishing bur, stone, rubber points, cups, and wheels.

Hand Instruments and Polishing Devises

In addition to rotary trimming instruments, there are a wide variety of hand instruments, polishing devises and agents, and techniques that can be used to finish a dental amalgam restoration. Commonly used hand instruments for trim-

ming composite acrylic include the finishing knife or scalpel and file, which can be used to successfully remove excessive amalgam and contour the restoration in areas, such as the proximal surface, that may be difficult to reach with a rotary instrument (Figure 35.3). The finishing knife is a sharp instrument that must be used with a secure finger rest. Only small increments of amalgam should be removed at any one time, and the operator will need to be careful not to injure the gingiva tissue, chip the amalgam, or remove the contact as pressure is applied to the instrument.

The finishing file can be placed against the proximal gingival cavosurface margin and moved from the facial to lingual to smooth rough amalgam. Finishing strips and sandpaper discs are available in various grits and are also used in the gingival margin area to finish and polish composite acrylic and amalgam restorations. The fine grit finishing strip usually provides the final finish. A small amount of tin oxide can be used with the finishing strip to provide as smooth a surface as possible. Finishing discs are used to finish margins in embrasure areas and facial and lingual surfaces. It is important to be careful not to cut the gingiva tissue by moving the disc too

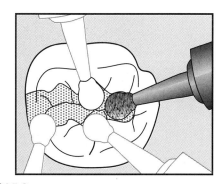

FIGURE 35.1

Dental files are used with composite resins to remove excess amalgam from the cavosurface margins.

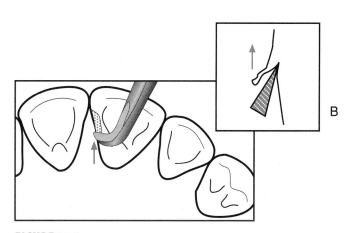

A

B

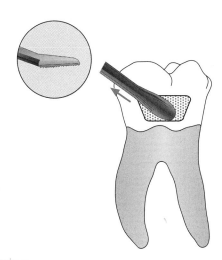

FIGURE 35.2

Round finishing burs and stones are used to anatomically contour amalgam and composite resin on occlusal surfaces.

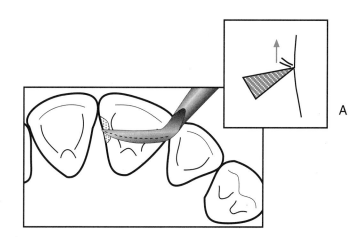

FIGURE 35.3

Gold knives or scalpels are used with (**A**) short scraping or (**B**) shaving strokes to remove excess composite resin.

close to the papilla. Procedures for the use of each of these instruments and devises are included in the following text.

Abrasive Agents

Flour of pumice and tin oxide are both used to polish the amalgam restoration. Water is added to the pumice to make a slurry mixture. The operator will dip the rubber cup or pointed brush into the wet pumice and apply pumice and polish into the grooves to polish the restoration (Figure 35.4). The pumice polish will be followed by using tin oxide in the same manner. Tin oxide is a more fine abrasive, which will provide a shiny restoration. It may be used wet or dry. It is important to remember when using rubber cups or any of these abrasives, they must be placed correctly to prevent ditching and overcontouring (Figure 35.5). Light, intermittent strokes must be used to prevent heat. Soft cup brushes and wheel brushes can be used to aid in polishing with tin oxide in concave areas. It is important that the cup rest lightly on the tooth surface to avoid ditching the restoration (Figure 35.6). After these abrasive agents are used the teeth will be sprayed and cleaned off with the air/water syringe and suction tip.

Restorative Problems and Corrections

The following descriptions along with Table 35.1 will provide insight into some of the problems and corrections that the operator may be faced with when trimming, finishing, and polishing a restoration:

Recontouring and Finishing Occlusal Surfaces
Marginal Overextension

Recontouring and finishing excessive amalgam at the cavo-surface margins on occlusal surfaces can be accomplished by using the flame-shaped bur in a low-speed handpiece. Tapered green stones can also be used when there is less extension of amalgam or as a follow up to using the bur. If the excess is small, a less abrasive, tapered white stone can be used. Abrasive discs and strips are also used to finish the amalgam restoration on the proximal surfaces.

Rotary finishing devises require that the operator use a modified pen-grasp and secure finger rest position while using the contra-angle and handpiece at a low speed. The side of the bur or stone is placed lightly on the tooth structure with the tip positioned on the amalgam. The tooth surface

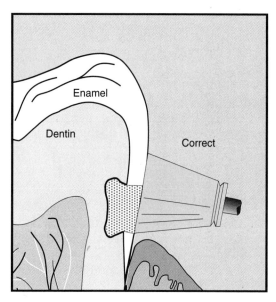

FIGURE 35.5

Place the rubber cup correctly to prevent ditching and removal of too much composite resin or amalgam material.

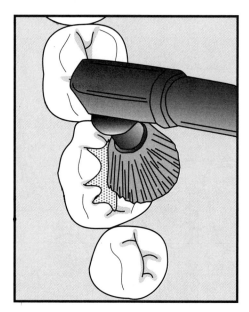

FIGURE 35.4

Soft cup brushes are used to polish with pumice, tin oxide, or polishing pastes.

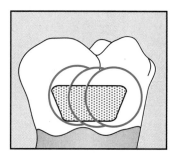

FIGURE 35.6

Rubber cups must be used with light intermittent strokes and placed correctly to prevent ditching and removal of too much composite resin or amalgam.

Flash

Dental amalgam or composite acrylic resin that has been undercarved leaving an extension of material over the cavo-surface margins, which must be removed

will help guide the bur smoothly over the **flash**. Using low to medium speed gently sweep or brush the bur over the amalgam until the excess has been removed. Remember to use intermittent strokes and light pressure, being sure not to leave the bur in one place too long. It is important not to overheat the metal alloy or cause removal of too much alloy or tooth structure.

Overcontoured/Undercarved Surfaces

Occlusal areas that are highly overcontoured can often be identified by observing smooth shiny marks or burnished spots on the amalgam. This is caused by the patient biting on the overcontoured restoration. High bites can also be identified by using articulating paper. The undercarved occlusal surface can be recontoured with a flame-shaped bur or stone and the anatomy redefined using the same procedures as for marginal overextensions. A pear-shaped bur may also be used for recontouring the occlusal surface of the amalgam. The developmental grooves and fossas can be recontoured and redefined by using a small round finishing bur or round stone. Using light, intermittent strokes the round bur is brushed through the grooves or fossas until there is appropriate contour and anatomical detail. These same procedures are used with the tapered and round white stone over the entire amalgam to finish a restoration that has been placed satisfactorily but needs to be smoothed and polished. When finishing a distoocclusal restoration, for instance, the occlusal is usually completed before the proximal.

Aesthetics

The philosophy or principle pertaining to beauty

Table 35.1

Trimming, Finishing, and Polishing

Problems	Corrections
Flash or overextension of the margins	Remove with flame-shaped finishing bur and smooth with stone and rubber points
Slight submarginal area	Remove small amount of enamel with small white stone
Grainy, open margin or submarginal area	Remove amalgam with spoon excavator and replace amalgam
Fossas, grooves, or ridges too high or improperly located	Recontour with round or flame-shaped finishing bur
Premature contact in centric occlusion	Same as above
Premature contact in lateral or protrusive movement	Same as above
Slight roughness	Smooth with flame-shaped finishing bur, stone, and rubber points on occlusion and sandpaper discs, rubber wheels, and points interproximally
Interproximal overhang	As above if possible or knife, amalgam file, and abrasive strips. May need to replace.
Overcontour/undercarved	Recontour with flame-shaped finishing bur, stone, and rubber points or wheels depending on location
Undercontour/overcarved	Replace unless slight
Location of contact	Recontour with flame-shaped finishing bur, stone, rubber points, wheels, discs, or abrasive strip if possible.
Lack of contact or gross location problem	Must be replaced
Aesthetics	Bleach tooth, change composite shade, recontour
Hard tooth tissue	Avoid abrasion of surrounding tooth structure
Soft tissue	Do not lacerate soft tissue
Overheating	Prolonged contact on the tooth will cause overheating and tooth trauma

Recontouring and Finishing Proximal Surfaces

Marginal Overextension and Overcontour

A marginal extension or overhang in the interproximal area may be difficult to detect. The operator may choose to have a radiograph taken to view these areas. It is important for the operator to examine these areas carefully. The amalgam may extend gingivally beyond the cavosurface margin and be overcontoured or it may extend proximally from the cavosurface margin and be overcontoured. In all cases the excess interferes with the gingival embrasure and causes pressure on the interdental papilla.

Round finishing burs and stones can be used to remove composite resin on the lingual surfaces and to contour the occlusal surfaces of amalgam and composite restorations (see Figure 35.2). Excessive dental amalgam and composite acrylic flash can be removed from the cavosurface margins with a flame-shaped or pointed finishing bur or stones using a low speed and a light, smooth stroke against the amalgam edge (Figure 35.7). The bur is placed from the facial surface and extended until the tip has reached the center of the tooth below the contact. At this point the bur is repositioned from the lingual aspect and the procedure is continued until the excess has been removed. Using the flame-shaped bur or stone to recontour anatomy and finish the facial and lingual proximal surface may be difficult because there is a lack of access to these areas. Finishing burs and stones can be used to finish composites and amalgam and also to reduce small amounts of tooth enamel to eliminate a submarginal area (Figures 35.8 and 35.9). Ditching may occur if the operator is not careful.

Proximal areas are difficult to reach, therefore, the operator may choose to use a finishing or sandpaper disc (Figure 35.10). This embrasure area can be recontoured and finished by placing the edge of the disc on the facial or lingual margin while moving the disc lightly (light intermittent strokes) in the same brushing motion over the amalgam or composite surface and away from the contact area. It is important not to remove the contact area or harm the soft tissue with the disc. The occlusal embrasure can be contoured using the same procedure.

Another alternative to using the bur is the use of an amalgam knife or scalpel (see Figure 35.3). Also called a finishing knife, the tip is placed on the amalgam ledge and pulled lightly away from the margin toward the contact using short scraping or shaving strokes to remove excess composite resin. The excess is carved away in small increments. This is continued until the excess has been removed and the tip of the blade has passed halfway. The same procedure is continued on the lingual surface until the blade has passed halfway and the overhang is removed and smooth.

Further finishing and removal of excess amalgam from the cavosurface margins can be accomplished with the dental or amalgam file using the same procedure. Finishing strips can also be used to provide a smooth amalgam surface.

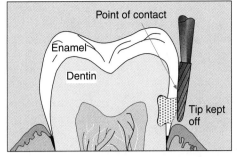
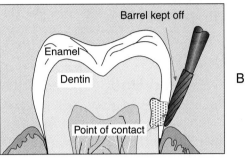
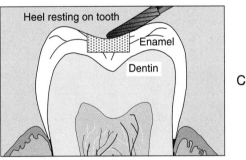

FIGURE 35.7

Correct placement of finishing bur or stone: (**A**) When finishing the occlusal cavosurface margin of a Class V restoration, for instance, the tip should be kept off the restorative material; (**B**) when finishing the gingival cavosurface margin of the restoration the barrel should be angled away from the restoration, and (**C**) when finishing the cavosurface margin of an occlusal restoration the barrel should be resting lightly on the tooth.

The finishing strip is placed into the gingival embrasure under the contact area and pulled lightly back and forth along the gingival margin on the amalgam restoration up to the contact area being careful not to cut the interdental papilla.

Recontouring and Finishing Facial and Lingual Surfaces

Marginal Overextension and Overcontour

If the restoration replaces a portion of the facial or lingual surface it may be necessary to recontour a convex or undercarved area on these surfaces. This can be accomplished by using a finishing disc. The angle of the disc against the amalgam is important because the buccal height of contour lies

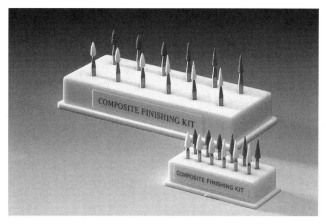

FIGURE 35.8

Finishing burs and stones are used to finish composite and amalgam restorations. (Courtesy SHOFU.)

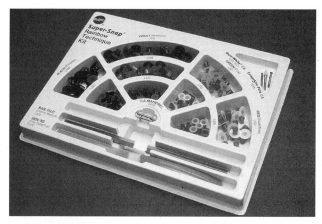

FIGURE 35.10

Proximal areas are difficult to reach, therefore the operator may choose to use a finishing sandpaper disc. (Courtesy SHOFU).

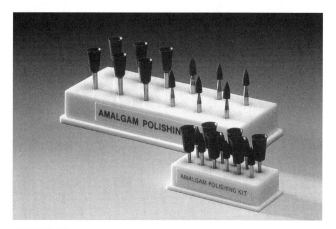

FIGURE 35.9

Rubber points and cups are used to further smooth and finish composite and amalgam restorations.

in the middle of the restoration. The outer edge of the finishing disc is moved with the disc turning slowly from the tooth surface to the center or height of contour of the restoration across each marginal surface in a light, brushing stroke. When polishing a Class V amalgam restoration do not try to finish both the occlusal and gingival margins at the same time because this will remove the convex height of contour. It is important not to cross the center because too much amalgam can be removed thus losing the contour of the tooth. Finishing and polishing is accomplished by using the medium or more abrasive finishing disc and progressing to a fine disc for a smooth finish. The disc is mounted with the abrasive surface facing away from the head of the contra-angle. The flame-shaped bur can be used if excessive recontouring needs to be completed. The procedure is the same as above but the operator must be careful not to ditch the amalgam or damage the hard or soft tissue. Gingival retractors may be needed to gain access in Class V areas that are close to or below the gingival margin.

Procedures for Finishing and Polishing Restorations

The purpose of polishing the restoration is to provide a smooth restoration that has a satin luster. The operator must use proper sequencing of polishing materials in order to accomplish a smooth shiny surface (Box 35.1 and Table 35.2). It is important to remember to use the rotary polishing devices with light intermittent strokes so as not to produce heat or damage the tooth. Polishing should remove any roughness or scratches. This is accomplished by using coarse abrasive materials and advancing to medium and fine agents. After the finishing bur is used, the operator will usually advance to the green stone and then to the white stone. The green stone is less abrasive than the bur but more abrasive than the white stone. The shape of the bur and stones will depend on the surface that is to be finished. In certain areas, as described, a sandpaper disc may be used (Figure 35.11). Rubber wheels and points can be used after the stones and discs. This will further define the finish and provide a smoother surface. Wheels and points also vary in abrasiveness.

Flour of pumice and tin oxide may be used with the occlusal brush and rubber cup for a progressively smoother finish. The brush is able to reach into the occlusal depressions where the rubber cup may not be able to reach. The operator may choose to mix the powdered flour of pumice and tin oxide with water. The tin oxide is often used dry. A prepared amalgam gloss paste is also available. The brush and rubber cup and points are dipped in the polishing agents and used to polish the restoration.

The darker rubber points are used in the concave surfaces such as the developmental grooves and fossas of the occlusal surface. As the points are placed in the depressions, the side of the points are lightly brushed against the facial and lingual inclined plane of the ridges and moved across the occlusal surface from the distal fossa to the mesial fossa. The

Box 35.1 *Procedure*
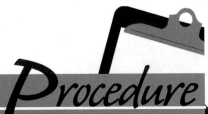

Procedure for Finishing and Polishing an Amalgam Restoration

1. Check the restoration and the occlusion.
2. Smooth the occlusal surface contours, fossae, and grooves with a round finishing bur using light brushing intermittent strokes (Figure 35.12).
3. Check the surface for rough areas and scratches.
4. Proceed smoothing the surface using the coarse to fine stone points and repeat any procedure if needed to remove deep scratches (Figure 35.13).
5. Finishing with stones.
6. Use the brown coarse rubber point and proceed to the fine green point for a smooth finish.
7. Finishing with rubber points.
8. Use the rubber cup and pumice with water to polish the surfaces of the amalgam using light intermittent strokes so as not to cause overheating and trauma to the pulp (Figure 35.14).
   a. With light pressure force the rubber cup into the depths of the grooves.
   b. Adapt the rubber cup to round or smooth the marginal ridges.
   c. Pumice with the rubber cup to a matte finish.
9. Use the bristle prophy brush and pumice to polish the grooves (Figure 35.15).
10. There will be a matte finish after the use of pumice.
11. Final luster can be provided by using a Robinson bristle brush (Figure 35.16).
    a. Use wet tin oxide or amalgam gloss for a final polish.
    b. As the heat dries the tin oxide the alloy will attain a "high shine."
12. The final polished restoration will have a smooth luster (Figure 35.17).

Table 35.2

Evaluation for Polishing Dental Amalgam

Polishing Dental Amalgam	4	3	2	0	X
Anatomy/contours.					
Marginal integrity.					
Surface smoothness.					
Contact replacement.					
Occlusion.					

The numeric criteria: 4 Excellent; 3 Good but some improvement can be made; 2 Below average, usable, needs to improve skill; 0 Unsatisfactory; X Not able to evaluate.

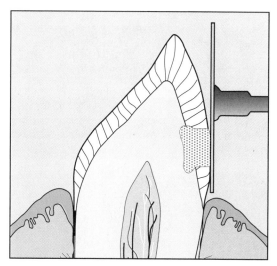

FIGURE 35.11

Brush the sandpaper disc across the restoration with light, intermittent strokes.

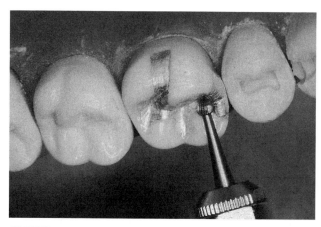

FIGURE 35.12

Smooth the occlusal surface contours, fossae, and grooves with a round finishing bur using light brushing intermittent strokes.

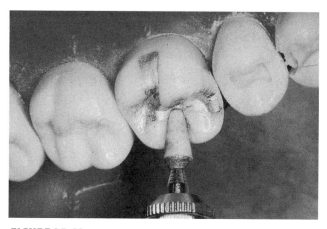

FIGURE 35.13

Proceed smoothing the surface using the coarse to fine stone points and repeat any procedure if needed to remove deep scratches.

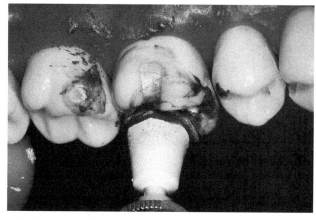

FIGURE 35.14

Use the rubber cup and pumice with water to polish the surfaces of the amalgam using light intermittent strokes so as not to cause overheating and trauma to the pulp.

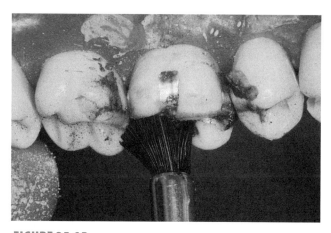

FIGURE 35.15

Use the bristle prophy brush and pumice to polish the groves.

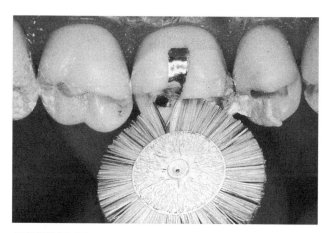

FIGURE 35.16

Final luster can be provided by using a bristle brush with wet tin oxide or amalgam gloss for a final polish.

points are followed with the rubber cup on the convex marginal ridges and incline areas of the occlusal surface.

The rubber cup will conform to the interproximal contours. During polishing, the cup holding one of the abrasive agents is brushed across the occlusal surface of the restoration until a satin luster appears. The more abrasive points and cups are followed by using finer rubber points and cups. The procedure is repeated until the scratches are removed and the restoration appears smooth with a luster finish. Pumice is usually used first with a rubber point and cup followed by tin oxide and a finer rubber point and cup.

The polishing brush with pumice or tin oxide may be used instead of the points and cups. The brush will often be trimmed to a point so as to reach into the depressions. Some operators prefer to use the brush rather than rubber cup because they believe that the rubber cup is often over used, causing the removal of a sufficient amount of enamel. The brush is dipped into the polishing agent and applied to the restoration. The brush needs to be run slowly to keep the pumice from flying off. Pumice provides a dull finish while the tin oxide will provide a high-luster polish. The polishing agents are removed from

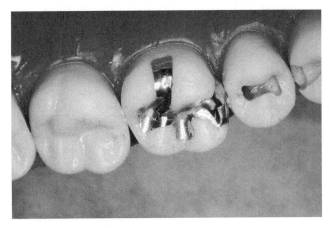

FIGURE 35.17

The final polished restoration will have a smooth luster.

the tooth surfaces with the air/water syringe spray and suction tip. The use of these instruments and agents should not damage the tooth structure during the polishing procedure.

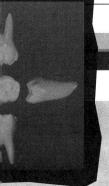

Points for Review

- Finishing and polishing
- Restoration problems and corrections
- Recontouring, finishing, and polishing guidelines
- Procedures for finishing and polishing restorations
- Evaluation for polishing dental amalgam

Self-Study Questions

1. It is important to use which of the following when polishing a restoration?
   a. Recontouring strokes
   b. Intermittent strokes
   c. Heavy strokes
   d. Heavy and then light strokes

2. The restorative material that has been left over the cavosurface margins that must be removed is called?
   a. Submarginal
   b. Ditch
   c. Flash
   d. Contouring

3. A ditch caused from overcarving or incomplete condensing at the cavosurface margin is called?
   a. Submarginal
   b. Overhang
   c. Undercarved
   d. Flash

4. Why are low speed, intermittent strokes, and light pressure used during finishing and polishing procedures?
   a. Prevent heat loss
   b. Provide a high shine
   c. Prevent weakened restorations
   d. All of the above

5. When polishing, which of the following sequence of instruments is used?
   a. Finishing burs, stones, abrasive discs, rubber points, prophy brush, rubber cup
   b. Stones, finishing burs, rubber points, abrasive discs, rubber cup, prophy brush
   c. Stones, rubber points, finishing burs, abrasive discs, prophy brush, rubber cup
   d. Finishing burs, abrasive discs, stones, rubber points, rubber cup, prophy brush

6. What trimming device is used on composite resins to remove excess from the cavosurface margins?
   a. Round stones
   b. Scalpel
   c. File
   d. B and c

7. What is the best device used to remove excess composite from lingual surfaces of anterior restorations?
   a. Flame-shaped and pointed finishing bur
   b. Round finishing burs and stones
   c. Sandpaper discs and rubber wheels
   d. Pointed prophy brush and cup

8. Polishing the dental restoration provides which of the following?
   a. Satin luster
   b. Smooth surface
   c. Surface hardness
   d. All of the above

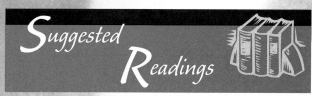

Suggested Readings

Ash MM: *Wheeler's dental anatomy, physiology, and occlusion*, ed 7, Philadelphia, 1993, WB Saunders.

Crimm G: *Operative dentistry*, Louisville, Kentucky, 1995, University of Louisville School of Dentistry.

Council on Dental Materials, Instruments, and Equipment: *Choosing intracoronal restorative materials*, 1994, *Journal of the American Dental Association*.

Jordan RE, Abrams L, Kraus B: *Kraus' dental anatomy and occlusion*, St Louis, 1992, Mosby.

Miyasaki-Ching C: *Chasteen's essentials of clinical dental assisting*, ed 5, St Louis, 1997, Mosby.

Spohn EE, Halowski WA, Berry TG: *Operative dentistry procedures for dental auxiliaries*, St Louis, 1981, Mosby.

US Department of Health, Education and Welfare: *Restoration of cavity preparations with amalgam and tooth-colored materials*, Castro Valley, Calif, 1979, Project ACORDE, Quercus Corporation.

Zwemer TJ: *Mosby's dental dictionary*, St Louis, 1998, Mosby.

Clinical Application of Dental Amalgam Restorations

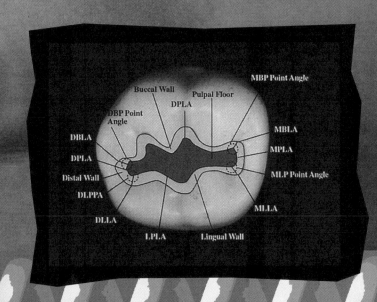

Chapter Outline

Learning Objectives

On completion of Chapter 36, the student should be able to do the following:

- Define key terms.

- Describe the placement techniques involved in the various amalgam cavity classifications.

- Finish and polish dental amalgam restorations.

- Identify the anatomic landmarks of listed teeth and explain their significance in the placement of dental amalgam.

- Explain the techniques used to prevent undercontoured and over-contoured restorations.

- List the evaluation criteria for dental amalgam and composite resin restorations.

- Identify the types of pins used for amalgam pin retention.

- Complete a self-evaluation chart for identified amalgam and composite restorations.

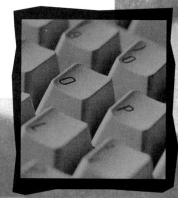

Key Terms

Condense	Overcontoured	Undercarved
Increments	Retention	Undercontoured
Overcarved	Trituration	

CLINICAL APPLICATION

Although dental amalgam is being challenged today by the new posterior composite materials, it is still one of the most commonly used restorative materials in dentistry. Composite acrylic resins have been used for more than 25 years in anterior teeth and are the primary restorative material of choice for all teeth in several countries and in many dental offices in the United States. However, the current composite materials do not perform as well as amalgam for all posterior teeth. Composite materials for posterior teeth are used primarily for restoration in low-stress areas.

Amalgam, which has been in use since 1528, still has a lower failure rate than other restorative material. Failure of amalgam restorations is usually the result of dimensional change, recurrent caries, fracture, tarnish, or corrosion. The strength and sitting time of amalgam are determined by the size and shape of the amalgam particles, the ratio of mercury to alloy, and the manipulation (mixing time and condensation) of the amalgam. Although the manufacturer controls the size and shape of the amalgam particles and the ratio of mercury to alloy if preproportioned mixes are used, the operator controls the trituration (mixing) time, condensation, and finishing and ensures a moisture-free working environment. Faulty manipulation and contamination of the material during insertion is believed to account for 40% of failed amalgam restorations. For this reason, it is important that the dental assistant and operator take care when working with dental amalgam.

Selection and Manipulation of Amalgam

The dentist usually chooses the type of dental amalgam to be used in the dental practice. However, the dentist and expanded-function dental specialist may want to discuss their personal preferences in the type of amalgam they use and the types of carving and finishing instruments and materials that work best for them. Dental personnel should understand that amalgam with a greater percentage of mercury is easier to mix and has a slower setting time, but the higher mercury content also weakens the amalgam and makes polishing the restoration more difficult. If preproportioned capsules are used, the mercury to alloy ratio has already been determined, and removing excess mercury will not be necessary. These capsules usually use less than 54% mercury, to increase the strength of the amalgam. However, this means that less working time is available, usually 2½ minutes from the time of trituration.

Trituration

Process of mixing the mercury and amalgam alloy into a homogenous mass.

Trituration

Trituration time varies, depending on the brand of alloy, the size of the mix, the mercury to alloy ratio, and the type of amalgamator used. Therefore it is important that the dental assistant always read the manufacturer's directions. Reading the directions helps the dental assistant understand the properties of the material and the trituration requirements and also enhances professional educational growth in the use of dental materials. If the mix is grainy, the amalgam is undertriturated and will be weak. If the mix is soupy, the amalgam is overtriturated and will be difficult to remove from the capsule. An overtriturated dental amalgam exhibits increased contraction, which increases the potential for leakage. It is important to check the time on the amalgamator if either of these conditions occurs.

Condensation

The operator examines the cavity preparation and the adjacent teeth before the dental amalgam is placed to view the preparation detail and the essential anatomic contours and contact areas. This also allows the operator to determine the type of pulpal protection necessary and the amount of dental amalgam needed. If a matrix band and wedge are to be used, they are placed and evaluated before trituration and condensation. It is crucial to stress again the importance of keeping the dental amalgam free of moisture contamination because of excessively delayed expansion. It is also important to emphasize that the matrix band must be placed properly; this is vital to the success of the restoration, because the band must withstand the pressure applied to it during condensation of the amalgam.

After essential precautions have been taken, the cavity preparation has been examined, and preliminary steps have been completed, the dental assistant triturates the amalgam and passes it to the operator in a carrier. It is important to maintain proper instrument-passing techniques during the placement, condensation, and carving procedures so that they can be completed smoothly and in a timely manner. Condensation should begin quickly to maintain the strength of the amalgam. However, if the operator begins carving too soon, the amalgam may be too soft and therefore difficult to **condense.** Amalgam at the proper condensation consistency is just firm enough to squeak as it is compressed and flows into the angles

Condense

To make more compact or solid.

when condensed firmly. If condensation lasts longer than 3 to 4 minutes, a new mixture should be used. Maximum strength is reached after 10 to 24 hours.

Note: It is important to tell the patient not to eat anything hard for 24 hours after completion of the procedure.

Dental amalgam should be inserted and condensed in small **increments** into the proximal box first if the preparation has an interproximal or Class II cavity preparation. The least accessible area of the preparation should be condensed first.

Increments

Small additions that increase the amount.

Small increments can be condensed more effectively, therefore the first placement should only partly fill the preparation. The amalgam is then inserted in small increments evenly over the pulpal floor until the cavity preparation has been filled. The smaller carrier and condenser are used first, then the larger placement and condensing instruments. Initially the condenser should be small enough to fit easily into the cavity preparation.

The amalgam is compressed forcefully with overlapping strokes so that the alloy is evenly condensed (Figure 36.1). The serrated condenser nib tip and side of the nib allow the operator to direct the strokes against the walls of the preparation (Figure 36.2). Tarnish and corrosion can be reduced and surface irregularities minimized if the amalgam is handled carefully; that is, the operator must avoid undertrituration, prevent moisture contamination, reduce the mercury content, and polish the restoration adequately.

The cavity preparation is slightly overfilled because the dental amalgam is adapted to the walls and over the cavosurface margins (0.5 mm) of the preparation. Consideration

Retention

A groove or undercut made in a cavity preparation to help hold the restoration and prevent it from moving.

must be given to the height of the cusps and marginal ridges if they are to be replaced. The amalgam also must be condensed firmly, with the operator making sure to compress the particles into the line and point angles and **retention** areas of the cavity preparation. The operator must be able to apply force sufficient to condense the amalgam and eliminate any air voids. This is accomplished by holding the condenser in a modified pen grasp with proper finger rest techniques and using forceful strokes.

Ineffective placement and condensation of the amalgam weaken the alloy bonding and could result in recurrent caries from voids around the cavosurface margins (open margins) and reduced strength in the porous alloy. Also, proper compression of the amalgam causes excess mercury to rise to the surface, where the mercury-rich amalgam can be removed during carving. Removal of excess mercury increases the strength of the amalgam and results in a better finished and polished restoration. Some operators do an initial burnish as soon as the preparation has been filled. Burnishing the amalgam alloy before carving also removes excess mercury by bringing it to the surface, allowing it to be removed during carving.

Carving

Carving is the removal of excess dental amalgam and the sculpturing of the restoration to replace the missing tooth structure and bring about proper form and function. Carving is a form of art in which the operator must maintain an image of the tooth and have the skills and knowledge essential to restore dentition. The ability to carve an amalgam restoration successfully is based on an understanding of the importance of each step in the restorative procedure. These steps include isolation, cavity preparation, pulp protection, and placement and finishing of the amalgam. The trituration and condensation of the amalgam affect the outcome of carving and polishing. If the material is undertriturated, the amalgam is grainy and weak. This condition or improper condensing of the alloy (or both) can result in air voids in the amalgam, which can prevent the alloy from bonding properly. It would be difficult during carving to eliminate pits, voids, and open margins and still have a smooth finished restoration. In such cases the amalgam must be replaced.

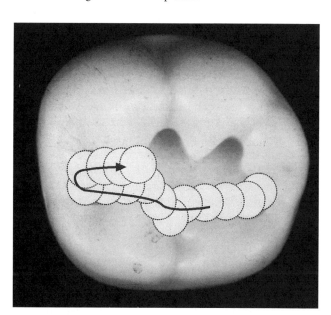

FIGURE 36.2

Overlapping strokes are used to condense amalgam.

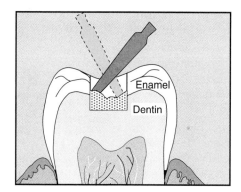

FIGURE 36.1

The amalgam is compressed forcefully with overlapping strokes so that the alloy is evenly condensed.

Removing the Mercury-Rich Layer of Amalgam

It is important to remove the mercury-rich layer of amalgam in the initial carving steps. The mercury is brought to the surface during the condensation, and this process can be enhanced by burnishing the amalgam before carving. Some burnishers commonly used for this procedure are the large round, the egg-shaped, and the acorn-shaped burnishers. If this procedure is done, the operator may begin by placing the burnisher against the tooth surface in the groove and burnishing the amalgam against the cavosurface margin of the cusp across to the area of the triangular fossa. Regardless of whether burnishing is done, the purpose of the preliminary step in carving is to remove the mercury-rich layer of amalgam.

Carving Techniques

The operator must not begin carving until the amalgam has reached the appropriate carving consistency, or resistance. This initial setting stage determines the ease with which the operator will be able to shape and contour the amalgam. The proper consistency has been reached if the operator can feel some resistance as the carver is guided across the tooth surface and amalgam. A light squeaking sound may be heard when the amalgam is ready to be carved. If no resistance is felt, the operator should wait briefly before checking again.

Many different kinds of carvers are available. The carvers and techniques described in this chapter vary according to the operator's preference and the type of design necessary for carving the contours of the particular restoration. Carvers should be sharp in order to remove the condensed amalgam. The operator uses a firm finger rest, holds the carver in the modified pen grasp, and places the heel or tip of the carver on both the tooth surface and the restoration while carving the amalgam.

The operator shapes the amalgam to the contours and anatomic form (grooves, ridges, fossae, and proximal embrasures) of the natural tooth by guiding the carver over the tooth surface along the cavosurface margin. Maintaining contact with the tooth surface while carving reduces the possibility of creating a submarginal area by ditching the amalgam below the cavosurface margin of the cavity preparation. When carving the occlusal surface, the operator must not let the tip of the instrument cross over the central developmental groove area of the restoration; this could ditch or undercut the opposite cavosurface margin. If ditching or overcarving occur, the problem cannot be solved by placing additional amalgam in the area; the amalgam must be removed and the procedure repeated.

A restoration that has been **overcarved** has had too much amalgam removed; this is also referred to as an **undercontoured** restoration (Figure 36.3). If the operator does not remove enough amalgam, the restoration is **undercarved, or overcontoured.** If the restoration has been undercarved and the amalgam has become too hard to carve, the operator can remove the excess amalgam with a bur or other abrasive device. Undercarving on the occlusal surface is detected when the occlusion is checked with articulating paper.

Carving continues until the restoration is contoured with the outline of the natural tooth form. After carving has been completed, the operator burnishes the amalgam by placing the burnisher on the tooth surface and the amalgam and lightly smoothing the surface of the restoration. This creates an even, smooth surface, which helps eliminate tarnish and

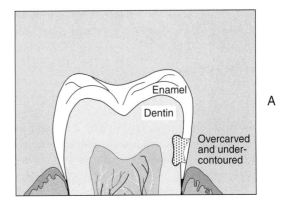

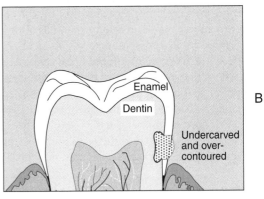

FIGURE 36.3

A, A restoration that has been overcarved has had too much amalgam removed; this is also referred to as an undercontoured restoration. **B,** If the operator does not remove enough amalgam, the restoration is undercarved, or overcontoured.

Overcarved
Too much amalgam has been removed.

Undercontoured
Contour does not extend far enough.

Undercarved
Not enough amalgam has been removed.

Overcontoured
Contour extends beyond the normal.

corrosion by removing irregularities. Burnishing also provides a tight, smooth cavosurface margin. When the burnishing procedure has been completed, the operator evaluates the margins for excess amalgam, or flash. The amalgam must be flush with the cavosurface margin; this is referred to as marginal integrity. Any flash noted is removed with the carver.

Problems in Amalgam Placement

Proper placement of the dental amalgam is vital to the success of the restoration. Amalgam that is not condensed properly has air voids, open margins, and submarginal areas. Improper condensation, as well as improper trituration, can result in a weak restoration that will fracture or an accumulation of food and calculus that can cause recurrent caries, tarnish, and corrosion. Improper condensation, trituration, or moisture control can cause overextension of the dental amalgam at the cavosurface margin or an overhang at the gingival margin. Dental amalgam has a very weak edge that breaks under the normal stress of chewing, and such breakage may ditch the amalgam at the cavosurface margin. Both a ditch and an overextension can cause a buildup of plaque and calculus, recurrent caries, and recession of the gingival tissue. An overextension can be caused by operator error or by the natural expansion of the amalgam alloy after a period of time (Figure 36.4). In such cases correction or replacement must be considered.

Examination of the Restoration

When examining the restoration, the operator checks the tooth surface and the restoration to make sure that the restoration is flush at the cavosurface margin and has no pits or irregularities at the margins or within the restoration. The occlusal, proximal, and facial and lingual anatomy must be continuous with the existing anatomic form. The cusps, planes, grooves, and marginal ridges must be restored. The restoration must closely resemble the original form of the tooth.

Because it is difficult to remove amalgam from the interproximal surfaces, these areas must be checked as soon as the matrix band is removed; this allows the operator to eliminate any excess amalgam while it can still be removed with a carver or explorer. The removal of the matrix band is also the time to check for any voids along the gingival floor in case the amalgam needs to be removed and replaced. The proximal contours need to be continuous with the existing anatomic form, and the contacts need to be confirmed by flossing, visual checking, and use of an explorer.

After the restoration has been placed, the operator examines the occlusal surface, proximal surfaces, and facial and lingual surfaces for any defect, such as an overextension of material, a submarginal area, overcontoured surface, undercontoured surface, or anatomic accuracy. The restoration is checked visually and with an explorer, dental floss, and articulating paper. In questionable cases, a radiograph of the interproximal area may be taken to detect any overhang or void.

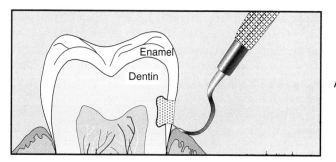

A

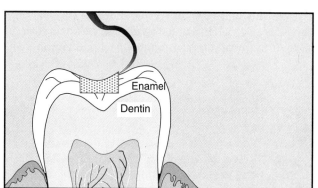

B

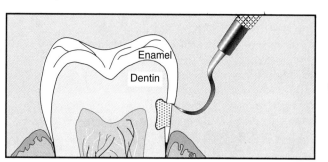

C

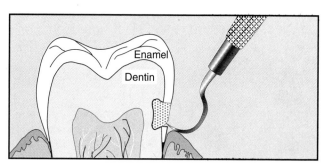

D

FIGURE 36.4

An overextension can be caused by operator error or by the natural expansion of the amalgam alloy after a period of time.

Marginal Overextensions and Overcontoured/Undercarved Surfaces

The operator checks the occlusal and proximal surfaces for overextension of dental amalgam along the cavosurface margins, taking care not to scratch or ditch the amalgam, by sliding the explorer from the tooth surface over the restoration along the cavosurface margins. The explorer and dental floss can be used interproximally to detect extensions of amalgam or overhang. Overextensions can make it difficult for the patient to brush and floss and eventually can cause tissue damage and bone loss. The operator should remove excess amalgam with a carver before the amalgam hardens.

To evaluate the occlusion, the operator asks the patient to slowly and carefully bring the teeth together to see if the bite feels high. The occlusion is examined with articulating paper to check occlusal contacts when the teeth are in centric occlusion and during excursive movements. The markings should be of equal density and evenly distributed on adjacent teeth. If the occlusion is correct, minimal finishing and polishing are needed to provide a smooth surface. If the occlusion is high, the operator must remove the excess material.

The facial and lingual surfaces may also need to be redefined. If an overextension exists, it may be removed with a pointed or flame-shaped stone. Facial or lingual grooves on these surfaces should be carved into the amalgam restoration and should run evenly from the tooth to the restoration. If a cusp has been replaced, the facial, lingual, and proximal surfaces should be mirror images of the natural tooth contours and embrasures. The occlusal embrasure involves the marginal ridge, which is rounded away from the matrix band toward the occlusal surface leaving a V shape between the restored tooth and the adjacent tooth. This ridge is not

---

Box 36.1   *Evaluation*

Evaluation of Amalgam and Composite Restorations

Condensation

All margins of the preparation are covered by amalgam.
Preparation is slightly overfilled.
Amalgam surface is shiny, with not voids or graininess.
Overlapping condensing strokes are visible.

Anatomy

The location, size, and depth of the fossae are correct.
The major grooves are distinct and located correctly.
Supplemental grooves in the adjacent enamel extend into the restoration.

Marginal integrity

No excess amalgam is seen beyond the margins.
No open margins are seen.
No submarginal areas are seen.
Amalgam does not extend beyond the cavosurface margin.

Surface smoothness

The amalgam is smooth.
No pits or voids are seen.
The amalgam has a dull luster.

Occlusion

The contacts are on the marginal ridge or in the fossae.
The occlusion of uninvolved teeth is unchanged.
The restoration does not feel too high to the patient.

Marginal ridges

The marginal ridge has been restored to the height of the adjacent or involved tooth.

The fossa has been established and the occlusal surface defined.

Contour and contact replacement

The marginal ridge has been rounded to form the occlusal embrasure.
The proximal contour is convex faciolingually.
The contact area is convex occlusogingivally from the marginal ridge through the contact area.
The contour is flat or slightly concave from the gingival border of the contact area to the cervical line.
The lingual embrasure is slightly larger than the facial embrasure.

Esthetics

The restoration blends with the shade of the surrounding tooth surface.
The restoration has no stains or metallic streaks.

Contour and incisal edge replacement

Incisogingival contours are present.
Faciolingual contours are present.
No submarginal areas are seen.
The contact is slightly facial to the faciolingual midline and in the incisal one third of the proximal surface.
The contact is tight enough to tug during the passage of floss.
No premature contact of the restoration occurs in centric occlusion.
No premature contact occurs during lateral or protrusive movement.

straight, nor does it have a knife-shaped edge. The facial, lingual, and gingival embrasures must also be checked for anatomic accuracy.

Submarginal Areas, Voids, and Undercontoured/Overcarved Surfaces

The operator also carefully examines the restoration and tooth with the explorer to detect any submarginal areas. If a submarginal defect is minimal, the operator can carefully remove a small amount of tooth enamel to make the margin of the tooth flush with the restorative material. If the defect has been caused by incorrect placement or condensation and is excessive, the restoration must be replaced.

Lack of contact between the restored tooth and the adjacent tooth can be caused by incorrect placement and adjustment of the matrix band, improper removal of the matrix band, ineffective condensation, or overcarving in the proximal areas. Because the contours of the tooth protect the gingival tissue and ultimately the alveolar bone structure, it is imperative that these contours be replaced as near to the natural tooth form as possible (see Chapter 10). If the undercontouring is significant enough to affect the well-being of the gingival tissue and alveolar bone, the restoration must be replaced.

Box 36.1 presents a general guideline for evaluating finished amalgam or composite restorations.

PLACEMENT OF AMALGAM

This chapter has reviewed the prerequisites for clinical restorative dentistry. Infection control and patient management procedures are important for the safety and well-being of the patient and dental personnel. A well-designed dental practice effectively uses team concepts, four-handed sit-down dental procedures, and expanded-function dental assistants to serve patients more efficiently. The knowledge and skills of allied dental personnel allow the dentist and dental assistants to work in a more supportive and effective environment. Restorative dentistry is a key element in a general dentistry practice. The dentist can serve a greater number of patients in a more relaxing environment by using appropriately trained dental personnel who can assume some of the operative procedures, thus allowing the dentist more time to perform procedures and services that require a higher level of skill. Whether the dentist or the expanded-function dental assistant performs the intricate restorative procedures, there must be a defined level of competency in the related areas. This chapter provides information to guide dental personnel who are assisting the dentist during advanced restorative procedures or who are personally restoring the tooth.

Preparation

An operative appointment begins with preparation of the clinical area, after which the dental amalgam or composite

instruments are set up, and the patient is greeted and placed in a comfortable supine position (see Chapter 19 for a list of amalgam instruments). The operator reviews the patient's records and then is seated in the appropriate working position. The chairside dental assistant is seated in position with the operator; the assistant aids in isolation of the teeth and passes essential instruments to the operator for removal of dental caries and placement of the restoration (see Chapter 20 for positioning procedures). Pulp protection is placed, and the cavity is cleaned and lightly dried with warm air. After these procedures, the amalgam restoration is started.

It is important to note that the instruments used must be able to fit into the cavity preparation. The size of the cavity preparation, therefore, determines the appropriate placement and condenser to be used for the procedures listed in Box 36.2.

Class I Amalgam Restoration

The Class I dental amalgam restoration described here is completed on the mandibular right permanent first molar, tooth #30 (Figure 36.5). The dentist and expanded-function dental assistant note the anatomic landmarks on the tooth before preparing it (Figure 36.6). This mental reflection and image help the operator to restore the tooth to a form closely resembling that of the natural tooth.

Review of Anatomic Contours

The tooth described in this Class I dental amalgam procedure is the mandibular right permanent first molar. It has five cusps: a mesiofacial cusp, a distofacial cusp, a distal cusp, a distolingual cusp and a mesiolingual cusp. The smallest cusp is the distofacial cusp, which is angled slightly toward the facial surface. The central developmental groove is in the center of the middle third of the occlusal surface. Seven grooves must be carved and contoured into the occlusal surface of the restoration: the mesial marginal groove, the mesial groove, the mesiofacial groove, the distofacial groove, the distal groove, the distal marginal groove, and the lingual groove. A mesial triangular fossa and distal triangular fossa are present.

Insertion and Condensation

Insertion and condensation of the amalgam are accomplished through the following steps:

1 The tip of the carrier is placed into the distal concavity of the preparation. With light pressure, the first increment of amalgam is inserted into the angle of the preparation. Continuing the light pressure, the operator flows the amalgam mass across the pulpal floor to the mesial angle.

2 The first increment is condensed quickly with a condenser small enough to reach into all areas of the cavity preparation (Figure 36.7). The operator begins condensation in the distal area, pressing the amalgam against the pulpal floor and the walls. Overlapping strokes are used as the

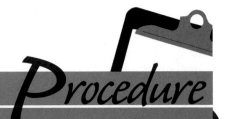

Box 36.2

Procedure for Amalgam Placement

Anatomic review

1. Review the anatomic form and anatomic structures.

Cavity preparation

1. Isolate the field of operation.
2. Prepare the cavity.
3. Examine the cavity preparation.
4. Remove debris with high-velocity evacuation.
5. Clean the cavity with warm water.
6. Gently dry the cavity.

Liner or base

1. Place the liner or base in the prepared cavity.

Trituration

1. Put mercury and alloy in a capsule if preencapsulated amalgam is not being used.
2. Put the capsule in the amalgamator.
3. Check the proper timing.
4. Push the start button.
5. Put in amalgam well or cloth.

Condensation

1. Use appropriate size carrier and condenser.
2. Eject small increments of amalgam.
3. Condense each increment firmly.
4. Overfill the cavity.

Carving

1. Remove excess amalgam.
2. Contour the amalgam to recreate the original form and function of the tooth.
3. Smooth and burnish the amalgam.
4. Remove the wedge, matrix, and rubber dam.

Finishing

1. Examine the restoration with an explorer.
2. Refine the anatomy and remove any excess amalgam with hand instruments and burs.

Polishing

1. Polish to a smooth, shiny finish.
   (Final finishing and polishing may be completed at the recall appointment.)

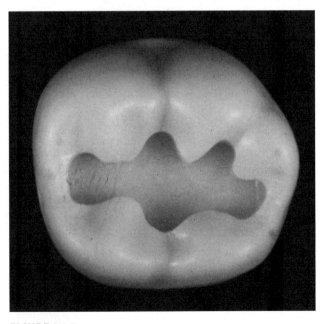

FIGURE 36.5

Cavity classification I (tooth #30).

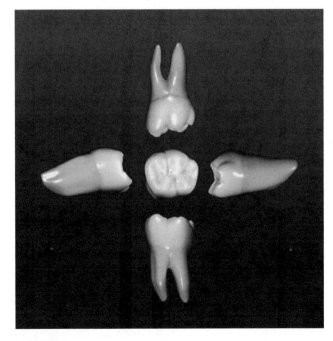

FIGURE 36.6

An advanced-function dental assistant must understand the nomenclature of all surfaces of each tooth: occlusal, buccal, distal, lingual, and mesial.

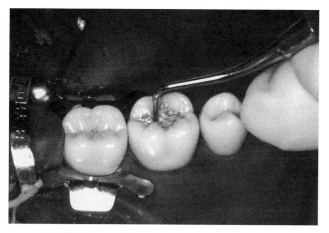

FIGURE 36.7

The amalgam is condensed in small increments.

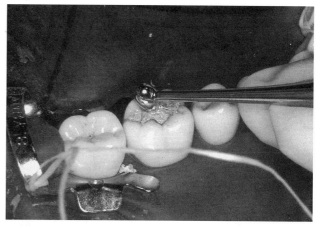

FIGURE 36.8

A burnisher is used to smooth the surface of the amalgam and to bring excess mercury to the surface for removal.

instrument is moved across the pulpal floor into the mesial concavity.

3 Following the same placement sequence, the operator continues to insert increments of amalgam proportional to the size of the cavity preparation until it is overfilled with amalgam.

4 The operator condenses the mass with pressure, using overlapping strokes to blend and bind each increment of amalgam. The amalgam is pressed and condensed into any extension or angle, as the operator continues to push the amalgam against the walls of the cavity preparation. This condensation should bring excess mercury to the surface, where it can be removed during the carving procedure.

Carving

Carving begins when the operator feels some resistance to pressure exerted on the amalgam with the carver:

1 The initial contouring of the dental amalgam can be accomplished with one of several burnishers. This procedure brings the excess mercury to the surface while contouring the dental amalgam into the extensions and grooves and against cavosurface margins (Figure 36.8).

2 The large discoid carver usually is used first and then the cleoid carver. The discoid carver is used for general shaping of the occlusion, and the sharp point on the cleoid carver allows the operator to form the grooves and fossae (Figure 36.9). The side of the carver is rested in the groove and against the tooth structure. With the side of the instrument on the tooth surface and the tip of the instrument angled toward the developmental depression, the carver is moved toward the triangular ridge and triangular fossa with sufficient pressure to shave away the amalgam. The assistant uses the suction tip to remove amalgam debris. The operator must make sure that the point of the instrument does not ditch the opposite side of the cusp incline by crossing over the central developmental

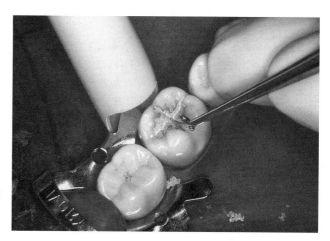

FIGURE 36.9

A discoid carver is used to form the grooves.

groove. This process is continued from the buccal and lingual surfaces until the carving is finished.

3 A burnisher can be used for final contouring and to achieve closed margins and a smooth finish on the amalgam.

4 Any scraps of amalgam are removed with the suction tip, and the completed restoration is examined. An explorer can be used to carefully examine the cavosurface margins, and articulating paper is used to check the occlusion (Table 36.1).

Simple Class II Amalgam Restoration

The Class II amalgam restoration described here is completed on the mandibular left permanent second premolar, tooth #20. The patient, operator, and dental assistant are positioned as described above, and all preparations essential for a Class II amalgam restoration are completed. A Class II cavity

Class I Amalgam Restoration	4	3	2	0	X

Evaluation for a Class I Amalgam Restoration

Amalgam condensation.
Anatomy.
Lack of flash.
Adaptation of margin.
Surface smoothness.
Occlusion.
Pulp protection.

The numeric criteria: 4 Excellent; 3 Good but some improvement can be made; 2 Below average, usable, needs to improve skill; 0 Unsatisfactory; X Not able to evaluate.

preparation is a continuation of the Class I preparation. The key difference is that a Class II cavity preparation extends into the proximal surface. Because of this extension and the lack of a proximal wall, a matrix band must be placed around the tooth. The carving of a Class II cavity preparation is more complicated and requires more time and skill than a Class I preparation because the marginal ridge, proximal surface, contact, and embrasures must be restored.

Review of Anatomic Contours

The mandibular left permanent second premolar has a variety of occlusal anatomic contours, and the locations of the cusps and grooves vary (Figure 36.10). The tooth described for this preparation has two cusps: one large facial cusp and one smaller lingual cusp. If the tooth has three cusps, the mesiolingual cusp is shorter and smaller than the distolingual cusp. The occlusal shape of the tooth is somewhat rectangular. From the occlusal aspect, the central developmental groove is located in the middle of the middle third and extends to the distal and medial triangular fossae. Five secondary grooves form the distal triangular fossa, and four form the mesial triangular fossa. The fossae form small depressions, or concavities, in the distal and mesial one third of the occlusal surface below the marginal ridges. Because the fossae and ridges are affected by the opposing maxillary cusps, they must be contoured properly to provide centric occlusion. It should also be noted that the marginal ridges are rounded to create the occlusal embrasure (Figure 36.11).

Review of Matrix Band Placement

The matrix band should be checked to ensure that it has been placed properly:

1 The matrix band must extend 1 to 2 mm occlusally to the anticipated marginal ridge height.
2 The matrix band must be tightly wedged and must extend 1 mm below the gingival cavosurface margin of the cavity preparation.

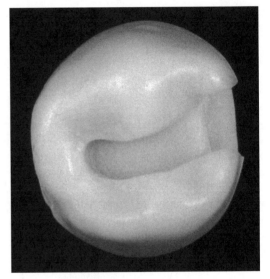

FIGURE 36.10
Cavity classification II (tooth #20).

3 The matrix band must be secure against the tooth gingivally and contoured sufficiently to provide a tight contact with the adjacent tooth. The band can be burnished and contoured with the round or football-shaped burnisher.
4 The inside of the cavity preparation must be checked with an explorer along the gingival cavosurface margin to make sure that the band is tight and that there are no openings that would allow amalgam to escape.
5 The facioaxial and linguoaxial retentive grooves in the dentin must be checked to confirm that no pulp protector has filled these grooves.

Insertion and Condensation

After the matrix band has been checked, the amalgam is inserted and condensed according to the following steps:

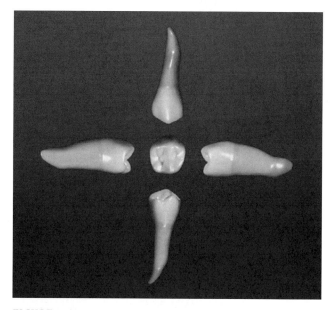

FIGURE 36.11

The anatomy of each of the surfaces of this tooth should be reviewed.

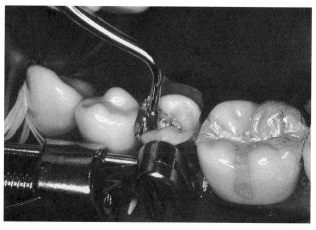

FIGURE 36.13

The amalgam is condensed into the retentive grooves and point angles.

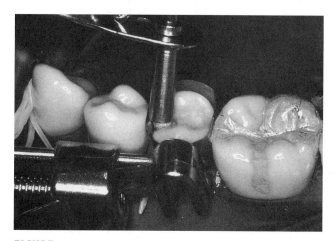

FIGURE 36.12

Small increments of amalgam are placed in the deepest area of the cavity preparation.

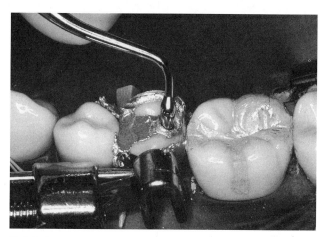

FIGURE 36.14

After condensing in the proximal area has been completed, placement and condensation in the occlusal area are begun.

1 The first small increment of amalgam is ejected into the deepest area of the cavity preparation by placing the tip of the carrier into the mesial gingivoproximal line angle (Figure 36.12). The purpose of this initial placement is to fill the critical area first. It also gives the operator a better view of this area while placing and condensing amalgam.

2 Only a small portion of this proximal area is filled with the first placement; this allows the operator to better condense the amalgam tightly into the small area.

3 A condenser with a small nib is used so that more force can be exerted in this small area. The condenser is used to direct the force toward the buccoaxial and linguoaxial line angles and against the cavity walls.

4 The amalgam is condensed into the retentive grooves and the buccoaxial and linguoaxial proximal point angles, which are the buccal and lingual corners where the matrix band meets tooth structure (Figure 36.13).

5 The proximal area is filled before condensing into the occlusal area is begun. Using overlapping strokes, the operator continues condensing firmly with the small condenser, changing to the larger round, flat-end condenser as more amalgam is inserted (Figure 36.14).

6 The operator inserts and condenses quickly and evenly (spending about $3\frac{1}{2}$ minutes, total) across the pulpal floor until all areas of the cavity preparation are overfilled.

Carving

Carving begins when the operator feels some resistance to pressure exerted on the amalgam with the carver:

1 Initial carving is begun by removing excessive amalgam in the proximal area and rounding the marginal ridges with an explorer (Figure 36.15).

2 Using the burnisher or discoid/cleoid carver, the operator begins initial carving of the grooves and the distal and mesial triangular fossae. With the side of the instrument placed on the tooth surface to prevent ditching, the instrument is guided over the contours of the occlusal surface. The carving is left shallow; carving to a finished depth is not done at this time.

3 The operator removes the matrix band and retainer by (1) loosening the band from around the tooth, (2) loosening the locking set screw, and (3) removing the band from the retainer (Figure 36.16). Because the amalgam is still weak, the band is carefully removed in the buccal or lingual direction. The band can be removed from the occlusal direction if a rocking motion is used as the band is lifted; however, if a tug is felt, the band should not be forced, because this could break the marginal ridge.

4 As soon as the band has been removed, the operator quickly examines and finishes the interproximal area from the facial and lingual aspects with an explorer or Hollenback carver (Figure 36.17). At this stage, the cavosurface margins can be further contoured and smoothed if necessary. The amalgam knife can be used to remove any flash.

5 The operator checks the occlusion with articulating paper and by asking the patient to "close very carefully" (Figure 36.18). Any overcontoured amalgam is removed and any irregularity refined. The presence of a void, fracture, or undercontoured area may require removal of the amalgam. If this is the case, the amalgam should be removed quickly with an excavator.

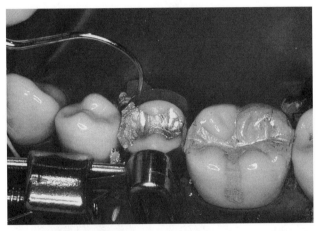

FIGURE 36.15

The marginal ridges are rounded with an explorer.

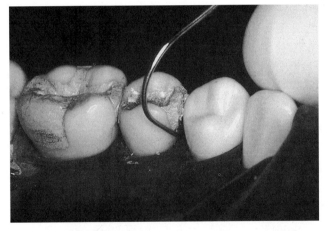

FIGURE 36.17

The proximal amalgam is removed first.

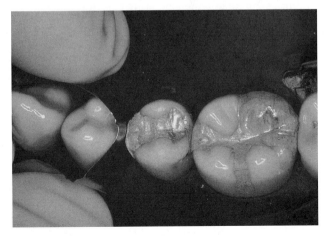

FIGURE 36.16

The matrix band is loosened from around the tooth and then removed.

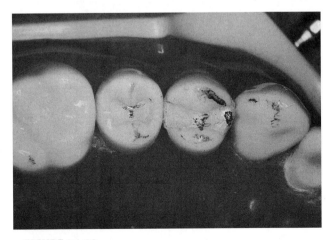

FIGURE 36.18

The bite is checked with articulating paper (occlusal view).

Complex Class II Amalgam Restorations

The degree of difficulty involved in restoring any tooth is determined by the amount of missing tooth structure and by the tooth's location in the oral cavity. Three of the more difficult, or complex, amalgam restorations are the three-surface, or mesioocclusodistal (MOD), preparation; the five-surface, or mesioocclusodistal plus buccal and lingual (MODBL) preparation; and an MODBL, cusp-removed, pin-retained preparation. These restorations are presented here in order of increasing difficulty, and each preparation is an extension of the one before it.

Restoration of an MOD Cavity Preparation

The mandibular right permanent second molar (tooth # 31) has an MOD cavity preparation (Figure 36.19). This Class II cavity preparation is more complex than the Class II preparation on tooth #20; it is an extension of the single-surface occlusal and the two-surface occlusoproximal preparations described previously. The MOD preparation extends into two proximal surfaces, therefore the matrix band must cover both proximal extensions of the cavity preparation below the gingival cavosurface margins. A wider MOD matrix band often is needed to ensure this coverage. Carving of this Class II amalgam restoration is further complicated by the size of the preparation, the additional anatomic contouring required, and the need to ensure that the matrix band is tight proximally. The operator must work quickly to place, condense, and carve the amalgam.

Review of Anatomic Contours

The mandibular right permanent second molar, tooth #31, is similar to the mandibular first molar except that it has four cusps (no distal cusp) and is smaller (Figure 36.20). The occlusal surface is more square than rectangular. It has well-defined cusps, and the mesiobuccal cusp is larger and more contoured than the others. The central developmental groove is centered faciolingually and terminates in the mesial and distal triangular fossae. The buccal and lingual grooves intersect with the central groove, creating a well-defined central triangular fossa. The marginal ridges are rounded and are located in the middle third of the tooth. The contact area is centered approximately in the mesial and distal one third and the buccal and lingual one third.

Review of Matrix Band Placement

Placement of the matrix band is always checked first:

1 Placement of the matrix band for a three-surface preparation is slightly more difficult than for a two-surface preparation. With an MOD preparation, the operator must make sure that the single matrix band extends sufficiently occlusally above the marginal ridge area and gingivally below the cavosurface margin on both the mesial and distal proximal surfaces. An MOD matrix band may be needed, which can reach into the gingival area and can be tightly wedged.

2 The band must be secure against the tooth gingivally and contoured sufficiently on both proximal surfaces to provide a tight contact with adjacent teeth.

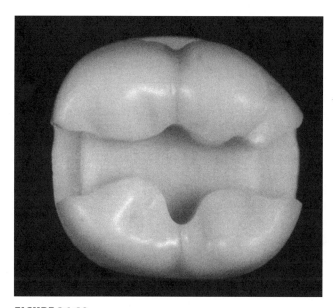

FIGURE 36.19

Cavity classification II: complex cavity preparation (tooth #31).

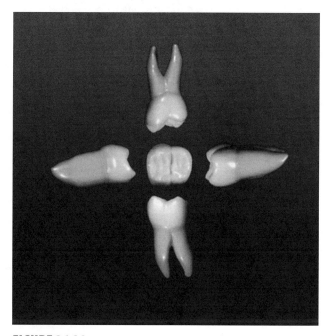

FIGURE 36.20

The morphology of tooth #31 should be reviewed before restorative procedures are begun.

3 The inside of the cavity preparation must be checked on both proximal extensions to ensure that the band is tight and no open areas exist through which amalgam can escape.

Insertion and Condensation

Insertion and condensation are accomplished in much the same way as with the restorations previously described:

1 The operator ejects a small increment of amalgam first into the distal proximal extension and then into the mesial proximal extension, making sure that any central depression has been filled before flowing the amalgam across the pulpal wall of the cavity preparation.

2 A condenser with a small nib is used first and then a larger one so that the hard-to-see areas are filled and condensed first, as described for a simple Class II restoration.

3 A three-surface preparation is larger than a two-surface preparation and often takes longer to fill, requiring the operator to insert and condense the amalgam quickly and evenly until the cavity preparation has been overfilled.

Carving

As with other restorations, carving is begun when the operator fees resistance to pressure exerted on the amalgam:

1 The carving procedures described previously and in Box 36.3 are followed.

2 Carving is done carefully but quickly because of the size of the preparation and the amount of time needed to complete the restoration.

3 It is imperative that the matrix band be removed carefully, especially with the two proximal extensions. The amalgam is loosened from around the marginal ridges and the matrix band and then, using a slight rocking motion, the band is lifted away. *If any tug is felt, the band should not be forced because this could break the marginal ridge.*

3 The distal proximal area and then the mesial area are quickly examined and finished with the explorer or Hollenback carver.

5 The occlusion is checked, and any overcontoured amalgam is removed and any irregularity refined.

Restoration of an MODBL, Cusp-Removed, Pin-Retained Cavity Preparation

This mandibular left permanent first molar (tooth #19) MODBL cavity preparation is complicated by the missing cusp and the placement of a pin. The procedure is consid-

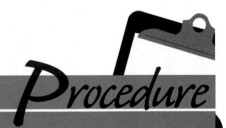

Box 36.3

Procedure for a Mesioocclusodistal (MOD) Restoration

1. **Place the rubber dam, remove debris, and place a liner or base.**
2. **Place the matrix band tightly from the facial surface.**
3. **Place wedges in both the mesial and distal interproximal spaces (Figure 36.21). Secure the matrix band tightly at the gingival floor of the cavity preparation and begin inserting amalgam into the deepest area of the preparation.**
4. **Using the condensation technique and the smallest condenser, forcefully compress the amalgam into angles and against the cavity walls.**
5. **Add increments of amalgam to the mesial, distal, and occlusal depressions.**
6. **Using overlapping strokes, add the increments quickly and evenly across the floor of the preparation.**
7. **As the preparation becomes overfilled (Figure 36.22), use the larger condenser and compress firmly across the amalgam.**
8. **After the preparation has been overfilled, use a football-shaped burnisher to begin contouring and to bring the mercury to the surface for removal (Figure 36.23).**
9. **Use an explorer to remove excess amalgam from the marginal ridge around the matrix band (Figure 36.24).**
10. **Carefully remove the matrix band from the facial and lingual areas.**
11. **Using an explorer and a carver, quickly remove excess amalgam from the proximal surfaces (Figure 36.25).**
12. **Refine the grooves with a Hollenback carver.**
13. **Refine the marginal ridge with a discoid/cleoid carver and the marginal ridges with an explorer (Figure 36.26).**

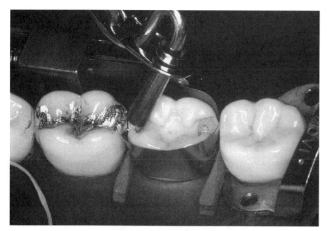

FIGURE 36.21

Wedges are placed gently.

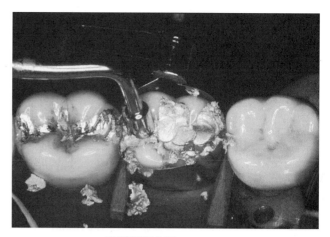

FIGURE 36.22

An overfilled restoration.

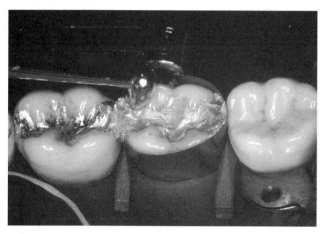

FIGURE 36.23

A football-shaped burnisher can be used to remove excess amalgam and bring mercury to the surface for removal.

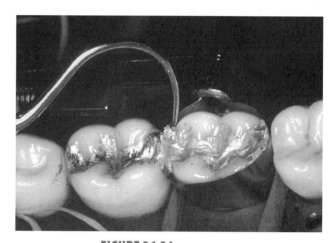

FIGURE 36.24

Excess amalgam is removed.

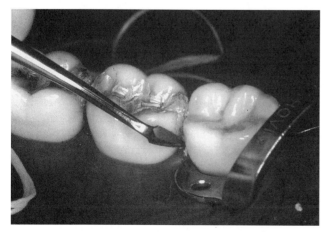

FIGURE 36.25

Excess flash is removed from the proximal surfaces.

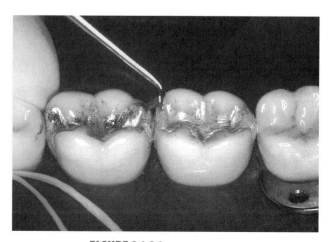

FIGURE 36.26

The marginal ridges are refined.

ered a complex Class II cavity preparation, but it is more complex than a Class II MOD preparation because of the missing cusp and the need to condense carefully and completely around the pin inserted for cusp replacement and support of the tooth structure support.

With this restoration the operator must create the proximal extensions, contacts, cavosurface margins, overall tooth contour, and anatomic replacement. Placement of the matrix band is more difficult because of the lack of tooth structure to help contour and support the band below the cavosurface margins. A wider matrix band usually is needed for this preparation to ensure extension of the band coverage.

Carving this type of complex amalgam restoration is complicated because of the restoration's size and anatomic contour and the need for a secure, contoured matrix band. The operator must work quickly to place, condense, and carve the amalgam. Expanded-function dental assistants may prefer to use an amalgam that sets more slowly to restore a cavity preparation of this complexity.

Pin Retention

The dentist may choose to restore a badly decayed or damaged tooth with a permanent gold crown or even a temporary stainless steel crown if the patient is unable to have the gold crown at that time. The dentist also may decide to restore the damaged tooth to useful function with an amalgam pin-retained restoration. A pin is a metallic peg or screw that is placed in the dentin of a tooth to provide retention for restorative dental material. One or more pins are used to anchor an amalgam core, on which a partial or full-cast restoration can be placed, or a temporary restoration can be placed to stabilize the remaining tooth structure. A pin-retained restoration can be an economic, permanent restoration for a tooth that is badly broken down, or it can maintain the tooth until further treatment is undertaken, such as endodontic treatment or removal.

Types of Pins Many types of pins are available in various sizes. The types most commonly used are (1) cemented pins, which are cemented into holes larger than the pin that have been drilled into the dentin; (2) friction-retained pins, which are driven into holes that are smaller in diameter than the pin; and (3) self-threading pins, the most popular type because they screw into holes that are slightly smaller in diameter than the pin (Figure 36.27). Cemented pins put less stress on the surrounding tooth structure, but self-threading pins have greater retentive strength.

Self-threading pins can be placed with a rotary-driven handpiece or, if accessibility is poor, they can be placed with a hand wrench method. The E-Z Place driver is a new hand instrument designed to turn a slow-speed latch-type contraangle by hand (Figure 36.28). The twist driver allows the operator to place pins in difficult areas and avoid getting the hand wrench tangled up in the gloves, and it provides tactile

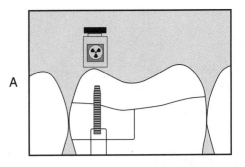

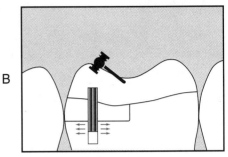

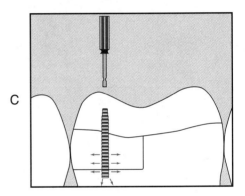

FIGURE 36.27
Retention pins can be (**A**) cemented, (**B**) tapped, or (**C**) screwed into place.

sense to ensure positive seating. The instrument is made of stainless steel and can be sterilized.

Before the pin is placed, the dentist evaluates the vitality of the tooth, its size, the location of the pulp, the thickness of the dentin, and the anatomy and occlusion of the tooth. These factors are important in determining if a pin-retained amalgam will be successful. The dentist places the pin or pins so as to avoid pulp involvement and lateral perforation. The procedure described below uses a self-threading pin.

Matrix Band Placement for Tooth with Missing Cusp

Placement of the matrix band for this type of restoration is more difficult than for the previously described Class II restorations because the matrix band must be secure while

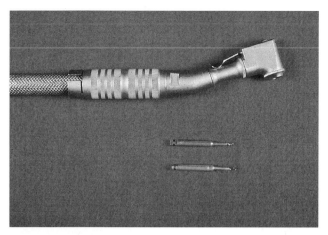

FIGURE 36.28

E-Z Place system. (Courtesy Dr. AG Podshadley ULSD, and Whip Mix Corp.)

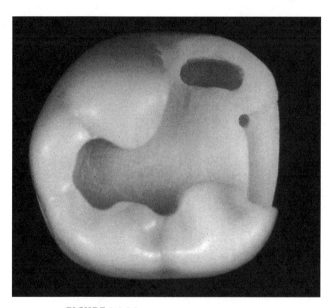

FIGURE 36.29

Anatomy of a Class II complex amalgam.

fitting tightly below the cavosurface margin of the entire missing distolingual cusp (Figure 36.29). The band must be wide enough to extend above the marginal ridges and below the gingival cavosurface margins, yet not impinge on the soft tissue. The wide matrix band material may need to be trimmed to fit appropriately.

1 The matrix band must fit tightly around the entire cervix of the tooth and extend 1 mm below the gingival cavosurface margin of the tooth preparation.

2 The band must not impinge on the soft tissue or catch any of the rubber dam, but it must be secure against the gingival surfaces of the tooth.

3 The matrix band must also extend 1 mm occlusal to the marginal ridge and cusp tips. It must be straight or parallel to the long axis of the tooth and be contoured sufficiently on both proximal surfaces to provide a tight contact with adjacent teeth.

4 A wedge is placed in each proximal embrasure. More than one wedge can be used to hold the band firmly. The wedges can be contoured, if necessary, and dental compound can be adapted to the lingual surface of the matrix band if additional support is needed.

5 The operator uses a mirror and explorer to examine the inside of the matrix band along the cavosurface margins of the cavity preparation to make sure the band is tight and has no open areas through which amalgam could escape.

Insertion and Condensation

Box 36.4 and Table 36.2 present procedures specifically related to an MODBL, cusp-removed, pin-retained restoration. This information does not cover all general techniques for matrix band placement, insertion, condensation, and carving of a Class II amalgam restoration.

Class V Amalgam Restoration

The Class V amalgam restoration described here is completed on the mandibular right permanent first molar (tooth #30) (see Figure 36.34). The patient is placed in a supine position, the operator sits at the 10 to 11 o'clock position, and the chairside dental assistant sits at the 3 o'clock position. After the teeth have been isolated, the preparation completed, and pulp protection placed, the operator and chairside dental assistant start the procedure.

Review of Anatomic Contours

The overall anatomy of the mandibular right permanent first molar is described on p. 910. However, the Class V amalgam restoration in this procedure is concerned with the facial, or buccal, contours. The facial surface is convex, and a mesiofacial groove extends into the cavity preparation (see Figure 36.35). This particular preparation is well above the cementoenamel junction and is not affected by the rubber dam. However, if the preparation were located more toward the gingival area, a retractor might be needed. In restoring this preparation, the operator's primary concerns are to ensure that the mesiofacial groove is carved into the amalgam restoration and that the restoration continues the convex facial contour.

Insertion and Condensation

Insertion and condensation proceed as follows:

1 Retention grooves will have been prepared in the dentin. The pulp protector used must not fill or interfere with these grooves, which help secure the amalgam. Using the small tip of the amalgam carrier, the operator inserts

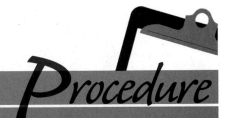

Box 36.4

Procedure

Procedure for a Mesioocclusodistal plus Buccal and Lingual (MODBL), Cusp-Removed, Pin-Retained Restoration

Especially for a restoration of this size and complexity, the rule is: *Work quickly and carefully!*

1. Clean the cavity preparation and check the pin.
2. Place the matrix band (Figure 36.30) and evaluate the occlusal height and gingival depth. Tighten the band securely, positioning it parallel to the long axis of the tooth, and contour the band for proximal contact.
3. Place the first increment in the most inaccessible area of the preparation, usually the gingival cavosurface margin area, the retentive groove, or around the retentive pin. Next, eject a small increment of amalgam into the distal proximal extension, across the pupal wall along the cavosurface margins around the pin, and into the mesial proximal area, making sure that any central depression is filled.
4. Use a small or medium condenser to thoroughly compress the amalgam into the preparation. Concentrate on condensing tightly around the pin using firm, overlapping strokes. It is extremely important to ensure that no voids are left around the pin, because this could weaken the restoration and cause it to fail.
5. Condense each increment completely before adding the next increment. Continue inserting and condensing the amalgam quickly and evenly until the cavity preparation has been overfilled.
6. The PKT #3 instrument can be used to begin shaping the major fossae, triangular ridges, and grooves (Figure 36.31). Remember to keep the side of the instrument on the hard tooth structure with the tip toward the central groove; this aids in shaping of the occlusal surface of the restoration and brings excess mercury to the surface for removal.
7. Use a #23 explorer to round and shape the distal and mesial marginal ridges and the linguoocclusal angles.
8. Use a discoid/cleoid carver to carve the grooves, fossae, and triangular ridges.
9. Examine the amalgam thoroughly before removing the matrix band. Compare the following features with those of adjacent teeth:
   - Contours and anatomic landmarks
   - Buccal and lingual contours (to make sure they are aligned with those of adjacent teeth)
   - Appearance of the embrasure
   - Cusp tips (to make sure they are about the same height as those of adjacent teeth)
   - Rounded form of the buccal and lingual proximal line angles
10. Carefully remove the matrix band from the contact that is looser and then from the tighter contact, holding the band straight.
11. After removing the band, quickly use a #23 explorer to remove excess amalgam from the proximal cavosurface margin (Figure 36.32).
    Use a Hollenback or interproximal carver to contour the lingual surface and grooves, to shape the embrasures, to remove gingival overhangs, and to finish carving the proximal margins.
12. Finish carving the occlusal surface with cleoid and Hollenback carvers.
13. Evaluate the carved restoration and refine any details.
14. Check the occlusion by (1) comparing the restored tooth with the adjacent teeth; (2) using articulating paper; and (3) checking for burnish marks on the amalgam made by occluding teeth. Also, the patient can identify pressure from high spots.
15. Finish and polish the restoration (Figure 36.33).

Table 36.2

Evaluation for a Class II Amalgam Restoration

Class II Amalgam Restoration	4	3	2	0	X
Amalgam condensation.					
Anatomy.					
Lack of flash or overhangs.					
Marginal integrity.					
Surface smoothness.					
Marginal ridge.					
Contact replacement.					
Matrix band and wedge placement.					
Occlusion.					
Pulp protection.					

The numeric criteria: 4 Excellent; 3 Good but some improvement can be made; 2 Below average, usable, needs to improve skill; 0 Unsatisfactory; X Not able to evaluate.

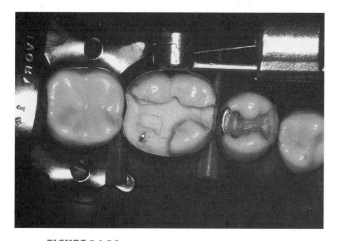

FIGURE 36.30

The matrix band and wedges are placed carefully.

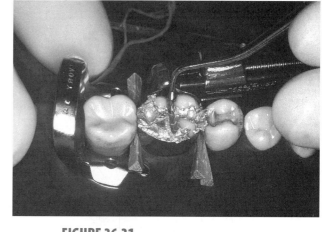

FIGURE 36.31

The fossae, ridges, and grooves are shaped.

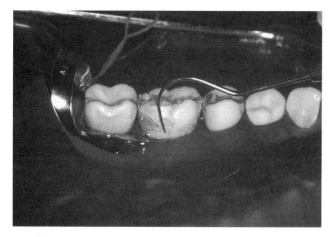

FIGURE 36.32

An explorer is used to remove excess amalgam from the proximal and lingual cavosurface margins.

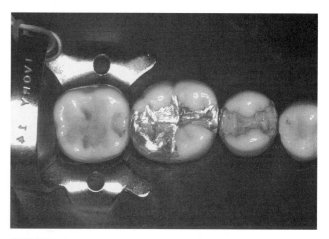

FIGURE 36.33

The restoration is finished with finishing burs, stone or rubber points, brushes, and rubber cups.

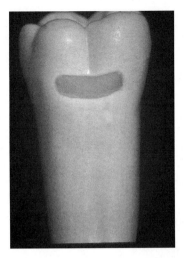

FIGURE 36.34

Class V amalgam restoration completed on the mandibular right permanent first molar.

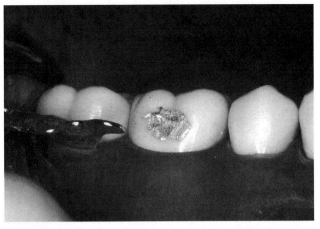

FIGURE 36.36

It is important to condense the first increment into the retentive grooves.

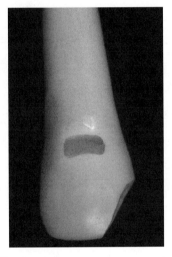

FIGURE 36.35

The facial surface is convex, and a mesiofacial groove extends into the cavity preparation.

the first increment of amalgam into the distal angle of the preparation. This first increment is very small because of the size of the Class V cavity preparation. The small amount also allows the operator to better view initial condensing. The alloy is expressed from the distal angle across the pulpal floor into the mesial angle.

2 Using the small condenser, the operator compresses the amalgam with firm pressure and overlapping strokes, directing the amalgam against the walls and line angles. This first increment must be condensed into the retentive grooves (Figure 36.36).

3 Following the same placement sequence, the operator inserts the increments of amalgam into the cavity prepara-

tion until all areas are completely full and the preparation has been overfilled to a level of 0.5 to 1 mm of excess amalgam. Overfilling the preparation allows sufficient condensation and provides enough excess amalgam that the mercury-rich layer can be removed, yet enough amalgam is left to carve a convex restoration.

Carving

The following steps are involved in the carving of this type of restoration:

1 A tapered burnisher can be used to adapt the margins and bring any excess mercury to the surface.

2 Carving should not be started until the amalgam has reached proper carving consistency. The amalgam should exhibit some resistance to the carver. The explorer can be used to help adapt the amalgam to the cavosurface margins and to begin initial removal of the amalgam along these margins. The Hollenback carver is used to continue carving. It is important to make sure that the amalgam is flush with the tooth structure. The restoration cannot be overcarved or undercarved.

Carving of a Class V amalgam restoration is completed in four steps because of the convex contours involved:

1 Occlusal cavosurface margin: When adapting and carving the occlusal cavosurface margin, the operator places the side of the instrument on the tooth surface and amalgam occlusal to the preparation so that the tip is angled facially (Figure 36.37). The instrument must be angled so that it touches the tooth surface and only the occlusal half of the restoration (Figure 36.38). The operator slides the instrument across the tooth, the marginal surface, and the amalgam from distal to mesial.

2 Gingival cavosurface margin: This margin is adapted and carved with the tip of the instrument on the tooth surface and the heel of the instrument angled away from the

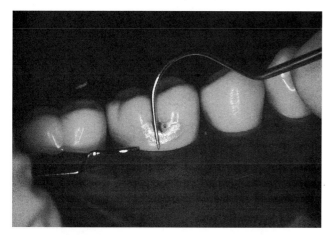

FIGURE 36.37

The occlusal surface is refined with an explorer.

restoration. The instrument is angled so as to touch the tooth surface and only the gingival half of the amalgam restoration.

3 Distal and mesial cavosurface margins: As the occlusal and gingival cavosurface margins are adapted and carved, the operator angles the instrument slightly to contour the distal and mesial cavosurface margins, always maintaining an instrument rest on the tooth structure. These procedures are continued until the restoration is complete (Table 36.3).

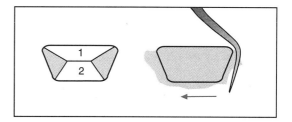

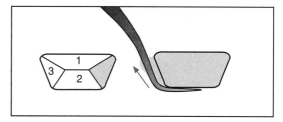

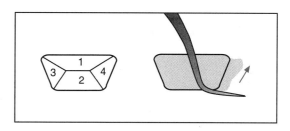

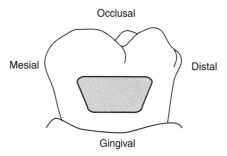

FIGURE 36.38

The instrument must be angled so that it touches the tooth surface and only the occlusal half of the restoration.

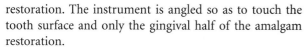

Evaluation for a Class V Amalgam/Composite Restoration

Class V Amalgam/Composite Restoration	4	3	2	0	X
Condensation.					
Contour.					
Lack of flash.					
Adaptation of margin.					
Surface smoothness.					
Esthetics.					
Pulp protection.					

The numeric criteria: 4 Excellent; 3 Good but some improvement can be made; 2 Below average, usable, needs to improve skill; 0 Unsatisfactory; X Not able to evaluate.

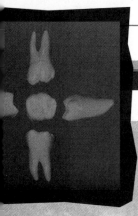

Points for Review

- Clinical application of amalgam restorations
- Placement of amalgam
- Problems encountered in amalgam placement
- Evaluation criteria for amalgam/composite restorations

Self-Study Questions

1. What problem will undercarving a Class V amalgam restoration cause?
   a. Bulky proximal
   b. Excessive contacts
   c. An area of potential plaque accumulation
   d. Malocclusion in excursive movements

2. Which of the following is the best way to begin condensation of amalgam?
   a. Use the largest condenser
   b. Alternate from large to small
   c. Use the smaller condenser followed by the large one
   d. Use the large condenser followed by the small one

3. In what area should condensation of a Class II amalgam begin?
   a. Distal area
   b. Gingival floor of the proximal box
   c. Central area
   d. It is not critical where condensation begins.

4. How should the carver be held during removal of excess amalgam?
   a. At a 90-degree angle to the cavosurface margin
   b. Parallel to the long axis of the tooth
   c. Contacting both tooth structure and amalgam
   d. Entirely on the amalgam

5. Which carving condition causes plaque retention?
   a. Overcontouring
   b. Overhangs
   c. Open margins
   d. All of the above

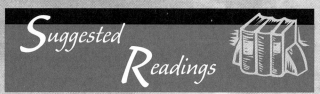

Suggested Readings

Ash MM: *Wheeler's dental anatomy, physiology, and occlusion,* ed 7, Philadelphia, 1993, WB Saunders.

Miyasaki CE: *Chasteen's essentials of clinical dental assisting,* ed 5, St Louis, 1997, Mosby.

Crimm G: *Operative dentistry,* Louisville, Ky, 1995, University of Louisville School of Dentistry.

Council on Dental Materials, Instruments, and Equipment: Choosing intracoronal restorative materials, *J Am Dent Assoc,* 1994.

Jordan RE, Abrams L, Kraus B: *Kraus' dental anatomy and occlusion,* St Louis, 1992, Mosby.

Spohn EE, Halowski WA, Berry TG: *Operative dentistry procedures for dental auxiliaries,* St Louis, 1981, Mosby.

US Department of Health, Education and Welfare: Restoration of cavity preparations with amalgam and tooth-colored materials: Project ACORDE, Castro Valley, Calif, 1979, Quercus Corp.

Zwemer TJ: *Mosby's dental dictionary,* St Louis, 1998, Mosby.

Direct and Indirect Composite Acrylic Resin Restorative Techniques

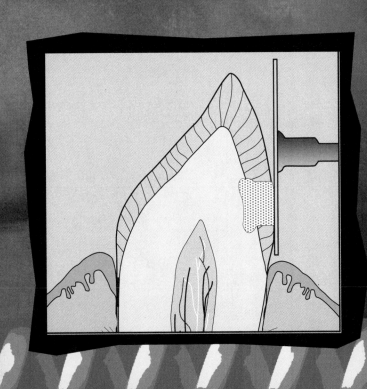

Learning Objectives

On completion of Chapter 37, the student should be able to do the following:

- Define key terms.
- Identify the armamentarium used for composite acrylic resin restorations.
- Define the procedures involved in Class III, Class IV, and posterior composite resin placement.
- Identify shade selection determinations.
- Place the matrix and wedge for composite restorations.

- Finish and polish composite resins.
- Place composite restorations.
- Contour and shape composite restorations.
- Identify the anatomical landmarks of the teeth and describe their significance to composite placement.

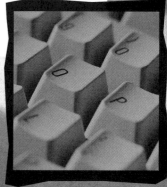

Key Terms

Composite	**Etchant**	**Shade Selection**
Direct Composite	**Indirect Composites**	

CLINICAL APPLICATION FOR DIRECT COMPOSITE ACRYLIC RESIN RESTORATIVE PROCEDURES

Composite

An acrylic resin restorative material that provides a lifelike, esthetic appearance.

Although dental amalgam is a strong restorative material and is easy to handle it lacks the major requirement for an anterior filling material. It does not have an esthetic quality. Therefore **composite** acrylic resins and glass ionomer restorative materials are primarily used for restoring anterior teeth. The following information will include placing composite acrylic resin materials in a Class III and Class IV anterior cavity preparation and a Class II posterior preparation. Refer to Chapter 15 for additional information on composite filling materials.

Clinical Application for Composite Restorations

Today, new microhybrid, light-activated composites and glass ionomer restorative materials are providing more lifelike and esthetic dental restorations. They can also be used for direct veneers, to repair cervical erosion, and also to provide repair to porcelain in the mouth. New color systems more accurately match natural tooth shades as well as simulate light refraction, fluorescence, and translucency of natural teeth.

Composite acrylic resin restorative material is available in chemically activated or light-activated two-paste systems. Composite can be applied direct, is easier to condense, and produces more realistic anatomical form. The direct techniques refer to the placement of the composite material directly into the cavity preparation where it is cured and bonded to the tooth structure. There are also indirect applications in which the restoration or inlay preparation is completed on the tooth, an impression is taken, a die is fabricated, and the composite is fabricated and cured in a dental laboratory and then cemented or bonded in place, finished, and polished in the mouth (see page 931). Glass ionomer restorations may be obtained in powder and liquid form or in a premeasured capsule form. It chemically adheres or bonds to the tooth structure, is radiopaque, does not irritate the pulp, and releases fluoride to help strengthen the tooth structure.

Armamentarium (Figure 37.1):

- Mirror
- Explorer (#19 Shepherd's hook)
- Probe
- Cotton forceps
- Mylar matrix strip
- Wedges
- Cotton pellets
- Bard-Parker scalpel and #12 Blade
- Etchant gel solution
- Primer and bonding agent
- Brush or applicator
- VLC light unit
- Anterior filling material
- Mixing pad, spatula, and plastic placement instrument or applicator
- Shade guide
- Round and pointed white poly-stones
- Finishing burs
- Finishing discs, course, medium, and fine with mandrel
- Finishing strips, coarse and fine

Procedure for Class III Composite Restoration

The Class III composite restoration described here will be completed on the maxillary left permanent central incisor, #9 (Figure 37.2). The armamentarium and supplies will be assembled and the patient, operator, and dental assistant will be in proper four-handed sit-down position.

Shade Selection

The **shade selection** will be determined before placement of the rubber dam and the cavity preparation will be completed. Light shades facilitate curing of the material whereas darker shades block the curing light transmission and cannot be cured in deeper

Shade selection

The determination of the color or shade to be used to restore a tooth using a composite resin material.

depths as lighter composites. Many operators use the lightest shade possible in posterior areas.

Prewedge Placement

A wedge is often placed between the teeth being restored in order to provide room for the matrix band and to produce a good proximal contact.

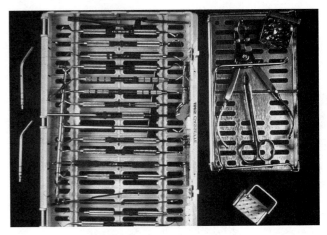

FIGURE 37-1

Composite resin cassette tray setup.

Matrix Placement

When placing the Mylar matrix strip the ends of the matrix must be long enough to grasp securely and pull firmly around the tooth. The gingival edge of the strip should be extended approximately 1 mm below the gingival cavosurface margin of the preparation and 1 to 1.5 mm above the incisal cavosurface margin. The strip must be wide enough to continue onto the enamel tooth surface and provide the proper form when the strip is pulled around the tooth.

Wedge Placement

The wedge will help to conform the matrix strip to the gingival half of the tooth. The top of the wedge must be level with the gingival cavosurface margin of the preparation and it must hold the matrix securely against the gingival proxi-mal surface of the tooth. The wedge should not interfere with access to the cavity preparation.

Incremental Composite Placement

It is important that small increments of composite is placed in the cavity preparation to reduce polymerization shrinkage at the cavosurface margin (approximately 0.5 mm thickness). After two or three small increments have been added to the preparation the remaining preparation should be filled by sloping the material. This reduces the amount of stress placed on the buccal and lingual walls while reducing shrinkage of the composite. Filling the preparation in one increment and curing it can cause postoperative sensitivity by causing the cusps to be pulled toward the center of the tooth.

Reetching, Sealing, and Postcuring the Restoration

After the restoration has been adjusted and finished it is important to reapply the **etchant** for 20 to 30 seconds and rinse for 30 seconds. Once the tooth has been dried, apply the bonding agent or sealant thinly over the restoration and cure to 30 to 40 seconds. This will help to fill in porous surfaces and allow additional curing for a stronger restoration.

Etchant
An acid based material applied to the cavity for abrasion purposes.

Review of Anatomical Contours

The labial surface of the central incisor is broad and flat with a convex labial embrasure on the mesial surface. The mesioproximal contact is located in the incisal third and appears slightly to the incisal-middle one third on this particular tooth. The size of the preparation will be determined by the extent of the carious lesion. If possible, the facial tooth structure will be maintained and a conservative preparation will be made from the lingual surface. This preparation, however, is large and includes the labial surface. Retention grooves will have been made. It is important that the operator makes a mental picture of the cavosurface margins in order to determine margin adaptation of the composite material.

Placement and Finishing

It is important that the operator follows the manufacturers directions for placement and finishing (Box 37.1 and Table 37.1).

Procedure for Class IV Composite Restoration

The Class IV composite restoration is an extension of the Class III as it also includes replacement of the incisal angle. The restoration described here is completed on the maxillary left permanent central incisor, #9, distoincisal surfaces. The anatomical contours are the same for this Class IV restoration as the Class III. The exception is that

A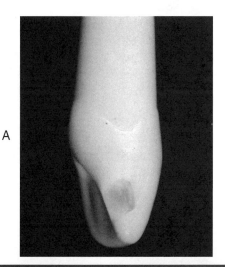

B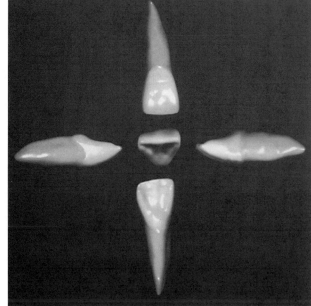

FIGURE 37-2

A, Cavity class III cavity outline. **B**, The center surface is incisal. Clockwise starting at top: labial, mesial, lingual, and distal.

Box 37.1   *Procedure*

Procedures for Placement and Finishing Class III Composite Resin

Placement

1. The shade should be selected before placing the rubber dam.
2. Examine, clean, and dry the preparation and apply base if necessary (Figure 37.3, *A*).
3. Apply etchant to the enamel for 15 seconds (Figure 37.3, *B*).
4. Rinse off etchant for 20 seconds and dry slightly.
5. Apply bonding agent and light cure for 20 seconds.
6. Place matrix strip and wedge.
7. Place increments of composite resin by direct injection into the cavity preparation (Figure 37.3, *C*).
8. Condense each increment firmly.
9. Cure each amount before adding the next.
10. Continue to condense the composite. Figure firmly.
11. Overfill the prep.
12. Pull the matrix slightly to the labial to adapt the composite to the cavosurface margin.
13. Pull the matrix and hold the lingual portion of the strip firmly against the lingual surface of the tooth. Do not pull too tightly and distort the natural contour.
14. Cure with the VLC unit for 30 seconds from the lingual and 30 seconds from the facial.

Finishing

15. A scalpel may be used to remove excessive flash interproximally from the labial aspect.
16. Remove only small amounts of flash at any one time with the scalpel and continue to the lingual aspect.
17. Finishing burs and fine diamonds can be used to finish the margins (Figure 37.3, *D*), contour interproximally, and refine the lingual anatomy.
18. Check the surface smoothness.
19. Use strips to remove remaining flash and contour gingival surface below the contact. Be careful not to touch the contacts.
20. Finish margins with discs.
21. Evaluate final finish, rubber points and cup may be used for final polish. Check the patients protrusive movement with articulating paper and adjust if necessary. Recure the surface of the restoration for 20 seconds for maximum hardness and wear resistance.

Table 37.1

Evaluation for a Class III Composite Resin Restoration

Class III Composite Restoration	4	3	2	0	X
Lack of flash.					
Adaptation of margin.					
Surface smoothness.					
Placement of wedge.					
Contact replacement.					
Contour.					
Aesthetics.					
Pulp protection.					

The numeric criteria: 4 Excellent; 3 Good but some improvement can be made; 2 Below average, usable, needs to improve skill; 0 Unsatisfactory; X Not able to evaluate.

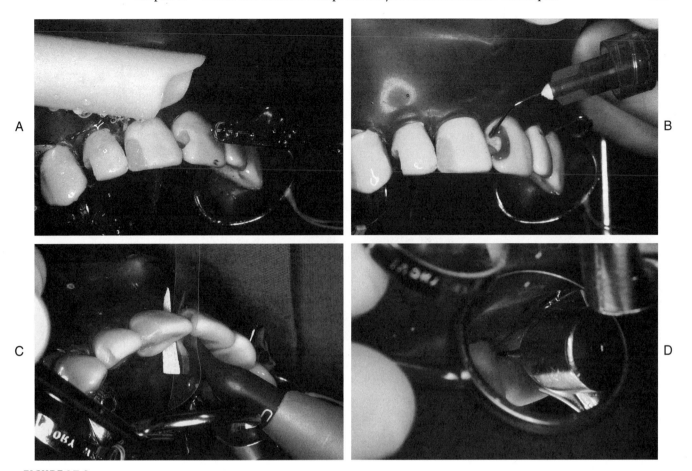

FIGURE 37-3

Placement and finishing. **A**, Examine, clean, and dry the preparation and apply base if necessary. **B**, Apply etchant to the enamel for 15 seconds. **C**, Place increments of composite resin by direct injection into the cavity preparation. **D**, Finishing burs and fine diamonds can be used to finish the margins, contour.

this restoration of the teeth will include replacing the incisal angle. All procedural steps must be completed as described for Class III. In addition, the following steps must be followed to replace the incisal angle (Box 37.2 and Table 37.2).

Procedure for Class V Restoration

Usually amalgam is the restorative material of choice for posterior Class V restorations, since aesthetics is not a major factor. Composite resin is the material used in anterior Class V restorations because of the appearance factor. The Class V restoration may appear rather simple to replace. However, it is unique in that it is often close to the gingival margin or below it (subgingivally) making access difficult. It is important to keep the restoration dry. If a rubber dam is used the hole will need to be punched slightly to the facial to allow greater access to this area.

A matrix is used to help form the facial convex contour. The material is placed in small increments and condensed tightly to ensure accurate cavosurface margin contact. Finishing and polishing are described in Chapter 35.

Procedure for Class II Posterior Composite Restorations

Since the mid 1970s many dentists have been using composite acrylic resin materials for posterior restorations. Although initial studies indicated high failure rates, some of the advantages of posterior composites have been their esthetic value, the ability to bond to tooth structure, low thermal conductivity, and the strengthening value of remaining tooth structure. These restorations can be completed in one appointment and are low cost when comparing them with gold or porcelain. They have no mercury vapors, are not corrosive, and do not cause galvanic currents as associated with amalgam restorations.

Composites have disadvantages such as low wear resistance in high stress areas, a higher coefficient of thermal expansion than tooth structure, and they exhibit polymerization shrinkage (2% to 6%). Composites have no antimicrobial properties and are not radiopaque as are glass ionomers. They provide lower compressive and tensile strength than amalgam, are porous, discolor over time, and composites are toxic to pulpal tissue. Although there are improvement in placement sensitivity, posterior composites and glass

Box 37.2

Procedure for Placement and Finishing Class IV Composite Resin

Placement

1. Class IV mesial view: examine (Figure 37.4, *A*).
2. Clean and dry the cavity preparation.
3. Prepare the etchant, bonding, and lining materials.
4. Mix the liner and place it in the cavity preparation (Figure 37.4, *B*).
5. Etch the enamel for 15 seconds.
6. Rinse off etchant for 20 seconds and dry the tooth slightly.
7. Apply bonding resin and cure for 20 seconds with VLC unit. Read manufacturers directions.
8. Place matrix strip and wedge.
9. Place composite resin by direct injection into the cavity or with a placement instrument in small increments and condense tightly (Figure 37.4, *C*).
10. Pull matrix strip to labial to form to cavosurface margin (Figure 37.4, *D*).
11. Continue to add small increments until overfilled.
12. Pull matrix strip tightly around tooth and hold securely while curing with the VLC unit (Figure 37.4, *E*).

Caution: Protect eyes with glasses or shield

Finishing

13. Examine the lingual and labial surfaces of the restoration.
14. Use the Bard-Parker scalpel to remove small increments of composite from the cavosurface margins.
15. Finish the lingual surface with the football-shaped finishing bur.
16. Finish the lingual cavosurface margins.
17. Finish the interproximal margins with flame-shaped finishing bur.
18. Finishing discs are used with a mandrel to smooth and finish the. incisal edge and distoincisal angle (Figure 37.5, *A*).
19. Finish the margins with finishing discs beginning with the coarse grit and finishing with the fine grit.
20. Use finishing strip to remove remaining flash and contour interproximal surface.
21. Examine the finished restoration by flossing the interproximal margins and contacts. Remove rubber dam and check protrusive movement and polish (Figure 37.5, *B*).

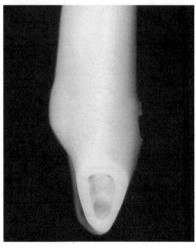
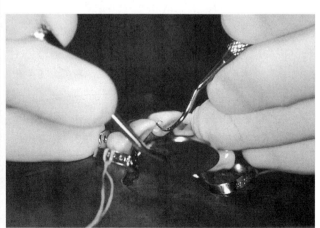

A   B

FIGURE 37-4

Placement. **A**, Class IV cavity preparation. **B**, Mix the liner and place it in the cavity preparation.

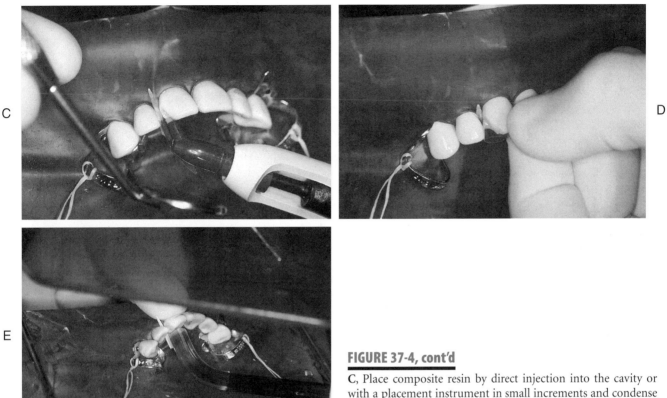

FIGURE 37-4, cont'd

C, Place composite resin by direct injection into the cavity or with a placement instrument in small increments and condense tightly. **D**, Pull matrix strip to labial to form to cavosurface margin. **E**, Pull matrix strip tightly around tooth and hold securely while curing with the VLC unit.

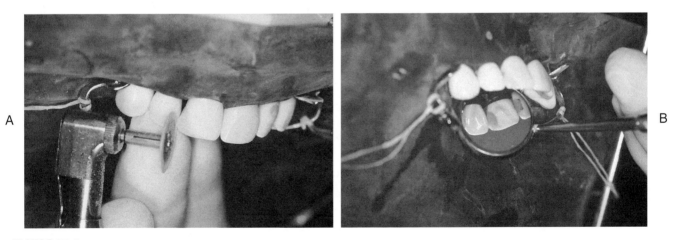

FIGURE 37-5

Finishing. **A**, Finishing discs are used with a mandrel to smooth and finish the incisal edge and distoincisal angle. **B**, Examine the finished restoration flossing the interproximal margins and contacts.

Table 37-2

Evaluation for a Class IV Composite Restoration

Class IV Composite Restoration	4	3	2	0	X
Lack of flash.					
Adaptation of margin.					
Surface smoothness.					
Placement of wedge.					
Contact replacement.					
Incisal edge replacement.					
Contour.					
Aesthetics.					
Pulp protection.					

The numeric criteria: 4 Excellent; 3 Good but some improvement can be made; 2 Below average, usable, needs to improve skill; 0 Unsatisfactory; X Not able to evaluate.

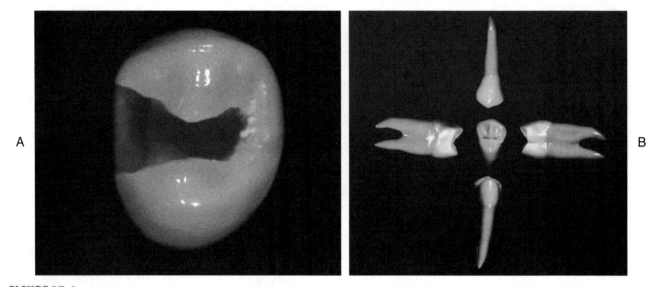

A   B

FIGURE 37-6

A, Class II posterior cavity preparation. **B,** Maxillary right permanent first premolar #5 anatomical surfaces. The center surface is occlusal. Clockwise starting at top: buccal, mesial, lingual, and distal.

ionomers have been considered technique sensitive and time consuming when compared with amalgam restorations.

Posterior composites are usually indicated for (1) Class V restorations, (2) Class VI restorations if the cusp tips are nonfunctional, (3) Class I restorations where there is minimal isthmus width (one third isthmus) and no heavy occlusal contact, (4) Class II restorations where there is also minimal isthmus width, minimal box depth, and no heavy occlusal contacts, and (5) veneers.

It is not recommended to use posterior composites (contraindications) when esthetics is not essential; patient oral hygiene is not good and particularly with composite acrylic resins: there is a high caries rate; there are heavy occlusal stress (molars) and wear facets on the teeth and bruxing; iso-

lation is poor; and subgingival areas make it difficult to properly isolate the teeth. See Figure 37.6, Box 37.3, and Table 37.3 to review anatomy and procedures for posterior composite resin restorations.

Veneer Restorations

Veneers can also be placed on the facial surface of a tooth to cover more severe problems such as stains, to close diastemas, repair fractures, and alter the contours of a tooth. Veneers are more resistant to stain than bonded or bleached teeth. Veneers are generally more expensive although they are more durable than bonding. Veneers can be direct, constructed in the mouth, or they can be constructed in a dental laboratory on models using composite resins or porcelain.

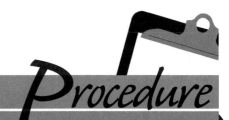

Box 37.3

Procedures for Posterior Composite Restorations

Placement

1. Select the shade.
2. Check the occlusion and place the rubber dam.
3. Prewedge and prepare the tooth (Figure 37.7, A).
4. Examine and clean the preparation.
5. Apply the liner and base.
6. Etch the cavity preparation, rinse and lightly dry (Figure 37.7, B).
7. Select a primer and bonding system (Figure 37.7, C).
8. Place the dentin adhesive.
9. Place the matrix and wedge and burnish the matrix to form a tight contact.
10. Select the composite system (some systems have the primer and bonding agent included).

11. Place the first increment of composite into the deepest area of the cavity preparation (Figure 37.7, D).
12. Continue to fill in increments until the cavity preparation is over filled.

Finishing

13. Begin contouring and finishing the restoration with a football-shaped finishing bur (Figure 37.8).
14. Contour the marginal ridges with a flame-shaped finishing bur.
15. Check the proximal contact with dental floss.
16. Final refining can be completed with the Bard-Parker scalpel.
17. Check the occlusion and make any necessary adjustments.
18. Reetch and seal the restoration.

Table 37.8

Evaluation for a Class III Posterior Composite Restoration

Class II Posterior Composite Restoration	4	3	2	0	X
Placement.					
Anatomy.					
Lack of flash.					
Adaptation of margin.					
Surface smoothness.					
Marginal ridge.					
Matrix and wedge.					
Contact replacement.					
Occlusion.					
Contour.					
Aesthetics.					
Pulp protection.					

The numeric criteria: 4 Excellent; 3 Good but some improvement can be made; 2 Below average, usable, needs to improve skill; 0 Unsatisfactory; X Not able to evaluate.

The operator must be able to reform the tooth's natural contour, shape, and surface smoothness to reflect the anatomy of adjacent teeth. However, it may be necessary to alter the appearance of individual teeth by closing a diastema, elongating, or shortening a tooth. The success of veneer treatment will be determined by good hygiene habits and refraining from biting on hard objects.

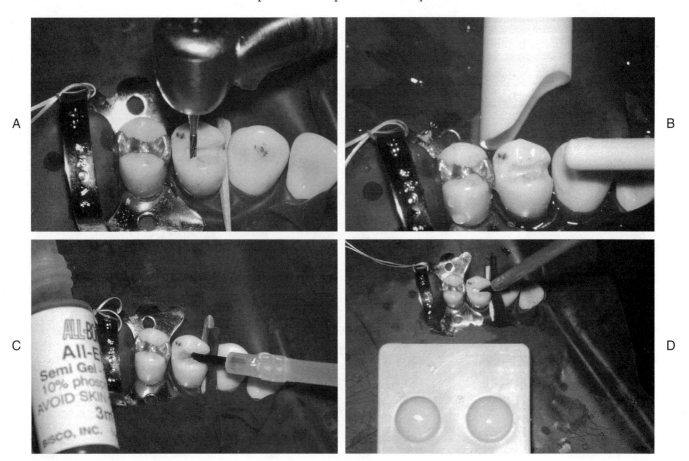

FIGURE 37-7

Placement. **A,** Prewedge and prepare the tooth. **B,** Etch the cavity preparation and rinse and lightly dry. **C,** Select a primer and bonding system. **D,** Place the first increment of composite into the deepest area of the cavity preparation angling the material over floor preceding up cavity wall. Continue to fill in increments until the cavity preparation is overfilled.

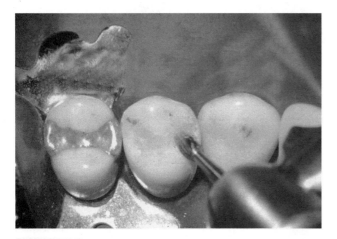

FIGURE 37-8

Begin contouring and finishing the restoration with a football-shaped finishing bur.

Procedures for Placement of Veneer Composites

Although the operator must have patience and skill, the **direct composite** acrylic resin veneer can eliminate time, laboratory costs, and provide greater operator control. Initial procedures include cleaning the involved teeth and selecting the appropriate shade. The dentist will decide on the amount of enamel to remove based on the amount and depth of stain or repair needed (Figure 37.9, *A*).

Direct composite

Placing and finishing the composite resin on the tooth.

Following the preparation of the tooth, the tooth is washed, dried, and etched for 15 to 30 seconds. After it is etched the operator will again wash and dry the tooth and apply a bonding agent. The bonding agent will be cured for 20 seconds. The composite resin is spread over the surface of the tooth with a stiff brush, a flat instrument, or by finger pressure. The resin is cured and additional resin is added as needed. The composite veneer is contoured with finishing burs, diamonds, and discs.

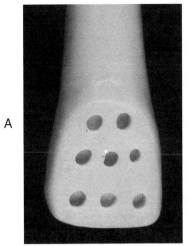

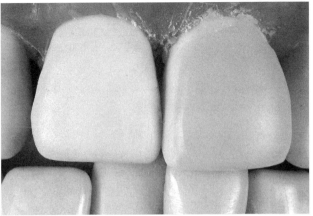

FIGURE 37-9

A, Tooth prepared for a veneer. **B**, Tooth restored with a veneer.

Following contouring of the veneer, it will be polished and the veneer will be recured (Figure 37.9, *B*).

CLINICAL APPLICATION FOR INDIRECT COMPOSITE ACRYLIC RESIN RESTORATIVE PROCEDURES

Indirect composites

Fabricating a composite resin restoration outside the mouth in a dental laboratory.

The public is becoming better informed about tooth-colored, esthetic restorations for posterior teeth. They are, therefore, increasingly demanding alternatives to traditional alloy restorations (Figure 37.10, *A*). Composite resin inlays and onlays are an esthetic direct or indirect restoration that is cemented into a cavity preparation. **Indirect composite** resin inlays and onlays are indicated for the restoration of posterior teeth when a carious lesion, defective restoration or tooth fracture is too involved for a direct composite resin but not enough for a crown. Their indications are similar to those for gold inlays and onlays with the addition of esthetics (Figure 37.10, *B*). Laboratory fabricated composite resin restorations give excellent esthetic and functional results and require only average technical skills by the operator.

Direct composite resins for posterior teeth exhibit several problems that are related to shrinkage from polymerization. The shrinkage results in gap formation, which causes marginal leakage, postoperative sensitivity and secondary caries. Wear resistance can be poor as a result of the voids in direct composite resins.

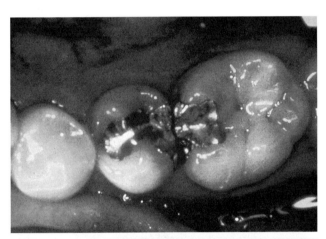

FIGURE 37-10

Clinical application for indirect composite restoration procedures using Concept. **A**, Teeth with alloy restoration. **B**, Teeth after placement of indirect composite restoration. (Courtesy Ivoclar.)

Advantages of Indirect Composite Resins

Indirect composite resins have several advantages over direct composite resins. The development of indirect composite resins allows the polymerization to occur outside of the mouth. The restoration is fabricated on a stone die or directly on the tooth, cured extraorally and then cemented into the cavity preparation with a composite cement. Because the polymerization shrinkage of the composite resin occurs outside of the mouth, the polymerization shrinkage that occurs is restricted to the luting cement. This shrinkage is insignificant. With good marginal adaptation of the restoration, the average marginal gap filled with luting cement is 50 to 100 microns. As a result, marginal leakage is improved and there is less postoperative sensitivity, marginal staining and secondary caries. Also, if the composite resin material is processed using heat and pressure, many of its physical properties are enhanced.

It should be noted in the chart that the patient was informed that this is an esthetic restoration with decreased longevity compared with full coverage or porcelain inlays and onlays. This composite resin material is more wear resistance, color stable and has increased diametrical tensile strength and compressive strength. Because it is fabricated outside of the mouth, there is more control over contour and contacts.

Fabrication of Indirect Composite Inlays

The following is a step by step guideline for the fabrication of an indirect inlay or onlays using Concept. Other indirect systems are similar and these steps can be easily modified to meet other techniques available (Boxes 37.4 and 37.5). Depending on state regulations, dental assistants may be able to perform many of the following procedures.

Box 37.4

First Appointment

1. Secure preoperative alginate impressions for both arches and a bite registration.
2. Anesthetize the patient.
3. Place rubber dam.
4. Prepare tooth.
   a. The principles of preparation are different from those of gold inlay or onlays preparations. It is a more conservative preparation and does not require the removal of undercuts. The chairside assistant can help maintain a clear field as the dentist removes any existing restoration and caries. The chairside assistant or advanced function personnel may assist with or complete the following procedures:
   b. Clean preparation and adjacent tooth using a prophy brush and a mixture of pumice and chlorhexidine.
   c. Place a noneugenol liner such as calcium hydroxide where the pulp may be compromised.
   d. Block out deep undercuts with a glass ionomer base.
   e. Cover remaining dentin with a chemically or light cured glass ionomer lining cement.
   f. Place a thin coat of dentin protector, which acts as a sealer, on the base and liner.
   g. Refinish the cavosurface margins with a high speed diamond to refine the preparation, smooth block out material and remove any dentin protector that may have been applied to the margins.
   h. Rinse and dry the tooth.
5. Remove rubber dam.
6. Check preparation for occlusal clearance (Figure 37.11).
7. Place retraction cord.
8. Secure final impression.
   a. A polyvinylsiloxane or polyether impression material can be used, allowing the laboratory to do three pours.

9. Select shade.
   a. Use shade guide. This step can be performed by the assistant and then checked by the doctor.
   b. If an error should occur, it should be toward the lighter side because the restoration can darken later with age and water absorption.
   c. Patient may desire stain in the pits and fissures for a more natural appearance.
10. Fabricate temporary.
    a. Suggestions for onlays are the use of either ion crowns or a stint and acrylic material using only a noneugenol cement to lute.
    b. It is recommended, for temporary inlays, to use a light cured semiflexible material that is easy to place and remove (for example, Fermit).
    c. Apply chlorhexidine beforehand to reduce sensitivity between appointments.
    d. Warn patient of the potential for sensitivity.
11. Send prescription and materials to laboratory.
    a. Prescription, in addition to routine information, should note shade selection, whether patient desires stain in pits and fissures and should request solid model contacts.
    b. Send the laboratory the following materials:
       Impression of prepared tooth
       Opposing cast
       Bite registration
12. Receive materials from laboratory.
    a. Check margins.
    b. Although they do not need to be as exact as with crowns, they should be close and accurate.
    c. Check if internal surface has been sandblasted by laboratory.

Box 37.5

Second Appointment

1. Anesthetize patient.
2. Remove provisional/temporary (Figure 37.12) and clean preparation with pumice.
3. Try in restoration.
   a. Place a piece of gauze in patients mouth for throat protection.
   b. Check color using water as a temporary adhesive.
   c. Check preliminary fit of restoration.
   d. Remove restoration.
4. Place retraction cord.
5. Place rubber dam.
6. Clean preparation.
   a. Use a prophy brush and a mixture of pumice and chlorhexidine.
7. Try in restoration.
   a. Check fit, margins and interproximal contacts.
   b. Pressure should not be applied when seating.
8. Clean preparation.
   a. Use a prophy brush and a mixture of pumice and chlorhexidine.
9. Place a clear matrix and wedge and retry restoration to check fit.
10. Prepare restoration.
    a. Etch the inside of the restoration with phosphoric acid for 1 to 2 minutes and rinse and dry restoration (Figure 37.13).
    b. Coat inside of restoration with a thin layer of a light cured methacrylate solvent-primer (for example, Special Bond II), which enhances bonding (Figure 37.14).
11. Etch preparation.
    a. Etch entire preparation and enamel with phosphoric acid for 30 to 60 seconds.
    b. Rinse and dry.
12. Apply primer and adhesive.
    a. Use a system with a primer and adhesive, for example, Syntac, Probond, All Bond.
13. Cement restoration.
    a. Use a dual cure cement, for example, Variolink, Enforce, Dual Cure.
    b. Cement should be applied to the internal surface of the restoration and into the preparation.
    c. Gentle but firm pressure should be used when seating the restoration (Figure 37.15).
    d. Hold the restoration with an occlusally placed blunt instrument while the excess cement is removed from the margins with a sable brush.
    e. While continuing to hold restoration in place, cure the center of the occlusal surface for 20 seconds.
    f. Cement is removed except for a small excess at the margins.
    g. The gingival embrasure can be cleaned using super-floss by sweeping once occlusogingivally below the gingival margins. Leave floss in place until the cement is completed by light curing.
    h. Stop removing cement when the chemical cure begins in order to avoid pulling cement from the margins and creating voids.
    i. Again, hold restoration in place with pressure with a blunt instrument and light cure one minute each from buccal, lingual, and occlusal.
    j. Let restoration stand 10 minutes.
14. Remove Mylar strip and wedge.
15. Remove remaining excess cement using the following instruments and materials:
    #12 scalpel blade to remove cement in gingival embrasure
    Finishing diamond or discs to remove cement from occlusal, facial and lingual embrasures
    Plastic finishing strips to smooth gingival margins.
16. Remove rubber dam and retraction cord.
17. Complete the occlusal adjustment of restoration.
    a. Use finishing burs.
18. Polish restoration.
    a. Smooth surface with pumice.
    b. Smooth with rubber points and cups.
    c. Final polish with resin polish paste or fine diamond paste.
19. Final check of margins and occlusion.
    a. Note: It is important that the dentist completes the final check and this is documented in the patients record.
20. Complete final cure of all surfaces.
    a. Light cure 1 minute each from buccal, lingual and occlusal.

Premolar inlay preparation guide, proximal view.

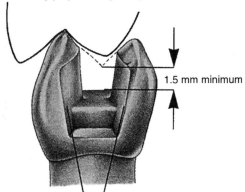

1.5 mm minimum

5°-15° divergence

FIGURE 37-11

Occlusal clearance must be approximately 1.5 mm minimum. (Courtesy Ivoclar.)

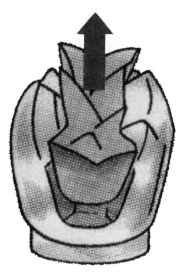

FIGURE 37-12

Remove provisional/temporary restoration. (Courtesy Ivoclar.)

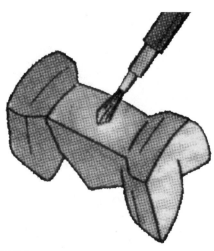

FIGURE 37-14

Coat inside of restoration with primer. (Courtesy Ivoclar.)

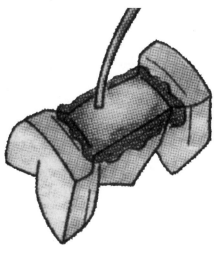

FIGURE 37-13

Etch the inside of the restoration with phosphoric acid for 1 to 2 minutes, rinse and dry. (Courtesy Ivoclar.)

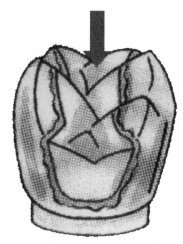

FIGURE 37-15

Cement restoration. (Courtesy Ivoclar.)

One of the many benefits of a composite restoration is the ease with which it can be repaired. The restoration and tooth are roughened and then etched for one minute. After rinsing and drying, primer and adhesive are applied, and the composite resin material is added, shaped and cured. Polishing is the same with any composite resin.

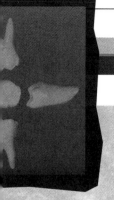

Points for Review

■ Clinical application for direct composite acrylic resin restorative procedures

■ Clinical application for composite restorations

■ Clinical application for indirect composite resin restorations

■ Clinical application for veneer restorations

Self-Study Questions

1. What are the indications for indirect composite resin restorations?
   a. Carious lesion in posterior teeth
   b. When a defective restoration is present
   c. When a tooth fracture is too involved for a direct composite but not enough for a crown
   d. All of the above
2. What are some of the advantages of indirect composite resins?
   a. Polymerization occurs inside the mouth
   b. Restoration can be fabricated on a die rather than the tooth
   c. Shrinkage does not occur
   d. Shrinkage is significant
3. What are some advantages of direct composite resins?
   a. Shrinkage does not occur when resin is cured inside the tooth
   b. Leakage does not occur
   c. Wear resistance is good
   d. Esthetic appearance

4. What is polymerization?
   a. Shrinkage
   b. Setting
   c. Luting
   d. Cementation
5. Shade selection should be which of the following?
   a. Darker
   b. Lighter
   c. Stained
   d. Both a and c

Suggested Readings

Ash MM: *Wheeler's dental anatomy, physiology, and occlusion*, ed 7, Philadelphia, 1993, WB Saunders.

Bowen RF, Marjenhoff WA: *Adhesion of composites to dentin and enamel*, 1993, C.D.A.J.

Council on Dental Materials, Instruments, and Equipment: Choosing intracoronal restorative materials, 1994, *Journal of the American Dental Association.*

Goldstein RE, Garber DA: *Complete dental bleaching*, 1995, Quintessence.

Sheets CG, Taniguchi T: Advantages and limitations in the use of porcelain veneer restorations, 1990, *Journal of Prosthetic Dentistry.*

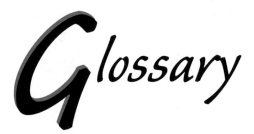

Glossary

ALARA Principle: The philosophy that radiation exposure to the patient must be as low as reasonably achievable.

Abscess: A local accumulation of pus, usually from a bacterial infection.

Abutment Teeth: The natural teeth that are prepared to support the partial denture.

Accreditation: The granting of approval by an official review board to an educational institution for meeting specific program or institutional requirements.

Activator or Catalyst: A chemical that reacts with a chemical initiator to start a reaction.

Acute: A disease or condition that begins abruptly with marked intensity and then subsides after a relatively brief period.

Adequate Diet: An eating pattern that includes a variety of foods and provides all nutrients essential for good health.

Adherent: The materials on which the adhesive is placed.

Adjustments: A modification or change on a bill.

Adverse Conditioning: A negative reinforcement method used to stop an undesirable behavior.

Aesthetics: The philosophy or principle pertaining to beauty.

Allergy: A hypersensitivity to immunogenic substances.

Allied Dental Personnel: The staff associated with the practice of dentistry, for example, dental assistant, dental hygienist, and dental laboratory technician.

Alloys: A mixture of two or more metals.

Alternative Dental Care Delivery Systems: Various choices or options for paying for dental care.

Alveoloplasty: Surgical preparation, shaping, and smoothing of socket margins and alveolar ridges after extraction of teeth; it is done to ensure optimal healing for the placement of dentures.

Analgesia: A reduction in pain without producing unconsciousness.

Anaphylaxis: A violent allergic reaction characterized by sudden collapse, shock, or respiratory and circulatory failure following the introduction of an allergen usually by injection or inhalation.

Anatomy: The study of the body and its parts.

Anesthesia: Total or partial loss of physical sensation.

Angulation: Moving the tooth root backward or forward to correct the tooth angle.

Antagonism: When the action of drugs together produces an undesirable effect.

Antibiotic: Drug to kill or inhibit the growth of bacteria.

Antigen: A foreign substance capable of inducing an immunologic response.

Antiinflammatory: Drugs that reduce inflammation.

Antipyretics: Agents that reduce fever.

Antiseptics: A chemical compound that inhibits bacterial growth and can be used on the surface of living tissue.

Aphthae: Canker sores.

Apicoectomy: Surgical removal of the apex of a tooth.

Appliance: A mechanical device for changing tooth position.

Apposition: The process by which the enamel and dentin matrices begin to receive deposits of calcium salts.

Apprenticeship: A specified term of study under the direct supervision of a professional practitioner.

Articulate: In orthodontics, to place teeth in their proper "bite" position for esthetic and functional purposes.

Aseptic: Free of viable microorganisms.

Aspiration: Ingestion of a foreign body into the airway tree; also, negative pressure in a hypodermic syringe.

Attachment Apparatus: The portion of the periodontium that connects the tooth to the bone (that is, the cementum, the periodontal ligament, and the alveolar bone).

Attenuation: The reduction of the energy of a beam of radiation as it passes through tissue or structures.

Autoclave: Chamber containing saturated steam generally at 121° C used for sterilization.

Autonomy: The ethical principle of respect for the individual and of the individual's right to pursue life, liberty, and welfare, as long as such decisions and actions do not adversely affect the life or welfare of others.

Axial Skeleton: The portion of the skeleton composed of the vertebral column, thorax, and skull.

Axial Wall: Surface within the cavity preparation parallel to the long axis of the tooth and named for the aspect where it is located.

Back Order: An unfilled order that will be available at a later date.

Bactericide: An agent that kills bacteria.

Bacteriostatic: An agent that inhibits bacterial growth.

Balanced Diet: An eating regimen that incorporates meals consisting of foods from several of the food groups at each meal.

Base: The main ingredient of a material or a type of cement placed on the pulpal floor of a cavity prep to form a base or bulk of material.

Baseplate (Record Base): A temporary denture base used to support the record rim material when determining the maxillomandibular relationships.

Basic Life Support: Artificial support of vital life processes; includes the ABCs: airway opening, breathing, and circulation of the blood.

Benefits: Entitlements or advantages that enhance the well-being of an employee and that are part of an employment agreement.

Bevel: The angle or slope of the sharp or working ends of a dental cutting instrument.

Biopsy: The removal of living tissues or cells for microscopic examination.

Bisecting Angle: The concept of directing the central x-ray perpendicular to the line that equally divides the angle formed by the image receptor and the long axis of the tooth.

Bruxism: The grinding of teeth while sleeping.

Buffer: An ingredient that neutralizes acid.

CD-ROM: Compact disk-read only memory. The disk resembles an audio CD and stores large amounts of data.

Calculus: Plaque that has mineralized (hardened) from calcium salts in the saliva.

Calories: A measure of energy in foods. They are obtained from the protein, carbohydrate, and fat in the diet.

Carcinogenic: Refers to cancer-causing substances.

Cardiopulmonary Resuscitation (CPR): Artificial ventilation of the lungs and pumping of the heart.

Career: A chosen occupation and pursuit in professional advancement.

Cassettes: Specially designed set-up tray used for organizing instruments and accessories for dental procedures and sterilization.

Casting: In dentistry, to form into a given shape; the result is a cast restoration, such as a gold crown or bridge.

Cavosurface Margin: The angle or junction where the walls of the preparation join the tooth surface.

Centric Occlusion: Occlusion of the opposing teeth when the mandible is in centric relation.

Centric Relation: The maxillomandibular relationship in which the condyles articulate with the disks when the articular complex is in its most anterorsuperior position against the articular eminence.

Cephalometrics: The science of measuring the cranial bones in the head.

Certification: A credential assuring that a person has met a level of competency required for particular functions.

Certified Dental Assistant (CDA): A credentialing title awarded to a dental assistant who has passed the examination given by the Dental Assisting National Board (DANB) and has maintained 12 hours of continuing education requirements yearly.

Chemotherapy: The treatment of disease with chemical agents.

Cholesterol: A fat-soluble substance that is manufactured only by animals, including humans, and therefore only present in animal-source foods.

Chronic: A disease or condition that develops gradually and persists for a long period.

Clamp: A devise used to secure the rubber dam material.

Collimation: The reduction of the dimension of a beam of radiation. The dimensions produced with rectangular collimation are $1\frac{1}{2}$ inches by 2 inches. Round collimation produces a circle 2.75 inches in diameter.

Complete Denture: A removable dental prosthesis that replaces the entire dentition and associated structures of the maxilla or mandible.

Composite: An acrylic resin restorative material that provides a lifelike, esthetic appearance.

Condense: To make more compact or solid.

Conical: A cone shape.

Consent: Permission given to someone to do something.

Contract: A voluntary agreement between two or more competent people involving the exchange of a specified service or product in return for a specific compensation (usually money).

Contraction: A shortening or reduction in size of an object.

Contraindications: An opposite or contrasting view.

Contrast: The difference in densities as visualized on a radiograph. High-contrast (short scale) images are produced using low kVp techniques (60 to 70 kVp). Low-contrast (long scale) images are produced using high kVp techniques (90 to 120 kVp).

Coronal Polishing: A cleansing and polishing of the coronal surfaces of the teeth by the use of motor-driven rubber cups, bristle brushes, and paste.

Corrosion: Chemical attack on a material causing deterioration.

Culture: The growth of living cells on an artificial media.

Curettage: A surgical procedure in which the infected portion of the gingival tissue lining, the sulcus, is removed.

Cylindrical: A cylinder or tube shape.

Cyst: An epithelial-lined, fluid-filled cavity.

Debridement: The removal of pulpal tissue and debris from the pulp canal of a tooth.

Deductible: The amount that the insured must pay.

Deferred Payment Plan: Payment plan for dental services in place of fee for service.

Deglutition: The act of swallowing.

Demineralization: A breakdown of the tooth structure with a loss of mineral content.

Denaturation: A process in which proteins lose their configuration and biologic activity.

Density: The overall darkness of a processed radiograph. Density is affected by kVp, mA, exposure time, TFD, and processing.

Dental Assistant (DA): A general term that refers to the chairside assistant, office assistant, office manager, laboratory assistant, expanded duty assistant, and specialty assistant, such as an orthodontic assistant or oral surgery assistant.

Dental Auxiliaries (DAUX): Dental assistants, hygienists, and laboratory technicians. The current term used is *allied dental personnel*.

Dental Auxiliary Utilization (DAU): The performance of dental procedures with the aid of allied dental personnel according to the accepted principles of practice, which have been determined through research.

Dental Caries: A bacterial disease of the teeth involving decay, disintegration, and destruction of the structure.

Dental Implant: A prosthetic device of alloplastic material implanted into the oral tissues beneath the mucosa and periosteal layer and within the bone to provide retention and support for a fixed or removable prosthesis.

Dental Prophylaxis: A professional cleaning (scaling and polishing) of the teeth, consisting of complete mechanical removal of all hard and soft deposits.

Dentistry: The healing art and science of treating dental diseases and replacing the teeth and supporting structures of the oral cavity.

Depressants: Drug used to reduce anxiety.

Detergents: Synthetic cleansing agents with soap characteristics.

Dew Point: The point of coolness at which moisture will form.

Diagnosis: An evaluation of existing conditions.

Diastema: A space between teeth.

Diastolic: The lowest pressure exerted against the arterial walls; the heart is at rest.

Die: A form used to fabricate a crown or bridge restoration.

Diet: The pattern or regimen of food intake.

Digestion: The breaking down of ingested food into particles small enough to be absorbed into the blood.

Dimension: The extent or size of an object or situation that is measurable.

Direct Composite: Placing and finishing the composite resin on the tooth.

Disbursements: An expenditure or payment.

Discount: A reduction in the cost, quantity, or value of products.

Discrimination: Acting on the basis of prejudice.

Disease: A condition of the body that displays a characteristic pathology.

Disinfectant: A substance that destroys vegetative state microbial pathogens.

Disk Operating System: Operating system software that functions as a supervisor of a computer and is essential before any application software can run on a computer. The disk operating system is the program first loaded into a computer at boot-up and controls other applications programs used. It also controls the printer, monitor, disk drives, and other equipment attached to the computer.

Drug Interaction: When two or more drugs, given concurrently, produce an altered pharmacologic response.

Dysgeusia: Change in the sense of taste.

Dyspnea: Difficulty breathing.

Edema: Swelling, usually caused by accumulation of fluid in the tissues.

Edentulous: Without teeth; loss of all of the natural teeth.

Eligibility: The act of being qualified.

Emergency Protocol: Preplanned roles and behaviors to be followed by those responding to a medical emergency.

Empty Habit: A habit that has no detectable cause and can be discontinued without psychologic trauma.

Endodontics: The branch of dentistry concerned with treatment of the pulp and surrounding periapical tissues.

Endosteal Dental Implant: Implant placed directly into the alveolar and basal bone of the maxilla or mandible, transacting only one cortical plate. Endosteal means "into the bone."

Etchant: An acid based material applied to the cavity for abrasion purposes.

Ethics: The branch of philosophy that encompasses moral conduct (right and wrong behavior), good and evil, duty, and judgment.

Etiology: The study of the cause or origin of a disease.

Evaluation: A process used to review past efforts to achieve goals and objectives.

Exodontia: Refers to the extraction of teeth.

Exothermic: Any reaction that produces heat.

Expanded Duty Dental Assistant (EDDA): A credential given to a dental assistant who has had additional training and therefore is allowed to perform certain intraoral procedures previously performed only by the dentist.

Expansion: An increase in the dimensions of an object.

Fabrication: Construction or molding of a prosthesis.

Facing: A veneer of any restorative material used on a prosthesis to simulate a natural tooth.

Fat: Several compounds that are insoluble in water but soluble in fat solvents such as ether and chloroform.

Filtration: The selective removal of lower energy photons from a beam of radiation. Aluminum is the material most commonly used as a filter in dental radiography.

Fixed Partial Denture: This type of denture is luted or securely retained to natural teeth, tooth roots, or dental implant abutments and is also called a bridge.

Flash: Dental amalgam or composite acrylic resin that has been undercarved leaving an extension of material over the cavosurface margins, which must be removed.

Flora: Organisms that reside in a particular area.

Fluoridation: The addition of fluoride to the public water supply as a public health measure aimed at reducing dental caries.

Fluorosis: An excessive intake of fluoride during the development and mineralization of the teeth, resulting in small white spots or severe brown staining with pitting of the tooth enamel.

Four-Handed Dentistry: Procedures practiced while the dentist and dental assistant work together.

Free-Way Space (Interarch Distance): The distance between the occluding surfaces of the maxillary and mandibular teeth when the mandible is in a specified position.

Frenectomy: The surgical removal of the frenum (median fold of mucous membrane connecting the inside of each lip to the gingivae tissue).

Fungicide: An agent capable of destroying fungi.

Germicide: An agent that destroys pathogenic microorganisms.

Gigabyte: A measure of capacity for disk drive storage.

Gingivectomy: A surgical procedure in which a portion of the gingival tissues is excised, or removed.

Gingivitis: A reversible, preventable inflammation of the gingiva, caused primarily by dental plaque.

Goals: General statements that translate the mission statement or philosophy of an institution into an attainable objective.

Granulocytopenia: Lack of neutrophils in the blood.

Hand-Over-Mouth-Exercise (HOME): A physical restraint used by dentists with small children to gain attention and protect the child during a temper tantrum.

Hardware: Computer equipment such as the monitor, keyboard, printer, or light pen.

Health: A state of complete physical, mental, and social wellbeing, not merely the absence of disease or infirmity.

Heimlich Maneuver: An emergency maneuver performed to expel a foreign body from the airway; a quick thrust is used to squeeze the upper abdomen and force residual air from the lungs, ejecting the object.

Hemorrhage: Flow of blood caused by trauma.

Hereditary: The genetic characteristics associated with parents and offspring.

Hierarchy: A system of arranging people or things in order of rank or importance; for example, from basic concepts to complex situations.

Hone: To sharpen or smooth a cutting edge.

Hormone: A chemical substance formed in one part of the body and transferred through the blood to affect another part of the body.

Hypersensitivity: A reaction or altered response of an individual to a drug.

Hypertension: An abnormal elevation of the blood pressure.

Immediate Denture: A complete denture or a removable partial denture fabricated for placement immediately after removal of the natural teeth.

Immunosuppression: The destruction or impairment of the immune response caused by chemotherapy or radiation therapy.

Impingement: To encroach or push against.

Implant: A prosthetic device implanted into the oral tissues beneath mucosa and periosteal layer and within bone to provide retention and support for a fixed or removable prosthesis.

Implant Abutment: The portion of a dental implant that serves to support and retain any prosthesis.

Implant Prosthodontics: The phase of prosthodontics concerning the replacement of missing teeth or associated structures by restorations that are attached to dental implants.

Implant Surgery: The phase of implant dentistry concerning the selection, planning, and placement of the implant body and abutment. Most implant systems in use today use a two-stage implant where the implant body is first surgically placed (Stage I) and covered by the oral tissues until healing is complete. Then it is uncovered with a second surgery (Stage II) to attach the abutment.

Implied Consent: Nonverbal and nonwritten consent given by one person to another by external actions and behavior. For example, a person who comes to the dentist for a checkup gives the dentist implied consent to conduct a standard dental examination.

Impression Coping: The component of a dental implant system that is used to provide a spatial relationship of an endosteal dental implant to the alveolar ridge and adjacent dentition or other structures. Impression copings can be retained in the impression or may require a transfer from intraoral usage to the impression after attaching the analog or replicas.

Increments: Small additions that increase the amount.

Indemnity Programs: A table of allowance or the set fees provided for specific treatment.

Indications: Signs or action signifying a symptom or action.

Indirect Composites: Fabricating a composite resin restoration outside the mouth in a dental laboratory.

Infectious: Capable of transmitting organisms that cause disease.

Inflammation: The protective response of the body's tissues to irritation or injury.

Informed Consent: Expressed consent, always at least verbal and usually written, that is freely given and based on a reasonable presentation and understanding of the facts.

Initiation: The first stage of tooth development often called the bud stage.

Initiator: Source of energy (chemical, light, heat) that starts a reaction.

Inlay: An overlay or thin layer of acrylic resin or ceramic used to cover the labial surface of a tooth.

Insured: The patient or person covered by the plan benefits.

Insurer: The administering agent who provides the prepayment coverage.

Interaction: The activity or behavior that takes place between people or things.

Intermediate Denture: A complete denture or removable partial denture fabricated for placement immediately following the removal of natural teeth.

Intermittent: Stopping and starting at intervals.

Internet: A massive integrated network of computer connections throughout the world that permits electronic communications with a PC.

Interproximal Space: The area or space between the teeth.

Interseptal Rubber Dam: The part of the rubber dam material that is positioned between the teeth.

Interview: A conversation between and employer and a potential employee for the purpose of assessing the qualification of a person for a job.

Inventory: A detailed list of all equipment and dental materials in stock.

Invert: To turn under the rubber dam material around the neck of the tooth to prevent moisture leakage.

Invoice: The detailed list of goods shipped or services provided and an accounting of all costs.

Isometry: Theory used in bisecting techniques recognizing that two triangles having equal angles and a common side are equal triangles.

Justice: The principle of fairness in the distribution of goods and deprivations and treating people fairly and equitably,

Land Area: The portion of a dental cast that extends beyond the impression's replica surface laterally; it defines the area between the end of the replica's surface and the cast.

Laser: The handpiece that converts electromagnetic radiation to frequencies of highly amplified and coherent visible radiation to cut hard and soft tissues.

Lateral or Distal: The portion of the body that is toward the side.

Leadership: A process of guiding office personnel to accomplish tasks. Leadership requires effective communication, instruction and motivation skills.

Liability: A legal obligation and responsibility.

Licensure: The legal document provided by a state law assuring that the practitioner is qualified to practice.

Ligate: To secure the rubber dam material with a small piece of the material itself, a double strand of dental floss, a wedge, or an anchor ring.

Line Angles: The junctions where two surfaces meet.

Liner: A material used to line or seal a cavity preparation to protect the pulp.

Long Axis: Horizontal or line measured from the crown of the tooth to the root tip.

Luxation: The dislocation or displacement of the condyle in the temporomandibular fossa or a tooth from the alveolus.

Malignant: Cancerous.

Malocclusion: Poor positioning of the teeth so that they do not meet correctly, interfering with efficiency.

Malpractice: Any professional misconduct or any unreasonable lack of skill, care, or judgment in the performance of professional duties. The word means "bad practice."

Matrix: The phase or part of a material that surrounds another phase to bind the material together.

Matrix Band: A band placed around the tooth to restore the form of the missing tooth structure or wall.

Matrix Retainer: A device that holds the matrix band in place around the tooth.

Maxillofacial: Pertaining to the jaws and face, particularly with reference to specialized surgery in this region.

Maxillofacial Prosthetics: The use of artificial materials to replace parts of the body, such as the eyes, ears, and nose, lost to surgical defects, trauma, or congenital defects.

Medial or Mesial: The portion of the body that is toward the midline.

Medicaments: Medical substances or agents.

Midline: The imaginary line that divides the right and left sides of the body.

Minerals: Certain inorganic elements essential in human nutrition.

Mobility: The degree of movement of the tooth within the socket, expressed by a number rating (0, 1, 2, 3) designating no mobility to extreme mobility.

Model: A replica of the mouth, usually in plaster or stone.

Motion Economy: Involves minimizing body motions to accomplish tasks.

Motivation: The ability to incite or impel oneself or others to action.

Mucositis: An oral inflammation.

Necrosis: The morphologic change indicating cell death caused by infection.

Negligence: An unintentional tort (wrongful conduct not involving a contract).

Nutrients: A substance required by the body for health and function and categorized into proteins, carbohydrates, fats, vitamins, minerals, and water.

Objective Fears: Fears caused by an actual experience or similar event.

Objectives: Further defines the goals by making them specific, measurable, and timely.

Obstruction: An object that blocks, impedes, or interferes with passage.

Obturator: A device used to restore the continuity of the hard or soft palate or both.

Occlude: To close or bring the teeth together.

Occlusion Rim (Record Rim): The occlusal surfaces fabricated on a baseplate (record base) to record the maxillomandibular relationship or to arrange teeth.

Olfaction: Examination using the sense of smell.

Onlay: A cast restoration that fits largely within the tooth and extends over the cusps; it replaces all or part of the occlusal surface.

On-the-Job Training: A type of informal training that takes place in the workplace rather than through an academic educational program of study.

Operating System: Operating system software that functions as a supervisor of a computer and is essential before any application sotfware can run on a computer. The disk operating system is the program first loaded into a computer at boot-up and controls other applications programs that are used. It also controls the printer, monitor, disk drives, and other equipment attached to a computer.

Operative: Refers to a dental procedure.

Operator: The individual who performs dental procedures directly on the patient. Depending on the procedure, this may be the dentist, expanded-function dental assistant, dental assistant, or dental hygienist.

Oral Assessment: An examination of the oral cavity for the purpose of detecting and diagnosing pathologic lesions

Organizing: A process to identify resources necessary to implement a plan, such as how business will achieve goals and objectives.

Orthodontics: The specialty of dentistry that deals with the causes, prevention, and correction of irregularities or malocclusion of the teeth and jaws.

Osseointegration: The process and resultant direct connection of the surface of an exogenous material and the host bone tissues, without intervening fibrous connective tissue present.

Osteoplasty: The surgical reshaping of bone.

Osteoradionecrosis (ORN): An infection, or necrosis, of the bones.

Osteotomy: The cutting of bone, usually by means of a saw or chisel.

Overcarved: Too much amalgam has been removed.

Overcontoured: Contour extends beyond the normal.

Overhang: Marginal overextension, additional material left at the gingival cavosurface margin caused from the matrix band not being wedged properly and from undercarving.

Oxidation: Loss of electrons by an atom or compound.

Palatal Augmentation (Drop) Prosthesis: A prosthesis that allows the hard or soft palate, or both, to be reshaped.

Palatal Lift Prosthesis: A prosthesis that helps in velopharyngeal closure by elevating an incompetent soft palate.

Palpation: Examination using the sense of touch.

Panoramic Radiograph: An x-ray that shows the entire dentition on a single film.

Parallel: Side by side or an equal distance apart.

Paternalism: Authorized decisions or actions on behalf of another person.

Pathogens: Organisms capable of causing disease in a host.

Percussion: Examination by striking an area and evaluating the sounds and sensations.

Pericoronitis: Inflammation and infection of the gingival tissue surrounding the crown of an erupting tooth.

Periodontal Diagnosis: The determination of the type of periodontal disease present, including its extent, distribution, and severity.

Periodontal Disease: The various diseases that affect the periodontium, especially gingivitis and periodontitis.

Periodontal Ligament: The connective tissue fibers that surround the root of the tooth and attach it to the alveolar process.

Periodontics: The branch of dentistry concerned with the cause, treatment, and prevention of periodontal disease.

Periodontitis: Inflammation of the periodontium that involves alveolar bone loss and deepening of the gingival sulcus (pocket).

Periodontium: The tissues that surround and support the tooth and anchor it to the bone.

Peripheral Nervous System: All nerves of the body.

Perpendicular: A line or plane at right angles or vertical to a given horizontal position.

Personnel: The dental assistant, dental hygienist, laboratory technician, or other employees.

Photon: A weightless packet of pure energy.

Physiology: How the body functions.

Plane of Occlusion: The surface of wax occlusion rim, which is contoured to guide the arrangement of denture teeth.

Planning: A process to formulate a program to accomplish specific goals or objectives, such as what the dental practice wants to accomplish.

Plaque: A collection of organized bacteria growing in a deposit of soft material on the surface of a tooth.

Point Angles: The junctions where three surfaces meet.

Policies: A course of action, guiding principle, or procedure designed to influence and determine decisions and actions.

Pontic: The artificial replacement for a missing tooth; pontics maintain space, stabilize the arch, and aid in proper occlusion.

Posterior Palatal Seal: The seal area at the posterior border of a maxillary prosthesis.

Premium: The charge paid for service or treatment.

Preventive Dentistry: Procedures in the practice of dentistry and community health programs that prevent the occurrence of oral diseases and abnormalities.

Primary (Deciduous): Children's teeth.

Primary Prevention: The application of preventive measures prior to the onset of disease.

Probation: The trial period during which one has to prove the ability to carry out the responsibilities of the job.

Procedures: A set of established forms or methods for administering the affairs of a business.

Prognosis: A prediction of the duration and course of a disease and the likelihood of its response to treatment.

Prophylaxis: Active protection against disease.

Prosthodontics: A special branch of dentistry that maintains oral function, comfort, appearance, and health by restoring natural teeth or replacing missing teeth and oral and maxillofacial tissue with artificial substitutes.

Provisional: A temporary restoration.

Proximal: The area or tooth next to a given point of reference.

Pulp Capping: Treatment of exposed pulp to maintain tooth vitality.

Pulpalgia: The clinical symptoms of pulpal pain.

Pulpectomy: Surgical removal of the complete pulp from the pulp chamber.

Pulpitis: Infection of the pulp that causes pulpal pain.

Pulpotomy: Surgical removal of the coronal pulp tissue only because of exposure of the pulp.

RDA: Recommended dietary allowances of the levels of nutrient intake based on age, sex, and activity of U.S. population.

Radiation: The transmission of energy by waves through space.

Radiation Caries: Decay, mostly at the cervical margins, caused by the loss of minerals that results from radiation therapy.

Radiation Therapy (Radiotherapy): The treatment of disease by ionizing radiation.

Radiograph: The visual image produced by exposing and processing radiographic film.

Radiography: The making of radiographs (electronic images) by passing radiation through an object of interest and capturing the resultant energy on an image receptor.

Radiology: The branch of health sciences that deals with the diagnostic and therapeutic uses of radiation.

Radiolucent: Permeable to radiation; luminous.

Radiopaque: Not allowing penetration of radiation.

Recall: A periodic patient appointment scheduled after initial treatment for preventative measures.

Receipt: A slip given to the patient when a payment is received for services.

Reciprocity: The granting of a license by credentials only, without the dentist having to take the usual examination.

Reconcile: Comparing office records with bank statements to affirm they are consistent.

Recontouring: To shape again.

Reference: A person who is in the position to recommend another person for a job.

Regeneration: The formation of new tissue to replace lost tissue.

Registered Dental Assistant (RDA): The dental assistant has fulfilled a state education or examination requirement to perform specific delegated advanced functions.

Registered Dental Assistant-American Medical Technologist (RDA-AMT): A credentialing title awarded to a dental assistant who has passed the examination given by the American Medical Technologist Examining Board (AMT) and has maintained 12 hours of continuing education requirements yearly.

Registration: A record of people who are licensed to perform specific functions.

Regulations: Criteria described in laws outlining what a practitioner can do under that act or statute.

Remineralization: A restoring of the lost mineral content of the tooth following demineralization, enhanced by the presence of fluoride.

Removable Partial Denture: A prosthesis that replaces one or more teeth in a partially dentate arch and is removable from the mouth.

Reorder Point: The point at which a dental item needs to be reordered to maintain a certain level of supplies.

Requisition: A formal written request for something needed.

Resection Prosthesis: A prosthesis that replaces the missing part of the mandible and associated teeth.

Resolution: The ability to discern two objects that are very close together.

Resorption: The loss of osseous (bone) tissue that occurs with periodontitis.

Resumé: A record of one's personal history and experiences provided for job application.

Retainer: A device used to preserve space in the dentition or to stabilize a bridge in the dental arch.

Retarder: A chemical that slows the rate of a reaction.

Retention: A groove or undercut made in a cavity preparation to help hold the restoration and prevent it from moving.

Retract: To draw or pull back as in holding back the cheek, lip, tongue or intraoral tissues as part of a dental procedure.

Retraction: The technique of withdrawing gingival tissue from around the tooth and holding it out of the way.

Retroprep: Preparations located on the apex of the tooth.

Root Planing: A procedure for smoothing roughened root surfaces that is performed after the scaling procedure.

Rotary Instruments: Power-driven instruments, often called dental drills, which are used to cut hard and soft oral tissue and other materials.

Rotate: The movement of a tooth in a circular direction.

Rubber Dam: A material used in the patient's mouth for protection, to ensure access and visibility in the operating field, and for efficient use of operating time.

Sanitize: To reduce the number of bacteria to a nonhazardous level.

Scaling: The removal of calculus from the tooth with various mechanical and hand instruments.

Schedule of Benefits: The type of service, benefits, and innetwork and out-of-network coverage.

Sealants: A plastic material (polymer) that bonds to the enamel tooth surface through mechanical locking, creating an effective barrier that prevents occlusal caries.

Sealer: A material used to seal the dentinal tubules to protect the pulp.

Secondary (Permanent): Adult teeth.

Sedative: A drug that causes a calming or unaroused effect.

Sedative or Obtundent: A medicated material that has soothing properties and decreases sensitivity.

Shade Selection: The determination of the color or shade to be used to restore a tooth using composite resin material.

Sit-Down Dentistry: Procedures provided by operators and chair-side assistants while sitting down in a zone.

Software: Generic term to describe the program instructions given to the computer. Software can be either (1) operating system software such as the disk operating system (DOS) or (2) application software such as word processing, database, electronic spreadsheet, graphics, or telecommunications.

Soluable: Being able to dissolve.

Solution: A single phase containing more than one component (for example, sugar dissolved in water).

Speech Aid (Bulb) Prosthesis: A prosthesis that restores a congenital defect of the soft palate.

Sphygmomanometer: A blood pressure cuff, used to indirectly measure the systolic and diastolic blood pressure.

State Dental Practice Acts: Statues that define the law and regulations that describe how the law is carried out. Each state regulates the dental procedures that can or cannot be delegated to allied dental personnel and any continuing education requirements essential for continued practice, licensure, or certification.

Statement: A letter or form providing the patient with a description of services, payments, and the balance owed on the accounts.

Statutes: The laws that give authority or licensure for individuals to practice in a profession.

Statutory Law: Law that is written and imposed by the legislature of various sovereign (lawful) governments.

Sterilization: The process that eliminates all living microorganisms.

Stethoscope: Medical device used to listen to various body sounds. Used with a sphygmomanometer to "hear" systolic and diastolic blood pressure sounds.

Storage Guidelines: The proper methods followed when storing and dispensing supplies.

Subjective Fears: Imagined fears that are not real.

Submarginal: A ditch caused from overcarving or incomplete condensing at the cavosurface margin, which must be corrected.

Subperiosteal Dental Implant: An eposteal (on top of the bone) dental implant that is placed beneath the periosteum and overlying the bony cortex.

Sugar: Carbohydrates classified as either monosaccharides or disaccharides, all having a sweet taste and being cariogenic.

Supernumerary: More than the normal number of teeth in the dental dentition.

Supplies: Equipment, instruments, and clinical, laboratory, and office materials needed to operate the dental practice.

Surgical Template: Guide used to assist in proper surgical placement and angulation of dental implants.

Systolic: The maximum pressure exerted against the arteries as the heart is working to pump blood through the constricted artery.

Tactile: The sense of touch.

Template: The plastic form used to mark the maxillary and mandibular dental arches on the rubber dam material.

Thermolable: Sensitive to heat.

Third-Party Coverage: The carrier or insurer.

Tincture: An alcoholic solution of a particular substance, such as tincture of iodine.

Tomography: Making an x-ray of a given plane by blurring out the images of other planes.

Tort: Wrongful conduct that violates common law but does not involve a contract. In law, the person who commits a tort is responsible to compensate the victim of the tort with damages to "make the victim whole."

Translation: The movement of a tooth forward or backward without tipping or rotating.

Transosteal Implant: A dental implant that penetrates both cortical plates and passes through the full thickness of the alveolar bone of the mandible. The term transosteal means "through the bone."

Treatise: A study or outcome of scientific investigation.

Trigeminal Nerve: The primary nerve of the oral cavity.

Trismus: Difficulty opening the mouth.

Trituration: Process of mixing the mercury and amalgam alloy into a homogenous mass.

USRDA: U.S. recommended daily allowances. A guide developed by the food and drug administration (FDA) for use in nutrition labeling of foods. Also called *daily value.*

Ulcerations: A break in the skin or mucous membranes.

Undercarved: Not enough amalgam has been removed.

Undercontoured: Contour does not extend far enough.

Varicose Vein: A dilated, tortuous vein that appears swollen and blue.

Vasodilator: Drug used to cause blood vessels to expand.

Vendor: The manufacturer's sales representative who sells dental products

Veneer: An overlay or thin layer of acrylic resin or ceramic used to cover the labial surface of a tooth.

Vertical Dimension at Rest: The postural position between the maxilla and the mandible in which the musculature is in a state of rest.

Vertical Dimension of Occlusion: The distance measured between two points when the occluding members are in contact.

Virulence: The relative ability of an organism to cause disease.

Vital Signs: Indicators of the state of the body's basic functions: pulse rate, respiratory rate, temperature, and blood pressure.

Vitalometer: An instrument used to measure the vitality of a tooth.

Vitamins: A class of nutrients that are essential components of the body's enzyme systems, usually required by the body in small amounts and present in minute quantities in foods.

Wedge: A wedge-shaped piece of wood or plastic that helps adapt the matrix band to the cervical position of the tooth structure; it also helps separate the teeth slightly, allowing for a tight margin.

Work Simplification: The process of simplifying and standardizing all dental tasks.

X-Radiation: A type of electromagnetic radiation that moves in divergent straight lines from the source at the speed of light, with a wavelength measured in angstroms (Å).

Xerostomia: Dry mouth.

Answers to Self-Study Questions

CHAPTER 1

1. D
2. D
3. A
4. B
5. B
6. C
7. B
8. A
9. A
10. D
11. D
12. A
13. C
14. A
15. C
16. A
17. A
18. A
19. B
20. A
21. B
22. B

CHAPTER 2

1. A
2. D
3. B
4. A
5. D
6. D
7. D
8. B
9. A
10. B

CHAPTER 3

1. A
2. C
3. A
4. B
5. C
6. C
7. A
8. C

9. E
10. D
11. D
12. D

CHAPTER 4

1. D
2. C
3. D
4. C
5. D
6. A
7. C
8. A
9. D
10. D
11. C
12. B
13. B
14. A
15. D
16. B
17. B
18. C
19. B

CHAPTER 5

1. C
2. C
3. C
4. B
5. C
6. A
7. C
8. B
9. B
10. B
11. A
12. B
13. A
14. C
15. B
16. B
17. D
18. C

19. B
20. D
21. C

CHAPTER 6

1. B
2. C
3. A
4. A
5. D
6. D
7. C
8. A
9. B
10. D
11. D
12. B
13. C
14. D
15. D
16. D

CHAPTER 7

1. C
2. B
3. D
4. A
5. B
6. D
7. B
8. A
9. D
10. C

CHAPTER 8

1. B
2. D
3. C
4. B
5. B
6. C
7. A
8. A
9. C
10. A

CHAPTER 9

1. C
2. C
3. D
4. B
5. B
6. D
7. B
8. D
9. D
10. C
11. B
12. C
13. D
14. A
15. B

CHAPTER 10

1. B
2. C
3. B
4. C
5. A
6. A
7. B
8. B
9. A
10. A
11. B
12. A
13. A

CHAPTER 11

1. B
2. E
3. A
4. E
5. A
6. C
7. E
8. E
9. D
10. B
11. A
12. B

943

CHAPTER 12
1. A
2. D
3. C
4. C
5. D
6. B
7. A
8. C
9. B
10. A

CHAPTER 13
1. D
2. C
3. D
4. B
5. C
6. B
7. A
8. C
9. B
10. B
11. A
12. C
13. A
14. B
15. C
16. A
17. A
18. A
19. B
20. D

CHAPTER 14
1. A
2. C
3. C
4. A
5. A
6. A
7. B
8. D
9. B
10. C

CHAPTER 15
1. A
2. C
3. B
4. C
5. B
6. C
7. A
8. C
9. D
10. A

CHAPTER 16
1. D
2. A
3. D
4. C
5. C
6. A
7. B
8. D
9. A
10. C
11. A
12. B

CHAPTER 17
1. A
2. A
3. E
4. B
5. E
6. B
7. C
8. C
9. E
10. E
11. A
12. C
13. C
14. E
15. A
16. C
17. D
18. A
19. C
20. C
21. E
22. E
23. A
24. E

CHAPTER 18
1. C
2. A
3. A
4. C
5. B
6. B
7. B
8. C
9. B
10. A

CHAPTER 19
1. B
2. A
3. B
4. A
5. D
6. C

7. B
8. A
9. C
10. C
11. A
12. C
13. D
14. A
15. D

CHAPTER 20
1. C
2. B
3. A
4. B
5. C
6. B
7. A
8. D
9. A
10. C

CHAPTER 21
1. B
2. D
3. B
4. C
5. C
6. A
7. A
8. D
9. B
10. B

CHAPTER 22
1. B
2. B
3. D
4. B
5. E
6. A
7. B
8. B
9. E
10. B
11. B
12. D
13. C
14. B
15. A
16. E

CHAPTER 23
1. B
2. B
3. A
4. D
5. A
6. C

7. D
8. C
9. A
10. B

CHAPTER 24
1. A
2. D
3. B
4. C
5. A
6. D
7. C
8. A
9. C
10. B

CHAPTER 25
1. B
2. E
3. A
4. D
5. B
6. A
7. C
8. B
9. A
10. B
11. A
12. B
13. B
14. C
15. A
16. A

CHAPTER 26
1. B
2. C
3. D
4. D
5. A
6. C
7. C
8. D
9. B
10. B
11. A
12. B
13. D
14. C
15. C

CHAPTER 27
1. B
2. C
3. B
4. A
5. B
6. A

7. B
8. D
9. C
10. B

CHAPTER 28

1. B
2. D
3. B
4. D
5. D
6. C
7. D
8. B
9. D
10. A
11. B
12. C
13. B
14. B
15. A
16. B
17. A
18. A

CHAPTER 29

1. B
2. C
3. C
4. A

5. A
6. B
7. D
8. A
9. B
10. A

CHAPTER 30

1. D
2. B
3. D
4. B
5. A
6. A
7. D
8. B
9. A
10. A

CHAPTER 31

1. E
2. A
3. E
4. A
5. E
6. E
7. B
8. B
9. A
10. B

CHAPTER 32

1. A
2. D
3. B
4. D
5. B
6. B
7. A
8. A

CHAPTER 33

1. D
2. D
3. A
4. B
5. C
6. C
7. C
8. A
9. B
10. D

CHAPTER 34

1. C
2. B
3. D
4. B
5. B
6. C

7. D
8. B
9. D
10. A

CHAPTER 35

1. B
2. C
3. A
4. C
5. A
6. D
7. B
8. D

CHAPTER 36

1. C
2. C
3. B
4. C
5. D

CHAPTER 37

1. D
2. B
3. D
4. B
5. B

$\boldsymbol{Index}$